The Occupational Environment — Its Evaluation, Control, and Management 3rd Edition

Edited by

Daniel H. Anna, PhD, CIH, CSP

A Publication of the American Industrial Hygiene Association®
Fairfax, VA

ISBN: 978-1-935082-15-6

AIHA®

2700 Prosperity Avenue, Suite 250
Fairfax, Virginia 22031

Tel: (703) 849-8888
Fax: (703) 207-3561
E-mail: Infonet@aiha.org
http://www.aiha.org

AIHA® Stock Number: BIHT10-566

Foreword

By John Howard, MD

I am pleased that the American Industrial Hygiene Association (AIHA®) has published the Third Edition of *The Occupational Environment—Its Evaluation, Control, and Management,* first published by the National Institute for Occupational Safety and Health (NIOSH) in 1973. Once again, *The Occupational Environment* will serve as a primary and comprehensive reference for occupational and environmental health practitioners and students throughout the world.

Today, we in the occupational safety and health community are challenged by having to know about, and respond to, hazards and risks that were largely unanticipated 40 years ago when the Occupational Safety and Health Act was enacted into law. Indeed, 40 years ago, an industrial hygiene practitioner might have had command of the entire body of knowledge in occupational hygiene without reliance on reference texts. Now, that achievement is only for the very few. The scope of risks in the occupational environment has multiplied and even the historical ones have become more complex to control. Now, most of us need to rely on a comprehensive resource like *The Occupational Environment.*

The Third Edition of *The Occupational Environment: Its Evaluation, Control, and Management* will assist professionals to address today's critical issues by including updated and new chapters on air contaminants, risk assessment, sampling, occupational exposure limits, biological monitoring, engineered nanoparticles, prevention through design, internationalization of hazard communication, and many other topics of interest. The ultimate achievement of The Occupational Environment will be in making the occupational environment as safe and healthful as it can be for the protection of workers.

I would especially like to acknowledge the contributions of the many expert chapter contributors, the editor, and the work of the AIHA, in developing the Third Edition. All of your efforts will help to ensure that the occupational and environmental health practitioners of now and of the future will be able to achieve the highest level of skill to address old and new problems in the occupational environment.

John Howard, MD
Director, National Institute for Occupational Safety and Health
U.S. Department of Health and Human Services
September 2011

Preface

By Daniel H. Anna, PhD, CIH, CSP

Since the publication of the Second Edition of *The Occupational Environment: Its Evaluation, Control, and Management* in 2003, the role of the industrial hygienist has continued to evolve and expand. The scope of responsibilities for most industrial hygienists now includes at least some aspects of safety, environmental, sustainability, quality, security, emergency response, or part of another ancillary discipline. But, even with all of these changes, one thing has remained constant — the need for qualified, trained professionals who can anticipate, recognize, evaluate, and control potential health hazards that arise in and from the workplace. The increasing reliance on technology, the expanding world of nanotechnology, the continuing globalization of business and industry, and the changing definition of "workplace" all contribute to the complexities of potential exposures and the challenges of assessing risk of exposure. Terms like exposure risk assessment and management have become part of the language used to describe traditional industrial hygiene responsibilities to a broader international audience.

The evolution of the profession played a role in the development of this edition, and, in turn, hopefully the revised content will play a significant role in preparing IHs for success in the continually evolving work environment. It was essential to incorporate changes because this book serves as a primary textbook for courses that help to prepare future IH, EHS and other related professionals. Beyond the classroom, this book has traditionally served as a fundamental reference for a broad range of topics within the scope of IH related competencies. But with the increasing complexities of the profession and the increasing scope of competencies required to protect worker health, this book can only serve as the starting point for many of the topics presented. In many chapters, the authors have added recommended resources to consult for additional information.

Nearly 120 authors contributed to this edition. New chapters were added to address nanotechnology, professional ethics, IH issues in construction, and the AIHA® Value Strategy. Almost half of the chapters were written or revised by new authors. Most of the other chapters had significant changes and updates to the content.

The most obvious physical difference in this edition is the split into two volumes. Many users of the previous edition commented on the book being "entirely too big" to transport. The decision to divide the book into two parts resulted from the user feedback and the fact that this edition has too many pages to reliably bind into a single volume. Separating the content was a tremendous challenge; countless iterations were considered. In the end the chapters were grouped loosely around chemical hazards, physical hazards and management/program aspects. Many of the relationships between chapter content and chapter location have been maintained from the previous editions. Although this edition is provided in two volumes, it should be considered a single book.

It is an honor to be associated with this edition, to be the first person to read all of the chapters, and to know how many people will benefit from the wealth of information contained in *The Occupational Environment — Its Evaluation, Control and Management.*

Acknowledgments

The most significant contributions to this book came from nearly 120 authors that voluntarily contributed chapters to this edition. Since the first edition of the AIHA Press version of "The Occupational Environment" was published in 1997, this book has become a primary reference for industrial hygienists and an essential textbook used in industrial hygiene and other EHS academic programs. Without their willingness to share their expertise and time to write and revise the technical chapters for this book, development of this outstanding resource for IH and other EHS professionals would not have been possible. A sincere thank you is also extended to the AIHA® Volunteer Groups, and countless AIHA® members and other affiliated professionals who provided thorough technical reviews of the chapters. The peer review process is an essential part of validating the technical content and, by default, the knowledge base for the profession. A special thank you also goes out to the authors and editor of the previous editions; they developed the framework for this and all future editions.

A few individuals from the AIHA® staff deserve individual recognition. Words cannot describe the significant contributions Katie Robert made to this project, including, among her other responsibilities, editing, formatting and preparing content for publication. Katie was an outstanding colleague and friend throughout this project. She kept the project progressing by using her amazing ability to balance "nagging" with an understanding about how my day job sometimes interfered with progress. Jim Myers worked long hours on the layout of the chapters and the design and overall appearance of the book. His work was especially appreciated during the last few months prior to publication as the number of submitted chapters increased and the deadlines shortened. Finally, thanks to Sheila Brown for assisting with the editing of some chapters when the backlog in the queue started to build.

Most of the work on this edition occurred while I was a faculty member at Millersville University. Thank you to the Faulty Grants Committee and the administration at Millersville University for recognizing the significance of this publication and providing some release time from my course load that allowed me to focus on this project. I also want to thank the many students who provided input about the book from their perspective; their comments helped shape many of the changes seen in this edition.

On a personal level, no one was more understanding about my time commitment to this project than my wife Laura. She provided encouragement from the beginning and continued support throughout the project, in spite of having to endure far too many stories, complaints, and frustrated moments. And, my son Nik, whose entire life has occurred during this project, has already said that he will be happy when there is nothing to review "before we go play."

About the Editor

Daniel H. Anna, PhD, CIH, CSP

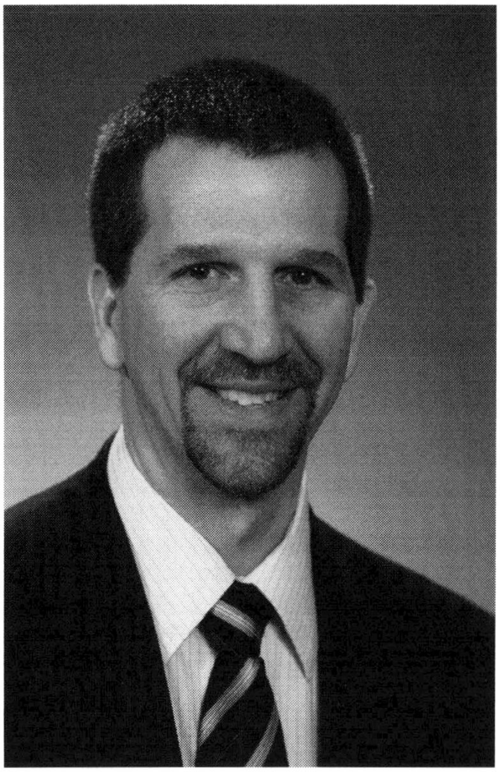

Dr. Anna is currently a Senior Industrial Hygienist and Assistant Group Supervisor at the Johns Hopkins University Applied Physics Laboratory (APL) in Laurel, MD. Prior to joining APL, he spent nearly 15 years at Millersville University (Millersville, PA), where he was a Professor and Program Coordinator in the Occupational Safety & Environmental Health program. In addition, he has worked an industrial hygienist in the petrochemical industry and as an independent consultant. Dr. Anna received a Bachelor of Science in Safety Science from Indiana University of Pennsylvania, a Master of Science in Industrial Hygiene from Texas A&M University, and a PhD in Industrial Health from the University of Michigan. Dr. Anna is a Certified Industrial Hygienist and a Certified Safety Professional. He has been an active member of AIHA® since 1991. He is a graduate of the inaugural Future Leaders Institute in 2005, and has served in leadership roles in the Central Pennsylvania Local Section, on several AIHA® technical committees, and as a Director and the Secretary on the AIHA® Board of Directors.

Contents

Section 3: Dermal, Biological, and Nanomaterial Hazard Recognition and Assessment

Volume 2

Section 4: Physical Agent Recognition and Evaluation

Section 5: The Human Environment

Section 6: Methods of Controlling the Work Environment

Section 7: Program Management

The Occupational Environment — Its Evaluation, Control, and Management 3rd Edition

Volume 1

AIHA
Protecting Worker Health

Outcome Competencies

After completing this chapter, the reader should be able to:

1. Define underlined terms used in this chapter.
2. Describe the contribution of key individuals in the development of the industrial hygiene profession.
3. Explain the role the history of civilization plays in the development of the industrial hygiene profession.
4. Discuss the role of governmental entities in the history of industrial hygiene.
5. Describe how the public health profession relates to industrial hygiene.
6. Explain the industrial hygiene paradigm of anticipation, recognition, evaluation, prevention and control.
7. Recognize the conflicts around, "whom do we serve?"
8. Recognize the need to continue to grow as a professional to not only survive but to be of greater service to those in need of our talents.

Key Terms

Agricola • Alice Hamilton • American Academy of Industrial Hygiene • American Board of Industrial Hygiene (ABIH)• American Conference of Governmental Industrial Hygienists (ACGIH®) • American Industrial Hygiene Association (AIHA®) • Benjamin W. McCready • Bernardino Ramazzini • certified industrial hygienist (CIH) • Charles T. Thackrah • Mine Safety and Health Administration (MSHA) • National Institute for Occupational Safety and Health (NIOSH) • Occupational Safety and Health Act • Occupational Safety and Health Administration (OSHA) • permissible exposure limits • Pliny the Elder • Sir Percival Pott • Threshold Limit Values® • Ulrich Ellenbog

Prerequisite Knowledge

None.

Key Topics

I. Origins of Industrial Hygiene

II. The U.S. Experience
   A. Anticipation and Recognition
   B. Evaluation
   C. Prevention and Control
   D. Occupational Disease Spurs Reforms
   E. Education and Professional Organizations

III. Public Health Roots

IV. Professional Recognition and Title Protection

V. The Future

VI. Summary

History and Philosophy of Industrial Hygiene

1

By Leigh Ann Blunt, John N. Zey, CIH, Alice L. Greife, PhD, CIH, and Vernon E. Rose, DrPH, CIH, CSP, PE

Origins of Industrial Hygiene

As with most professions, identifying the origin of the practice of industrial hygiene is difficult, if not impossible. The early chroniclers of occupational hazards and control measures such as Agricola, who, in 1556, described the prevalent diseases and accidents in mining, smelting, and refining and prevention measures including ventilation might be designated as founders of the profession. The contributions of Plinius Secundus (Pliny the Elder) should also be considered, who, in the first century AD, wrote "minimum refiners . . . envelop their faces with loose bladders, which enable them to see without inhaling the fatal dust."(1) If their works were read, thus influencing others to control work hazards, they deserve the title, at least posthumously, of industrial hygienists.

But there were others who simply identified problems. It has been suggested a special honor in the field of occupational medicine is owed to Hippocrates (c. 460–370 BC). His writings include the first recorded mention of occupational diseases (e.g., lead poisoning in miners and metallurgists) and provide more frequent allusions to this class of ailments than those of any other author prior to Ramazzini.(2)

In 1713, Bernardino Ramazzini published the first book considered to be a complete treatise on occupational diseases, *De Morbis Artificum Diatriba*.(3) From his own observations he accurately described scores of occupations, their hazards, and resulting diseases. Although he recommended some specific as well as general preventive measures (workers should cover their faces to avoid breathing dust), most of his control recommendations were therapeutic and curative. While he had a vast knowledge of the literature of his time, it has been suggested that many of the works he cited were of questionable scientific validity, and some were more myth than science and should have been recognized as such even in Ramazzini's time. Because of his prestige, these "fanciful notions must have received wide acceptance . . . and because his book was so admired, Ramazzini's influence may have stifled progress in his field during a period when great advances were being made in other branches of medicine."(2)

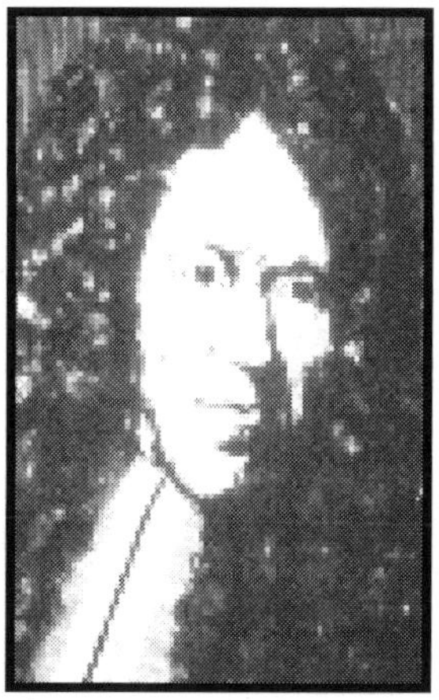

Figure 1.1 — A portrait of Bernardino Ramazzini — the father of occupational medicine.

Nevertheless, his cautions to protect workers and his admonition to any doctor called on to treat patients of the working class to ask "What occupation does he follow?" earned him the designation "Father of Industrial Medicine."

For almost 100 years following Ramazzini's work, no significant additions to the literature on occupational medicine were published. In 1814 Matthieu Orfila, a renowned toxicologist of Spanish descent, published the first of five editions of *Traité de Toxicologie*, which has been identified as "the first book devoted entirely to toxicology as an experimental science different from pharmacology."[4] Not since Paracelsus noted that it was the dose of a material that made it a poison, had there been such a substantial influence on the field of toxicology. While Paracelsus' ideas were not popular among the medical profession in his time, Orfila was highly regarded and is often referred to, along with Paracelsus, as the father of modern toxicology. Orfila's work in toxicology furthered the field of forensics with his studies about the decomposition of the human body and exhumations. Upon Orfila's death in 1853, an obituary was published in the *Association Medical Journal* that lauded his extensive career and lamented the loss of "this truly good man."[5] The obituary summed up his great contribution to science with the following words: "Before the appearance of Orfila's work, Toxicology had few cultivators, no teachers in the schools, and little claim to be regarded as a science: now, it is zealously studied in all countries, taught in every school, and simplified the by the labours of many eminent men, as to be practically available, by every educated practitioner, in the detection of crime, and in the preservation of life."[5]

In the nineteenth century two physicians, Charles T. Thackrah in England and Benjamin W. McCready in America, began the modern literature on the recognition of occupational diseases. McCready's book, On the Influence of Trades, Professions, and Occupations in the United States, in the Production of Disease, is generally recognized as the first work on occupational medicine published in the U.S.[6]

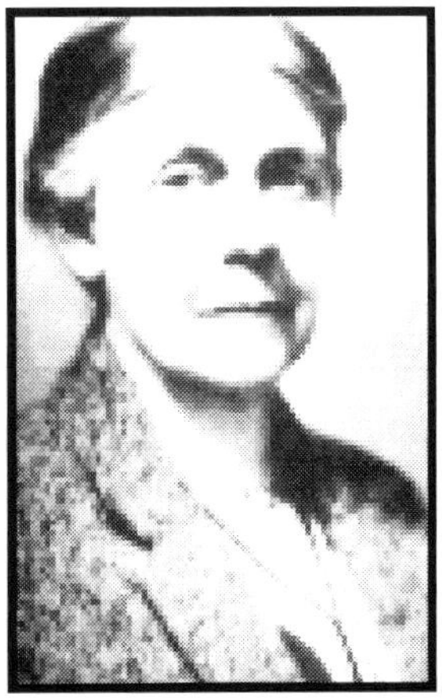

Figure 1.2 — Dr. Alice Hamilton.

The recognition of a causal link between workplace hazards and disease was a key step in the development of the practice of industrial hygiene. The observations by physicians, from Hippocrates to Ramazzini and extending into the twentieth century, of the relationship between work and disease are the foundation of the profession. But recognition of hazards without intervention and control, i.e., without prevention of disease, should not qualify one as an industrial hygienist.

The crystallization of the practice of the profession can be traced to simultaneous developments in Great Britain and the United States in the late nineteenth and early twentieth centuries. While legislation controlling working conditions was enacted in England beginning in 1802, the early laws were considered totally ineffective, as "no proper system of inspection or enforcement was provided."[7] The British Factories Act of 1864, however, required the use of dilution ventilation to reduce air contaminants, while the 1878 version specified the use of exhaust ventilation by fans. The real watershed in industrial medicine and hygiene, however, came in the British Factories Act of 1901, which provided for the creation of regulations to control dangerous trades. The development of regulations created the impetus for investigation of workplace hazards and enforcement of control measures. In the U.S. in 1905, the Massachusetts Health Department appointed health inspectors to evaluate dangers of occupations, thus establishing government's role in the emerging field of occupational health.

It has been suggested industrial hygiene did not "emerge as a unique field of endeavor until quantitative measurements of the environment became available."[8] But in 1910 when Dr. Alice Hamilton went, in her own words, "as a pioneer into a new, unexplored field of American medicine, the field of industrial disease"[9], worker exposures to many hazards (e.g., lead and silica) were so excessive and resulting diseases so acute and obvious, the "evaluation" step of industrial hygiene practice required only the sense of sight and an understanding of the concept of cause and effect. This "champion of social responsibility" for worker health and welfare not only presented substantial evidence of a relationship between exposure to toxins and ill health, but also proposed concrete solutions to the problems she encountered.[10] On an individual basis, Dr. Hamilton's work, which comprised not only the recognition of occupational disease, but the evaluation and control of the causative agents, should be considered as the initial practice of industrial hygiene, at least in the U.S.[11,12]

It should be appreciated that many of the early practitioners of industrial hygiene were physicians who, like Alice Hamilton, were interested not only in the diagnosis and treatment of illnesses in industrial workers, but also in hazard control to prevent further cases. These physicians working with engineers and other scientists interested in public health and environmental hazards took the knowledge and insights developed over several millennia from Hippocrates to Ramazzini, Thackrah and McCready, and began the process of deliberately changing the work environment with the goal of preventing occupational diseases.

When considering what or who can be designated as representing the origin of the profession or deserving of the title "Founder of Industrial Hygiene, Alice Hamilton stands out. Hamilton made truly remarkable contributions through the course of her life. She received her M.D. at the University of Michigan in 1893.(9) She was the first female faculty member at Harvard University, although, she was never promoted and was not allowed to participate in graduation ceremonies. In 1910, she was selected by the governor of Illinois to serve on the Commission for Occupational Diseases.(9,10) She would later write that since the time of that appointment "I have been following the trail of lead, mercury, nitric acid, carbon disulphide, carbon monoxide, explosives, aniline dyes, benzol and a long list of chemicals with complicated names which are interestingly varied in their uses and in the effects on that more or less unconscious victim, the worker."(13) She was recognized for her work through the U.S. Bureau of Labor, demonstrating the morbidity and mortality data associated with lead exposures.(9) Her autobiography, Exploring the Dangerous Trades, provided insight into the terrible conditions that workers endured to produce the nation's goods.(11,12,14) Additionally, her article, "Lead poisoning in American Industry" was the second of four scientific articles published in the inaugural edition of the *Journal of Industrial Hygiene* in May of 1919.(15)

Along with her knowledge and passion, Hamilton demonstrated a natural ability to lead, motivate, and actuate change in an era devoid of regulatory controls.(16) With very few material resources, "Hamilton was able to motivate businessmen to change their operations by appealing to their best instincts — their innate desire to do the right thing. She made her case with persistence, persuasiveness, sincerity, and carefully collected and presented hard data."(16) It is perhaps fitting that the woman who dedicated her life to the health and safety of others, lived to be 101 years old.

The underlying philosophy and ultimate outcome of the profession is the protection of people from hazards in the workplace. It began when one person recognized a work hazard and took steps not only for self protection, but also for protection of fellow workers. This is the origin and essence of the profession of industrial hygiene.

The U.S. Experience

The events presented in Table 1.1 illustrate many of the historical milestones relevant to the development and progression of industrial hygiene. While the concepts which formed the art and science of industrial hygiene flourished in many countries, the U.S. provided the fertile ground for the development of the profession as it exists today.

As the industrial revolution, propelled by the Civil War, progressed in the nineteenth century, individuals began to observe serious health and safety problems (recognition). They also considered the effects on workers (evaluation) and made changes in the work environment (control) to lessen the effects observed. Although these efforts may have resulted in improved worker health and safety, their application was not recognized as the practice of industrial hygiene until the early-1900s. The 1920s saw very little activity aimed at workplace safety and health, with progress stifled by anti-labor sentiments.(17) However, changes were starting to take root as "The devastation of the Depression of the 1930s, the massive unemployment, the growth in labor militancy, and the pledge of Roosevelt's Administration to give a 'New Deal' to the American people gave a new importance to the Department of Labor."(17) Perhaps of most significance was Roosevelt's appointment of Francis Perkins as the U.S. Secretary of Labor and the first woman to be a member of the Cabinet.(17) In 1935, it was Perkins who appointed Dr. Alice Hamilton as a "special advisor on technical problems in connection with the prevention of industrial diseases."(18) Perkins declared publicly that "the most liberal of our compensation laws is only a partial substitute for lost wages, so that industrial injuries and diseases always bear down heavily upon the unfortunate victims."[18] Her commitment to the safety and health of workers and strong beliefs in a fair compensation system stemmed from the tragic day in 1911 when the Triangle Shirtwaist Fire in New York City claimed the lives of 146 people, mostly young women.

Throughout history, many events helped shape the profession of industrial hygiene. Today, industrial Hygiene is defined by AIHA® as the "science and art devoted to the anticipation, recognition, evaluation, prevention, and control of those environmental

Table 1.1 — Historical Events in Occupational Health and Safety

1,000,000 BC	Australopithecus used stones as tools and weapons. Flint knappers suffered cuts and eye injuries; bison hunters contracted anthrax.
10,000 BC	Neolithic man began food-producing economy and the urban revolution in Mesopotamia. At end of Stone Age, grinding of stone, horn, bone, and ivory tools with sandstone; pottery making, linen weaving. Beginning of the history of occupations.
5000 BC	Copper and Bronze Age—metal workers released from food production. Metallurgy—the first specialized craft.
370 BC	Hippocrates dealt with the health of citizens, not workers, but did identify lead poisoning in miners and metallurgists.
50 AD	Plinius Secundus (Pliny the Elder) identified use of animal bladders intended to prevent inhalation of dust and lead fume.
200 AD	Galen visited a copper mine, but his discussions on public health did not include workers' disease.
Middle Ages	No documented contributions to the study of occupational diseases.
1473	Ellenbog recognized that the vapors of some metals were dangerous and described the symptoms of industrial poisoning from lead and mercury with suggested preventive measures.
1500	In *De Re Metallica* (1556), Georgius Agricola described every facet of mining, smelting, and refining, noting prevalent diseases and accidents, and means of prevention including the need for ventilation. Paracelsus (1567) described respiratory diseases among miners with an excellent description of mercury poisoning. Remembered as the father of toxicology. "All substances are poisons . . . the right dose differentiates a poison and a remedy."
1665	Workday for mercury miners at Idria shortened.
1700	Bernardino Ramazzini, "father of occupational medicine," published *De Morbis Artificum Diatriba*, (Diseases of Workers) and examined occupational diseases and "cautions." He introduced the question, "Of what trade are you?"
1775	Percival Pott described occupational cancer among English chimney sweeps, identifying soot and the lack of hygiene measures as a cause of scrotal cancer. The result was the Chimney-Sweeps Act of 1788.
1830	Charles Thackrah authored the first book on occupational diseases to be published in England. His views on disease and prevention helped stimulate factory and health legislation. Medical inspection and compensation were established in 1897.
1911	On March 25 of this year, the Triangle Shirtwaist Factory fire claimed the lives of 146 people, mostly women. This event spawned the development of what is now the American Society of Safety Engineers (ASSE).
1919	First Issue of the Journal of Industrial Hygiene published.
1963	Clean Air Act
1976	Toxic Substances Control Act created.
1986	Emergency Planning and Community Right to Know Act created.
1990	Clean Air Act revised and expanded
2006	Mine Improvement and New Emergency Response (MINER) Act

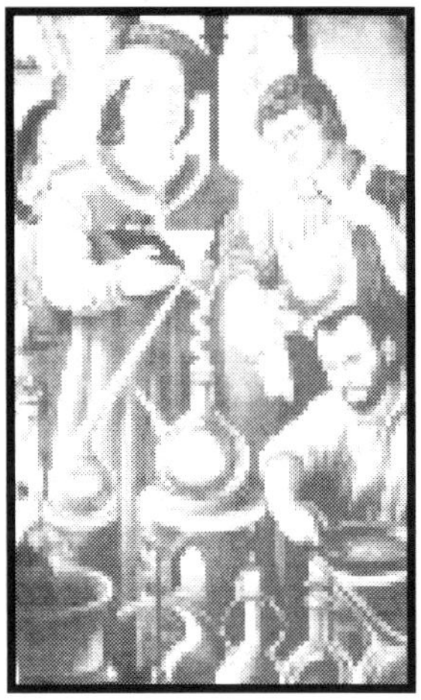

Figure 1.3 — A portrait of Paracelsus (1567) who is remembered as the father of toxicology.

factors or stresses arising in or from the workplace which may cause sickness, impaired health and well being, or significant discomfort among workers or among citizens of the community." Only in the last decade has the notion of anticipation and prevention been formally included in the definition of industrial hygiene.

Anticipation and Recognition

Anticipation and recognition of the potential for occupational health problems is a prerequisite for the implementation of industrial hygiene activities. Therefore, early attempts at defining the scope and magnitude of occupational health problems were very important to the subsequent efforts of evaluation and control. The Illinois Occupational Disease Commission's survey of the extent of occupational health problems in the state of Illinois in 1910 was the first such survey undertaken in the U.S.[19] Dr. Alice Hamilton was a member of the commission and served as its chief investigator. Two years later, she presented her survey of lead hazards in American industry. Although other states formed commissions to identify problems, it was many years before there was an organized effort to develop information about the scope of the industrial health problems in the working population in America.

The Division of Industrial Hygiene in the United States Public Health Service (USPHS), later to become the National Institute for Occupational Safety and Health (NIOSH), revived interest in assessing the extent of health hazards. Beginning in the 1960s the USPHS conducted surveys in a number of states and metropolitan areas for the purpose of identifying the extent of worker exposure to occupational health hazards. The results of these studies were used to determine the need for occupational health specialists in the governmental agencies and for setting priorities for government inspection and consultation programs.[20] These efforts culminated in NIOSH's National Occupational Hazard Survey conducted in the early 1970s. This project involved walk-through surveys in more than 5000 randomly selected workplaces in the United States and for the first time provided a comprehensive assessment of workplace hazards and the extent of their control for a large segment of the working population. A subsequent NIOSH study, the National Occupational Exposure Survey, provided additional insight on the magnitude of worker exposure to hazards.[21] These studies were used by NIOSH to set priorities for research and for developing recommended standards.

Concurrent with the development of occupational hazard information was the recognition that information on the incidence of occupational illnesses in the U.S. work force was not available. Prior to the passage of the Occupational Safety and Health Act (OSH Act) in 1970, the sources of occupational disease incidence data were limited primarily to the information developed in several state health and labor departments such as California, New York, and Michigan. The California reports of occupational illnesses were thought to be the most comprehensive and reliable; consequently, they were often used for projections of the national problem. The passage of the OSH Act gave the U.S. Department of Labor the responsibility for developing a national occupational injury and illness reporting system. The system includes a requirement for employers to record occupationally related injuries and illnesses with separate categories for dermatitis, lung disorders due to dusts, lung disorders due to chemicals, systemic effects, physical agent disorders, repeated trauma disorders, and "all other" illnesses. A sample of employers report their experience, which is used to develop state and national estimates. For many years skin disorders were the most frequently reported illnesses, but in the late 1980s repeated trauma, which includes musculoskeletal problems such as carpal tunnel syndrome and back disorders, became the leading category of illness.

It is widely recognized occupational diseases are underreported in this system for a variety of reasons beyond a conscious decision not to record. Many occupationally related diseases can also be caused by non-occupational exposures (e.g., lung cancer and tobacco). Also, when a disease has a long latency period before it can be diagnosed, its relationship to early work exposures may be obscure. In some cases work factors may worsen a preexisting condition. And, as a relatively new discipline, the recognition of workplace illnesses can be hampered by a limited knowledge base. It is unlikely a worker's illness will be recognized as work related if epidemiologic or toxicological studies have not documented cause and effect, i.e., exposure to a toxin and illness.

Concurrent with studies to estimate hazard distribution and incidence of occupational illness were specific epidemiologic studies designed to link cause and effect. Two key studies firmly established the specialty of occupational epidemiology first practiced by Sir Percival Pott in the late eighteenth century. One study could be considered an extension of his work, which linked a byproduct of coal combustion (soot) with scrotal cancer in chimney sweeps. In the twentieth-century study, the epidemiologists who looked at the mortality distribution of U.S. steelworkers found a population whose health was better than expected when compared with the overall U.S. population (the healthy worker effect).[22] However, when subpopulations, specifically coke oven workers, were considered, excesses of respiratory and kidney cancer deaths were uncovered. The complexity of environmental exposures surrounding these workers precluded the identification of any one specific causative agent and led to the designation of coal tar pitch volatiles (CTPV) as the surrogate hazard to be controlled. Documentation of excess mortality in coke oven workers led to promulgation of the Occupational Safety and Health Administration (OSHA) regulation on coke oven emissions.[23]

The second major occupational epidemiologic study focused on asbestos. Reports of cases of lung disease due to asbestos exposure began to accumulate beginning in 1906. By 1938 the USPHS had studied workers in asbestos textile plants and had recommended a tentative limit for asbestos dust in the textile industry of 5 million particles per cubic foot (mp/ft^3), determined by the impinger technique.[24] In the late 1940s, workers manufacturing asbestos products in England were observed to have a frequency of bronchogenic cancer greater than expected as compared with the general male population. These findings led to the study of U.S. insulation workers exposed to airborne asbestos fibers and the documentation of an excess of bronchogenic cancers in this population.[25] These and other studies led to the promulgation of OSHA's first emergency temporary standard in 1971 and first complete health standard in 1972.[26] The hazards of asbestos also firmly established toxic tort (product liability) lawsuits as a force to control workplace hazards.

In occupational epidemiologic studies, one test for concluding the existence of cause and effect is the presence of an exposure-response relationship. When industrial hygiene exposure data are not available, substitute measures such as "high, medium, and low" are utilized. However, where historical exposure data are available or can be estimated, risk-assessment evaluation can be more objective and lead to occupational exposure limits which define the expected reduction in the incidence of illness. Use of risk-assessment tools to estimate illness reduction from lowering workplace exposure limits has been applied by OSHA since the benzene standard was promulgated in 1987.[27]

At the present time, industrial hygiene efforts in the U.S. are guided by hazard rather than disease considerations. At the national and state levels, information on worker exposure to hazards by various industry categories is available and is used to set priorities for governmental investigations and research. Within industry, the concept of hazard recognition vis-a-vis illness is seen as important in developing programs focused on prevention. Consequently, the emphasis on anticipation and recognition of potential occupational health problems primarily involves the industrial hygiene practice of hazard or risk determination, where hazard or risk combines the inherent toxicity of a substance or agent and the likelihood for exposure.

Evaluation

Although the use of the senses, including sight, smell, and sometimes taste, were important in the early years of the practice of industrial hygiene, the transition to a science required the development of more sophisticated sampling methods to aid in the evaluation of problems. One of the first such sampling methods, developed by researchers at Harvard University in 1917, was the color-indicating detector tube for measuring airborne levels of carbon monoxide.[28] Dust exposure in mining and other industries was an early industrial hygiene concern and generated the need to measure airborne concentrations of particulates. In 1922, Greenberg and Smith developed their impinger, and in 1938, Littlefield and Schrenk modified the design and developed the midget impinger.[8] The subsequent development of the hand-operated pump for dust sampling with midget impingers gave the industrial hygienist flexibility in collecting breathing zone samples to better characterize occupational exposures. The associated analytical method of counting and sizing particles with a microscope, thus yielding concentrations of million particles per cubic foot, was the standard method for characterizing particulate exposures until 1953, when the application of the membrane filter allowed exposures to be evaluated on a mass per volume basis.[29]

The early application of impingers, using water as the collection medium, was for dust sampling. Gas and vapor monitoring required the development of a variety of sampling media for use in midget impingers and later in the more efficient fritted-glass bubblers. In 1970, a major breakthrough in sampling methodology occurred when NIOSH developed the charcoal sampling tube and provided support for development of the battery-operated pump.[30] Concurrent with the development of these active sampling devices was Palmes' work in 1973 on a passive dosimeter for nitrogen dioxide. Subsequent commercialization of the passive dosimeter concept led to a modest revolution in the scope of industrial hygiene sampling. These technological developments greatly enhanced the art of personal sampling and allowed the industrial hygienist even greater flexibility in characterizing worker exposure to hazardous conditions.[31]

At the same time sampling methods were being developed, the application of new analytical technology to industrial hygiene assessments was taking place. In the early 1930s, technical articles described the use of gas chromatography for evaluating samples of airborne organic vapors. In later years other forms of technology were employed at a rapid pace. Today samples are analyzed using atomic absorption, high pressure liquid chromatography, mass spectroscopy, and other sophisticated instrumentation and techniques.

As industrial hygienists learned more about the environment and further refined their techniques for measuring hazardous exposures in the workplace, the need to compare measurements with unacceptable exposure levels became apparent. In 1929, several industrial hygienists in the USPHS recommended upper limits for exposure to quartz-bearing industrial dusts based on studies in the Vermont granite industry.[32] The publication of workplace exposure limits was greatly enhanced by the formation of the American Conference of Governmental Industrial Hygienists (ACGIH®) in 1938. In 1939, ACGIH®, in cooperation with the American Standards Association, developed the first list of maximum allowable concentrations (MACs) to limit worker exposure to airborne contaminants. In 1943, Dr. James Sterner published the MAC list in Industrial Medicine, followed by Warren Cook's publication (also in Industrial Medicine) in 1945 of a MAC list for 140 substances with sources and bases for the recommendations. In 1947, ACGIH® began publication of its MAC list, and converted to the term threshold limit values (TLVs®) in 1948.[33] Today, even with major responsibility for standards-setting vested with the federal government, the role of ACGIH® in developing exposure guidelines is a valuable tool in protecting the health of workers.

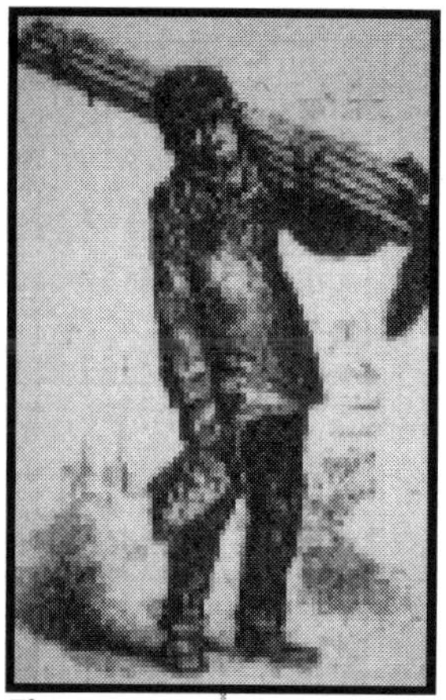

Figure 1.4 — A London chimney sweep (mid-1700s).

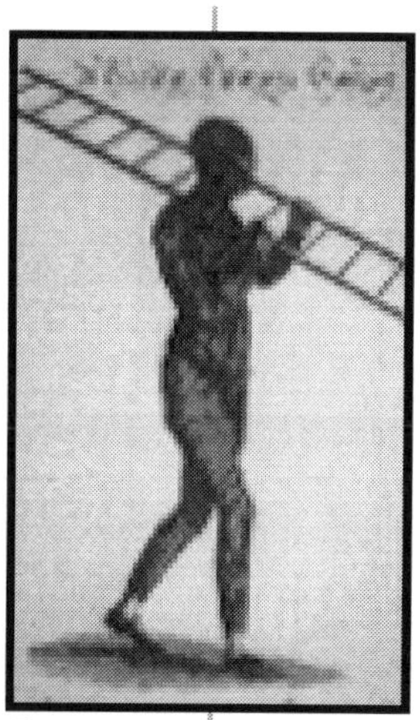

Figure 1.5 — A German chimney sweel (mid-1700s). Note the tight-fitting personal protective clothing. There were no reported problems of scrotal cancer among the German workers.

Prevention and Control

Prevention of occupational disease and injury is arguably the primary end-goal of industrial hygiene. The prevention of hazards in the workplace becomes possible through the anticipation of hazards based on past experiences and knowledge. While prevention of a hazard trumps control measures every time, it is often difficult to accurately predict the potential hazards of new and emerging technologies. When the pairing of anticipation and prevention do not succeed, the combination of recognition, evaluation and control become imperative.

Control of occupational health problems can take several forms. Industrial hygienists most often employ the technological approach, i.e., engineering measures such as substitution with less hazardous substances or implementation of local exhaust ventilation. Where these techniques cannot eliminate or reduce the hazard sufficiently, administrative measures and personal protective equipment are also utilized. These concepts, which can also be shuffled to the categories of control "at the source, in the environment, and at the worker," were first introduced, in a comprehensive form, in 1473 by Ulrich Ellenbog.[8] He suggested three methods of control still applied today: use dry coal instead of wet coal to avoid production of toxic "fumes," work with windows open, and cover the mouth to prevent inhalation of noxious "fumes."[8] The history of two specific control measures, industrial ventilation and respirators, should be of special interest to practicing industrial hygienists.

Agricola, in his 1561 publication, *De Re Metallica*, emphasized the need for ventilation of mines and included many illustrations of devices to force air below ground.[34] The first recorded design of a local exhaust ventilation system, however, was by the Frenchman D'Arcet in the early 1800s. To control noxious fumes he led an exhaust duct from a hood at a furnace into a chimney with a strong draft. The induced airflow carried the fumes away from the source.

The British window tax of 1696, which was not repealed until 1851, resulted in dark and under ventilated factories. The first legislation regulating conditions in factories was the British Factory and Workshops Act of 1802, which required ventilation in workplaces. The Act of 1864 required sufficient ventilation to render gases and dusts as harmless as possible, but it was 1867 before an inspector was given authority to require fans or other mechanical devices to control dust. Although the British Factories Act of 1897 required the use of ventilation for certain operations, little was published on techniques until the late 1930s. It has been suggested the main reasons for the lack of published information probably were "attempts on the part of industry to keep their trade secrets, and the lack of interest on the part of universities and colleges."[8] In 1951, ACGIH® published the first edition of *Industrial Ventilation: A Manual of Recommended Practice*. The regularly updated manual is a compilation on design, maintenance, and evaluation of industrial exhaust ventilation systems. The manual has found wide acceptance as a guide for official agencies, as a standard for industrial ventilation designers, and as a textbook for industrial hygiene and other hazard control courses.

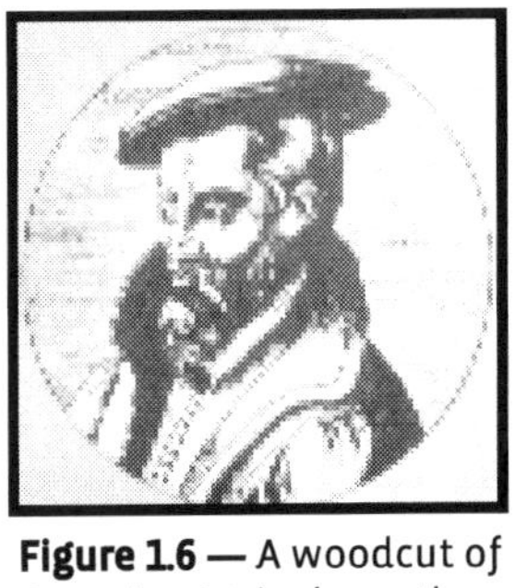

Figure 1.6 — A woodcut of Georgius Agricola, author of *De Re Metallica*.

As noted earlier, the concept of respiratory protective devices (e.g., animal bladders) to reduce exposure to airborne contaminants dates back to at least 50 AD. There is no record of worker acceptance of these early "respirators" nor of their effectiveness as personal protective devices, but in all likelihood, they didn't score high in either category. The same can probably be said for other devices which have fallen by the wayside over the centuries: scarves, shawls, handkerchiefs, magnetic mouthpieces, magnetized screens, wet sponges, and breathing tubes. It should come as no surprise Leonardo da Vinci (1452–1519) considered the problems of respiratory protection when he recommended the use of a wet cloth to protect against chemical warfare agents. He also devised two underwater breathing devices, one being a snorkel consisting of a breathing tube with an attached float.[35] Ramazzini wrote a critical review of the inadequate respiratory protection available in his time (c. 1700). Shortly thereafter, the first descriptions appeared of the ancestors of today's atmosphere-supplying devices, such as open- and closed-circuit self-contained breathing apparatus and hose masks.

In the 1800s, the realization of the separate natures of particles and gases or vapors led to great advances in respirators. A particulate-removing filter encased in a rigid container was developed in 1814 and was the predecessor of modern filters for air-purifying respirators. The ability of activated charcoal to remove organic vapors from air was discovered in 1854 and was almost immediately put to use in respirators. The most rapid advances in respiratory protection grew out of the use of chemical warfare agents in World War I. Research on gas sorbents for use in military masks and high efficiency particulate filters was accelerated by the introduction of different gases and highly toxic particulate matter on the battlefield. Since the 1920s, the major advances in respirator design include resin-impregnated dust filters, which use electrostatic force fields to remove dust particles from air, and the ultra high-efficiency (HEPA) filter from paper containing very fine glass fibers.[35] Other advances include the use of more flexible and durable (synthetic) materials for face pieces, and the combination of a battery-operated air mover with a respirator for use as a lightweight air-supplied respirator (i.e., the powered air purifying respirator).

A different approach to control involves the application of governmental powers to assist, motivate, and require employers to maintain safe and healthful work environments. In the United States, legal protection of industrial workers was for the most part, until 1971, the responsibility of state and local governments. The development of state governmental responsibilities in occupational health took place as early as 1905, when inspectors in the Massachusetts Health Department investigated workplace dangers. In 1913, the first formal governmental program, the New York Department of Labor's Division of Industrial Hygiene, was established. The Office of Industrial Hygiene and Sanitation was formed in the USPHS in 1914 and subsequently underwent many reorganizations before becoming NIOSH in 1971.[36]

During the 1920s and early 1930s, industrial hygiene activities were initiated in five state health departments (Connecticut, Maryland, Mississippi, Ohio, and Rhode Island). The Social Security Act of 1935 made federal resources (money and industrial hygienists) available to states to aid in the development of industrial hygiene programs.[37] By 1936, 12 more state health department programs were initiated, and the USPHS recommended a "large industrial state" should have at least one chief industrial hygienist with a salary of $6,000. The minimum qualifications of this specialist called for a chemical engineering degree, two years' graduate work in industrial hygiene, three years of experience, and, in addition to a wide range of scientific and technical knowledge, "the ability to establish contacts with plant executives; ability to enlist cooperation of plant executives, foremen and laborers; initiative; tact; good judgment; and good address."[38]

World War II provided significant impetus for the development of state and local government industrial hygiene programs. By 1946, 52 programs were operational in 41 states. However, the withdrawal of federal resources after the war led to a steady decline in both number and activity of these programs. By the late 1960s, while there were a number of states with programs, most involved only one or two professionals. The exceptions to this situation were found in the large industrial states such as Massachusetts, New York, Pennsylvania, Michigan, and California.

As in most countries, national legislation to control hazards in the workplace first focused on mining. The U.S. Bureau of Mines was established shortly after the turn of the century, but it was 1941 before the Bureau was authorized to conduct inspections in mines. A number of mining tragedies in the mid-1960s led to the passage of the Metal and Nonmetallic Mine Safety Act and the Coal Mine Safety and Health Act in 1966 and 1969, respectively. These mining laws were superseded by the comprehensive Mine Safety and Health Act of 1977. This law created the Mine Safety and Health Administration (MSHA) within the U.S. Department of Labor. MSHA regulates and conducts inspections in mines and related industries.

Federal safety and health activities in general industry were not initiated until passage of the Walsh-Healey Public Contracts Act in 1936. This legislation authorized federal occupational safety and health standards for government contractors. The Department of Labor adopted existing American Standards Association (now the American National Standards Institute, or ANSI) safety and

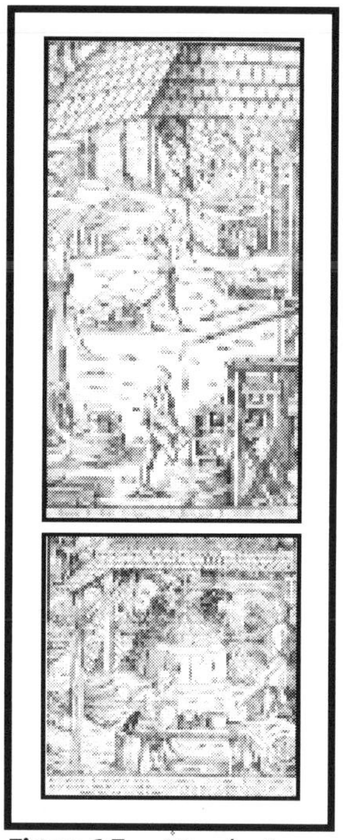

Figure 1.7 — Woodcuts depicting foundry workers at a smeltery.

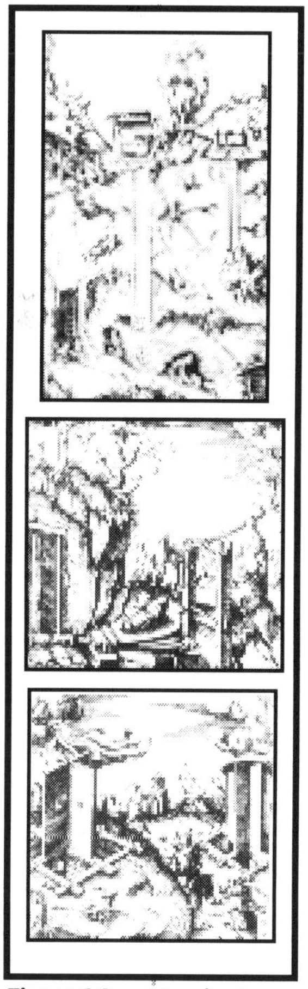

Figure 1.8 — Woodcuts showing ventilation systems for mines.

health standards and the ACGIH® TLVs® as Walsh-Healey standards.

In the late 1960s, the U.S. Congress became concerned with the comprehensive problem of occupational safety and health in the workplace. A number of congressional hearings resulted in the documentation of the seriousness of workplace deaths, injuries, and illnesses, and the lack of consistent and comprehensive safety and health programs at the state and local level to prevent such problems. Consequently, the Occupational Safety and Health Act[39] was passed in 1970 and created OSHA within the U.S. Department of Labor and NIOSH in the Department of Health and Human Services. OSHA was given the responsibility to promulgate standards and conduct inspections in most workplaces, while NIOSH was to conduct research and recommend health and safety standards to OSHA.

The initial health standards adopted by OSHA were the existing Walsh-Healey standards. These included the 1968 ACGIH® TLVs® minus the 21 chemicals for which there were ANSI standards.[38,40] The exposure limits for these substances are known as permissible exposure limits (PELs). Subsequent to these initial standards, OSHA began promulgating comprehensive health standards for a variety of chemicals including asbestos, benzene, coke oven emissions, and lead. In addition to a PEL, these comprehensive standards include requirements such as medical monitoring, administrative control measures, respirator selection, training, and record keeping.

Challenges to the regulation of two hazards ultimately led to U.S. Supreme Court decisions on the need for OSHA to quantify risk reduction and the cost-benefit of its regulatory actions. OSHA's 1978 regulation to reduce the PEL for benzene from 10 to 1 ppm was remanded by the Court because of its belief OSHA did not justify the PEL reduction would substantially reduce the risk to the health of exposed workers. The Court rejected the notion lower exposure is better and required OSHA to quantify the risk at current conditions of exposure and then document the proposed standard would substantially reduce risk to an acceptable level. In describing an acceptable level of risk, the Court suggested the risk of job-related death caused by injury or illness over a working lifetime would be an appropriate level of acceptability. This risk was estimated to be 1 in 1000, and this value has become OSHA's target in determining acceptable PELs for chemical substances. In reviewing the 1978 OSHA standard for cotton dust, the U.S. Supreme Court decided the OSH Act required OSHA to consider the technical and economic feasibility of new standards, but a cost-benefit analysis was not required.

In January 1989, OSHA promulgated a new regulation amending its existing Air Contaminants standard.[41,42] This reduced 212 PELs and established 164 new ones. OSHA stated it had reviewed health, risk, and technical/economic feasibility for the 428 substances considered in this rulemaking and found the new PELs substantially reduced a significant risk of material health impairment among American workers and were technologically and economically feasible. OSHA estimated benefits would accrue to 4.5 million workers and would result in the reduction of over 55,000 occupational illness cases annually. If not prevented, it was projected these illness cases would eventually result in approximately 700 fatalities each year.

Several industrial organizations and the AFL/CIO had a different perspective and successfully convinced the U.S. Court of Appeals the regulations should be vacated and remanded to OSHA. The court ruled (1) OSHA failed to establish existing exposure limits in the workplace represented significant risk of material health impairment or the new standards eliminated or substantially lessened the risk; (2) OSHA did not meet its burden of establishing the new PELs were either economically or technologically feasible; and (3) there was insufficient explanation in the record to support across-the-board, four-year delay in implementation of rule.[43]

The court stated "the inadequate explanation made it virtually impossible for a reviewing Court to determine if sufficient evidence supports the agency's conclusion."[43] The court indicated it could easily believe OSHA's claim of going through detailed analysis for each of the substances was not possible given the time constraints set by the agency for this rulemaking. The court determined OSHA's approach to this rulemaking was not consistent with the requirements of the OSH Act.

The end result was a major setback to efforts to formally update the PELs. However, benefits from the rulemaking effort remain after the court decision and include (1) adoption and continued use of the revised PELs by several state health protection programs; (2) informal adoption by some industrial organizations; (3) sensitization by many parties to the inadequacies and obsolescence of the existing PELs; and (4) plans by OSHA to initiate another effort to revise PELs for a group of substances (fewer than 428) where some commonality can be identified, and where the objections identified by the court can be avoided. Although the "revised" PELs were vacated in 1993, OSHA has yet to develop and implement a procedure for updating their antiquated list of PELs.

Reestablishing state authority for occupational safety and health was also an important goal of the OSH Act. States were encouraged to enact their own legislation and to develop programs at least as stringent as OSHA's. State programs approved by OSHA would receive 50% of their operational costs from the federal government. However, 25 years later fewer than half of the states reasserted their control over workplace hazards.

In addition to standards setting and enforcement, the OSH Act also included a provision to provide free consultation services to small businesses. These services are found in all 50 states and offer management confidential advice on safety and health problems.

While some may argue with the details of the content or the implementation of the OSH Act, most would agree with an early OSHA administrator that "its impact on working life in the United States cannot be overestimated."[44] The growth in the membership of the American Industrial Hygiene Association (AIHA®) demonstrated the impact on the number of practitioners in the profession. In 1970, AIHA® membership numbered 1,649 and within 10 years had tripled. It cannot be scientifically proven these additional practitioners (as well as those who entered the occupational safety profession) have improved the health and well-being of the American worker. But the attention paid to workplace hazards by this greatly expanded number of professionals is one factor contributing to a safer U.S. workplace.

Occupational Disasters Spur Reforms

Sentinel social events have often served as impetus for improvements in occupational working conditions. High profile tragedies captured the hearts and empathy of the public, leading to demands for reform. Individuals often responded with books, articles, poems, or songs that served as an exposé on some of the poor working conditions or on the effects of occupational disasters.[45–50]

Mining. Mining and mining disasters deserve special recognition in any discussion about the history of working conditions faced by employees. Historically, mining has been one of the most hazardous occupations with single incidents responsible for the loss of hundreds of miners. NIOSH maintains a website that chronicles over 700 mining disasters, defined as those incidents involving five or more fatalities.[51] Whether the death toll numbered in the dozens or in the hundreds, the memory lives on in the surrounding region.[48,49]

Nineteen disasters (each involving at least 5 deaths) were recorded in 1907, including the worst mining disaster in the history of the U.S.[51] On December 6, 1907, 362 miners were killed in a series of explosions at the Monongah No. 6, in Monongah, West Virginia. Twelve days later, 239 miners died in an explosion in Jacobs Creek, Pennsylvania when the Darr mine exploded.[51]

The phrase "mining towns" was used to designate the almost total control held over miners and their families by the mining companies.[50] Companies owned the houses miners lived in, along with the only grocery store near the mine. Mine companies also charged the miners for the tools they used. The following describes the miners' plight:

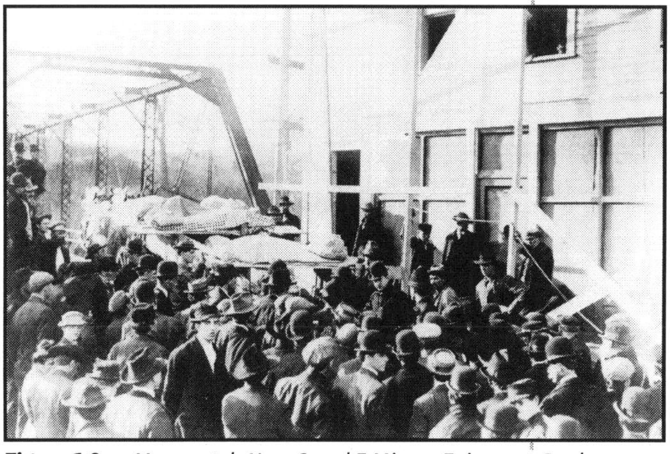

Figure 1.9 — Monongah Nos. 6 and 7 Mines. Fairmont Coal Company., Monongah, West Virginia. Removing the dead. Scenes after explosion.

Life in coal towns was not idyllic. Tom Lowry, a retired miner and former resident of the now abandoned Cumberland Plateau coal town of Wilder-Davidson, succinctly put it: "The company just about owned you." Mrs. Della Mullins, a coal miner's wife, concurred by saying: "Mining companies were king of the hill. You stooped and you bowed." Indeed, the mining company controlled nearly every essential aspect of community life, from work, shopping, education, retail merchandising, and medical care. The company store became the hub of coal mining community life, while nondenominational and generic wooden frame churches were the general rule for religious expression. The company provided schools and medical facilities as well. Social conditions were feudal and the coal operator was the law-giver.[50]

The Hawk's Nest incident is another sentinel event.[45] In the 1940s, a tunnel was drilled through a mountain of rock in southern West Virginia. The mountain consisted of a high percentage of crystalline silica, but the company often ignored protective measures such as wet drilling, due to the increased time for drilling and resulting loss of profit.[45] As a result, exposures to crystalline silica were so high that miners who had the highest exposures died from acute silicosis within a few months to a few years of starting work in the tunnels.[45,52] Silicosis, a chronic disease that normally develops over 20 or more years of exposure. The exposure levels to crystalline silica were so high that many developed silicosis within a year after their initial exposure and it is believed that over 500 workers died as a result of exposure while digging the tunnel.[35] *The Hawk's Nest Incident*, by Chernick details the terrible working conditions for workers who were assigned to work inside the tunnel.

The hazards of the mining industry are extensive and include black lung disease, asbestos, silicosis, lead, mercury, noise, falls, radon gas, and fire and explosion hazards. Protecting workers in such dangerous environments has been a daunting task. Advancements in the mining industry include the passage of laws in Pennsylvania in 1869 requiring two exits from all mines, and the creation of the Bureau of Mines in 1907 by the U.S. Department of Interior to investigate accidents, review hazards, and recommend improvements.[53] As a result of the incident at Hawk's Nest, the Air Hygiene Foundation (AHF) was founded in 1936."[52] Formation of the AHF led to the establishment of ACGIH® (1938), AIHA® (1939) and the initial development of TLVs®."[52] Additionally, the Federal Mine Safety Act was passed in 1977 to set and enforce safety standards in the industry and led to the creation of the Mine Safety and Health Administration (MSHA) in 1978.

Even with regulatory improvements and a focus on mine safety, mining continues to be a very hazardous occupation.[54,55] In January 2006, 12 miners were killed following an explosion in the Sago Mine in West Virginia. Media attention highlighted the dangers as a country watched the rescue turned recovery mission on the nightly news. This was followed by yet another incident in 2007 at Utah's Crandal Canyon Mine. The death toll reached nine, including the deaths of three rescue workers attempting to free the trapped miners. On June 15, 2006, President George W. Bush signed the Mine Improvement and New Emergency Response (MINER) Act of 2006, legislation that MSHA calls "the most significant mine safety legislation in 30 years."[56] The MINER Act specifies requirements for emergency response procedures and increases the civil and criminal penalties for companies in violation of standards. On May 5, 2010, one of the worst mine disasters, based on the of number of fatalities, occurred once again in West Virginia, where 29 miners were killed.[55]

Pollution. Other important events have impacted workers, community members, and society in general, and have helped to spur the public into action. This includes the London Fog, in which over 1,000 London residents died during a year-long pollution episode. The pollution from industrial facilities made the air quality much worse than it would otherwise have been.[57]

Similarly, in 1948, the people of Donora, Pennsylvania fell victim to a deadly smog that killed 20 people and caused another 6,000 to become ill.[58] Contributing to the pollution were several manufacturing plants, including a zinc smelting plant, a steel production facility, and a sulfuric acid plant. A study by an industrial hygiene team revealed high atmospheric levels of sulfur dioxide, soluble sulfates and fluorides. Emissions from the plants, together with an unusually heavy fog and a calm atmospheric period, converged to create the disaster. Bill Schempp, a Donora firefighter at the time, described the smog by saying "If you chewed hard enough, you could swallow it. It almost got to the point where it was claustrophobic, it was so dense and thick. You couldn't see a thing."(58) In the end, the events at Donora resulted in the passage of the Clean Air Act by Pennsylvania in 1955, and ultimately paved the way for the U.S. Clean Air Act in 1970.(58)

Radiation. Another example of poor early work conditions is the radium dial painting studios in the northeastern U.S. at the turn of the 20th Century. An Austrian physicist and owner of the early radium studios, Sabin A. von Sochocky, created a formula for the radioactive luminous radium paint.(12) Radium was required for use in military instrument dial faces during World War I and for the newly developed wristwatch. The Radium Luminous Material Corporation targeted girls and young women ages 15–25 to work in the studios. These well-paying jobs were considered ideal for women because the work was less physically demanding and female workers were assumed to have strong manual dexterity.(12) The trained work practice for dial painters was to lip point their brushes to obtain the fine point necessary for such intricate work. Many of the girls died and others suffered horrible disfigurement as a result of their exposure.(12)

Another advancement, this time in the shoe industry, involved radiation exposure to workers as well as the general public. For a period of time beginning in the 1930s through the 1950s, shoe stores across the country marketed a Shoe-Fitting Fluoroscope to help ensure proper shoe fitting. The machine required customers to place their feet in the machine for an x-ray of their feet inside their new shoes. A study published in 1950(59) revealed an across the board lack of maintenance and inspection of the machines, and concluded, "In view of the probability of improper use and because of uncertain knowledge as to the danger of cumulative small dosage of x-ray, it is clear that a very good case can be made for the removal of these devices from commercial shoe stores. This is particularly true in view of the lack of proof of their merit as scientific devices for fitting shoes."(60) Due to elapsed time and the inability to ascertain actual exposures, it is difficult to link the Shoe-Fitting Fluoroscopes with cases of cancer.(61)

In 1986, one of the worst industrial disasters in history occurred at Chernobyl, Ukraine. An explosion of a reactor resulted in the accidental release of a massive amount of radiation from cesium-137. It is difficult to quantify the number of deaths directly attributed to the incident, but there are fears that thousands of cancer deaths may continue to occur as a result of radiation exposures. "The Chernobyl accident also resulted in widespread contamination in areas of Belarus, the Russian Federation, and Ukraine inhabited by millions of residents."

Chemical Exposures. Bhopal, India is the site of what has been called the worst industrial accident in the world. In December 1984, 41 metric tons of gas composed largely of methyl-isocyanate (MIC) was released into the atmosphere from a Union Carbide plant.(63,64) MIC, an ingredient used in pesticides, has a TLV®-TWA of 0.02 ppm and an LC_{50} of 5 ppm for rats.(65) With a vapor density greater than the density of air, the chemical hovered at ground level traveling with the prevailing wind patterns.(65) The cloud of lethal gas that drifted over the adjacent town killed approximately 2,800 people overnight and injured an estimated 170,000.(66) The incident at Bhopal brought about significant change in chemical process safety and resulted in new OSHA and EPA regulations. Bhopal led to the creation of the Emergency Planning and Community Right to Know Act (EPCRA) in 1986.(53) Additionally, it led to the eventual formation of the U.S. Chemical Safety and Hazard Investigation Board (CSB) in 1998 to independently investigate chemical accidents.

Education and Professional Organizations

Growth of Industrial Hygiene Academic Programs in the U.S.

With the increased awareness of workplace hazards, as well as government oversight, the need for trained experts grew. Harvard University is recognized as the first academic institution to offer research in industrial hygiene leading to an advanced degree, although MIT offered a course in industrial hygiene prior to the program at Harvard.[67,68] Many of the early leaders in industrial hygiene were graduates of Harvard.[67]

Following Harvard, academic programs were developed at the University of Pittsburgh, the University of North Carolina, and Johns Hopkins University.[20] Also among the first to develop IH programs were the University of Cincinnati and the University of Iowa.[69,70] The growth in academic industrial hygiene programs was slow for the first 50 years after Harvard. That changed in 1970 after passage of the OSH Act on December 29, 1970.[20,67,71] After the OSH Act passed, the number of IH programs grew to over 200 by 1979. There was a subsequent decline in the number of academic IH programs; a survey conducted in 1987 identified 106 programs.[67] By 2011, the evolution of academic programs to include safety, environmental, and other "non-traditional" IH topics has resulted in a wide variety of program names and descriptions, making it difficult to determine the exact number academic IH programs. The Academy of Industrial Hygiene has identified nearly 60 universities in the U.S. offering at least one degree, concentration area, or significant coursework in industrial hygiene.

As with any profession, quality of academic programs available is essential for developing competent and prepared professionals. ABET, Inc is the premier accrediting body for industrial hygiene and safety programs. Originally founded in 1932 as the Engineers Council for Professional Development (ECPD), the organization was renamed the Accreditation Board for Engineering and Technology in 1980, and then changed its name to ABET, Inc. in 2005. Comprised of thirty professional and technical societies, ABET accredits individual degree programs based on general and program specific criteria.[72,73]

ABET has four accreditation commissions: the Applied Science Accreditation Commission (ASAC), Computing Accreditation Commission (CAC), Engineering Accreditation Commission (EAC), and Technology Accreditation Commission (TAC). ASAC was created in 1983 (originally called the Related Accreditation Commission) and is the commission responsible for accrediting industrial hygiene, safety and environmental safety & health programs.[74] Guidance on accrediting these programs is provided to ABET by AIHA® and the American Society of Safety Engineers (ASSE).

General accreditation requirements include the development of specific program educational objectives and outcomes, qualified faculty, appropriate facilities and institutional support, and curricular integrity to include student coursework in math and basic and applied sciences. Additional program specific criteria are set forth by the lead societies. According to ABET's 2010 Annual Report, there were seven undergraduate and 28 graduate programs accredited by ASAC/ABET under the disciplinary area of industrial hygiene, nine bachelor degrees and two masters programs under the disciplinary area of safety, and two undergraduate programs under the disciplinary area of environmental, safety and health.

Research

Research is a significant resource for the practice of industrial hygiene. Professional organizations encourage members to actively engage in lifelong learning and many offer avenues for publishing in journals and professional magazines.

Given the wide variety of research activities, the National Institute for Occupational Safety and Health (NIOSH), a division of the Centers for Disease Control and Prevention (CDC), looks closely at workplace safety and health issues. In an effort to focus on the challenges in today's workforce, NIOSH develops and promotes a National Occupational Research Agenda (NORA) which focuses on eight unique and varying sectors of the workforce. The sectors are based on areas with common workplace concerns and each has a NORA Sector Council, which is responsible for identifying specific research agendas for that sector. The sectors defined by NORA include the following: Agriculture, Forestry and Fishing; Construction; Healthcare and Social Assistance; Manufacturing; Mining; Services; Transportation, Warehousing and Utilities; and Wholesale and Retail Trade.

In addition to NORA, NIOSH recognizes that for research to provide true benefits to the workplace and society, it must translate into practice. As a result, NIOSH has also developed Research to Practice (r2p) as a priority. NIOSH describes r2p as "a collaborative process between NIOSH and its partners that combines the generation of knowledge with the adoption of that knowledge in the workplace to reduce worker injury and illness."

A development that has turned into a national movement is the Prevention through Design Initiative. As explained by Manuele, safety through design was initiated in the National Safety Council in the early 1990s.[75] More recently, NIOSH has given credence to this movement by establishing a specific PtD initiative.[76] The PtD initiative fits in nicely to the valuing the profession that AIHA and other organizations have supported for the past several years.[77]

Development of Professional Associations

It has been suggested that "one can date the emergence of the profession of industrial hygiene by the formation of our professional societies."[78] In 1938, 76 industrial hygienists representing 24 states, 3 cities, 1 university, the USPHS, the U.S. Bureau of Mines, and the Tennessee Valley Authority convened in Washington, D.C., to formally establish the National (later to become the American) Conference of Governmental Industrial Hygienists. ACGIH® was established to "coordinate activities in federal, state, local, and territorial organizations and agencies; to help the public health service carry out its mission; and to develop state industrial hygiene units in a rational manner."[79] By 2010, ACGIH® membership had reached over 3,000.[80]

In 1939, AIHA® was formed. At the first meeting of the AIHA® Board of Directors, four major goals of the association were enunciated.

1. The advancement and application of industrial hygiene and sanitation through the interchange and dissemination of technical knowledge on these subjects.
2. The furthering of the study and control of industrial health hazards through determination and elimination of excessive exposures.
3. The correlation of such activities as conducted by diverse individuals and agencies throughout industry, educational, and governmental groups.
4. The uniting of persons with these interests.[81]

AIHA® membership has grown from 160 members in 1940 to more than 10,200 members in 2011.[82] AIHA® also has 73 local sections throughout the U.S. and in 3 other countries, which foster the interaction of industrial hygienists. The *AIHA® Journal* first appeared in 1946, while *ACGIH's® Applied Occupational and Environmental Hygiene* (originally appearing as Applied Industrial Hygiene) debuted in 1986. The individual journals from AIHA® and ACGIH® ceased publication in 2003 and were replaced by a joint peer-reviewed journal titled the *Journal of Occupational and Environmental Hygiene* (JOEH).

AIHA® and ACGIH® were also founding members of the International Occupational Hygiene Association (IOHA). Membership in IOHA is limited to occupational hygiene professional associations, which by 2011 included associations located in Australia, Belgium, Brazil, Canada, Columbia, Denmark, Finland, France, Germany, Hong Kong, Ireland, Italy, Japan, Malaysia, Mexico, The Netherlands, New Zealand, Norway, Poland, Southern Africa, Spain, Sweden, Switzerland, Taiwan, the United Kingdom (BIOH and BOHS), and the U.S. IOHA is recognized as a "Non Governmental Organization" (NGO) by both the International Labour Organization and the World Health Organization. As a NGO to these two international bodies, IOHA serves as the voice of the occupational hygiene profession at the international level.

In 1960, AIHA® and ACGIH® created the American Board of Industrial Hygiene (ABIH) to develop voluntary professional certification standards for industrial hygienists and to implement a certification program.[83] The initial group of certified industrial hygienists (CIHs) has grown from 18 in 1960 to more than 6600 at the end of 2010. In 1966, the diplomates of the ABIH certification program activated the American Academy of Industrial Hygiene (AAIH) as a professional organization. As stated in their bylaws, the purpose of AAIH was to provide leadership in advancing the professional field of industrial hygiene, by raising the level of competence of industrial hygienists and by securing wide recognition of the need for high quality industrial hygiene practice to ensure healthful work conditions in the various occupations and industries.[84]

The major activities of AAIH included promotion of the recognition of industrial hygiene as a profession by individuals, employers, and regulatory agencies and the accreditation of academic programs in industrial hygiene in cooperation with the Accreditation Board of Engineering and Technology. AAIH sponsored the annual Professional Conference on Industrial Hygiene to provide a forum for exploring professional issues, especially those encountered by more experienced industrial hygienists.

In the mid 1990s, an effort was made to unite the four industrial hygiene organizations (AAIH, ABIH, ACGIH® and AIHA®). After considerable exploration of options and their impact, the ACGIH® and the ABIH® decided to remain as independent organizations. However, the membership of the AAIH and AIHA® voted, with over 90 percent positive in each case, to merge the Academy into the AIHA®. In 1999, the Board of ABIH voted to dissolve the AAIH, for its reformation as the Academy of Industrial Hygiene (AIH) within AIHA®. In January 2000, the American Academy of Industrial Hygiene merged with AIHA® and the AIHA® membership approved a change to the bylaws creating the Diplomate membership category. The Diplomate member category was created to recognize members who were both Full members of AIHA® and Certified Industrial Hygienists in good standing with the American Board of Industrial Hygiene.

Public Health Roots

It has been postulated the "[f]irst Public Health Revolution unfolded in nineteenth-century Europe as that society sought to address the adverse health effects of squalid living conditions: poor sanitation, poor housing, dangerous work environments and air pollution."(85) There is ample evidence the roots of industrial hygiene extend into the field of public health. The public health philosophy of protection and enhancement of the health and well being of groups of people through preventive rather than curative measures applies as well to industrial hygiene.

The Institute of Medicine has defined public health as "what we, as a society, do collectively to assure the conditions in which people can be healthy."(86) Thus, when industrial hygienists implement a control measure to reduce a worker's exposure to a toxin, they are practicing the art and science of public health. Those who practice in the field of public health are well aware throughout the history of public and especially occupational health, two major factors have shaped our solutions: the availability of scientific and technical knowledge and the content of public values and opinions. The Institute of Medicine has recognized the lack of agreement about the public health mission as reflected in the division in some states of traditional public health functions "such as water and air pollution control, to separate departments of environmental services, where the health effects of pollutants often receive less notice."(86) Although industrial hygiene functions are now most often found combined with safety programs in labor rather than public health departments, the concepts of injury prevention, whether on or off the job, have strong public health underpinnings. Thus, safety and hygiene are intertwined.

The first professional journal to address industrial hygiene concerns was the *Journal of the American Public Health Association*. In 1914, the journal announced a new department on industrial hygiene and sanitation to put the readers "in touch with the latest information in this very recently new field of Public Health work," and a review article on industrial hygiene and sanitation was published.(87) In the same year, the association created an industrial hygiene section, and at the annual meeting a special symposium on industrial hygiene was held. Alice Hamilton served as vice chairman of the new section and succeeded to the chairmanship in 1916.(88)

As noted earlier, in 1914, the USPHS established an office of industrial hygiene and sanitation, which 57 years later became NIOSH. NIOSH is part of the federal Centers for Disease Control and Prevention, which encompasses most of the public health functions of the federal government. Prior to the OSH Act of 1970, most state and local government industrial hygiene units were found in public health agencies.

Industrial hygiene graduate level academic training in the United States has since its inception been associated with schools of public health. In 1918, the Harvard Medical School established a Department of Applied Physiology, which in 1922 became the Department of Physiology and the

Department of Industrial Hygiene in the School of Public Health. In the late 1930s, state public health agencies used Social Security funds to train industrial hygienists in schools of public health at Harvard, the University of California, Columbia University, The Johns Hopkins University, the University of Michigan, and Yale University. Today industrial hygiene academic programs are found in at least 18 of the 27 accredited schools of public health.

Professional Recognition and Title Protection

As the profession of industrial hygiene and occupational health and safety changes, so do the perceptions of what constitutes an individual who is qualified to practice industrial hygiene. It is an issue which has been debated within the profession for many years. In the early 1990s, AIHA® became more proactively involved with this issue. This increased interest was a result of several events, most notably an expanding requirement by federal and state regulators mandating all individuals have additional training and certification for many single-substance issues (e.g., asbestos and lead).

Starting with the adoption of an official position statement on title protection in 1994, AIHA® began working to assist local sections and state government affairs organizations with efforts to enact title protection legislation in the individual states. AIHA's® original model bill included definitions for CIH and the now discontinued Industrial Hygienist in Training (IHIT). The model bill adopted in 2001 also included a definition for the title Certified Associate Industrial Hygienist (CAIH) and included the Certified Safety Professional (CSP). The result of these efforts was the passage of legislation in numerous states that defined IH titles and/or protected these titles from being used by unqualified individuals. It should be noted that there is a difference between "defining and/or recognizing" a title and "protecting" a title. In many cases the legislation "defines and/or recognizes" various titles; however only those titles that are accredited are "protected." By the end of 2010, 19 states had some form of professional recognition/title protection enacted into law. On the federal level, AIHA® works to see federal regulations and legislative efforts do not restrict the profession. All regulatory and congressional activities are monitored to assure the profession is protected. When possible, AIHA® seeks to add language recognizing the certified industrial hygienist as a competent, qualified, and knowledgeable occupational health and safety professional.

While title protection will not eliminate new credentialing organizations, it provides the industrial hygiene professional with legal recognition and protection. It will also be of assistance in future regulatory efforts on both the federal and state levels as AIHA® seeks to have this profession recognized as a leader in the field of protecting workers. In 2011, the AIHA® Registry Programs LLC began offering credentials that provide a means to validate a person's knowledge and skills in a specialized area of practice through a demonstration of competency. Each registry program is based on a body of knowledge relevant to the specialty area of practice and developed by subject matter experts. These Registry Programs focus on promoting sound skill development by professionals who are not certified, those at the operator or technician level and by supporting industrial hygiene skills and knowledge within allied professions.

The Future

To not only remain viable but also to achieve increased recognition and acceptance of their work, it is apparent industrial hygienists must, as do most professions, continue to reevaluate and, where necessary, redesign the scope and content of their practice. Today in many organizations the hygienist is called upon to provide support to the entire arena of environment, safety and health. Hygienists must continue to expand the scope of their practice to include environmental health considerations, especially those arising from the workplace. The skills and knowledge involved in the recognition, evaluation, and control of air, and even water, pollution problems as well as those of hazardous wastes are not dissimilar to the skills and knowledge applied to traditional industrial hygiene problems. Indeed, many of the early environmental health practitioners, especially addressing air pollution, radiological health and hazardous waste problems, were industrial hygienists.(89) The first air pollution disaster in the U.S., the Donora, PA, smog of October 1948, resulted in the death of 20 people and to some degree affected almost 6000 persons.[90] The investigation of the incident involved a multidisciplinary team of physicians, nurses, engineers, chemists, meteorologists, housing experts, veterinarians, and dentists under the direction of a USPHS industrial hygienist George D. Clayton. Industrial hygienists must become more effective in providing comprehensive rather than one-issue services.

Safety cannot be seen as some distinct area of practice separate from industrial hygiene. The significant overlap between health and safety in many activities (e.g. confined space entry or product stewardship) is well recognized. And, the reality is that protecting a worker from chronic health hazards does little if the worker is killed or seriously injured on the job. In a walk through survey, a competent hygienist should be able to recognize a wide range of traditional safety hazards as well as potential exposures.

This concept of expanding skills and knowledge needed by the industrial hygienist underscores the need to not only be technically competent, but also be able to communicate (verbally and in writing) effectively and to develop productive working relationships with management, unions, other health and safety professionals and, above all, workers. Just as they were in 1936, these skills are essential for success, especially when addressing non-traditional workplaces and hazards.[36]

Finally, as a profession and as individuals, industrial hygienists must demonstrate their services, in addition to preventing industrial and environmental health and safety problems, provide a tangible, positive contribution to the individual worker, the community, and the employer. The ability to demonstrate the value of industrial hygiene within the business context is essential to successfully protecting worker health. As professionals the job cannot be limited to meeting minimum government standards, but more importantly it must enhance the organization. Enhancement does not happen automatically or necessarily through chance. It must be a goal with plans developed with the participation, and as appropriate, approval of involved and affected parties (management and workers), implemented and then measured to determine the level of achievement.

Summary

This chapter reviews the history of industrial hygiene with an emphasis on the significant milestones, including the U.S. experience. In addition to a chronological listing of developments, the profession's history is also viewed in the context of its tenants of practice: anticipation, recognition, evaluation, prevention and control. The considerable impact of the OSH Act on the growth of the profession and its practice is described. A review of several of the occupational disasters that helped instigate reform is provided. A historical review of the professional organizations is presented. In considering the philosophy of the practice of the profession, its public health roots are apparent. The public health philosophy of protection and enhancement of the health and well being of groups of people through preventive rather than curative measures applies as well to the practice of industrial hygiene. As the importance of the profession grew, AIHA® recognized the need to ensure the practice of industrial hygiene was limited to qualified professionals. AIHA's® effort in title enhancement and protection has resulted in increased recognition of the profession by federal and state legislators and regulators. The future of industrial hygiene will be shaped by the leadership of practitioner through professional engagement, life-long learning, and a dedication to improving health and safety in the workforce, the community, and at home.

References

1. **Patty, F.A.:** Industrial hygiene: retrospect and prospect. In *Patty's Industrial Hygiene and Toxicology*, Vol. 1, 3rd edition. New York: John Wiley & Sons, 1978. pp. 1–21.
2. **Goldwater, L.J.:** *Historical Highlights in Occupational Medicine*. (Readings and Perspectives in Medicine, Booklet 9). Durham, NC: Duke University Medical Center, 1985. pp. 1–14.
3. **Ramazzini, B.:** *Diseases of Workers*. New York: Hafner Publishing Co., 1964.

4. **Borzelleca, J.F.:** The Art, the Science, and the Seduction of Toxicology: An Evolutionary Development. In *Principles and Methods of Toxicology*, 4th edition. Philadelphia, PA: Taylor and Francis, 2001. pp. 1–22.
5. **Association Medical Journal:** *Death of Orfila*. Vol.1, no. 11, March 18, 1853. p. 228. From http://www.jstor.org/stable/25494474.
6. **McReady, B.W.:** *On the Influence of Trades, Professions and Occupations in the United State, in the Production of Disease* (transactions of the Medical Society of the State of New York, Vol. III). Albany, NY: Medical Society of the State of New York, 1837.
7. **Luxon, S.G.:** A history of industrial hygiene. *Am. Ind. Hyg. Assoc. J. 45*:731–39 (1984).
8. **Brown, H.V.:** This history of industrial hygiene: a review with special reference to silicosis. *Am. Ind. Hyg. Assoc. J. 26*:212–26 (1965).
9. **Hamilton, A.:** *Exploring the Dangerous Trades*. Fairfax, VA: AIHA®, 1995. p. 1.
10. **Clayton, G.D.:** Industrial hygiene: Retrospect and prospect. In *Patty's Industrial Hygiene and Toxicology*, Vol. 1, part A, 4th edition. New York: John Wiley & Sons, 1991. p. 1–13.
11. **Hamilton, A.:** *Exploring the Dangerous Trades: The Autobiography of Alice Hamilton*, MD. Fairfax, VA: AIHA®, 1995.
12. **Clark, C.:** *Radium Girls: Women and Industrial Health Reform, 1910–1935*. Chapel Hill, NC: The University of North Carolina Press, 1997.
13. Dr. Alice Hamilton Celebrates 100th Birthday: Famed Industrial Toxicologist is Honored for Her Work in Mines and Factories. *New York Times*, Feb 28, 1969, p. 35.
14. **American Chemical Society:** National historic chemical landmarks: Alice Hamilton and the development of occupational medicine. 2002. Retrieved June 2, 2011 from http://portal.acs.org/portal/acs/corg/content?_nfpb=true&_page Label=PP_ARTICLEMAIN&node_id=924&content_id=WPCP_007617&use_sec=true&sec_url_var=region1&__uuid=b4fe1ddb-291f-4944-9806-b32edf68f9c7.
15. **Smith, D.R.:** Celebrating a Milestone in EOH: The Pioneering First Issue of the Journal of Industrial Hygiene, May 1919. *Arch. Env. Occup. Health 65(4)*:240–242 (2010).
16. **D'Orsie, S.M.:** Leadership Without Authority: The Example set by Dr. Alice Hamilton. Professional Safety, 32-35 (August 2004).
17. **Rosner, D. and G. Markowitz:** Research or Advocacy: Federal Occupational Safety and Health Policies During the New Deal. *J. Soc. Hist. 18(3)*:365–81 (2001).
18. To Advise Miss Perkins. *New York Times*, October 26, 1935, p. 13.
19. **Corn, J.K.:** Historical aspects of industrial hygiene-I: Changing attitudes toward occupational health. *Am. Ind. Hyg. Assoc. J. 39*:695–99 (1978).
20. **Rose, V.E.:** The development of occupational hygiene in the United States-a history. *Ann. Am. Conf. Gov. Ind. Hyg. 15*:5–8 (1988).
21. **Greife, A., et al.:** National Institute for Occupational Safety and Health-general industry occupational exposure databases: their structure, capabilities, and limitations. *Appl. Occup. Environ. Hyg. 10*:264–69 (1995).
22. **Redmond, S.K., A. Ciocco, J.W. Lloyd, and H.W. Rush:** Long-term mortality of steel workers. VI. Mortality from malignant neoplasms among coke oven workers. *J. Occup. Med. 13*:53–68 (1971).
23. "Coke Oven Emissions," Code of Federal Regulations, Title 29, Section 1910.1029. 1977.
24. **National Institute for Occupational Safety and Health (NIOSH):** Criteria for a Recommended Standard. Occupational Exposure to Asbestos (DHEW/NIOSH pub. HSM72-10267). Washington, DC: Government Printing Office, 1972. p. V-4.
25. **Selikoff, I.J., J. Chung, and E.C. Hammond:** Asbestos exposure and neoplasia. *J. Am. Med. Assoc. 188*:22 (1964).
26. "Asbestos," Code of Federal Regulations, Title 29, Section 1910.1001. 1972.
27. "Benzene," Code of Federal Regulations, Title 29, Section 1910.1028. 1987.
28. **Lamb, A.B. and C.R. Hoover:** U.S. Patent 1321 062 (1919).
29. **Goetz, A.:** Application of molecular filter membranes to the analysis of aerosols. *Am. J. Pub. Health 43*:150–59 (1953).
30. **White, L.D., D.G. Taylor, P.A. Mauer, and R.E. Kupel:** A convenient optimized method for the analysis of selected solvent vapors in the industrial atmosphere. *Am. Ind. Hyg. Assoc. J. 31*:225–32 (1970).
31. **Rose, V.E. and J.L. Perkins:** Passive dosimetry-a state of the art review. *Am. Ind. Hyg. Assoc. J. 43*:605–21 (1982).
32. **National Institute for Occupational Safety and Health (NIOSH):** Criteria for a Recommended Standard. Occupational Exposure to Crystalline Silica (DHEW/NIOSH pub. 75-120). Washington, DC: Government Printing Office, 1975. p. 62.
33. **Baetzer, A.M.:** The early days of industrial hygiene-their contribution to current problems. *Am. Ind. Hyg. Assoc. J. 41*:773-777 (1980).
34. **Felton, J.S.:** *History. In Occupational Health & Safety*, 2nd edition. LaDou, J. (ed.). Itasca, IL: National Safety Council, 1994. pp. 17–31.
35. **National Institute for Occupational Safety and Health (NIOSH):** *A Guide to Industrial Respiratory Protection*. Pritchard, J.A. (ed.). (DHEW/NIOSH pub. 76-189). Washington, DC: Government Printing Office, 1976. p. 5–8.

36. **Cralley, L.J.:** Industrial hygiene in the U.S. Public Health Service (1914–1968). *Appl. Occup. Environ. Hyg. 11*:147–55 (1996).
37. **Bloomfield, J.J.:** Development of industrial hygiene in the United States. *Am. J. Pub. Health 28*:1388–97 (1938).
38. **Sayers, R.R. and J.J. Bloomfield:** Industrial hygiene activities in the United States. *Am. J. Pub. Health 26*:1007–96 (1936).
39. "Occupational Safety and Health Act," Pub. Law 91-596, Section 2193. 91st Congress, Dec. 29, 1970; as amended, Pub. Law 101-552, Section 3101, Nov. 5, 1990.
40. "Limits for Air Contaminants," Code of Federal Regulations, Title 29, Section 1910.1000. 1971. Tables Z-1 (chemicals) and Z-3 (mineral dusts).
41. "Limits for Air Contaminants," Code of Federal Regulations, Title 29, Section 1910.1000. 1971. Table Z-2.
42. "Limits for Air Contaminants; Final Rule." Federal Register, January 19, 1989.
43. AFL/CIO v. OSHA, U.S. Court of Appeals, 11th Cir., July 7, 1992.
44. **Corn, M.:** The progression of industrial hygiene. *Appl. Ind. Hyg. 4*:153–57 (1989).
45. **Cherniack, M.:** *The Hawk's Nest Incident; America's Worst Industrial Disaster.* New Haven, CT: Yale University Press, 1989.
46. **Hanig, J., (Producer) and D. Davis (Director):** *Song of the Canary.* New Day Film. 1979. http://www.newday.com/films/Song_of_the_Canary.html. [Accessed on May 26, 2009.]
47. **Public Broadcasting System (PBS):** Triangle Fire. 2011. http://www.pbs.org/wgbh/americanexperience/films/triangle/player/. [Accessed on July 12, 2011.]
48. **Isom, Y.D.:** The Scofield Mine Disaster in 1900 was Utah's worst. Utah History to Go, 1995. http://historytogo.utah.gov/utah_chapters/mining_and_railroads/thescofieldminedisasterin1900wasutahsworst.html. [Accessed June 2, 2011.]
49. **Clement, M.:** Mine explosion victims remembered. Fayetteveille Online Features. May 26, 2000. http://freepages.history.rootsweb.ancestry.com/~pfwilson/mine_explosion_victims_remembered.htm. [Accessed June 2, 2011.]
50. **Jones, J.:** Social Control, Social Displacement and Coal Mining in the Cumberland Plateau, 1880–1930. 1999. http://www.netowne.com/historical/tennessee/index.htm. [Accessed August 28, 2010.]
51. **National Institute for Occupational Safety and Health (NIOSH):** Historical Mine Disasters (Incidents with 5 or more fatalities. http://www.cdc.gov/niosh/mining/statistics/disasters.htm. [Accessed June 1, 2011.]
52. **Stalnaker, C.:** Hawk's Nest Tunnel: A forgotten tragedy in safety's history. *Prof. Safety (7)*:27–33 (2006).
53. **Goetsch, D.L.:** *Occupational Safety and Health for Technologists, Engineers and Managers.* Upper Saddle River, NJ: Prentice Hall, 1998.
54. **National Public Radio:** A bitter saga: The sago mine disaster. Scott Simon Host, January 7, 2006. http://www.npr.org/templates/story/story.php?storyId=5134307. [Accessed June 2, 2011.]
55. **Mine Safety and Health Administration (MSHA):** MSHA news release MSHA announces series of pubic meetings to bolster transparency in investigation of upper big branch mine explosion, May 5, 2010. Mine Mine Safety and Health Administration. http://www.msha.gov/MEDIA/PRESS/2010/NR100506a.asp. [Accessed June 2, 2011.]
56. **Mine Safety and Health Administration (MSHA):** The Miner Act. http://www.msha.gov/mineract/mineractsinglesource.asp. [Accessed June 2, 2011.]
57. **Bell, M.L. and D.L. Davis:** Reassessment of the Lethal London Fog of 1952: Novel indicators of acute and chronic consequences of acute exposure to air pollution. *Env. Health Persp. 109(3)*:389–94 (2001).
58. **Templeton, D.:** Cleaner air is legacy left by Donora's killer 1948 smog. Pittsburgh Post Gazette. Post-Gazette.com magazine. (October 29, 1998).
59. **Lewis, L. and P.E. Caplan:** The shoe-fitting fluoroscope as a radiation hazard. *California Med. 72*:26–30 (1950).
60. **Lewis, L. and P.E. Caplan:** The shoe-fitting fluoroscope as a radiation hazard. *California Med. 72*:26–30. p.30 (1950).
61. **Smullen, M.J. and D.E. Bertler:** Basal cell carcinoma of the sole: possible association with the shoe fitting fluoroscope. *Wisc. Med. J. 106(5)*:275–78 (2007).
62. **Nuclear Regulatory Commission (NRC):** (2006). Backgrounder on chernobyl nuclear power plant accident. 2006. http://www.nrc.gov/reading-rm/doc-collections/fact-sheets/chernobyl-bg.html. [Accessed on July 11, 2007.]
63. **Brelis, D.:** India's night of death, More than 2,500 people are killed in the worst industrial disaster ever. *Time*, 22–26, 31. December 17, 1984.
64. **Rosenblatt, R.:** All the World Gasped: A Tragic Gas Leak Offers a Parable of Industrial Life. *Time*, 20-21. December 17, 1984.
65. **Willey, R.J.:** *Process Safety Progress.* Volume 18, Issue 4. New York: John Wiley & Sons, Winter 1999. pp. 195–200.

66. **U.S. Environmental Protecting Agency (EPA):** Methyl isocyanate. Technology Transfer Network Air Toxics Web Site. http://www.epa.gov/ttn/atw/hlthef/methylis.html. [Accessed June 2, 2011.]
67. **Clayton, G.D.:** Industrial Hygiene: Retrospect and Prospect. In *Patty's Industrial Hygiene*, Fifth edition, Vol 1. Harris, R. (ed.). John Wiley and Sons, 2000.
68. **Rose, V.E.:** History and Philosophy of Industrial Hygiene (Chapter 1). In *The Occupational Environmental: It's Evaluation, Control and Management*, 2nd edition. DiNardi, S. (ed.). Fairfax, VA: AIHA® Press, 2003. pp. 2–19.
69. **University of Cincinnati, Department of Environmental Health:** Our History. http://www.eh.uc.edu/dept_history.asp. [Accessed June 2, 2011.]
70. **Yaffe, C.D.:** Clyde M. Berry. In *Some Pioneers in IH.* Cincinnati, OH: ACGIH®, 1984.
71. **Rentos, P.E. and T.C. Purcell:** The United States professional occupational work force: needs and demands. In *Training and Education in Occupational Hygiene: An International Perspective.* Annals of the American Conference of Governmental Industrial Hygienists. Vol 15. Cincinnati, OH: ACGIH, 1988.
72. **ABET, Inc.:** Going Global: Accreditation takes off worldwide. ABET 2008 Annual Report for ABET Fiscal Year 2007–2008. Baltimore, MD: ABET, 2008.
73. **ABET, Inc.:** Criteria For Accrediting Applied Science Programs: Effective for Evaluations During the 2010-2011 Accreditation Cycle. Baltimore, MD: ABET, Inc., 2009. http://www.abet.org/formsorg/forms.shtml#For_Applied_ Science_Programs_Only. [Accessed on August 5, 2010.]
74. **ABET, Inc.:** History: More than 75 years of quality assurance in technical education. http://www.abet.org/history.shtml. Baltimore, MD: ABET, 2010. [Accessed on August 5, 2010.]
75. **Manuele F.:** Prevention Through Design (PtD): History and Future. *J. Safety Res. 39*:127–30 (2008).
76. **National Institute for Occupational Safety and Health (NIOSH):** Prevention through Design Plan for the National Initiative. (DHHS - NIOSH) pub. No. 2011-121. Cincinnati, OH: NIOSH, 2011.
77. **American Industrial Hygiene Association (AIHA®):** *A Strategy to Demonstrate the Value of Industrial Hygiene.* AIHA®. http://www.aiha.org/votp_new/study/index.html. [Accessed on June 3, 2011.]
78. **Corn, J.K.:** Historical review of industrial hygiene. *Ann. Am. Conf. Gov. Ind. Hyg. 5*:13–17 (1983).
79. **Corn, J.K.:** *Protecting the Health of Workers: The American Conference of Governmental Industrial Hygienists 1938–1988.* Cincinnati, OH: ACGIH®, 1989. p. 8.
80. **American Conference of Governmental Industrial Hygienists (ACGIH®):** Homepage. 2010. http://www.acgih.org/home.htm. [Accessed on May 30, 2011.]
81. **American Industrial Hygiene Association (AIHA®):** *The American Industrial Hygiene Association: Its History and Personalities 1939–1990.* Fairfax, VA: AIHA®, 1994. p. 3.
82. **American Industrial Hygiene Association (AIHA®):** About AIHA; Homepage. http://www.aiha.org/ABOUTAIHA/Pages/default.aspx. [Accessed on May 30,2011.]
83. **American Board of Industrial Hygiene (ABIH):** Bulletin of the American Board of Industrial Hygiene. Lansing, MI: ABIH, 1996.
84. **American Board of Industrial Hygiene (ABIH):** Roster of the American Board of Industrial Hygiene. Lansing, MI: ABIH, 1996.
85. **McMichael, A.J.:** *Planetary Overload.* Cambridge, UK: Cambridge University Press, 1993. p. 63.
86. **Institute of Medicine:** The Future of Public Health. Washington, DC: National Academy Press, 1988. p. 1.
87. **American Public Health Association (APHA):** Industrial Hygiene and Sanitation. [Announcement] Am. J. Pub. Health, vol. 4 (1914).
88. **Harris, R.L.:** "The Public Health Roots of Industrial Hygiene." Paper presented at the Professional Conference in Industrial Hygiene, Nashville, TN, October 14, 1996.
89. **Rose, V.E.:** Industrial hygiene-coping with change. *Am. Ind. Hyg. Assoc. J. 56*:853 (1995).
90. **Clayton, G.D.:** Air pollution; U.S. Public Health Service pioneering studies; genesis of the Environmental Protection Agency. *Appl. Occup. Environ. Hyg. 12*:7–10 (1997).

Outcome Competencies

After completing this chapter, the reader should be able to:

1. Define the underlined terms used in this chapter.
2. Describe the rationale for developing and adhering to a professional code of ethics.
3. Discuss the history of the professional code of ethics for industrial hygiene.
4. Compare and contrast the two codes of ethics that are most relevant to the practice of industrial hygiene.
5. Explain the enforcement process used by ABIH.
6. Apply the ethical decision making model to case scenarios.
7. Demonstrate ways to operationalize the ethical behaviors in challenging cases.

Key Terms

American Board of Industrial Hygiene (ABIH) • aspirational code • care-based principle • code of ethics • enforceable code • ethical dilema • Kantian principle • member ethical principles • utilitarian principle

Prerequisite Knowledge

Prior to beginning this chapter, the reader should review the following chapters.

Chapter Number	Chapter Topic
1	History and the Philosophy of Industrial Hygiene

Key Topics

I. Rationale for Professional Codes of Ethics
II. Current Industrial Hygiene Ethical Codes and Guiding Principles
III. ABIH and the Enforcement Process
IV. Avoiding Ethical Conflicts
V. Resolving Ethics Issues — A Decision Making Model
VI. Exhibiting Leadership When Confronting Ethical Issues
VII. Working to Resolve Ethical Issues — Introduction to Case Studies
VIII. References
IX. Appendix A: Case Studies in the Application of Professional Ethics to the Practice of Industrial Hygiene

Industrial Hygiene Professional Ethics

2

Thomas C. Ouimet, MPH, MBA, CIH, CSP; Ann Bracker, MPH, CIH; Alan Leibowitz, CIH, CSP; David C. Roskelley, MSPH, CIH, CSP and Jeff V. Throckmorton, CIH

Rationale for Professional Codes of Ethics

As collective technical knowledge has grown over the past century, there has been a steady movement toward specialization in technical fields. This trend has led to the development of professions, or groups that have acquired highly technical specialized knowledge, through academic study, internships and sometimes a mentoring process. Members of professions have traditionally received prestige, respect and social status in society and are often better compensated than occupations that are not considered professions.

Because their knowledge is specialized and difficult for lay people to acquire, professions are self-governing and society has allowed them a great deal of autonomy in the way they operate, certainly more than it allows the practitioners of trades or managers of businesses. Members of a profession typically set their own standards of practice, regulate entry into their profession, discipline their own members, and function with fewer constraints than others. This is the case in the field of industrial hygiene where professionals develop sampling methodologies, set occupational exposure standards, create entry requirements, i.e., set criteria for sitting for the American Board of Industrial Hygiene (ABIH) certification exam, and discipline members through the ABIH ethics review process. In many areas in which IHs practice, the profession has defined acceptable practice standards. This autonomy is justified because society in general does not possess the specialized knowledge of the profession and therefore is not in a position to create standards for practitioners, define practices or discipline members. Only members of the profession who possess the specialized knowledge, can perform these functions. In return for this autonomy, society has high expectations for members of professions. Members of

Why do Ethics come into play and why are ethics important?

Certain behavior in society is regulated. Stealing and physically abusing others are examples of behavior that society has strict laws prohibiting. Many aspects of an industrial hygienist's professional life are dictated by various government regulations. On the opposite end of the spectrum from regulated behavior is free will, where there are no constraints over how one behaves. In this domain, people are all free to do whatever they wish and act according to their free will. Ethics comes into play in between these two domains — regulated behavior and free will. It belongs to the domain where no regulations (i.e., "the law") apply but, if certain actions were taken, some closely held values would be subverted or be diminished in some way. It is in this middle ground that ethical issues arise and difficult decisions about how to behave are made. Difficult professional ethical decisions must be guided by an understanding of our collective professional values as well as our personal values. If someone does not make good professional ethical choices, their careers and profession suffers.

History — Industrial Hygiene Professional Code of Ethics

In 1968, the first Code of Ethics for Professional Practice was developed by the American Academy of Industrial Hygiene (AAIH) Ethics Committee. The officers and councilors of the Academy accepted the code that year without taking further action. This code was further refined in the mid-1970s with the assistance of the American Board of Industrial Hygiene (ABIH) and after receiving comments from the Academy membership in 1978 was voted on and adopted. The code provided standards of ethical conduct to be followed by industrial hygienists as they practice their profession and serve employees, employers, clients, and the general public. This code was adopted in 1981 by the AIHA® and ACGIH®, thus extending coverage to most industrial hygiene practitioners.

In 1991, the four industrial hygiene organizations organized the Code of Ethics Task Force and charged them with revising the code, supplementing it with supporting interpretive guidelines, recommending methods to educate members about ethical conduct and recommending disciplinary procedures and mechanisms for enforcement. The leadership felt that industrial hygiene practice had changed since 1978 (the numbers of members practicing as consultants was increasing dramatically) and this raised new ethical issues for the profession that should be addressed in the code.

The report of the task force was presented to the four boards in October 1993, a final draft of a revised code of ethics was presented at the 1994 American Industrial Hygiene Conference and Exposition (AIHce), and by January 1995, all four organizations had approved the new code. In 1995, the industrial hygiene organizations approved the formation of the Joint Industrial Hygiene Ethics Education Committee (JIHEEC), the purpose of which is to conduct educational activities for industrial hygienists and promote an understanding of the code of ethics within the industrial hygiene community. A formal ethical complaint review and disciplinary process could not be agreed upon and was not established.

Beginning in 2006, a Joint Ethics Task Force was established and consisted of representatives of the four original chartering organizations (AIHA®, ACGIH®, AIH, and ABIH), the JIHEEC, and an attorney with experience in writing professional codes of ethics. The primary goal of this task force was to revise and renew the existing code of ethics, with a special emphasis placed upon enforcement. The need to sharpen and refine code language and wording were considered a key component of the task force's mission.

This effort resulted in the development of two new codes, the "American Board of Industrial Hygiene Code of Ethics," and the "Joint Industrial Hygiene Associations Member Ethical Principles," both of which were adopted in May of 2007 and presented to the general membership at the 2007 AIHce in Philadelphia. The membership-based organizations (AIHA®, ACGIH®, and AIH) recognizing that they were not in an enforcement position, adopted the joint code, leaving the issue of enforcement to ABIH.

professions are expected to serve the public good, to set higher standards of conduct for their members than are required of others, and to enforce a higher degree of discipline on themselves than others do. The trade-off granted by society is that it imposes less social control on the condition that the profession is self-regulating and self-disciplinary.

The standards to which members of a profession are to hold themselves are expressed in a professional code of ethics. The code is written and enforced by an organization representing the profession. In the case of industrial hygiene, the professional is the Certified Industrial Hygienist (CIH) and the organization representing the profession for code enforcement purposes is the ABIH. The rationale is that the profession itself is in the best position to know how its members should behave, the areas where ethical lapses can occur, and is most likely to become aware of violations of the standards it sets. In addition, the profession is in the best position to censure or dismiss from its ranks those who do not live up to the profession's standards. The autonomy and benefits that society bestows upon members of the profession are only justifiable if the members live up to this code and the profession adequately disciplines itself.

To fulfill its obligation to society, it's essential for the profession's ethical code to meet certain requirements. It must identify behavior that is unacceptable and that if expressed by a practitioner would lead to sanctioning by the profession. In other words, the code cannot just be a set of ideals but must identify unacceptable behavior and be enforceable. The code must also address those aspects of the profession that create the greatest opportunity for its members to act unethically or in a manner inconsistent with the public good. It cannot simply focus on unlawful behavior or ethical breaches that apply widely in society. Finally, the code must be focused on promoting the public good and particularly the interests of those served and impacted by the profession.

Current Industrial Hygiene Ethical Codes and Guiding Principles

There are several ethical codes and guidelines which are of particular significance to the practicing industrial hygienist. These are the "American Board of Industrial Hygiene Code of Ethics," and the "Joint Industrial Hygiene Associations Member Ethical Principles." Another code, the "International Code of Ethics for Occupational Health Professionals," established by the International Commission on Occupational Health is also of interest as it serves as an example of another type of code, an aspirational code, for the practicing industrial hygienist.

There are different ways in which professional codes can be interpreted and used. This is a significant consideration, one which needs to be established early on in the mind of the practitioner in the application of any code. That is, how do you best use a professional code? Should a code be the law? Should it be a set of guidelines? Is it a means by which the profession establishes a baseline standard of practice? Or is it the intention of the code to "raise the bar," for the profession or be aspirational? A professional code can be all of these things. In the most pure sense, however, a professional code is a definition of the baseline "standard of care" for the profession.

As practicing industrial hygienists, and certainly as certified industrial hygienists, there are two codes with which we should be most familiar: The "American Board of Industrial Hygiene Code of Ethics," and the "Joint Industrial Hygiene Associations Member Ethical Principles," both of which were adopted in May of 2007. These documents are available on the AIHA® and ABIH websites. The former, the ABIH code, is enforceable and binding upon all CIHs as well as applicants seeking to take the CIH exam. The latter, the "Joint Association" principles, have been adopted by AIHA®, ACGIH®, and the Academy, and establish guidelines for the members of those organizations. It is intended to be complementary to the enforceable code, set expectations and standards for the members of these associations, educate members as well as the public, and help all industrial hygiene practitioners understand their ethical responsibilities. Both codes describe an expectation that individuals will maintain high standards of integrity and professional conduct, accept responsibility for their actions, continually seek to enhance their professional capabilities, practice fairness and honesty, and encourage others to act in a professional manner consistent with the certification standards and responsibilities set forth in the codes. Each code is divided into two sections. The first describes an industrial hygienist's responsibility to professional organizations (AIHA®, ACGIH®, AIH, and ABIH), the profession, and the public and the second describes responsibilities to clients, employers and employees.

In a 2006 communication with ABIH, Richard Goldberg, an attorney who specializes in the development of codes of ethics for professional organizations, discussed the logic behind having two separate codes. The ABIH, is a credentialing organization, and therefore serves important public and professional protection purposes. It must carefully regulate the use of its certifications and related public representations. The conduct of a certificant or candidate may bear directly on his/her fitness to practice with an ABIH certification. A primary method of such regulation is the adoption of a code of ethics which permits the organization to discipline certificants and candidates who violate conduct rules. The need to regulate the conduct and activities of association members, although important, is not as compelling. In contrast to ABIH certificants, IH associations' members do not represent themselves to the public as being certified or otherwise qualified by the organization to practice (i.e., having met specific, validated professional skills and knowledge requirements). Rather, the professional associations operate to support and develop the profession, including the promotion of applicable practice standards. To support this mission and better the profession, the IH associations have developed a body of guidelines and principles intended to promote appropriate professional behavior and development of their respective memberships.

A detailed comparison between the code and member ethical principles is beyond the scope of this section. However, a brief inspection of the two documents will reveal that they are almost identical, with one difference being that the "Joint Association" member ethical principles contains a few more sections. Careful comparison will also reveal that there are a number of subtle differences in wording between the two documents. This comes from the fact that some ethical concepts may be desirable, but tricky to enforce within the framework of an administrative review, the setting in which the enforceable ABIH code has to live. One example of this difference is found in the inclusion of paragraphs C.2 and C.3 of the "Joint Association" ethical principles, copied below:

C.2. "Inform appropriate management representative and/or governmental bodies of violations of legal and regulatory requirements when obligated or otherwise clearly appropriate."

C.3. "Make reasonable efforts to ensure that the results of industrial hygiene assessments are communicated to exposed populations."

The use of words such as "appropriate," "otherwise clearly appropriate," "reasonable efforts," and so on do not present a strong foundation for an enforceable code and therefore will not be found in the code.

But once one has entered the world of "ethical principles" as opposed to enforceable code elements, what is appropriate in the standard? And how far does one go? Some codes contain statements that would be difficult if not impossible for the professional to comply with 100% of the time. These are intended to describe behavior to which professionals should aspire. A code that contains statements of this type, which can be quite thought provoking as well as controversial, is the "International Code of Ethics for Occupational Health Professionals," established by the International Commission on Occupational Health.

The International Commission on Occupational Health, founded in 1906, claims 2,000 professionals in 93 countries. Arguably more robust than the "Joint Association" ethical principles, it consists of 18 pages and twenty six "shall" statements, including explanatory language in an introduction and preface. It is not an enforcement-based code, and the wording of it would make it potentially problematic to serve as such. It is also broader in scope, addressing the concept of an "occupational health professional." Its phrasing and considerations could be considered more "worker focused." It is mentioned here as it represents a different and more globally-based view of ethical considerations for the "occupational health professional." The code itself is found at the web site for the International Commission on Occupational Health, and may be freely reproduced as long as the source is indicated. Two excerpts from it follow which reflect its more aspirational elements:

- "Occupational health professionals must request that a clause on ethics be incorporated in their contract of employment."
- "...occupational health professionals must regularly and routinely, whenever possible, visit the workplaces and consult the workers and the management of the work that is performed."

It is an interesting document for individuals who are seeking a wider perspective on the issue of ethics for IH professionals, especially if looking at an international venue.

ABIH and the Enforcement Process

To enforce the code, the ABIH has established a formal ethical complaint review and disciplinary process. However, before initiating an ethics review it is hoped that every effort will be made to resolve the ethical concern privately between the parties involved. The administrative review process can be both detailed as well as time consuming, and can represent a substantial effort on the part of ABIH. Although it is necessary and important to police and maintain the integrity of the profession, ABIH hopes that members will use both wisdom and judgment in any filing action. It is a serious matter, and treated as such.

The ABIH ethical review process is triggered by a written complaint. Anyone can submit the form, including a member of the general public. Although members of the public can submit complaints, experience has demonstrated that the process is most efficient when individual familiar with the profession are involved in the complaint process. The complaint form, along with an explanation of ethics complaint review process can be found on ABIH's web site. The multiple stage administrative review includes a thorough collection and review of facts and interviews with involved and affected individuals.

What happens when a filing has occurred? In the simplest version, the ABIH Executive Director (ED) and/or a five member ethics review committee can choose to accept or reject a complaint. If accepted for consideration, the ED and/or the ethics review committee can then weigh the matter, and recommend, after review and investigation, a variety of actions ranging from case dismissal to revocation of certification. The complainant as well as the accused are kept abreast of findings as the investigation proceeds and have the chance to provide additional information throughout the proceeding. The five members on the ethics review committee are not members of the ABIH board. In the event that an appeal (of certain parts of the process) is requested, a three member appeals committee comprised of ABIH board members can be formed.

After a through ethical complaint review, the following disciplinary actions may be imposed on a CIH, Certified Associate Industrial Hygienist (CAIH) or applicants seeking to take the CIH exam:

- Specified corrective actions
- Ineligibility for certification or recertification
- Private reprimand and censure
- Public reprimand and censure
- Probation, including conditions on conduct
- Suspension of certification
- Revocation of certification

Avoiding Ethical Conflicts

Few people set out to commit ethical violations. One ethicist, Rushworth Kidder, has noted, "The single largest problem in ethics is the inability to recognize ethical issues."[5] Professionals may be most vulnerable to not correctly recognizing potential ethical breaches as well as ethical malfeasance when practicing in professional areas that are not well defined, in areas of unfamiliar professional territory, and where extensive professional judgment and interpretation is necessary. In these situations practitioners must tread cautiously with heightened awareness of potential ethical entanglements. Communication with trusted colleagues can also be of value.

One thing that practitioners can do to avoid ethics entanglements as well as complaints (beyond using good ethical and professional behavior) is to communicate, early on, what they can and can't do, and what services and outcomes can be expected. This requires the practitioner to carefully think through not only the technical issues of a project, but also the expectations and relationships of the various parties involved and to make sure there is a common understanding of these issues between all parties.

Resolving Ethical Issues — A Decision Making Model

Resolving an ethical issue can be a challenge. Sometimes a great deal can be at stake. Decisions of this type can have long-term consequences to one's career and even end a career. Although the decision making process is difficult it can be made easier by following a process which involves a series of thoughtful and sequential steps. This helps identify the key individuals involved, frame the questions to be addressed, and clarify values. A number of ethical decision models exist and we will review the steps often found in these models. First, it's critical to highlight two important aspects of the ethical decision making process — the importance of studying and understanding our ethical code and guiding principles and the importance of consulting trusted colleagues.

The code and principles should be considered distilled wisdom from the industrial hygienists that have preceded them. These documents are intended to identify what are unethical behaviors and the boundaries of appropriate ethical behavior. It is therefore essential that practicing IHs understand their obligations under the code and the restrictions it places on their actions. Each person must seek to express the principles outlined in these documents in all their professional activities. The code and ethical principles are the first place to turn when confronted with an ethical decision and any professional decision they make must be consistent with them. However, the code and principles will not address all of the ethical issues that arise in a career. In these situations the IH must have a good understanding of the underlying professional values held within each element of code or ethical principle and do the hard work of working through an ethical decision-making process to its end point.

Access to a trusted colleague is an invaluable resource when confronting an ethical decision. Ethical decision-making can be very stressful and frequently the decision maker is emotionally involved. Having access to a second opinion, or an outsider's view of the situation, can lead to valuable insights and a better ethical decision. For that second opinion, a trusted, very experienced colleague with a strong commitment to the profession should be chosen. A candid, insightful views or opinions of the situation may be needed to facilitate the decision-making process. It is important to share the facts honestly as well as the context in which the actions occurred. It is also imperative that all confidential information be protected, particularly the identity of the individual whose behavior is being questioned. Some professionals create reciprocal relationships where the two professionals consult one another from time to time when issues arise.

An ethical decision can be overwhelming even with the support of a colleague. To enhance the chance of making a good decision it is important to follow a thoughtful process. A number of ethical decision-making models exist that can assist. These models contain many similarities in the steps they recommend as well as the approach to evaluating potential decisions or actions. The following steps to evaluating options, extracted from several models, will assist in making ethical decisions:

1. Gather facts carefully, including the context in which the action occurred, and define as clearly as possible the ethical issue.
2. Identify who will be impacted by the decision.
3. Refer to the code of ethics, guiding principles and other professional guidelines and relevant laws/regulations for guidance.
4. Clarify the personal and professional values as they relate to the situation.
5. Formulate alternative courses of action and define the outcomes for parties impacted by the decision.
6. Evaluate the potential courses of action by: (1) reviewing the practical consequences of each action; (2) evaluating the action to determine if it could be universally applied; and (3) evaluating the action against the resolution principle (do what you want others to do to you).
7. Make a decision and act accordingly.

At Step 5 in the process, one will typically arrive at two courses of action that appear equal in merit but will vary in their impact on others. The problem is to decide how to proceed. Philosophers have defined two major approaches to making this type of decision or handling ethical dilemmas — the ends-based approach or applying the utilitarian principle (act in a manner that does the greatest good for the greatest number of people) and the rule-based approach or applying the Kantian principle (act in a manner consistent with the individual's highest sense of principle).[1] The first approach looks at the merits of the end result or the consequence of the action and the second looks at the merits of the act itself and if the act is honorable, disregarding completely the end results or consequences of the action. A third approach, applying the care-based principal, is based on the application of the "golden rule" found in many religious texts (act toward others as you would like them to act toward you if your roles were reversed). It typically encourages actions that are more compassionate. After arriving at potential courses of action each of the three principles is applied to each action being considered and its outcome (or the decision regarding the appropriateness of the action after applying the principle) is weighted against the outcomes or decisions reached when each of the other resolution principles are applied to the same action. Different conclusions regarding the appropriateness of a potential action are often reached when applying these different principles. However, by looking at a potential action through these three different lenses a more complete picture of the potential positive and negative impacts from a given decision are identified. In addition, this weighing and evaluation of outcomes from applying these different principals forces an assessment of our individual and professional values, and by doing so, helps to clarify the issues and move us toward a satisfactory resolution.

Since individuals weigh values differently, professionals may reach different decisions regarding how to proceed when faced with an ethical dilemma. This is to be expected. The process is designed to help clarify personal values and identify a line of reasoning that seems most relevant and persuasive to the issue at hand.

There is one more question that should be asked when faced with a difficult ethical decision. Is there another, perhaps a more creative solution, to the dilemma? In other words, is there a third choice that is not initially apparent? One should always hold this possibility in his/her minds as they analyze potential actions. Sometimes, when following the rigorous process just described, a third path forward is uncovered that is an honest compromise.

Exhibiting Leadership When Confronting Ethical Issues

Successful resolution of an ethical issue not only depends on following a resolution process and confiding with colleagues, it also requires leadership skills and in some instances moral courage. This is particularly true when there is a conflict between the demands of the professional code or the professional obligations and the demands placed on IHs by a client, an employer or perhaps even the culture in which they are practicing. For example, what are the responsibilities of an IH who believes that a needed change in a work place will not be made, perhaps due to economic constraints of the employer or maybe a cultural difference in what is perceived to be necessary? In these situations, do IHs say to themselves, "I have discharged my responsibilities by recognizing, evaluating, and recommending controls— it's someone else's responsibility to see they are implemented"? Or should they believe their ultimate responsibility is to see worker and community health protected?

Industrial hygienists clearly have an obligation not to do what is immoral — to knowingly cause harm or to allow others to remain in conditions where they are at imminent risk of injury or loss of life. But this is not the situation they typically find themselves. In most situations, practicing IHs are obligated to employ their knowledge to accurately characterize the work environment and warn against unsafe work conditions. However, final judgments regarding how to respond to warnings or recommendations are typically the responsibility of management. The IH's input is only one part of the relevant information that must go into that managerial decision. However, the IH is obligated to make his or her views and concerns understood and must insist that employee health and safety is protected when clearly threatened.

An IHs chances for success in inspiring action to improve work place conditions increases significantly when they demonstrate effective leadership skills. Industrial hygienists must communicate effectively with decision-makers as well as employees and take every opportunity to educate and inform both management and labor regarding work place hazards and their control. They must also model responsible behavior at all times and encourage this behavior in both management and labor consistently.

Industrial hygienists must also learn to be persuasive when communicating with management and labor regarding work place hazards. It's the ability to make that persuasive case that distinguishes industrial hygiene leaders from advisors. Leaders of organizations in general want to do the right thing. Ethical lapses most often occur through a lack of understanding of the issues or where judgment becomes clouded in the pursuit of profits or other goals. When the IH demonstrates leadership by being able to identify and clearly articulate the issue and potential consequences of a particular action, or in some cases inaction, the "right" decision is most often made. The following steps provide valuable guidance on making a persuasive case:[8]

- Begin by giving your audience a specific reason to listen — what problem or question of theirs will you solve or address.

- Keep supporting data simple and only use the most impressive — three or five (not four) points are best.
- Answer anticipated difficult questions the audience is likely to have as part of the second half of the presentation.
- Relate all arguments back to the key questions you are answering — avoid extraneous points of interest.
- Conclusions, solutions, answers should appear near the beginning of the presentation, but repeat key themes during the course of the presentation.
- Be respectful of opposing views — allowing discussion provides opportunities to strengthen the message

To maintain credibility, it's important for IHs to raise only those issues that represent true risks to individuals and the organization. Professionals achieve credibility when they can focus on the important issues and not act as alarmist naysayers at all levels of risk or potential exposure. Highly credible individuals are much more likely to be successful when attempting to persuade others.

When discussing issues with ethical ramifications within organizations, it's also important to focus the discussion on how different courses of action will impact important organizational values. For example, in most businesses preserving financial resources and maintaining a good reputation are highly held values. Demonstrating the impact from making a poor choice on a business' financial position or reputation can be an effective approach to making a persuasive case for taking action to address a potential employee, operational or community harm.

Industrial hygienists are faced with additional challenges when they practice in multinational organizations where cultural differences must be factored into each decision and culturally relevant solutions developed to address issues that arise. In the international environment, professionals often encounter practices that are different but no less ethical than their more familiar approach. When working around the world, it's important to focus on desired behaviors. Then programs and practices consistent with local resources and values can be developed to address program needs. While cultural sensitivity is important, it is essential that such awareness not be taken as license for moral ambiguity. In an ethical organization the life of every employee, customer, partner and community member must be valued at the same high level. They should not be exposed to any unreasonable risk beyond what can be properly managed and where necessary risk mitigation strategies are applied consistently throughout the organization. A good test for acceptance of risk is to ask whether an individual would allow his or her child or spouse to perform the task as currently practiced.

In good organizations the need for these discussions should decrease over time as leadership becomes familiar with the issues and precedents are established for difficult decisions. Establishing an effective management system is the best way to insure consistent, reproducible behaviors and practices that are essential elements of an organizational ethics' program. Such systems identify proper behaviors and establish mechanisms to insure these behaviors are followed. Over time most organizations develop systems to address each area where moral choices are required and define a solution or procedure to assist in reaching the best decision.

A cultural problem may exist within an organization if the leaders must be constantly convinced to take the ethical path. It is in such an organization where the most difficult and potentially extreme decisions may be required of the industrial hygienist. Each practitioner must be prepared to address issues that potentially violate their professional and personal values. Kidder refers to "moral courage" when discussing the ability to act as needed in response to ethical challenges. He describes three requisites to acting with moral courage: "a commitment to moral principles, an awareness of the danger in supporting those principles and a willing endurance of that danger."[6] An ethical industrial hygiene practitioner must be aware of the potential repercussions of any decision and must be have the tenacity to see those with real consequences through to their proper outcome.

Working to Resolve Ethical Issues — Introduction to Case Studies

Some of the ethical values highlighted in the industrial hygiene professional organization's ethical codes and principles are summarized

Table 2.1 — Operationalizing Industrial Hygiene Ethical Values

Ethical Values	*Ethical Behavior at Work*	*Case Study*
Follow recognized science	Stick to the facts Use NIOSH/EPA procedures, accredited labs	Nano- Lippy
Counsel parties factually	Use reliable sources Communicate findings to all affected parties Communicate clearly as to roles and responsibilties	MWF- Bracker IAQ- Throckmorton
Avoid conflicts of interest	Don't accept gifts to influence outcome Disclose potential conflicts of interest Take on only as much work as you can complete	COI- Rice
Practice only in areas of competence	Only work in areas where you are qualified Seek training, certification or registration in these areas	IAQ- Throckmorton
Act with integrity	Behave in a manner that reflects well on profession Respect the confidentiality of sensitive information Don't misrepresent yourself, or engage in fraudulent activities	Ambitious Professional- Burke

in Table 2.1. Frequently, the ethical behavior that should be adopted as an industrial hygienist can be clearly identified. Examples of "operationalized" ethical behaviors associated with the profession's ethical values are summarized in the table. In other cases, the ethical response may be less clear. For example, the profession instructs IHs to "follow recognized science." What should we do when the science is incomplete or ambiguous? We are advised to "counsel parties factually." What facts should be shared — those with regulatory implications or those published in guidance documents? They are instructed to practice in our areas of competence. What should be done when emerging issues arise that may be outside of their area of expertise?

The case studies provided in the appendix address one or more of the profession's core ethical values. As you read the case studies, think about how you would respond to the dilemmas. Identify the ethical behaviors that all industrial hygienists should observe. In addition, identify the ethical responses that are not so straight-forward. Think about how your organizational affiliation (corporate, consulting, academic, government, labor) and your role within an organization may have a bearing on your approach. Evaluate the ways in which your personal values may influence your response to an ethical dilemma. And lastly, think about how you could have avoided the ethical dilemma in the first place.

A mature understanding of our professional responsibilities comes with experience, practice and dialog. Our profession and its individual practitioners will best flourish as members clearly communicate with each other regarding ethical questions and issues. It is hoped that this chapter can assist in facilitating this dialog.

References

1. **Appelbaum, D. and S. Lawton:** *Ethics and The Professions.* Englewood Cliffs, NJ: Prentice-Hall, 1990.
2. **De George, R.:** *Business Ethics.* New York, NY: Macmillan, 1990.
3. **George, B. and D. Gergen:** *True North: Discover Your Authentic Leadership.* San Francisco, CA: Jossey-Bass, 2007.
4. **Johnson, W.B. and C. Ridley:** *The Elements of Ethics: For Professionals.* New York, NY: PalGrave Macmillan, 2008.
5. **Kidder, R.:** *How Good People Make Tough Choices: Resolving the Dilemmas of Ethical Living.* New York, NY: Harper, 2003.
6. **Kidder, R.:** *Moral Courage.* New York, NY: Harper, 2006.
7. **Lawrence, J.:** *Argument for Action: Ethics and Professional Conduct.* Brookfield, VT: Ashgate, 1999.
8. **Kotick, R.:** *The Executive Speaker — Presentation Skills,* Course book used during a training program in Washington DC in January 2001.

Appendix A: Case Studies in the Application of Professional Ethics to the Practice of Industrial Hygiene

CASE STUDY 1

Conflict of Interest Case Study: Moral Questions for Industrial Hygienists

J. Nicholas Rice, CIH

A version of this case study appeared in *The Synergist*, November 2009, p. 24

As professional industrial hygienists, we put our skills and judgments into the service of workers, employers, clients, and the public. In turn, we are granted a trust to carry out our duties to protect worker health with professional integrity. Failures to avoid, disclose, or appropriately manage conflict of interest situations violate professional relationships and may tarnish the trust placed with the industrial hygiene profession.

The Joint Industrial Hygiene Associations Member Ethical Principles and the ABIH Code of Ethics have provisions related to conflict of interest and the appearance of impropriety. A conflict of interest might be described as a situation in which one has a personal or financial interest sufficient to appear to influence the objective exercise of his or her duties as a professional, public official, or employee. A conflict of interest involves the actual, apparent, or potential abuse of trust. It does not necessarily indicate impropriety or wrongdoing; rather, it raises a moral question. Possible responses include disclosure of the conflict, recusing oneself from the conflict, or managing the conflict.

The scenario presented below explores a conflict of interest that industrial hygienists may face.

Scenario: Choosing a Lab

Jack, an industrial hygienist working for Chemo Pharmaceutical Manufacturing, is tasked with selecting an industrial hygiene lab to conduct analysis of air and surface samples related to a new chemotherapy drug. Jack has narrowed the lab selection to two vendors — IH Analysis Lab and NJ Pharma Labs.

Jack's evaluation reveals that IH Analysis has new liquid chromatography tandem mass spectrometry equipment that is necessary to conduct the specialized analysis and is able to exceed the minimum detection limit required. Jack knows of IH Analysis Lab's exceptional technical expertise as his niece is a laboratory technician there. A small company— just seven employees— that rewards staff with quarterly bonuses based on profit and business growth, IH Analysis Lab is competitive in price and turn around time.

NJ Pharma Lab, a vendor that Chemo Pharmaceutical Manufacturing has used for three years, has older liquid chromatography tandem mass spectrometry equipment that could be used for the specialized analysis. Nonetheless, NJ Pharma is able to meet the minimum detection limit required. NJ Pharma is competitive in price and turn around time.

Jack decides to hire IH Analysis as the exclusive provider of industrial hygiene lab services based on their newer analytical equipment and ability to exceed the requirement for minimum detection limit. IH Analysis Lab's business volume will increase 25 percent with the new business from Chemo Pharmaceutical Manufacturing. Jack has not disclosed that his niece works for IH Analysis Lab.

Questions

- Is a conflict of interest present? If so, is it a real conflict or a perceived conflict?
- Is the relation of Jack and his niece and their respective employment a concern for either company?
- Would the conflict be any different if IH Analysis employed Jack's wife instead of his niece?
- Would the conflict be any different if IH Analysis employed Jack's neighbor?
- What is the financial cost/gain to Chemo Pharmaceutical with respect to Jack's conflict?
- What is the financial cost/gain to IH Analytical Lab with respect to the conflict?
- Was Jack's professional judgment influenced by the conflict?

- Would Jack be happy if his colleagues or the local paper became aware of the conflict?
- Should Jack inform his employer even if he doesn't believe the situation violates his employer's guidelines?
- Is disclosure sufficient?
- How could have the conflict of interest have been prevented?

CASE STUDY 2

The Ambitious Professional: What You Don't Know Can't Hurt

John P. Burke, CIH, CSP
This article appeared in *The Synergist*, September 2007, page 53

Jane Richards, CIH, left the Friday interview really hoping she would be selected for the new assignment within her company, the Axis Corporation. Richards had been performing safety and health work for Axis at one of their smaller plants for almost four years and she knew that the new assignment was a career-boosting one. If nothing else, Jane was ambitious about her career. Prior to working for Axis, Jane worked as safety coordinator for two years at a small toll manufacturer. At both Axis and her old plant, several hazardous chemicals were processed and handled regularly in relatively large quantities, so Jane taught herself industrial hygiene air sampling and did quite a bit of it. Seeing industrial hygiene certification as an important feather in her career advancement cap Jane did the necessary studying and passed the board certification exam.

On Monday afternoon following her interview, Richards got the call she was waiting for, and immediately accepted the new assignment as safety and health manager at Axis' largest plant. At the new plant there was a significant amount of industrial hygiene work to be done due to the nature of the manufacturing operation. After a couple of weeks in the new job she realized that the traditional safety-related management aspects required almost all of her attention. Injury incident rates were increasing, and there were several very serious incidents at the plant in the last few months related to deficiencies in the existing electrical, lock out/tag out and confined space programs. She would definitely need help in the IH area. She had several discussions with her new supervisor and the plant manager and finally they approved her hiring someone internally at the plant to assist her. After interviewing several internal candidates Richards selected Mike Jones, known as one of the plant's better laboratory technicians.

Jones had no technical background in IH practice, but before he knew it he was being asked to begin air monitoring for some of the chemicals regularly handled by the process workers. He did what he could to schedule meetings with Richards to get her input and advice, but usually Jane was short on time since she was being pushed by her boss and other managers for the safety-related reports and meetings. The managers also wanted to know what Richards was doing about the employee exposure concerns regarding the most toxic chemicals they use. Richards knew that if she didn't meet these manager's requests her career was in jeopardy and she was not about to let that happen. The result was that Jones received very little technical input from Richards and relied mostly upon what he could find on the Internet regarding air monitoring techniques. Jones purchased a few air sampling pumps and associated equipment and started his air sampling campaign.

After a few weeks the results started coming in, and Jones did his best to interpret them and put together some reports for Richards to review. The good news for her was that the summary reports indicated that exposures were low, relative the occupational exposure limits. Although Richards had not performed formal IH qualitative assessments of the operations being sampled, the results seemed to align with what she saw while passing by the operations on her way to meetings or while performing other safety activities. Richards hurriedly scheduled Jones to attend the next manager meeting and do a presentation on the results. She knew that this would be a good demonstration to the managers that she had control of the situation. Richards was also happy that Jones had managed to pick up the air sampling so quickly and knew that this would continue to free up time for her to concentrate on her other safety responsibilities.

After a year and half of proceeding like this, Richard's facility was audited by a professional environmental consultant hired by

Axis' corporate safety office. One of the auditors, Jim Callahan was a very experienced CIH who had spent over 20 years in the chemical processing industry. The first day of the audit, Richards assigned Jones to Callahan, and they sat down together to review industrial hygiene records. Callahan first read Jones' last six monitoring reports then asked for some selected monitoring records from each sampling campaign. It wasn't long before Callahan noticed problems.

First, he noted that the monitoring log sheets were not standardized and basic sampling information like pre and post calibration, air flow rate, sample start and stop times, and sampling methodology were not being recorded. No information was recorded either about what exactly the worker did during the shift. An AIHA®-accredited lab was being utilized but chain of custody forms for the samples were not being maintained. Many eight-hour time-weighted average results were being calculated from three-hour samples, and information about what the worker was doing during the non-monitored shift period was not recorded. Work area samples were used to calculate some TWA results even though they were not representative of breathing zone samples.

After completing his full review Callahan was convinced, that given the lack of documentation, the samples could not be treated as valid assessments of worker exposure. When he discussed his findings with Jones, he could see the disappointment on Jones' face as he replied, "I thought I was doing the right things and didn't know what else I had to do." Callahan continued his discussion with Jones to find out as much as he could to find the root causes of the problem and identify appropriate corrective actions.

The next step was his meeting with Richards, and by the time of the meeting Callahan had a pretty good picture of what had happened and why. Callahan proceeded to point out the audit deficiencies to her and there was dead silence when he stated his conclusion that most if not all of the monitoring data was not valid. Richards immediately tried to deflect the blame to Jones stating that she told him to ask questions and not do anything he was unsure about. Her final comment was, "I am not going to let a non-professional like Mike Jones ruin my career."

Questions

- Which aspects of the scenario present ethical issues?
- What ethical principles apply to this scenario?
- What could the professional Industrial Hygienist have done with respect to the occupation exposure issues that would have helped eliminate or minimize the problem?
- If confronted with similar issues in your job what actions would you take?

CASE STUDY 3

Potential Harm, or Hysteria?: An Ethical Dilemma

Jeff V. Throckmorton, CIH

A version of this case study appeared in *The Synergist*, November 2008, Page 28

Having successfully passed his CIH examination, Bill is among the latest group of ABIH-certified industrial hygienists. Although he works for a large industrial firm, he has always wanted to augment his income with some side consulting work. Recently he was contacted by Impenetrable Construction (IPC), a home builder with a problem. An upscale home IBC built and sold a few years ago has been determined to have water intrusion in one of the wall sections. A physical examination of the inside of an exterior wall, accessed by removing facade stonework, demonstrated that the plywood underlayment was wet, that the nails were rusted completely through, and that the wood was covered with a "blackish material." It appeared, however, that water intrusion into the adjoining wall cavity was limited. IPC is scrambling to figure out what happened, and fix any leaks; wanting only to stop water intrusion, it is not planning to have any remediation work performed.

The homeowner has become increasingly concerned that his home is contaminated with mold and his young family is at risk. The Internet is a fertile source of information as he explores sites warning him of the dangers and hazards of toxic black mold.

Meanwhile, IPC hires Bill to take air samples. IPC believes there is no danger to building occupants, since the mold is seemingly limited to one wall section and essentially trapped in the wall cavity and exterior plywood layer. IPC also strongly indicates to Bill that it does not consider the home structure to have been damaged significantly. IPC is hoping for a definitive report demonstrating that no possibility exists of hazardous exposure to building occupants and that the building has suffered to significant damage. According to IPC, talk of mold and any accompanying hazard is an exaggeration.

The homeowner is looking to Bill for assurance that he and his family are perfectly safe from mold, black or otherwise, now or in the future. They are also worried about possible damage to their home, and the need for remedial corrective action.

Bill has submitted two bulk samples of the plywood to the lab for analysis, and the lab reports a mix of cladosporium and mycelial fragments for each of the samples. He also takes four air samples inside of the house and two outside; the results being unremarkable. Because IPC has hired him, Bill cannot give his results to the homeowner, even though they have asked for an assurance of safety and have also queried him regarding damage to the home.

Bill faces several issues as he prepares his report. IPC is a huge homebuilder, and Bill is hoping to get future work from them. IPC has made it clear that it considers mold issues to be largely based upon hysteria and wants a clear statement from Bill that no potential risk or harm to the structure exists. Bill can't talk directly to the homeowner without approval from IPC, but he is aware that the home suffered some damage, as evidenced by the crumbling, rusted nails. He is also aware that he is not an architectural expert. Sensing a dilemma, he turns to JIHEEC's ethical principles guidance.

Questions

- If you were in Bill's position, how would you handle this situation?
- How should Bill address the homeowners concerns, and what can he say? In short, how should be summarize his qualitative and quantitative findings?
- How could Bill have avoided this ethical dilemma before he began the work?

CASE STUDY 4

The Industrial Hygiene Report — An Ethical Dilemma

Anne Bracker, MPH, CIH
A version of this article appeared in *The Synergist*, June/July 2008, Page 38

Javier is an industrial hygiene consultant for a non-union machine shop. The company's twenty nine employees tend grinding, milling and drilling machines. The computer numerically controlled (CNC) machines use several water based metal working fluids (MWF).

The company asks Javier to complete an industrial hygiene survey to insure that they are in compliance with Occupational Safety and Health Administration (OSHA) standards. The scope of work is limited to the collection of air samples and the reporting of results.

Although OSHA had considered promulgating a comprehensive metalworking standard, the rulemaking process has stalled. Therefore, the most relevant OSHA standards appear to be the oil mist 5 mg/m^3 permissible exposure limit (PEL) and the hazard communication standard. Based on his review of the literature, Javier does not expect the exposures at this plant to exceed the OSHA PEL.[1]

During Javier's walkthrough of the facility he notes that the employer has not implemented many of the recommended "best practices" for machining with metalworking fluids.[2–5] For example, the high speed wet grinding machines do not have mist extraction, the company does not have a centralized coolant management program and some of the sumps are contaminated with tramp oil. Javier is aware that many of the "best practices" were developed because water-based metalworking fluids can become highly contaminated with harmful microbial agents. Mists from these machines may lead to occupational asthma and other lung diseases; even when the OSHA PEL is <u>not</u> exceeded. He knows that many employers mistakenly believe compliance with the PEL is synonymous with a "clean bill of health."

During his survey, one of the employees confidentially tells Javier that he was diagnosed with asthma after he started working at the plant. The employee is worried because a co-worker has breathing problems as well. The employee is pleased that Javier has been asked to complete an industrial hygiene survey. He tells Javier that he plans to ask his employer for a copy of Javier's industrial hygiene report. He plans to give the report to his primary care physician.

Not surprisingly, the air sampling results Javier gets back are well below the OSHA PEL.

When Javier starts to write his industrial hygiene report he is confronted with an ethical dilemma about the type of report to submit. Should he:

1. Limit the report to a discussion of his sampling methods and results, noting clearly that this was the scope of the contract.
2. Include an additional section in his report that encourages the employer to implement multiple interventions so that machining with metalworking fluids "best practices" are met.
3. Provide the employer with best practice guidance resources as a report attachment- without making reference to the specific interventions he would propose.
4. Take a different approach: ______________________________?

Javier identifies the following issues. The employer had made it clear that he wanted to limit the scope of work to compliance with OSHA regulations. Javier hopes to work for this employer on future projects and he is pleased that a small employer sought his services. If he develops a relationship he may have more opportunities in the future to recommend enhanced controls. On the other hand, he is concerned that the employer's failure to implement "best practices" could put workers at an increased risk for developing or exacerbating lung diseases such as asthma. A report that specifically addresses "best practices" may protect the asthmatic employee and his co-workers from future exposures.

If confronted with a similar issue at your job, what actions would you take?

References

1. **Piacitelli GM et al.:** Metalworking fluid exposures in small machine shops: an overview. *Am. Ind. Hyg. Assoc. J. 62(3)*:356–70 (2001).
2. **Occupational Safety and Health Administration (OSHA):** *Metalworking Fluids: Safety and Health Best Practices Manual.* available at: http://www.osha.gov/SLTC/metalworkingfluids/metalworkingfluids_manual.html [Accessed March 28, 2008].
3. **National Institute for Occupational Safety and Health (NIOSH):** *Criteria for a Recommended Standard: Occupational Exposure to Metalworking Fluids.* DHEW (NIOSH) Publication No. 98-102, NIOSH, Cincinnati, OH, 1998.
4. **Organization Resources Counselors (ORC) Inc.:** *Management of the Metal Removal Fluid Environment.* Washington, DC: ORC, 1999.
5. **Health and Safety Executive (HSE):** *Machining with Metalworking Fluids.* Control of Substances Hazardous to Health (COSHH) Essentials MW Publication Series (4/2006).

CASE STUDY 5

Nanomaterials Case Study: What Do We Tell Workers When We Don't Have the Answers?

Bruce Lippy, PhD, CIH, CSP

This case study appeared in *The Synergist,* September 2009, p.23

Nanomaterials are widely believed to have begun a promising new revolution in manufacturing. But as most industrial hygienists are aware, engineered nanoparticles have been shown in animal studies "to reach the alveolar region; avoid macrophage engulfment; cause oxidative stress, inflammation, and fibrosis; and translocate into the blood."[(1)] NIOSH has raised concerns about what prevention and control actions should be taken while toxicological research is ongoing.[(1)]

Given the incomplete state of toxicological knowledge, a major ethical question must be posed about what workers manufacturing these products should be told about the risks they face. As a 2007 article in *Professional Safety* noted, "Making ethical decisions is not easy — especially when the situation involves multiple points of view, conflicting objectives, incomplete knowledge or ambiguity."[(2)] With $88 billion worth of products containing nanomaterials reportedly sold in 2007, there are clearly many workers potentially exposed.[(3)] Their numbers have been projected by the U.S. government to grow to 2 million worldwide over the next 15 years.[(4)]

Material Safety Data Sheets (MSDSs) are required for nanomaterials that meet the definitions of hazardous chemicals under OSHA's Hazard Communication standard. MSDSs from suppliers are the preferred source of risk information for nanotechnology firms, according to a survey of firms in Massachusetts.[5]

The National Institute for Occupational Safety and Health (NIOSH) appears to maintain the most complete collection of MSDSs for engineered nanomaterials and recently analyzed 60 of them from 33 different manufacturers for technical sufficiency.[6] The researchers only rated 5 percent as "good" while 55 percent were rated as "in need of serious improvement."[6] Over half contained Occupational Exposure Limits (OELs) for the bulk material without providing guidance that the OEL may not be protective for the nanoscale material. Eighty percent "failed to recognize the material as being nano in size or list a particle size distribution showing the nano size range" and a higher percentage "lacked toxicologic data specific to the nanomaterials." Eight percent failed to "suggest any type of engineering controls or mechanical ventilation."

These findings corroborated a similar analysis of a subset of the same MSDSs presented at an international conference sponsored by the EPA in October 2008.[7] The earlier analysis also noted that of those MSDSs that recommended local exhaust ventilation, 25 percent recommended a face velocity greater than 100 feet per minute even though NIOSH has indicated that standard fume hoods operated at that rate tend to create too much turbulence to fully contain nanoparticles, which when dry are extraordinarily buoyant.[7] The earlier study also reported that not one of the MSDSs reported that nanoparticles pose a much greater flammability risk. As the British Health and Safety Executive warned, "An increasing range of materials that are capable of producing explosive dust clouds are being produced as nanopowders."[8]

Ethical Scenario

Marie, a Certified Industrial Hygienist working for a large, international manufacturer of single-walled carbon nanotubes, arguably one the most toxic nanomaterials in animal studies, has just been assigned to run the company's product stewardship program. She is troubled that their MSDS for the single-walled carbon nanotubes lists the OSHA PEL for synthetic graphite (15 milligrams per cubic meter) even though NIOSH has stated that "...the occupational exposure limit for graphite should not be used to allow extensive exposure to carbon nanotubes that appear far more toxic than graphite."[1] OSHA does not have specific requirements about warning language for nanomaterials so the company is not in violation of 29 CFR 1910.1200. Given the world-wide economic downturn, there is strong pressure from management not to take voluntary steps that will depress sales further. Discussions of plant closings have been circulating.

1. Is it unethical for Marie to not include stronger warning language in the MSDS?
2. How should the lack of definitive toxicological research be handled in an MSDS?
3. If Marie worked as a field IH in a branch office and was not in charge of the program, what would she be ethically obligated to do?
4. If the firm sold carbon nanotubes in Europe, too, where the precautionary principle holds much stronger philosophical sway, would it have bearing on her ethical duties?

References

1. **Schulte, P., C. Geraci, R. Zumwalde, M. Hoover, and E. Kuempel:** Occupational Risk Management of Engineered Nanoparticles. *J. Occup. Env. Hyg. 5(4)*:239–49 (2008).
2. **Nichols, N., G.V. Nichols, and P.A. Nichols:** Professional Ethics: The importance of teaching ethics to future professionals. *Prof. Safety July*:37–41 (2007).
3. **Woodrow Wilson International Center for Scholars:** New Nanotech Products Hitting the Market at the Rate of 3–4 per Week. http://www.nanotechproject.org/news/archive/6697/. April 2008. [Accessed on July 22, 2010.]
4. **U.S. National Nanotechnology Initiative:** Frequently Asked Questions. http://www.nano.gov/html/facts/faqs.html. April 2008. [Accessed on July 22, 2010].
5. **Lindberg, J.E. and M.M. Quinn:** A Survey of Environmental, Health and Safety Risk Management Information Needs and Practices among Nanotechnology Firms in the Massachusetts Region. PEN Research Brief Number 1. http://www.nanotechproect.org/publications/archive/a_survey_environmental_health_safety/. December 2007. [Accessed on July 22, 2010.]

6. **Crawford, C. and L. Hodson:** Guidance for preparing good MSDSs for engineered nanomaterials. Poster session presented at the American Industrial Hygiene Conference and Expo, June 2009.
7. **Lippy, B.E.:** MSDSs fail to communicate the hazards of nanotechnologies to workers. Paper presented at the International Environmental Nanotechnology Conference. Chicago, Illinois, 2008.
8. **Pritchard, D.K.:** Literature Review — Explosion Hazards Associated with Nanopowders. HSL/2004/12. Health and Safety Lab. Health and Safety Executive. Buxton, U.K.: Harpur Hill, 2004.

Outcome Competencies

After completing this chapter, the reader should be able to:

1. Define underlined terms used in this chapter.
2. Identify conditions that caused the development of the OSH Act.
3. Recognize legal aspects of industrial hygiene practice.
4. Relate the role of occupational hygiene in providing professional services to employers.
5. Recognize the role of the occupational hygienist as an expert witness.
6. Recall the general duty clause.
7. Explain the phrase "...free from recognized hazards."

Key Terms

Federal Rule 702 • general duty clause • negligence • Notice of Contest • occupational safety and health (OSH) standards • Occupational Safety and Health Act • Occupational Safety and Health Review Commission • product liability • strict liability • tort • variance

Prerequisite Knowledge

None.

Key Topics

I. Federal Laws
   A. Establishment of OSHA
   B. Citations
   C. EZ Trial
II. State Programs for Health and Safety
   A. Youth Worker Safety and Health
   B. Workers' Compensation
   C. Employee or Independent Contractor
III. State Laws which Affect Industrial Hygienists
   A. Civil and Criminal Law
   B. Contract Law
   C. Tort Law
   D. State Professional Regulations and Certifications
IV. The Industrial Hygienist and Safety Professional as an Advisor
V. The Industrial Hygienist and Safety Professional as an Expert Witness
   A. New Federal Rule 702 — Testimony by Experts
   B. Ethical Obligations
VI. References

Legal Aspects of Industrial Hygiene

3

Margaret Norman and Dan Napier, CIH, CSP

The U.S. has been experiencing rapid advances in technology, changes in society, and the effects of global economic forces. Hazards to workers and the general public increase at a rapid pace with these advances. Laws also develop and change to protect the worker and the general public.

The Industrial Hygienist (IH) in the workplace contributes to safety and health by ensuring that Federal, State and local laws and regulations are known and followed by workers and employers. They conduct scientific research to provide data on possible hazards and about harmful substances in the environment and in the workplace. Industrial hygienists also serve on government advisory panels and contribute to the development of regulations which involve Health and Safety.[1] To complete these tasks, they must understand existing laws and regulations.

Major sources of law affecting Industrial Hygiene and Safety professionals are:

1) Federal codes, rules, and regulatory agencies
2) State laws and regulations
3) Case laws interpreting Federal, State and local laws

The laws that affect the practice of industrial hygiene start with the Federal Laws. They are found primarily in, but not limited to, two major areas. The Occupational Safety and Health Administration (OSHA) Codes and Environmental Protection Agency (EPA) Codes are most salient to the profession. Knowledge and understanding of these two large bodies of regulation is important. They are Title 29, Chapter 15, Occupational Safety and Health Act and 40 CFR: Protection of the Environment. Title 29 sets Standards which define exposures, testing methods, and safety and health parameters in detail. The OSHA standards do not typically protect all workers from all exposures; they provide a starting point as an enforceable level for worker protection. In some cases, state regulations can be more rigorous than the Federal OSHA Standards.

Federal Laws

Establishment of OSHA

Congress enacted the Occupational Safety and Health (OSH) Act of 1970 "to assure so far as possible every working man and woman in the nation safe and healthful working conditions."[2] The OSH Act established a nationwide, federal program to protect workers from harm on the job. The Act was intended to protected almost the entire work force from job-related death, injury and illness.

The OSH Act established the Occupational Safety and Health Administration (OSHA) within the Department of Labor, the National Institute for Occupational Safety and Health (NIOSH), and the National Advisory Committee on Occupational Safety and Health (NACOSH). OSHA is responsible for developing and enforcing workplace safety and health regulations. Two kinds of obligations under 29 USC 654 (a) require the employer to take steps for the occupational safety and health of their employees. First, the "General Duty Clause" requires an employer to make the workplace free from recognized hazards which could cause death or serious physical harm to employees. Second, the employer is to comply with occupational safety and health standards established under the chapter. This has become known as the "general duty clause"[3] These duties require the employer to make the workplace safe. OSHA enforces these safety standards and obligations by inspecting facilities, and reviewing documents and work plans and by citing violators. The citations bear various penalties. Employers who experience standards that are difficult to meet with available technology can apply for a variance.[4] If an employer can show that the process that they are using does not expose workers to greater risk of injury the condition may be provided with a variance.[5] For anyone who is involved advising those cited by OSHA or participating in the Appeals process, required reading would be *Occupational Safety and Health Law*.[6]

The Occupational Safety and Health Review Commission (OSHRC) is the agency that hears appeals and accepts applications for variances to code.[7] NIOSH was established to conduct research and to provide information, education and training related to occupational safety and health.[8] NACOSH was established to advise the Secretaries of Labor and Health and Human Services on occupational safety and health programs and policies. The 12-person advisory committee is composed of persons with experience in occupational safety and health.[9]

Inspections by OSHA

OSHA Compliance Safety and Health Officers (CSHO) conduct workplace inspections based on the following priorities.[10]

1. **Imminent Danger Situations** — These include incidents that could cause death or serious injury; an accident about to happen. CSHOs will ask employers to correct these hazards immediately, or to remove endangered employees. Before leaving the workplace, the CSHO will advise all affected employees of the hazard and will post an imminent danger notice if the employer refuses to voluntarily correct the situation or remove the employees from exposure.
2. **Fatalities or Catastrophes** — A fatality or catastrophe must be reported to OSHA within eight hours. A catastrophe is defined as an event that results in the hospitalization of three or more employees. Hospitalization is defined as being admitted for a 24 hour period.
3. **Complaints** — Complaints that allege "serious" hazards or violations receive a high priority. It should also be noted that complaints are categorized as formal and non-formal which also affects priority. Formal complaints generally receive an inspection, and can be filed by employees or their representatives. Non-Formal complaints are generally handled through the Phone and Fax procedure which is described later in this chapter.
4. **Referrals** — Hazard information from another government agency, individuals, organizations or the media receive consideration for inspection.
5. **Follow-ups** — These inspections are intended to check for abatement of violations cited during previous inspections.
6. **Planned or programmed inspection** — The Site Specific Targeting (SST) list constitutes a portion of OSHA's planned inspection activity. OSHA also uses National Emphasis Programs, Special Emphasis Programs, Regional Emphasis Programs and Local Emphasis Programs to target workplaces for inspection. In addition, OSHA conducts recordkeeping audits of a percentage of those employers participating in the OSHA Data Initiative which forms the basis for the SST.

Investigations and Inspections

The OSHA Field Operations Manual outlines the procedures and policies of workplace inspections and points out the following important steps.[11] For low-priority hazards, with permission of a complainant, OSHA may telephone the employer to describe safety and health concerns, following up with a fax providing details on alleged safety and health hazards. OSHA may also use the "Phone and Fax" method of complaint processing for complaints filed by parties other than a current employee or their representative. The employer must respond in writing within five working days. If the response is adequate, OSHA generally will not conduct an on-site inspection.[10]

Onsite Inspections — Before the inspection, OSHA CSHOs research the inspection history, research operations and processes and the standards that apply. They decide what protective equipment and testing instruments are appropriate and bring them to the inspection. By law and regulation CSHOs are not allowed to provide advanced notice of an inspection. The punishment is a maximum $1000 fine or imprisonment for not more than 6 months or both.

Presentation of Credentials — The CSHO presents credentials which include a photograph and a serial number. Since the search is pursuant to administrative powers, there is no probable cause requirement. The OSH Act specifically authorizes inspections so it is not difficult to obtain a warrant. There is a constitutional right of individuals to be free from warrantless administrative searches, but there are exceptions–plain view, emergency, and consent. Most administrative inspections are conducted with consent.

Opening Conference — The CSHO explains why the workplace was selected, the scope of inspection, walk-around procedures, employee representation and employee interviews. The employer selects someone to accompany the CSHO. An authorized representative of the employees has the right to go along.

Walk-around — During the inspection, the CSHO and representatives will walk through the portions of the workplace covered by the inspection, looking for hazards, and inspecting for violations.

Closing Conference — When the inspection is completed, the CSHO meets with the employer and the employee representatives to discuss the findings, and actions that the employer may take following an inspection.

Statute of Limitations — OSHA must issue a citation and proposed penalty within 6 months of the violation's occurrence.[11]

Citations

OSHA citations are issued after a very formal process. The workplace inspection begins with a formal conference and ends with a conference. The citations are issued and sent to the employer after the citations have been finalized and the fines have been determined.

Citations are issued for violating OSHA standards. The citation describes OSHA requirements allegedly violated, lists any proposed penalties and gives a deadline for correcting the alleged hazards. Violations are: a) other than serious b)serious c) willful, d)repeated e)failure to abate. Penalties range from up to $7,000 for each serious violation and up to $70,000 for each willful or repeated violation.[10] The employer must post the citation in a conspicuous place accessible to the employees.

A citation may contain several items. Each of the items carries a penalty. For instance in a recent OSHRC case, there were only two citations.[12] One contained 13 items each of which carried a penalty of $600 for each item. The second citation contained eight items labeled "other than serious." No penalty was proposed for those items.

The period of time stated in the citation for an employer to correct the alleged violation is called the abatement period.[10] The employer must fix the hazard, certify that the hazard is fixed, notify employees that the hazard is fixed, document the hazard correction and send proof to OSHA. If any movable equipment was cited, warning tags or a copy of the citation must be affixed. The employer must provide abatement documentation, abatement plans, and progress reports for some violations.[10] No further abatement certification is required for items which the employer permanently corrects during the inspection.

Contesting the Workplace Citation

Since some citations carry either a small penalty or none at all, an employer may wish to simply abate the conditions which have been cited and pay the fine. However, there may be reasons to contest the citations. If an employer disagrees with any part of the OSHA citation — the alleged violation, the abatement period, or proposed penalty — it must notify OSHA in writing of that disagreement within 15 working days (Mondays through Fridays, excluding Federal holidays) of receiving the citation. This written notification is called a "Notice of Contest." Employers have the right to contest OSHA citations and/or penalties before the Occupational Safety and Health Review Commission (OSHRC), an independent Federal agency created to decide contests of citations, abatement or penalties resulting from OSHA inspections.

OSHRC is comprised of three members appointed by the president with the "advice and consent of the Senate."[13] The Review Commission is an administrative court, with established procedures for conducting hearings, receiving evidence and rendering decisions by its Administrative Law Judges (ALJs).[7] Administrative Law Judges are appointed for life and serve in the various Regional offices around the country. Decisions of the commission are reported online.[7]

The "Notice of Contest" does not have to be on any particular form. It has to include the information regarding whether the penalty, the citation, abatement date is in contest. The notice of contest must be delivered in writing to the Area Director of the OSHA office that mailed the citation. Prior to filing a notice of contest, employers may request within the 15 day period, an informal conference with the Area Director to discuss the citations and penalties. The Area Director may enter into an Informal Settlement Agreement with the employer to resolve any issues. OSHA may also make use of an Expedited Informal Settlement Agreement which for certain citations will be mailed along with the citations to the employer. In essence, it offers a penalty reduction if the employer agrees to fully abate the items noted and pay the penalty.

Failure to file the "Notice of Contest" within the 15 day period will prevent the cited employer from claiming any further right of appeal. OSHRC has developed their Rules of Procedure which are to be followed.[14] The rules determine such things as when an employer can request the evidence that the Agency has collected, or what evidence can be produced during the hearing.

The U.S. Department of Labor regulations at Regulations 29 CFR Regulations §2200.22 indicates that an attorney is not necessary even for a corporation. "Any party or intervenor may appear in person, through an attorney, or through another representative who is not an attorney. A representative must file an appearance in accordance with §2200.23. In the absence of an appearance by a representative, a party or intervenor will be deemed to appear for himself. A corporation or unincorporated association may be represented by an authorized officer or agent."[15] Many industrial hygiene practitioners have developed a practice that focuses on OSHA defense.

Pleadings and Discovery — No later than 20 days after the Notice of Contest is sent to the Commission, the Secretary must file a complaint. The employer then has 20 days to file a motion for a more definite statement or an answer which is a brief, simple statement denying the allegations in the complaint which the party intends to contest. Affirmative defenses must be made at the same time. The most common errors are that the answer is either incomplete or filed late. Approximately 90% of all cases are settled without a hearing, so settlement negotiations are important. Sometimes, mediation is employed to facilitate a settlement. Employees are entitled to notice of a proposed settlement.

EZ Trial

Cases involving employers with few OSHA citations and under $20,000 in fines may be set for EZ Trial procedures. The Chief Administrative Law Judge makes the decision as to whether the procedure will be under EZ Trial or not. The procedures prohibit pre-trial discovery, do not use the Federal Rules of Evidence and requires parties to negotiate over pre-trial settlement. Trials can take place more quickly, and the decision can still be appealed to the full commission.[16] There are some problems with EZ Trial process. Since the employer is not entitled to pre-trial discovery, they are not getting full information about the case before going to trial. Without the Federal Rules of Evidence, hearsay evidence can be introduced to the detriment of the employer. Also employers believe that since it is an "EZ trial" they have a greater chance of winning and do not accept a settlement. Apparently this is an error on their part which could result in greater penalties than a settlement.[17]

Regular Hearings not set for EZ Trial

In the event that an early settlement cannot be reached, the parties need to prepare for trial. This is done through a process called Discovery. Interrogatories which are written questions can be sent to either party. Depositions are taken under oath, in front of a court reporter. Questions are asked and the deponent answers them. The information is recorded for use in the court proceedings. Requests for documents or photographs are frequently made during discovery. The ALJ hears the case following the

Procedural Rules of the OSHRC. The Federal Rules of Civil Procedure cover any items not covered in the OSHRC rules. The Federal Rules of Evidence apply to these hearings.

Hearings under EZ Trial or Regular Trial

If an employer does not appear at the hearing, a default is taken. That means that the employer loses if they do not show up, and the original citation and penalties apply. Some employers have claimed that since penalties under the Act are assessed solely by administrative process, the Act is in violation of the seventh amendment which provides for trial by jury. There is no right to a jury trial in OSHRC cases.[6] This issue was addressed by the Supreme Court in Atlas Roofing Co. v. OSHRC, 430 U.S. 442 (1977)[18], where the Court held that the process of administrative adjudication established by the Act does not violate the seventh amendment right to jury trial.[6]

During the trial, the employer can testify, and can call other witnesses. Both lay witnesses and expert witnesses may be called. Lay witnesses or percipient witnesses are those who have seen something relevant and can testify to it. Expert witnesses must be qualified to render an opinion and ALJ must decide whether their testimony is admissible. After each side has examined and cross examined witnesses, they can rest their case. The ALJ may direct both sides to brief any issue. That means that a written document citing authorities and discussing a certain issue must be filed. Usually that is not done with EZ Trial. After considering all testimony and briefs, the ALJ can render their decision.

Post Hearing

The written decision of the ALJ becomes a final order of the commission unless there is direction for review. There are provisions for Judicial Review which can go all the way to the U.S. Supreme Court.

In a recent case[19], a contractor was cited for failing to provide protective equipment to 11 workers exposed to asbestos, failing to tell them they were exposed to asbestos, failing to have a safety plan, and having them work at night to escape detection. A gas explosion injured the workers. The contractor contested the citations. The ALJ upheld the citations which claimed 28 violations and penalties totaling nearly $1.5 million. The decision was appealed to the Commission which ruled that it was only single violation of each standard and reduced the proposed penalties by more than 80 percent. OSHA itself then appealed that decision and asked the U.S. Court of Appeals to reverse the OSHRC commission decision. In this landmark case the Supreme Court upheld OSHA's egregious penalty policy. As a result of this case OSHA modified several regulations making them amenable to citing and penalizing instance by instance.

State Programs for Health and Safety

The OSH Act of 1970 encourages states to develop and operate their own job safety and health programs. These plans may cover both private and public sector employment or may be limited to public sector employment only. OSHA approves and monitors these state plans and provides up to 50 percent of an approved plan's operating costs.[20] The states must set job safety and health standards that are at least as effective as comparable federal standards. The states also have the ability to develop standards covering hazards not addressed by federal standards.

States must conduct inspections without advance notice, to enforce these safety and health standards. They must cover state and local government employees and operate occupational safety and health training and education programs. OSHA helps to fund assistance to employers to identify and correct workplace hazards in addition to compliance assistance for employers and employees.

If a state's plan has been granted final approval, a so-called "18(e) determination", by OSHA, OSHA relinquishes its authority to cover occupational safety and health matters covered by the state. Sixteen states have received final 18(e) approval. A total of 27 states have approved plans in operation, with five of those covering public sector only.[20]

Some IHs and safety professionals work for companies that operate in more than one state, so it is important to ascertain which agencies are responsible for enforcement of safety and health regulations in each state and know where to find those regulations.

Youth Worker Safety and Health

Workers under the age of 18 are a substantial part of the work force according to the Bureau of Labor Statistics of the U.S. Department of Labor. Their injury rate is higher than adult workers even though they are legally barred from working in the most dangerous industries which are mining, manufacturing and construction. It is thought teens are injured more frequently than adult workers because of inexperience, reluctance to ask questions, and poor training. As a professional in occupational health and safety, it is important to make an extra effort to educate young workers about safety, risks and be sure that they understand and follow directions.

Fair Labor Standards Act (FLSA) sets limits on the hours youth under the age of 18 may work and the occupations in which young workers may be employed. The U.S. Department of Labor's Employment Standards Administration's (ESA) Wage and Hour Division, through its enforcement and administration of the FLSA, has primary responsibility for the protection of young workers. All OSHA rules also apply to young workers. All states have rules concerning the employment of young workers. When federal and state standards are different, the rules that provide the most protection to young workers apply.[21]

Workers' Compensation

State Programs for Worker Compensation

When an employee is injured through accident, or work related illness, they need medical care and replacement for their lost wages. Employees of private companies or state and local government agencies are covered under their state workers' compensation laws. Workers' compensation benefits are not administered by a government agency. They are administered mainly by private insurance companies and those employers who are allowed to self insure their workers' compensation liability. Most states also have a competitive state insurance agency for employers. Insurance companies that offer worker's compensation coverage will often employ an industrial hygienist to investigate accidents and exposures, to inspect companies and to review safety programs and records as a condition of coverage. This is considered "loss control work."

Companies with an extremely high net worth and income or small companies in the same industry group who pool their liability, sometimes are self insured. The process of self insuring requires an evaluation of the self insured applicant's injury and illness prevention program. A compliance inspection by a private, independent, registered professional safety engineer, certified industrial hygienist, or certified safety professional is part of the application process in most states. The self insured applicant must be in compliance with state safety and health regulations and financial responsibility requirements.[22]

The workers compensation system provides benefits to both employees and employers. Employees are entitled to receive prompt, effective medical treatment for on-the-job injuries no matter who was at fault and, in return, are prevented from suing their employers over those injuries. There are exceptions to "no fault" because employees who engage in drugs or alcohol, or other misconduct in the workplace that results in injury may not be covered. Workers' comp insurance provides six basic benefits: medical care, temporary disability benefits, permanent disability benefits, supplemental job displacement benefits or vocational rehabilitation and death benefits.

In exchange for these benefits, the worker cannot bring a civil action against the employer for pain and suffering or other damages, except in cases of intentional acts. In most states, a worker injured by the intentional action of his or her employer can sue the employer for the harm in addition to filing for workers' compensation. Intentional employer behavior like assault, intentional infliction of emotional distress, or known exposure to hazardous conditions could result in greater liability for the employer. Instead of allowing an additional lawsuit, some states have included in their workers' compensation law an additional monetary award or penalty when an employer acts either willfully or maliciously to injure an employee or is reckless about their safety.

When an employer becomes aware of a work-related injury or illness, it is expected to begin providing benefits to the injured worker. Sometimes a dispute may arise between the claims administrator and the injured worker over benefits. Each state has its own Worker Compensation Agency or Appeals Board to resolve the disputes. These boards are administrative law hearings, and less formal than a court of law. An expert witness often testifies in these cases. A doctor may testify about the injury or illness but industrial hygiene and safety professionals may be called upon to testify as expert witnesses as to what constitutes hazardous workplace procedures or known exposure to hazardous conditions.

Employee or Independent Contractor

An emerging legal issue in the workplace is the distinction between employee and independent contractor. Employers sometimes classify employees as independent contractors so that they, the employer, do not have to pay payroll taxes, the minimum wage or overtime, comply with other wage and hour law requirements such as providing meal periods and rest breaks, or reimburse their workers for business expenses incurred in performing their jobs. Employers do not have to cover independent contractors under workers' compensation insurance, and are not liable for payments under unemployment insurance, disability insurance, or social security. Potential liabilities and penalties are significant if an individual is treated as an independent contractor and later found to be an employee, from a tax standpoint as well as worker compensation and civil liability.

The Internal Revenue Service (IRS) makes the determination about whether a worker is an independent contractor or an employee using issues of control. They consider evidence which falls into three categories — behavioral control, financial control, and the type of relationship itself. Behavioral control covers facts that show whether the business has a right to direct or control how the work is done through instructions, training, or other means. Financial control covers facts that show whether the business has a right to direct or control the financial and business aspects of the worker's job. The financial aspect includes whether or not the worker can make a profit or take a loss on the work and whether they own equipment used. The distinction between independent contractor and employee has been considered by the U.S. Supreme Court and by state courts as well. There is no absolute definition, and there are a number of factors to consider.

OSHA applies to employees, not independent contractors. In contesting citations, employers will sometimes claim that a worker is an independent contractor. In OSHA cases, factors developed by the Department of Labor are used to determine whether the person is an employee or not. This "economic reality" tests whether a contractor is an independent business person or the employer controls the workers' ability to make money. Various factors are considered including ownership and control of the workplace and equipment, profit or loss of the individual and whether individual judgment and planning are necessary. The test is very similar to the factors the IRS uses.

Working as a professional in the Health and Safety field, it is wise to follow the law carefully. Maintain worker compensation insurance, make the proper deductions for taxes and maintain Errors and Omissions or professional liability insurance.

State Laws which Affect Industrial Hygienists

Laws affecting industrial hygienists and safety professionals vary from state to state. Code sections may be similar, but court cases which interpret those codes can differ. The legislature in a state can develop a law but a court case can interpret that law narrowly or in a way that broadens the law. The following is a general outline of law in categories that are likely to affect industrial hygienists and safety professionals.

Civil and Criminal Law

Civil law involves non-criminal problems such as contract disputes, property ownership disputes, consumer laws, divorce, and child custody. It also includes personal injury and property damage. The outcome of a civil law case is that the winning side may be awarded money or property.

Criminal cases are filed by federal, state or local prosecutors because of crimes that have been committed. The outcome of a criminal case is that if the defendant loses, he may be fined or serve a prison term and in some states there is a death penalty for certain crimes.

Contract Law

Leases of office space, purchases of supplies, and retainer agreements with clients are all examples of contracts. State contract law governs written and sometimes oral agreements between persons and/or between businesses. A contract is a legal document containing agreements that can be enforced in a court of law.

If a breach of contract is settled in court of law, the prevailing or winning party can receive money damages, including compensatory, liquidated and sometimes punitive damages. If the contract includes a provision for attorney fees and costs the prevailing party may also be awarded those fees and costs. A breach of a contract occurs when either side refuses to perform their part of the contract.

Compensatory damages can be awarded to the prevailing party. These are awarded in an amount that would put the plaintiff in the same position as if the contract had been performed. Liquidated damages are a predetermined amount to be awarded in case there is a breach. These are often included in construction contracts as a per day penalty for late completion of the project. Usually the liquidated damages must be a realistic amount. In some contracts, a bonus may be included for early completion using the same structure as the as the liquidated damages.

Specific performance, when the party is forced to complete their contractual commitments, is an equitable remedy that can be awarded for breach of contract. Generally a contract to perform industrial hygiene services is a personal services contract so a court could not order specific performance in the event the contract is breached. However, a court could award damages if a breach occurred.

The most important contract which affects the industrial hygiene and safety professional is the agreement that sets the work to be done, what the pay will be, and terms and conditions which apply. It is important to be specific about what the industrial hygienist will do, and what will not be done. A professional should not begin work without a written agreement that is specific, complete and appropriate for the job. Employers sometimes have provisions in an employment contract with a professional regarding whether they can work for a competing company in the same field. A contract case involving Industrial Hygienists is Occusafe v. EG&G Rocky Flats which involved industrial hygienists who signed employment contracts not to work for a competitor of Occusafe for 6 months after leaving Occusafe (non-compete agreements) because industrial hygienists in that area were scarce. Seven of the industrial hygienists left and went to work for a competitor. Occusafe sued for damages for breach of contract. It was decided that the "non compete clause" was valid, and the case was sent back to the lower court to decide damages.[23]

A Retainer Agreement, Services Contract, or the Terms and Conditions must be signed by the appropriate person in the company hiring the professional. Each client and situation is unique so the document must be tailored appropriately. A sensible plan would be to have a knowledgeable attorney prepare a template for a contract to use as a starting point. Costs for permits, lab tests, rental of equipment, additional personnel as well as travel expenses and other costs are among the many terms that must be included. Decisions about indemnity, insurance, liability and time of completion of the contract need to be agreed upon. The appropriate court and which state laws would govern in case of a dispute should be identified. Be assured that the items left out or vaguely worded are the ones which typically result in a dispute.

If the client wants to change the terms of the contract after the job has started, those changes need to be agreed upon in writing by both parties to the contract. Thorough records and documentation should be maintained and all problems or difficulties should be communicated in writing. Contract disputes between the professional and the client can often be avoided by clear and complete contracts and by good communication during the job.

Tort Law

A tort is an injury to another person, to their business or to their property that results in damage. The injured person can recover the cost of medical treatment if they are injured, lost wages for the period of injury, pain and suffering, loss of earnings capacity. Future costs of medical care may be sought.

Generally torts are divided into three major groups, intentional torts, negligent torts, and strict liability torts which includes product liability.

Intentional torts include assault, battery, intentional infliction of emotional distress, intentional misrepresentation and fraud. These are acts which result in damage and injury committed either deliberately or recklessly. An industrial hygienist or safety professional would be committing an intentional tort by submitting fraudulent data which results in damage. The damage can result in physical damage to a person's health. It could also be fraud that results in someone paying for tests that were never made, or falsely interpreted. Those situations are intentional torts. There are other intentional torts that could be committed such as misrepresenting qualifications, concealing hazardous conditions, disposing of hazardous substances in an illegal manner.

Negligence is a failure to use ordinary care through either an act or omission. A person does not exercise the amount of care that a reasonable person would use under the same circumstances or they do something that a reasonable person would not do under the same or similar circumstances which results in harm. Negligence liability is imposed when a duty of due care is owed by the defendant to the person injured or to all persons who are foreseeably endangered by his conduct with respect to all risks that make the conduct unreasonably dangerous. For example, it would be considered negligence if an industrial hygienist that had been retained to measure hazardous exposures at a workplace discovered high levels of a toxic substances, but then failed to complete reports and warn employees in a timely manner to prevent the employees from being exposed. The industrial hygienist had a duty to those persons, but he breached the duty and they were damaged. That is negligence which can result in a lawsuit demanding damages.

Under the strict liability theory, a person or company is responsible for damage as a result of actions or products that caused harm. Even if the damage was caused without the intent to do harm. For example, under strict liability if a demolition company imploded a building that resulted in a cloud of dust and debris that killed pets in a nearby pet store, the company is fully responsible for all damages even if it took all possible precautions to avoid harm.

Product liability is a type of strict liability as applied to products in the stream of commerce. Strict liability for products causing injury can be caused by manufacturing defects, design defects or poor labeling and failure to warn.

State Professional Regulations and Certifications

Industrial hygienists can be certified by professional agencies. Certified Industrial Hygienists (CIH) are certified by the American Board of Industrial Hygiene (ABIH). Industrial hygienists could have licenses or state certifications, such as the regulated California asbestos training certification and certified mold remediation consultants. Some states have certifications for hazardous material managers and certified environmental consultants. In addition, some states provide "title protection." The Minnesota statute states the reason for title protection as follows:

> "The purpose of the Industrial Hygienist and Safety Professional Title Protection Act is to provide legal recognition to the profession of industrial hygiene and safety, to assure the public that individuals representing themselves as industrial hygiene and safety professionals meet minimum qualifications, and to further public health and safety."[24]

It is necessary to check each state to see what regulations apply to professional designations, what the continuing education requirements are, and whether there is title protection and regulation. In most states enforcement of title protection is done without the requirement of proving that anyone has been damaged by the deceptive use of the titles. An injunction can be issued to prevent the person from continuing to advertise themselves deceptively.

An example of title protection occurs the Commonwealth of Virginia, where the code prohibits persons from using the letters or words "Industrial Hygienist in Training," "IHIT," "Certified Associate Industrial Hygienist," "CAIH," "Certified Industrial Hygienist," "CIH," or a variation of those words, to represent that the person does possesses the applicable certification issued by ABIH. Professional certifications issued by the Board of Certified Safety Professionals (BCSP) also are protected under this code.[25,26] Indiana's title protection provides that a violation is a misdemeanor.[27,28]

The Industrial Hygienist and Safety Professional as an Advisor

Expert advice and information are provided by industrial hygiene and safety professionals to employers, to unions, to attorneys and sometimes to individuals. Whether they are in-house personnel or in private practice they evaluate health hazards, recommend measures to ensure maximum employee protection and keep informed of the standards and practices of that industry. Industrial hygienists and safety professionals can conduct a "base line survey" of a facility and advise what steps need to be taken to comply with standards and regulations before any accidents or illnesses occur.

If an employer is cited by either OSHA or a state run program, the professional is consulted regarding the merits of the citation, and helps determine what needs to be done. Initially, it is necessary to determine whether the citation is accurate and if a violation has occurred as alleged in the citation.

A citation may have been issued because there is a standard required of the employer and the employer did not comply. The professional will be able to examine the site of the accident and determine whether the standard applies in this case and whether the abatement proposed is feasible. A decision needs to be made about whether it is possible to have the citation re-characterized. The answers to all of these questions may help to resolve the matter prior to an OSHRC hearing. If not, decisions must be made about whether the case should go to trial. The professional can provide valuable information and insight on these issues.

Where a serious injury or illness has occurred, civil lawsuits are a possibility. In some circumstances relatives of the worker or the community at large have been injured. The safety and health professional advises the company and their attorneys about relevant standards and practices that may have been violated. The professional's advice is valuable in deciding how to handle the case and can be helpful in settlement negotiations.

The Industrial Hygienist and Safety Professional as an Expert Witness

An industrial hygienist is sometimes called upon to act as a witness in a Civil Case, a Criminal Case or a Worker Compensation case. The prescient or fact witness who has information which is relevant to the case can only testify about what they have personally seen. They do not give opinions or their own personal view of the matter.

Attorneys began to use "expert witnesses" prior to the 1920's in an attempt to influence a judge or jury. Frye v. United States was a case that was appealed to the Court of Appeals of the District of Columbia in 1923.[29] Frye had been convicted of murder, and was appealing on the grounds that he had not been allowed to present necessary evidence that proved his innocence. An expert witness would have testified to the results of a "deception test" involving systolic blood pressure. The expert claimed that it was possible to tell if a person was lying based on their blood pressure readings which went up if a person was lying, angry or deceptive. The trial judge had refused to allow the testimony and refused to allow a demonstration of the test in the courtroom.

The attorney for the defendant claimed that it was necessary to have a skilled or expert witness to explain technical theories to the judge and jury. The Appeals Court held that it is difficult to decide where a scientific theory crosses the line between experiment and fact. Stating that courts "will go a long way in admitting expert testimony deduced from a well-recognized scientific principle or discovery, the thing from which the deduction is made must be sufficiently established to have gained general acceptance in the particular field in which it belongs."[29] In deciding that the "deception test" had not gained standing and scientific recognition adequate to justify using it in court, the Appeals Court agreed that the expert testimony should not have been admitted into evidence.

The Frye case was long used to help determine whether scientific or technical evidence could be admitted. But in 1993, two minor children born with birth defects and their parents sued Merrill Dow Pharmaceuticals, Inc., alleging that the defects were caused because the mother had taken Benedictine, a prescription drug marketed by Dow. In a Summary Judgment Motion, the defendants (Daubert) presented their expert's affidavit which stated that after reviewing published scientific literature on the subject, maternal use of Bendectine was not a risk factor for human birth defects. The petitioners in their objection to the Summary Judgment Motion had responded with the testimony of eight other well credentialed experts, who based their conclusion that Bendectin can cause birth defects on animal studies, chemical structure analyses and re examination of previously published human statistical studies.

The trial court determined that this evidence did not meet the applicable "general acceptance" standard for the admission of expert testimony. The Court of Appeals agreed and affirmed, citing Frye v. United States for the rule that expert opinion based on a scientific technique is inadmissible unless the technique is "generally accepted" as reliable in the relevant scientific community.[29]

The U.S. Supreme Court held that the Federal Rules of Evidence, not Frye v. U.S., provide the standard for admitting expert scientific testimony in a federal trial.[30] This is a liberal standard that uses Rule 402 as the baseline:[31] "All relevant evidence is admissible, except as otherwise provided by the Constitution of the United States, by Act of Congress, by these rules, or by other rules prescribed by the Supreme Court pursuant to statutory authority. Evidence which is not relevant is not admissible."

New Federal Rule 702 — Testimony by Experts

Federal Rule 702 states that "If scientific, technical, or other specialized knowledge will assist the trier of fact to understand the evidence or to determine a fact in issue, a witness qualified as an expert by knowledge, skill, experience, training, or education, may testify thereto in the form of an opinion or otherwise, if (1) the testimony is based upon sufficient facts or data, (2) the testimony is the product of reliable principles and methods, and (3) the witness has applied the principles and methods reliably to the facts of the case."[31]

Note that Daubert v. Merrell Dow Pharmaceuticals was a federal case and the rule referred to is one of the Federal Rules of Evidence. States have different statutes and rules which vary considerably. Following the Daubert case in 1993, almost all states adopted rules of evidence nearly identical to the Federal Rule of Evidence No. 702 that was cited in that case. Federal Rule 702 was amended in 2007, but not all states have amended their Evidence Rule to conform with the revisions. Individual states determine if they follow Daubert's reasoning or rely solely on cases in their own jurisdiction.

An effective expert witness needs to know what the standard is in the jurisdiction in which they are testifying. Depending on the type of expert testimony they will be offering, and the scientific or economic basis for it, there is almost always a pre-hearing inquiry to determine if the testimony will be admissible or not. Testimony is taken, usually in the form of questioning the expert on the basis for their opinion as well as their qualifications. Written briefs challenging or supporting the evidence that will be given are also submitted. That inquiry is not held with the jury present. Sometimes the challenges to the testimony are heard long before trial.

The attorney who is offering the testimony of the expert or the one who is challenging the expert testimony may make motions in connection with the testimony in addition to the pre-hearing inquiry. If the testimony or the studies on which it may be based are new or unusual, there will be more time spent to determine whether it will be admissible or not.

Industrial hygienists can serve as experts in two different ways. The first is as a consulting expert who provides scientific information by collecting, testing, analyzing studies and statistics and forming an opinion as to that evidence; which is used to evaluate the case or to inform the attorney as to how to manage the evidence. The IH also could be used as the forensic and trial expert who gives that opinion and its basis to the judge and jury.

The consulting expert can make assessments of conditions and provide opinion for the attorney or insurance company to aid informed decisions regarding the case. Generally, their information is protected by Attorney-Client privilege and is not available to the opposing side.

The IH who is a forensic or trial expert may testify at trial, or depositions where they provide sworn statements of their opinions and interpretations of conditions. The deposition is then used to provide judge or jury with information to help them understand the basis for their opinions. The expert needs to be prepared to explain their background, training, education, and experience and to be comfortable with cross examination about that information.

Because the credibility of an expert witness is vital to success, they must keep careful records of certifications, classes taken, lectures given and the date and expiration of credentials. A successful expert witness was recently discredited because her certification had expired and she had neglected to renew it.

Ethical Obligations

Health and safety professionals must know and understand the laws that affect their practice but they also must comply with the ethical guidelines set by their Professional Organizations. The ABIH[32] sets ethical principles for how to practice and counsel parties regarding health and safety risks. In the ABIH code is also a reminder that personal and business information must be kept confidential. Standards for conflict of interest and disclosures are also included. An Industrial Hygienist should perform services only when qualified. Cautions about being truthful and accurate in professional advertising are also included. In addition AIHA and ACGIH developed and approved a "Joint Industrial Hygiene Associations Member Ethical Principles" document and the Board of Certified Safety Professionals promotes a "Code of Ethics and Professional Conduct" for CSPs.[33,34]

As Adrian Zaccaria, vice chairman of Bechtel recently stated, "Business success and ethical conduct go hand in hand. If customers don't trust us, they don't hire us. When you are asked — directly or indirectly — to violate your code of conduct, you must shut the conversation down immediately."[35] In short, the profession clearly points the IH to a path of clearly defining issues, neither to overstate nor understate a risk or exposure to the workforce or the public. For the professional in health and safety, ethical behavior, understanding and compliance with laws and regulations are absolute requirements. A reputation for honesty, integrity and knowledge are essential to an IH and safety professional.

References

1. American Industrial Hygiene Association. http://aiha.org
2. 29 U.S.C §651 (b)
3. 29 U.S.C.A. §654 (a)
4. **Ashford, N. and C. Caldart:** *Technology, Law and the Working Environment.* Washington, D.C.: Island Press, 1996.
5. Variance procedures: http://www.osha.gov/OshDoc/data_General_Facts/VarianceFactS.pdf.
6. **Rothstein, M.A.:** *Occupational Safety and Health Law.* 2nd edition. St. Paul, MN: Thompson West, 2010.
7. The U.S. Occupational Safety and Health Review Commission. http://www.oshrc.gov/
8. The National Institute for Occupational Safety & Health. http://www.cdc.gov/niosh
9. National Advisory Committee on Occupational Safety and Health. http://www.osha.gov/dop/nacosh/nacosh
10. **Occupational Safety and Health Administration:** *OSHA Inspections.* OSHA Pub. No. 2098, 2002.
11. **Occupational Safety and Health Administration:** *OSHA Field Inspection Reference Manual.* CPL 02-00-148, 2009.
12. Secretary of Labor, Complainant, v. OSHRC Docket No. 02-0051 Joel Patterson Air Conditioning
13. How OSHRC Works. The U.S. Occupational Safety and Health Review Commission. http://www.oshrc.gov/about/how-oshrc.html
14. Rules of Procedure. The U.S. Occupational Safety and Health Review Commission. http://www.oshrc.gov/procrules/procrules.html
15. DOL Regulations (Standards - 29 CFR)§2200
16. Guide to EX Trial Procedures. The U.S. Occupational Safety and Health Review Commission. http://www.oshrc.gov/ publications/e-ztrial/e-ztrial.html
17. **Montoya, V.:** OSHA Review Commission's E-Z Trial: Backdoor Authoritarianism? Reg. 21(3):9–11 (1998).
18. Atlas Roofing Co. v. OSHRC, 430 U.S. 442 (1977)
19. Occupational Safety and Health Review Commission (OSHRC) in Secretary of Labor v. Ho, OSHRC No. 98-1645, 98-1646 (OSHRC, Sept. 29, 2003).

20. http://www.osha.gov/dcsp/osp/index.html
21. **Wage and Hour Division:** Child Labor. U.S. Department of Labor. http://www.dol.gov/esa/whd/childlabor.htm
22. Division of Workers' Compensation — Answers to frequently asked questions about workers' compensation for employers. California Department of Industrial Relations. http://www.dir.ca.gov/dwc/faqs.html
23. Occusafe v. EG & G Rocky Flats, 1995, No. 93-1469.
24. Minnesota Statute, Industrial Hygiene & Safety Profession, § 182A.
25. Virginia Labor Code, §§ 40.1-140
26. Virginia Labor Code, §§ 40.1-141
27. Indiana Code; Prohibitions against use of title, § 24-4-11-10
28. Indiana Code; Prohibitions against use of title, § 24-4-11-11
29. Frye v. United States, 1923, 54 App D.C. 46, 293 F 1013
30. Daubert v. Merrell Dow Pharmaceuticals, 509 U.S. 579 (1993)
31. Federal Rules of Evidence, Ithica, NY: Legal Information Institute, 2009.
32. American Board of Industrial Hygiene Code of Ethics. American Board of Industrial Hygiene. http://abih.org/downloads/ABIHCodeofEthics.pdf.
33. Joint Industrial Hygiene Associations Member Ethical Principles. Academy of Industrial Hygiene. http://www.aiha.org/academy/Documents/MemberEthicalPrinciples52107.pdf
34. Code of Ethics and Professional Conduct. Board of Certified Safety Professionals. http://www.bcsp.org/pdf/ethics.pdf
35. **Zaccaria, A. and Bechtel Corporation:** Ethics at all Cost. Address to Ethics & Compliance Officers. April 30, 2009.

Outcome Competencies

After completing this chapter, the reader should be able to:

1. Define underlined terms used in this chapter that are germane to understanding occupational exposure limits (OELs).
2. Select resources for obtaining OEL values.
3. Describe the differences between the various OELs.
4. Summarize the factors evaluated in setting an OEL.
5. Explain limitations of OELs.
6. Calculate workplace exposures.

Key Terms

action level • airborne particulate matter • biological exposure indices (BEI®) • carcinogen classification system • ceiling • maximum allowable concentrations (MAKs) • new chemical exposure limits (NCELs) • notice of intended change (NIC) • permissible exposure limit (PEL) • recommended exposure limit (REL) • short-term exposure limit (STEL) • skin notation • threshold limit value® (TLV®) • time-weighted average (TWA) • workplace environmental exposure limit (WEEL)

Prerequisite Knowledge

Prior to beginning this chapter, the user should review the following references for general content:

Academic Discipline	Reference Citation
Occupational hygiene	*Threshold Limit Values® for Chemical Substances and Physical Agents—Biological Exposure Indices®*, ACGIH®
Toxicology	*Toxicology Primer*, Kamrin
Toxicology	*Casarett & Doull's Toxicology—the Basic Science of Poisons*, Klaassen

Prior to beginning this chapter, the reader should review the following chapters.

Chapter Number	Chapter Topic
1	History and the Philosophy of Industrial Hygiene
5	Occupational Toxicology
6	Occupational Epidemiology
8	Occupational and Environmental Risk Assessment/ Risk Management
9	Comprehensive Exposure Assessment
10	Modeling Inhalation Exposure
20	The Skin and the Work Environment

Key Topics

I. Introduction
   A. The Question from the Health, Safety, and Environmental Team
   B. Objectives and Terminology
   C. Physiology of the Respiratory Tract and Skin

II. Goals and Limitations of OELs

III. Terminology Used in OELs

IV. Groups That Recommend OELs
   A. Inhalation Exposure Limits
   B. Biological Exposure Limits
   C. Physical Agent Exposure Limits

V. Important Considerations in the Development of OELs
   A. Identification of the Hazard
   B. Routes of Exposure
   C. Review and Evaluation of the Chemical-Specific Toxicology Data
   D. Carcinogen Classification System and Risk Models

VI. Other Issues Impacting OELS

Occupational Exposure Limits

4

Dennis Klonne, PhD, DABT

Introduction

The Question for the Health, Safety & Environmental Team

The toughest question faced by the occupational health, safety, and environmental affairs professional is, "We know we are exposed to this chemical (or physical or biological) agent, but is it safe for us at this level?"

This question is often raised at safety meetings, training sessions, new process reviews, high-level management meetings, and other gatherings both inside and outside the workplace. Although it may be difficult to answer, it deserves a response. However, the answer must always be given with the caveat that it is the best answer that can be given based on current data and the application of best professional judgment. There is no black and white answer to this question.

Objectives and Terminology

The objective of this chapter is to make the reader aware of resources for occupational exposure limits (OELs), to understand the basic terminology used in OELs, and to develop an appreciation of the factors that are evaluated in setting an OEL. The reader should not expect to be able to develop an OEL after reading this chapter, because that is best left to teams of occupational hygienists, toxicologists, occupational physicians, and others who have many years of experience and have developed expertise in this area.

Following is some terminology that is defined for its specific use in this chapter.

OEL. This term is used in a generic sense, as opposed to limits with specific acronyms that are set by specific groups, such as the TLV® (Threshold Limit Value) set by ACGIH® (American Conference of Governmental Industrial Hygienists) or the WEEL (Workplace Environmental Exposure Level) set by AIHA® (American Industrial Hygiene Association).

Agent. An agent may be physical (e.g., radiation, noise), chemical, or biological (e.g., virus, bacteria, mold spore, plant fragment) in nature. Although in this chapter chemical agents principally are discussed, because they are the most common agent in the industrial setting, the same principles generally apply to physical or biological agents.

Workplace Health Professional. As used here, this is a generic term encompassing many different disciplines, including but not limited to occupational hygiene, safety, toxicology, industrial medicine, environmental and process engineering, and so forth.

There are many books available to help obtain information on specific chemicals. However, the use of computerized online databases should be included in any serious search because the most recent published data will likely be cited in the journals included in those databases. The National Library of Medicine's (NLM's) online databases contain more than 18 million references. In the Additional Resources section of this chapter, additional online resources are listed. Especially useful is the downloadable version of the *NIOSH Pocket Guide to Chemical Hazards.*

Physiology of the Respiratory Tract and Skin

A review of the basic physiology of the respiratory tract and skin can be found elsewhere in this book as well as in several references.[1–11] Therefore, basic knowledge in these areas is assumed, and only some specific ideas, directly applicable to topics in this chapter, are discussed here.

Physiology of the Respiratory Tract

The upper respiratory tract consists of the nasopharynx and is the portal of entry for many toxicants. Its geometry provides for turbulent airflow, which helps to trap particles greater than about 5 µm by inertial impaction. Because its surface area is covered by a mucus layer, and because the incoming air is humidified to approximately 100% relative humidity in this region, it is also a site where soluble gases and vapors may be trapped. The olfactory (i.e., nasal) epithelium also provides an early warning system with its ability to detect odors. However, individual ability to detect odor varies greatly, and a phenomenon known as olfactory fatigue decreases the ability to detect odors over time. That is, the threshold for detecting the odor is raised over time. It should further be noted that odor does not correlate with toxicity. That is, compounds with a very low odor threshold and very disagreeable odor, such as mercaptans or thiols, may be detected at levels very much lower than that producing toxicity, whereas compounds such as carbon monoxide are never detected by odor even up to concentrations that cause death. For further information on odor thresholds, see references 12 and 13. Another important component of the nasopharyngeal region (and in the conducting airways of the lung) is the cilium. The hair-like cilia keep mucus flowing upward to clear the upper respiratory tract. However, some chemicals (e.g., cigarette smoke) may paralyze the cilia, resulting in increased accumulation of mucus and decreased clearance of toxicants.

The conducting airways, consisting of the trachea and bronchi, have many bifurcations (splits) that are potential sites of impact and deposition for toxicants. The increased branching of these airways into the lung results in a decreased airflow due to increasing total cross-sectional area with resultant differences in particle deposition throughout the lower respiratory tract. Particles in the 1–5 µm range are deposited in this region of the lung primarily by sedimentation. Again, mucociliary transport is an important route of toxicant elimination that works by trapping the vapor or particle in the mucus layer then moving it upward to be expectorated or swallowed. If swallowed, the route of exposure then becomes oral, instead of the initial inhalation route of exposure.

The lungs are designed for maximum transport and absorption. The alveolar/blood barrier is only a few cells thick, and the lung is highly vascularized and perfused. Furthermore, the lung has a very large surface area (approximately 300 to 1000 ft^2 [27.87 to 92.9 m^2]), especially in comparison with that of the skin (approximately 20 ft^2 [1.86 m^2]). Submicron particles and vapors are deposited in this alveolar region of the lung by simple diffusion. For most calculations of respiratory volume during a normal workday, a value of 10 m^3 can be used.

Physiology of the Skin

The outer skin (epidermis) is the principal barrier (approximately 0.2 mm thick) blocking entry of foreign chemicals into the body. The layer of dead cells (stratum corneum) is the principal component in this role and is replaced about every 2–4 weeks. Passage of chemicals through this layer to the dermis (which is approximately 2 mm thick) can result in the systemic uptake of the chemical and its distribution through the body. Chemicals that have both lipid and water solubility pass through the skin the easiest; those that are mostly lipid-soluble pass easier than those that are mostly water-soluble. Many chemicals are known to pass through the skin readily and are used as carriers for drugs (e.g., dimethyl sulfoxide). However, chemicals that pass through the dermal barrier can carry other toxic chemicals with them, producing illness in workers despite the fact that the workplace concentrations are well below the OEL. Similarly, chemicals that de-fat or dry out the skin can also compromise the dermal barrier and thereby allow other chemicals to pass into the body in toxic amounts. The most common skin-related complaints in the workplace are dermatitis, which is a localized inflammation and is reversible; corrosion, which is a destruction of the skin and results in irreversible scarring; and sensitization, which is a reversible allergic reaction but which produces potentially irreversible changes in immune cells thereby causing future reactions to the chemical at extremely low exposures. Phototoxicity and photosensitization occur less frequently and result from the interaction of chemicals with sunlight (ultraviolet radiation) and the cells in the skin.

Goals and Limitations of OELs

The question asked at the opening of this chapter—whether a chemical is safe at a particular level—is the reason for OELs. Although some people think that only a zero exposure level is safe or question the need for OELs, the real world dictates the precision at which the question is answered. The OELs are quite simply there to protect worker health. Although zero exposure should be a goal to strive for, it is generally not a reality of the industrial environment. When no safe level is thought to exist (e.g., very potent carcinogens, lethal viruses), then extreme measures such as engineering controls and use of personal protective equipment must be taken to ensure that there is indeed no exposure.

The Occupational Safety and Health Act of 1970 (OSH Act)[10,11,14,15] was enacted

> "to assure so far as possible every working man and woman in the nation safe and healthful working conditions by authorizing the Secretary of Labor to set mandatory occupational safety and health standards . . . (and) by providing medical criteria which will assure insofar as practicable that no employee will suffer diminished health, functional capacity, or life expectancy as a result of his work experience."[14]

Although this is indeed a desirable goal, ACGIH® [16] recognizes that OELs may not protect all people in all cases.

> "Threshold Limit Values® (TLVs®) refer to airborne concentrations of substances and represent conditions under which it is believed that nearly all workers may be repeatedly exposed, day after day, over a working lifetime, without adverse health effects.
>
> ACGIH® recognizes that there will be considerable variation in the level of biological response to a particular chemical substance, regardless of the airborne concentration. Indeed, TLVs® do not represent a fine line between a healthy versus an unhealthy work environment or the point at which material impairment of health will occur. TLVs® will not adequately protect all workers. Some individuals may experience discomfort or even more serious adverse health effects when exposed to a chemical substance at the TLV® or even at concentrations below the TLV®. There are numerous possible reasons for increased susceptibility to a chemical substance, including age, gender, ethnicity, genetic factors (predisposition), lifestyle choices (e.g., diet, smoking, abuse of alcohol and other drugs), medications, and pre-existing medical conditions (e.g., aggravation of asthma or cardiovascular disease). Some individuals may become more responsive to one or more chemical substances following previous exposures (e.g., sensitized workers). Susceptibility to the effects of chemical substances may be altered during different periods of fetal development and throughout an individual's reproductive lifetime."[16]

Thus, it is already stated that not all people are protected all the time. There are even many instances when a single individual is protected until a change in physiological state suddenly occurs (e.g., pregnancy, acute liver disease), and then the OEL is no longer protective. There are also examples in which hobbies can render an OEL unprotective, such as the case of a foundry worker who likes to target-shoot in the evening, or a person who works in a solvent production plant by day and strips and refinishes furniture at night.

Being cognizant of the limitations of OELs requires the practicing workplace health professional to be ever vigilant for the individual(s) who may suffer adverse effects, even if the OEL is always maintained. It should always be remembered that OELs such as the TLV® or WEEL do not have the force of law and are recommendations or guidelines, not boundaries between safe and unsafe conditions for all workers. Their proper implementation requires people with appropriate training to continually observe and monitor both the employees and the work environment.

The goal of OELs is to protect workers over their entire working lifetime, which is approximately 40 years. This has traditionally been applied to the 8 hours/day, 5 days/week work schedule. With the concept of the flexible workweek (e.g., four 10-hour workdays), the traditional workweek may well apply to a smaller percentage of the work force. When this is the case, people engaged in these unusual work shifts should be monitored carefully, and in some instances the OEL may have to be adjusted to a lower level to account for the increased time of continuous exposure and the decreased time for metabolism and elimination between exposures. There are several ways to make such an adjustment to the OEL, ranging from relatively simple to very complicated procedures. Paustenbach[17] provides an extensive review of several approaches. The need to adjust the OEL varies by the toxicity endpoint; there may be no need to adjust a value set for irritation effects, whereas a systemic toxicant with a moderately long biologic half-life would need to be decreased to maintain the same body burden from an unusual work shift as that from a standard work shift. More involved procedures may require extensive pharmacokinetic data—information that is often not available. However, the "reward" for developing such data may be a higher value for the OEL than that calculated using simpler procedures that utilize more conservative assumptions to compensate for the lack of data. Again, Paustenbach[17] provides a detailed treatment and sample calculations of several models, whereas Appendix A provides examples for two of the simpler models.

It is also very important to remember that the basis for the OEL varies from chemical to chemical. The goal for one chemical may be simply to avoid unpleasant odor, whereas for another it may be to prevent irreversible reproductive effects or cancer. This should always be considered by the workplace health professional because the relative importance of overexposures is very much affected by the toxicity endpoint. Thus, it is of utmost importance for the practicing professional to read the documentation for the OEL to understand the basis of the level and the strength of the supporting data. It is strongly recommended that every practicing occupational hygienist read the introduction section of the TLV® booklet[16] because it eloquently describes both the goals and limitations of OELs.

One final point with regard to OELs: OELs typically are meant to apply to a work force that, on average, is healthier than the general public. Because of activities that require some degree of physical exertion, generally the workforce consists of a subpopulation that is healthier than the U.S. population in general. Furthermore, in industrial settings it has been the practice to exclude the very young and very old, as well as those with infirmities and physical impairment, because of the nature of the work. This phenomenon is typically referred to as the healthy worker effect. Therefore, OELs are not meant to apply to the general population and are not to be used as community-based standards. Furthermore, the application of some set safety factor (e.g., divide the OEL by 100) to produce a community-based standard from an OEL is equally inappropriate.

Terminology Used in OELs

A fairly standard terminology has come to be used with regard to OELs. All the terms used in this chapter (except action level) are derived from the definitions given in the TLV® booklet[16] but are provided here for the sake of completeness and as points of discussion. The reader is also referred to glossaries in Plog[11], AIHA®[18], and in Accrocco.[19]

Time-Weighted Average (TWA). This is the fundamental concept of most OELs. It is usually presented as the average concentration over an 8-hour workday within the context of a 40-hour workweek. However, this implies that concentrations will be both above and below the average value during the work shift. The ACGIH® TLV® committee has recommended excursion limits to prevent concentrations from severely exceeding the TLV®-TWA. The proposed excursion limits are that exposures should typically not exceed the TLV®-TWA by more than threefold and for a period not exceeding 30 minutes during the workday. Even if the TWA is not exceeded for the work shift, in no case should the excursion be more than fivefold the TLV®-TWA value. These guidelines should encourage employers to minimize the frequency and severity of peak exposures that occur during the work shift. Examples of calculations germane to the concept of the TWA appear in Appendix A. See also Chapters 7 and 10.

Short-Term Exposure Limit (STEL). STELs are recommended when even short-duration exposures to high concentrations of a chemical are known to produce acute toxicity. It is the concentration to which workers can be exposed continuously for a short period of time without suffering from (1) irritation, (2) chronic or irreversible tissue damage, (3) dose-rate-dependent toxic effects, or (4) narcosis of sufficient degree to increase the likelihood of accidental injury, impaired self-rescue, or materially reduced work efficiency. A STEL is defined as a 15-minute TWA exposure that should not be exceeded at any time during a workday, even if the overall 8-hour TWA is within limits, and it should not occur more than four times per day. There should be at least 60 minutes between successive exposures in this range. If warranted, an averaging period other than 15 minutes also can be used. Again, these guidelines are to encourage employers to minimize the severity of peak exposures and to maximize the time between such exposures to provide sufficient recovery time for employees during the work shift.

Ceiling (C). The concentration that should not be exceeded during any part of the working exposure. In conventional occupational hygiene practice, if instantaneous monitoring is not feasible, then the ceiling can be assessed by sampling over a 15-minute period, except for chemicals that may cause immediate irritation, even with exposures of extremely short duration.

Action Level. This is the concentration or level of an agent at which it is deemed that some specific action should be taken. The action can range from more closely monitoring the exposure atmosphere to making engineering adjustments. In general practice the action level is usually set at one-half of the TLV®.

Skin Notation (skin). The skin notation denotes the possibility that dermal absorption may be a significant contribution to the overall body burden of the chemical. That is, the airborne OEL may not be adequate to protect the worker because the compound also readily penetrates the skin. Other toxicity endpoints on skin such as irritation, dermatitis, and sensitization are not sufficient to warrant the skin notation. In practice, the skin notation is given to compounds with a dermal LD_{50} less than 1000 mg/kg, or if there are other data indicating that repeated dermal exposure results in systemic toxicity.

Airborne Particulate Matter. The ACGIH® TLV® committee has divided this general category into three classes based on the likely deposition within the respiratory tract. Although past practice was to provide TLV®s in terms of total particulate mass, the recent approach is to take into account the aerodynamic diameter of the particle and its site of action. Inhalable particulate matter (IPM) TLV®s are designated for compounds that are toxic if deposited at any site within the respiratory tract. The typical size for these particles can range from submicron size to approximately 100 µm. Thoracic particulate matter TLVs® are designated for compounds that are toxic if deposited either within the airways of the lung or the gas-exchange region. The typical size for these particles can range from approximately 5 to 15 µm. Respirable particulate matter (RPM) TLVs® are designated for those compounds that are toxic if deposited within the gas-exchange region of the lung. The typical size for these particles is approximately 5 µm or less. It should also be noted that the term "nuisance dust" is no longer used because all dusts have biological effects at some dose. The term "particles (insoluble or poorly soluble) not otherwise specified" is now being used in place of "nuisance dusts." However, the TWA of 10 mg/m^3 for IPM is still used, whereas a value of 3 mg/m^3 for RPM is now recommended. Further discussion of the intended application of this classification is provided by ACGIH®.[16]

Notice of Intended Change (NIC). This term is unique to ACGIH®. Chemicals appearing on the NIC list for at least 1 year serve as notice that a chemical has a TLV® proposed for the first time or that a current TLV® is being changed. This procedure allows ample time for those with data or comments to come forth.

The TLV® booklet[16] should be consulted for a more complete discussion of these terms and several others that are not discussed here.

Groups that Recommend OELs

Many sources of OELs for chemicals are available to the practicing workplace health professional. It is a good idea to gather as many of the lists as possible to keep a compendium of OELs for quick reference. This section will briefly describe some of the groups that recommend OELs and provide an indication of whether they have the force of law in the United States. Of course, OELs recommended by groups outside the U.S. do not have the force of law here but provide guidance of a similar quality to that of groups based within the U.S.

One other point should be noted about OELs that do not have the force of law behind them. Although they are merely recommendations and are not legally binding, one would be well advised to have a very strong case regarding why those recommendations were not followed if litigation arose because the limits were routinely exceeded. It should be remembered that groups that promulgate OELs are considered to be learned bodies consisting of individuals from many different health-related professions, that come together to reach some level of consensus and recommend the OEL. They therefore carry much more weight in a litigation situation than one or two health professionals within a single company or agency.

Inhalation Exposure Limits

Table 4.1 summarizes several of the groups that recommend OELs. Additionally, several of the groups that recommend community-based limits that are not necessarily applicable to the occupational setting are discussed to alleviate confusion.

The original list of approximately 400 permissible exposure limits (PELs) adopted in 1970 under the OSH Act came from the 1968 list of TLV®s and the standards of the American National Standards Institute (ANSI).[9,11,20,21] However, since that time only about two dozen limits have been changed or adopted because the regulatory process of having these values made into law is very difficult and contentious. An attempt was made in 1989 to adopt 428 chemicals from the 1989 TLV® list as legally binding PELs, but legal proceedings by various groups ultimately resulted in the overturning of adopted values in 1992.

The recommended exposure limits (RELs) from the National Institute for Occupational Safety and Health (NIOSH) are published as criteria documents that could serve as the scientific basis for compounds that could then be evaluated by the Occupational Safety and Health Administration (OSHA) for setting PELs. However, because of the breakdown in the PEL process, these documents remain as recommended limits without the force of law. Nevertheless, they are

Table 4.1 — Summary of Various Inhalation Exposure Limits

Type of Limit	*Recommending Body*	*Legally Binding?*
Permissable exposure limit	Occupational Safety and Health Administration	Yes
Recommended exposure limit	National Institute for Occupational Safety and Health	No
Threshold limit value	ACGIH®	No
Workplace Environmental Exposure Level	AIHA®	No
New chemical exposure limit	Environmental Protection Agency (EPA)	Yes
Maximum allowable concentration (translated)	Deutsche Forschungsgemeinschaft (Commission for the Investigation of Health Hazards of Chemical Compounds in the Work Area) (Germany)	No
Occupational exposure limit	Health and Safety Commission & Health and Safety Executive (Britain)	No
Emergency Response Planning Guide	AIHA® (community-based standard, not an OEL)	No
Reference concentration	EPA (community-based standard, not an OEL)	Yes

comprehensive documents that provide a wide spectrum of use and toxicology information. The *Pocket Guide to Chemical Hazards* published by NIOSH is indispensable to anyone dealing with OELs or chemical exposures and provides a concise summary of such information as physicochemical properties, respirator selection, personal protective equipment, health hazards, and so forth for about 400 chemicals.[22] It should also be noted that NIOSH states that its RELs, given as TWAs, are appropriate for a 10-hour workday in the context of a 40-hour workweek.

ACGIH® is undoubtedly the first and foremost authority on OELs. Its publications include the TLV® booklet[16], the documentation of the TLV®s[23], and a compendium of exposure values from ACGIH®, OSHA, NIOSH, and the German maximum allowable concentrations (MAKs).[24] The TLV® committee started in 1941, adopted its first list of exposure limits in 1946, and has since developed TLV®s for approximately 650 chemicals and physical agents. Again, these ACGIH® publications are a must for anyone dealing with exposures to chemical or physical agents.

The AIHA® WEEL™ committee started in 1980 with the goal of providing OELs, on request of AIHA® members, for chemicals for which the ACGIH® TLV® committee was not considering setting TLVs®. There are currently approximately 110 WEELs, and AIHA® provides a summary list of the limits and a volume of documentation for them.[25]

Environmental Protection Agency (EPA) new chemical exposure limits (NCELs) are promulgated under Section 5 of the Toxic Substances Control Act. They are set by an individual company (or group of companies) entering into an agreement with EPA for chemicals to be produced for commerce under the Significant New Use Rules or Pre-Manufacturing Notification.[26] The author of this chapter is not aware of any published list of these values.

The German Commission for the Investigation of Health Hazards of Chemical Compounds in the Work Area, which develops the MAKs, is probably the best known foreign group recommending OELs. Their publication and thought process is similar to that of ACGIH, but some significant differences do exist. Some examples of differences are the designation of compounds causing chemical sensitization, presenting potential for embryo/fetal toxicity, or which are considered to be mutagens. Currently about 800 chemicals are reviewed in the handbook.[27] Again, this publication is a must for anyone dealing with chemical exposures both because of the number of compounds reviewed and the additional designations just described.

Great Britain has several hundred OELs, some approved by the Health and Safety Commission having the force of law and others that serve as recommendations made by Britain's Health and Safety Executive.[28] These OELs also carry designations such as the skin notation and sensitization potential.

AIHA®s Emergency Response Planning Guidelines are community-based values that are recommended in the event of a large chemical spill that may result in exposure of the general public.[29] Although they provide an excellent summary of the expected inhalation toxicity of compounds at various concentrations, they are not workplace recommendations and will not be discussed further here.

EPA Reference Concentrations (RfCs) are also community-based values that take into account the entire spectrum of the general population assumed to be exposed to the compound for 24 hours/day for a lifetime. The values can be found in the EPA's Integrated Risk Information System (IRIS) database, which can be obtained from EPA (http://www.cfpub.epa.gov/ncea/iris/index.cfm) or accessed online through NLM. Data for 189 chemicals listed on the priority air pollutant list will ultimately be reviewed. The RfCs are not workplace limits, so they will not be discussed further here.

One additional source of OELs is the manufacturers/formulators of chemicals. Larger chemical companies may have an internal group that sets OELs for the compounds manufactured or formulated in their plants. These internal OELs should appear on the company material safety data sheet. If a company purchases a chemical for formulation, the workplace health professional responsible for exposures to the chemical within the plant should contact the manufacturer and request information on the documentation of its internal OEL.

Biological Exposure Limits

ACGIH® has recommended biological exposure indices (BEIs) for nearly 50 chemicals or classes of chemicals.[16,23] A BEI® has been defined by ACGIH® as a level of a determinant (which is either the actual chemical, a metabolite, or a biochemical change produced by the chemical) that is likely to be observed in a specimen (such as blood, urine, or exhaled air) collected from a worker who was exposed to a chemical and who has similar levels of the determinant as if he or she had been exposed to the chemical at the TLV®. That is, because the BEI® takes into account exposures from all sources (inhalation, dermal, and oral), it is indexed to reflect the level of the determinant if a person were exposed only via inhalation. As with airborne OELs, the values are not exact numbers that dictate healthy versus unhealthy exposures or exposure levels. As with the TLVs®, the BEIs® are recommended for 8-hour days in the context of a 40-hour workweek.

BEI®s are the best technique available for determining the actual body burden of a chemical by all routes of exposure. This is particularly useful when skin exposures to a chemical are significant and when merely monitoring the airborne concentration of a chemical would not provide a reliable indicator of potential exposure. However, BEIs® require that metabolism and pharmacokinetic data from humans be established.

Other issues also impact the BEIs®. The collection of the specimen has much better acceptance if it is noninvasive (urine or breath) than if it is invasive (blood collection). The sources and routes of the exposure also are not known, because an endpoint of total exposure is being evaluated. For instance, inhibition of cholinesterase from an organophosphate could occur via air and skin during production at the workplace, via air and skin at home during application to lawns or gardens, and orally from water or food that have trace residues in them. The workplace health professional must then conduct an investigation to determine what the various sources of the exposure are and then make recommendations on how to limit the total exposure.

Physical Agent Exposure Limits

ACGIH® has recommendations for several physical agents listed in their TLV® booklet.[16] Additional information (and references) on several physical agents such as ionizing and nonionizing radiation, biological agents, heat stress, noise, electromagnetic fields, and so forth is also available.[7,9,11,30–32] Unlike many of the TLVs® for chemicals, the recommendations for physical agents are derived primarily from human data. Extensive epidemiological data for agents such as ionizing radiation have been gathered from large populations for some 40 years (i.e., atomic bomb survivors from World War II), whereas other data have been gathered due to more recent health concerns (e.g., microwave radiation).

Important Considerations in the Development of OELs

The purpose of this section is to help the reader gain an appreciation for the types of data evaluated in setting an OEL and to be aware of the issues surrounding the use of these data. With this awareness the reader should be more able to appraise the strengths and weaknesses of the data used to set an OEL. Again, it is not the intent of this section or this chapter to provide the reader the wherewithal to begin setting OELs. Additional references are also available that provide historical perspectives as well as information on the level setting process.[1,11,20,33–36]

Identification of the Hazard

Although hazard identification may at first seem to be apparent to the point of being overly simplistic, in practice it can be the source of significant consternation. It should be recognized that the type of toxicity hazard changes with the physical form of the chemical, which is in turn a function of the chemical process that it is involved in or its end use. For example, an isocyanate monomer in paint may produce a vapor hazard during production or high temperature curing; an aerosol inhalation hazard (spray process) or dermal hazard (brush-on) at room temperature; and during these various processes one must be cognizant that the toxicity of the prepolymer or polymer may be significantly different from that of the monomer. Another factor to consider is that the primary chemical of interest may present very different hazards when in different formulations. Every chemical mixture has its unique physical and chemical hazards due to such differences as solvents, stabilizers, surfactants, that result in differences in vapor pressures, impurities, reactivity, and so forth. Exacerbation (potentiation) of toxicity, masking of toxicity, or different manifestations of toxicity can occur for the same chemical of interest when put in different formulations. Again, constant monitoring and observation of exposed workers by the workplace health professional can help prevent problems of a serious nature.

Related to this is the situation in which two or more chemicals, each with proposed OELs, are present together in the exposure atmosphere. Again, the combination of the chemicals may have no untoward effect at all, the effect may be additive, there may be potentiation of the effect (an effect that is greater than additive), or in rare instances the presence of one chemical may actually decrease the toxic effects of another. However, there is a standard practice of adjusting the exposure limit based on whether the multiple chemicals are expected to have additive or independent effects. ACGIH provides detailed examples in the TLV® booklet[16], and examples of these calculations are provided in Appendix A.

Routes of Exposure

The primary route of exposure in an occupational setting is generally via inhalation, but this obviously depends on such factors as the production method, uses, physicochemical properties, and so on. Some chemicals primarily have their effect at the portal of entry (e.g., upper respiratory tract irritants) and may produce a spectrum of effects ranging from irritation to tumors. Other chemicals exert their toxic effects at a remote site from the portal of entry, that is, systemically. Examples of this include chemicals that produce neurotoxic effects, effects on the fetus, liver tumors, and so forth when the route of exposure is either via inhalation or the skin. Even when the apparent route is via inhalation, the skin may actually serve as the principal route of exposure. Compounds with the skin notation in the TLV® booklet[16] should be monitored carefully in the workplace as they have demonstrated the potential to be absorbed dermally in toxicologically significant amounts. Effects at the portal of entry include irritation and necrosis, whereas allergic responses are actually systemically mediated.

Review and Evaluation of the Chemical-Specific Toxicology Data

Data that are used in setting OELs for human workers are generally derived from laboratory animals. A discussion of toxicological principles and the use of animals for extrapolation to humans can be found later in this book as well as in other sources, ranging from basic treatment of the topics[1,4,20,37,38] to very detailed discussions.[2,7,8,39–42] Therefore, no lengthy discussion on this topic will ensue here, but the reader is reminded that not all effects in animals can be extrapolated to humans, and that experience and professional judgment are necessary to weigh the relative importance of these effects. The detailed methodology or protocol typically used for conducting these studies also will not be discussed here. However, the reader is referred to information found elsewhere in this book and also to several other sources for more complete details.[8,43–45]

Physicochemical Properties

Some important information can be gleaned just from the physicochemical data on the chemical. For instance, vapor pressure data provide information on the propensity for a chemical to volatilize and result in appreciable airborne concentrations. The expected saturated vapor concentration can be calculated, and an initial assessment of potential hazard via this route can be gained by comparing the value to inhalation toxicology data (e.g., a product with very high volatility and high toxicity via the inhalation route will likely present an inhalation hazard in open industrial processes). Octanol:water partition coefficients provide some insight as to the potential for the compound to accumulate in biological systems (e.g., a high coefficient means the compound has a propensity to accumulate in biological systems). Solubility data provide an indication of the potential to cross the dermal barrier. Odor information provides some indication of whether the chemical has potential warning properties.

Acute Toxicity and Irritation Data

Acute toxicity data primarily provide a relatively crude estimate of toxicity, with death as the principal endpoint, usually being assessed in an animal model after 14 days following a single dose of the chemical. Data are typically available for oral and dermal routes of exposure, with data via the inhalation route available somewhat less frequently. Acute toxicity data are often performed to meet regulatory requirements for classification of a chemical for labeling, transport, and commerce. The data serve as a rough comparison of the relative toxicity of chemicals to one another, and this may often be the only information available for low-production or new chemicals or chemical intermediates. Comparison of acute toxicity values for a single chemical by various routes also gives an indication of the relative absorption by those routes. Acute toxicity information, particularly the inhalation data, may also be useful in the assessment of whether a chemical should be considered for a ceiling or STEL. Listings of different toxicity classification schemes are presented in Appendix B, Tables 4.B1 through 4.B4.

Irritation studies are performed to determine the potential for a chemical to produce damage to the eye or skin from direct contact. They are typically performed in rabbits and involve material applied directly to the eye or skin, with measures employed to maintain contact, then a follow-up period of up to 21 days. These data are often used for hazard classification for handling and transport. They can also impact the decision on whether to set a ceiling or STEL for a chemical.

Sensitization Studies

These studies are used to determine whether a chemical has the potential to cause an allergic reaction, most often in the skin. There are several different protocols for doing these studies in guinea pigs, ranging from painting the chemical on the skin to mimic the workplace, to using subcutaneous injections as a stringent evaluation for any sensitizing potential. This information can be very important because sensitized individuals may not be protected by the OEL, and they may react at much lower concentrations of the chemical or biological agent. The reaction is not that considered consistent with the expected toxicity of the agent, but is instead consistent with a wide spectrum of agents that produce allergic reactions. The reaction can range from mild dermatitis to anaphylactic shock and death. Thus, the workplace health professional should be vigilant for allergic-type reactions in workers and immediately remove those individuals from exposure. If this is more than a very rare event, then the OEL and occupational hygiene practices must be closely scrutinized.

Metabolism and Pharmacokinetics

Metabolism and pharmacokinetic data provide information on the uptake, distribution, excretion, and biotransformation of a chemical. Information can be obtained on whether a chemical is rapidly metabolized and eliminated or whether it is bioaccumulated (i.e., whether 16 hours without exposure at work is enough time to eliminate the chemical from the body); whether the chemical produces toxic metabolites and what their possible relevance for humans might be; what the critical doses at target organs are; and what doses exceed the normal metabolic capability and thereby produce non-physiological responses. These studies are critical to understanding and interpreting many of the toxicology studies performed on a chemical. Unfortunately, although they often are performed to some degree for agricultural and pharmaceutical chemicals, these studies only rarely are performed for commodity or industrial chemicals. This is related to the technical difficulty and high cost of performing them.

Genotoxicity

These data are derived from a wide variety of studies using models as diverse as bacteria, mammalian cells, insects, and whole mammals. Many of the test systems have been modified to be very sensitive so that false negatives are minimized. However, the disadvantage to this approach is that it may lead to an increased number of false positives. Thus, evaluation of genotoxicity data requires experience and expertise to know which assays are designed to demonstrate any genotoxic potential by amplifying effects and circumventing normal uptake and metabolic processes. Often, a weight-of-the-evidence approach is used to evaluate the genotoxicity data as a whole, because there are bound to be a few equivocal or even positive findings when several of these studies have been performed. However, these data can have a substantial impact on the determination of the relevance of tumorigenic effects. These data may determine whether a threshold (or nongenotoxic) mechanism is assumed for a carcinogenic effect with the resultant use of a safety factor approach, or if a nonthreshold (genotoxic) mechanism is assumed and a more severe model is used for the risk assessment (see later section on Carcinogen Classification System and Risk Models for further explanation of these terms and this approach).

Reproductive/Developmental Toxicity

The severe and debilitating birth defects resulting from the administration of thalidomide to pregnant women served as the impetus for the routine evaluation of the teratogenic potential of chemicals. This was an example of a drug, taken voluntarily, that was therapeutic to the expectant mother but uniquely toxic to the fetus. With women of reproductive age now being commonly employed in the workplace, the impact of these studies is obvious. Developmental and reproductive toxicity studies are performed to evaluate the potential of agents to produce structural or functional deficits in the offspring during pregnancy and the postnatal period, until development is complete, as well as to evaluate the behavioral and functional aspects of parental animals and their offspring to successfully mate and reproduce.

Developmental Toxicity (teratology) studies are most commonly conducted in rats and rabbits and employ a forced oral administration of the chemical to the dam during the time when embryo/fetal toxicity is likely to produce a teratogenic effect (during the period of organogenesis). Endpoints for the dam include general growth and appearance and an assessment of successful maintenance of the pregnancy (without spontaneous abortions, early deliveries, and dead or resorbed fetuses). The fetuses are collected just before actual birth and evaluated for such endpoints as growth and the development and appearance of internal organs and bones. One aspect of these studies is the requirement that the highest dose administered be maternally toxic. This may produce some degree of toxicity to the fetus, often exhibited as decreased maturity of the skeleton (delayed ossification), extra or fused ribs, and so on. This effect should be factored into the evaluation of these studies and its impact on the OEL. However, many agents known or suspected to be human teratogens or developmental toxicants, producing either physical defects, growth retardation, or learning or behavioral deficits are readily encountered outside the workplace (radiation, therapeutic drugs, alcohol, cigarettes, viruses such as rubella and herpes, excesses of vitamin A or D, lead, etc.). Additionally, nearly 10% of all pregnancies are expected to result in some sort of birth defect. This makes the evaluation of workplace exposures and their contribution to normal pregnancy outcome an extremely difficult task.

Reproductive effects of chemicals are often evaluated in rats, with the exposure customarily being via the diet or water for two consecutive generations. The endpoints evaluated include the reproductive success of parental males and females, the care of the neonates, the viability and development of the offspring, their reproductive success, and the development of their offspring through weaning. Other endpoints include observations of growth and appearance and histological evaluations. Often concern is highest for the female for reproductive effects of agents, but it should be remembered that effects on the male are also well documented in the workplace setting (e.g., dibromochloropropane and male sterility).

Neurotoxicity

Although behavioral evaluations for neurotoxicity have been informally performed for some time[46], formalized guidelines only recently have been promulgated by EPA.[47] This study battery consists of evaluations for effects from acute (single dose) and subchronic (90-day) dosing as well as evaluations for developmental effects, with dams being dosed from gestation to 10 days after birth and pups evaluated through about 10 weeks of age. The evaluated endpoints include effects on growth, behavior, development, activity levels, and nervous system morphology. Considerations in the review of these studies are that the top dose must result in toxicity in all the studies, so some limited effects may be expected in the animals or offspring at the top dose. Although many chemicals have neurotoxic effects (e.g., narcosis due to solvents), these effects are ordinarily readily reversible. The objective of these studies is really to identify chemicals that produce irreversible effects on adults or offspring. True neurotoxic effects have been demonstrated for such chemicals as methanol and methyl isobutyl ketone. Lead serves as an example of a chemical that is still being feverishly evaluated for its potential to affect the learning and behavior of children following fetal exposure, and some researchers propose that there may be many chemicals, as yet unscreened, that also have this potential.

Subacute/Subchronic Toxicity

Subacute studies are defined here as studies with exposure lasting up to 2 weeks; subchronic studies as studies ordinarily lasting from about 15 days up to 6 months. These studies are generally 14, 28, or 90 days in duration and are conducted in mice, rats, or dogs. The endpoints of toxicity generally include survival, general health parameters (e.g., growth and clinical signs), extensive blood evaluations (hematological and biochemical), urinary evaluations, and the general appearance of internal organs coupled with fairly extensive microscopic evaluations. The objective of these studies is to provide information on target organs, reversibility of effects, potential for bioaccumulation, and so on. These studies very often serve as the longest-term studies available for a chemical, and as such they are often the critical study on which the OEL is based. Ninety days has been a common duration for subchronic studies for several decades, but because the state of the science has evolved greatly over this period there is a wide spectrum in the quality of these studies.

Chronic Toxicity and Oncogenicity

As a rule, the longest duration animal toxicology studies that are typically performed on chemicals are the chronic studies. These studies are almost always performed for agricultural chemicals, quite often for pharmaceuticals, and also for many of the high-volume industrial or commodity chemicals. They are much less frequently performed on the tens of thousands of industrial chemicals that have more limited distribution or lesser economic value. These studies may include a 1- or 2-year toxicity study with dogs, an 18- or 24-month oncogenicity study with mice, and/or a 24-month chronic toxicity and oncogenicity study with rats. The endpoints generally include survival, general health parameters (e.g., growth and clinical signs), extensive blood evaluations (hematological and biochemical), urinary evaluations, and extensive microscopic evaluations of internal organs. The objective of these studies is to determine if repeated exposures over long durations, approaching the complete lifetime for the rodents, produce cancer or other types of toxicity.

Although these studies are the best available information for assessing the toxic potential of lifetime exposures to chemicals, they are not without their limitations.(7,43,48,49) The reader should be aware of the various limitations and realize that they may have a very significant impact on the strength of the data set for the OEL. Some of the issues that affect these studies include the use of excessively high doses that may alter the normal metabolism, distribution, and excretion of the chemical; molecular mechanisms in the animal that do not directly extrapolate to humans, such as kidney tumors in male rodents from alpha-2u-globulin; liver tumors from peroxisomal proliferators; and differences in metabolism between animals and humans. Such considerations may warrant a smaller safety factor for the final OEL than what might otherwise be necessary.

Human Use and Experience

Although data from human use would be the most useful for setting an OEL, there is often a paucity of information and/or the quality of the information is not sufficient to be of practical use. Except for rare cases when adequate human data exist to factor heavily in setting an OEL for a chemical with systemic toxicity, data from humans are probably most often used for OELs based on avoidance of irritation. That is, in the course of normal use and production there is enough information to determine an irritation threshold, incorporate a safety factor, then determine whether more complaints arise.

Epidemiology data also serve as a source of human toxicity information. However, the number of well-controlled epidemiology studies useful for setting an OEL is surprisingly small. Many of the older studies, or even more recent reports for that matter, have poor control group data and too many confounding variables, because people in the workplace are rarely exposed to a single chemical and rarely have homogeneous personal habits. Additionally, there are often poor exposure concentration data to correlate with the human findings, and the myriad anecdotal reports shed little light on the topic. Somewhat related to this are the situations in which accidental exposures have occurred in the workplace or in the general public. Again, there are generally little or no reliable exposure concentration data and too many anecdotal reports; and when the exposure concentrations are available, they are typically so high that they are not useful for setting OELs.

References

References are often overlooked in the evaluation of the strength of the data that support an OEL. The references should be judged on such considerations as whether they appeared in refereed journals, the studies reported were performed at reputable labs, the work was amply described or performed to specific guidelines or regulations, and so forth.

Rationale

The rationale is ultimately the most important section of the OEL document because it brings together all the data; it is where the data are discussed and weighted for relative importance and the OEL is derived. Unfortunately, it is too often the only section of the document that gets read, if anything other than the actual value is scrutinized at all. This section should summarize the pertinent physicochemical properties of the compound (e.g., warning properties from odor, vapor pressure, potential for bioaccumulation); note the location of the effect (portal or systemic); show important toxicity endpoints or types of effects (e.g., odor or irritation versus teratogenic effect); determine the relevance of the routes of exposure, doses, and so forth used in the animal studies (e.g., whether all studies are via gavage doses, or at or above the maximum tolerated dose); determine the relevance of the effects observed in animals for humans (e.g., certain kidney tumors in male rats, whether genotoxic or nongenotoxic); differences in the susceptibility between animals and humans, and so on. Additionally, such factors as uses of the chemical and structural similarities to other chemicals may have a significant impact in the evaluation. Finally, experience and professional judgment are employed to weight all the information, apply an appropriate safety factor based on the strength of the available data, and recommend the OEL.

Carcinogen Classification Systems and Risk Assessment Models

Several different carcinogen classifications have been developed by organizations such as EPA, the International Agency for Research on Cancer, and ACGIH®.[48,50] However, for the discussion here the system used by ACGIH® for the TLVs®[16] is selected because it has an expanded classification system that uses all the available data and also considers the lack of data, in an attempt to account better for the weight of the evidence. The system used by ACGIH® can be summarized as follows.

A1: Confirmed Human Carcinogen. A chemical must have human data to support this classification. Examples include nickel subsulfide, bis(chloromethyl) ether, benzene, arsenic, and chromium VI compounds.

A2: Suspected Human Carcinogen. This designation requires relevant animal data in the face of conflicting or insufficient human data. Examples include diazomethane, chloromethyl methyl ether, and carbon tetrachloride.

A3: Confirmed Animal Carcinogen with Unknown Relevance to Humans. To have this designation a chemical must have caused cancer in animal studies by nonrelevant routes of exposure or mechanisms (e.g., kidney tumors produced in male rats from many hydrocarbons, para-dichlorobenzene, etc.; hormone-mediated thyroid tumors from compounds such as the ethylene bisdithiocarbamates {note: this class of chemicals is not listed in the TLVs}) or at excessive doses, and so on. Furthermore, human data are available that are in contradiction to the results in animals. Examples include nitrobenzene, crotonaldehyde, and gasoline.

A4: Not Classifiable as a Human Carcinogen. This classification is given to chemicals for which there are inadequate data to say whether it is a potential human carcinogen. It is typically applied to chemicals for which an issue of carcinogenicity has been raised but for which there are insufficient data to answer the question. Examples include pentachloronitrobenzene, phthalic anhydride, and acetone.

A5: Not Suspected as a Human Carcinogen. This classification is given to chemicals that have strong supporting data in humans to show that they are not carcinogens. Data from animals also can be used to support this classification.

Examples of chemicals receiving this designation are elemental nickel and caprolactam.

There are even more risk assessment models from which to choose than there are carcinogen classification systems. However, a few methods are more common than the others.[2,8,39,40,48,49,51–53] The most common approach for setting OELs has been the use of a safety factor (SF) of some multiple applied to the no-observable-effect level (NOEL) of interest. This approach involves determining the lowest NOEL or NOAEL (no-observable-adverse-effect level) in the most sensitive species (or if the data allow, in the most appropriate species), strain, and sex from a critical study or set of studies. From this NOEL a safety factor (often ranging from 10 to 1000) is divided into the NOEL to determine the OEL for workers. This additional SF is applied to obtain greater confidence and further assurance that the health of the worker will be protected. The actual SF depends on many considerations, but the type of toxic effect and the duration of the longest study often have the most impact. This SF approach is also used for air, food, and water contaminants.

Another method currently being assessed for use by several regulatory agencies, most notably EPA, is the so-called benchmark dose approach. This approach fits a curve to all the available data from a given study type (e.g., subchronic studies in rats). A benchmark dose is the dose that is calculated from the curve to affect some predetermined percentage of animals, ordinarily from 1 to 10% of the animals (effective dose ED_1 or ED_{10}). The lower-bound confidence value for that benchmark dose will then have the SFs applied to it to estimate the acceptable exposure level. This method has the advantage of using all the data and fitting a curve to it instead of using just a single NOEL value to select the acceptable exposure level. This method has gained increasing acceptance in regulatory use and will likely become more commonly used for OELs.

An approach used for some carcinogens that are assumed not to have a threshold (i.e., a genotoxic chemical for which only zero exposure results in zero risk) a model called the linearized multistage is employed. Because zero exposure is often not achievable, a level of acceptable risk must be decided on. For the general public a risk of 1×10^{-6}, or 1 in 1,000,000, is considered acceptable by EPA. For workers, OSHA appears to have used a range of 10^{-3} to 10^{-4} as acceptable.[17] When evaluating these risk assessment calculations from the linearized multistage approach, it should be remembered that, assuming that it is the appropriate calculation to use (i.e., the chemical is a potent genotoxin that is relevant for humans), there are multiple conservative assumptions built into the model. It has been estimated that, at least in some instances, the linearized multistage model may overstate the actual risk by up to several orders of magnitude.[54–58] However, new approaches that use all the available mechanistic and dose-response data should greatly enhance the cancer risk assessment process in the future.[59–61]

Other Issues Impacting OELs

Setting workplace OELs is not an exact science. It requires knowledge, experience, and professional judgment. There is plenty of room for honest disagreement. However, knowing that workplace exposures are not likely to approach zero in the foreseeable future, it represents the best mechanism currently available to protect worker health and safety.

OELs are not values that are etched in stone. Always staying below the value does not guarantee good health for all workers, and going above the limit does not mean that workers will necessarily suffer toxic effects. There is sufficient biological variability in the work force, sufficient analytical variability in the instrumentation used for the collection and analysis of samples, sufficient lack of reliable data, and sufficient uncertainty on the part of those making the recommendations to state with confidence that the values will not always be 100%

correct. Thus, it is always incumbent on the practicing workplace health professional to observe the work force carefully and not just blindly rely on values that have been proposed by various groups of professionals.

It quite often happens that new toxicology data become available for chemicals over the course of many years after the OEL is recommended. It may be that none of the data are that significant alone and therefore may not warrant immediate attention. However, the total of available new data may have an impact on an OEL and require adjustment of the value. Although all OEL-setting groups will reevaluate an agent if significant new data arise, it is sometimes difficult to tell exactly when that point occurs. It is obvious when some data grab headlines, encourage sudden extensive publications, or prompt symposia. It is less obvious in other situations. Therefore, it would be desirable for all the OELs to be updated on some routine basis, with complete new literature searches and documentation prepared. Although this is the procedure followed by the AIHA® WEEL committee (review required every 10 years) with only about 100 OELs, it is obvious that it would be a daunting task for ACGIH® or the MAK commission with more than 600 chemicals. Thus, the important point is that some OELs may be quite old, and only by reviewing the documentation for the OEL can one gain an appreciation for its age, the strength of the data supporting it, and the approach used to set a safety factor and ultimately the OEL. All of these factors may change over time and could have a significant impact on an OEL that would be recommended according to present-day practice.

In theory, making recommendations for OELs is a scientific process that uses the best available toxicology and human experience data. However, the reality is that these decisions are not made in a scientific vacuum, and social, economic and political influences are present to varying degrees, sometimes intentionally and sometimes not. Several papers have called into question the independence of the TLVs and the review process. The authors have proposed that the use of unpublished corporate data and the undue influence by industry on the level-setting process have resulted in TLVs that are not protective for workers.[62,63] For more than 55 years ACGIH has been promulgating OELs, now called TLVs®. The TLVs® traditionally have ranked as some of the best OEL data available, but with the limitation that truly informed decisions cannot be made with very limited or outdated data sets. This problem would only have been exacerbated if there had been no contact with industry, the owner of the majority of toxicology data. Allegations of political influence notwithstanding, there is always an inherent unfairness in applying current-day standards to procedures that were novel and cutting edge for their time. Paustenback[64] presents a more comprehensive discussion of these issues surrounding the TLVs®.

The original approach was likely framed by the question of whether it was better to make OEL recommendations with limited data to provide some guidance for worker protection or to make no recommendation at all. We have reframed this issue by our current willingness to apply large safety factors.

There are currently approximately 75,000 chemicals on the Toxic Substances Control Act inventory[65], and the number grows every year. There are only a few thousand OELs at most to help guide the practicing workplace health professional. Thus, the question arises as to how to approach some sort of level setting for new chemicals or existing chemicals without much available toxicity data. Some companies or groups have proposed using systems in which the amount and quality of the toxicity data can have very drastic effects on the OEL. Although there can be many variations, the system works roughly as follows. A chemical that is being prepared for commercial production must have a base set of data such as the acute toxicity and irritation battery and some genotoxicity tests. The safety factor used in setting the provisional OEL would be extremely high, resulting in an extremely low OEL. When the chemical begins commercial production, certain types of toxicology studies are required based on the production volume of the chemical. As production volume increases and more revenue is generated and more people become involved in production, more toxicology data must be generated. Additionally, as more toxicity data become available and confidence increases in the provisional OEL (and the safety factor should typically decrease with the result that the OEL becomes higher), then the engineering controls and personal protective equipment requirements should become less onerous and cumbersome. Thus, in this system there is linkage between the production volume, the amount of available toxicology data, and the safety factors applied in setting the OEL. This approach is now being used in Europe and on a voluntary basis in the United States, whereby certain toxicology data sets are required based on the production volume of the chemical.

A similar system being used by several pharmaceutical companies is the performance based exposure control limit. Data on toxicity, structure-activity relationships, and so forth are used to assign chemicals to various health hazard categories that have defined engineering control strategies. A seminal paper on this approach was published by Nauman et al.[66] Also, the United Kingdom has presented its approach in detail. Specific toxicology phrases accepted by the European Union[67] are used in conjunction with the potential for the chemical to become airborne to recommend a control strategy for maintaining inhalation exposures at safe levels.[68] A complete discussion of the U.K. approach can be found in a special issue of the *Annals of Occupational Hygiene*.[69]

New approaches for fostering the generation of toxicology data and establishing default controls for limiting airborne exposure to chemicals have become more popular during the last 15 years. This trend will likely become even more prevalent in the future. Worker protection can only be enhanced by programs that use more stringent exposure controls as defaults and then offer the possibility of reduced controls as base sets of toxicology data required for proper hazard evaluations and recommendations of OELs become available.

Summary

The makeup of the workplace has changed substantially over the last several decades. Women proved during the war years that they were every bit as capable as their male counterparts in the workplace environment of heavy industry. Their numbers have increased over the years in all workplace settings. Furthermore, approaching the workplace as simply consisting of production plants is also no longer possible. Office environments contained within sealed buildings have added a new dimension to the role of the workplace health professional. Additionally, laws mandating equal access for the physically infirmed or disabled have substantially changed the makeup of the work force. Thus, the idea that the work force is made up entirely of healthy adult men is no longer valid in many scenarios. These changes have raised many questions regarding the appropriateness of current OELs in protecting all workers. It is obvious that issues regarding reproduction and effects on the fetus and the newborn have become a primary concern in the workplace. Moreover, issues regarding the indoor environment of office buildings and the broader spectrum of the health status of this work force have spawned numerous groups concerned with indoor air quality. Now and in the future, all these issues will have to be dealt with by groups recommending OELs, as well as the workplace health professionals responsible for the health of the work force in these environments.

Additional Resources

Online Databases

The National Library of Medicine has an extensive system of computerized databases and data banks. It can be accessed at http://www.nlm.nih.gov. The NLM includes Medline bibliographic listings at www.nlm.nih.gov/databases/databases_medline.html. It also includes several other databases that may be of special interest: TOXNET (http://toxnet.nlm.nih.gov) is comprised of several databases including HSDB® (Hazardous Substances Data Bank); IRIS (Integrated Risk Information System); GENE-TOX (Genetic Toxicology); CCRIS (Chemical Carcinogenesis Research Information System); DART® (Development and Reproductive Toxicology); TRI (Toxic Chemical Release Inventory); ChemIDplus® (Chemical Identification); Genetox (Genetic Toxicology), TOXLINE® (Toxicology Information Online) and ITER (International Toxicity Estimates for Risk). For more information contact NLM, 8600 Rockville Pike, Bethesda, MD 20894 (phone: 888-346-3656.)

Other useful sites include NCI's CANCER-LIT® (http://www.cancer.gov/search/cancer_literature), the RTECS® database of the Canadian Centre for Occupational Health and Safety (http://www.ccohs.ca/products/rtecs), MSDS-Search National Repository (http://www.msdssearch.com/msdssearch.htm), Vermont Safety Information Resources (http://hazard.com), and the HazDat Database of ATSDR (http://www.atsdr.cdc.gov/hazdat.html). The NIOSH site of the Centers for Disease Control and Protection has the Pocket Guide to Chemical Hazards (NPG) in a downloadable format at http://www.cdc.gov/niosh/npg/. This is an indispensable guide for the practicing industrial hygienist.

A discussion of the OEL process in many countries around the world is available at http://osha.europa.eu/en/good_practice/topics/dangerous_substances/oel/members.stm/#uk.

References

1. **Schaper, M.M.:** "General Toxicology." Paper presented at the 11th Annual AIHA Toxicology Symposium, San Antonio, TX, 1996.
2. **Klaassen, C.D.:** "Mid-America Toxicology Course." University of Kansas Medical Center, Kansas City, KS, 1997.
3. **West, J.B.:** *Respiratory Physiology—The Essentials*, 2nd ed. Baltimore, MD: Williams & Wilkins, 1979.
4. **Loomis, T.A.:** *Essentials of Toxicology*, 3rd ed. Philadelphia: Lea & Febiger, 1978.
5. **Casarett, L.J., and J. Doull:** *Toxicology—The Basic Science of Poisons.* New York: Macmillan, 1975.
6. **Hayes, A.W.:** *Principles and Methods of Toxicology.* New York: Raven Press, 1982.
7. **Klaassen, C.D.:** *Casarett & Doull's Toxicology—The Basic Science of Poisons*, 5th ed. New York: McGraw-Hill, 1996.
8. **Hayes, A.W.:** *Principles and Methods of Toxicology*, 3rd ed. New York: Raven Press, 1994.
9. **Clayton, G.D., and F.E. Clayton:** *Patty's Industrial Hygiene and Toxicology*, vol. 1, 4th ed. New York: John Wiley & Sons, 1991.
10. **National Institute for Occupational Safety and Health:** *The Industrial Environment—Its Evaluation and Control.* Washington, D.C.: U.S. Government Printing Office, 1973.
11. **Plog, B.A.:** *Fundamentals of Industrial Hygiene*, 3rd ed. Chicago: National Safety Council, 1988.
12. **American Industrial Hygiene Association (AIHA):** *Odor Thresholds for Chemicals with Established Occupational Health Standards.* Fairfax, VA: AIHA, 1993.
13. **Amoore, J.E., and E. Hautala:** Odor as an aid to chemical safety: Odor thresholds compared with threshold limit values and volatilities for 214 industrial chemicals in air and water dilution. *J. Appl. Toxicol. 3*:272-290 (1983).
14. **Miller, J.:** "Workshop on Setting Exposure Limits." Course presented at the 9th Annual AIHA Toxicology Symposium, Baltimore, MD, 1994.
15. Occupational Safety and Health Act of 1970, Pub. L. 91-596, 91st Congress December 29, 1970.
16. **American Conference of Governmental Industrial Hygienists (ACGIH):** *2008 TLVs® and BEIs®—Threshold Limit Values for Chemical Substances and Physical Agents—Biological Exposure Indices.* Cincinnati, Ohio: ACGIH, 2008.
17. **Paustenbach, D.J.:** Pharmacokinetics, and unusual work schedules. In R.L. Harris, editor, *Patty's Industrial Hygiene*, vol. 3, 5th ed. (pp. 1787-1901). New York: John Wiley & Sons, Inc., 2000.
18. **American Industrial Hygiene Association (AIHA):** *Emergency Response Planning Guidelines and Workplace Environmental Exposure Levels Handbook.* Fairfax, VA: AIHA, 2007.
19. **Accrocco, J.O.:** *The MSDS Pocket Dictionary.* Schenectady, NY: Genium Publishing, 1988.
20. **Hathaway, G.J., N.H. Proctor, J.P. Hughes, and M.L. Fischman:** *Proctor and Hughes' Chemical Hazards of the Workplace*, 3rd ed. New York: Van Nostrand Reinhold, 1991.
21. **Mackison, F.W., R.S. Stricoff, and L.J. Partridge, Jr.:** *Occupational Health Guidelines for Chemical Hazards* (DHHS [NIOSH] pub. 81-123). Cincinnati, OH: National Institute for Occupational Safety and Health, 1981.
22. **National Institute for Occupational Safety and Health (NIOSH):** *NIOSH Pocket Guide to Chemical Hazards.* Available at http://www.cdc.gov/niosh/npg/npg.html (November 24, 2002).
23. **American Conference of Governmental Industrial Hygienists (ACGIH):** *Documentation of the Threshold Limit Values Biological Exposure Indices*, 7th ed. Cincinnati, OH: ACGIH, 2001.
24. **American Conference of Governmental Industrial Hygienists (ACGIH):** *2008 Guide to Occupational Exposure Values.* Cincinnati, Ohio: ACGIH, 2008.
25. **Workplace Environmental Exposure Level Committee:** *2007 Workplace Environmental Exposure Level (WEEL) Complete Set.* Fairfax, VA: American Industrial Hygiene Association, 2007.
26. **Abel, M.T., S. Ahir, M.C. Fehrenbacher, R.S. Holmes, J.B. Moran, and M.A. Puskar:** "EPA's New Chemical Exposure Limits Program." Paper presented at the American Industrial Hygiene Conference and Exposition, Kansas City, MO, 1995.

27. Deutsche Forschungsgemeinschaft (DFG) (ed.) **MAK- und BAT-Werte-Liste 2008** Maximale Arbeitsplatzkonzentrationen und Biologische Arbeitsstofftoleranzwerte. Mitteilung 44 MAK-Werte-Liste (DFG) (Volume 44). Available in the United States from Wiley-VCH online at http://www.wiley-vch.de/publish/en/books/bySubjectCH00/bySubSubjectCH37/3-527-32303-1/?sID=pnfvoajvp09f1e6q76fv56ljh1
28. **Health and Safety Executive:** EH40/2005 Workplace Exposure Limits: Containing the List of Workplace Exposure Limits for use with the Control of Substances Hazardous to Health Regulations 2002 (as amended) Environmental Hygiene Guidance Note EH40 HSE Books 2005 ISBN 0 7176 2977 5. HSE Books, PO Box 1999, Sudbury, Suffolk, CO10 2WA. Or available at www.hsebooks.co.uk
29. **Emergency Response Planning Committee:** *2007 Emergency Response Planning Guidelines (ERPG) Complete Set.* Fairfax, VA: American Industrial Hygiene Association, 2007.
30. **Harris, R.L. (ed.):** *Patty's Industrial Hygiene,* vol. 2, 5th ed. New York: John Wiley & Sons, 2000.
31. **Goldberg, R.B.:** "Electromagnetic Fields (EMFs): Bioeffects and Potential Health Concerns." Paper presented at the 11th Annual AIHA Toxicology Symposium, San Antonio, TX, 1996.
32. **International Agency for Research on Cancer (IARC):** *Solar and Ultraviolet Radiation* (IARC Monographs on the Evaluation of Carcinogenic Risks to Humans, vol. 55). Lyon, France: IARC, 1992.
33. **Klonne, D.R.:** "Occupational Exposure Limits-the Practical Implementation of Toxicology in the Workplace." Paper presented at the 8th Annual AIHA Toxicology Symposium, Asheville, NC, 1993.
34. **Klonne, D.R.:** "Inhalation Exposure Assessment and the Role of Occupational Exposure Limits." Paper presented at the 10th Annual AIHA Toxicology Symposium, Boston, MA, 1995.
35. **Doull, D., G.L. Kennedy, Jr., L.K. Loury, R.S. Ratney, D.H. Sliney, and W.D. Wagner:** "Threshold Limit Values (TLVs): How, Why, and Current Issues." Course presented at the American Industrial Hygiene Conference and Exposition, New Orleans, LA, 1993.
36. **Workplace Environmental Exposure Level Committee:** "Establishing, Interpreting and Applying Occupational Exposure Limits: Current Practices and Future Directions." Course presented at the American Industrial Hygiene Conference and Exposition, Dallas, TX, 1997.
37. **Kamrin, M.K.:** *Toxicology—A Primer on Toxicology Principles and Applications.* Chelsea, MI: Lewis Publishers, 1988.
38. **Ottoboni, M.A.:** *The Dose Makes the Poison — A Plain Language Guide to Toxicology.* Berkeley, CA: Vincente Books, 1984.
39. **Cralley, L.J., L.V. Cralley, and J.S. Bus:** *Patty's Industrial Hygiene and Toxicology,* vol. 3, part B, 3rd ed. New York: John Wiley & Sons, 1995.
40. **Calabrese, E.J.:** *Principles of Animal Extrapolation.* New York: John Wiley & Sons, 1983.
41. **Hardman, J.G., L.E. Limbird, P.B. Molinoff, et al.:** *Goodman & Gilman's The Pharmacological Basis of Therapeutics,* 9th ed. New York: McGraw-Hill, 1996
42. **Homburger, F.:** *Safety Evaluation and Regulation of Chemicals 2—Impact of Regulations—Improvment of Methods.* Basel, Switzerland: Karger, 1985.
43. **Environmental Protection Agency (EPA):** *Pesticide Assessment Guidelines,* rev. ed., by B. Jaeger (TS-769C). Washington, DC: EPA, 1984.
44. **Environmental Protection Agency (EPA):** *New and Revised Health Effects Test Guidelines* (TS-792). Washington, D.C.: EPA, 1983.
45. **Organization for Economic Cooperation and Development (OECD):** *OECD Guidelines for Testing of Chemicals.* Paris, France: OECD, 1981.
46. **Irwin, S.:** Comprehensive observational assessment: Ia. A systematic quantitative procedure for assessing the behavioral and physiologic state of the mouse. *Psychopharmacologia 13*:222-257 (1968).
47. **Environmental Protection Agency (EPA):** *Pesticide Assessment Guidelines* (Neurotoxicity series 81, 82, and 83). Washington, D.C.: EPA, 1991.
48. **Clayton, G.D., and F.E. Clayton:** *Patty's Industrial Hygiene and Toxicology,* vol. 2, part A, 4th ed. New York: John Wiley & Sons, 1993.
49. **National Research Council:** *Issues in Risk Assessment.* Washington, D.C.: National Academy Press, 1993.
50. **International Agency for Research on Cancer (IARC):** *IARC Monographs on the Evaluation of Carcinogenic Risks to Humans. Supplement 7—Overall Evaluations of Carcinogenicity: An Updating of IARC Monographs, Volumes 1 to 42.* Lyon, France: IARC, 1987.
51. **Baker, S.:** "Fundamentals of Risk Assessment." Paper presented at the 9th Annual AIHA Toxicology Symposium, Baltimore, MD, 1994.
52. **Cohen, S.M.:** "Chemical Carcinogenesis: Implications for Dose and Species Extrapolation." Paper presented at the 11th Annual AIHA Toxicology Symposium, San Antonio, TX, 1996.

53. **Keller, J.G.:** "Risk Assessment for Industrial Hygienists." Paper presented at the 11th Annual AIHA Toxicology Symposium, San Antonio, TX, 1996.
54. **Hoel, D.G., and Portier, C.J.:** Nonlinearity of dose-response functions for carcinogenicity. *Environ. Health Perspect. 102(suppl.)*:109-113 (1994).
55. **Sielken, R.L., Jr., and D.E. Stevenson:** Another flaw in the linearized multistage model upper bounds on human cancer potency. *Reg. Toxicol. Pharmacol. 19*:106-114 (1994).
56. **Andersen, M.E., and K. Krishnan:** Physiologically based pharmacokinetics and cancer risk assessment. *Environ. Health Perspect. 102(suppl.)*:103-108 (1994).
57. **Lovell, D.P., and G. Thomas:** Quantitative risk assessment and the limitations of the linearized multistage model. *Human Exp. Toxicol. 15*:87-104 (1996).
58. **Crump, K.S.:** The linearized multistage model and the future of quantitative risk assessment. *Human Exp. Toxicol. 15*:787-798 (1996).
59. **Butterworth, B.E., R.B. Conolly, and K.T. Morgan:** A strategy for establishing mode of action of chemical carcinogens as a guide for approaches to risk assessments. *Cancer Lett. 93*:129-146 (1995).
60. **Wiltse, J.A., and V.L. Dellarco:** U.S. Environmental Protection Agency's revised guidelines for carcinogen risk assessment: Evaluating a postulated mode of carcinogenic action in guiding dose-response extrapolation. *Mutat. Res. 464*:105-115 (2000).
61. **Andersen, M.E., M.E. Meek, G.A. Boorman, et al.:** Lessons learned in applying the U.S. EPA proposed cancer guidelines to specific compounds. *Toxicol. Sci. 53*:159-172 (2000).
62. **Castleman, B.I., and G.E. Ziem:** Corporate influence on threshold limit values. *Am. J. Ind. Med. 13*:531-559 (1988).
63. **Roach, S.A., and S.M. Rappaport:** But they are not thresholds: A critical analysis of the documentation of threshold limit values. *Am. J. Ind. Med. 17*:727-753 (1990).
64. **Paustenbach, D.J.:** The history and biological basis of occupational exposure limits for chemical agents. In R.L. Harris, editor, *Patty's Industrial Hygiene*, vol. 3, 5th ed. (pp. 1903-2000). New York: John Wiley & Sons, 2000.
65. **Environmental Protection Agency (EPA):** What is the TSCA Chemical Substance Inventory? Retrieved from http://www.epa.gov/opptintr/newchems/pubs/invntory.htm (November 23, 2008).
66. **Naumann, B.D., E.V. Sargent, B.S. Starkman, et al.:** Performance-based exposure control limits for pharmaceutical active ingredients. *Am. Ind. Hyg. Assoc. J. 57*:33-42 (1996).
67. **Brooke, I.M.:** A UK scheme to help small firms control health risks from chemicals: Toxicological considerations. *Ann. Occup. Hyg. 42*:377-390 (1998).
68. **Maidment, S.C.:** Occupational hygiene considerations in the development of a structured approach to select chemical control strategies. *Ann. Occup. Hyg. 42*:391-400 (1998).
69. **British Occupational Hygiene Society (GOHS):** *Annals Occ. Hyg. 42(6)*:355-422 (1998).
70. **Brief, R.S., and R.A. Scala:** Occupational exposure limits for novel work schedules. *Am. Ind. Hyg. Assoc. J. 36*:467-469 (1975).

Appendix A

Calculations for OELs

This appendix contains calculations often required for assessing contaminant levels in workplace atmospheres. The first equation converts parts per million to milligrams per cubic meter for vapors.[16,C6]

Changing Parts Per Million to Milligrams per Cubic Meter of Air

$$\text{OEL}\left[\frac{\text{mg}}{\text{m}^3}\right] = \frac{\text{OEL (ppm)} \times \text{MW (grams)}}{24.45}$$

or

Changing Milligrams Per Cubic Meter to Parts Per Million

$$\text{OEL (ppm)} = \frac{\text{OEL}\left[\frac{\text{mg}}{\text{m}^3}\right] \times 24.45}{\text{MW (grams)}}$$

Example 1. If the measurement of the vapor phase of toluene is 25 ppm, what is the measurement in milligrams per cubic meter? Assume 25 ppm of toluene and that 92 g/mole is the gram molecular weight (MW) of toluene.

$$\text{OEL}\left[\frac{\text{mg}}{\text{m}^3}\right] = \frac{\text{OEL (ppm)} \times \text{MW (grams)}}{24.45}$$

$$= \frac{25 \text{ ppm} \times 92}{24.45}$$

$$= 94 \frac{\text{mg}}{\text{m}^3}$$

Approaches for Multiple Agents in the Workplace

Systems are often very dynamic in the work environment. Sometimes exposure to more than one agent is possible. Different approaches are used to evaluate the following situations: additive effects, for agents with similar toxicological effects; independent effects, for agents with different toxicological effects; and a mixed atmosphere assumed to be similar to a liquid mixture. The reader is referred to reference 16 for further discussion.

Additive Effects

If it is reasonable to conclude that the chemicals present in the workplace could add, one on the other, to the total effect, then it is also reasonable to consider adding the exposure assessments to derive a total exposure assessment. An example would be the presence of three chemicals, X, Y, and Z, each having a similar toxicological effect on the same target organ, the liver. The total value (TV) is determined based on the concentration (C) and the threshold limit value (TLV) of each of the chemicals using the following equation:

$$\text{TV} = \frac{C_1}{\text{TLV}_1} + \frac{C_2}{\text{TLV}_2} + \cdots + \frac{C_n}{\text{TLV}_n}$$

Example 2. Assume 25 ppm of toluene with a TLV of 50 ppm; 25 ppm of mixed xylenes with a TLV of 100 ppm; and 75 ppm, of ethylbenzene with a TLV of 100 ppm. Substituting into the equation, it becomes

$$\text{TV} = \frac{C_1}{\text{TLV}_1} + \frac{C_2}{\text{TLV}_2} + \cdots + \frac{C_n}{\text{TLV}_n}$$

$$= \frac{25 \text{ ppm}}{50 \text{ ppm}} + \frac{25 \text{ ppm}}{100 \text{ ppm}} + \frac{75 \text{ ppm}}{100 \text{ ppm}}$$

$$= 0.50 + 0.25 + 0.75$$

$$= 1.50$$

The generally used standard for the total value is 1.00. It could be judged from this evaluation that the exposure may have an additive impact above acceptable limits, and the exposure should be reduced.

Independent Effects

Workplace atmospheric mixtures also may be comprised of agents with different toxicological effects and target organs. That is, the effects are not considered to be additive. In this situation the exposure assessment is simpler but still uses the acceptable total value of 1.0.

$$TV_1 = \frac{C_1}{TLV_1}$$

$$TV_2 = \frac{C_2}{TLV_2}$$

$$TV_n = \frac{C_n}{TLV_n}$$

Example 3. Assume 25 ppm of toluene with a TLV of 50 ppm and 0.1 mg/m³ of cotton dust with a TLV of 0.2 mg/m³. Substituting into the equation, it becomes

$$TV_{toluene} = \frac{25\ \text{ppm}}{100\ \text{ppm}}$$

$$= 0.25$$

$$TV_{cotton\ dust} = \frac{0.1\ \frac{mg}{m^3}}{0.2\ \frac{mg}{m^3}}$$

$$= 0.50$$

It could be judged from this evaluation that the exposures may not have exceeded acceptable limits.

Synthetic Limit for Mixtures

Another approach to the issue of mixtures is to create a synthetic OEL. This is done for mixtures of liquids when the relative percentage of the components is known, and when it can be assumed that all the components evaporate so that the atmospheric vapor concentration is similar in relative composition to the liquid. The synthetic OEL is calculated using the decimal fraction (f) of each of the mixture components and the TLV of each component.

$$OEL = \frac{1}{\frac{f_1}{TLV_1} + \frac{f_2}{TLV_2} + \cdots + \frac{f_n}{TLV_n}}$$

Example 4. Assume 25% component by weight of toluene with TLV of 188 mg/m³, 25% component by weight of mixed xylenes with a TLV of 434 mg/m³, and 50% component by weight of ethylbenzene with a TLV of 434 mg/m³. Substituting into the equation, it becomes

$$OEL = \frac{1}{\frac{f_1}{TLV_1} + \frac{f_2}{TLV_2} + \frac{f_3}{TLV_3}}$$

$$= \frac{1}{\frac{0.25}{188} + \frac{0.25}{434} + \frac{0.5}{434}}$$

$$= \frac{1}{0.001330 + 0.00058 + 0.00115}$$

$$= \frac{1}{0.00306}$$

$$= 327\ \frac{mg}{m^3}$$

Each component contributes the following amount to the overall occupational exposure limit of 327 mg/m³:

Toluene:	0.25 × 327 mg/m³ = 82 mg/m³ or 21.8 ppm
Xylenes:	0.25 × 327 mg/m³ = 82 mg/m³ or 18.9 ppm
Ethylbenzene:	0.50 × 327 mg/m³ = 164 mg/m³ or 37.8 ppm

The total of these contributions results in a synthetic OEL of 78.5 ppm for the mixture.

Modifying OELs for Unusual Work Shifts

OELs usually are set for an 8 hour/day, 5 day/week, 40-hour workweek. Changes in the hours per day or hours per week worked may warrant a modification of the OEL to maintain the same body burden on which the OEL was predicated. An extensive review of different models is available,[17] and examples of modifications using the models of Brief and Scala[17,70] and OSHA[17] are provided here. Both models incorporate the number of hours worked per day (h) into the modification of the OEL. The reader should become familiar with the myriad details contained in these references before making modifications to the OEL.

Brief and Scala model:

$$\text{OEL Reduction Factor (RF)} = \frac{8}{h} \times \frac{24 - h}{16}$$

$$\text{Modified OEL} = \text{OEL RF} \times \text{OEL}$$

OSHA model:

$$\text{Modified OEL} = \text{OEL} \times \frac{8}{h}$$

Example 5. Compound Z is an acute systemic toxicant with a moderate half-life (OSHA Category 4 chemical; an acutely toxic chemical, see reference 17) with a WEEL=100 mg/m³.

Group 1 workers are working 10 hour/day, 4 days/week, for a 40-hour workweek:

Using the Brief and Scala model:

$$\text{OEL Reduction Factor (RF)} = \frac{8}{10} \times \frac{24 - 10}{16}$$

$$= 0.70$$

$$\text{Modified OEL} = 0.70 \times 100 \frac{mg}{m^3}$$

$$= 70 \frac{mg}{m^3}$$

Using the OSHA model:

$$\text{Modified OEL} = 100 \times \frac{8}{10}$$

$$= 80 \frac{mg}{m^3}$$

Group 2 workers are working 10 hour/day, 7 days/week, for a 70-hour workweek followed by 2 weeks without exposure. For this example both models are adjusted to modify the OEL based on working more than 40 hours per week. H represents the number of hours worked per week.

Using the Brief and Scala model:

$$\text{OEL Reduction Factor (RF)} = \frac{40}{H} \times \frac{168 - H}{128}$$

$$= \frac{40}{70} \times \frac{168 - 70}{128}$$

$$= 0.44$$

$$\text{Modified OEL} = 0.44 \times 100 \frac{mg}{m^3}$$

$$= 44 \frac{mg}{m^3}$$

Using the OSHA model:

$$\text{Modified OEL} = \text{OEL} \times \frac{40}{H}$$

$$= 100 \times \frac{40}{70}$$

$$= 57 \frac{mg}{m^3}$$

Appendix B

Toxicity Classification Schemes

There are many different toxicity classification schemes available throughout the world. Even within the United States there are several different schemes for the various regulatory agencies that deal with shipping and handling of various classes of chemicals. Toxicity classification schemes are inexact, at best, at categorizing the acute toxicity and primary irritation of chemicals because of the different protocols used, the number of dose groups used, animal variability, vehicles for dosing, and so forth. However, they do provide at least some indication of comparative acute toxicity and/or irritation and provide some useful information to those unfamiliar with the toxicity of the chemicals that they handle as part of their job.

Provided here are four classification schemes, some of which are used by regulatory agencies. They at least provide some indication of the relative differences in the approaches used, and they are schemes that will likely be encountered by workplace health professionals.

Table 4.B1— Combined Tabulation of Toxicity Classes

Toxicity Rating	*Common Term*	*LD_{50} Single Oral Dose (Rats)*	*Vapor Exposure Mortality*[A]	*LD_{50} Skin (Rabbits)*	*Probable Lethal Dose for Humans*
1	extremely toxic	1 mg or less/kg	<10 ppm	5 mg or less/kg	a taste, 1 grain
2	highly toxic	1–50 mg	10–100	5–43 mg/kg	1 teaspoon, 4 cc
3	moderately toxic	50–500 mg	100–1000	44–340 mg/kg	1 ounce, 30 g
4	slightly toxic	0.5–5 g	1000–10,000	0.35–2.81 g/kg	1 pint, 250 g
5	practically nontoxic	5–15 g	10,000–100,000	2.82–22.59 g/kg	1 quart
6	relatively harmless	15 g and more	>100,000	22.6 or more g/kg	>1 quart

Source: H.C. Hodge and J.H. Sterner, "Tabulation of toxicity classes." *Am. Ind. Hyg. Assoc. Q. 10*:93 (1949).
[A]Inhalation 4 hours, 2/6-4/6 rats

Table 4.B2— Warnings and Precautionary Statements—EPA (FIFRA)

Hazard Indicators	*Toxicity Categories* I	II	III	IV
Oral LD_{50}	up to and including 50 mg/kg	from 50–500 mg/kg	from 500–5000 mg/kg	>5000 mg/kg
Inhalation LC_{50}	up to and including 0.2 mg/L	from 0.2–2 mg/L	from 2–20 mg/L	>20 mg/L
Dermal LD_{50}	up to and including 200 mg/kg	from 200-2000 mg/kg	from 2000–20,000 mg/kg	>20,000 mg/kg
Eye effects	corrosive; corneal opacity not reversible within 7 days	corneal opacity reversible within 7 days; irritation persisting for 7 days	no corneal opacity; irritation reversible within 7 days	no irritation
Skin effects	corrosive	severe irritation at 72 hours	moderate irritation at 72 hours	mild or slight irritation at 72 hours

Source: *Code of Federal Regulations* Title 40, Part 162.10 (h)

Table 4.B3— OSHA Health Hazard Definitions

Acute oral LD_{50}	highly toxic; $LD_{50} \le 50$ mg/kg	toxic; 50 mg/kg < $LD_{50} \le 500$ mg/kg
Acute dermal LD_{50}	highly toxic; $LD_{50} \le 200$ mg/kg; 24 hrs	toxic; 200 mg/kg < $LD_{50} \le 1000$ mg/kg
Inhalation LC_{50}	highly toxic; $LC_{50} \le 200$ ppm $LC_{50} \le 2$ mg/L; 1 hr	toxic; 200 ppm; < $LC_{50} \le 2000$ ppm 2 mg/L ≤ LC_{50} < 20 mg/L
Carcinogen	If IARC "carcinogen"; or if National Toxicology Program "carcinogen" or "potential carcinogen"; or OSHA regulated carcinogen	
Corrosive	visible destruction of, or irreversible alterations in living tissue by contact; 4 hrs	
Irritant	not corrosive; reversible inflammatory effect on living tissue by contact; 4 hrs; skin score: 5	
Sensitizer	substantial portion of exposed people or animals develop allergic reaction	

Source: *Code of Federal Regulations* Title 29, 1910.1200. Appendix A

Table 4.B4— Acute Toxicity Rating Criteria

Acute Toxicity Rating	*Oral[A] Liquids, Solids*	*Dermal Liquids, Solids*	*Inhalation Gases, Vapors (ppm) Dusts, Fumes, Mists (mg/L)*	*Skin Irritation Liquids, Solids*	*Eye Irritation Liquids, Solids*
	LD_{50} RAT (mg/kg)	LD_{50} Rabbit (mg/kg)	LC_{50} Rat 1-hr Exposure	4-hr Exposure[B]	
4	0–1	0–20	0–0.2 mg/L	not applicable	not applicable
3	>1–50	>20–200	>0.2–2 mg/L >20–200 ppm	severely irritating and/or corrosive	corrosive; irreversible corneal opacity
2	>50–500	>200–1000	>2–20 mg/L 200–2000 ppm	primary irritant sensitizer	irritating or moderately persisting > 7 days with reversible corneal opacity
1	>500–5000	>1000–5000	>20–200 mg/L >200–2,000 ppm	slightly irritating	slightly irritating but reversible within 7 days
0	>5000	>5000	>200 mg/L >10,000 ppm	essentially nonirritating	essentially nonirritating

[A]The oral route of exposure is highly unlikely in a workplace setting. If situations are encountered in which the oral LD_{50} value would indicate a significantly different rating, toxicity values for the other routes of entry may be considered more appropriate when assigning the rating.
[B]Note animal species and duration of exposure if different from that recommended.

Source: National Paint & Coatings Association (Hazardous Materials Identification System® HMIS®; Label Master); Washington, DC

Outcome Competencies

After completing this chapter, the reader should be able to:

1. Define underlined terms used in this chapter.
2. Apply the fundamentals of chemistry and biology to the specialized discipline of toxicology as related to occupational health.
3. Classify toxic materials based on physical states and potential adverse interactions or effects (toxic responses).
4. Describe the concepts of dose-response and time-response and the factors that influence the potential for toxic responses to occur.
5. Summarize the fate of toxic substances that contact and/or enter the body as a result of occupational exposures (toxicokinetics).
6. Describe the potential mechanisms of adverse effects of toxic substances that contact and/or enter the body as a result of occupational exposures (toxicodynamics).
7. Understand the basic structure and function of the following target organ systems as they relate to the most common toxic substance exposures in the workplace: respiratory, dermal, cardiovascular, renal, nervous, hepatic, reproductive, blood, immune; as well as carcinogenesis.
8. Discuss the application of toxicological data to establish occupational exposure limits.
9. Discuss the risk assessment paradigm.
10. Discuss emerging issues in occupational toxicology, that include nanotechnology, toxicogenetics, industrial accident response planning, and non-traditional occupational exposures.

Key Terms

ADME • axonopathies • BEIs • BBB • carcinogenesis • CNS • demyelination • dermatoxicants • dermis • glomerulus • hepatotoxicants • hematoxicants • nephrotoxicants • neuropathy • neurotoxicants • PNS • pulmonotoxicants • REACH • risk assessment • SKIN notation • TLV® •target organs

*Note to readers: There are additional key terms underlined within the chapter.

Prerequisite Knowledge

Prior to beginning this chapter, the reader should review the following chapters:

Chapter Number	Chapter Topic
4	Occupational Exposure Limits
6	Occupational Epidemiology
8	Occupational and Environmental Health Risk Assessment/Risk Management
10	Modeling Inhalation Exposure
19	Biological Monitoring
20	The Skin and the Work Environment
44	Emergency Planning and Crisis Management in the Workplace

Key Topics

I. Introduction
   A. History of Toxicology
   B. Types of Toxicology
   C. Routes of exposure
   D. Absorption, Distribution, Metabolism, Excretion (ADME)
   E. Toxicity
   F. Dose Response
II. Target Organ Toxicology
   A. Inhalation Toxicants
   B. Dermal Toxicants
   C. Cardiovascular Toxicants
   D. Nephrotoxicants
   E. Neurotoxicants
   F. Hepatotoxicants
   G. Reproductive Toxicants
   H. Hematotoxicants
   I. Immunotoxicants
   J. Carcinogenesis
III. Exposure Level Setting
   A. Exposure Standard Organizations
   B. Threshold Limit Values (TLVs)
   C. Workplace Environmental Exposure Levels (WEELs
   D. Environmental Protection Agency (EPA)
IV. Emerging Issues
   A. Nanotechnology
   B. Toxicogenomics
   C. Industrial Accident Response Planning (terrorism, natural disaster, continuity of operations)
   D. Non-traditional Occupational Exposures
V. Occupational Human Health Risk Assessment
VI. Environmental Risk Assessment
VII. Sources of Toxicological Data
VIII. References

Occupational Toxicology

5

Kenneth R. Still, PhD, CIH, CSP, CHMM; Warren W. Jederberg, MS, CIH and William E. Luttrell, PhD, CIH

Introduction

The mantra for industrial hygienists to "anticipate, recognize, evaluate and control"[1,2] potential exposures to harmful materials, requires them to apply the principles, methodologies and data from many disciplines within the biological, physical and social sciences. Among the chief disciplines that contribute to the information used to address the full-spectrum of potential impacts on worker health is the discipline of toxicology. Indeed, a brief review of the history of toxicology and industrial hygiene/ occupational health reveals that they developed together and are intertwined. It could be said that their futures will continue to be interdependent as many of the incentives for new directions in toxicology research are spawned as a consequence of the addition of new materials and methods in commerce and the workplace. Today, it is widely recognized that exposures outside of the workplace can have a profound impact on worker health and susceptibility to further adverse outcomes. Contaminants in foods, chemicals used in hobbies, and environmental contaminants are only some of the current public health concerns involving chemicals.

Toxicology dates to early mankind who used natural products from animals and plants to sustain their existence. These natural products remain in existence today, from animal venoms to plant compounds. The timeline for toxicology can be traced back to 3000 BC, for these early uses and by 1500 BC, there is evidence that hemlock, opium, arrow poisons and certain metals were frequently used to poison enemies or for state executions. This timeline can be broken down into a series of eras beginning with antiquity (3000 BC–90 AD), followed by the Middle Ages (476 AD–1453), the Renaissance Period (14th–16th centuries), the Age of Reason (17th –18th centuries) and the Age of Modern Toxicology (19th century to modern day).[3,4] The science of toxicology has changed dramatically since the discipline was formally described by Philippus Aureolus Theophrastus Bombastus von Hohnenheim-Paracelsus (1493–1541). Paracelsus conceived of a key principle of the science of toxicology: "all substances are poisons; there is none which is not a poison. The right dose differentiates a poison from a remedy."[4–6] Whether this axiom is applied in basic acute lethality studies, or is extended to the applied science of chemical risk assessment, Paracelsus' maxim forms the bulwark for all aspects of toxicology. A Renaissance man, Paracelsus formulated other views that remain an integral component of modern toxicology. He promoted the idea that experimentation is essential in understanding the effects of exposure to chemicals and emphasized the distinction between therapeutic and toxic properties of chemicals. An in-depth historical account of the entire evolution of toxicology can be found in *Casarett and Doull's Toxicology*.[4]

The popular definition of toxicology is "the study of poisons." However, the modern scientific definition is much more descriptive: toxicology is the study of adverse effects of agents on living organisms and a toxicologist studies the nature of those effects and the probability of their occurrence. The study of toxicology falls into

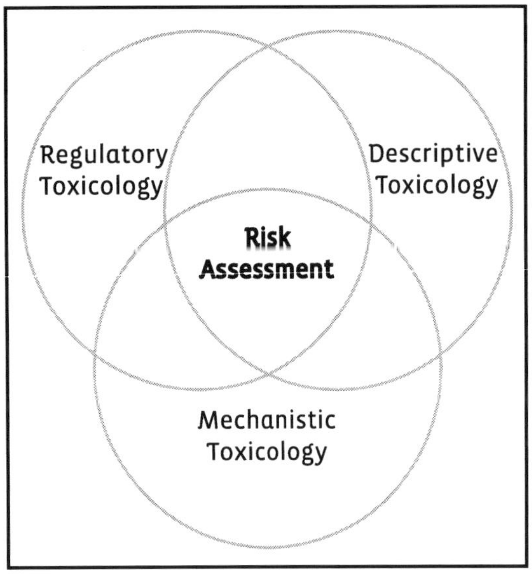

Figure 5.1 — Venn diagram showing relationship between the three primary categories of toxicology and risk assessment. (Modified from *Casarett and Doull's Toxicology*, 7th edition, Reprinted with permission).

primarily three categories: mechanistic, descriptive and regulatory[7]. The overlap of these three areas provides the basis for risk assessment as shown in Figure 5.1.

Mechanistic toxicology concerns itself with the identification and characterization of cellular, biochemical, and molecular mechanisms that are utilized by chemicals to exert toxic effects on living organisms. Descriptive toxicology addresses primarily toxicity testing, while regulatory toxicology addresses those areas for decision making that become law or impinge on the safety of humans via the environment or both consumable and non-consumable products. These three primary categories can be further broken down into sub-categories based upon specialty. For example, environmental toxicology (addresses chemical impact on biological systems in the environment); ecotoxicology (a specialized area of environmental toxicology that addresses the impact of chemicals on the ecosystem, particularly on population dynamics); forensic toxicology (addresses the medical and legal aspects of chemical impact on living organisms); clinical toxicology (specifically addresses the outcomes of chemical impacts on organisms); occupational toxicology; industrial toxicology; reproductive toxicology, developmental toxicology and military toxicology (also known as deployment toxicology) are additional examples.[7-10]

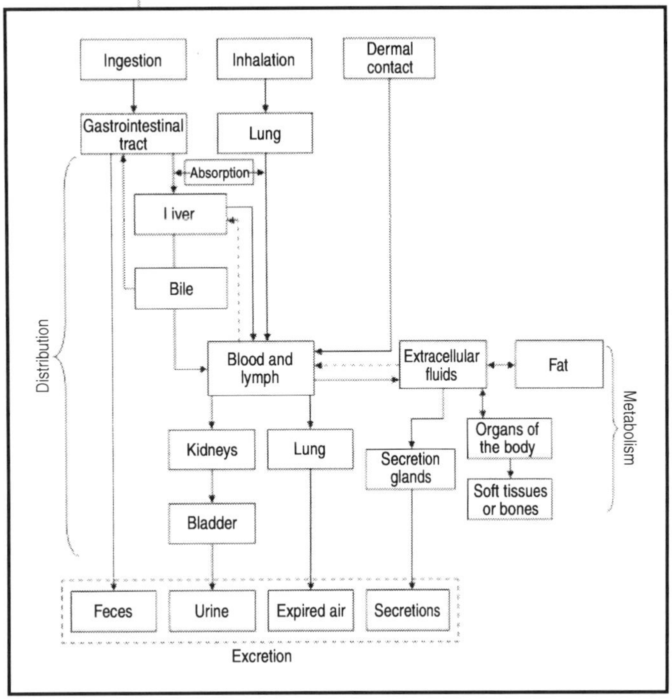

Figure 5.2 — Routes and modes of entry. (Source: C.D. Klaassen, *Cassarett and Doull's Toxicology*, 6th edition (New York: McGraw-Hill, 2001); reprinted with permission).

Exposure to chemicals is of major concern. The route and site of exposure as well as the duration and frequency of the exposure must be elicited. The major routes of entry include pulmonary, dermal, and gastrointestinal systems. Additional routes of entry include: injection [i.e., intraperitoneal (i.p.), intravenous (i.v.), intramuscular (i.m.), subcutaneous] and other parenteral avenues. As a result of exposure to a chemical, the absorption, distribution, metabolism and excretion (ADME) process is begun (Figure 5.2).

Toxicants are classified by target organ interaction. The more common interactions include:

- *Hepatotoxicants* – cause damage to the liver (e.g. Acetaminophen, Ethyl Alcohol)
- *Nephrotoxicants* – damage to kidneys (e.g. Cadmium, Mercury)
- *Neurotoxicants* – damage to the nervous system (e.g. Lead, Mercury)
- *Immunotoxicants* – damage to the immune system (e.g. Toluene)
- *Hematoxicants* – damage to the circulatory system (e.g. Benzene)
- *Dermatoxicants* – damage to the skin (e.g. Magnesium Chromate)

- *Pulmonotoxicants* – damage to the lungs (e.g. Asbestos)
- *Carcinogens* – agents that increase cancer risk (e.g. Hexavalent Chromium)

The "toxicity" of a material is its inherent ability to cause damage to living organisms or tissues. The "hazard" of a material takes into account the probability of biologic organisms being exposed to the toxic material. Terms such as "highly toxic," "moderately toxic," and "nontoxic" are of little value to the worker unless used in relation to common experience. Table 5.1 presents a common scheme for classification of materials as related to their oral toxicity in humans where the lethal dose (LD_{50}) is the concentration of the test material at which 50% of the exposed organisms died.[11] Caution must be exercised in the interpretation of data such as those presented in Table 5.1. Although a compound may be "highly toxic," it may not present a significant hazard, if the probability of exposure is very low. In contrast, material of low toxicity may present a significant hazard under the proper exposure conditions. For example, a small amount of water in the lung can cause severe problems.

Some examples of materials in these toxicity categories are shown in Table 5.2.

Toxicity information provided on the Material Safety Data Sheet (MSDS), or other sources, must include the test species and conditions under which the data were collected to be relevant for the toxicologist and industrial hygienist. For example, using the Department of Defense's (DoD's) Hazardous Materials Information System (HMIS)[12–14], the definition of "Highly Toxic" is:

(1) A chemical that has a median lethal dose (LD_{50}) of 50 milligrams or less per kilogram of body weight when administered orally to albino rats weighing between 200 and 300 grams.
(2) A chemical that has a median lethal dose (LD_{50}) of 200 milligrams or less per kilogram of body weight when administered by continuous contact for 24 hours (or less, if death occurs within 24 hours) with the bare skin of albino rabbits weighing between 2 and 3 kilograms each.
(3) A chemical that has a median lethal concentration (LC_{50}) of gas or vapor in air of 200 parts per million (ppm) or less by volume, or 2 milligrams per liter or less of mist, fume, or dust, when administered by continuous inhalation for 1 hour (or less, if death occurs within

Table 5.1 — Relative Ranking of Toxic Materials Based on Oral Toxicity in Humans[11,modified]

Toxicity Class	*Lethal Dose for a 70 kg person*	*Relative amount for Average Adults*
Practically non-toxic	>15,000 mg/kg	More than 1 quart
Slightly Toxic	5,000–15,000 mg/kg	Between 1 pint and 1 quart
Moderately toxic	500–5,000 mg/kg	Between 1 ounce and 1 pint
Highly toxic	50–500 mg/kg	Between 1 teaspoon and 1 ounce
Extremely toxic	5–50 mg/kg	Between 7 drops and 1 teaspoon
Supertoxic	<5 mg/kg	Less than 7 drops

Table 5.2 — Some Representative Chemical Agents with Various Toxicities. (Modified from *Casarett and Doull*, 7th Ed. Reprinted with permission.)

Agent	*LD_{50} (mg/kg in Test Animals)*	*Toxicity Rating*
Ethyl alcohol	10,000	Slightly Toxic
Sodium chloride (Table Salt)	4,000	Moderately Toxic
Ferrous sulfate (Iron Tablets)	1,500	Moderately Toxic
Morphine sulfate	900	Moderately Toxic
Phenobarbital sodium	150	Highly Toxic
Picrotoxin	5	Extremely Toxic
Strychnine sulfate	2	Supertoxic
Nicotine	1	Supertoxic
Tetrodotoxin	0.1	Supertoxic
Dioxin	0.001	Supertoxic
Botulinum	0.00001	Supertoxic

1 hour) to albino rats weighing between 200 and 300 grams each, provided such concentration or condition, or both, are likely to be encountered by man when the chemical is used in any reasonably foreseeable manner.

(4) A chemical that is a liquid having a saturated vapor concentration (ppm) at 68.5°F (20.5°C) equal to or greater than ten times its LC_{50} (ppm), if the LC_{50} value is 1000 ppm or less when administered by continuous inhalation for 1 hour to albino rats weighing between 200 and 300 grams each, provided such concentration, or condition, or both, are likely to be encountered by man when the chemical is used in any reasonably foreseeable manner.

Definitions 1–3 are also used by OSHA (29 CFR 1910.1200, appendix A) to define a "toxic chemical."

Other terms which are used in common sources relate to the cancer causing potential of a material. ACGIH® provides definitions of terms in its publication entitled *Threshold Limit Values® (TLVs®)* and *Biological Exposure Indices (BEIs®)*.[15] Other organizations that also evaluate carcinogenicity are discussed later in this chapter. A chemical is listed as a "Confirmed Human Carcinogen" when there is "weight of evidence from epidemiologic studies of, or convincing clinical evidence in, exposed humans". The designation of "Suspected Human Carcinogen" is applied when "the agent is carcinogenic in experimental animals at dose levels, by route(s) of administration, at site(s), of histologic type(s), or by mechanism(s) that are considered relevant to worker exposure and available epidemiologic studies are conflicting or insufficient to confirm an increased risk of cancer in exposed humans." The term "Animal Carcinogen" is applied when animal studies at high doses resulted in cancers; available epidemiologic data do not reveal increased cancers among exposed individuals; and available evidence suggests that cancer probably will not occur in humans except under "uncommon or unlikely routes of exposure." "Not Classifiable as a Human Carcinogen" means that for a particular agent, there is insufficient data to adequately address the issue. "Not Suspected as a Human Carcinogen" means that based on adequate epidemiologic studies, there is no evidence that the material will cause cancer in humans. It must be remembered that for substances where no data have been collected, there are no designations. The AIHA® Emergency Response Planning Committee (ERPG) and the Workplace Environmental Exposure Levels (WEEL) Committee also use comparable terminology.[16]

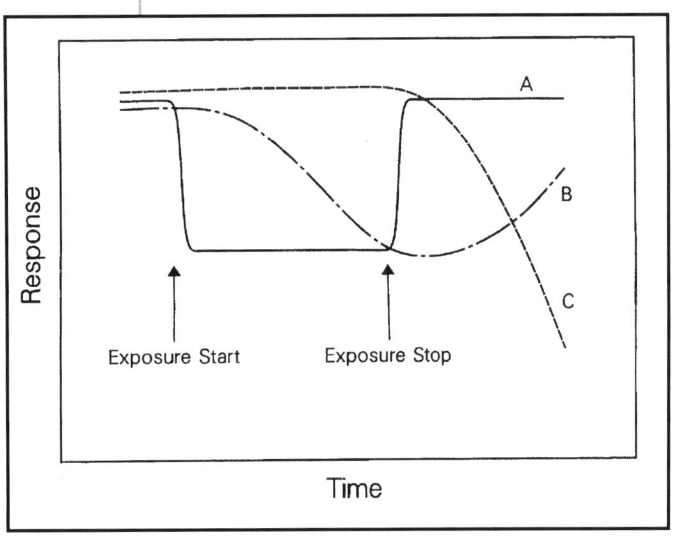

Figure 5.3 — The dose-response relationship (Source: C.D. Klaassen, *Cassarett and Doull's Toxicology*, 6th edition. (New York: McGraw-Hill, 2001); reprinted with permission.

Uses of Toxicology Principles

One of the most fundamental principles of toxicology is the dose-response curve. This curve or relationship displays the fact that a high dose of a xenobiotic has a greater effect than a low dose. The magnitude of the exposure can be expressed as dose, concentration, duration of exposure, or some other expression of exposure, and it is depicted along the x axis. The magnitude of the effect can be expressed as response, number of animals with a certain outcome, or some other expression of effect, and it is depicted along the y axis as a cumulative percent response.

Most dose-response curves are sigmoid shape (Figure 5.4). In the first part of the curve, the flat portion, an increase in dose produces no effect. This is the subthreshold phase. The lowest dose that produces an observable or measurable effect is the threshold. Beyond the threshold point, the curve rises steeply and enters a linear phase where the increase in response is proportional to the increase in dose. The slope of this linear phase should be of great interest to the industrial hygienist, because if the slope is high, it is an indication that there is a sudden increase in response with a small increase in exposure. In the last part of the curve, the curve flattens out showing a maximal response. At this point, all the exposed individuals or all the susceptible individuals have shown the effect.[11] Figure 5.4 demonstrates the LD_{50} determination using the dose response curve.

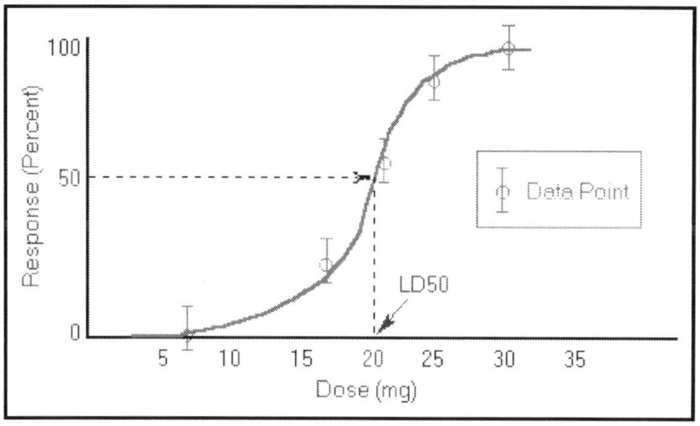

Figure 5.4 — Dose response curve for LD_{50} determination. (Source: Toxicology Tutor, National Library of Medicine)

Another fundamental principle of toxicology involves exposure considerations. The amount of a substance needed to cause an adverse effect varies widely among different materials. For example, botulism toxin can cause death in humans with just a few micrograms being ingested, whereas many other chemicals are essentially harmless following doses that are received in grams. The intrinsic toxicity of a substance is important, but it is the associated degree of risk caused by the exposure circumstances that can be critical in determining if workers become over exposed. A very toxic chemical when carefully handled is less hazardous than a relatively nontoxic substance that is improperly handled. A key element in assessing the degree of risk for any chemical is the exposure that can potentially occur. Toxic effects of a chemical are produced only if the chemical or its metabolites reach the appropriate receptors in the body at a concentration and for a length of time sufficient to cause the toxic effects. Exposure considerations such as route of administration, the dose, and the duration and frequency of exposure all will determine if toxic effects actually occur.[12] Exposure circumstances need further study when any of the following conditions exist: (1) uptake routes include both the lung and skin; (2) acute toxicity data from animal studies show extreme toxicity due to very low LD_{50} values; (3) chronic toxicity data shows lethality, carcinogenicity, or embryotoxicity; (4) warning properties of the substance, such as odor or irritation threshold, are at levels substantially higher than typical exposure levels; (5) the substance is a gas, respirable aerosol, or a highly volatile liquid; (6) very large quantities are used over periods of time; (7) there is a large number of workers potentially exposed to the substance (>125); or if any of the following conditions exist: open process, manually operated, frequent intervention in the process during service or maintenance, regular leaks and spills, absence of ventilation or inadequate ventilation.[8] The principles of toxicology are needed to assess the significance of a toxic effect. When does a toxic effect become significant? When does a pathophysiologic change indicate a disease process? Body defense mechanisms, such as mucociliary clearance and inflammation, normally occur in response to environmental stresses. A disease is likely to occur if the body defense mechanisms become overwhelmed by the environmental stressors. However, some changes that occur in response to chemical exposures do not cause diseases. In these cases, the significance is not completely known. For example, is hyperplasia or hypertrophy considered a normal physiologic adaptation to a stress or should it be considered a pathologic process? Often a worker can be exposed to a toxin and show no sign of illness. Does normal biologic adaptation cause an unacceptable effect on the body? Is there a limit to which the body can compensate for toxic effects? Looking at it from another point of view, is there a certain amount of stress that is beneficial to the body? In other words, can a low-level exposure to a substance ever cause a beneficial effect? Hormesis is an area of study that reports beneficial effects of low-level exposures to a substance, while higher exposures cause disease. Currently, there are no clear cut answers to these questions.[11]

Types of Toxicological Tests

Toxicology testing has always been important in determining potential toxicity of a chemical. However, because of the Toxic

Substances Control Act (TSCA), the Environmental Protection Agency may require data on mutagenic, carcinogenic, teratogenic, synergistic, or behavioral effects by using epidemiologic, in vitro, or laboratory animal methods whenever an unreasonable risk to health or environment may exist and there is not sufficient data to determine the risk. The principles of toxicology have contributed to several fundamental assumptions that underlie all toxicity testing. First, the effects observed in laboratory animals are often the same effects observed in humans. Second, the degree of adverse effect increases as the dose or exposure increases. As a general principle, if the absorption, distribution, metabolism, and excretion of a material are similar in humans and a particular animal species, test results in that species are generally predictive of toxicity of the material in humans. However, since there are usually important differences in these characteristics, toxicology studies must be carefully interpreted.[12]

Target Organ Toxicology

A chemical exposure may cause a local or systemic effect. A local effect occurs at the site of exposure to the chemical. For example, an acid spill on the skin can cause reddening at the site of contact. Systemic effects occur at locations other than at the site of exposure. For example, the majority of occupational exposures occur through inhalation, but many of the effects are seen at sites other than in the lung. In this section of the chapter, we are going to focus primarily upon chemical exposures that will result in systemic effects, but we will also mention local effects especially after exposure of the skin and respiratory tract. Not only will we look at inhalation and dermal toxicants, but also toxicants that have their target organ of toxicity in other parts of the body, such as cardiovascular, renal, nervous, hepatic, reproductive, blood, and immunity type tissues. Systemic effects can also include carcinogenesis.

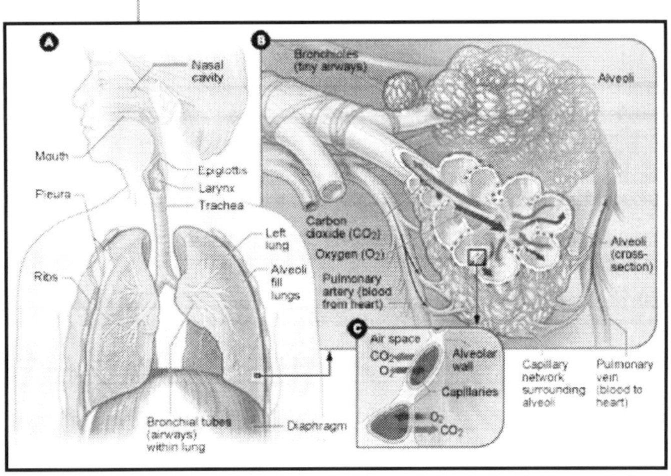

Figure 5.5 — The Respiratory System—A shows the location of the structures of the respiratory system in the body. B is an enlarged view of the airways, alveoli, and capillaries. C shows the location of the capillaries and alveoli undergoing gas exchange. (Source: National Institutes of Health, accessed from http://www.nhlbi.nih.gov/health/dci/images/lung_anatomy.jpg).

Inhalation Toxicants

Structure and Function of the Respiratory System

The major components of the respiratory system include the nasal cavity, pharynx, larynx, trachea, primary bronchi, bronchioles, and alveoli or air sacs. The nose has coarse hairs that help remove larger particulates as air enters the respiratory tract. Figure 5.5A shows the location of the respiratory system structures in the body. Ciliated epithelial cells and mucous cells are found throughout the respiratory tract except in alveoli. The thick, sticky, mucous layer that is on the surface of the respiratory tract is produced by the mucous cells. This mucus layer traps the particulates within the inhaled air. Cilia like structures move the mucous with trapped particulates from the respiratory tract toward the throat where it is swallowed.[17]

The functional unit of the respiratory system is the alveolus, which is depicted in Figure 5.5B. It is composed of a single layer of cells surrounded by a network of capillaries. The close association of these cells allows the passage of materials, such as oxygen and carbon dioxide, between the bloodstream and the lung. Oxygen is supplied to the bloodstream and gases produced by cellular metabolism, such as carbon dioxide, are removed. The gases are transported between the bloodstream and the lung by passive diffusion. This occurs due to the concentration gradient for each gas between the blood and air. It is also through the alveolus that toxic materials can be absorbed into the blood. Particulates can accumulate in the alveolus.

As described above, the exchange of oxygen and carbon dioxide between the bloodstream and the lungs is the primary function of the respiratory system. Figure 5.5C shows the location of gas exchange between the capillaries and the alveoli. The respiratory system also performs other functions as well, including defense mechanisms and metabolism of toxic substances.

There are specific and nonspecific defense mechanisms that the respiratory system uses to protect itself from inhaled substances and microorganisms. Nonspecific mechanisms are primarily responsible for removing particulates by the action of cilia, hairs, mucus-secreting cells. These actions result in the trapping of substances, especially particulates, before they reach the alveoli. Smoking decreases the ciliary activity, which can result in particulates staying in the lungs longer, potentially having a more intense toxic effect locally and systemically. Particulates 5–30 micrometers in diameter are trapped in the nasopharyngeal region. Particles 1–5 micrometers are trapped primarily in the region between the trachea and the bronchioles. Many particles 1 micrometer or less in diameter reach the alveolus. Once in the alveolus many of these particles are engulfed and destroyed by macrophages by phagocytosis. The macrophages are then carried to the upper regions of the respiratory tract by the mucociliary escalator to the nasopharyngeal region to be swallowed or expectorated. Particles are also phagocytized by neutrophils. In addition to phagocytosis, macrophages also present the foreign substances to lymphocytes. This can result in the initiation of the immune response and the production of specific antibodies. Some lymphocytes become natural killer cells which can interact directly with the xenobiotic and destroy it.

Several enzymes that are responsible for metabolizing drugs are found in the respiratory system. They are similar to those found in the liver and they will either detoxify or activate various toxic substances. These enzymes occur throughout the respiratory tract.

Examples of Inhalation Toxicants

Irritants. Primary irritants have an effect on the respiratory tract by direct contact, resulting in mechanical or chemical reaction. Secondary irritants cause systemic effects. An example of a primary irritant is ammonia, which is a highly water soluble compound. High exposure results in nasal and throat irritation because of the chemical reaction taking place at the epithelium. An example of a secondary irritant is hydrogen sulfide gas. Not only does it have respiratory effects, but it is toxic to the nervous system. It can cause unconsciousness, known as "knockdown," in those acutely exposed to high concentrations.[18] Irritants can also be classified as sensory or pulmonary irritants.[19] Sensory irritants cause a response in the nose, and result in burning and painful sensations, nasal inflammation and hypersecretion, and vasodilation and obstruction. Pulmonary irritants stimulate receptors in the pulmonary conducting airways and alveoli, and result in inflammation, bronchoconstriction, edema, cough, and mucous hypersecretion, as well as rapid shallow breathing. Some materials, such as isocyanates and machining fluid mixtures can cause both sensory and pulmonary irritant type responses.[20] Irritants are commonly found in the workplace and include bleaching agents, ammonia, sulfuric and hydrochloric acids, isocyanates, volatile organic compounds, and oxides of nitrogen and sulfur. Due to its water solubility, ozone is easily captured in the mucosa of the nasopharynx and in the acinar region at the junction of the conducting airways and the alveoli, causing an inflammatory response in exposed workers that results in cough, shortness of breath, dry throat, and wheezing.[21] Removing workers from or limiting exposures usually resolves symptoms.[22]

Sensitizers. Initial exposure to low concentrations of a sensitizer usually does not result in an adverse reaction. However, with repeated and intermittent exposures, some individuals will begin to develop severe responses. Sensitization usually takes repeated exposures over days to weeks. Sensitization to biogenic substances, metals, cutting oils, machining fluids, and low molecular weight proteins can result in asthma-like inflammation, bronchoconstriction and mucus hypersecretion.[23] Usually antigen (hapten) formation, antibody production, and an antigen/antibody reaction occur following subsequent exposure(s). Disocyanates are low molecular weight aromatic and aliphatic compounds. Toluene diisocyanate (TDI), methylene bisphenyl isocyanate (MDI), and hexamethylene diisocyanate (HDI) are the most common diisocyanates. Often diisocyanates as a group are referred to as isocyanates.[24] Over-exposure to these compounds usually results in occupational asthma. Isocyanates are classified as haptens, which are compounds too small to directly stimulate specific antibody responses. Haptens must conjugate to host proteins to become immunogenic. The increasing prevalence of respiratory hypersensitivity and asthma in the workplace has made it the most common form of occupational lung disease.[25] Individuals with pre-existing asthma or hypersensitivities may exhibit adverse respiratory symptoms to exposure levels much lower than regulated exposure limits. A recent case involving latex allergy in health care workers demonstrated that even when sensitized individuals stopped using latex gloves, respiratory symptoms persisted while remaining in the work environment due to elevated airborne latex allergen as a result of continued use by others, entrapment of the powder in the ventilation systems with continued dispersion throughout the building.[22,26]

Agents That Cause Pneumoconiosis. This is a classic example of the development of disease as a result of chronic inhalation over-exposure to dusts with disease latency spanning years to decades. Common pneumoconioses include coal workers' pneumoconiosis (coal dust), siderosis (iron), stannosis (tin), baritosis (barium), and asbestosis (asbestos). Mortality due to pneumoconiosis, including asbestosis, has decreased between the years of 1968 and 2000.[27] Pneumoconiosis diseases are characterized by pulmonary fibrosis. Human and animal studies have demonstrated an immune component to chronic beryllium disease and to some forms of silicosis.[28,29] Hard metal lung disease occurs from chronic exposures to aerosolized tungsten carbide and cobalt. Interstitial lung diseases have been associated with nickel, chromium, and iron when chronic exposures to aerosols or dusts are common.[22,30] In the case of hexavalent chromium (Cr^{6+}), inhalation of compounds containing this valence of chromium has been associated with a wide variety of respiratory disorders, including loss of lung function, perforated nasal septum and lung cancer.[31]

Food Additives. Bronchiolitis obliterans is a pulmonary disease that involves the plugging of bronchiole airways with fibrous tissue. In 2000, several workers in a microwave popcorn plant were diagnosed with this condition that was later attributed to inhalation exposure to diacetyl, a ketone used for artificial flavoring.[32]

Agents That Cause Building Related Illnesses. Chronic exposures to volatile organic hydrocarbons, molds, and bacteria that originate from specific structural elements and routine building operations can lead to a variety of exposure-related illnesses defined as building related illness or sick building syndrome. When an identified toxicant in a building is the cause of the illness, the term "building related illness" is often used to describe the illness. When the toxicant is undetermined, but is known to be within the envelope of a building, the term "sick building syndrome" is often used to describe the illness. Depending on building materials, formaldehyde and terpenes that are slowly released from construction woods and carpeting account for most of the volatile organic hydrocarbons in office buildings. A related phenomenon to sick building syndrome is damp building syndrome. Multiple symptoms are associated with the presence of mold and fungi in water damaged buildings. "Farmer's lung", which is associated with molds in hay, cotton, and sugar cane, is characterized by airway hypersensitivity and production of IgG antibodies against specific antigens found in mold. Hypersensitivity and immune processes similar to farmer's lung, and reactions to certain mold-derived toxins or mycotoxins, likely mediate the effects seen in sick building syndrome and damp building syndrome.[22,33]

Dermal Toxicants

Structure and Function of the Skin

Contact with the skin is the second most common pathway for exposure to toxic materials, only second to inhalation. The three major layers of the skin are: (1) the epidermis or the outer layer; (2) the inner and thicker layer, the dermis; and (3) the fatty or subcutaneous layer. Figure 5.6 shows the layers of the skin and other important anatomical structures.

The stratum corneum, which means cornified layer, is the outermost layer of the epidermis. Several layers of cells from the underlying basal layer make up the stratum corneum. The cells of the basal layer divide continuously with the older cells moving toward the stratum corneum. The epidermis does not contain blood vessels. The cells of the basal layer receive their oxygen and nutrients from the blood vessels in the underlying dermis. The cells of the epidermis migrate to the surface of the epidermis where they degenerate and die. Keratin, a protein, forms from proteins reacting with enzymes located in the dying cells. The rough, impermeable nature of the epidermis is due to the presence of keratin. It is very insoluble and is resistant to other substances and conditions such as changes in pH, heat, and cold. A toxic material must penetrate the stratum corneum in order to be absorbed by the skin. If a substance can penetrate the stratum corneum, it will move easily through the other layers in the skin and is absorbed into the blood very quickly.(17)

The second layer of the skin is the dermis. Connective tissue is the primary component of the dermis. Blood vessels are located throughout the dermis and supply nutrients to the cells of the dermis and the epidermis. Hair follicles, sweat glands, and sebaceous glands are found in the dermis. Smooth muscles, known as arrector pili muscles, are associated with the hair follicles. Contraction of these muscles due to the release of epinephrine cause "goose bumps" often in response to feeling cold or strong emotions.

The subcutaneous layer provides a cushion to underlying structures. It also allows the dermis to connect to the underlying tissues such as muscle.

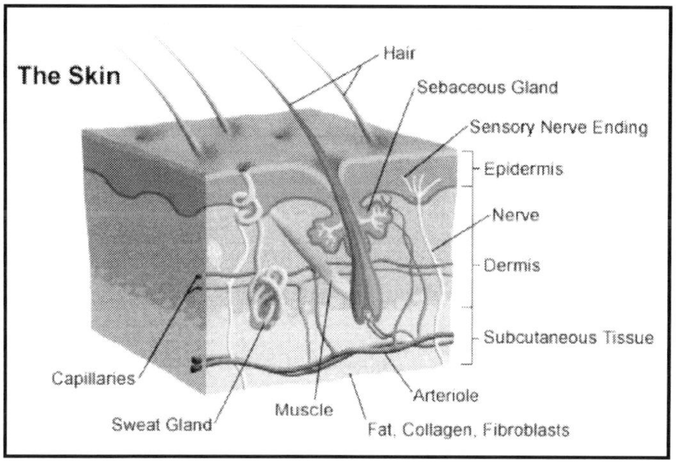

Figure 5.6 — The Skin (Source: Stanford School of Medicine, accessed from http://cancer.stanford.edu/information/cancerDiagnosis/images/ei_0390.gif)

Examples of Dermal Toxicants

Corrosive and Drying Substances. Acids, such as sulfuric and nitric acids, as well as strong bases, such as sodium hydroxide, are toxic substances that break down the outer layers of the epidermis. When a chemical burn occurs, toxic substances, which are usually poorly absorbed, are more readily absorbed through the damaged skin. Repeated exposures to soaps, detergents, and organic solvents can cause water loss and dryness of the skin. Organic solvents dissolve skin surface lipids and remove lipids in the cells. This will enhance the absorption of other toxic substances. Metals, such as chromium and arsenic, alter cell protein structure, resulting in skin damage. These are examples of local effects, since the symptoms appear only at the point of contact between the toxic substance and the skin.(17)

Substances That Cause Systemic Effects. Toxic substances that pass through the skin may cause systemic effects, in addition to local effects. For example, dermal contact with carbon disulfide can affect the nervous system and heart. Carbon tetrachloride passing through the skin can adversely affect the liver, kidneys, and nervous system. Dermal exposure to organophosphate pesticides can result in symptoms associated with the gastrointestinal tract, renal system, and nerve-muscle function. Therefore, there are workplace chemicals that can not only alter the structural and functional character of the skin, but they can be absorbed into the blood and cause systemic effects. This has resulted in the use of the "Skin Notation" in the Threshold Limit Values® (TLVs®) published by the American Conference of Governmental Industrial Hygienists® for chemicals with potential for systemic toxicity from cutaneous exposure.(34)

Agents That Cause Contact Dermatitis. The symptoms of contact dermatitis are found in the area of the skin that has had exposure to the chemical agent. Irritant contact dermatitis reactions include corrosion, acute irritation and cumulative irritation, being the result of direct physical and chemical properties of the agent.(35) The following substances are associated with irritant contact dermatitis: pesticides, oils, greases, alkalis and acids, soaps, and some plant matter, as well as nickel, chromium, mercury, gold, phenol, and some of their compounds. Allergic contact dermatitis is caused by a type IV cell-mediated hypersensitivity reaction. It is easily distinguished from irritant contact dermatitis by its appearance well beyond the area of direct contact and it occurs 12–24 hours after exposure.[36] Workers who have skin exposure to metals, plastics, rubbers, pharmaceuticals, jewelry, and explosives frequently experience allergic contact dermatitis.[35]

Agents That Cause Photosensitization. Contact photosensitization is the most common occupational phototoxic reaction. The photoactive chemical coming into contact with the skin is absorbed and then sunlight (ultraviolet A) activates the chemical. Tetracycline, nalidixic acid, eosin and acridine dyes, anthracene, and some plants will cause this reaction. Contact photosensitization has been seen in farmers, asphalt workers, and miners.[36]

Agents That Cause Urticarial Reactions. Urticaria is a vascular reaction of the skin resulting in the appearance of wheals that are redder or paler than surrounding skin and is extremely itchy.[37] This reaction may result from direct contact or it may be a type I hypersensitivity reaction that includes the release of substances that act on the vascular system.[36] Aspirin, curare, azo dyes, benzoates, and other compounds use the nonimmunologic mechanism. Chloro-2,4-dinitrobenzene, diethyltoluamide, penicillin, and some plants and animal toxins use the immunologic process.[39]

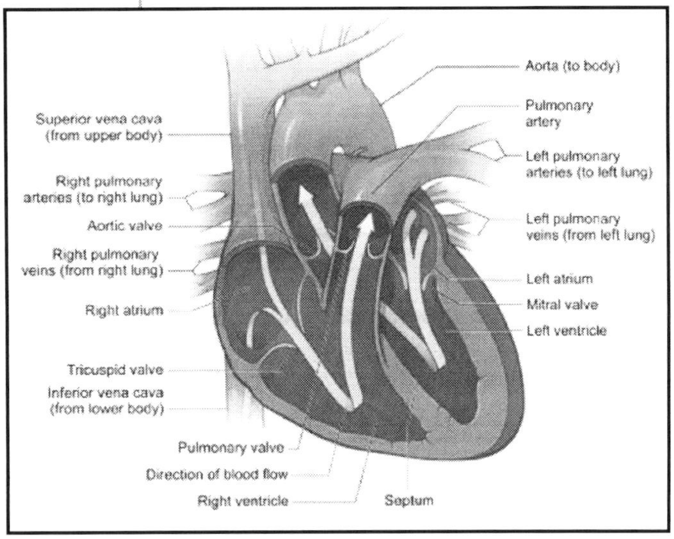

Figure 5.7 — The Heart and Major Blood Vessels. This is a cross-section of the heart and its inside structures. The direction in which oxygen-poor blood flows from the body to the lungs is shown by the blue arrow. The direction in which oxygen-rich blood flows from the lungs to the rest of the body is shown by the red arrow. (Source: National Institutes of Health, accessed from http://www.nhlbi.nih.gov/health/dci/images/ heart_interior.gif)

Agents That Cause Occupational Acne. Coal-tar pitch, creosote, greases, and oils can cause acne in exposed workers. Chloracne, a difficult form of acne to treat, may be caused by halogenated aromatic hydrocarbons, including dibenzofurans and polychlorinated biphenyls (PCBs), as well as dioxins and chlorobenzenes.[36]

Cardiovascular Toxicants

Structure and Function of the Cardiovascular System

The heart and blood vessels are responsible for transporting oxygen and nutrients through the blood to the cells throughout the body. Waste products from cellular metabolism are picked up by the blood and taken to various organs for elimination. Various active and passive transport mechanisms allow oxygen, nutrients, waste products, and xenobiotics to pass into and out of the blood.[17]

The heart consists of four chambers: the right and left ventricles and the right and left atria. The atria are smaller and have thinner walls than the ventricles. Blood low in oxygen from the systemic circulation goes into the right atrium. Oxygen-rich blood goes into the left atrium from the lungs. At exactly the right time the atria deliver their blood to the corresponding ventricle. The right ventricle pumps blood through the pulmonary artery to the pulmonary circulation in the lungs. The pulmonary circulation contains capillaries that are in association with the alveoli of the lungs, allowing the diffusion of gases such as oxygen, carbon dioxide, or airborne toxicants, between the blood and inhaled air. Blood rich in oxygen returns to the left atrium through the pulmonary veins and then the left atrium pumps the blood into the left ventricle. The left ventricle sends the blood through the aorta to the systemic circulation which reaches all the tissues of the body. Figure 5.7 shows the inside of the heart and the direction of blood flow, as described above.

Once in the pulmonary or systemic circulation, blood travels in arteries. The arteries become smaller in size, eventually forming arterioles. These are small-diameter arteries that provide blood to the capillaries. These structures have a single layer of flattened cells that make up their walls. The capillaries change slowly into small diameter venules, which eventually change into larger veins that ultimately return blood to the right atrium of the heart.

There are billions of capillaries in the vascular system. They are the primary site of exchange of substances between the blood and tissues. Active and passive transport mechanisms through the capillary endothelial cells allow the movement of nutrients, gases, and toxic materials from or into the blood. Gases, lipid-soluble substances, and water-soluble substances move primarily by diffusion. Nutrients, nonlipid-soluble substances use active transport or facilitated transport. Toxic substances are also transported by these mechanisms, depending on molecular size. The rate of absorption and subsequent toxicity of a foreign substance can be affected by the competition for protein-carrier molecules that are used by essential nutrients, such as amino acids. In order for a toxic substance to have a toxic effect, it must be absorbed and reach the target tissues in sufficient concentrations. The following mechanisms tend to oppose distribution to target tissues—binding to plasma proteins, distribution to storage sites, and specialized cellular barriers, such as the brain blood barrier.(17)

Control of the Heart

The heart must maintain its continuous rhythmic contractions. Specialized cardiac muscle cells in the sinoatrial (SA) node initiate the contraction of the right atrium. The SA node is the pacemaker for the heart, providing intrinsic control of the heart. It sends action potentials to the muscle cells of the right and left atria causing their contraction. The atrioventricular (AV) node is in the lower part of the right atrium. The AV node passes action potentials to specialized cardiac muscle cells in the atrioventricular bundle or bundle of His. It divides into the left and right bundle branches. These branches eventually divide into many small conducting Purkinje fibers. The Purkinje fibers transmit

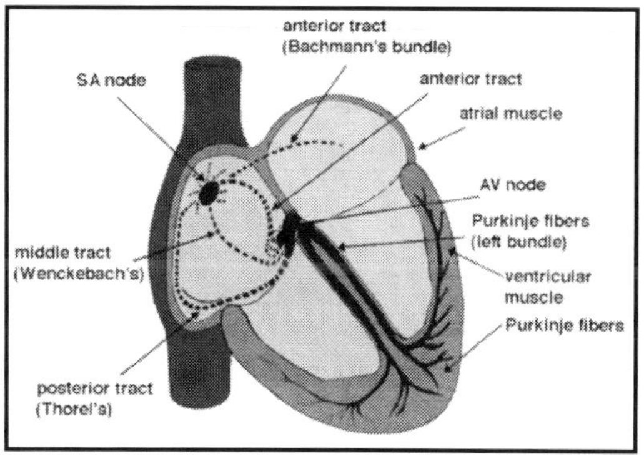

Figure 5.8 — The Conduction System of the Heart (Source: University of Minnesota, accessed from http://www.vhlab.umn.edu/atlas/phystutorial/graphics/fig5.gif).

action potentials to the muscle cells of the ventricles. A change in cell membrane permeability to sodium (Na^+), potassium (K^+), and calcium (Ca^{2+}) result in the initiation of an action potential in the SA node.(17) Figure 5.8 shows the conduction system of the heart.

There is also extrinsic control of the heart rate. The nerves of the autonomic nervous system affect the heart rate. Stimulation of the parasympathetic nervous system or vagus nerve will affect the SA node, atrial muscle fibers, AV node, and some of the muscle fibers of the ventricles where acetylcholine is released. Parasympathetic stimulation will result in a decrease in heart rate and a decrease in the strength of atrial and ventricular muscle contraction. Stimulation of the sympathetic nervous system will result in the release of norepinephrine in the SA node and the ventricles, causing an increase in the heart rate and the strength of contraction. Toxic materials can affect both the intrinsic and extrinsic control mechanisms of the heart, resulting in a change in heart rate or a change in the strength of contraction, or both.

Examples of Cardiovascular Toxicants

Substances can adversely affect the heart by having a direct effect on the cardiac tissues or by producing their effect indirectly by altering the functions of other systems in the body, such as the nervous system. Therefore, toxic substances can affect the heart by changing the metabolism of cardiac tissues, or by affecting the neural control of the heart by altering nerve cell functioning. The symptoms of cardiotoxicity are the same in both cases—change in the strength of contraction, change in rhythm of contraction, or both. Arrhythmias are any changes in the normal rhythmic beat of the heart. These can result from changes in the rate at which action potentials are generated or the rate at which conduction of the action potential occurs. Tachycardia is an increase in heart rate, while slowing of the heart rate is brady cardia. Atrial fibrillation is irregular unsynchronized contractions of the atrium, which leads to irregular filling of the ventricles with blood. Ventricular fibrillation is rapid and randomized excitation of the ventricles, which can be life threatening, due to inefficient contraction of the ventricles.[17]

Metals. Various metals affect the strength of contraction and the conduction of the electrical signal through the heart. Barium can cause tachycardia by interfering with calcium diffusion. Manganese and nickel affect calcium, changing the generation of the action potential. Lead can cause arrhythmias and decrease the strength of contraction by interfering with energy metabolism and ATP synthesis in the heart. Lead, cadmium, and cobalt interfere with cellular metabolism in cardiac cells, decreasing the strength of contraction. Lead, arsenic, and cobalt can cause cardiomyopathy. Cobalt, formerly used as a foam stabilizer in beer, was known to induce endemic cardiomyopathy in chronic alcoholics.[39]

Organic Solvents. These substances have both direct and indirect effects on the heart. They interfere with the generation and conduction of the action potential, causing a change in heart rate and strength of contraction. They also disrupt the generation of the action potential in the nerve cell membrane. This depresses the activity of the Central Nervous System (CNS), which affects the cardioregulatory center in the brain, affecting sympathetic and parasympathetic innervation of the heart. Arrhythmias and decreased contractility of the heart may occur. Toluene and ketones, such as acetone, can cause arrhythmias due to the depression of parasympathetic activity. Halogenated hydrocarbons, such as methylene chloride, can cause arrhythmias and decreased contractility by depressing the parasympathetic activity of the CNS.[17] Halogenated alkanes, such as 1,1,1-trichloroethane, can depress the heart rate, strength of contraction, and action potential conduction. Some of these compounds can sensitize the heart to arrhythmias caused by beta-agonists, such as endogenous epinephrine and common heart medications. Fluorocarbons (freons) have also been reported to have a similar sensitizing effect on the heart.[40] Therefore, a variety of solvents cause tachycardia, including chlorinated hydrocarbons, such as trichloroethylene (TCE), aromatic solvents (xylene, toluene), aliphatic hydrocarbons (naphthas, gasoline), and fluorocarbon refrigerants.[41]

Carbon Monoxide. CO can have both a direct and indirect effect on the heart. Acute exposure to CO will cause a decreased oxygen supply to cardiac tissue by direct binding to hemoglobin or a decreased oxygen supply to nerve tissues of the CNS. Elevated CO and decreased oxygen levels results in tachycardia. Low oxygen levels in the blood causes the cardioregulatory center to malfunction, resulting in arrhythmias.

Particulate Matter. Disturbances in heart function can occur after exposure to particulate matter with a median mass diameter of 2.5 micrometers (PM 2.5) or less. One possible mechanism involves the production of cytokines, protein-like substances that serve as cellular signaling molecules. Cytokines can induce inflammatory changes that may result in heart disturbances.[42]

Agents That Cause Changes in Blood Vessels. When in physiological concentrations, chromium has a positive effect on the cardiovascular (CV) system. A chromium deficiency is associated with an increase risk for atherosclerosis (fatty plaque build-up in the walls of large and medium-sized arteries).[41] Lead and other heavy metals may block calcium channels causing the CV system to be unable to maintain normal blood pressure, resulting in hypertension. If in sufficiently high concentrations, common organic solvents can depress the CNS to an extent that will result in circulatory collapse and shock. Nitrated aliphatics, such as trinitroglycerin, can produce circulatory depression. Chronic exposure to carbon monoxide can damage vascular endothelial cells, resulting in accelerated atherosclerosis.[43] Exposure to carbon disulfide is another classic example of an industrial toxin associated with accelerated atherosclerotic disease in workers.[44] It may be mediated by carbon disulfide reacting with essential sulfhydryl groups, resulting in enzyme inhibition. A more direct toxic effect has been observed with allyl amine whose metabolite, acrolein, may produce damage to vessels walls.[45]

Nephrotoxicants

Structure and Function of the Renal System

There are two bean-shaped kidneys near the posterior wall of the abdomen. There are two major areas in the kidney—the cortex and the medulla. The outer part is the cortex and the inner part is the medulla. Renal pyramids are in the medulla with urine passing from the tips of the pyramids to the renal pelvis, a funnel-like structure. After narrowing, the renal pelvis becomes the ureter, which connects the kidney to the urinary bladder. Figure 5.9 shows the structure of the kidney. The nephron, which is shown in Figure 5.10, is the functional unit of the kidney. It is located in both the cortex and the medulla. There are over a million of these structures in the kidney. A nephron has the following components: renal corpuscle, a proximal convoluted tubule, a Loop of Henle, and a distal convoluted tubule. The distal convoluted tubule connects to the collecting duct, which takes the urine to the renal pelvis area where it goes into the ureter. A renal corpuscle has two primary components—Bowman's capsule and the glomerulus. The glomerulus is a ball-like collection of capillaries. Blood and all of its components reach the renal corpuscle of the nephron. The liquid portion of blood is filtered from the glomerulus into Bowman's capsule. It then goes to the proximal convoluted tubule and then into the Loop of Henle. The Loop of Henle has a descending and an ascending limb. Both limbs of the Loop of Henle are surrounded by a dense blood supply called the peritubular capillaries. The ascending limb turns into the distal convoluted tubule, which then empties into the collecting duct. About 25 percent of the cardiac output goes to the kidneys, which is about 1.3 liters of blood per minute. Therefore, the kidneys have a high perfusion rate. Due to this high perfusion rate, any toxins in the blood will be delivered to the kidneys in large amounts.[17]

The primary function of the kidneys is to remove metabolic waste from the body and to maintain homeostasis of the body. These functions are accomplished by the nephrons, which involves the absorption and excretion of solutes and water from the blood to the nephrons and vice versa. The structure of the nephron is shown in Figure 5.10. Characteristics of the solute, such as molecular size, electrical charge, lipid-water solubility, and active and passive transport mechanisms determine which substances will be transported from the blood into the

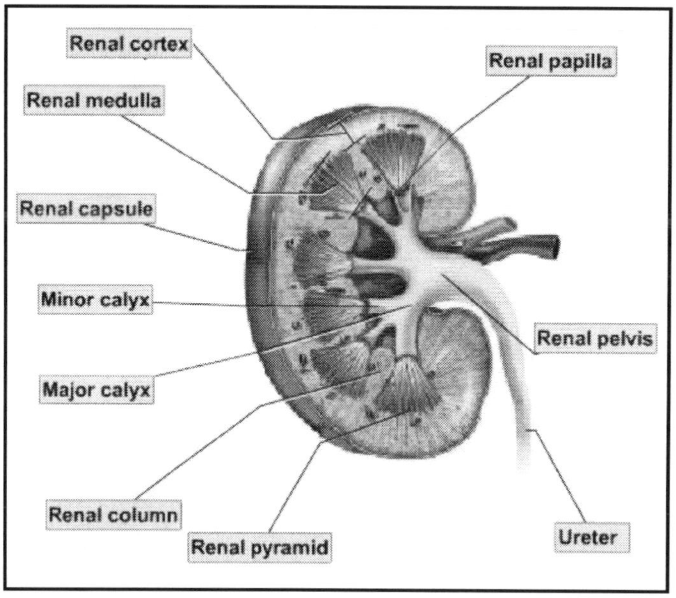

Figure 5.9 — The Kidney (Source: Comprehensive-Kidney-Facts.com, accessed from http://www.comprehensive-kidney-facts.com/images/KidneyAnatomy.jpg).

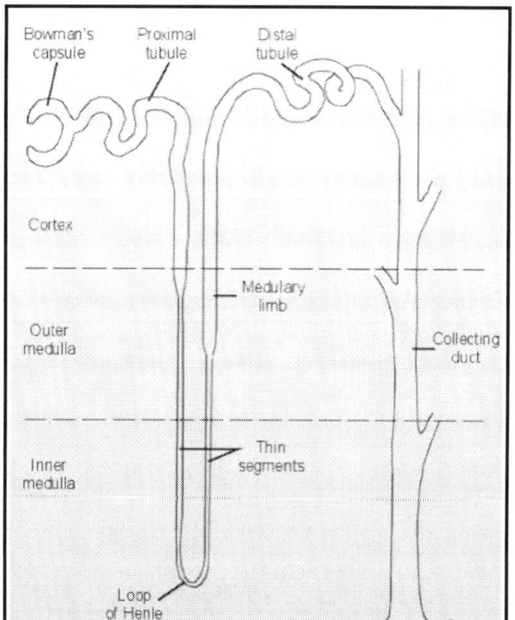

Figure 5.10 — The Nephron (Source: Bellarmine University).

kidneys and reabsorbed from the kidneys back into the blood. Small molecular size solute particles and water will pass into the nephron easily. Large molecules, such as proteins (like albumin), will not easily pass through the walls of Bowman's capsule. Therefore, normally, only a very small amount of protein will enter the kidneys. Substances that enter the kidneys can be reabsorbed by active or passive transport mechanisms. Water and solutes are primarily reabsorbed by the proximal convoluted tubule. Proteins, amino acids, glucose, as well as sodium, potassium, and chloride ions are actively transported from the proximal convoluted tubule to the peritubular capillaries. Lipid-soluble, water-soluble, and small size toxicants can easily pass into the nephron. If they are not reabsorbed as they pass through the nephron, they will be excreted in the urine. Lipid-soluble toxicants are reabsorbed easily. Unbound metals like cadmium and mercury are reabsorbed by active transport mechanisms in the cells of the proximal convoluted tubule. These metals can then bind to metallothionein, which can then have an adverse effect.

In addition to removing metabolic waste, the kidneys maintain the blood pH between 7.2 and 7.4. If blood pH decreases, acidosis can occur, which can result in increased heart and respiratory rates. The kidneys play a role in maintaining blood pH by removing excess hydrogen ions. Renin is also secreted by the kidneys, which is involved in regulating blood pressure. Renin is released into the blood where it interacts with angiotensin, another protein, which stimulates contraction of arteriolar smooth muscle. This results in contraction and an increase in blood pressure. So by regulating ion and water balance in the body and blood pressure, the kidneys help maintain homeostatis.

Examples of Nephrotoxicants

The kidneys are a metabolic site for the deactivation of some toxic substances. There are several mechanisms that facilitate the accumulation of toxic substances in the kidneys, including a high blood flow and the presence of active and passive transport mechanisms that are normally involved in the excretion and reabsorption of ions, amino acids, glucose, and metabolic wastes. These same transport mechanisms are used to increase the accumulation of toxic substances, such as heavy metals, which compete for the same carrier molecules.

Heavy Metals. Lead, mercury, and cadmium accumulate in the kidneys and adversely affect the proximal convoluted tubules of the nephrons. Cadmium binds with proteins in the blood and is able to freely pass into the glomerular filtrate of the kidneys. The cadmium-protein complex is absorbed into the cells of the proximal convoluted tubule where noncomplexed free cadmium is formed as a result of cellular metabolic processes. The free cadmium now binds with intracellular metallothionein or with other intracellular proteins, such as enzymes and components of the cell membrane. Binding of cadmium to proteins other than metallothionein disrupts normal cellular metabolism and can result in cell death. Mercury also can cause the death of proximal convoluted tubule cells. It inhibits enzymes in the mitochondria, which are involved in the production of ATP. ATP is essential for normal cell functions and in particular intracellular metabolism. If it becomes absent, the cell will eventually die. Lead is rapidly transported into the cells of the proximal tubules, where it is stored. Storage in the nucleus and interaction with nuclear DNA may explain the carcinogenic effect of lead. Like mercury, lead also binds with enzymes associated with mitochondria and ATP production. Lead also alters calcium homeostasis. Heavy metals typically inhibit essential enzymes by blocking sulfhydryl groups.[46]

Organic Substances. Chloroform and carbon tetrachloride have the potential to cause cellular dysfunction in the kidney, due to the formation of phosgene during its metabolism. Nephrotoxicity results in damage to the cell membrane and subsequent cell death. The binding of chloroform to DNA may be associated with its cancer-causing potential in the kidneys. Ethylene glycol (antifreeze) may cause renal failure through the formation of oxalic acid from its metabolism. The oxalic acid reacts with calcium in the lumen of the nephron, forming an insoluble calcium oxalate precipitate. This obstructs the normal flow of urine through the nephron, leading to renal failure. Other nephrotoxicants are hexachlorobutadiene and trichloroethylene. These compounds are conjugated with glutathione in the liver and then eliminated in the kidney, finding their way into the tubular cell. There they are cleaved with the formation of a sulfur derivative of the parent compound, which is cytotoxic.[47]

Neurotoxicants

Structure and Function of the Nervous System

The central nervous system (CNS) and the peripheral nervous system (PNS) are the two major divisions of the nervous system of the body. The brain and the spinal cord are the structures of the CNS. All other nerves outside the CNS are in the PNS. Afferent and efferent nerves make up the PNS. Afferent or sensory nerves carry sensory information, such as touch or pain, to the CNS. Efferent or motor nerves transmit information from the CNS to the muscles and glands. Efferent nerves can be a part of the somatic motor nervous system or the autonomic nervous system. Skeletal muscles are stimulated by the somatic motor nerves. The autonomic nervous system can be divided into the sympathetic and parasympathetic nervous systems. The autonomic nervous system transmits information from the CNS to organs and glands, such as the heart, gastrointestinal tract, blood vessels, salivary glands, pancreas, and adrenal glands.[17]

Cells of the nervous system include the neuron and supporting cells called the neuroglia or glia cells. Figure 5.11 shows the neuron and associated structures. The neuron is the basic functional unit of the nervous system. It serves as the receptor for internal and external stimuli. It transmits information to the CNS and carries signals to muscles and glands. The neuron consists of a cell body (soma), the axon, and dendrites. The cell body contains the nucleus, endoplasmic reticulum, Golgi complex, and mitochondria. Dendrites are short, branching processes that carry impulses toward the cell body. The axon is a single fiber that carries impulses away from the cell body. Axons of sensory nerves transmit information to the CNS. Axons of motor nerves carry information to muscles and glands. Glia cells include astrocytes, oligodendrocytes, and Schwann cells. Astrocytes are an essential component of the blood-brain barrier, as described below. Oligodendrocytes in the CNS and Schwann cells in the PNS have cell processes that surround the nerve cell axons, facilitating the transmission of nerve impulses along the axon. The cell processes wrap around the axon forming concentric layers of cell membrane called a myelin sheath. These axons are considered myelinated nerves. If myelin is not surrounding an axon, it is considered an unmyelinated nerve. Myelin is a good insulator, not allowing movement of sodium and potassium ions into or out of the axon, which helps maintain the membrane potential and the initiation of the action potential.

The cell membrane of the neuron has a change in permeability upon receiving a stimulus, such as sensation of heat or pain, causing the movement of sodium and potassium ions across the cell membrane. An electrical charge is generated and it is called the action potential. It travels along the nerve cell and will eventually reach the end of the axon, where it causes the release of a neurotransmitter, a chemical substance. This specific chemical substance will initiate a response in another nerve cell, muscle, or gland. Acetylcholine and norepinephrine are two well known neurotransmitters. As shown in Figure 5.11, the synapse is where the neuron interacts with another cell. The

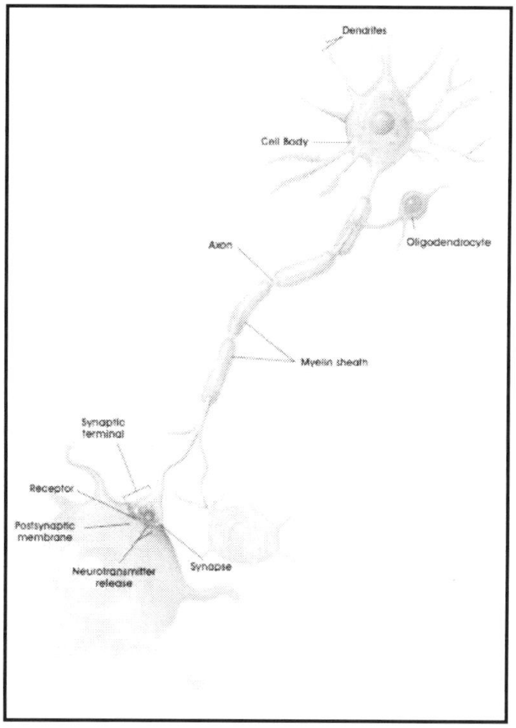

Figure 5.11 — The Neuron and Associated Structures (Source: National Institutes of Health — Stem Cell Information, http://stemcells.nih.gov/ info/scireport/chapter8.asp.).

end of the axon is the presynaptic terminal. The cell membrane of the stimulated tissue is the postsynaptic membrane. The synaptic cleft is the space between these two structures. The presynaptic terminal releases the neurotransmitter and it diffuses across the synaptic cleft, and binds to receptors on the postsynaptic cell membrane. This initiates a response in the affected tissue. To keep the affected tissue from being constantly stimulated, the neurotransmitter is broken down rapidly by enzymes, or it is reabsorbed by the presynaptic terminal quickly.

The blood-brain barrier (BBB) consists of the close association between brain capillaries and astrocytes, the specialized cells of the nervous system. The BBB decreases the type and amount of toxicants that can be transferred from the blood to the brain. It reduces the absorption of toxicants because of the closely packed endothelial cells of the capillaries; the astrocytes; and the low protein content of the interstitial fluid. The endothelial cells of the BBB have few or no pores between them, reducing the movement of substances from the blood through the capillaries. However, lipid-soluble compounds, such as ethanol, can still easily diffuse through the cell membrane and into the interstitial fluid around the brain. Water-soluble substances, such as glucose, are transported across the BBB by carrier-mediated transport. The cellular processes of the astrocytes surround the capillaries. Being high in lipid content, the cell membrane of the astrocyte is an effective barrier to the movement of water-soluble molecules through the BBB. If a toxic substance is able to pass through the BBB, further movement towards the brain is decreased because of the low protein content in the interstitial fluid. Transport of water-insoluble substances through the aqueous interstitial fluid requires the presence of proteins. Methyl mercury will pass through the BBB because it uses a carrier-mediated process. Mercuric chloride is not lipid soluble, so it is unable to readily cross the BBB. Organophosphate pesticides will penetrate the BBB easily due to their lipophilic nature.

Examples of Neurotoxicants

The structure of the neuron can be damaged by toxic substances. The damage can be classified as neuronopathy, axonopathy, or myelinopathy, all of which can result in toxicity. Toxic substances can also affect neurotransmission between the pre-synaptic terminal and the postsynaptic membrane by disrupting normal events.

Neuronopathy. Toxic substances can interact with the nerve cell body which will cause the entire nerve cell, including the dendrites and axons, to degenerate. Ultimately, the entire neuron is destroyed (neuronopathy). Various mercury compounds, trimethyltin, aluminum, manganese, methanol, carbon monoxide, and hydrogen cyanide will cause neuronopathy. Mercury-containing waste from various industries can find its way into lakes, rivers, and the oceans. There it is converted to an organic mercury compound, methylmercury, which bioaccumulates in the food chain. Organic mercury compounds are easily absorbed through the gastrointestinal tract. A major case of human poisoning as a result of exposure to methylmercury occurred in Minamata, Japan, after the bay became contaminated with mercury-containing waste. Since organomercurials are lipid-soluble compounds, they will easily pass through the blood-brain barrier (BBB) into the CNS. At low doses, ataxia, the loss of muscle coordination and control, results. At high doses, methylmercury can cause generalized neuronopathy.[48] A tragic case of delayed cerebellar disease and death was reported in a research chemist following accidental exposure to dimethylmercury.[49] This compound is more lipid soluble and therefore more dangerous than methylmercury. Lethal tissue concentrations resulted from transdermal absorption through a permeable latex glove. The monovalent (mercurous) and divalent (mercuric) inorganic salts of mercury have neurologic toxicity. Divalent compounds are more toxic than monovalent compounds.[50] Severe cases of poisoning occur through accidental and intentional ingestion. The phrase "mad as a hatter" originated from workers in the hat industry being exposed to inorganic mercury. The symptoms displayed by these workers included depression, moodiness, insomnia, confusion, and tremors.[51] The elemental form of mercury also has neurologic toxicity. Elemental mercury is easily absorbed through the lungs as a vapor. Acute inhalation of high concentrations of mercury vapor has a corrosive effect on lung tissue, causing bronchitis and interstitial pneumonitis, as well as nervous system effects of tremor and excitability. Chronic inhalation of lower concentrations of mercury vapor leads to neurasthenic symptoms that include headache, fatigue, dizziness, memory loss, and depression. As intoxication becomes more severe, erethism (withdrawal, memory loss, excitability, and depression), tremor, and gingivitis are predominant symptoms along with diffuse polyneuropathy.[46] Trimethyltin, sometimes known as organotin, can pass through the blood-brain barrier and enter the brain where it leads to diffuse neuronal injury. This organometal compound most easily damages neurons in a very specific area of the brain, the hippocampus and surrounding areas. Aluminum has been associated with Alzheimer's disease. It may have an adverse effect on cell membrane integrity, causing a lack of proper ion distribution and disrupting normal nerve cell function. Manganese is a toxicant that can also be found in industrial waste that is released into ambient air and into bodies of water. High concentrations of manganese can cause damage in the CNS, especially the brain. Neuropsychiatric symptoms can occur that include irritability, difficulty in walking, and speech abnormalities. Parkinson-like symptoms, such as tremors and spastic contractions of skeletal muscles, can occur. Exposure to methanol can result in nerve damage causing blindness or death. Depending on the level of exposure, symptoms may progress to temporary or permanent blindness. Carbon monoxide and hydrogen cyanide interfere with aerobic metabolism, depriving nerve cells of oxygen that maintains normal cell function and integrity. Metabolic processes in the nerve cells are disrupted, which leads to cell death.[51]

Axonopathy. Damage to axons is axonopathy and is most often in the peripheral nervous system with resulting sensory and motor dysfunction. Axonopathies are usually categorized as either proximal or distal. Proximal axonopathies result in the swelling of proximal axons with the formation of giant axonal swellings. Abnormal changes in distal portions of axons can result in distal axonopathies. It often includes the degeneration of myelin. Since the damage often appears first in the axon terminal, distal axonopathies are sometimes called "dying-back neuropathies." Axons that innervate the hands and feet are usually affected first by chemicals that cause axonopathies, resulting in loss of feeling and motion. Acrylamide, carbon disulfide, n-hexane, and organophosphate insecticides cause axonopathy. Acrylamide is a vinyl monomer that produces distal axonopathies primarily by inhibiting axonal transport.[51] Workers in the Vulcan rubber and viscose rayon industries have had exposure to carbon disulfide.[52] In prolonged low doses this compound can induce psychiatric disturbances. At higher exposures it can result in a toxic encephalopathy. In addition to CNS effects, exposure to carbon disulfide can cause a distal axonopathy that is identical to that caused by hexane. If exposure continues, sensory and motor symptoms will develop as a result of chronic axonopathy. When exposed to high concentrations of n-hexane repeatedly, individuals develop a progressive sensorimotor distal axonopathy. Methyl n-butyl ketone (2-hexanone) causes the same neuropathy, since they both form the same ultimate toxic metabolite, 2,5-hexanedione. When animals are exposed to n-hexane and methyl n-butyl ketone at the same time, there is synergistic interaction between these two compounds. Some organophosphate compounds can cause distal axonopathies that result in delayed neuropathy. This is in addition to acute inhibition of acetylcholinesterase throughout the body, especially in synapses. These compounds include tri-o-cresyl phosphate (TOCP) and leptophos.[52] During the 1920s and 1930s, "Ginger Jake" paralysis was linked with ingestion of ginger extract contaminated with trace amounts of TOCP. Another outbreak of distal axonopathy occurred in Morocco when olive oil contaminated with TOCP was consumed.[53] Delayed neuropathy can be readily reproduced in hens, usually with a delay of eight to ten days after exposure.[52] It is likely that the organophosphate axonopathy is due to the inhibition of an esterase enzyme different from acetylcholinesterase known as the "neurotoxic esterase" or the "neuropathy target esterase" (NTE).

Meylinopathy. Normal function of the nervous system can be disrupted if there is damage to myelin. Damage to myelin can result in blockage of an action potential completely, or it may delay or reduce the amplitude of an action potential. When this occurs, symptoms can include numbness, weakness, and paralysis. Toxicants exist that cause the separation of the myelin lamellae, called intramyelinic edema, and cause the loss of myelin, called demyelination. Triethyltin, hexachlorophene, and lead are demyelinating agents. An incident occurred in France in 1954, in which over 1000 people were exposed to triethyltin in a contaminated oral antibacterial preparation. Over 100 people died of acute toxicity over the course of six to eight weeks following ingestion. Intramyelinic edema resulted in extremely severe, persistent headache, visual disturbance, impaired consciousness followed by coma and death.[54] An antimicrobial agent very similar to triethyltin, hexachlorophene, is also highly lipid soluble and has similar effects upon myelin. Lead exposure can result in peripheral neuropathy because of segmental demyelination in the peripheral nervous system. Swelling and other morphological changes are seen in Schwann cells. An effect of lead on the membrane structure of myelin and myelin membrane fluidity has been shown in rats.[55] Cumulative exposure to inorganic lead was found to be related to performance on neuropsychological tests.[56] Lead exposure is known to have an adverse effect on the intellectual abilities of children.[57]

Neurotransmission Toxicity. Toxic substances can disrupt normal events during neurotransmission between the presynaptic terminal and the postsynaptic membrane. These toxic substances can be categorized according to their mechanisms of action, including: blocking agents, depolarizing agents, stimulants, depressants, or anticholinesterase agents. Blocking agents can bind to the presynaptic terminal and prevent the release of neurotransmitter. In the case of botulism, the bacterium *Clostridium botulinum* toxin binds to the presynaptic terminal and prevents the release of acetylcholine at the neuromuscular and peripheral nervous system synapses. A blocking agent can also bind to the postsynaptic membrane and prevent the binding of the neurotransmitter. Curare is a competitive postsynaptic acetylcholine antagonist at the neuromuscular junction.[58] Atropine, a substance found in the plant *Atropa belladonna,* is a muscarinic blocker, since it binds to muscarinic receptors, blocking the binding of acetycholine. Atropine is, therefore, an anticholinergic compound. Atropine exposure can cause tachycardia, dilation of the pupils, dilation of bronchioles, decrease in peristalsis, and decrease in saliva and other secretions. The resting membrane potential that normally exists across the cell membrane is maintained by an energy-dependent ATP sodium-potassium pump, which transports sodium ions out of the cell and potassium into the cell. Depolarizing agents can eliminate the resting membrane potential by altering the permeability of the cell membrane towards sodium and potassium ions. The organochlorine insecticide dichlorodiphenyl trichloroethane (DDT) depolarizes the presynaptic neuron membrane partially, causing it to be in an almost continuous state of excitation with the release of neurotransmitter in response to weak stimuli. Individuals with exposure may develop persistent tremors, irritability, hypersensitivity to external stimuli, and dizziness. Stimulants can exert an effect by increasing the sensitivity of neurons to stimuli or by inhibiting the reabsorption of neurotransmitters. Nicotine is a stimulant that increases the excitability of neurons. It binds to and stimulates a subset of receptors that normally bind acetylcholine, called nicotinic receptors. These receptors are found in the CNS and the neuromuscular junction. Caffeine (1,2,7-trimethylxanthine) is a stimulant of the CNS. By preventing the breakdown of cyclic AMP, it affects the active transport system that maintains the sodium/potassium concentration gradient across the cell membrane.[58] Cocaine is a strong stimulant of the CNS causing euphoric and addictive effects. Depressants of neurotransmission cause adverse effects mainly by interfering with the maintenance of the resting membrane potential and the generation of the action potential. Volatile organic toxicants, aromatic organic solvents, and alcohols all impair neurotransmission and are strong CNS depressants. Volatile organic solvents commonly found in the workplace, such as carbon tetrachloride, chloroform, and methylene chloride, are very lipophilic and easily absorbed through the myelin sheath and cell membrane of neurons. The term, solvent neurotoxic syndrome, describes the major symptoms of the CNS when affected by exposure to a mixture of volatile organic solvents. They include difficulties in concentration, forgetfulness, headaches, irritability, insensitivity, personality disorders, mental disabilities and suicidal tendencies.[59] This syndrome has also been called painters' syndrome, chronic toxic encephalopathy, or psycho-organic syndrome. Compounds that have one or more benzene rings in their structure are aromatic organic solvents and they also have depressant effects on the CNS. This group of compounds includes benzene, toluene, and xylene. The other group of organic solvents that strongly depress the normal function of the CNS is alcohols. Methanol and ethanol are most commonly encountered in the workplace.

Anticholinesterase agents bind directly to the enzyme, acetylcholinesterase, and inhibit it from breaking down acetylcholine. This affects nerves, ganglion, and muscles throughout the body that are stimulated by the neurotransmitter acetylcholine. This results in an increased and prolonged stimulation of the postsynaptic membranes due to the increased amount of acetylcholine. Abdominal cramps, blurred vision, miosis, and increased salivation and sweating are indications of cholinergic excess and are easily reversed by atropine which blocks muscarinic receptors.[50] Also, a compound called pralidoxime (2-PAM) helps accelerate the reversal of acetylcholinesterase inhibition.[51] Organophosphate pesticides and carbamate insecticides are the most common anticholinesterase agents.

Organophospahte compounds, which include parathion, malathion, diazinon, soman, sarin, etc., bind tightly to the enzyme. In the case of parathion, the binding is prolonged, but eventually is reversible. With the nerve gas agents, soman and sarin, the binding is irreversible. Acute and severe organophosphate poisoning is characterized by an increase in secretions—four classic symptoms including salivation, lacrimation, urination, and defecation (SLUD). These symptoms can progress to muscular twitching, extreme weakness, and paralysis. Carbamate insecticides, which include carbaryl, Aldicarb, and Sevin, also bind to acetylcholinesterase and inhibit the breakdown of acetylcholine. In this case, the carbamate-enzyme complex is not stable and readily disassociates, resulting in reversible inhibition of acetycholinesterase.[48]

Hepatotoxicants

Structure and Function of the Hepatic System

The liver is the largest single organ in the body. It has two lobes, which consist of many lobules. The anatomical features of the liver lobule are shown in Figure 5.12. The lobule, which is the functional unit of the liver, consists of cords of liver cells surrounding a central vein. Venous blood reaches the liver from the lower extremities, kidneys, spleen, and the gastrointestinal (GI) tract. The blood from the GI tract that reaches the liver through the hepatic portal vein is nutrient-rich, but oxygen-poor. This blood passes into the hepatic sinusoids between the lobular cords of liver cells. Here the venous blood is mixed with oxygen-rich and nutrient-poor blood from the hepatic artery, which is the other major source of blood for the liver. The blood from the sinusoids finds its way to the center of the lobule and to the central vein, which eventually exits the liver through the hepatic veins.[17]

Lipophilic substances, such as organic solvents, are easily absorbed by the liver. If they are not biotransformed into water-soluble substances, which allows them to be removed from the liver, they will accumulate in the liver. If toxicants become concentrated in the liver, damage can occur. Protein-carrier molecules in the cell membrane can transport copper and iron ions into the hepatocyte, the liver cell, for use in normal cell function. Toxic metals, such as mercury and lead, can compete with these essential metals for the protein-carrier molecules in the cell membrane, and thereby be easily absorbed into the liver. There are two other

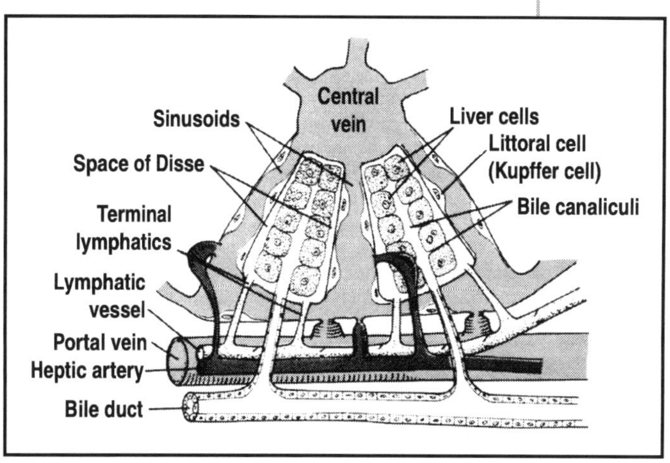

Figure 5.12 — A Liver Lobule.

mechanisms that allow toxicants to be absorbed into the hepatocyte. Blood enters the sinusoids between strands of hepatocyes. The layer of endothelial cells lining the sinusoids is discontinuous with fenestrae or pore like structures. These openings allow larger molecules in the blood to pass through the endothelial lining into the hepatocyte. As a result, it is easier for toxic materials that are bound to blood proteins to pass through the endothelial lining and be absorbed by the hepatocyte. Metallothionein, an intracellular protein, is also present in the liver cell. It has a high affinity for toxic metals such as cadmium, mercury, and lead. Therefore, when bound to metallothionein, the protein-metal complex does not easily leave the cell through the cell membrane. Due to these mechanisms, toxicants can reach higher concentrations in the liver cell than in surrounding tissue.(17)

There are six major metabolic functions of the liver: interconversion of carbohydrates, fats, and proteins; removal of excess nitrogen; storage; destruction of red blood cells; synthesis of substances for metabolic activities; and detoxification. The liver can interconvert carbohydrates, fats, and proteins, depending on the needs of the body. If glucose levels are low, glucose can be generated from amino acids, which are the components of proteins. The liver will convert protein and carbohydrate to fat when blood glucose levels are normal. The liver will metabolize excess amino acids, creating ammonia. It is converted to urea in the liver and then excreted by the kidneys. Substances such as carbohydrates, fats, proteins, and fat-soluble vitamins A, D, E, and K, and metabolically important metals, are stored in the liver. Since red blood cells have a life span of approximately 120 days, as they degenerate they are engulfed by macrophages throughout the body. Macrophages in the liver are known as Kupffer cells and are active in destroying red blood cells. A protein, bilirubin, is a byproduct of red blood cell destruction in the liver. It is metabolized by the liver and its metabolites are excreted in the bile to the small intestine or removed by the kidneys. The liver also synthesizes several different substances that are important to vital functions. It synthesizes glycogen, which is stored in the liver for use when glucose levels are low. The liver produces albumin, the most common glycoprotein in the blood. Albumin is released into the blood to maintain proper osmotic pressure. Proteins involved in blood clotting, prothrombin and fibrinogen, are synthesized in the liver. Heme, an organic compound containing iron and nitrogen, is produced in the liver and then used in developing reticulocytes to form hemoglobin. Bile is also synthesized in the liver and stored in the gall bladder and is used in digestion and absorption of fats in the small intestine. The liver metabolizes endogenous substances from normal processes as well as toxic substances that enter the body through ingestion, inhalation, or dermal absorption. Several oxidation-reduction metabolic processes are involved that convert toxins to more water-soluble and less toxic forms. Being more water-soluble increases excretion by the kidneys. In some situations, the metabolic conversion can result in increased toxicity, resulting in bioactivation instead of detoxification. In addition to engulfing degenerated red blood cells, the macrophages of the liver, Kupffer cells, can engulf and destroy foreign substances that are too large to pass through cell membranes or are lipid insoluble.

Examples of Hepatotoxicants

Workplace chemicals can cause liver toxicity by a variety of mechanisms, including liver cell death and fatty liver (steatosis), immune-mediated damage, cirrhosis/fibrosis, biliary damage, and by cancer.

Agents That Cause Liver Cell Death and Fatty Liver. Cell death can occur by apoptosis or necrosis. Apoptosis, also known as programmed cell death, occurs in response to cellular signals that initiate specific death pathways. Apoptotic cells shrink with the nucleus condensing and then fragmenting. Small bud-like "apoptotic bodies" pinch off the cells and are ingested by Kupffer cells. There is very little cellular debris and no leaking of intracellular contents. Due to this, there is no inflammatory response to apoptosis. Necrotic cells swell. Plasma membranes allow leakage of intracellular liver enzymes. Necrotic cells release chemical signals that attract an influx of inflammatory cells. Hepatitis is the term used for this influx of inflammatory cells in association with cellular necrosis. There are three primary patterns of necrotic death: focal, zonal and panacinar. Focal death is the death of just a few cells in a defined area. Zonal death is centrilobular, midzonal or periportal in nature. An example of zonal death is the centrilobular necrosis seen in livers of animals and humans exposed to toxic levels of carbon tetrachloride. Panacinar cell death is massive cell death. Fatty liver (steatosis) is characterized by an increase in hepatic lipid content and is often in conjunction with hepatocellular necrosis. Steatosis is readily visible as round vesicles of fat that fill the cytoplasm of hepatocytes. It is reversible once exposure stops and is a clear marker of potential hepatotoxicity. Carbon tetrachloride is known to cause extensive centrilobular necrosis of the liver. Inhalation of high levels of carbon tetrachloride has been shown to cause elevated serum enzyme levels[60], steatosis and centrilobular necrosis.[61] Liver fibrosis or cirrhosis can develop after acute and chronic exposure.[62] Carbon tetrachloride is bioactivated to a more reactive metabolite (free radical) by phase I enzymes. CYP2E1 is the predominant metabolizing enzyme in humans. Alcohol consumption will increase the levels of CYP2E1 in hepatocytes, so individuals who drink alcohol are much more likely to develop liver toxicity following exposure to carbon tetrachloride than those who don't drink alcohol. CYP2E1 bioactivates carbon tetrachloride to the reactive trichloromethyl radical. In the presence of oxygen, the trichloromethyl radical forms another reactive metabolite, the trichloromethylperoxy radical. The peroxy radical can cause significant cellular toxicity through destruction of intracellular membranes. This is called lipid peroxidation. Steatosis is the result of blocked transport of lipids due in part to lipid peroxidation. After this occurs, soluble liver enzymes begin to appear in the plasma, and necrosis is seen in the centrilobular hepatocytes. "Fibroblast-like" cells in the sinusoid, called Ito cells, begin producing large amounts of collagen, leading to fibrosis in the affected regions of the liver. 1,1,2,2-tetrachloroethane is one of the most toxic of the chlorinated hydrocarbon solvents. Workers with high exposure to this compound usually present with jaundice, pale stools and tenderness over the upper abdomen. Autopsy shows livers to be markedly reduced in size. Microscopic examination shows extensive centrilobular necrosis. The mechanism of toxicity for 1,1,2,2-tetrachloroethane is also lipid peroxidation due to free radical formation.[63]

Agents That Cause Immune-Mediated Damage. First, exposure to a new chemical occurs. The chemical is bioactivated in the liver to a reactive metabolite that binds to a specific protein in hepatocytes. The immune system does not recognize the modified protein and treats it as a foreign substance by forming antibodies against the metabolite-protein complex (protein adduct). If a second exposure occurs, the reactive metabolite again binds to the protein forming more of the protein adduct. Now, cells containing the protein adduct are attacked by the new antibodies formed after the first exposure. Liver toxicity occurs as hepatocytes are destroyed by the body's own immune system.[63] For example, "halothane hepatitis" was found to occur most often in patients who had previously been given halothane as an anesthetic agent. Halothane hepatitis is characterized by severe hepatocellular necrosis. Halothane is metabolized by CYP2E1 to reactive metabolites that bind to cellular macromolecules. With oxygen present, halothane is converted to trifluoroacetyl chloride (TFAC).[64] This then binds to proteins, including CYP450 enzymes, producing modified cellular proteins called TFAC-antigens. When the next exposure to halothane occurs, the immune system mounts a defense against the newly formed TFAC-antigens.

Agents That Cause Cirrhosis/Fibrosis. The replacement of functioning hepatocytes with fibrotic tissue is cirrhosis. Chronic, repeated exposure to hepatotoxicants causes hepatocyte death which stimulates the deposition of collagen by activated Ito cells. It is hypothesized that trinitrotoluene (TNT) is metabolized to reactive metabolites that bind to liver proteins[65] and produce oxidative stress.[66] The production of reactive oxygen species (ROSs), including superoxide radicals, may be the mechanism for activating the Ito cells to begin producing extracellular matrix.

Agents That Cause Biliary Damage. The reduction in bile volume or reduced secretion of bile components, such as bilirubin, into bile is known as cholestasis. Some toxicants can cause blockage of the canaliculi (bile ducts), causing bilirubin to accumulate in blood or urine, leading to jaundice. Some hepatotoxicants can cause direct damage to the bile ducts. Methylene dianiline (MDA) causes cholestasis and damage to biliary structures. It is hypothesized that MDA is metabolized to a reactive metabolite that is excreted through the bile.[67] Reactive metabolites would concentrate in biliary ducts causing necrosis of biliary epithelial cells.

Agents That Cause Cancer. Malignant neoplasms can arise from hepatocytes (hepatocellular carcinoma), bile duct cells (cholangiosarcomas) or from sinusoidal cells (angiosarcomas). Occupational exposure to high levels of vinyl chloride has been found to increase the incidence of liver angiosarcomas. After inhalation, vinyl chloride (VC) enters the bloodstream and is quickly distributed to the liver and kidneys. Once in the liver, VC is bioactivated by CYP2E1 to 2-chloroethylene oxide, a reactive metabolite capable of binding to DNA and RNA. This can cause mutations that can result in cancer.[68] Up to 70% of the metabolites of VC migrate out of the hepatocyte into the sinusoid. This may explain why the primary tumor associated with VC overexposure is not derived from hepatocytes, but from the endothelial cells that line the blood vessels or sinusoids (angiosarcoma).[63]

Reproductive Toxicants

Anatomy and Physiology of the Male Reproductive System

The structures of the male reproductive tract include the testes, epididymis, ductus deferens, seminal vesicles, urethra, prostate gland, and bulbourethral gland. The testes are divided into lobules that contain seminiferous tubules, where sperm cells develop. These tubules are surrounded by tissue that contains interstitial cells called cells of Leydig. These cells secrete testosterone, the male hormone. The seminiferous tubules join with the efferent ductules, which then join the epididymis.[17]

As the result of mitotic and meiotic cell divisions in the seminiferous tubules, spermatogenesis occurs. First, spermatogenia or germ cells mitotically divide to produce additional spermatogenia and primary spermatocytes. Second, the primary spermatocytes divide meiotically to produce two secondary spermatocytes. Now, each of the two secondary spermatocytes undergo the second meiotic division to produce four smaller cells called spermatids. These cells become smaller and develop flagellum. After these changes occur in the spermatids, they become sperm cells or spermatozoan. Sertoli cells are also located in the seminiferous tubules. They regulate spermatogenesis, as well as provide metabolic and structural support for the germ cells, secrete fluid for sperm transport, and form part of the blood-tubule barrier in the testis.

The secretion of hormones and the nervous system are involved in regulating the development of sperm and the function of the male reproductive system. Gonadotropin-releasing hormone (GnRH) is released from neurons in the hypothalamus of the brain. GnRH causes luteinizing hormone (LH) and follicle-stimulating hormone (FSH) to be released from the anterior pituitary. LH causes the secretion of testosterone from the cells of Leydig, which is essential for spermatogenesis. FSH interacts with the Sertoli cells, causing spermatogenesis.

Anatomy and Physiology of the Female Reproductive System

The ovaries, fallopian tubes, and the uterus are components of the female reproductive system. The egg is released from the ovary into the fallopian tube where it may be fertilized. If it is fertilized, then it may implant in the uterus.

Ovarian follicles are in the ovary and contain oocytes, which are structures analogous to spermatogenia. At birth the oocyte has begun the first meiotic division, but it is stopped at an early stage. These are the primary oocytes. Granulosa cells surround the primary oocyte in a single layer. Primodial follicles consist of primary oocytes and granulosa cells. There are about 300,000 to 400,000 primodial follicles at birth. After the beginning of puberty, primordial follicles change in response to hormones secreted during the monthly cycle. Each month a follicle enlarges to form a Graafian follicle. After the first meiotic division is completed the follicle ruptures releasing the egg. This is known as ovulation. The second meiotic division is initiated but is not completed. At fertilization the second division is completed. Fertilization usually occurs in the upper third of the fallopian tube. The uterus has three layers: external serous layer; middle layer or myometrium; and the innermost layer called the endometrium. During the menstrual cycle and pregnancy, the endometrium changes a great deal.

The pituitary gland and specialized cells in the ovary secrete hormones that control ovulation and changes in the endometrium of the uterus. These hormones have cyclic levels. Changes in the hormone levels cause ovulation to occur on average every 28 days. An increase in FSH in the blood causes one follicle to grow large enough to rupture and release an egg cell. The follicle secretes estrogen, which causes changes in the endometrium. Increased levels of LH actually cause ovulation to occur. Cells of the ruptured follicle now form the corpus luteum. This structure secretes another hormone, progesterone, along with estrogen. Both of these hormones help to prepare the endometrium for the potential implantation of a fertilized egg. The corpus luteum degenerates, if pregnancy does not occur, and then the cycle begins again.

Examples of Reproductive Toxicants

Substances in the workplace can have potential effects on reproduction in humans. General reproductive effects, gender differences, and fertility effects have been seen with specific chemicals in the occupational setting.

Agents That Effect General Reproductive Outcomes. 2-bromopropane (2BP) exposure has been found to have multiple reproductive effects in males and females working in the electronics industry.[69] A cluster of women performing switch assembly in an electronics factory experienced amenorrhea (lack of menstruation).[70] A high incidence of bone marrow effects as well as secondary amenorrhea accompanied by increased circulating FSH and LH levels and hot flashes were found in these women. Six of eight exposed men showed effects as well—two with azoospermia (no measurable sperm) and four with oligospermia (low sperm count) and reduced sperm motility. Studies in rats have shown 2BP to cause destruction of ovarian follicles in all stages of development.[71] In male rats, spermatogonia have been the target of 2BP.[72] A study to determine the effect of low-dose fuel (primarily JP-8 jet fuel) and solvent exposures (toluene, benzene) on female U.S. Air Force personnel was conducted. Pre-ovulatory LH levels were found to be significantly lower among women whose total hydrocarbon levels were above the median. This suggested that some compounds in fuels and some solvents may act as reproductive endocrine disruptors, but confirmation is still needed.[73] It is well understood that when ethanol is consumed during pregnancy at levels that produce a blood alcohol concentration of 150–200 mg/dL, a developmental toxic effect may occur (fetal alcohol syndrome). A legal blood alcohol content limit for driving in the U.S. is <0.08 g/dL, which equates to 80 mg/dL.[74] However, usually in the occupational setting exposure is by inhalation. For exposures up to 600 ppm ethanol, the predicted blood alcohol levels would be less than 1 mg/dL.[75] Therefore, when the data for ethanol in the workplace was reviewed, there was no evidence that occupational exposure to ethanol is a developmental toxicity hazard.[76]

Toxicants That Have Different Gender Effects. Exposure to xenobiotics are often assumed to have similar effects on reproductive processes in the male and female, but there are cases in which one sex may be susceptible and the other not. Therefore, gender differences should always be considered. For example, in the case of chemicals that destroy germ cells in the early stages of meiotic division, extensive damage may cause irreversible ovarian failure in females, but reversible reductions in spermatogenesis in males. Within the ovary the oocyte is arrested in prophase of the first meiotic division, and once destroyed, no more are formed. However, within the testis, spermatogonia can divide by mitosis to maintain a continuously renewable source of these cells.[69] Exposure to di-n-butyl phthalate (DBP) during gestation and lactation specifically impaired the androgen-dependent development of the male reproductive tract, suggesting that DBP is not estrogenic but antiandrogenic in the rat.[77] In the female rat, effects of DBP have been reported in pregnant rats. Effects included impaired implantation in mated females.[78] 2,3,7,8-tetrachlorodibenzo-p-dioxin (TCDD) has been found to possibly influence the sex ratio in children with more females born than males, but more research is needed.[79,80]

Agents That Effect Fertility. Inability to produce a clinically recognizable pregnancy after one year of unprotected intercourse is the definition of infertility.[81] Traditionally, it has been linked with female health problems. However, evidence indicates that spermatogenesis (production of round spermatids) and spermiogenesis (cellular differentiation of spermatids into spermatozoa) are highly susceptible to many toxic substances in the workplace. The following substances are known to have an effect on fertility: 1,2-dibromo-3-chloropropane (DBCP), glycol ethers, metals, styrene, lead, trimethyltin, inorganic arsenic, and perfluoroalkyl acids. Men working in a pesticide factory with exposures to 1,2 dibromo-3-chloropropane (DBCP), a nematocide, were found to be suffering from infertility.[82] Workers with sperm counts less than one million had been exposed at least three years, while workers exposed for only three months had normal sperm counts. Sperm motility in workers exposed longer was also reduced and there was an increase in abnormal morphology of sperm. FSH levels were significantly elevated among the workers exposed for longer durations. In an animal study, DBCP produced severe atrophy of the testes with degenerative changes in the seminiferous tubules and reduction in number of sperm cells.[83] In a large shipbuilding facility a study was completed among men handling paints containing glycol ethers.[84] Semen analysis indicated that glycol ethers caused a decline in sperm counts.[85] Testicular atrophy was seen in mice exposed to 2-methoxyethanol (2-ME).[86] Studies have been conducted to determine the potential for welding exposures to affect fertility because of the metals involved, the heat and low doses of ultraviolet radiation. Mild steel workers showed a moderate decline in several semen parameters, as well as an increase in FSH.[87] Major components in welding fumes are iron, zinc, and manganese; while chromium, nickel, copper, cadmium and lead are present in trace quantities.[88] The metals in welding fumes may be producing testicular damage and decreased semen quality. Therefore, welding has the potential to produce reproductive effects, but a more comprehensive study is needed. A study in plastics workers has provided evidence that low-level styrene exposure may deteriorate spermatogenesis.[89] In an animal study, the metabolite of styrene, styrene oxide, has been shown to produce reproductive and developmental toxicity and maternal toxicity.[90] A study was conducted in men employed by ten companies with potential lead exposures (two smelters, three battery companies, three copper alloy foundries, a hospital, and a security company).[91] The median sperm concentration was decreased by 49% in men with blood lead concentration above 50 micrograms/dL. A threshold slope least square regression identified a blood lead concentration of 44 micrograms/dL as a potential threshold for sperm reduction. Trimethyltin (TMT) caused a decrease in maternal weight in pregnant rats and became more pronounced with increasing dose. Litter sizes were decreased for groups treated with the highest dose of TMT.[92] A variety of species have shown embryotoxic effects after exposure to inorganic arsenic. Malformations of the skeleton, neural tube (developing brain), and eyes have been reported in animal studies.[93]

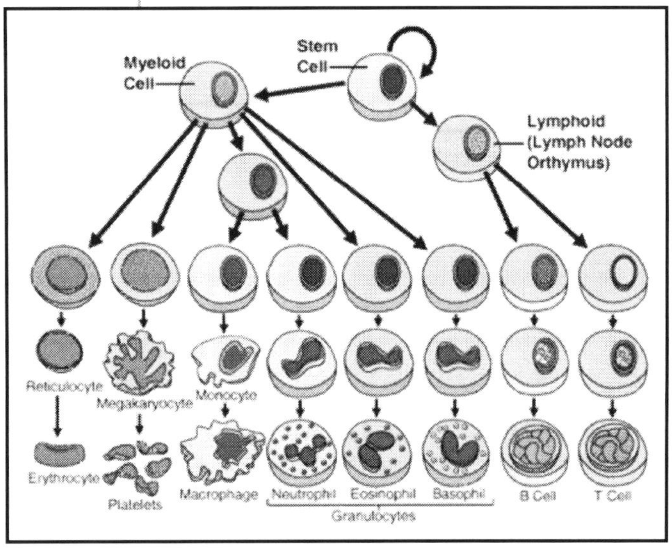

Figure 5.13 — Differentiation of Blood Cells (Source: National Biological Information Infrastructure, accessed from (http://www.nbii.gov/portal/server.pt/community/basic_genetics___cell_biology/401/cell_differentiation/564).

Hematotoxicants

Components of the Blood

The blood is composed of cellular material in a non-cellular liquid, called plasma. The cells are derived from non-differentiated stem cells found in the bone marrow, as depicted by Figure 5.13. The stem cells differentiate into red blood cells or erythrocytes, white blood cells or leukocytes, and platelets or thrombocytes. Leukocytes can be divided into granulocytes and agranulocytes. Neutrophils, eosinophils, and basophils are granulocytes. Neutrophils make up 60–70 % of all leukocytes. Neutrophils phagocytize bacteria and foreign matter in the blood. Eosinophils make up only 1–4 % of leukocytes. They are involved in inflammation. Basophils make up 0.5–1 % of leukocytes. They release histamine, promoting inflammation, and heparin, which prevents blood clotting. Lymphocytes and monocytes are agranulocytes. Lymphocyes make up 20–30 % of leukocytes. They are involved in the immune response by producing antibodies, which kill microorganisms, are involved in allergic responses, reject tissue grafts, and control cancerous cells. Monocytes have the largest size of all leukocytes. They make up 2–8 % of all leukocytes. They migrate out of the blood, become larger, and are then called macrophages. They phagocytize bacteria, cell fragments, and other tissue debris. The erythrocyte is the most numerous of all blood cells. They carry oxygen from the lungs to all the cells throughout the body. They also carry carbon dioxide from the tissues to the lungs for exhalation. The transport of oxygen and carbon dioxide is facilitated by hemoglobin, an iron containing molecule found in the erythrocyte. Thrombocytes are small cell fragments consisting of cytoplasm with a cell membrane. They come from megakaryocytes in the bone marrow. Each cell fragment has granules which contain chemicals involved in blood clotting. The plasma of the blood is about 92% water and 8% other materials, such as proteins, ions, nutrients, gases, and waste products. Albumin, globulin, and fibrinogen are the most abundant proteins in the blood. Fibrinogen is involved in blood clotting. Blood formation is known as hematopoiesis. It occurs primarily in the bone marrow, which is in the medullary cavity of bone. All blood cells originate from a single multipotential cell known as a stem cell or hemocytoblast.[17]

Examples of Hematotoxicants

Mature blood cells as well as immature blood cells in the bone marrow can be adversely affected by toxic substances. The effects that result are dependent upon the type of substance, length of exposure, and concentration. A transient decrease in production of one or more types of cells with recovery after exposure ends occur. Also exposures may result in persistent, long-term decrease in the number of cells. Changes in the type and number of circulating blood cells include anemia, granulcytopenia, thrombocytopenia, lymphocytopenia, or pancytopenia.

Agents That Cause Anemia. A decrease in the number of red blood cells (RBCs), a decrease in the size of RBCs, a decrease in RBC hemoglobin content, or a combination of any of these, is defined as anemia. Microcytic anemia is a decrease in the size of RBCs. Toxins, excessive blood loss, and nutritional deficiencies can cause anemia. Toxins can interact directly with RBCs or interact with precursor cells in the bone marrow. Some insecticides bind to the surface of the RBC, forming a RBC/insecticide complex that is recognized as a foreign substance by the immune system. It is destroyed by this defense mechanism. Other toxins, such as benzene, lead, methylene chloride, nitrobenzene and naphthalene are capable of destroying RBCs directly by interfering with cell membrane integrity and ion balance. Since oxygen is transported bound to hemoglobin, any toxic substance that decreases the synthesis of hemoglobin may cause anemia. Lead decreases hemoglobin synthesis by interfering with the synthesis of the globin portion of hemoglobin. Lead also inhibits the use of iron in the heme portion of hemoglobin. Therefore, lead inhibits the synthesis of hemoglobin, resulting in a decrease in the oxygen-carrying capacity of the blood. The brain and the heart are the first to demonstrate symptoms due to a decrease in oxygen availability. Normal nerve and heart cell functions are disrupted with arrhythmias possible. Shortness of breath, pale skin, and fatigue may occur. Aplastic anemia occurs when toxic chemicals, such as carbon tetrachloride, chlordane or benzene, affect the cells of the bone marrow directly, suppressing the production of RBCs. Benzene acts primarily upon the stem cells in the bone marrow, inhibiting their differentiation into mature RBCs. Other toxic substances, such as mercury and cadmium, may adversely affect the functioning of the kidneys, decreasing the secretion of erythropoietin, which is normally released in response to low oxygen levels in the blood to stimulate bone marrow to produce more RBCs. This is known as nephrotoxicity-induced anemia.

Agents That Induce Hypoxia. When inadequate amounts of oxygen are delivered to the tissues, hypoxia occurs. Oxygen transport capability of RBCs can be adversely affected by some chemicals. If carbon monoxide is inhaled, it will bind with hemoglobin forming carboxyhemoglobin. Since the affinity of hemoglobin for carbon monoxide is more than 225 times greater than that for oxygen, carbon monoxide will displace oxygen in the RBCs. As a result, the oxygen-carrying capacity of the blood is significantly decreased. Oxygen reaching tissues becomes decreased with the smooth muscle of blood vessels unable to contract, resulting in a drop in blood pressure. With a drop in blood pressure, the heart rate increases. Dizziness, fainting, headaches, muscular weakness, and nausea can occur. Normally the hemoglobin molecule contains an iron atom in the ferrous state (Fe^{2+}). Certain toxins, such as sodium nitrite, hydroxylamine hydrochloride, or nitrobenzene, will convert the ferrous atom to the ferric atom (Fe^{3+}). This converts hemoglobin into methemoglobin (MetHb). MetHb does not carry oxygen to body tissues. Symptoms just as with exposure to carbon monoxide occur. Some toxic substances produce symptoms that appear to be chemically-induced hypoxia without changing the oxygen-carrying capacity of the blood. For example, hydrogen cyanide or hydrogen sulfide interferes with the ability of cells to use oxygen. This is cytotoxic hypoxia.

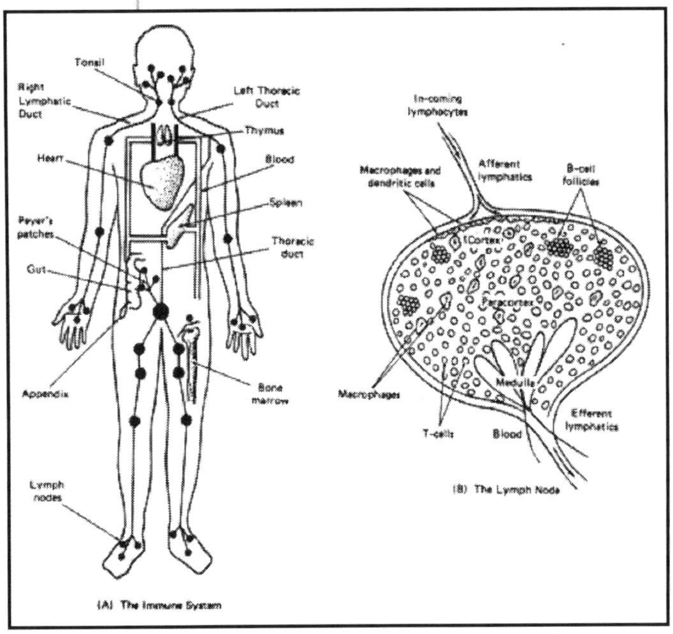

Figure 5.14 — The Immune System and The Lymph Node (Source: *Todar's Online Textbook of Bacteriology* by Kenneth Todar, PhD, accessed from http://www.textbookofbacteriology.net/immune.html).

Granulocytopenia, Lymphocytopenia, and Thrombocytopenia. Granulocytopenia, lymphocytopenia, and thrombocytopenia are the decrease in granulocytes, lymphocytes, and thrombocytes, respectively. They occur due to suppression of stem cell proliferation and differentiation. Benzene, carbon tetrachloride, and trinitrotoluene can suppress the stem cells for these blood cells. Some pesticides (DDT) and dinitrophenol only affect the production of white blood cells. Thrombocytopenia results in slower clotting of the blood. Granulocytopenia and lymphocytopenia result in a depression of the immune system.

Agents That Cause Leukemia. Exposure to benzene may cause a total suppression of all stem cells, resulting in pancytopenia, which is anemia, leukocytopenia, and thrombocytopenia together. This is followed by a sudden increase in white blood cells above and beyond normal values, called leukemia.

Immunotoxicants

Structure and Function of the Immune System

Cells of the lymphatic system and cells of the blood, as well as antibodies are the major components of the immune system. The actions of these three components are integrated in a manner to remove or destroy microorganisms and other environmental factors that can cause illness and disease.[17] The components of the immune system and the lymph node are illustrated in Figure 5.14.

Liquid from the blood is filtered through the walls of capillaries into the space between cells, known as interstitial space. Most of this liquid is reabsorbed into the blood, but a small amount remains in the interstitial space and eventually moves into lymphatic vessels. The liquid moves into lymphatic capillaries that are anatomically similar to blood vessel capillaries, since they both are a single cell thick. This liquid is call lymph and it ultimately is returned to the bloodstream by either the right lymphatic duct or the thoracic duct, which empties into the heart. As the lymph travels through the lymphatic vessels it passes through structures called lymph nodes. Dense populations of lymphocytes and other cells are in the lymph nodes, forming lymph nodules. Between the lymph nodules are sinuses that contain macrophages. The lymphocytes and macrophages serve as an effective filter for microorganisms and cellular debris in the lymph. If microorganisms are present, the lymphocytes proliferate quickly. They can leave the lymph nodules and travel to other lymph nodes throughout the body. The spleen and the thymus are also part of the lymphatic system. Lymphocytes and macrophages are in the spleen and serve to remove and destroy microorganisms as the blood passes through the spleen. Lymphocytes are produced and mature in the thymus. These lymphocytes will enter the blood and eventually find their way to other lymphatic tissues in the body, including other lymph nodes and the spleen.

Other cells found in the blood and originating in the bone marrow, including lymphocytes, macrophages, and neutrophils are also part of the immune system. They have already been discussed in the section on hematotoxicants in this chapter. Lymphocytes further differentiate into T cell lymphocytes and B cell lymphocytes. Specialized T cells, known as natural killer (NK) cells, can recognize and destroy virus-infected cells and cancer-like cells. Neutrophils and macrophages can phagocytize and destroy bacteria in a nonspecific manner. A more specific response is provided by the T and B lymphocytes in the form of antibody production.

T cells, B cells, and macrophages interact with each other to cause the production of antibodies that are perfectly specific for a foreign substance or an antigen. Macrophages present antigens to T cells, which interact with B cells. This stimulates the B cells to divide and form plasma cells, which synthesize the antibody specific for the antigen.

Examples of Immunotoxicants

These toxic substances suppress the immune response, resulting in individuals becoming more susceptible to illnesses and disease. Various aspects of the immune system can be adversely affected, such as the inhibition of the production of leukocytes in the bone marrow, inhibition of the proliferation of leukocytes in response to an antigen; inhibition of cellular mechanisms involved in producing antibodies.

Halogenated Aromatic Hydrocarbons. This group of organic compounds include polychlorinated biphenyls (PCBs), polybrominated biphenyls (PBBs), polychlorinated dibenzo-p-dioxins (2,3,7,8-tetrachlorodibenzo-p-dioxin or TCDD), and dibenzofurans. These compounds cause atrophy of the thymus, decrease in all blood cell types, decrease in antibody production, and they promote tumor growth. PCBs are known to atrophy the spleen, reduce the number of circulating lymphocytes, and decrease antibody production. TCDD causes the atrophy of lymphoid organs, inhibits lymphocyte development and maturation, and inhibits the development and maturation of B cells with resultant decrease in antibody production. Dibenzofurans have similar effects on the immune system as TCDD. Individuals poisoned by contaminated rice with TCDD had a decreased number of circulating T cells and recurring respiratory infections.

Polycyclic Aromatic Hydrocarbons. These compounds include anthracene, benzanthracene, benzo[a]pyrene, dimethylbenz[a]anthracene, and methylcholanthrene. All of these compounds are carcinogenic, which may be due to their immunosuppressive characteristics. Benzo[a]pyrene (BaP) suppresses the division of B cells and their differentiation into plasma cells, with the resultant suppression of antibody production. 7,12-dimethylbenz[a]anthracene (DMBA) may be carcinogenic because it suppresses antibody production, natural killer cell activity, and tumor resistance.

Heavy Metals. High concentrations of lead, arsenic, mercury, and cadmium will cause immunosuppression. Lead causes the decrease in the production of antibodies. Arsenic suppresses the immune system by inhibiting circulating lymphocyte proliferation, decreasing formation of plasma cells, with a resultant decrease in antibody production. Mercury binds and inhibits enzymes involved in antibody synthesis in B cells. Mercury can also cause an autoimmune response in the kidney. Since mercury is stored in the kidney, it forms a protein-mercury complex that is recognized as a foreign substance by the immune system. As a result, the immune system attacks the kidney tissue in which it is stored. This autoimmune disease of the kidney is glomerular nephritis, which can result in kidney failure. Cadmium causes decreased lymphocyte proliferation and suppression of macrophages and antibody production.

Pesticides. High doses of organophosphate pesticides decrease antibody production. Parathion suppresses antibody production, natural killer cell and macrophage activity. It causes the atrophy of the thymus and it decreases the proliferation of lymphocytes in response to antigens. Organochlorine pesticides (DDT) decreases antibody production.

Organic Solvents. Toluene has little effect on the immune system, but it will reduce the effect of benzene, by competing with it for the metabolic enzymes needed for bioactivation. Nitrobenzene and 2,4-dinitrotoluene suppress antibody production. 2,4-dinitrotoluene also suppresses natural killer cell and macrophage activity.

Carcinogenesis

Chromosome Structure and Function

Deoxyribonucleic acid (DNA) along with histones make up most of the structure of chromosomes. Long strands of nucleotides make up DNA. Each nucleotide has a sugar (deoxyribose in the case of DNA), a base, and a phosphate group, as shown in Figure 5.15. Histones are proteins that are involved in regulating genes on the chromosomes. There are two strands of nucleotides bound together forming a double-helix that make up the structure of DNA. The strands of nucleotides are bound together by hydrogen bonds between bases in each strand. Adenine and guanine, which are purines; and thymine and cytosine, which are pyrimidines, are the four bases found in DNA. The bases in one strand bind to the bases in the other strand in a particular manner. Adenine binds to thymine; cytosine binds to guanine.

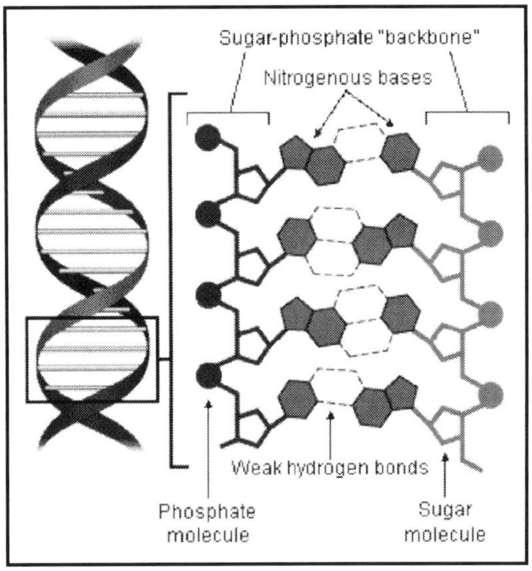

Figure 5.15 — Deoxyribonucleic Acid (DNA) Structure (Source: University of California at Berkley, accessed from http://www.evolution.berkeley.edu/evosite/history/dna2.shtml).

Somatic cells have two sets of chromosomes (diploid), while sex cells have one set of chromosomes (haploid). Portions of DNA, along the chromosome strands, consisting of thousands of nucleotides, contain the genes. Genes are responsible for the synthesis of structural and functional proteins. During protein synthesis the double helix of DNA separate, allowing the exposed sequence of bases to provide a code for the synthesis of the specific protein. The DNA code first directs the formation of messenger RNA (ribonucleic acid), which has bases that are complementary to the bases in the exposed portion of DNA. The messenger RNA carries the genetic information in the nucleus to the ribosome in the cytoplasm of the cell so protein synthesis can begin. Codons or base triplets on the mRNA specify the amino acids to be used in the protein being synthesized. So, the sequence of codons in mRNA will determine the amino acid sequence in the protein. Each amino acid is carried to the proper position by another type of RNA, transfer RNA (tRNA), which has the same code of the mRNA. mRNA and tRNA interaction result in a specific protein molecule being formed.[17]

Examples of Carcinogens

It is believed that as high as 90% of all cancers are due to exposure to environmental agents, including chemical agents. Cancer is characterized by uncontrolled division and growth of cells. They divide rapidly and invade normal tissues, consuming enormous amounts of energy and displacing cells that perform normal functions. Exactly how cancer is initiated is not totally understood.

Definitions. Any cancer-causing substance, chemical or physical, such as benzene, cadmium, asbestos, or certain types of radiation, is a carcinogen. A new (neo) growth (plasia) is a neoplasm. An enlarged mass of cells is a tumor. Tumors are benign or malignant. Benign tumors are usually encapsulated by fibrous tissue, have uncontrolled, but slow growth of cells that do not invade surrounding tissues. Malignant tumors are not encapsulated and invade normal surrounding tissues, have rapid growth and their cells metastasize to other parts of the body. Different forms of neoplasm can be classified according to the type of tissue in which they originated. Benign tumors usually have the suffix "oma". A benign tumor originating from the dermal papillae is called an epidermal papilloma. Mesothelioma, lymphoma, and melanoma are notable exceptions to the suffix "oma" emplying a benign tumor. A malignant tumor that originated from epithelial cells is called a carcinoma and a malignant tumor from bone or muscle is called a sarcoma. For example, an adenoma is benign, while an adenocarcinoma is malignant. A fibroma is benign, but fibrosarcoma is malignant.

Mechanisms of Action. Toxic substances that interact directly with DNA or affect DNA replication are genotoxic carcinogens. The somatic cell mutation theory says that genotoxic carcinogens interact with DNA and produce mutation of the genes controlling cell division, resulting in uncontrolled growth of nondifferentiated cells, forming a tumor. The single-hit theory or one-hit theory of carcinogenesis says that a genotoxic carcinogen at any exposure level can cause a single genotoxic event that results in irreversible damage to a critical segment of the DNA responsible for controlling cell division. Epigenetic carcinogens promote the development of cancer without directly interacting with the DNA of cells by causing the loss of cell communication, hormone imbalances, or cellular damage and excessive regeneration. The multiple-hit theory of carcinogenesis says that a series of mutations has occurred in affected cells and that the appearance of a tumor is due to the cumulative effect of the series of mutations over many years. A small number of random discrete changes in cell structure and function can account for the steady rise in cancer mortality with age.[94]

Stages of Development. The development and growth of tumors involves three distinct stages: initiation, promotion, and progression. The initiation stage is an irreversible change in the DNA structure caused by genotoxic agents. Promotion occurs when tumor growth is stimulated without the carcinogen interacting with DNA. The initiating and promoting carcinogens may or may not be the same agent. Removing the promotor carcinogen can result in stopping tumor growth. Tetrachlorodibenzo-p-dioxin (TCDD), androgens, and estrogens may promote cancer development in the liver. Like initiation, progression is also irreversible. Once the cancerous cells enter this stage, removal of the carcinogen has no effect on cell growth and development. Progressor agents may affect the DNA by inhibiting DNA repair. Progressor agents include arsenic salts, asbestos fibers, benzene, benzoyl peroxide, and 2,5,2',5'-tetrachlorobiphenyl.

Occupational Carcinogens. Chemical substances in the workplace have been associated with cancer development in workers. Asbestos fibers cause two types of cancer: bronchogenic carcinoma (lung cancer) and malignant mesothelioma (cancer of connective tissue). Frequency of occurrence of lung cancer among people exposed to asbestos is affected by smoking cigarettes. For example, a 5-fold increase in lung cancer incidence was found among asbestos workers, an 11-fold increase among cigarette smokers, and a 55-fold increase among asbestos workers who were cigarette smokers.[95] Other potential carcinogens in the workplace include: fiberglass, wood dust, various metals, benzene, and formaldehyde. Due to contamination with TCDD, organophosphate pesticides can be carcinogenic. Vinyl chloride causes cancer of the liver.

Identification and Classification of Carcinogens. The International Agency for Research on Cancer (IARC), part of the World Health Organization, was one of the first organizations to identify and classify chemicals according to their carcinogenicity. Other organizations have established lists of chemicals that are either known or suspected human carcinogens, including the Environmental Protection Agency (EPA), the Chemical Manufacturers Association (CMA), the ACGIH® and the Occupational Safety and Health Administration (OSHA). The National Toxicology Program (NTP) publishes the Report on Carcinogens (RoC) which lists substances that are either known to be carcinogens or may reasonably be anticipated to be human carcinogens.[96]

Exposure Level Setting

As shown in the Figure 5.1, Venn diagram risk assessment determination utilizes the three main divisions of toxicology: descriptive, mechanistic, and regulatory. For worker and public health safety concerns exposure standards are established primarily by three different types of organizations: regulatory, consensus and private industry. Regulatory organizations are governmental agencies, either federal, state, county, or city that may use the standards developed by consensus or guideline establishing organizations as the starting point for legal limits. These organizations are private groups that use knowledge of a specific industry and their injury and illness records or results from scientific studies to establish standards that are protective of worker health. In many cases the consensus standards are more restrictive than the legal standards. Regulatory agencies develop exposure limits based on risk and exposure assessments using the consensus level as the beginning but then expand these consensus levels into limits that carry the weight of law. Regulatory limits are designed to protect a much wider population than the consensus standards and include older and younger individuals, pregnant women, hypersensitive/hyposensitive individuals, immuno-compromised individuals, and other individuals not considered in the general working population. Private industry groups may have unique chemicals that are used in their processes and consequently develop occupational exposure limits for their personnel. In many cases these private industries will adopt existing consensus standards or will develop limits that are more restrictive than regulatory standards. However, if there are no existing standards then the industry may opt to develop their own set of standards.

There are numerous consensus organizations which produce and publish standards for their respective organizations. Many of these have had their consensus standards enacted directly into law, either in total or partially. Examples of the more common occupational exposure limit guidelines or consensus standard setting organizations include ACGIH®, the American National Standards Institute (ANSI), AIHA®, National Academy of Sciences/National Research Council (NAS/NRC), National Institute of Occupational Safety and Health (NIOSH), and others. Regulatory agencies who establish exposure limits that are supported by legal enforcement include the Occupational Safety and Health Admini stration (OSHA), the Environmental Protection Agency (EPA), the Department of Transportation (DOT), and others. International organizations, both governmental and private, also develop and publish exposure standards which are mostly recommended values and have no legal support in the United States. Organizations such as Germany's MAK Commission, the International Organization for Standardization (ISO), the World Health Organization (WHO), and many others recommend exposure levels for their respective areas. Most of these international standards are simply recommended values although some carry the force of law within signatory nations.

Many of the consensus organizations publish their values under specific names and the names often are trademarked for that organization. ACGIH® publishes the Threshold Limit Values (TLVs®) and the Biological Exposure Indices (BEIs®) for occupational exposure to common industrial chemicals.[15] TLVs® and BEIs® are not consensus standards, by definition of the consensus process, because TLV® and BEI® values are based on a review of existing peer-reviewed scientific literature by committees with experts in the respective fields. This organization annually publishes TLV® and BEI® values and has for many years. AIHA® annually produces Workplace Environmental Exposure Levels™ (WEEL™) which are also health-based chemical exposure limits for which there is no published guidance for health professionals.[16] WEELs™ are developed by committee using scientifically sound state-of-the-art risk assessment procedures. The WEEL™ Committee coordinates the development of WEEL™ values with the TLV® Committee to avoid duplication of effort in occupational exposure level development.

Another important organization which releases exposure values based upon scientific review by committee is the NAS/NRC. This organization functions through sub-committees for the review and development of position recommendations and is an advisory body to the U.S. government for a wide area of research, including chemical toxicology and radiological protection. The National Academy of Sciences has provided overall guidance for chemical risk assessment as further developed and applied by U.S. regulatory agencies.[97–99] The National Research Council of the National Academy of Sciences has published numerous reports addressing the development of occupational exposure limits (OELs) for confined and non-confined workplaces and for various activities and groups.[100–124] In the area of chemical toxicology, the NAS/NRC has evaluated the science behind the Emergency and Continuous Exposure Limits for Selected Airborne Contaminants, which established Emergency Exposure Guidance Levels (EEGLs), Short-Term Public Emergency Guidance Levels (SPEGLs), and Continuous Exposure Guidance Level (CEGLs) for a small number of chemicals of concern. Specific definitions for these exposure levels can be found in the respective references. The Department of Defense (DOD) and the National Aviation and Space Administration (NASA) were the original requesters of the services of the NAS/NRC in this regard. Best known in radiation are the volumes entitled Biological Effects of Ionizing Radiation (BEIR), which have carefully evaluated the status and quality of the science on setting radiation standards, especially considering low-level exposures.[125] EPA requires New Chemicals Exposure Limits (NCELs) for certain chemicals under TSCA 8(e) and 5(e) consent orders. They are generally developed in conjunction with specified work practices, engineering controls, and PPE requirements. There are approximately 100 NCELs to date.[126]

The EPA establishes standards for air contaminants, water contaminants, hazardous wastes, and toxic chemicals. EPA is charged with protecting community public health including the most susceptible individuals, and the environment in general. When EPA was created, there were fewer standards for environmental protection than for worker protection. Consequently, EPA had to develop standards or use those set by the National Institute for Environmental Health Sciences (NIEHS). EPA regulations are found in Title 40, Code of Federal Regulations (CFR).

The EPA has the broadest scope of standard setting of all U.S. government agencies because they are responsible for all aspects of hazardous waste, the manufacture of toxic chemicals, air pollution, water and groundwater protection, and radiation from naturally-occurring radionuclides. EPA has established standards for water quality and treatment under the Clean Water Act (CWA); hazardous waste operations under the Resource, Conservation, and Recovery Act (RCRA); past hazardous waste practices under the Comprehensive Environmental Restoration, Compensation, and Liability Act (CERCLA or "Superfund"); the Superfund Amendments and Reauthorization Act (SARA); and air releases under the Air Pollution Control Act (APCA) and, environmental radiation. Historically EPA is less involved in environmental radiation except for recommended public exposure levels to radon.

EPA conducts much of the necessary research itself, unlike the relationship that exists between OSHA and NIOSH. EPA standards have been promulgated by the agency, although inputs from the National Institute for Environmental Health Sciences (NIEHS) and the Agency For Toxic Substances and Disease Registery (ATSDR) have been used in setting standards. The EPA must consider the public at large not just occupationally-exposed workers. Workers are generally healthier, young adults, and aware of potential exposures. The public consists of people with greater susceptibility to injury from chemical and physical exposures; infants, children, the elderly, and the ill especially. These individuals need to be protected by EPA standards more so than workers who are protected by the OSHA standards. Furthermore, unlike workers, these individuals are not in control of their exposures. Numerous questions regarding exposure limit development have been raised: How protective should exposure standards be? Should individuals who are genetically predisposed to harm or with compromised immune systems be protected? Should only a statistical portion of the entire population be protected, for example the lower 5% to upper 95%? These questions have yet to be answered.

How can the general public or workers in general be assured that promulgated standards are protective of their health?

Currently a cost-benefit ratio philosophy is used to help make these decisions. Based on this philosophy there will always be a few individuals who fall outside the parameters that are set, regardless of the limits. However, it is believed that health-based standards are protective of the large majority of the population. When regulatory and consensus organizations develop standards, the uppermost concern is protecting the most individuals.

Private industry also establishes standards for their specific companies or groups of similar industries. These standards do not have the effect of law, may not be based upon scientific consensus, and are usually developed by company health and management professionals. The foundation for establishing any occupational exposure limit (OEL) is based on historical or current risk assessments. Paracelsus stated that "all substances are poisons; there is none which is not a poison. The right dose differentiates a poison from a remedy." This then is the foundation for establishing any OEL. Commonly, the OEL is regarded as a level of exposure to any airborne contaminant that is considered safe to nearly all workers. Individual susceptibility plays a role in response to the OEL levels; there may be adverse health effects at or below the established OEL. OELs are developed by various organizations and companies, and are primarily based upon the risk model discussed in the NAS/NRC book *Risk Assessment in the Federal Government: Managing the Process.*[98] This model incorporates risk assessment, risk characterization and risk management. Additional discussion regarding risk and exposure assessment can be found in other chapters of this book. The concepts of the time-weighted average (TWA), short-term exposure limit (STEL) and ceiling limits (CL) as discussed in the exposure assessment chapter are also pertinent when developing an OEL. Duration of exposure is of considerable concern when developing OELs which can be based on these concepts. As defined in the *ERPG™/WEEL™ Handbook*[16], the eight-hour TWA is the most frequently used exposure guideline used in the OSHA PELs and the ACGIH® TLVs®. The STEL represents a time-weighted average exposure that should not be exceeded for any 15-minute period. The STEL is referenced in the OSHA PEL-STEL and the ACGIH®'s TLV®-STEL. Finally, the ceiling limit is the maximum allowable human exposure limit for an airborne substance which is not to be exceeded even momentarily. Again, these ceiling limits are used in the OSHA PELs and the ACGIH® TLVs®. Frequently ceiling OELs are used for fast acting substances such as hydrogen fluoride or ozone; STELs are used with irritants such as formaldehyde or sulfur dioxide; and, TWAs are associated with slow acting irritants and chronic disease agents such as benzene, vinyl chloride or silica.

The ACGIH® TLVs® also may contain notations for skin and sensitizer. The skin designation refers to "the potential significant contribution to the overall exposure by the cutaneous route, including mucous membranes and the eyes, by contact with vapors, liquids, and solids."[15] The notation for sensitization refers to "the potential for an agent to produce sensitization, as confirmed by human or animal data."[15] These two aspects are not covered in a numerical OEL, but need to be considered in the management of occupational health risk. In general, OELs are not reduced to account for these two aspects, but must be considered by the industrial hygienist when developing protective measures.

Emerging Issues in Occupational Toxicology

Introduction

As has been previously discussed, on the order of 43% of the chemical compounds in commerce in the United States have not been adequately evaluated for toxicity.[127] In addition to new chemical compounds and new methods being developed to assess the toxicity of these substances, changes in the occupational environment require new approaches to assessing the risks associated with their use. Also, impacting the interpretation and use of new toxicity data are changes in the demographics of the workforce, shifting patterns in the kinds of work being done and the locations where these activities occur. The composition of the workforce is changing and will continue to change as traditional industrial economies migrate to new technologies and new areas and other economies become more "industrialized." These changes will also require changes in the assumptions on the potentially exposed populations, the length of exposure (changes in work shifts, and the time which is spent in the workforce), and potential confounding exposures.[128,129]

Nanotechnology

Among the emerging issues of concern to toxicologists and occupational health professionals are the development, manufacturing, use and environmental fate of nanoparticles. This technology requires an evaluation strategy that includes not only traditional toxicology, but a clearer understanding of the total impact of the physical, chemical and biological characteristics of these materials. As the breadth and scope of application of nanoparticles in research, medicine and industry increases, and their complexity evolves, they represent and will continue to represent a challenge to the toxicologist, occupational health specialist, medical practitioner, environmental professional and regulatory authorities.[130–134] Although a strategy for the evaluation and control of these materials in the workplace has been described[135] based on the application of traditional approaches, ongoing efforts are being made by the National Institute for Occupational Safety and Health (NIOSH) and others to continuously compile and make available to the occupational health profession new data in this evolving arena.[136] The nanotechnology topics page on the AIHA® website lists a number of links to useful sites for the practicing occupational health professional.

Toxicogenomics

The term "toxicogenomics" was coined to describe the application of genomic tools to toxicology.[137,138] In a joint meeting of the Committee on Toxicity, Committee on Mutagenicity and Committee on Carcinogenicity on the use of genomics and proteomics in toxicology, it was concluded that: there is great potential for the use of proteomics and genomics in toxicological risk assessment; the techniques may be used as adjuncts to conventional toxicology studies (particularly where specific proteins are known to be casually related to the toxicity); and there is a need for more research and validation before these techniques can be routinely used in regulatory toxicological assessment.[139,140] Similar conclusions resulted from an International Programme on Chemical Safety (IPCS) workshop on toxicogenomics and risk assessment held in Berlin in 2003.[141] The basic approach involves identifying early activation/suppression of genes and their protein products resulting from the exposure of the organism to potentially toxic materials.[142–144] While such techniques look at the sub-cellular events associated with toxic insult, there does not yet exist sufficient data to differentiate those events from cellular responses that may not be specific or may be a consequence of normal variation within the genome of test species and humans.[142–145] Also, regulatory agencies have not yet determined the use of such data in the formal risk assessment process.

Industrial Accident Response Planning

Recent events and regulations have made it imperative that industrial organizations, federal, state and local entities be aware of the potential for disasters involving the release of toxic materials either as the result of accidents or intentional activities.[146–148] They should also be aware that the roles of the industrial hygienist and other occupational health professionals in the preparation for and response to such incidents is being defined.[149–151] These topics are beyond the scope of this chapter. However, many of these roles require the understanding and use of toxicologic data from a wide variety of resources.[149,150] Whatever source the practitioner uses, the practioner must be aware of the limits of the guidelines presented and cautious about interpreting and applying them in circumstances different than those for which they were designed (e.g., population exposed, meteorological conditions, physical characteristics of material, geography, the presence of more than one toxic material, etc.)[150,152,153] The problems associated with determining acute hazard rating for materials for which no standard has been developed have been defined[154] and further show the need for standard toxicologic data sets for all industrial compounds.

Non-traditional Occupational Exposures

As mentioned previously, shifting demographics in the work force and evolving technologies will result in new and un-assessed exposures to a variety of confounding chemical, physical and biological stressors. Traditional industrial plants may become the exception and occupational health professionals will need to be more informed on the impacts of exposures on more varied populations in much less controlled environments than previously seen. The U.S. Department of Labor is not currently collecting accident/ injury statistics on such exposures. Indeed, developing a strategy to do so is a monumental task.

Occupational Human Health Risk Assessment

As shown in Figure 5.1, risk assessment uses aspects of mechanistic, descriptive and regulatory toxicology when addressing people, animals and the ecosystem. The risk assessment process is a critical function essential for making decisions relative to establishing risk reduction procedures and for formulating appropriate exposure levels from potentially hazardous chemicals. These decisions are based on quality science that guides sound judgments which result in effective risk characterization and risk management. Risk assessment is the process of characterizing the resultant risk from chemical releases which may affect human health or the environment. More expressly stated, risk assessment is using science to quantify personal risk, i.e., the technical assessment of the nature and magnitude of risk. The modern day use of the risk assessment process has its roots in the insurance industry. The use of actuarial processes for determination of insurance premiums gave rise to the use of comparable processes to determine the amount of personal risk in numerous scenarios, but especially in human health concerns from occupational and environmental settings. The currently used risk assessment process has only been defined in the last 25 years. In comparison to other sciences, risk assessment is a neophyte.

Risk assessment is the process of using factual basis to delineate the health effects of exposure to humans, and, effects to individuals, populations and communities of organisms in the environment, to potentially hazardous materials.

Risk Assessment Process

The risk assessment process for chemicals, including mixtures[155], involves four primary steps[97,98,156–161]: hazard identification, dose-response assessment, exposure assessment, and risk characterization. These four steps are necessary for a complete risk assessment.

Hazard Identification

This step of the process involves gathering and evaluating data on the types of health effects that may be produced by a hazardous chemical. Inclusive in this step are the conditions under which the material may produce injury or disease. Hazard identification incorporates the identity of the contaminant suspected of posing health hazards, a quantification of the concentrations at which the contaminants are present in the environment, a description of the specific forms of toxicity that can be caused by the contaminants of concern (e.g. neurotoxicity, carcinogenicity, hepatotoxicity, etc.), and an evaluation of the conditions under which these forms of toxicity might be expressed in exposed humans. These data are gathered from three primary sources: environmental monitoring, epidemiological studies, and animal studies conducted in the laboratory. Hazard identification is not risk assessment; it is simply determining whether it is scientifically correct to infer that toxic effects observed in one setting will occur in other settings. For example, if a chemical is found to be carcinogenic in laboratory animal studies, will this chemical likely have the same result in humans. Of the four steps to the risk assessment process, hazard identification is the most easily recognized in the actions of regulatory agencies such as the Environmental Protection Agency (EPA).[162–164]

Dose-Response Assessment

Dose-response assessment involves describing the quantitative relationship between the amount of exposure to a chemical and the extent of toxic injury. It is the evaluation of the conditions under which the toxic properties of a chemical might be manifested in exposed people. Particular emphasis is placed on the quantitative relationship between the dose and the toxic response. This step may include an assessment of variations of response, for example the differences in susceptibility between infants and adults. Simplistically stated, the dose-response assessment is the process of characterizing the inherent toxicity of a chemical and involves determining the adverse effects and how much of the chemical is required to produce the adverse effect. The observed adverse effect is usually termed the toxic endpoint, i.e., a biological effect used as an index of the effect of a chemical/substance on an organism. The route of entry into the body and the disposition of the chemical in the body are of paramount importance to the dose-response step of the process. The usual routes of entry for humans are inhalation, ingestion and skin absorption as shown in Figure 5.2. These routes of entry to the body and the ultimate excretion avenues are the major areas of concern and identification for the determination of exposure to hazardous materials. These four areas of concern, absorption, distribution, metabolism and excretion, are the major variables influencing the toxicity of chemicals. Dose is either absorbed or effective. Absorbed dose is the amount of risk agent that is absorbed by the lungs, gastrointestinal tract, and skin; effective dose, also called internal dose, is the amount of a risk agent reaching a tissue or an organ where it will inflict damage. In toto, dose-response describes the relationship that exists between the degree of exposure to a chemical (i.e., the dose) and the magnitude of the effect (response) in the exposed organism. No chemical present, yields no response! Once in the body, the general mechanism of chemical toxicity is interference with some important cellular reaction, the details of which will vary with the individual chemical. The chemical may react with key cellular molecules, changing their properties causing damage or rendering them ineffective; or, the chemical may substitute for a normal body chemical and lead to formation of unusual new by-products which may be more or less toxic than the parent chemical and prevent formation of normal products.

Exposure Assessment

The third step in the risk assessment process is exposure assessment. This step specifies the population that might be exposed to the agent of concern, identifies the routes through which exposure can occur, and estimates the magnitude, duration, and timing of the doses that humans may receive as a result of their exposure to the chemical of concern. The first determinant of the exposure assessment is to identify the concentration of chemical to which organisms are exposed. This may be accomplished by direct measurements, use of models, or by analogy. Analogy is often used by collecting exposure measurement on a small group of workers and then applying those values to other segments of the worker population. Particular attention must be given to various grouping of workers in a given area and exposed to a specific chemical. Some groups in a worker population may be especially susceptible to adverse health effects. For example, pregnant women, very young and very old people, and health impaired individuals may be particularly important in evaluating the exposure assessment.

Risk Characterization

This, the final step in the risk assessment process, is the complete integration of information from the preceding three steps, i.e., hazard identification, dose-response assessment and exposure assessment. During this phase the collected information is used to develop a qualitative or quantitative estimate of the likelihood that any of the hazards associated with the chemical of concern will be realized in exposed people. If exposure data are not available, hypothetical risk can be characterized by the integration of hazard identification and dose-response data. Risk is generally characterized based upon the two very general categories of chemicals: non-carcinogens and carcinogens. Definitive procedures are used for determining risk of each category, but will not be covered in this chapter. Ultimately risk characterization is the process of estimating the incidence of a health effect under various conditions of exposure. It is during this phase that any resultant uncertainties encountered during the preceding steps are taken into account and described.

Environmental Risk Assessment

The intent of this section is to review the potential impact of environmental toxicants on the overall human health risk in occupational venues. The specifics of Environmental and Human Health Risks as required by the

U.S. Environmental Protection Agency for evaluating/identifying sites for remediation or other activities are covered elsewhere in this book (see Chapter 8). Though much of the toxicity data used in such evaluations are applicable to overall human health risk, their interpretation must be tempered by the specific limitations of the exposure scenario represented by the work force of interest.

Contaminants in the environment have become widely recognized as potentially impacting human health whether at the workplace, at home, or during recreational activities. Thus, the scope of exposure scenarios for the worker has broadened greatly as awareness of the potential impacts of multiple stressors (chemical, biological, and physical) has become recognized. Exposure to xenobiotics outside of the traditional industrial workplace and under unusual circumstances (responses to natural, man-made, and technological disasters) must now be considered in evaluating the overall exposure of workers. Representative of the kinds of processes that must be employed and the interpretation of data are the studies done by the U.S. Army Center for Health Promotion and Preventative Medicine.[165] Because deployable forces may be exposed in industrial, urban, and other environments under the a variety of global conditions, consideration is given to an overall approach to prioritizing chemicals that incorporates not only traditional risk assessment approaches, but recognizes the potential intentional use of these materials in destroying, disruption or delaying force objectives. A similar approach could be used in evaluating the potential for disruption of work force objectives. Indeed, as is pointed out in the beginning of this section and generally accepted, toxic industrial chemicals and compounds abound in any environment and represent confounders to traditional occupational exposures. While there are on-going efforts to standardize the kinds of data that are collected and disseminated through the registration, evaluation, authorization and restriction of chemicals (REACH) program, complete harmonization has not been achieved.[166] The REACH program is intended to include provision for the collection of basic data for those chemicals that have not been sufficiently covered by existing requirements. However, agreement has not yet been reached on the proper use of a variety of toxicological techniques [structure activity relationships, genetic tools, in vitro analysis, physiologically based pharmacokinetic (PBPK) modeling, etc.] in publishing information to the end user and database entries are not critically evaluated under REACH.

Attempts to establish universally accepted methods for evaluating the potential toxicological outcomes of exposure to multiple chemicals have also illustrated the difficulties with finding applicable data representative of the exposures experienced by workers at the work site and during other activities.[167–170]

Representative studies of the contamination of water supplies and food stuffs with compounds that may or may not have additive, synergistic or canceling effects on the toxicants seen in the workplace, illustrate the complexity of the problem that toxicologists, environmentalists, regulators and occupational health professionals must address in performing adequate human health risk assessments for workers.[171–175]

Sources of Toxicological Data

It has been estimated that the U.S. imports or produces close to 7.1 trillion pounds of some 3,000 chemicals at over 1 million pounds each per year. This is from some 100,000 chemicals in commerce. Of these, 43% have no toxicity testing data and only seven percent have a full set of basic data.[176–178] Thus, the challenge to the practicing Industrial/ Occupational Hygienist to find sufficient data to assess potential health hazards in the workplace can be daunting.

Sources fall into three broad categories: Material Safety Data Sheets (MSDS), books, journals and websites (including databases). Though MSDSs are required to be available for every material in the workspace, their usefulness in assessing the health risk of the worker can be very limited and requires some expertise to interpret and may not include essential toxicologic information.[179–182] Because the data contained on MSDSs vary in quantity and quality, efforts are being made to standardize the information and format for MSDSs in both the US and globally.[183] There are many commercially available MSDS databases. Some books that are useful and commonly available include (NOTE: These texts are frequently updated):

(1) *Casarett and Doull's Toxicology: The Basic Science of Poisons*, 5th edition. Klaasen, C.D., M.O. Amdur, and J. Doull (eds.). New York: McGraw-Hill, 1996,

(2) *Patty's Industrial Hygiene and Toxicology*, 4th edition. Clayton, G.D. and F.E. Clayton (eds.). New York: John Wiley and Sons, 1991.

(3) *Sax's Dangerous Properties of Industrial Materials*, 11th edition. Lewis, R.J. (ed.). New York: John Wiley and Sons, 2004.

Also readily available are publications from professional organizations and governmental agencies. Good examples are the *Threshold Limit Values (TLV®) for Chemical and Physical Agents and Biological Exposure Indices (BEIs®)* of the American Conference of Governmental Industrial Hygienists (published annually), and the National Institute of Occupational Safety and Health (NIOSH) Pocket Guide to Chemical Hazards (NIOSH Publication No. 2005-151). These are also updated regularly. However, the information provided in those publications is for very specific uses and does not provide detailed toxicology.

With the proliferation of the Internet and the growing social awareness of the impact of chemicals in the workplace and the environment as a whole, the ability to obtain toxicologic information by "web surfing" continues to increase. However, as can be seen from the following examples (Table 5.3, all searches were performed on July 22, 2008) from some of the most common search engines, the data can be overwhelming. If the searcher is unfamiliar with the logic used to optimize such efforts, they may find the Internet an inefficient way to find data, particularly if they need it in a very timely manner. By focusing on sites maintained by government and academic organizations/agencies, the volume of data may be reduced and the value of the data found improved. The result of a search of the ToxNet site for "Benzene Toxicity" is illustrated in Figure 5.16 and demonstrates this idea (search was conducted August 24, 2010). Many of the non-government sites that are found by such searches are sponsored by organizations that have a vested interest in how the data are perceived and caution must be used in relying solely on the data from any one site. The following Internet sources are provided to help the reader narrow their effort to authoritative and readily available sources:

Internet websites (US Government):

- Agency of Toxic Substances and Disease Registry at www.atsdr.cdc.gov.
- Environmental Protection Agency (EPA) Ecological Toxicity (ECOTOX) at www.epa.gov/ecotox/.
- National Institute of Occupational Safety and Health (NIOSH) at www2.cdc.gov/nioshtic-2/nioshtic2.htm (This is a publication search website).

Table 5.3 — Internet Search Examples

Search Phrase:	*MSN Search® Hits:*	*Google® Hits:*	*Yahoo® Hits:*
Toxicology of Cobalt	79,100	316,000	284,000
Toxicology of Benzene	183,000	503,000	690,000
Toxicology of Formaldehyde	132,000	394,000	535,000
Toxicology of Hydrogen Sulfide	9,740	242,000	212,000

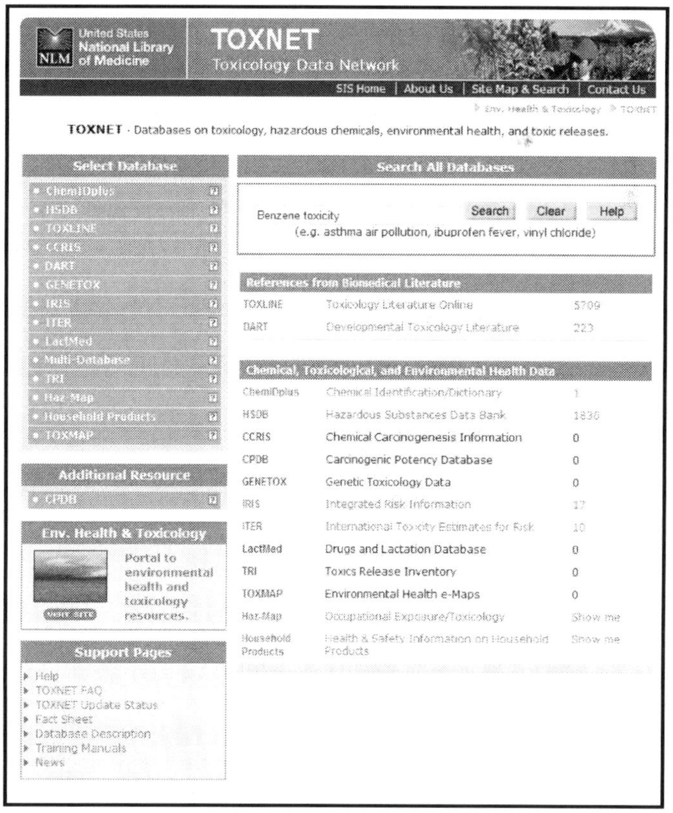

Figure 5.16 — Result of TOXNET Query.

- National Library of Medicine at toxnet.nlm.nih.gov.
- National Toxicology Program (Department of Health and Human Services) at ntp-server.niehs.nih.gov/
- Registry of Toxic Effects of Chemical Substances (RTECS) at www.cdc.gov/niosh/srchpage.html
- U.S. Coast Guard at: www.chrismanual.com

Internet Websites (Non U.S. governments):

- Australian Government Department of Health and Aging (NICNAS) at www.nicnas.gov.au/publications/car/default.asp
- European Chemical Substances Information System (EU ESIS) at ecb.jrc.it/esis
- Global Information Network on Chemicals (Ministry of Health, Labor and Safety, Japan) at wwwdb.mhiw.go.jp/ginc/html/db1.html
- International Programme on Chemical Safety (IPCS INCHEM) at www.inchem.org
- International Programme on Chemical Safety (IPCS Intox) at www.intox.org/databank/index.htm
- Substances in Preparation in Nordic Countries (Norway, Sweden, Denmark, and Finland) at www.spin2000.net/spin.html

A comprehensive list of sources has been compiled and is available to members of the American Industrial Hygiene association at www.aiha.org/webapps/taxonomy/portal.htm titled "Essential Resources for Industrial Hygiene — Chapter 4 Occupational Toxicology" written by W.E. Luttrell.

Conclusion

Regardless of the source, without some familiarity with basic principles of toxicology, interpretation of data as it applies to any given exposure scenario can be difficult. Part of the purpose of this chapter is to introduce the practicing Industrial/Occupational Hygienist or other Occupational/Preventive Medicine specialist with enough information to know when they need to consult with someone with more expertise in the area of applied toxicology.

References

1. **Plog, BA:** Overview of Industrial Hygiene. In *Fundamentals of Industrial Hygiene*. Plog, B.A, J. Niland, and P.J. Quinlan (eds.). Itasca IL: National Safety Council, 1996. pp 3–32.
2. **Rose, V.E.:** History and Philosophy of Industrial Hygiene. In *The Occupational Environment, Its Evaluation, Control, and Management*, 2nd Edition. DiNardi, S.R. (ed). Fairfax, VA: AIHA Press, 2003. pp 4–18.
3. Toxicology Timeline; http://www.toxipedia.org/display/toxipedia/Toxicology Timeline. [Accessed August 2010].
4. **Gallo, M.A.:** History and Scope of Toxicology. In *Casarett and Doull's Toxicology—The Basic Science of Poisons*, 6th edition. Klaassen, C.D. (ed). New York: McGraw-Hill, 2001. pp 3–10.
5. **James, R.C.:** General Principles of Toxicology. In *Industrial Toxicology: Safety and Health Applications in the Workplace*. Williams, P.L. and J.L. Burson (eds). New York: Van Nostrand Reinhold, 1985. pp 7–26.
6. **Lu, F.C. and S. Kacew:** *Lu's Basic Toxicology — Fundamentals, Target Organs, and Risk Assessment*, 4th edition. Washington, D.C.: Taylor & Francis, 2002.
7. **Klaassen, C.D.:** *Casarett and Doull's Toxicology, The Basic Science of Poisons*, 7th edition. McGraw Hill, 2008.
8. **Niesink, R.J.M.:** Occupational Toxicology. In *Toxicology — Principles and Applications*. Niesink, R.J.M., J. de Vries, and M.A. Hollinger (eds.). Boca Raton, FL: CRC Press, 1996.
9. **Still, K.R., G.B. Briggs, P. Knechtges, W.K. Alexander; and C.L. Wilson:** Risk Assessment in Navy Deployment Toxicology. *Hum. Ecolog. Risk Assess. 6*:1125–1136 (2000).
10. **Still, K.R., W.W. Jederberg, G.D. Ritchie, and J. Rossi, III:** Exposure Assessment and the Health of Deployed Forces. *Drug Chem. Toxicol. 25(4)*:383–401 (2002).
11. **Gochfeld, M.:** Principles of Toxicology. In *Environmental Medicine*. Brooks, S., M., Gochfeld, M.G., J. Herzstein, R.J. Jackson, and M.B. Schenker (eds.). St. Louis, Mo.: Mosby-Year Book, Inc., 1995.
12. **Logan, D.C.:** Toxicology. In McCunney, R.J. (ed): *A Practical Approach to Occupational and Environmental Medicine*, Boston: Little, Brown and Company, 1994.
13. **Lu, F.C.:** *Basic Toxicology — Fundamentals, Target Organs, and Risk Assessment*, 3rd edition. Washington, D.C.: Taylor & Francis, 1996
14. DoD 6050.5L
15. **ACGIH®:** *TLVs® and BEIs® Based on the Documentation of the Threshold Limit Values for Chemical Substances and Physical Agents & Biological Exposure Indices* (2007). Cincinnati, OH: ACGIH ®, 2007.

16. **AIHA®:** *The AIHA 2007 Emergency Response Planning Guidelines and Workplace Environmental Exposure Level Handbook.* Fairfax, VA: AIHA®, 2007.
17. **Kent, C.:** *Basics of Toxicology — Preserving the Legacy.* New York: John Wiley & Sons, Inc., 1998.
18. **Agency for Toxic Substances and Disease Registry (ATSDR):** *TOXFAQs™ for Hydrogen Sulfide.* July 2006.
19. **Alarei, Y., G.D. Nielsen, and M.M. Schaper:** Animal Bioassays for Evaluation of Indoor Air Quality. In *Indoor Air Quality Handbook.* Spengler, J.D., J.M. Samet and J.F. McCarthy (eds.). New York: McGraw-Hill, 2001.
20. **Castranova, V., D.G. Frazer, L.K. Manley, and R.D. Dey:** Pulmonary alterations associated with inhalation of occupational and environmental irritants. *Int. Immunopharmacol. 2(2-3)*:163–172 (2002).
21. **Parks, S., and D.W. Paul:** Ozone exposure: a case report and discussion. *J. Okla. State Med. Assoc. 93(2)*:48–51 (2000).
22. **Wagner, J.G., and M.L. Millerick-May:** Respiratory Toxicology. In *Toxicology Principles for the Industrial Hygienist.* Luttrell, W.E., W.W. Jederberg and K.R. Still (eds.). Fairfax, VA: AIHA®, 2008.
23. **Petsonk, E.L.:** Work-related asthma and implications for the general public. *Environ. Health Perspect. 110(4)*:569–572 (2002).
24. **National Institute for Occupational Safety and Health (NIOSH):** *Alert: Preventing Asthma and Death from Diisocyanate Exposure*, DHHS (NIOSH) Publication No. 96-111, 1996.
25. **American Lung Association:** Occupational Lung Disease Fact Sheet. http://www.lungusa.org [Accessed on July 3, 2009].
26. **Amr, S., and M.E. Bollinger:** Latex allergy and occupational asthma in health care workers: Adverse outcomes. *Environ. Health Perspect. 112*:378–381 (2004).
27. **Attfield, M.D., J.M. Wood, V.C. Antao, and G.A. Pinheiro:** Changing patterns of pneumoconiosis mortality—United States, 1968–2000. *MMWR 53(28)*:627–632 (2004).
28. **Amicosante, M., and A.P. Fontenot:** T cell recognition in chronic beryllium disease. *Clin. Immunol. 121(2)*:134–143 (2006).
29. **Huaux, F.:** New developments in the understanding of immunology in silicosis. *Curr. Opin. Allergy Clin. Immunol. 7(2)*:168–173 (2007).
30. **Nemery, B.:** Metal toxicity and the respiratory tract. *Eur. Respir. J. 3(2)*:202–219 (1990).
31. **Cohen, S.R., D.M. David, and R.S. Kramkowski:** Clinical manifestations of chromic acid toxicity: Nasal lesions in electroplate workers. *Cutis. 13*:558–568 (1974).
32. **Kreiss, K., et al.:** Clinical bronchiolitis obliterans in workers at a microwave-popcorn plant. *N. Engl. J. Med. 347(5)*:330–338 (2002).
33. **Sweeney, P.J.:** Farmer's lung: a clinical account of a disease probably caused by fungi. *Ulster Med. J. 21(2)*:150–154 (1952).
34. **ACGIH®:** *2009 TLVs® and BEIs®—Threshold Limit Values for Chemical Substances and Physical Agents and Biological Exposure Indices.* Cincinnati, OH: ACGIH, 2009.
35. **Weber, L.W., and J.T. Pierce:** Development of Occupational Skin Disease. In *The Occupational Environment: Its Evaluation, Control and Management*, 2nd edition, DiNardi, S.R. (ed.). Fairfax, VA: AIHA®, 2003.
36. **Rice, R.H., and D.E. Cohen:** Toxic Responses of the Skin. In *Casarett & Doull's Toxicology—The Basic Science of Poisons*, 6th edition. Klaassen, C.D. (ed.). New York: McGraw-Hill, 2001.
37. "Cutaneous Toxicity: Toxic Effects on Skin." [Online] Available at: http://pmep.cce.cornell.edu/profiles/extoxnet/TIB/cutaneous-tox.html. [Accessed August 2010].
38. **Jederberg, W.W.:** Dermal Toxicology. In *Toxicology Principles for the Industrial Hygienist.* Luttrell, W.E., W.W. Jederberg and K.R. Still (eds.). Fairfax, VA: AIHA®, 2008.
39. **Porth, C.M.:** *Pathophysiology: Concepts of Altered Health States*, 7th edition. Philadelphia, PA: Lippincott Williams & Wilkins, 2005.
40. **Taylor, A.E.:** Cardiovascular effects of environmental chemicals. *Otolaryngol. Head Neck Surg. 114*:209–211 (1996).
41. **Weber, L.W.D., J.D. Pierce, and J.T. Pierce:** Systemic Effects: Cardiovascular and Renal Toxicity. In *Toxicology Principles for the Industrial Hygienist.* Luttrell, W.E., W.W. Jederberg and K.R. Still (eds.). Fairfax, VA: AIHA®, 2008.
42. **Dockery, D.W., et al.:** An association between air pollution and mortality in six U.S. cities. *N. Engl. J. Med. 329*:1753–1759 (1993).
43. **Durante, W., F.K. Johnson, and R.A. Johnson:** Role of carbon monoxide in cardiovascular function. *J. Cell Mol. Med. 10*:672–686 (2006).
44. **Kristensen, T.S.:** Cardiovascular diseases and the work environment. A critical review of the epidemiologic literature on chemical factors. *Scand. J. Work Environ. Health 15*:245–264 (1989).
45. **Yousefipour, Z., K. Ranganna, M.A. Newaz, and S.G. Milton:** Mechanism of acrolein-induced vascular toxicity. *J. Physiol. Pharmacol. 56*:337–353 (2005).
46. **Kone, B.C., R.M. Brenner, and S.R. Gullans:** Sulfhydryl-reactive heavy metals increase cell membrane K^+ and Ca^{2+} transport in renal proximal tubule. *J. Memb. Biol. 113*:1–12 (1990).
47. **Sullivan, L.P., and J.J. Grantham:** *Physiology of the Kidney*, 2nd Edition. Philadelphia, PA: Lea & Febiger, 1982.

48. **Luttrell, W.E.:** Neurotoxicology. In *Toxicology Principles for the Industrial Hygienist.* Luttrell, W.E., W.W. Jederberg and K.R. Still (eds.). Fairfax, VA: AIHA®, 2008.
49. **Nierenberg, D.W., et al.:** Delayed cerebellar disease and death after accidental exposure to dimethylmercury. *New Eng. J. Med. 338(23)*:1672–1676 (1998).
50. **So, Y.T.:** Nervous System. In *Environmental Medicine.* Brooks, S.M., M. Gochfeld, J. Herzstein, R.J. Jackson, and M.B. Schenker (eds.). St. Louis, MO: Mosby-Year Book, Inc., 1995.
51. **Stine, K.E., and T.M. Brown:** Neurotoxicology. In *Principles of Toxicology.* New York: CRC, Lewis Publishers, 1996.
52. **Anthony, D.C., T.J. Montine, W.M. Vanentine, and D.G. Graham:** Toxic Responses of the Nervous System. In *Casarett and Doull's Toxicology—The Basic Science of Poisons.* Klaassen, C.D. (5th ed.). New York: McGraw-Hill, 2001.
53. **Lu, F.C., and S. Kacew:** Toxicology of the Nervous System. In *Lu's Basic Toxicology—Fundamentals, Target Organs, and Risk Assessment,* 4th edition. New York: Taylor & Francis, 2002.
54. **Boyer, I.J.:** Toxicity of dimethyltin and other organotin compounds to humans and to experimental animals. *Toxicol. 55*:253–298 (1989).
55. **Dabrowska-Bouta, G., et al.:** Chronic lead intoxication affects the myelin membrane status in the central nervous system of adult rats. *J. Mol. Neurosci. 13*:127–139 (1999).
56. **Lindgren, K.N., V.L. Masten, D.P. Ford, and M.L. Bleecker:** Relation of cumulative exposure to inorganic lead and neuropsychological test performance. *Occup. Environ. Med. 53*:472–477 (1996).
57. **Needleman, H.L.:** Childhood lead poisoning. *Curr. Opin. Neurol. 7*:187–190 (1994).
58. **Malachowski, M.J., and A.F. Goldberg:** Target Organ Effects. In *Health Effects of Toxic Substances.* Rockville, MD: Government Institutes, Inc., 1995.
59. **Winder, C.:** Occupational Toxicology of the Nervous System. In *Occupational Toxicology,* 2nd edition. Winder, C., and N. Stacey (eds.). Boca Raton, FL: CRC Press, 2004.
60. **New, P.S., G.D. Lubash, L. Scherr, and A.L. Rubin:** Acute renal failure associated with carbon tetrachloride intoxication. *JAMA 181*:903–906 (1962).
61. **Norwood, W.D., P.A. Fuqua, and B.C. Scudder:** Carbon tetrachloride poisoning. *Arch. Ind. Hyg. Occup. Med. 1*:90–100 (1950).
62. **Belyaev, N.D., V.C. Budker, L.V. Derly, I.A. Smolenskaya, and V.M. Subbotin:** Liver plasma membrane-associated fibroblast growth: Stimulatory and inhibitory activities during experimental cirrhosis. *Hepatology 15*: 525–531 (1992).
63. **Harris, A.J.:** Hepatic Toxicology. In *Toxicology Principles for the Industrial Hygienist.* Luttrell, W.E., W.W. Jederberg and K.R. Still (eds.). Fairfax, VA: AIHA®, 2008.
64. **Kenna, J.G., J.L. Martin, H. Satoh, and L.R. Pohl:** Factors affecting the expression of trifluoroacetylated liver microsomal protein neoantigens in rats treated with halothane. *Drug Metab. Dispos. 18*:788–793 (1990).
65. **Leung, K.H., M. Yao, R. Stearns, and S.H. Chiu:** Mechanism of bioactivation and covalent binding of 2,4,6-trinitrotoluene. *Chem. Biol. Interact. 97*:35–51 (1995).
66. **Glass, K.Y., C.R. Newsome, and P.B. Tchounwou:** Cyto-toxicity and expression of c-fox, HSP70, and GADD45/153 proteins in human liver carcinoma (HepG2) cells exposed to dinitrotoluenes. *Int. J. Environ. Res. Public Health 2*:355–361 (2005).
67. **Kanz, M.F., A. Wang, and G.A. Campbell:** Infusion of bile from methylene dianiline-treated rats into the common bile duct injures biliary epithelial cells of recipient rats. *Toxicol. Lett. 78*:165–171 (1995).
68. **Bolt, H.M., H. Kappus, R. Kaufmann, K.E. Appel, A. Buchter, and W. Bolt:** Metabolism of 14 C-vinyl chloride *in vitro* and *in vivo.* *IARC Sci. Publ. 976*:151–163 (1976).
69. **Hoyer, P.B.:** Reproductive toxicology: current and future directions. *Biochem. Pharmacol. 62*:1557–1564 (2001).
70. **Kim, Y., K. Jung, T. Hwang, G. Jung, J. Kim, H. Kim, et al.:** Hematopoietic and reproductive hazards of Korean electronic workers exposed to solvents containing 2-bromopropane. *Scand. J. Work Environ. Health 22*:387–391 (1996).
71. **Yu, X., M. Kamijima, G. Ichihara, W. Li, J. Kitoh, Z. Xie, et al.:** 2-Bromopropane causes ovarian dysfunction by damaging primordial follicles and their oocytes in female rats. *Toxicol. Appl. Pharmacol. 159*:185–193 (1999).
72. **Omura, M., Y. Romero, M. Zhao, and N. Inoue:** Histopathological evidence that spermatogonia are the target cells of 2-bromopropane. *Toxicol. Lett. 104*:19–26 (1999).
73. **Reutman, S.R., G.K. Lemasters, E.A. Knecht, R. Shukla, J.E. Lockey, G.E. Burroughs, et al.:** Evidence of reproductive endocrine effects in women with occupational fuel and solvent exposures. *Environ. Health Perspect. 110*:805–811 (2002).

74. **Heng, K., S. Hargarten, P. Layde, A. Craven, and S. Zhu:** Moderate alcohol intake and motor vehicle crashes: the conflict between health advantage and at-risk use. *Alcohol. 41*:451–454 (2006).
75. **Pastino, G., B. Asgharian, K. Roberts, M. Medinsky, and J. Bond:** A comparison of physiologically based pharmacokinetic model predictions and experimental data for inhaled ethanol in male and female B6C3F1 mice, F344 rats and humans. *Toxicol. Appl. Pharmacol. 145*:147–157 (1997).
76. **Irvine, L.F.:** Relevance of the developmental toxicity of ethanol in the occupational setting: a review. *J. Appl. Toxicol. 23*:289–299 (2003).
77. **Mylchreest, E., R.C. Cattley, and P.M.D. Foster:** Male reproductive tract malformations in rats following gestational and lactational exposure to di(n-butyl)phthalate: an antiandrogenic mechanism? *Toxicol. Sci. 43*:47–60 (1998).
78. **Ema, M., E.M. Miyawaki, and K. Kawashima:** Effects of dibutyl phthalate on reproductive function in pregnant and pseudopregnant rats. *Reprod. Toxicol. 14*:13–19 (2000).
79. **Mocarelli, P., et al.:** Paternal concentrations of dioxin and sex ratio of offspring. *Lancet 355*:1858–1863 (2000).
80. **Mattie, D.R.:** Reproductive and Developmental Toxicology. In *Toxicology Principles for the Industrial Hygienist.* Luttrell, W.E., W.W. Jederberg and K.R. Still (eds.). Fairfax, VA: AIHA®, 2008.
81. **Baranski, B.:** Effects of the workplace on fertility and related reproductive outcomes. *Environ. Health Perspect. 101(2)*:81–90 (1993).
82. **Whorton, D., R.M. Krauss, S. Marshall, and T.H. Milby:** Infertility in male pesticide workers. *Lancet 2*:1259–1261 (1977).
83. **Torkelson, T.R., S.E. Sadek, V.K. Rowe, J.K. Kodama, H.H. Anderson, G.S. Loquvam, and C.H. Hine:** Toxicologic investigations of 1,2-dibromo-3-chloropropane. *Toxicol. Appl. Pharmacol. 3*:545–559 (1961).
84. **Sparer, J., L.S. Welch, K. McManus, and M.R. Cullen:** Effects of exposure to ethylene glycol ethers on shipyard painters. I. Evaluation of exposure. *Am. J. Ind. Med. 14*:497–507 (1988).
85. **Welch, L.S., S.M. Schrader, T.W. Turner, and M.R. Cullen:** Effects of exposure to ethylene glycol ethers on shipyard painters. II. Male reproduction. *Am. J. Ind. Med. 14*:509–526 (1988).
86. **Paustenbach, D.J.:** Assessment of the developmental risks resulting from occupational exposure to select glycol ethers within the semiconductor industry. *J. Toxicol. Environ. Health 23*:29–75 (1988).
87. **Bonde, J.P.:** Semen quality and sex hormone among mild steel and stainless steel welders: a cross sectional study. *Br. J. Ind. Med. 47*:508–514 (1990).
88. **Kumar, S., S.S.A. Zaidi, A.K. Gautam, L.M. Dave, and H.N. Saiyed:** Short communication: Semen quality and reproductive hormones among welders—a preliminary study. *Environ. Health Prevent. Med. 8*:64–67 (2003).
89. **Kolstad, H.A., J.P. Bonde, M. Spano, A. Giwercman, W. Zschiesche, D. Kaae, et al.:** Change in semen quality and sperm chromatin structure following occupational styrene exposure. *Int. Arch. Occup. Environ. Health 72*:135–141 (1999).
90. **Sikov, M.R., W.C. Cannon, D.B. Carr, R.A. Miller, R.W. Niemeier, and B.D. Hardin:** Reproductive toxicology of inhaled styrene oxide in rats and rabbits. *J. Appl. Toxicol. 6*:155–164 (1986).
91. **Bonde, J.P., et al.:** Sperm count and chromatin structure in men exposed to inorganic lead: lowest adverse effect levels. *Occup. Environ. Med. 59*:234–242 (2002).
92. **Paule, M.G., K. Reuhl, J.J. Chen, S.F. Ali, and W. Slikker, Jr.:** Developmental toxicology of trimethyltin in the rat. *Toxicol. Appl. Pharmacol. 84*:412–417 (1986).
93. **Willhite, C.C., and V.H. Ferm:** Prenatal and developmental toxicology of arsenicals. *Adv. Exp. Med. Biol. 177*:205–228 (1984).
94. **Ashley, J.B.:** The two "hit" and multiple "hit" theories of carcinogenesis. *Br. J. Cancer 23(2)*:313–328 (1969).
95. **Selikoff, I.J., E.C. Hammond, and J. Churg:** Asbestos exposure, smoking, and neoplasia. *J. Am. Med. Assoc. 204*:106–112 (1968).
96. **U.S. Department of Health and Human Services:** *Report on Carcinogens*, 11th edition. Washington, D.C.: Public Health Service, National Toxicology Program, 2005.
97. **National Academy of Sciences (NAS):** *Risk Assessment in the Federal Government: Managing the Process.* National Academy Press, Washington, D.C.: NAS, 1983.
98. **National Academy of Sciences (NAS):** *Science and Judgment in Risk Assessment.* National Research Council. Washington, D.C.: National Academy Press, 1994.
99. **General Accounting Office (GAO):** Chemical Risk Assessment, Selected Federal Agencies" Procedures, Assumptions and Policies. GAO-01-810. Washington, D.C.: General Accounting Office, 2001.
100. **National Research Council of the National Academies:** Emergency and Continuous Exposure Limits for Selected Airborne Contaminants, Vol. 1. Washington, D.C.: National Academy Press, 1984.

101. **National Research Council of the National Academies:** Emergency and Continuous Exposure Limits for Selected Airborne Contaminants, Vol.2. Washington, D.C.: National Academy Press, 1984.
102. **National Research Council of the National Academies:** Emergency and Continuous Exposure Limits for Selected Airborne Contaminants, Vol. 3. Washington, D.C.: National Academy Press, 1984.
103. **National Research Council of the National Academies:** Toxicity Testing: Strategies to Determine Needs and Priorities. Washington, D.C.: National Academy Press, 1984.
104. **National Research Council of the National Academies:** Emergency and Continuous Exposure Limits for Selected Airborne Contaminants, Vol. 4. Washington, D.C.: National Academy Press, 1984.
105. **National Research Council of the National Academies:** Emergency and Continuous Exposure Limits for Selected Airborne Contaminants, Vol. 5. Washington, D.C.: National Academy Press, 1984.
106. **National Research Council of the National Academies:** Emergency and Continuous Exposure Limits for Selected Airborne Contaminants, Vol. 6. Washington, D.C.: National Academy Press, 1984.
107. **National Research Council of the National Academies:** Criteria and Methods for Preparing Emergency Exposure Guidance Level (EEGL), Short-Term Public Emergency Guidance Level (SPEGL), and Continuous Exposure Guidance Level (CEGL) Documents. Washington, D.C.: National Academy Press, 1986.
108. **National Research Council of the National Academies:** Emergency and Continuous Exposure Limits for Selected Airborne Contaminants, Vol. 7. Washington, D.C.: National Academy Press, 1987.
109. **National Research Council of the National Academies:** Emergency and Continuous Exposure Limits for Selected Airborne Contaminants, Vol. 8. Washington, D.C.: National Academy Press, 1988.
110. **National Research Council of the National Academies:** Guidelines for Developing Spacecraft Maximum Allowable Concentrations for Space Station Contaminants. Washington, D.C.: National Academy Press, 1992.
111. **National Research Council of the National Academies:** Guidelines for Developing Community Emergency Exposure Levels for Hazardous Substances. Washington, D.C.: National Academy Press, 1993.
112. **National Research Council of the National Academies:** Spacecraft Maximum Allowable Concentrations for Selected Airborne Contaminants, Volume 1. Washington, D.C.: National Academy Press, 1994.
113. **National Research Council of the National Academies:** Spacecraft Maximum Allowable Concentrations for Selected Airborne Contaminants, Volume 2. Washington, D.C.: National Academy Press, 1996.
114. **National Research Council of the National Academies:** Spacecraft Maximum Allowable Concentrations for Selected Airborne Contaminants, Volume 3. Washington, D.C.: National Academy Press, 1996.
115. **National Research Council of the National Academies:** Spacecraft Maximum Allowable Concentrations for Selected Airborne Contaminants, Volume 4. Washington, D.C.: National Academy Press, 2000.
116. **National Research Council of the National Academies:** Methods for Developing Spacecraft Water Exposure Guidelines. Washington, D.C.: National Academy Press, 2000.
117. **National Research Council of the National Academies:** Standing Operating Procedures for Developing Acute Exposure Guideline Levels for Hazardous Chemicals. Washington D.C.: National Academy Press, 2001.
118. **National Research Council of the National Academies:** Acute Exposure Guideline Levels for Selected Airborne Chemicals. Volume 1. Washington, D.C.: National Academy Press, 2001.
119. **National Research Council of the National Academies:** Acute Exposure Guideline Levels for Selected Airborne Chemicals. Volume 2. Washington, D.C.: National Academy Press, 2002.
120. **National Research Council of the National Academies:** Acute Exposure Guideline Levels for Selected Airborne Chemicals. Volume 3. Washington, D.C.: National Academy Press, 2003.
121. **National Research Council of the National Academies:** Acute Exposure Guideline Levels for Selected Airborne Chemicals. Volume 4. Washington, D.C.: National Academy Press, 2004.
122. **National Research Council of the National Academies:** Spacecraft Water Exposure Guidelines for Selected Contaminants. Volume 1. Washington, D.C.: National Academy Press, 2004.
123. **National Research Council of the National Academies:** Acute Exposure Guideline Levels for Selected Airborne Chemicals. Volume 5. Washington, D.C.: National Academy Press, 2006.

124. **National Research Council of the National Academies:** Spacecraft Water Exposure Guidelines for Selected Contaminants. Volume 2. Washington, D.C.: National Academy Press, 2006.
125. **National Research Council of the National Academies:** BIER Reference: Health Risk from Exposure to Low Levels of Ionizing Radiation (BEIR Phase 2), Committee to assess Health Risks from Exposure to Low Levels of Radiation, Washington, DC: National Academy Press, 2006.
126. 40 CFR 700 Subchapter R—Toxic Substances Control Act, Section 5 and 5(e) and Section 8 and 8(e)
127. **Jederberg, W.W.:** Sources of Chemical Hazard Information. In *Toxicology Principles for the Industrial Hygienist.* Luttrell, W.E., W.W. Jederberg, and K.R. Still (eds.). Fairfax, VA: AIHA, 2007. pp. 395–397.
128. **Lopez, K.:** "The Three Changing Faces of the U.S. Workforce." *Occupational Health & Safety.* January 2005.
129. "The American Workforce: 2004-14 – Projected Changes in Labor Force Participation, Industry Employment, Occupational Employment, Detailed Occupations." [Online] Available at: http://careers.stateuniversity.com/pages/838/American-Workforce-2004-14.html. [Accessed August 2010].
130. **Dreher, K.L.:** Toxicology Highlight: Health and Environmental Impact of Nanotechnology: Toxicological Assessment of Manufactured Nanoparticles. *Toxicol. Sci. 77*:3–5 (2004).
131. **Oberdörster, G., et al.:** A report from the ILSI Research Foundation/Risk Science Institute Nanomaterial Toxicity Screening Working Group: Principles for characterizing the potential human health effects from exposure to nanomaterials: elements of a screening strategy. *Part. and Fibre Toxicol. 6*:2–8 (2005).
132. **Borm, P.J.A., et al.:** The potential risks of nanomaterials: a review carried out for ECETOC. *Part. and Fibre Toxicol. 3*:11 (2006).
133. **Committee on Toxicology:** Committee on Toxicity of Chemicals in Food, Consumer Products and the Environment, The Toxicology of Nanoparticles used in Healthcare and Update on Nanomaterial Toxicology. *TOX/2006/28.*
134. **Medina, C., M.J. Santo-Martinez, A. Radomski, O.I. Corrigan, and M.E. Radomski:** Nanoparticles: pharmacological and toxicological significance. *Br. J. Pharmacol. 150*:552–558 (2007).
135. **Schulte, P., C. Geraci, R. Zumwalde, M. Hoover, and E. Kuempel:** Occupational Risk Management of Engineered Nanoparticles. *J. Occ. Env. Hyg. 5*:239–249 (2008).
136. **Miller, A.L., M.D. Hoover, D.M. Mitchell, and B.P. Stapleton:** The Nanoparticle Information Library (NIL): A Prototype for Lining and Sharing Emerging Data. *J. Occ. Env. Hyg. 4*:D131–D134 (2007).
137. **Nuwaysir, E.F., M. Bittner, J. Trent, J.C. Barrett, and C.A. Afshari:** "Microarrays and toxicology: The advent of toxicogenomics." *Mol. Carc. 24*:153–159 (1999).
138. **Ankley, G.T., G.P. Daston, S.J. Degitz, N.D. Denslow, R.A. Hoke, S.W. Kennedy, A.L. Miracle, E.J. Perkins, J. Snape, D.E. Tillitt, C.R. Tyler, D. Versteeg:** Toxicogenomics in Regulatory Ecotoxicology. *Env. Sci. Tech. 40 (13)*:4055–4065 (2008).
139. **Committees on Toxicity, Mutagenicity and Carcinogenicity of Chemicals in Food, Consumer Products and the Environment:** Joint Statement on a Symposium Held by the Three Committees on the use of Genomics and Proteomics in Toxicology. [Online] Available at: http://cot.food.gov.uk/ pdfs/TOX-2004-02.PDF. [Accessed August 2010].
140. **Barlow, T., J. Battershil, B.R. Jeffery, F.D. Pollitt, C.S.M. Tahourdin:** MEETING REPORT: Report of a symposium on the use of genomics and proteomics in toxicology. *Mutagenesis 18(3)*:311–317 (2003).
141. **Workshop Report:** Toxicogenomics and the Risk Assessment of Chemicals for the Protection of Human Health (Summary). [Online] Available at: www.who.int/entity/ipcs/methods/en/toxicogenomicssummaryreport.pdf. [Accessed August 2010]
142. **Rockett, J.C.:** Use of genomic data in risk assessment. *Genome Biology 3(4)*4011.1–4011.3 (2002).
143. **Thomas, R.S., et al.:** Application of Genomics to Toxicology Research. *Env. Health Persp. 110*:919–923 (2002).
144. **Corvi, R.:** Genomics: An *In Vitro* Toxicology Point of Review. *ATLA 30*:129–131 (2002).
145. **Boedigheimer, M.J., et al.:** Sources of variation in baseline gene expression levels from toxicogenomics study control animals across multiple laboratories. *BMC Genomics 9*:285 (2008).
146. **Cavender, F., S. Phillips, M. Holland:** Development of Emergency Response Planning Guidelines (ERPGs). *J. Med. Tox. 4(2)*:127–131 (2008).
147. **Karasik T.:** "Toxic Warfare." Santa Monica CA: Rand Corp, 2002.
148. FM 3-11.9/MCRP 3.37.1B/NTRP 3-11.32/AFTTP(I), II. Chemical Warfare Agents and their properties. In: *Potential Military Chemical/Biological Agents and Compounds,* January 2005

149. **Ripple, S.D.:** Emergency Planning in Crisis Management in the Workplace. In *The Occupational Environment: Its Evaluation, Control and Management*, 2nd edition. DiNardi, S.R. (ed.). Fairfax, VA: AIHA, 2003. pp. 984–995.
150. **Jederberg, W.W.:** Toxicology in Emergency Response Planning. In *Toxicology Principles for the Industrial Hygienist*. Luttrell, W.E., W.W. Jederberg, and K.R. Still (eds.). Fairfax, VA: AIHA, 2008. pp. 329–338.
151. **AIHA®:** White Paper — Industrial Hygienist's Role and Responsibilities In Emergency Preparedness and Response [Online]. http://www.aiha.org/news-pubs/govtaffairs/Documents/whitepaper09_EPRWhitePaper_Final.pdf. [Accessed August 2010].
152. **AIHA®:** *2007 Emergency Response Guidelines & Workplace Environmental Exposure Levels Handbook*. Fairfax VA. AIHA Press, 2007.
153. **Department of Transportation (DOT), Transport Canada (TC):** *The 2008 Emergency Response Guidebook*. Neenah, WI: J.J. Keller & Assoc., 2008.
154. **Simmons. F., D. Quigley, D. Freshwater, H. Whyte, L. Boada-Clista, and J.C. Laul:** Determining Acute Health Hazard Ratings in the Absence of Applicable Toxicological Data. *J. Occ. Env. Health 4*:841–847 (2007).
155. **U.S. Environmental Protection Agency (EPA):** Guidelines for the Health Risk Assessment of Chemical Mixtures. *Federal Register 51 (185)*:34014–34025 (1986).
156. **Hallenbeck, W.H.:** *Quantitative Risk Assessment for Environmental and Occupational Health*. Boca Raton, FL: Lewis Publishers, 1993.
157. **Timbrell, J.A.:** *Principles of Biochemical Toxicology*. New York: Taylor & Francis, 1996.
158. **Williams, P.L. and J.L. Burson:** *Industrial Toxicology, Safety and Health Application in the Workplace*. New York: Van Nostrand Reinhold. 1985.
159. **Klaassen, C.D. (ed.):** *Casarett and Doull's Toxicology—The Basic Science of Poisons*, 5th edition. McGraw-Hill, Inc., 1996.
160. **National Research Council:** *Issues in Risk Assessment*. Washington, D.C.: National Academy Press, 1993.
161. **Fischhoff, B., A. Bostrom, and M.J. Quandrel:** Risk perception and communication. *Ann. Rev. Pub. Health 14*:183–203 (1993).
162. **U.S. Environmental Protection Agency (EPA):** Risk Assessment Guidance for Superfund, Volume 1, Human Health Evaluation Manual, Part A, Interim Final. EPA/540/1-90/002, Office of Emergency and Remedial Response. Washington, D.C.: U.S. EPA, 1989.
163. **U.S. Environmental Protection Agency (EPA):** Exposure Factors Handbook, Final Report. Washington, DC, Exposure Assessment Group, Office of Health and Environmental Assessment. Washington, D.C.: U.S. EPA, 1989.
164. **U.S. Environmental Protection Agency (EPA):** Guidelines for Exposure Assessment Federal Register 57: 22888–22938. Washington, D.C.: U.S. EPA, 1992.
165. **Hauschild, V.D. and G.M. Bratt:** Prioritizing Industrial Chemical Hazards. *J. Tox. Env. Health 68*:857–876 (2005)
166. **Foth, H. and A.W. Haye:** Concept of REACH and impact on the evaluation of chemicals. *Hum. Exper. Toxicol. 27*:5–21(2008).
167. **Monosson, E.:** Chemical Mixtures: A review of the evolution of toxicology and chemical regulation from a single chemical approach to a science and regulatory process that must address complex chemical mixtures. Military Waste Cleanup Program, 2003 (On line: www.rachel.org/files/document/Chemical_Mixtures.pdf) [Accessed August 2010].
168. **Mumatz, M.M., D.B. Tully, H.A. El-Masri, and C.T. DeRosa:** Gene Induction Studies and Toxicity of Chemical Mixtures. *Env. Health Pers. 110*:947–956 (2002).
169. **Monosson, E.:** Chemical Mixtures: Considering the Evolution of Toxicology and Chemical Assessment. *Env. Health Pers. 113*:383–390 (2005).
170. **Vyskocil A, et al.:** A Web tool for the Identification of Potential Interactive Effects of Chemical Mixtures. *J. Occ. Env. Hyg. 4*:281–287 (2007).
171. **Safe, S.H.:** Polychlorinated Biphenyls (PCBs): Environmental Impact, Biochemical and Toxic Responses, and Implications for Risk Assessment. *Crit. Rev. Toxicol. 24(2)*:87–149 (1994).
172. **Harrison, W.N., S.M. Bradberry, and J.A. Vale:** Chemical Contamination of Private Drinking Water Supplies in the West Midlands, United Kingdom. *Clin. Tox. 38(2)*:137–144 (2000).
173. **Teague, J.K.:** Research Article: Volatile organic compounds in Beech Creek, a tributary of Lake Columbia, Arkansas. *BIOS 76(1)*:15–21 (2005).
174. **Armitage, J.A. and F. Gobas:** A Terrestrial Food-Chain Bioaccumulation Model for POPs. *Env. Sci. & Tech. 41(11)*:4019–4025 (2007).
175. **Wright, C.:** Analytical methods for monitoring contaminants in food – An industrial perspective. *J. Chronog. 1216(3)*:316–319 (2009).

176. **U.S. Environmental Protection Agency (EPA):** *Chemical Hazard Data Availability Study: What Do We Really Know About the Safety of High Production Volume Chemical?* Washington, D.C.: Office of Pollution Prevention and Toxics, April 1998.
177. **Chemical Profiles:** High Production (HPV) Chemicals. [Online] www.scorecard.org/chemical-profiles/def/hpv.html. [Accessed August 2010].
178. **U.S. Environmental Protection Agency (EPA):** Chemical Hazard Data Availability Study: High Production Volume (HPV) Chemicals and SIDS Testing Office of Pollution Prevention and Toxics. Office of Pollution Prevention and Toxics. Washington, D.C.: U.S. EPA, 1998. [Online] www.epa.gov/hpv/pubs/general/hazchem.htm [Accessed July 22, 2008].
179. **AIHA®:** *Position Statement: Material Safety Data Sheet.* American Industrial Hygiene Association. [Online] Available at www.aiha.org/1documents/GovernmentAffairs/P-MSDS-09-02-2005.pdf. [Accessed August 2010].
180. **Jederberg, W.W.:** Issues with the Integration of Technical Information in Planning for and Responding to Non-Traditional Incidents. *J. Toxicol. Environ. Health 68(11–12)*:877–888 (2005).
181. **Silk, J.C.:** Hazard Communication. In *The Occupational Environment, Its Evaluation, Control, and Management*, 2nd edition. DiNardi, S.R. (ed). Fairfax, VA: AIHA, 2003.
182. **Kopstein, M.:** Potential Uses of Petrochemical Products Can Result in Significant Benzene Exposures: MSDSs Must List Benzene as an Ingredient. *J. Occ. Environ. Hyg. 3*:1–8 (2006).
183. **Grumbles, T.G.:** "Hearing on Material Safety Data Sheets and Hazard Communications," United States Senate Committee on Health, Education, Labor and Pensions Subcommittee on Employment, Safety and Training held March 25, 2004 [Online] Available at http://help.senate.gov/imo/media/doc/grumbles.pdf. [Accessed August 2010].

Outcome Competencies

After completing this chapter, the reader should be able to:

1. Define and apply the terminology used in this chapter.
2. Explain how risk is related to the results of epidemiological studies.
3. Recognize and appropriately apply the appropriate study type based on the study population and the outcome of concern.
4. Discuss the significance of epidemiological surveillance in the identification of potential work-related health problems.
5. Describe the process of estimating exposure from workplace data, including reconstructing from historical information.
6. Describe the role industrial hygienists play in conducting epidemiological studies.

Key Topics

I. Introduction
II. Terminology
III. Concept of Causation
IV. Expressing Risk
V. Study Types
   A. Case Series
   B. Cross-sectional Study
   C. Cohort Study
   D. Case-Control Study
   E. Summary of Study Types
VI. Industrial Hygiene and Retrospective Epidemiology Studies of Past Exposures
VII. Review Available Data and Information
VIII. Exposure Assessment Study Design and Conduct
IX. Industrial Hygiene Records Systems for Future Study Use
X. Conclusion
XI. References

Key Terms

causation • cohort • exposure assessment • exposure reconstruction • incidence • odds ratio• person-time • prevalence • risk • retrospective exposure assessment • work history

Prerequisite Knowledge

Prior to beginning this chapter, the user should review the following references for general content:

Academic Discipline	Reference Citation
Introduction to Epidemiology	**Rothman, K.J.:** *Epidemiology: An Introduction.* New York: Oxford University Press, 2002.
Occupational Epidemiology	**Checkoway, H., N.A. Pearce, and D. Kriebel:** *Research Methods in Occupational Epidemiology,* 2nd Edition. New York: Oxford University Press, 2004.
Epidemiological Terminology	**Last, J.M.:** *A Dictionary of Epidemiology,* 4th Edition. New York: Oxford University Press, 2000.

Prior to beginning this chapter, the user should review the following chapters:

Chapter Number	Chapter Topic
4	Occupational Exposure Limits
7	Principles of Evaluating Worker Exposure
41	Program Management
45	Risk Communication
46	Developing an Occupational Health Program

Occupational Epidemiology

6

Thomas W. Armstrong, CIH, PhD; Ernest P. Chiodo, MD, JD, MPH, MS, CIH; Robert F. Herrick, ScD, MS, CIH; and Christopher P. Rennix, ScD, MS, CIH

Introduction

Epidemiology is a discipline of science that explores the distribution of disease or injuries in populations with the ultimate goal of defining causation. The term epidemiology originates from the Greek term "epidemos" which means "upon the people." The term is a reference to the original use of the word referring to infectious diseases afflicting large segments of a population, including bubonic plague which caused the Black Death in 14th century Europe. Epidemiology developed as a scientific discipline along with the development of mathematics during the 17th century. One of the early victories in the use of epidemiology was the ability of the English physician John Snow to show that cholera was spread by contaminated water. Over time, the principles of epidemiology were used outside of infectious diseases and began to be applied to occupational exposures.

While some adverse outcomes appear to be obvious, like a head injury from an object striking an unprotected head, most times the cause is more complex. Epidemiology provides a framework for evaluating relationships even when the actual cause will remain unknown. The context under which the type of epidemiology is defined is based on the population under study and the source of the risks. Thus, occupational epidemiology is the study of the working population and the risks for illness and injury associated with the work environment.

The practice of occupational epidemiology is a team effort. Data on exposures and workplace stressors are collected, organized, analyzed, and interpreted by industrial hygienists (IH). Occupational histories, details on behavioral and genetic risk factors, and screening examinations are a function of the occupational health nurse. Clinical evaluation of the worker's health in response to their job, exposures, and risks falls under the occupational physician. The occupational epidemiologist reviews population-level data, like morbidity and mortality statistics, for trends in outcomes that might indicate a problem or support a successful injury prevention program. Because epidemiology uses the comparison of groups as a measure of risk, unusual or rare outcomes may be lost in the statistical noise and the team has to communicate their observations and investigate these cases. There are many examples where the astute physician, nurse, or industrial hygienist has provided the initial evidence that led to new information about an occupational hazard.

The primary objective of this chapter is to provide industrial hygienists with sufficient information about occupational epidemiology to clearly describe their roles in conducting studies, aid in the collection of workplace data to improve exposure assessments, and provide context for the interpretation of study findings. The materials in this chapter are presented in two sections — basic occupational epidemiologic concepts and historical exposure reconstruction. Many occupational hazards have been studied and the results published in the peer-reviewed literature. This chapter will also provide industrial hygienists with the basic tools to evaluate these studies and to use them as guides for understanding the results of their own workplace assessments.

In 1987, Checkoway et al.[1] constituted a task force from the AIHA's® Occupational Epidemiology Committee to describe the roles of industrial hygienist in conducting occupational epidemiology studies. This chapter updates that seminal work and provides more information that was not included in the journal article. Checkoway et al.[7] provides a more detailed description of the studies and methods discussed in this chapter and should be consulted to obtain additional information about occupational epidemiology. Other resources for general epidemiologic concepts, methods, analysis, and interpretation of study results are provided at the end of the chapter.

Terminology

Risk – The chance that an event will occur or a person in a group will get the outcome of interest.

Absolute risk – The number of cases or people with an outcome in a population over a period of time.

Relative risk – The risk for an outcome in an exposed group or population compared to the risk in the unexposed.

Odds – The number of individuals with the outcome divided by the number without the outcome in the same exposure group.

Odds ratio – The odds in the exposed divided by the odds in the unexposed for the outcome of interest.

Prevalence – The number of individuals with an outcome in a population over a specified period of time; includes existing and new cases.

Incidence – The number of individuals with an outcome in a population over a specified period of time that were outcome-free at the beginning of the time period, i.e. new cases.

Person-time – The amount of time a person is at risk to develop an outcome, usually beginning at the time of first exposure to the suspected agent or risk.

Incidence rate – The number of incident individuals divided by the total person-time at risk in a population.

Case series – A descriptive study of common factors shared by a series of people with the same or similar outcome.

Cross sectional study – A study that compares the prevalence of an outcome between groups that are divided by exposure status.

Cohort study – A longitudinal study that follows groups that are divided by their exposure status compares the risk for an outcome between the groups.

Case-control study – A study that evaluates groups that are divided by their disease status to compare the level(s) of exposure between the groups.

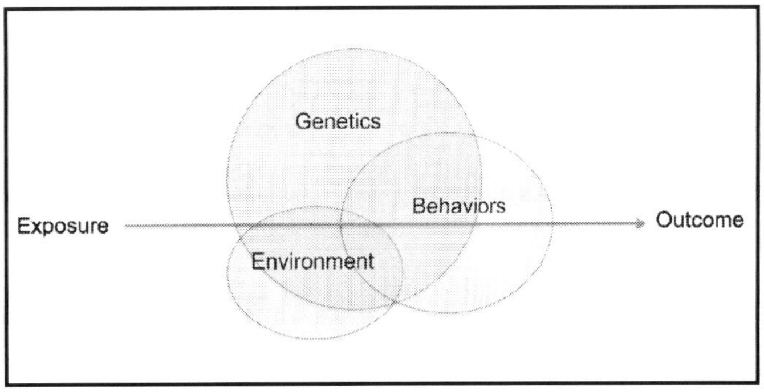

Figure 6.1 — Exposure-Outcome model.

Concept of Causation

The goal of epidemiology is to discover the causes of the outcome. When the causes are not revealed by a study, then a secondary goal is to quantify the risks for an outcome. By knowing and understanding the causal process, interventions can be implemented, medical screening can be used at the appropriate time, and the workers can make better decisions regarding their risk for the outcome. The problem is that most outcomes of interest in an occupational setting have multiple causes and the gene-environment interaction varies with each individual. A simple model of exposure-outcome is illustrated in Figure 6.1.

For an exposure to be considered part of the casual pathway, it must precede the outcome with sufficient time for the casual mechanism to be completed. A worker's genetic make-up, personal behaviors, and the environment outside of the exposure of interest influence the body's response to an exposure. For IHs, this concept is well understood. For example, hearing loss has been associated with exposure to high noise levels, some organic solvents, and smoking.[3,4,5] The workplace IH is responsible for recognizing and anticipating hazardous operations, assessing the exposure, recommending controls to prevent, eliminate, or reduce exposure, and to evaluate the effectiveness of these measures. Without any knowledge of behaviors outside of the workplace or a person's genetic history, it is possible that an increase in some individual's hearing thresholds will be erroneously attributed to occupational exposure. Epidemiology can assist in the understanding of the causation model for hearing loss and assess the impact of the gene-environment interaction on the risk for developing hearing loss in an occupationally exposed population.

Outcomes in occupational health are usually classified as acute or chronic. Acute illnesses and injuries have a shorter causal pathway, increasing the likelihood that the root causes can be identified. Chemical pneumonitis in an air conditioning repairperson logically leads us to ask about recent activities that include welding or gas soldering around refrigerant gases, much like asking who ate the potato salad during a gastroenteritis outbreak investigation. Chronic disease usually results from long-term exposure to occupational and non-occupational stressors. The longer the time between the beginning of exposure and the detection of the outcome, the harder it is to separate the contributions from each source. Going back to the air conditioning repairperson, a diagnosis of lung cancer after 30 years of exposure to cadmium in silver solder and a pack-a-day smoking habit makes it very difficult to attribute the cause to either exposure.[6,7] Epidemiology methods can be used to study the exposure-response model including competing risks from other sources.

Cause can be divided into two groups — necessary and sufficient. Rothman[8] described necessary cause as a component of the causal pathway that must be present for the outcome to develop. For instance, berylliosis requires exposure to beryllium, making it necessary for the causal pathway to be complete. If all of the components in the casual pathway are present at the right time and under the right conditions, then there is sufficient cause for the health outcome.

One of the misconceptions about causation with respect to epidemiology is that an epidemiologic study will prove that an exposure or group of exposures caused someone's illness. This might be possible with acute outcomes, but the probability decreases with time as other casual pathways come into play. In most epidemiologic studies, the risk for a specific outcome in the exposed population is compared to the risk for disease in the unexposed population. These are group risks, not individual risks. More sophisticated studies will include information that is also related to the outcome and the exposure, such as age, gender, tobacco use history, alcohol use history, a family history of cancer, and some hobbies. Ignoring these factors may bias the study results if the distribution of the factors is different between the study groups. If the comparison group (non-repairpersons) is the engineering staff at the company and their prevalence for tobacco use is significantly lower than the repairpersons, then not including that factor in the study would bias the study towards the exposed group.[7] Specific study types designed to control the influence of these factors on the overall risk will be discussed later.

Expressing Risk

There are several ways to express the level of risk resulting from a particular exposure. While absolute risk can be measured in a population, it doesn't provide much information upon which action might be taken. If the risk in a group that is exposed to an agent that is suspected to be in the causal pathway is higher compared to a group that does not have that exposure or that outcome, then factors in the causal pathway may be actionable to reduce the risk. The methods used to compare exposed and unexposed groups include risk ratios, standardized ratios and regression analysis. The first level of analysis is very basic — "Is the observed risk higher than would be expected?" This level of analysis can be elegantly illustrated in a simple 2 by 2 table (Table 6.1). The table is used to calculate the risk of the outcome in the exposed (a/(a+c)) and the unexposed (b/(b+d)).

Table 6.1 — Example of 2 by 2 table

		Exposed *Yes*	*No*	*Totals*
Outcome	Yes	a	b	
	No	c	d	
	Totals	a + c	b + d	

$$\text{Relative Risk} = \frac{\text{Risk in exposed}}{\text{Risk in unexposed}} = \frac{(^{a}/_{(a+c)})}{(^{b}/_{(b+d)})} \quad (6\text{-}1)$$

For example, in a population of industrial workers, 15 new cases of dermatitis are observed in the clinic during annual physical exams. The industrial hygienist suspects it may be due to contact with a new cleaning solvent. The epidemiologist constructs a cohort of all 100 workers in the industrial area of the plant where the solvent was available for use and divides the cohort based on use of the solvent. In 100 workers, the number of workers that used the solvent was 30, including 8 of the cases (Table 6.2).

Table 6.2 — Risk for contact dermatitis

		Solvent user		
		Yes	*No*	*Totals*
Contact	Yes	8	7	15
dermatitis	No	22	63	85
	Totals	30	70	100

Some of the risk measures associated with a diagnosis of contact dermatitis that can be calculated from the table include:

a. Incidence — the number of new cases in the total population at risk.
   Incidence = 15/100 = 0.15 or 15% or 15 per 100 persons
b. Incidence in the exposed — the number of cases in the exposed population
   Risk = 8/30 = 0.27 or 27% or 27 per 100 exposed persons
c. Incidence in the unexposed — the number of cases in the unexposed population
   Risk = 7/70 = 0.1 = 10% or 10 per 100 unexposed persons
d. Relative risk = Incidence in the exposed/Incidence in the unexposed
   Relative Risk = 0.27/0.10 = 2.7

The relative risk for contact dermatitis in workers who used the solvent was 2.7 times greater than those who did not use the solvent. The study does not prove that the solvent caused the dermatitis; it shows the increased risk. If exposure to the solvent was eliminated and the <u>incidence</u> of this type of dermatitis decreased to levels seen in the unexposed population, then that information would contribute to the causal model. If the solvent exposure was eliminated and the incidence did not decrease, then it's possible that the solvent was a surrogate for another exposure in the plant that still needs attention.

This level of analysis works well for acute types of outcomes or studies in very large populations, but can easily be overcome by confounding. Confounding introduces bias into a study when a risk factor for the outcome is also independently associated with the exposure. In occupational studies, age is a routine confounder. The risk for many occupational diseases and injuries are associated with increasing age and the longer you live, the more exposure you accumulate and the more chances you have to acquire the outcome.

The next level of analysis that an epidemiologist may use replaces the population denominator with person-time. <u>Person-time</u> is the time that a person is at risk for exposure and usually begins when a person is first exposed or first employed. Because time is now part of the risk model, rates can be used to express risk. Incidence becomes incidence rate or the number of new cases of an outcome per unit of person-time, like 3.2 cases of leukemia per 100,000 person-years. The incidence rate by itself does not really convey whether the observed rate is higher than would be expected in the population. A comparison is needed to put the rate into context.

If the general population rate for a disease is known, it can be applied to the exposed population to find the number of expected cases. The ratio of the observed number cases to the expected is called the standardized mortality or morbidity ratio (SMR). Age is a strong confounder for many occupational diseases and injuries, so age-specific rates are used when calculating the expected case totals. To calculate the expected number of cases using the age distribution of person-time in the study population, the standard population rates are used for each age strata. If the observed number of cases exceeds the number of expected cases, that might indicate an increased risk. Because SMRs are calculated using the age distribution of the study population, SMRs for one study cannot be compared to SMRs from other studies.

For example, in a hypothetical population of workers at an university, the annual physical exams included audiometric testing. Hearing loss is associated with exposure to high levels of sound pressure. To determine if the number of temporary threshold shifts (TTS) was higher than would be expected in the general population, the rate of TTS in the university workers was compared to the rate of TTS in the general population. Rates in the general population can be obtained from government agencies, journal articles, and special interest groups. For instance, the age-specific rates for some cancers can be obtained from the National Cancer Institute publications. To calculate the SMR:

$$\text{SMR} = \frac{\text{Observed cases (A)}}{\text{Expected cases (D)}} \times 100 \qquad (6\text{-}2)$$

Where:

Expected cases (D) = Person-time for each strata (B) × Age-specific rate (C)

While the overall SMR is less than 100 (shown in Table 6.3), there is some concern about the 20–29 age-group and additional studies may be required to evaluate their apparent excess risk.

By stratifying on exposure, subgroups, like specific shops or occupations might be missed due a small number of cases. Subgroup analysis may provide insight to actions taken that reduced the observed cases as a measure of a successful intervention. When there are just a few exposure groups and one confounder or risk factor, stratified analysis is usually sufficient. When the model becomes more complex or exposure is going to be used as a continuous variable in the model, there are statistical computer programs specifically designed to provide the risk estimates.

Study Types

The study type is dictated by the circumstances, the budget, and the willingness of the population or groups and management to participate. Computerized records that include employment information, workplace exposures, medical surveillance results, and health histories can significantly reduce the cost of any study. There are two time periods to consider — retrospective and prospective.

Retrospective studies have the advantage of knowing the outcomes for the study and the task is to reconstruct the exposure period for the study population. The study period must start at a time when all of the participants were free of the outcome of interest and when first exposure can be ascertained. Most occupational epidemiology studies are retrospective because they seek to answer the question "Did exposure to agent X increase the risk for disease Y?" If there were a strong suspicion that agent X was associated with disease Y, then exposure to agent X should be limited or eliminated. Prospective occupational cohort studies try to anticipate the likely outcomes of a known exposure and follow the population over time, making them ideal for determining the success of interventions. Exposure, injury, and illness metrics used by industries to track compliance and health and safety performance are actually a type of epidemiology study. They identify a population that is free of the outcome at the time the follow-up starts and count the instances that occurred. By focusing on the targeted population as the "exposed" (e.g. received training), the incidence rates can be compared to the unexposed population or to the baseline rates to determine success.

All studies have some weaknesses that limit the ability to reach a definitive or fully accurate conclusion. Incomplete follow-up of all study members may introduce bias if the loss is not randomly distributed across the study population. In workplaces with significant turnover, follow-up can be problematic as workers change jobs or leave the

Table 6.3 — Example of SMR calculation

	Study Cohort		*Reference Population*		
Age	*Observed (A)*	*Person-years (B)*	*Rate per 100 (C)*	*Expected (D)*	*SMR*
20–29	20	2000	0.5	10	200
30–39	10	2000	0.8	16	63
40–49	5	1000	1.2	12	42
50+	15	500	3	15	100
Total	50			53	94.3

company. For prospective studies, the size of the study at the beginning must have a sufficient number of participants to allow for some loss to follow-up but still have enough power at the study end to conduct the analysis. Prospective studies are better suited for relatively acute responses, whether it is for the intended outcome or an intermediate outcome in the exposure-outcome model. For instance, if the goal was prevention of permanent threshold shifts due to exposure to occupational noise, the temporary threshold shifts could be used as an intermediate outcome instead of waiting until the damage is irreversible to conclude a study.

There are four study designs that are used frequently in occupational settings and selection of the most appropriate type is based on the question being asked.

Case Series

The most basic study type is the case series, also called the "astute clinician." The case series is not really a study in a traditional sense in that it is typically qualitative and is based on clinical observations in a single patient or group of patients that share a similar condition. The question "Where do you work?" is the beginning of this type of study. By interviewing to obtain retrospective information or following the group prospectively, hypotheses can be developed that can be tested with a more formal study. Several of the historical occupational medicine discoveries were based on the case series design including scrotal cancer in chimney sweeps, breast cancer in nuns, and angiosarcoma in vinyl chloride monomer workers.
Occupational health clinics provide this level of analysis as part of their normal function. When the occupational health nurse unexpectedly notices a cluster of hearing loss or impaired lung function in a group of workers from the same shop, a natural hypothesis is created that something in the shop is different and a quick survey of the shop by an industrial hygienist can either confirm the hypothesis or lead to a more in-depth study.

Cross-sectional Study

A cross-sectional study is focused on the prevalence of an outcome in a population that has a risk for exposure to a suspected agent in the outcome causal pathway at the time the survey is conducted. This type of design works well for acute illnesses and injuries or when evaluating the effectiveness or success of an intervention. The advantages of a cross-sectional study include simple design and execution, ability to use of intermediate conditions rather than the final outcome, and being able to compare the results to other populations with similar risks and exposures. For example, as part of a Contingency Operations Plan, an influenza vaccination program was begun at the plant to reduce lost workdays and to evaluate the effectiveness of the immunization plan. At the end of the influenza season, you surveyed all of the workers were surveyed to determine who was diagnosed with influenza and who had received their flu shots. The results could be compared to previous years lost workday metrics, other plants that do or do not have immunization plans, and to the local population influenza prevalence. Cross-sectional studies are subject to recall bias and may exclude workers that left before the collection of the data. Another limitation is that the timing of exposure and the outcome may not be related. In the contact dermatitis example before, there was no attempt to find out if any of the cases preceded the solvent use.

Cohort Study

While the results of a case series or cross-sectional design might give rise to a suspicion or hypothesis, the cohort study design can be used to test a hypothesis or to determine the magnitude of the problem. Cohort studies are used to compare the risk for an outcome in an exposed group or groups to an unexposed, lesser-exposed group, or a larger population in which the exposure is rare. The hypothesis being tested is that exposure to a suspected agent is associated with the outcome. When the exposure cannot be measured directly, surrogates of exposure may be used, such as time job title. As discussed earlier, retrospective cohort studies look at historical exposures and prospective cohort studies anticipate exposures that may be associated with the outcome. Depending on the causal model being used and the populations being studied, additional information at the group or individual levels may be required if these factors are part of the causal model. If this additional information were not included in the study, it is possible that the factor may not be randomly distributed between the groups and may bias the outcome estimates.

Cohort studies also incorporate a time variable through the use of person-time in calculating rates, making them more suited for the study of chronic outcomes. Because the initiation of the disease process is usually unknown, the date of first hire or first exposure can be used to begin the person-time counter. The time to complete the casual pathway is called the induction period and the time from the completed pathway to the clinical diagnosis of the disease is called the latent period.[8] Rothman calls the combined periods the empirical induction time. To provide an accurate estimate of the risk due to the suspected exposure, the time since first exposure (the start of the casual process) to the earliest detection of the outcome (the end of the latent period) must be incorporated into the study. For example, if the annual medical surveillance report for a plant listed the types of cancer detected within the population, a lung cancer case in a 55 year-old male smoker seems reasonable. Lung cancer can take up to 30 years to develop and most workers begin their working life at around age 20 and most people who smoke began in their teens. Also, a significant portion of this person's early working life did not benefit from the protections provided by occupational health and safety regulations. A cohort study that only included those with at least 20 years of employment would eliminate any earlier cases that might be due to other causes, allowing the study to focus on the workplace exposures. The early cases may be the result of an exposure to another agent or, at the individual level, due to a genetic mutation that reduced the induction period. These cases may warrant a separate investigation to determine possible associations with the occupational environment.

One of the most important parts of a cohort study is selecting the appropriate comparison group. The comparison group should be as close in composition as the exposed group except for the exposure. Analysis of the groups should establish the similarities, especially for recognized risk factors and age. In peer-reviewed journal articles, cohort studies almost always include a demographic table that establishes the comparability of the study groups. Groups that are not comparable across a risk factor, like age or race, may be biased because any difference in risk may not be solely due to the exposure. The best sources for the comparison group include another shop with similar skill levels, another plant, or a union for the trades being investigated where the suspected agent is not used. Industrial hygienists can assist the epidemiologist in locating and assessing the exposure in the comparison group.

Case-Control Study

Case-control studies are the primary tool in occupational epidemiology for understanding the casual pathway for an outcome. In the cohort study, the study is based on the difference in risk between exposure groups. In a case-control study, the focus is on the differences in risk based on outcome status, those with the outcome or "case" and those free of the outcome or "control." Case-control studies are best suited for rare outcomes where a comparable cohort study would need to be extremely large to accumulate enough cases to conduct the study. The primary cost of doing any study is data collection. Electronic databases have reduced this cost immensely over the years, but additional data, such as nutritional status, family history, other non-workplace exposures and activities, and risky behaviors, may be needed to fully evaluate the impact exposure has on the risk for the outcome. To collect that level of information for all cohort study participants could make case-control studies a more cost-efficient alternative.

Because case-control studies are based around the cases, the distribution of potentially confounding factors is not random and must be controlled. This may be accomplished by matching controls to each case on those factors. While the goal is to reduce the impact of confounding on the risk estimates, matching is a forced association and the confounding variable cannot be part of the analysis. To keep as many risk factors in the study model as possible, epidemiologists test for confounding before selecting factors to avoid unnecessary matching. For example, if a study matches on birth year, age cannot be included in the study risk model. Matching cases and controls using the birth year controls several factors simultaneously because of the potential for shared experiences.

Examples of these shared experiences could include changes in exposures due to regulation, changes in the general work environment and management practices, and lifestyle changes over the years.

The risk estimate used in a case-control study is the odds ratio, which is a good approximation of the relative risk when the outcome is rare in the population. The odds ratio is calculated by dividing the odds for the outcome in the exposed to the odds for the outcome in the unexposed. Because the outcome is dichotomous, statistical software with logistic regression functions should be used to obtain the risk estimates for the study model factors.

In each of the models, exposure is considered to be the primary risk for the outcome. Industrial hygienists fulfill an extremely valuable service to occupational epidemiology studies by providing an accurate exposure assessment and to provide context to the study when describing the plausibility of the exposure-outcome model.

Summary of Study Types

See Table 6.4 below.

Industrial Hygiene and Retrospective Epidemiology Studies of Past Exposures

There have been many texts and articles published in past and recent years that discuss the role of industrial hygiene and retrospective exposure assessments in occupational

Table 6.4 — Comparison of Study Types[2,8,9]

Study Type	*Strengths*	*Limitations*
Case Series	- Descriptive - No comparison group - Hypothesis generating	- Analysis limited to commonalities between the cases - Unable to test hypothesis - Doesn't provide a rate
Cross-sectional	- Hypothesis generating - Can be used to compare over time or between other groups - Easy to conduct	- Lacks time component for exposure to outcome model - Subject to recall bias
Prospective Cohort	- Reduces recall bias - Can capitalize on available electronic data - Can explore multiple outcomes for the planned exposures - Best when exposure to suspected agent is rare in the general population	- Finding an appropriate comparison group - Study attrition rate may require a very large study - Unplanned changes in work practices or elimination of the exposure may shut down the study - Time to conduct study can be very long for chronic outcomes
Retrospective Cohort	- Can explore multiple outcomes for exposures - Can be less expensive than a prospective cohort - Effects of confounding reduced with good comparison group selection - Best when exposure is rare in the general population - Provides a direct measurement of the risk in the population	- Subject to recall bias and exposure misclassification - Distribution of risk factors assumed to be random in exposed and unexposed groups - Cost dependent upon the amount of information that must be collected for the entire cohort
Case-control	- Relatively small size permits more resources for data collection - Can explore multiple exposure models for an outcome - Best when outcome is rare in the population - Usually less expensive than cohort studies	- Control selection critical to study - Very sensitive to uncontrolled confounding - Subject to recall bias and exposure misclassification

epidemiology studies. Two studies[1,9] are particularly drawn upon in this summary. The latter includes a recent bibliography of essential references for occupational exposure reconstruction. Estimation of past exposures is often a core part of retrospective occupational epidemiology study designs. Thus, industrial hygiene support to occupational epidemiology projects should include early stage engagement as a study team member and participate in decisions of overall study goals, study design, personnel available, budget and timelines. Once these are defined, the industrial hygiene exposure assessment may be more successfully undertaken. For the study as a whole to succeed, the exposure assessment approach must provide the data needed to meet the study goals. A study whose goal is improving the information available about dose-response of a substance from occupational exposure will likely need a rather rigorous quantitative exposure assessment. Alternatively, a study seeking to identify if a hazard exists may require only a qualitative assessment. An exposure assessment study, whether qualitative or quantitative, is likely to proceed in a loosely sequential order. Table 6.5 which was adapted from Viet, et al.[10] summarizes many of the stages and components to consider in a retrospective assessment. Additional discussion follows. Examples given below are largely drawn from experiences in published studies[11], and unpublished work currently underway.

Table 6.5 — Industrial hygienist roles and activities by study stage

Study Stage	*Industrial Hygienist Roles and Activities*
Study Design and Startup	
General study design	Evaluate literature on exposure assessment approaches suitable for the proposed epidemiology study design and goals. Evaluate past studies, if any, for similar populations and exposures. Review the diseases(s), exposure agent(s) of interest, and the time period(s) of exposure. Review possible confounders and effect modifiers, and metrics of exposure to be developed during the exposure assessment work.
Feasibility verification	Evaluate the scope of supporting information needed. Investigate a sample of the broad types of records and information available, which includes any relevant monitoring data. Determine and discuss the likelihood that available information is adequate to support the study exposure assessment objectives.
Study budget, timeline	Develop resource estimates, time required, key deadlines, and budget for the exposure assessment. Consider personnel, equipment, laboratory analysis support, travel and expenses, as appropriate. Include the review processes, data handling procedures (e.g., data confidentiality), and preparation of final manuscripts/reports and publications.
Scope of reconstruction activity	Identify the investigation criteria that will be used in the reconstruction effort (e.g., in the case of medical surveillance, all workers who were exposed above an agent's exposure limit action level for at least 30 days in the prior calendar year.)
Exposure assessment protocols	Identify the procedures that will be used to apply the project criteria in consistent and objective manner.
Study Conduct	
Data search and assembly	Where data are sparse or limited to a few exposure groups, incorporate a comprehensive baseline survey, as possible. Assemble, review, extract, and summarize records relevant to the exposure assessment for the study design, considering work histories, facility changes, exposures of concern and confounders, and other aspects. Evaluate the information sources available to apply the project criteria. Collect the information about the process or interview facility managers and workers. Identify and contact any expert sources that you may need for advice or information (e.g., medical staff, engineers, other researchers.) *The IH may need to develop ad hoc solutions to missing information and other barriers. Review and comments by other team members or selected experts may also need to be sought.

Table 6.5 — Industrial hygienist roles and activities by study stage (continued)

Study Stage	*Industrial Hygienist Roles and Activities*
Study Conduct	
Develop exposure estimates	Select exposure metrics and group exposures. Develop estimates for each worker or group of similar workers.
Perform data quality activities	"Validate" the exposure assessment to the extent possible and as stipulated in the protocol. Provide input into uncertainty and sensitivity analyses.
Study Data Analysis and Reporting	
Data analyses, reports and manuscripts	Deliver the exposure assessments in a format useful for the planned analyses (per protocol and feasibility). This may require various exposure metrics be generated. Provide an accurate assessment of the exposure assessment assumptions, strengths, and limitations. Support/prepare reports or publications.
Maintain documentation	Document the exposure assessment and revisions, including any assumptions made during the exposure assessment.* Document the QA/QC processes and procedures as planned in the protocol. Provide sufficient details in files and reports for others to follow and verify the work, or to build on it in subsequent studies. *Appropriate documentation will aid in report writing, QA/QC auditing, and support for any future, follow-up studies.

Review Available Data and Information

In retrospective occupational epidemiology, the level of detail about work histories and historical exposure information must be reconciled. The quantity, time span, and quality of exposure monitoring data are prime concerns for the industrial hygiene part of the exposure assessment. Measurements of exposure, without their survey purposes and operations conditions, are less than ideally informative. Information for retrospective assessments often is broader than just exposure monitoring. Table 6.6 lists the broad categories of information often sought.[1,10] These are discussed in more detail in this text. The extent of the search for and assembly of this broad range of information is dependent on the study goals and resources.

Table 6.6 — Categories of Information to Evaluate for Retrospective Exposure Assessment

1. Job and task descriptions. Include duration and frequency of main tasks with potential exposure to study substances of concern. Note which may be logically combined into similar Job/Task/Time/Exposure matrices.
2. Changes in raw materials, intermediates, additives and products over time for the relevant job/task groups in the study.
3. Process descriptions, and floor layouts, with particular emphasis on changes back through time in equipment and flow. Consider changes in rest/break areas as well.
4. Production records to track changes in quantities over time.
5. Exposure control system changes, such as installation and maintenance of new general or local exhaust or other means of reducing exposures.
6. Industrial hygiene monitoring records, including personal, area, and biological monitoring.
7. Usage of chemical protective clothing and use of respiratory protective equipment.
8. Environmental spill and discharge reports for contaminants of concern in the study.

1. *Job title and task information.* Ideally, personnel records provide sufficient discrimination of job titles, and work area assignments. However, these often need to be supplemented by interviews or other means to develop sufficient detail for quantitative assessments that consider work area and task pattern and time period differences in the work force under study. Organizations that implemented exposure assessment strategies of Homogeneous Exposure Groups (HEG)[12]or Similar Exposure Groups (SEG)[13,14] may have more details in

their records than for organizations that have not implemented these strategies or similar approaches. HEG or SEG assessments may extend back to the later 1980's in organizations that were developers of or early adopters of these systematic approaches. The early records of these assessments may form a basis for extrapolation backwards in time. Most of the HEG and SEG techniques described in the literature[13,14] although mainly for prospective assessments, have remarkable utility for retrospective assessments. They may provide a logical base for forming similar Job/Task/Time/Exposure matrices.

Example: Gaps in work histories (if any) should be resolved in consistent manner. For one completed study some missing work history segments were completed using several approaches. The electronic records were supplemented where necessary by looking for any archived paper records, which included medical records and personnel files. Note that medical records may be privileged information, and may contain disease diagnostic information, neither of which the exposure assessor should access. For some study subjects, review of prior and post jobs showed consistency in the type of work, which allowed for "filling in" the gap. However, blue-collar entry preceding a gap, with white-collar jobs afterward proved more difficult. One approach in such cases could be to "split the difference" by assigning one-half of the gap to the prior and the other half to the subsequent job.

2. *Raw materials, intermediates, additives and products over time for the relevant job/task groups in the study.* The current operations may or may not be relevant over the time periods of interest for the exposure assessment. If the operation has not been the same back through time, the exposure assessment becomes more challenging. Location of records of changes or interviews with long service employees (current and or retired) can be important. Both process engineers and operations employees may have valuable information than can be elicited in well-planned interviews. Day to day practices may not always have matched the intent of the process engineering designs.

   Example: Interviews with retired employees proved to be an important component in understanding the nature of operations that took place more than 20 years ago. Group interviews often lead to individuals challenging others recall, but yielding a consensus from the jogged memories of all. For a retrospective study in the petroleum industry, a retired industrial hygienist, who started his career in the operations of interest in 1953, confirmed the available data with respect to surveys and hazard controls for the significant issues of the eras investigated. Other experiences show that individual worker's interviews are highly variable in quality. Not many decades ago, workers seldom had access to reliable information about hazards in their workplaces. Hazard communication, once implemented, has made a difference in this, but not uniformly or ideally in all areas of the world. In some countries, current workers may be reluctant to give their opinions about hazards due to fears over the possible job loss. In some study designs such as hospital based case-control series, such worker interviews may be the most readily available information. Nevertheless, additional efforts may be needed to further develop the hazard inventory and nature of the exposure potential.

3. *Process descriptions, and floor layouts.* The particular interest is to find any time periods where there were redesigns of the process, or changes in the spacing and layout of the flow of materials. These could alter the nature of tasks and the intensity or frequency of exposure. Consider changes in rest/break areas as well. Where personnel take smoking breaks, coffee/tea breaks or where they eat may have changed over time.

   Example: During efforts to estimate exposures retrospectively, the blueprints for a company showed that designs for multiple locations followed essentially the same designs in similar blocks of time. This gave additional confidence in using data from given locations to estimate exposures at such "sibling" sites. Although this will not always be the case, industry technology and practices, especially that which enhances profits, often rapidly spread within a company and often within competitors too.

4. *Production records to track changes in quantities over time.* In some production processes, exposure may relate the production volume, such as to the number of batches produced, or the volume of material packaged. The number of workers assigned or their work hours (overtime, other shift patterns) may have changed with production.

   Example: Although only broad company average data were available for the eras investigated, more limited records for individual sites showed a fairly narrow divergence from the overall average.[11] This too helped confirm the utility of using data from available locations to fill in data for the sibling operations.

5. *Exposure control system changes. Installation and maintenance records for new general ventilation or local exhaust ventilation systems may have altered exposures.* These may be identified in engineering blueprints (item 3 above). Otherwise, for major changes in controls of exposure, employees there at the time may provide insights into the nature of the changes. Quantitative insights are harder to establish, and are probably seldom highly reliable. If engineering controls greatly reduced irritants or obnoxious odors, the changes will often be remembered if the right personnel can be located and asked questions in a structured way.

6. *Industrial hygiene monitoring records.* Monitoring data of reliable quality are obviously a key piece of information needed for retrospective exposure assessments. Information needed to put the data into context includes the reason for the survey and the design of the survey. The different survey rationale, such as regulatory (OSHA) compliance, investigation of release sources for exposure control selection, short-term samples of specific task exposures, or "random" samples to determine long-term average exposure may per interpreted differently. In some operations, the most likely highest exposed jobs were selectively surveyed. This may be an efficient strategy for regulatory compliance investigations, but such data must be interpreted cautiously since it may be biased high in relation to other jobs and for a metric such as a long-term average. Recent eras may present more measurement data than are available for the earlier years. The context of the sample and the broader operational; changes may also be harder to establish for the earlier years of the study. A range of approaches have been used to bridge gaps in available information. Statistical modeling based on the available data is one approach. Simulating past conditions and measuring the exposures is another possibility, but this may be difficult to complete with certainty, given historic materials, process equipment, and work practices may not be available. Mathematical modeling of exposure can help estimate past exposures, and may help improve the extrapolation back from current conditions and current exposures.[15] Statistical analysis tools, including Bayesian approaches[14] can aid in the interpretation of available data. Bayesian techniques have evolved that can combine prior knowledge about a scenario with limited data to yield an integrated interpretation of the total information. The Bayesian approaches have been utilized in retrospective exposure assessments.[16]

   Examples: Some industries compile data across organizations using standardized methods and job tiles. These may be valuable additions to a given company's own monitoring records. For example, several studies of petroleum marketing and distribution workers[11,17,18] have made use of European compilations of data[19] to supplement the available local data. In compilations of data, information about the sampling and analytical methods is important. Other issues include comparability of any job titles used across different companies (any within a company across locations and time), and information about the surveys that generated the data (e.g., worst case, random, full-shift samples or short-term).

7. *Usage of chemical protective clothing and use of respiratory protective equipment.* The quantitative impact of these controls, lacking biological monitoring results, can be particularly difficult to determine. However, they remain as important considerations. Workplace protection factors may consider the relative reliability of the protective equipment programs. Back through time, the quality of the programs was arguably not the same as in current practice.

   Example: In many situations, respiratory protective equipment (RPE), even in a plant producing a known human carcinogen, was significantly less than ideal in the mid-1970s. In addition, fit testing was often less than ideal, and devices were available in limited sizes. Heat and humidity made routine wear difficult (as it still may be). Although supervision had the responsibility for enforcing usage, this was sporadic at best. Following the OSHA Respiratory Protection Standard, several aspects of respiratory protection have undoubtedly improved, at least in major industries that take worker health seriously. Overall, reliable respiratory protection programs, in less than IDLH conditions, or with obnoxious odor/irritation circumstances, are frequently difficult to interpret as significantly reducing exposure very far back in history. RPE is low in the hierarchy of control priorities for good reason.

8. *Environmental spill and discharge reports.* For contaminants of concern in a study, such records may provide some insight into the general environmental contamination levels in the operations, and the nature and frequency of spills and other releases.

Exposure Assessment Study Design and Conduct

The design and conduct of the exposure assessment itself may progress somewhat during the review of information sources discussed above. As mentioned before, the epidemiology goals and the exposure assessment methods should be compatible. A significant part of this interaction is with respect to the exposure metrics needed to meet the study goals. Examples and brief discussion of a broad range of exposure metrics is given in Table 6.7. Additional details on the metrics and their use are available elsewhere.[10] Fewer resources and less information may be needed to complete a study design calling for a dichotomous "ever exposed, never exposed" rating than for a study that requires quantitative estimates for each study subject.

Table 6.7 — Exposure Metrics for Consideration in Study Design and Conduct

General Category	*Examples*	*Comments*
Dichotomous: Ever Exposed, Never Exposed	1. Occupationally exposed versus not exposed occupationally. 2. Ever employed in a relevant industry.	Suitable for a hazard identification study. Not suitable for a study intended to provide quantitative dose-response data for risk assessment and standards setting. Requires a workable definition of what level constitutes "not exposed."
Job or Task Ranking	Array of jobs (or tasks) from the study in order or approximate potential for exposure.	Will require some quantitative insights for reliable ordering.
Duration of Exposure	Length of employment in an exposed job, task, or industry.	May put high level and low level exposures in same category. Clerical and administrative workers for example may have no significant occupational exposure. However, this may be circumvented by defining included and excluded job categories.

Table 6.7 — Exposure Metrics for Consideration in Study Design and Conduct (continued)

General Category	*Examples*	*Comments*
Ordinal Scales	1. No, low, medium or high exposure. 2. Exposure ranges such as: No exposure <10% of the relevant OEL 10% to <100 % of the OEL > 100% of the OEL	Could be for jobs or for tasks. Could consider task frequency and duration as well as relative task intensity.
Intensity or Average Exposure	1. Job or task Time Weighted Averages. 2. Average radiation exposure. 3. Average decibel exposure.	Could consider task frequency and duration as well as relative task intensity.
Lifetime Average Exposure Intensity	Average exposure in ppm, mg/m³ or other metric for the agent under study.	Includes unexposed and low exposure jobs in the averaging.
Lifetime Cumulative Exposure	Duration x intensity, such as ppm-years.	Could consider only duration exposed above a chosen intensity, such as years exposed above 10% of the OEL.
Peak Exposure	1. Highest average exposed job. 2. Highest exposure ever received in career.	
Peak Exposure Frequency	Number of "peak" exposures per day, week, or year.	Requires definition of a biologically significant peak intensity and duration.
Dermal Exposure	1. Applied exposure via frequency, surface area and loading estimates. 2. Absorbed dermal dose.	For some hazards, often those with very low vapor pressure, the dermal route assessment may be a prime part of the study. Modeling and current measurement techniques have been used in studies.
Internal exposure, total exposure	Dose received or retained.	For some hazards, combination of ingestion, inhalation and dermal absorption can be important contributors to the received dose. Then, an integrated total exposure assessment process should be considered.
Confidence Ratings	1. High confidence (good supporting data). 2. Moderate confidence (such as some gaps in data). 3. Low confidence (speculative, little information available).	Although not directly an exposure metric, confidence ratings may be useful to see if results change as the more uncertain data are selectively dropped out of a "sensitivity check" analysis. If the reasons for the confidence score are retained, these may suggest productive areas to clarify to improve the study.
Data Validation	1. Comparison of historic estimates to reserved historical data. 2. Comparison of exposure scores provided by different experts for an overlapping subset set of work histories.	Validation has become an expected but often difficult aspect of study conduct. At one level, validation is simply verifying accuracy of data transfer from original records to the final study database. At another level, validation tries to assure the exposure estimates are at least reliable, compare reasonably to relevant data, and are provided with sufficient detail for study replication.

Industrial Hygiene Records Systems for Future Study Use

Current industrial hygiene exposure assessment strategies[14] include suggestions on retention of information for future studies and updates. An industrial hygiene sampling database by itself is a key part of the overall information. Key data elements for this aspect have been outlined in several publications.[20,21] However, it is also important to assure that organizational practices allow for sufficient retention of the broader information outlined in Table 6.6. Personnel records and tracking of individuals' major work assignments and exposures is almost as crucial for future studies as are the results from exposure surveys designed to measure relevant metrics for the hazard, such as typical, long term average exposures. For some hazards, there may be additional interest in the variability in exposure, including between worker differences and short-term acute exposures.

Conclusion

The purpose of conducting a health surveillance program is to identify, monitor, and reduce the severity and frequency of occupational disease, illness, and injury. The methods of epidemiology provide some of the analytical tools to quantify risks due to occupational exposures. The level of precision in linking exposure to a specific outcome is directly proportional to the quality and precision of the exposure assessment. Industrial hygienists provide a unique opportunity for epidemiologic studies in that exposures can be directly assessed for and assigned to all individuals in a study. Industrial hygienists also provide a context to the occupational epidemiology study for the assignment of exposure groups and how the study results relate to the workplace environment.

References

1. **Checkoway, H., et al.:** Industrial Hygiene Involvement in Occupational Epidemiology. *Am. Ind. Hyg. Assoc. J. 48(6)*:515–523 (1987).
2. **Checkoway, H., N.A. Pearce, and D. Kriebel:** *Research Methods in Occupational Epidemiology*, 2nd edition. New York: Oxford University Press, 2004.
3. **Burr, H. et al.:** Smoking and height as risk factors for prevalence and 5-year incidence of hearing loss: a questionnaire-based follow-up study of employees in Denmark aged 18-59 years exposed and unexposed to noise. *Int. J. Audiol. 44(9)*:531-9 (2005).
4. **Campo P. and K. Maguin:** Solvent-induced hearing loss: mechanisms and prevention strategy. *Int. J. Occup. Med. Environ. Health. 20(3)*:265-70 (2007).
5. **Ferrite S. and V. Santana:** Joint effects of smoking, noise exposure and age on hearing loss. *Occup. Med. (Lond). 55(1)*:48-53 (2005).
6. **Bernard, A.:** Cadmium & its adverse effects on human health. *Indian J. Med. Res. 128(4)*:557-64 (2008).
7. **Bruske-Hohlfeld, I.:** Environmental and occupational risk factors for lung cancer. *Methods Mol Biol. 472*:3-23 (2004).
8. **Rothman, K.J., S. Greenland:** *Modern Epidemiology*, 2nd edition. Philadelphia: Lippincott-Raven Publishers, 1998.
9. **Gordis, L.G.:** *Epidemiology*, 4th edition. Philadelphia, PA, Saunders Elsevier, 2009.
10. **Viet, S.M., M.R. Stenzel, et al., (eds.):** *Guideline on Occupational Exposure Reconstruction*. Fairfax, VA: AIHA, 2008.
11. **Armstrong, T.W., et al.:** Retrospective Benzene and Total Hydrocarbon Exposure Assessment for a Petroleum Marketing and Distribution Worker Epidemiology Study. *Am. Ind. Hyg. Assoc. J. 57(4)*:333–343 (1996).
12. **Hawkins, N.C., et al.:** A Strategy for *Occupational Exposure Assessment*. Akron, OH: AIHA, 1991.
13. **Mulhausen, J.R. and J. Damiano (eds.):** *A Strategy for Assessing and Managing Occupational Exposures*, 2nd edition. Fairfax, VA: AIHA Press, 1998.
14. **Ignacio, J.S. and W.H. Bullock (eds.):** *A Strategy for Assessing and Managing Occupational Exposures*, 3rd edition. Fairfax, VA: AIHA Press, 2006.
15. **Keil, C.B., C.E. Simmons, and T.R. Anthony (eds.):** *Mathematical Models for Estimating Occupational Exposure to Chemicals*, 2nd edition. Fairfax, VA, AIHA Press, 2009.
16. **Ramachandran, G.:** A Bayesian Approach to Retrospective Exposure Assessment. *Appl. Occup. Environ. Hyg. 14(8)*:547–557 (1999).
17. **Lewis, S.J., et al.:** Retrospective estimation of exposure to benzene in a leukaemia case-control study of petroleum marketing and distribution workers in the United Kingdom. *Occup. Environ. Med. 54(3)*:167–175 (1997).
18. **Glass, D.C., et al.:** Retrospective exposure assessment for benzene in the Australian petroleum industry. *Ann. Occup. Hyg. 44(4)*:301–320 (2000).
19. **CONCAWE:** Review of european oil industry benzene expsoure data (1986–1992). Brussels, CONCAWE: 7/94 (1994).
20. **Lippmann, M., et al.:** Data elements for occupational exposure databases: guidelines and recommendations for airborne hazards and noise. *Appl. Occup. Environ. Hyg. 11(11)*:1294–1311 (1996).
21. **Rajan, B., et al.:** European Proposal for Core Information for the Storage and Exchange of Workplace Exposure Measurements on Chemical Agent. *Appl. Occup. Environ. Hyg. 12(1)*:31–39 (1997).

Essential References for Retrospective Exposure Assessment Study Design and Conduct [adapted from Ref 10]

Armstrong, B.K., E. White, et al.: *Principles of Exposure Measurement in Epidemiology.* New York: Oxford University Press, 1992.

Benke, G., M. Sim, et al.: Beyond the job exposure matrix (JEM): the task exposure matrix (TEM). *Ann. Occup. Hyg. 44(6)*:475–82 (2000).

Bond, G.G., D.F. Austin, et al.: Use of a population-based tumor registry to estimate cancer incidence among a cohort of chemical workers. *J. Occup. Med. 30*: 443–448 (1988).

Bouyer, J. and D. Hemon: Studying the performance of a job exposure matrix. *Int. J. Epidemiol. 22 Suppl. 2*:S65–71 (1993).

Ignacio, J.S. and W.H. Bullock: *A Strategy for Assessing and Managing Occupational Exposures*, 3rd edition. Fairfax, VA: AIHA®, 2006.

Burgess, W.A.: *Recognition of Health Hazards in Industry.* New York: John Wiley & Sons, Inc., 1995.

Checkoway, H., N.A. Pearce, and D. Kriebel: *Research Methods in Occupational Epidemiology*, 2nd edition. New York: Oxford University Press, 2004.

Checkoway, H. and E.A. Eisen: Developments in Occupational Cohort Studies. *Epidemiol. Rev. 20*:100–111 (1998).

Cullen, A.C. and H.C. Frey: Probabilistic *Techniques in Risk Assessment: A Handbook for dealing with Variability and Uncertainty in Models and Inputs.* New York: Plenum Press, 1999.

Esmen, N.: Retrospective industrial hygiene surveys. *Am. Ind. Hyg. Assoc. J. 40(1)*:58–65 (1979).

Fritschi, L., J. Siemiatycki, et al.: Self-assessed versus expert-assessed occupational exposures. *Am. J. Epidemiol. 144(5)*:521–27 (1996).

Fritschi, L., L. Nadon, et al.: Validation of expert assessment of occupational exposures. *Am. J. Ind. Med. 43(5)*:519–22 (2003).

Gardiner, K.: Needs of Occupational Exposure Sampling Strategies for Compliance and Epidemiology. *Occup. Environ. Med. 52*:705–708 (1995).

Goldberg, M.S., J. Siemiatycki, et al.: Inter-rater agreement in assessing occupational exposure in a case-control study. *Br. J. Ind. Med. 43(10)*:667–76 (1986).

Hernberg, S.: *Introduction to Occupational Epidemiology.* Chelsea, MI: CRC Press, 1992.

Hoar, S.K., A. Blair, et al.: Agricultural Herbicide Use and Risk of Lymphoma and Soft-Tissue Sarcoma. *J. Am. Med. Assoc. 256*:1141 (1986).

Kauppinen, T.P.: Assessment of Exposure in Occupational Epidemiology. *Scand. J. Work Environ. Health 20*:19–29 (1994).

Mannetje, A., J. Fevotte, et al.: Assessing exposure misclassification by expert assessment in multicenter occupational studies. *Epidemiology 14(5)*:585–592 (2003).

McGuire, V., L.M. Nelson, T.D. Koepsell, H. Checkoway, and W.T. Longstreth: Assessment of Occupational Exposures in Community-Based Case-Control Studies. *Ann. Rev. Public Health 19*:35–53 (1998).

Morgan, M.G. and M. Henrion: *Uncertainty.* Cambridge, U.K.: Cambridge University Press, 1990.

National Research Council: *Assessing the Human Health Risks of Trichloroethylene.* National Academies Press: Washington D.C., 2006

Paustenbach, D.J.: The Practice of Exposure Assessment: A State-of-the-Art Review. *J. Toxicol. Env. Health Part B: Critical Reviews 3(3)*:179–291 (2000).

Rappaport, S.M. and T.J. Smith (eds.): *Exposure Assessment of Epidemiology and Hazard Control.* Chelsea, MI: Lewis Publishers, 1991.

Rothman, K.J., S. Greenland: Modern *Epidemiology*, 2nd edition. Philadelphia: Lippincott-Raven Publishers, 1998.

Schlesselman, J.J.: *Case-Control Studies: Design, Conduct, Analysis.* New York: Oxford University Press, 1982.

Semple, S.E., F. Dick, et al.: Exposure assessment for a population-based case-control study combining a job-exposure matrix with interview data. *Scand. J. Work Environ. Health 30(3)*:241–48 (2004).

Seixas, N.S. and H. Checkoway: Exposure Assessment in Industry-Specific Retrospective Occupational Epidemiology Studies. *Occup. Environ. Med. 52*:625–633 (1995).

Smith, T., S. Hammond, et al.: Health effects of gasoline exposure. I. Exposure Assessment for U.S. distribution workers. *Environ. Health Perspect. 101(6)*:13–21 (1993).

Steenland, K., L. Stayner, and A. Greife: Assessing the feasibility of retrospective cohort studies. *Am. J. Ind. Med. 12(4)*:419–30 (1987).

Stewart, P.A., A. Blair, et al.: Estimating historical exposures to formaldehyde in a retrospective mortality study. *Appl. Ind. Hyg. 1(1)*:34–41 (1986).

Stewart P.A., A. Blair, M. Dosemeci, and M. Gomez: Collection of Exposure Data for Retrospective Occupational Epidemiology Studies. *Appl. Occup. Environ. Hyg. 6(4)*:280–289 (1991).

Stewart, P.A. and W.F. Stewart: Occupational case-control studies: II. Recommendations for exposure assessment. *Am. J. Ind. Med. 26(3)*:313–26 (1994).

Stewart, P.A. and M. Dosemeci: A Bibliography for Occupational Exposure Assessment for Epidemiologic Studies. *Am. Ind. Hyg. Assoc. J. 55*:1178–1187 (1994).

Stewart P.A., W.F. Stewart, E.F. Heineman, M. Dosemeci, M. Linet and P.D. Inskip: A Novel Approach to data Collection in a Case-Control Study of Cancer and Occupational Exposures. *Int. J. Epidemiol. 25*:744–752 (1996).

Stewart P.A., W.F. Stewart, J. Siemiatychi, E.F. Heineman and M. Dosemeci: Questionnaires for Collecting Detailed Occupational Information for Community-Based Case Control Studies. *Am. Ind. Hyg. Assoc. J 59*:39–44 (1998).

Stewart P.A., C. Rice, P. Beatty, B. Wilson, W.F. Stewart, and A. Blair: A Qualitative Evaluation of Questions and Responses from Five Occupational Questionnaires Developed to Assess Exposure. *Appl. Occup. Environ. Hyg. 17(6)*:444–453 (2002).

Symanski, E., L.L. Kupper, et al.: Comprehensive evaluation of long-term trends in occupational exposure: Part 1. Description of the database. *Occup. Env. Med. 55(5)*:300–309 (1998).

Walker, A.M.: *Observation and Inference: An Introduction to the Methods of Epidemiology.* Newton Lower Falls, MA: Epidemiology Resources Inc., 1991.

Willett, W.C. and G.A. Colditz: Approaches for Conducting Large Cohort Studies. *Epidemiol. Rev. 20*:91–99 (1998).

Existing Relevant Guidelines

Guidelines for Good Epidemiology Practices for Occupational and Environmental Epidemiologic Research, Chemical Manufacturers Association, Epidemiology Resource Information Center. 1991.

EPA Guideline for Exposure Assessment, FRL - 4129-5, 169 pages (oriented toward Risk Assessment).

Framework for evaluating epidemiologic studies for quantitative risk assessment, Table 1, Diesel Emissions and Lung Cancer, Epidemiology and Quantitative Risk Assessment, Special Report, Health Effects Institute, June 1999, 1 page.

Guide for Evaluating Epidemiologic Studies, in Occupational Health, Recognizing and Preventing Work-related Disease, 3rd edition, Little Brown and Co, 1994, 1 page.

Diesel Rulemaking — four-tiered hierarchy used by MSHA for evaluating the weight of evidence from epidemiologic studies based on among other factors the quality of the exposure assessment, published in the Federal Register Volume 66, Number 13, January 19, 2001.

TLV® Documentation outline — Human Studies, TLV® Committee Operations Manual, ACGIH®.

IARC — Introduction to all volumes — Sections 7, 8, 12 — Exposure data, Studies of cancer in humans, and Evaluation.

Other Relevant References

Boleij, J., E. Buringh, D. Heedrik, and H. Kromhout: *Occupational Hygiene of Chemical and Biological Agents.* Amsterdam, the Netherlands: Elsevier Science Ltd., 1995.

Bond, G.G.: Ethical Issues Relating to the Conduct and Interpretation of Epidemiologic Research in Private Industry. *J. Clin. Epidemiol. 44(suppl 1)*:29S–34S (1991).

Finkelstein, M.M. and D.K. Verma: Exposure Estimation in the Presence of Nondetectable Values: Another Look. *Am. Ind. Hyg. Assoc. J. 62(2)*:195–198 (2001).

Greife, A.L., R.W. Hornung, L.G. Stayner, and K.N. Steenland: Development of a model for use in estimating exposure to ethylene oxide in a retrospective cohort mortality study. *Scand. J. Work Environ. Health 14(1)*:29–30 (1988).

Hornung, R.W. and L.D. Reed: Estimation of average concentration in the presence of non-detectable values. *Appl. Occup. Environ. Hyg. 5*:48–51 (1990).

Hornung, R.W., et al.: Statistical model for prediction of retrospective exposure to ethylene oxide in an occupational mortality study. *Am. J. Ind. Med. 25*:825–836 (1994).

Hulka, B.A., T.C. Wilcosky, and J.D. Griffith (eds.): *Biological Markers in Epidemiology.* New York: Oxford University Press, 1990.

Outcome Competencies

After completing this chapter, the reader should be able to:

1. Define the underlined terms used in this chapter.
2. Differentiate the four general principles of occupational hygiene: anticipation, recognition, evaluation, and control.
3. Develop and evaluate the objectives for a workplace monitoring event.
4. Plan a walkthrough survey and workplace monitoring prior to collecting any samples.
5. Develop a sampling strategy that includes the who, what, where, when, and how many.
6. Describe methods for interpreting sampling results.
7. Describe other workplace evaluations, such as ambient monitoring, biological monitoring, medical surveillance, and biological effect monitoring.
8. Integrate professional judgment into decision making.

Key Terms

Administrative controls • anticipation • chain of custody • compliance • control • control measures •engineering controls •evaluation • hazard • noncompliance • permissible exposure limits (PELs) • personal protective equipment (PPE) • recognition • regulatory standards • sampling strategy • short-term exposure limit (STEL) • significance • stressors • survey • time-weighted average (TWA) • toxicity • voluntary guidelines

Prerequisite Knowledge

Prior to beginning this chapter, the user should review the following chapters:

Chapter Number	Chapter Topic
1	History of Industrial Hygiene
3	Legal Aspects of Industrial Hygiene
4	Occupational Exposure Limits
5	Occupational Toxicology
9	Comprehensive Exposure Assessment

Key Topics

I. Introduction

II. General Principles of Occupational Hygiene
   A. Anticipation
   B. Recognition
   C. Evaluation
   D. Control

III. The Exposure Assessment
   A. Determining the Purpose and Scope of the Exposure Assessment
   B. Familiarization with Process Operations
   C. Preliminary Assessment (Qualitative)
   D. Workplace Monitoring (Quantitative Evaluation)
   E. Interpretation of Sampling Results

IV. Summary

Principles of Evaluating Worker Exposure

7

Sheryl A. Milz, PhD, CIH

Introduction

The purpose of this chapter is to provide the occupational hygienist with an understanding of the general principles of evaluating worker exposures in the industrial environment. Occupational hygiene has been defined as the science and art of anticipating, recognizing, evaluating, and controlling health hazards in the workplace[1] and therefore the role of the occupational hygienist is to anticipate, recognize, evaluate, and control these hazards.[2] After anticipating and/or recognizing a potential hazard, the industrial environment should be evaluated to determine the magnitude of the anticipated/recognized stressors. Effective control of the work environment can then be accomplished in a more efficient and effective manner. It is important to note that the evaluation or exposure assessment may have purposes other than controlling exposures in the workplace. Other purposes include compliance determinations; program management from initiatives implemented based on exposure levels (e.g., respiratory protection, hearing conservation, medical surveillance); epidemiologic studies; health complaint investigations; risk assessment; and proposed change evaluations (e.g., adding new chemicals or modifying existing processes).[2]

The general principles discussed in this chapter are drawn from traditional evaluation methodologies and reflect the current practice of occupational hygiene. This chapter does not discuss "cutting-edge" evaluation methods or provide checklists and how-to methods. This information can be found in other chapters. Instead, this chapter focuses on the evaluation process.

Traditionally, most effective workplace evaluations have used a multidisciplinary, knowledge-based approach. Occupational hygiene, chemistry, engineering, health physics, medicine, epidemiology, toxicology, and nursing disciplines, as well as management and manufacturing expertise, have contributed to this approach. Successful evaluations of the work environment in the past would integrate the knowledge of these various disciplines and develop control strategies for potential risks. However, it is not always possible or even practical to assemble such a diverse multidisciplinary group in the occupational setting. Therefore, the occupational hygienist must be familiar with these other disciplines and their potential contributions to the solutions of specific problems. The occupational hygienist must be willing to get expert opinions from other professionals, as necessary, in evaluating the workplace environment.

General Principles of Occupational Hygiene

Occupational hygiene is the science and art "dedicated to the <u>anticipation</u>, <u>recognition</u>, <u>evaluation</u>, and <u>control</u> of environmental factors arising in or from the workplace that may result in injury, illness, impairment, or affect the well-being of workers and members of the community."[3] The definition suggests a sequence for the occupational hygiene decision making process. When a hazard is anticipated and recognized, its magnitude can be determined by exposure assessment. Exposure assessment typically begins with a qualitative evaluation to prioritize exposures. Semi-quantitative (mathematical modeling) or quantitative (workplace monitoring) methods may then be utilized depending on the purpose of the exposure assessment and the desired certainty of the result.[1] The process is not always so straightforward and direct and often requires feedback from multiple sources of information. For example, in the recognition phase, hazards may be found that were not anticipated or those anticipated may not be found. Exposure estimates made for the purpose of prioritizing activities can be refined by actual exposure measurements and additional information. Newly implemented controls need to be evaluated to determine effectiveness and possibly to reset the priorities. In an effective occupational hygiene program, information collection, analysis, and decision making go on continuously and simultaneously.

Anticipation

Health hazard control has become more difficult and complex, necessitating the anticipation of hazards during the development of facilities, processes, and products. Problems discovered after development may be too costly to fix, both technologically and economically, to continue implementation. If the hazards had been anticipated during development, the project could either have been abandoned sooner, or the hazard could have been dealt with in a less costly manner. Anticipation is therefore an expectation of potential health hazards and is generally more difficult for the entry-level, inexperienced occupational hygienist since skills in anticipation generally increase with experience. The experienced occupational hygienist needs the ability to recognize potential health hazards, as well as knowledge of scientific developments, new technologies, and regulatory requirements and a general awareness of other activities that may impact worker health in order to effectively anticipate health hazards.

Recognition

Recognition is the acknowledgement of health hazards in the workplace. However, the difference between anticipation and recognition is not always clear. One means of distinguishing anticipation and recognition suggests that anticipation occurs during the conceptual phase of an operation while recognition occurs during existing operations. This is a somewhat arbitrary distinction since anticipation can also occur with existing operations and recognition can occur during the conceptual phase.

Recognition typically requires the collection of available information along with the application of occupational hygiene principles. The recognition of potential or existing health hazards evolves as the occupational hygienist becomes familiar with the processes; creates and maintains an inventory of physical, chemical, and biological hazards; reviews the different job activities of the work area; and studies control measures. With the information collected during the recognition phase, a workplace characterization can be developed. The characterization usually includes information on the workplace (physical environment), the work force (workers), and the agents (chemical, physical, and biological agents). The characterization often results in defining "exposure groups" (i.e., workers performing the same tasks in a similar fashion and therefore receiving similar exposures).

Evaluation

Evaluation is the process of examining an operation to determine the extent to which health hazards are present. Key skills necessary for evaluation are observation and judgment as well as technical knowledge in science and math. Both observation and judgment are developed and refined as a result of training and experience and therefore utilize "art" as well as science. The application of the occupational hygienist's experience is used together with quantitative measurements, if available, to determine the magnitude of the stressors, which are stimuli that disrupt the homeostasis of an organism and therefore represent potential adverse impacts on the health of workers. In the absence of quantitative measurements, the occupational hygienist can utilize semi-quantitative methods such as mathematical modeling to estimate the magnitude of stressors. The stressor measurements/estimates are then analyzed and tested for significance (e.g., determining the importance and meaningfulness of the results). Judging significance can involve both subjective decisions based on the occupational hygienist's experience as well as objective decisions based on statistical analyses.

In the early years of the occupational hygiene profession, evaluation was concentrated on the "dangerous trades" where elevated exposures and high disease rates were common. Today, occupational hygienists focus on many varied issues including indoor air quality in office environments, repetitive motion concerns with keyboarding operations, and management of hazardous waste operations, among others. The primary objective of evaluation is to determine the magnitude and significance of health hazards in the workplace using quantitative, semi-quantitative, and qualitative methods. Health hazards can cause an absence of well-being and their effects may be quite diverse, such as decreases in lung function and cancer. Health hazards may result from exposure to gases, vapors, aerosols, biological agents, noise, ionizing or nonionizing radiation, and temperature extremes. The remainder of this chapter will present the evaluation process for an occupational environment.

Control

The final principle of occupational hygiene is the control of health hazards in the work space in order to provide a healthful working environment. Control is defined as the adjustment or regulation of an operation to meet a standard or guideline, the reduction or prevention of contaminant release, and the ability to contain a stressor. Current occupational hygiene practice prioritizes controls in the order of engineering controls, administrative controls, and personal protective equipment (PPE). Engineering controls encompass the use of process change, substitution, isolation, ventilation, and source modification in order to control worker exposures by reducing the quantity of contaminants released into the work space. Administrative controls encompass the use of management involvement, training, job rotation, reduction of exposure time, preventive maintenance, and housekeeping in an effort to control worker exposures. PPE involves the use of devices (e.g., gloves, eye protection, respirators) designed to protect individuals from hazards in the workplace. Controls are discussed in detail in later chapters in this book.

The Exposure Assessment

Exposure assessment is the determination or estimation (qualitative or quantitative) of the magnitude, frequency, duration, and route of exposure. It identifies and defines any exposure that occurs or is anticipated to occur in human populations.[4] Therefore, it can be a complex task that requires analyzing any contact between people and hazardous substances.[4] During evaluation, the occupational hygienist may collect quantitative measurements (e.g., workplace monitoring), perform semi-quantitative estimation (e.g., mathematical modeling), or perform qualitative assessment to determine the magnitudes of the health hazards previously recognized. Both recognition and evaluation can be performed simultaneously if the hazards had previously been anticipated.

In this chapter the exposure assessment will be divided into five steps: 1) determining the purpose and scope of the survey; 2) becoming familiar with process operations; 3) performing the preliminary, qualitative survey; 4) performing workplace monitoring (quantitative evaluation); and 5) interpreting the sampling results. These steps may be performed consecutively (one after the other) or for steps 2, 3, and 4, simultaneously (at the same time).

Determining the Purpose and Scope of the Exposure Assessment

The reasons for performing an exposure assessment are many and varied, as noted in the introduction to this chapter. Types of evaluations may include: 1) a comprehensive exposure assessment to identify and quantify health hazards throughout a designated work area or limited to a single operation; 2) an assessment of compliance with various occupational health standards and guidelines; 3) an assessment of exposures in response to complaints; 4) an assessment of exposures for medical and epidemiological studies; and 5) an assessment of the effectiveness of engineering and administrative controls.

Comprehensive Exposure Assessment

In a comprehensive exposure assessment, the primary objective is to determine the acceptability of exposures to health hazards to all workers on all days in a designated work area or for a specific operation such as batch production, spill response, pilot projects, and maintenance activities. The acceptability determination is based on the identification and quantification/estimation of exposures to stressors in the workplace. The walkthrough survey can be used to identify the stressors while workplace monitoring, mathematical modeling, or qualitative assessments can be used to quantify/estimate the exposure levels. A well-maintained exposure database that includes worker tracking is a useful tool for describing measured exposures over time.

Compliance Survey

In a compliance assessment, exposures to stressors are quantified and evaluated against some health standard such as an Occupational Safety and Health Administration (OSHA) permissible exposure limit (PEL) or a guideline such as the American Conference of Governmental Industrial Hygienists (ACGIH®) Threshold Limit Value (TLV®). Compliance is defined as acting in accordance with health and safety regulations, whereas noncompliance is the failure to act in accordance with health and safety regulations. The occupational hygienist working on behalf of an organization is interested in documenting compliance with the standards or guidelines. The occupational hygienist working as a compliance officer for OSHA or state agency is interested in documenting noncompliance with the standards. Demonstration of noncompliance requires that an exposure exceed the standard with an acceptable degree of certainty, usually a 95 percent confidence. Demonstration of compliance requires that an exposure be below the standard with an acceptable degree of certainty, again usually a 95 percent confidence. Therefore, in a compliance assessment, maximum risk employees (those with the highest exposure potentials) are usually monitored to determine compliance so that the organization can reasonably be certain that all exposures, whether evaluated or not, are below the standard. This "traffic cop" approach does little to contribute to the process of fully judging health hazards in the workplace.

Monitoring performed by compliance officers in order to detect noncompliance is usually conducted in situations where noncompliance is most likely to occur. The monitoring is not intended to conclude that the results of the evaluation describe typical conditions of the workplace. A significant overexposure identified by a compliance officer is of concern because of the possible citation and penalty that could result. However, the noncompliance may indicate a possible weakness in the surveillance, evaluation, and control activities of the current occupational hygiene program, or the apparent overexposure could be a highly rare, atypical event. Current occupational hygiene standards allow re-evaluation of noncompliance when the employer can demonstrate through documentation and rigorous statistics that ongoing evaluations of the exposure to the health hazards have indicated the exposures are under control. This re-evaluation allowance is an incentive for an organization to administer ongoing comprehensive assessments rather than performing monitoring in the compliance assessment mode.

Complaint Response

Employee complaints occur even in organizations that have implemented comprehensive exposure assessment and workplace monitoring. The occupational hygienist will need to respond to these complaints, not only because the hazards may be real and require some corrective action, but also because the complainant believes the hazard is real, which creates anxiety. The evaluation of a complaint should include interviewing the complainant about the reported hazard and visiting the workplace for a walkthrough in order to demonstrate that the complaint is taken seriously and to obtain the necessary information to perform an evaluation. It is important to recognize that the cause of the health hazard in the complaint could be something other than what the complainant reported. For example, an individual may claim to be affected by one substance when another substance is actually the cause. Additionally, complaints may be registered even when exposures are within acceptable limits, such as when materials have a low odor threshold. At the conclusion of the evaluation, the complainant should always be informed of the results so as to demonstrate that all potential health hazards are considered potentially serious.

Medical and Epidemiological Studies

Both physician and epidemiologists have a need to know and understand worker exposure levels in order to fully evaluate the effect of exposures on workers either individually (the physician) or as a group (the epidemiologist). Past exposures have often had to be developed using an appropriate modeling scheme or on a qualitative, subjective basis such as job titles and job descriptions. This quantification of past exposures is often extremely difficult and error-prone, resulting in large uncertainties in study conclusions. However, as comprehensive occupational hygiene surveys and monitoring strategies have been implemented, exposure information has become available to perform epidemiological studies relating these exposures to health effects documented in medical surveillance programs.

Engineering and Administrative Control Effectiveness

The effectiveness of engineering and administrative controls can be assessed separately or as a part of a comprehensive exposure assessment. The simplest case would entail collecting before and after samples in an area where the engineering control is implemented. For example, air samples could be collected in the same locations before and after a local exhaust ventilation system is installed. Or for older systems, the samples could be collected with the ventilation system operating and with the ventilation system not operating. Another example would be collecting sound level measurements before and after an enclosure is installed around a noisy piece of equipment. For administrative controls, sampling could be performed over time during certain work practices, such as collecting process samples to ensure exposures are not increasing. Other evaluations may require a more elaborate sampling strategy.

Familiarization with Process Operations

After the purpose of the exposure assessment has been determined, the next step is for the occupational hygienist to become familiar with the processes that are the focus of the survey. The familiarization process entails collection of information about the process under study and its exposure conditions. This information may include: 1) the physical facility layout; 2) a process description with individual steps; 3) an inventory of all the stressors associated with the process, including raw materials, intermediates, support materials such as lubricating oils, by-products, and final products along with the health hazards associated with each; 4) the job classifications of the workers involved in the process; 5) the health status of the workers involved in the process; 6) a listing of the control measures in use with the process; 7) the results from past evaluations; and 8) any other hazards associated with the process.

Physical Facility Layout

An initial orientation to an industrial process should begin with an understanding of the general physical layout of the facilities. The location of the particular building or buildings of interest in relation to other structures in the area, the general terrain surrounding the facilities, and the physical arrangement of the facility itself all allow the occupational hygienist to put the general environmental condition of the facility in perspective. The facilities themselves then need to be examined. This examination can be done with the use of blueprints, engineering drawings, piping and electrical diagrams, and any other documents available. Additionally, the ventilation system should be examined to determine airflow patterns in the facility. Airflow patterns can be determined by observing the physical arrangement of ventilation equipment in and on the building. It is not uncommon, even in modern buildings, to discover arrangements of air supply systems in the vicinity of exhaust streams from separate locations within the building, making recirculation of contaminated air a potential problem. The occupational hygienist may find it necessary to take photographs or to create their own sketches of the facility from personal observations and interviews instead of relying on the documents provided.

Process Description

The occupational hygienist must also become familiar with all the processes within a facility. Engineering drawings and specifications may be available, but these are usually more detailed than needed by the occupational hygienist. A simple block flow diagram with descriptions of the individual activities is usually sufficient. The occupational hygienist needs to understand what stressors are involved as well as a description of the process including process temperatures and pressures. This information can be obtained by interviewing the process operators, by personal observations, by reviewing technical manuals or written procedures, and by reviewing purchase, inventory, or other records.

A walk-through tour of the facility is an important part of the process description in order for the occupational hygienist to verify and/or modify their documentation. The walk-through also gives the occupational hygienist an opportunity to look for potential sources of health hazards. Many potentially hazardous operations can be detected by visual observation. For example, dusty operations and fume-generating operations can be spotted easily. However, visibility does not equate to hazard level since dust particles not seen by the naked eye are usually more hazardous than visible dust particles because they are more likely of respirable size (see Chapter 12).

Beyond the raw materials, intermediates, support materials, products, and byproducts, basic industrial processes may generate many of the air contaminants found in occupational environments. The following are some examples:

- **Welding fumes:** In addition to metal fumes and oxides generated by the welding action, contaminants of concern include welding rod and road coating decomposition products, oxides of nitrogen, ozone, and combustion products.
- **Combustion products:** A wide range of substances make up this category, including carbon monoxide, oxides of nitrogen, diesel exhaust, particulates, ash, smoke, acrolein, acid gases, and polynuclear aromatic hydrocarbons.
- **Foundry emissions:** Common emissions are siliceous dust, oil mist, core and core rosin decomposition products, metal fumes, carbon monoxide, and polynuclear aromatic hydrocarbons.
- **Smelting:** Smelting air contaminants are similar to foundry emissions and include combustion products, metal fumes, sulfur dioxide, and metals (e.g., arsenic).

In addition to the general categories of air contaminants listed above, physical agents are also of concern. Some of the more common physical agents and their respective sources are:

- **Noise:** Sources include a variety of industrial machinery, engines, furnaces, pneumatic systems and other compressed air tools, and releases (see Chapter 24).
- **Ionizing radiation:** This physical stressor can result from the use of radioisotopes, high voltage machinery, x-ray equipment, and process control equipment (e.g., level controls and thickness gauges) as well as natural radiation (see Chapter 26).
- **Nonionizing radiation:** This physical stressor can result from welding and other sources of ultraviolet energy, thermal sources of infrared radiation, radar equipment, microwave ovens, and various high-frequency sources (see Chapter 25).
- **Heat:** Sources of thermal stresses include furnaces, smelting and casting operations, drying ovens, and glassmaking (see Chapters 27 and 28).

Stressor Inventory

A complete inventory of all chemicals, raw materials, intermediates, byproducts, waste products, and final products must be obtained during the exposure assessment and should be maintained and updated as changes occur. The inventory should also include potentially hazardous physical agents as well as stressors such as welding fumes and combustion products, which do not have material safety data sheets (MSDSs), but still need to be evaluated. Inventories of chemicals, along with the compilation of MSDSs for all chemicals utilized, are required by the Hazard Communication Standard (29 CFR 1910.1200) and state "right-to-know" laws. A review of MSDSs is a good starting point for the stressor inventory. However, the occupational hygienist should also verify by direct observation which chemicals are actually present in the workplace. Ideally, all chemicals seen in the workplace should have an MSDS on file and all MSDSs in the file should be represented by a chemical in use somewhere in the facility. Given the complexity of industries and the number of chemicals potentially available in a facility, documenting the stressor inventory, while straightforward, may be extremely difficult. The information sources, such as MSDSs and purchase records, may be decentralized throughout the facility and the materials themselves may be stored in multiple locations. Therefore, developing the stressor inventory is not necessarily a simple task.

Toxicological information. After the stressor inventory is complete, the occupational hygienist needs to determine the toxicities of all the stressors on the inventory. Other factors being equal, higher priority may be given to operations using materials with higher toxicities. However, the toxicity of a stressor is not the sole criterion in judging the natures of the health hazards associated with a process. Put very basically, "toxicity" and "hazard" are not synonymous. Toxicity is the ability of a stressor to cause damage to living tissue. It is a property of the stressor just like the material's boiling point, vapor pressure, or viscosity. However, hazard is the likelihood of illness or injury associated with the use of a stressor and, as such, is much more influenced by the conditions of use rather than by the toxicity of the stressor. Highly toxic materials can be handled quite safely with little hazard; minimally toxic materials can be used in poorly controlled ways that result in a moderate hazard. The nature of the process in which the stressor is used or generated, the possibility of reaction with other agents (chemical and physical), the work practices, and effective control measures all relate to the potential hazard associated with each use of a material.

For physical agents, biological agents, and pure chemicals, toxicity data is readily available in a number of standard textbooks and secondary source documents. For example, such information can be found in a number of reference books and scientific journals as well as in the *NIOSH Pocket Guide to Chemical Hazards*; the TLV® documentation published by ACGIH®; the Workplace Environmental Exposure Level (WEEL™) documentation published by the American Industrial Hygiene Association® (AIHA®); and the Z37 standard published by the American National Standards Institute (ANSI). The information may also be available from toxicologists, technical information centers, and manufacturers. The Toxic Substances List, published by the National Institute for Occupational Safety and Health (NIOSH), contains abbreviated summaries of toxicological information for more than 8,000 substances. Additionally, there are extensive computer-aided libraries of chemical hazard data and the Internet is providing access to a wide range of sites that maintain information on the hazardous properties of materials. In the absence of any specific information on mixtures of formulations, the occupational hygienist will need to rely on information provided by the supplier or manufacturer in the form of the MSDS. If completed correctly, the MSDS should provide information on the effects of overexposure to the extent that they are known. Additional information on toxicology is presented in Chapter 5.

OELs. The stressor inventory may also include any occupational exposure limits (OELs) for each stressor. OELs can be divided into three categories: regulatory standards, voluntary guidelines, and "local limits." Regulatory standards are issued by a governmental body (e.g., OSHA) that is authorized by law to issue and enforce compliance with these standards. Employers are required to comply with regulatory standards. On the other hand, guidelines are published for voluntary use using a consensus process by organizations such as ACGIH® and ANSI. Voluntary guidelines are used at the discretion of the employer. Unfortunately, the majority of stressors are not covered by regulatory standards (e.g., PELs) or voluntary guidelines (e.g., TLVs®) and therefore organizations may develop "local limits" for use in exposure assessment.[1]

Job Classifications

Since the occupational hygienist's efforts will be devoted to evaluating the potential exposure of specific workers to specific stressors while engaged in specific tasks, it will be necessary for the occupational hygienist to become familiar with the various categories of jobs and activities required of each category within a facility.

Job Activities. Ultimately, exposure is directly related to the job activities or tasks performed by the worker. Therefore, the occupational hygienist must become familiar with the workers' job activities and their consequent exposure potentials. A logical starting point for this effort is the formal job description. Even with a formal, well-defined job description, the occupational hygienist should consider talking to the employees and the employees' supervisors. Although the worker and the supervisor would be expected to be able to reliably describe worker activities, the supervisor may not know individual's work routines, and the worker may know only a portion of the process operations. It is not uncommon for the occupational hygienist to end up with three different versions of a job based on inputs from the formal job description, the worker, and the worker's supervisor. The occupational hygienist may need to observe the operation in order to adequately describe the job activities and to reach agreement between the provided job descriptions.

Health Status of Workers

A source of information often overlooked during the familiarization step is the overall health status of the workers. Even in organizations where there is periodic evaluation of workers' health (e.g., medical surveillance), there may not be a mechanism for the occupational hygienist to receive a summary of this information. However, medical surveillance data summarized by department or process may indicate the presence of an unrecognized health hazard and lead to further evaluation and possible control measures. Logs of first aid, OSHA 300 log recordable incidents, and lost workdays resulting from workplace injuries can be of great assistance in identifying common stressors present at the facility.

Control Measures

The familiarization process would not be complete without documenting the various control measures utilized and their apparent effectiveness. Control measures encompass the methods of eliminating or minimizing exposures to health hazards. These methods may include local exhaust and general ventilation; process isolation or enclosure; shielding from heat, ionizing radiation; ultraviolet light, or any other forms of radiant energy; administrative controls; protective clothing; respiratory protection; and other controls. A walk-through tour may be necessary to determine the apparent effectiveness of the controls and may include simple ventilation checks (see Chapter 38) or collecting sound level measurements (see Chapter 21). Other evidence of a lack of effective control may include a layer of dust on all horizontal surfaces when utilizing dusty operations or the presence of non-operational fans.

Past Evaluations

A final resource in the familiarization step could include the review of past occupational hygiene or related evaluations. During this review the occupational hygienist should determine: 1) how much time has elapsed since the last evaluation; 2) whether the process, equipment, or workforce has substantially changed; 3) whether significant problems, potential or real, have been identified, and 4) whether the indicators of problems (e.g., worker or neighborhood complaints, increased absenteeism, etc.) have increased.

Identify Potential Hazards

The occupational hygienist can now apply the fundamentals of the profession to identify potential hazards associated with the jobs to be evaluated. As part of the summation of the familiarization step, the occupational hygienist should interview selected workers and supervisors to confirm the information collected on the facilities, chemicals, job activities, work procedures, controls, and personal protective equipment. Getting the workers involved in the familiarization step of a survey will facilitate acceptance of the findings and implementation of any recommendations.

Preliminary Assessment (Qualitative)

An experienced occupational hygienist often can evaluate — quite accurately and in some detail — the magnitude of certain chemical and physical stressors associated with an operation without benefit of any instrumentation. In fact, the professional uses qualitative evaluation every time an assessment is made, whether it is intended to be the total effort of the work or a preliminary inspection prior to quantitatively evaluating stressor exposures. Qualitative evaluation can be applied by anyone familiar with the operation, from the worker to the occupational hygienist, to ascertain some of the potential problems associated with operation.

During a qualitative walk-through evaluation, many potentially hazardous operations can be detected visually. Operations that produce large amounts of dust and fumes can be spotted and generally will warrant implementation of additional controls. Additionally, the sense of smell can be used to detect the presence of many gases and vapors. Unfortunately, the odor threshold concentration — that is, the lowest concentration that can be detected by smell — is greater than the OEL for many substances. Therefore, when these types of materials are detected by odor, an elevated concentration is present in the area. Some materials, most notably hydrogen sulfide, can cause olfactory fatigue (e.g., numbing of the olfactory nerve endings) to the extent that even dangerously high concentrations cannot be detected by odor. Therefore, odor cannot be relied upon as a warning property for most materials.

Although it is usually possible to determine the presence or absence of potentially hazardous physical agents at the same time of the qualitative evaluation, rarely can the potential hazard be evaluated without the aid of mathematical modeling or instrumentation. As a minimum, however, the sources of physical agents such as radiant heat, abnormal temperatures and humidities, excessive noise, improper or inadequate illumination, ultraviolet radiation, microwaves, and various other forms of radiation, can be noted.

An important aspect of the qualitative evaluation is an inspection of the control measures implemented. In general, the control measures include such features as shielding from radiant or ultraviolet energy, local exhaust and general ventilation, administrative controls, and respirators or other personal protective equipment. General measures of the effectiveness of these controls include the presence or absence of accumulated dust on the floors, ledges, and other horizontal surfaces; the condition of the ventilation ductwork (e.g., any holes or other signs of deterioration); whether the ventilation appears to provide adequate control of contaminants; the consistency of work practices; and the manner in which personal protective equipment is used by the workers.

Workplace Monitoring (Quantitative Evaluation)

Although the information obtained during the walk-through inspection of a facility is important and useful, the occupational hygienist needs to document exposure levels either by measurement or by semi-quantitative methods such as mathematical modeling. This chapter will discuss quantitative measurements. Mathematical modeling is discussed in Chapter 10.

The sampling strategy developed for the quantitative measurement depends on the reason for the evaluation, which may one or more of the following:

- Documentation of worker exposures;
- Documentation of health and safety regulation compliance;
- Identification of the source(s) of contaminant release;
- Assistance in the design and/or evaluation of control systems; and
- Correlation of disease or injury with exposures to specific stressors.

The sampling objectives can be condensed into two major categories: sampling for engineering testing, surveillance, or control; and sampling for compliance, health research, or epidemiological purposes. A sampling program for engineering purposes should be designed to yield the specific information desired. For example, the occupational hygienist could collect samples before and after a change in ventilation to determine whether the change has had the desired effect. However, occupational hygiene is primarily concerned with the health effects of exposure, comparing sampling results with exposure guidelines, determining compliance with health codes or regulations, or defining as precisely as possible environmental factors for comparison with observed health effects.

The purpose of evaluation is to develop information that will lead to decisions that will reduce or eliminate health risks to workers. Sampling only produces data, which must then be converted into information to be of value in the decision making process. The type of data collected is dependent on the purpose of the evaluation. The purpose is the basic question that must be answered before the sampling strategy can be developed and is the most important step of the evaluation. Too often the purpose is phrased too simply (e.g., "What is the welder's exposure?"). This purpose is not detailed enough to design a sampling strategy. A more meaningful question would be, "What is the exposure distribution of the welders in Department A on the first shift doing MIG-welding on stainless steel A10 materials?" Included in the question is the distinction of either an exposure distribution determination or a compliance determination, the definition of the similar exposure group, the location, description of time and space, and the definition of task, relevant process conditions, and materials. Other chapters within this book discuss specific evaluation methods for an exposure assessment.

Stressor Selection

The familiarization step should provide all the information necessary to identify potential stressors to which the workers might be exposed and to prioritize these stressors in terms of exposure significance in order to select stressors for sampling. The prioritization of the stressors is usually based on the probability of an overexposure and/or the consequences of an overexposure should it occur. The stressors may include chemical, physical, and biological agents as well as ergonomic and psychological stressors.

Concentration Estimation

It is helpful to both the occupational hygienist and the laboratory analyst if a reasonable estimate of the contaminant concentrations to be measured can be made. The walk-through survey, discussions with plant personnel, degree of familiarity with similar operations, and examination of past data from the facility all serve as input to the estimate of contaminant concentrations, the occupational hygienist can select sampling equipment, size and/or type of collection media, and plan sampling times in accordance with the amount of material likely to be collected. Knowing the likely levels of contaminants also may facilitate the occupational hygienist's selection of specific monitoring equipment or the choice of equipment for collection of samples for subsequent analyses.

Sampling and Analytical Method Selection

The typical occupational hygienist does not usually analyze the environmental samples collected in the field, unless direct-reading instruments are utilized. And yet, it is important to note that the use of accurate, sensitive, specific, and reproducible analytical methods is equally as important as the proper calibration of the sampling equipment. Therefore, communication between the occupational hygienist and the analytical laboratory is important. For example, the occupational hygienist needs to be aware of analytical limitations such as minimum amount of material needed to be effectively analyzed, allowable volumetric sampling rates, and necessary sample duration. Similarly, if the occupational hygienist is aware of the presence of materials in the environment that may interfere with the analytical procedure, the analyst may be able to eliminate those materials prior to the analysis.

In evaluating the occupational environment, the concentration of the contaminant in the air is generally quite small, often in the nanogram per cubic meter or parts-per-billion (ppb) range. Thus, a sufficient quantity of sample may have to be collected to enable the analyst to accurately determine this small amount of material. Specific analytical procedures are discussed elsewhere in the book.

Principles. When available, validated methods of analysis should always be used. Fortunately, many methods have been validated under various situations and conditions by various recognized agencies. NIOSH has developed and validated a series of methods for most of the materials with exposure limits; these have been published in their *Manual of Analytical Methods*. Similarly the OSHA laboratory in Salt Lake City, Utah, has compiled a set of sampling and analytical methods optimized for their compliance officers to use with the OSHA enforcement program.

Many of the guides from various organizations contain recommended methods of analysis from the perspective of the issuing organizations. The American Public Health Association (APHA) has published a manual on methods of air sampling and analysis,

ACGIH® publishes references on air sampling instrumentation, and the American Society for Testing and Materials (ASTM) has undertaken the validation of testing methods for the evaluation of ambient air quality. All of these methods, even those focused on air pollution applications, can be used with minor modifications for evaluation of contaminant levels in the workplace. The occupational hygienist should refer to the above-listed organizations as well as OSHA and NIOSH to determine the best sampling and analytical method for the contaminants of interest.

This does not mean that methods other than the standard and proven methods cannot be used. In fact, it is often desirable and productive to explore development of specialized methods that suit the investigator, since these efforts may result in new methodologies. The problem of using other-than-standard methods is that they may not have been validated under conditions that are representative of the occupational environment. Thus, these other methods need to be tested, standardized, calibrated against known concentrations, and therefore validated in order to be a reliable method for documenting contaminant levels in the occupational environment.

Specificity, selectivity, and other considerations. In evaluating a worker's exposure, or in the working environment, the instrument must be able to provide the necessary sensitivity, selectivity, accuracy, and reproducibility, preferably with instantaneous, or at least rapid results. Detailed discussions of instruments used for sampling particulates or gases and vapors as well as direct-reading instruments for chemicals and for physical agents such as noise are in other chapters in this book (see Chapters 8, 14, 17, 19, 24–28). ACGIH® also publishes a reference book on air sampling instruments.

The use of continuous monitoring devices to evaluate the work environment has increased tremendously in recent years. In general, many industries install these instruments in areas where exposures to certain gases or vapors may vary considerably or where the presence of the contaminant would be a concern. In the latter application, the instrument serves more as a "leak detector" or alarm rather than as an exposure monitor. Examples include the use of carbon monoxide detectors in tunnels or plant areas where the gas is produced, monitors for chlorinated hydrocarbons such as in the production of trichloroethylene, and monitors for certain, specific alcohols. Many of the continuous detecting and recording instruments can be equipped to sample at several locations throughout the facility and record the general air concentrations to which workers may be exposed during a work shift. Many large facilities have added computerized equipment to the recorders so that the data can be made available and summarized for instant review.

Limitations. Apart from deliberate tampering with samples (which is usually easily detected by an experienced occupational hygienist), other factors can influence or otherwise affect the representativeness of samples, and therefore, their usefulness in the decision process. Compromises of sensitivity, selectivity, accuracy, stability, and reproducibility may limit the interpretation of the sampling/analytical result. For example, if an analytical method must be used that produces a result specific to a particular portion of the chemical (e.g., the carboxyl group) rather than the chemical itself (e.g., methyl ethyl ketone), then the occupational hygienist must take into consideration the presence of other chemicals that may contain the same portion as the chemical of interest.

The basic question "What was measured?" must be kept in mind to know whether the result can be applied as intended. If the measurement represents an unusual event, it is probably not useful in characterizing the long-term average exposure of workers. However, the measurement may be useful in determining if engineering controls are needed to prevent an infrequent but excessive exposure. Additionally, the occupational hygienist must combine workplace observations with the measurements in order to properly interpret the results. For example, measurements collected during the summer months when the windows are open would be expected to be lower than measurements collected during winter when the windows are closed.

Equipment Selection

The choice of a particular sampling instrument depends on a number of factors: 1) the type of analysis or information required; 2) the efficiency of the instrument;

3) the reliability of the instrument under various field use conditions; 4) the portability and ease of use of the instrument; and 5) the personal choice of the occupational hygienist based on past experience and other factors. No single universal sampling instrument is available, and it is doubtful that one will ever be developed. The current trend is to develop a greater number of specialized instruments. Examples include direct-reading gas and vapor detectors with detection of individual chemicals by specialized sensors. Even with multi-chemical capabilities, these specialized instruments are not universal samplers (see Chapters 8–14).

Calibration. Calibration of instruments is necessary to ensure that data collected in the field is representative of worker or environmental concentrations and is discussed in detail in this book (see Chapters 15 and 16). Results obtained during workplace monitoring are no more accurate than the accuracy of the instruments used to collect the data. To maintain accuracy, the sampling instruments need to be calibrated against a standard airflow measuring device before and after field use to establish the sampling airflow rate in order to determine the total volume of air sampled. This air volume is then used to estimate the contaminant concentration in the work space, both personal and environmental. Adjustments to the sample volume may be required if temperature and pressure are different between the calibration conditions and the sampling conditions. Final airborne concentrations must then e corrected to standard temperature and pressure for comparison with occupational exposure limits.

Direct-reading instruments, including colorimetric indicator (e.g., detector) tubes, must also be calibrated. The calibration for these instruments is against a known concentration of the chemical of interest. Calibration gases of known concentrations can be purchased by the occupational hygienist to calibrate these instruments prior to use in the field. Additionally, many direct-reading instruments require factor calibration at a central laboratory or by the manufacturer.

Personal Protective Equipment Selection

The final category of equipment to be selected by the occupational hygienist is personal protective equipment. Too often, field investigators arrive to perform extensive air sampling without any personal protection. The occupational hygienist may rationalize absence of PPE by not being in a position where overexposure is likely or being in that position for "only a short time." However, the occupational hygienist needs to wear the same PPE that is required for the workers so as not to send the message that use of PPE is not important since the health professional does not use it. Therefore, the occupational hygienist needs to include proper PPE during the workplace monitoring preparation.

Sampling Strategy Preparation

A sampling strategy is an overall plan or framework for sampling that may include the type and number of samples to be collected, the methods to be used and their accuracy, and the objectives for the sampling. The sampling strategy is prepared so that ultimate decision making will be based on correct and complete workplace monitoring. The decision making regarding exposure levels and necessary controls can then be made with the required level of confidence and with minimum cost and effort. However, data too often are collected with insufficient thought given to how they will be used. Basic strategy development will be discussed later in this chapter, and a detailed discussion of the statistical basis for a sampling strategy is discussed in Chapter 7.

Sampling strategy development is complicated by the tremendous variability of occupational exposures. For example, air contaminant concentrations in the workplace vary with time, both long-term and short-term, and with location. Workers' movements also vary throughout the work space, and these movements can affect the air contaminant concentrations. All of this variability generally results in an exposure profile, described statistically by a lognormal distribution with a geometric standard deviation typically between 2 and 5. Compared to this environmental variability, the sampling and analytical error is small.

The sampling strategy should be completed before any workplace monitoring is conducted and should describe how to collect the required information efficiently in the time allotted. The elements of the plan should include who, what, where, when, and how many. The why would have been determined with the objectives for the evaluation. Additionally, the sampling and analytical methods for the contaminants of interest need to be included in the sampling strategy, as well as the methods selected for data analysis. The sampling strategy needs to answer the following questions:

- Where to sample?
- When to sample?
- How long to sample?
- Whom to sample?
- How many samples to collect?
- How should the samples be obtained?

Where to sample. Sampling locations for air samples are divided into two types: general area and personal. General area samples may be collected at a specific operation or just within the work space. Personal samples are collected in the worker's breathing zone. The location is dictated by the type of information needed, and more than one sampling location may be necessary. The most frequent location is the personal sample in the worker's breathing zone in order to determine worker exposure levels throughout a work shift. However, when the purpose of the workplace monitoring is to determine the source of contamination or to evaluate engineering controls, general area samples may be more appropriate.

When to sample. When to sample is also determined by the information required as well as by the type of operation being sampled. Multiple shift operations should be sampled each shift, since airborne concentrations may differ for each shift. Similarly, samples should be collected during both summer and winter months, particularly in areas with large temperature gradients.

How long to sample. Minimum sampling time is usually determined by the length of time necessary to obtain a sufficient amount of the contaminant for laboratory analysis. Therefore, the sampling time is dependent on the sensitivity of the analytical procedure and the concentration of the contaminant in the workspace. However, total sampling time should preferably encompass an entire work shift or at least the total length of the operation if the operation lasts less than a full shift. Multiple samples can be used to measure the entire work shift as long as the minimum sampling time is exceeded. Full-shift sampling is required to determine compliance with occupational exposure limits.

Whom to sample. Whom to sample is dependent on the purpose of the workplace monitoring. If compliance with the occupational exposure limit is the objective, then the maximum risk employees should be sampled. Maximum risk employees are the workers with the highest potential exposures. If comprehensive exposure assessment is the objective of the workplace monitoring, then a random sample of employees in each exposure group should be sampled. See Chapter 7 for a more detailed description of comprehensive exposure assessment.

How many samples to collect. The number of samples to collect is also dependent on the purpose of the workplace monitoring. With a comprehensive exposure assessment strategy, a minimum of six samples per exposure group may be necessary before a decision of acceptability can be made. If time and budget constraints limit the number of samples that can be collected, semi-quantitative methods such as mathematical modeling may provide less biased results when only a few samples can be collected. However, there is no set rule regarding the number of samples to collect. The occupational hygienist needs to use personal experience to plan a sampling strategy to collect the optimal number of appropriate samples within budgetary constraints.

How should the sample be obtained. The choice of instrumentation depends on the portability and ease of use of the instrument, the efficiency of the instrument and the testing and analytical method, the reliability of the instrument under various conditions of field use, and the type of analysis or information required, among others. The choice of instrumentation and testing and analytical procedures is ultimately dependent on the capabilities of the analytical laboratory.

Sample Collection

The sampling strategy, once established, should be followed so as not to bias the results or compromise the integrity of the conclusions. However, the occupational hygienist may need to adjust the sampling strategy if the planning assumptions/information have changed or were originally incorrect. For example, if the amount of materials has been increased due to an increased throughput then the occupational hygienist may need to decide to increase the number of samples collected per worker so as not to overload the sampling media. A phased sampling scheme is another option when developing a sampling strategy that plans for adjustments based on the first set of sampling results.

Prior to beginning the workplace monitoring, the occupational hygienist needs to understand the sampling procedures and needs to ensure all necessary equipment and supplies are operating properly and ready for field use. It is the responsibility of the occupational hygienist or other field investigator to perform the monitoring competently so as not to compromise future interactions with the workers and their supervisors.

While performing the workplace monitoring, the occupational hygienist or other field investigator needs to be aware of the impact the sampling has on the work environment and especially on the monitored workers' routines. To limit the impact on the work environment, the sampling should be coordinated in advance with the workers and their supervisors. On the day of sampling, the occupational hygienist needs to explain the purpose and activities of the monitoring event to the workers to ensure sampling results will be representative of actual working conditions. The sampling equipment then needs to be mounted of each worker in a manner that least affects the worker's routines. The workers themselves can be asked to actively participate in the monitoring event by informing the occupational hygienist whenever the sampling pump stops running or of any other deviation in the sampling equipment.

The occupational hygienist or other field investigator also needs to keep a written record or all events occurring during the workplace monitoring event (e.g., field notes). This written record is useful in interpreting the sampling results, especially when there is a delay in receiving the results from the analytical laboratory. However, the occupational hygienist needs to avoid interference with normal work routines and to ensure monitored workers do not change routines due to being observed.

Record keeping. Along with the field notes, other information needs to be collected for each workplace monitoring event. This information should include the sample number, sample duration, airflow rate, PPE utilized, and type of ventilation, among others. Standardized sampling forms minimize the possibility of not recording important information needed for developing conclusions. Record keeping is discussed in detail in Chapter 41.

Handling samples. For reliable results from the workplace monitoring event, the samples need to be clearly labeled prior to the monitoring event to ensure proper identification in the field, at the analytical laboratory, and in the report. Additionally, transit times and temperatures should be written the limits allowed for the sample type and analysis. A written chain of custody is recommended to ensure that the analytical result is matched with the correct sample.

Sampling/Analytical Procedures

The selection of the measurement method (e.g., the combination of sampling and analysis) depends on the requirements of the sampling strategy and on the purpose of the workplace monitoring. Some considerations in the selection of the measurement method include the duration of sampling, the sensitivity of the method, the freedom from interference, the time to result, the intrusiveness, and the accuracy.

Duration of sampling. The sample duration is dependent on the averaging time of the occupational exposure limit. For standards reported as eight-hour time-weighted averages (8-hr TWAs), field samples should consist of a single eight-hour sample or several consecutive samples totaling eight hours. Short-term or instantaneous (i.e., grab) samples are not as satisfactory for estimating full-shift exposures due to the assumptions and extrapolations that are necessary. For short-term exposure limits (STELs) or ceiling standards, 15-minute samples or instantaneous samples are collected. The measurement method needs to be sensitive enough to detect the amount of material capable of being selected in 15 minutes.

Sensitivity. The limit of detection for the analytical method needs to be less than the occupational exposure limit of interest. The lower the limit of detection, the more sensitive the analytical method.

Freedom from interferences. The occupational hygienist needs to be aware of other substances in the sampled air that may interfere with the chemical of interest during the analysis. Interference may bias the result and make it unusable. The analytical laboratory should be able to inform the occupational hygienist of possible interfering substances and should offer guidance for selecting the most appropriate measurement method when interference is possible.

Time to result. The time from collection of samples to receipt of analytical result is generally not urgent when evaluating long-term health hazards — although once received the results should be interpreted and reported to the customer in a timely manner, such a within 10 working days. For acute hazards or urgent evaluations, the time from collection of samples to receipt of analytical results becomes critical. If direct-reading instruments are not available, the occupational hygienist may want to consider contracting with a laboratory that can provide results within 24 hours of receiving the samples. The report to the customer should also be expedited, such as within two working days after receipt of results.

Intrusiveness. Workers are likely to alter their behavior, consciously or subconsciously, when they are being observed or monitored. To the extent that a worker's exposure is related to the worker's actions, any change in behavior can affect the representativeness of the evaluation. Measurement methods that require the close presence of the field investigator are more likely to influence the result than samples collected with unobtrusive devices worn by the workers as they go about their normal working routine.

Accuracy. The more accurate the measurement method, the more representative the results will be to predict exposure. However, due to the large environmental variability, sampling and analytical imprecision rarely make a significant contribution to the overall error in the final result. Even highly imprecise methods, such as fiber counting, do no add much to the variability of results (e.g., do not add much to the width of the confidence limits), given that variability exists between workers performing similar activities and over time.

Interpretation of Sampling Results

The initial interpretation step is to calculate airborne concentrations from the raw data provided by the analytical laboratory, if the laboratory does not report the results in concentration units already. The concentrations can then be averaged over specific time periods (such as eight hours or 15 minutes) for comparison with occupational exposure limits or other measures of acceptability. When sample periods do not correspond to the averaging time of the occupational exposure limit, some assumptions must be made about the unsampled portions of the work period. Finally, some test statistics could be calculated in order to make inferences and to possibly define the statistical reliability of the data.

Professional judgment is a necessary part of every interpretation, even when statistical techniques are used. Before the occupational hygienist determines that workers are exposed to hazardous levels of materials, the following information is necessary: 1) the precise nature of the material or physical agent involved; 2) the intensity or magnitude of the exposures (e.g., the concentration of the contaminant); and 3) reliable knowledge of the duration of the exposure. In many cases, adverse effects from exposure to health hazards do not appear until the exposure has continued for several years. An important purpose of the occupational health standards is to protect against the future appearance of symptoms.

Statistical tests establish, for occupational hygiene, if sampling results are less than occupational health limits. However, professional judgment is also necessary to apply experience and field observation to the results.

Time-Weighted Average Exposures

When worker exposures are compared against occupational exposure limits such as OSHA's permissible exposure limits, the exposures need to be expressed as 8-hr TWAs. The best sampling strategy for standard comparison consists of full-shift integrated personal sampling. Short-term sampling for personal exposures adds more variability to the results due to the numerous assumptions necessary for the unsampled periods. General area sampling is not a recommended method for evaluating worker exposures.

Short-Term Exposures

Short-term sampling is not a precise method for estimating an 8-hr TWA unless the full eight-hour shift is monitored. However, short-term samples are useful for measuring peak concentrations for comparison with STELs and/or ceiling limits. STELs are expressed as 15-minute average exposures, and thus 15-minute personal samples are needed for comparison. Ceiling limits are generally instantaneous values, but when direct-reading instruments are not available, 15-minute personal samples can also be used.

Standard Comparison

Both a compliance sampling strategy and a comprehensive exposure assessment sampling strategy require collection of workers' 8-hr TWA exposures for direct comparison with occupational exposure limits, often expressed as 8-hr TWAs. For materials without an occupational exposure limit, a "local limit" should be established, based on relevant information, before the evaluation of exposures is conducted.

Occupational exposure limits are promulgated/developed by many organizations. The regulatory standards are the OSHA PELs. Unfortunately, most of the PELs are in need of updating, but the revision process can be long and cumbersome. Other occupational exposure limits are voluntary guidelines and include TLVs® from ACGIH®, recommended exposure limits (RELs) from NIOSH, and Workplace Environmental Exposure Levels (WEELs™) from AIHA®, among others.

Individual states may implement a state sponsored occupational safety and health program under provisions of the federal Occupational Safety and Health Act. These state plans are required to be "at least as effective" as the federal standards. Some states with state plans have implemented federal standards, while others have adopted more stringent standards or have promulgated standards for conditions not covered by federal regulations. Consequently, occupational hygienists must be aware of the standards applicable in their states and that the federal standards are minimum legal requirements.

Results Comparison

In additional to comparing results to occupational exposure limits, the occupational hygienist needs to compare the results to previous results collected for the same exposure groups/operations. In this context the occupational hygienist can determine if exposures have increased or decreased over time. Controls may be necessary for operations where exposures are increasing even these exposures may be under the occupational exposure limits.

Summary

Evaluation by exposure assessment is just one part of the overall effort in determining occupational health hazards. Such evaluation is valuable only if all environmental factors relating to workers' potential exposure are included. In evaluating worker exposure to toxic dusts, fumes, mists, gases, vapors, physical agents, and/or biological agents, a sufficient number of samples must be collected for the proper duration to permit the assessment of daily TWA exposures and evaluate peak exposure concentrations when needed. No matter why the exposure assessment was conducted, "a well-designed study is scientifically defensible, produces valid data, leads to a better understanding of disease, and results in improved public health."[5] All of this evaluation is necessary to meet the goal of an employer's exposure management program, which should be to minimize the number of workers who potentially have unacceptable exposures.[2]

It is essential that the proper instrument be selected for the particular hazard and that it be calibrated to ensure proper operation. Calibration can involve either airflow determination or measurement of known concentrations of the material of interest. For those samples to be analyzed in a laboratory, a method must be used that is accurate, sensitive, specific, and reproducible for the contaminant of interest. Adequate field notes during the workplace monitoring event are a necessity. The occupational hygienist should not rely on memory after monitoring is complete to provide the necessary details for report preparation.

Occupational hygiene has often been described as an art and a science – meaning that science alone will not lead to the end results, but must be augmented with professional judgment. In some occupational hygiene activities it is possible to follow a fixed set of rules, but in others judgment must guide decisions. Judgment will grow from experience and must be continually examined, analyzed, and tested, so as not to become a highly subjective opinion. Further, the foundation for, and the process of applying good judgment must be documented effectively so that it is understood and accepted by others. Finally, regardless of the analytical approach to quantify data, sound professional judgment is always a part of all phases of an evaluation: planning, conducting, analyzing, interpreting, drawing conclusions, and recommending decisions.

References

1. **Ignacio, J.S. and W.H. Bullock (eds.):** *A Strategy for Assessing and Managing Occupational Exposures*, 3rd edition. Fairfax, VA: AIHA Press, 2006.
2. **Ramachandran G:** *Occupational Exposure Assessment for Air Contaminants*. Boca Raton, FL: Taylor & Francis, 2005.
3. **American Industrial Hygiene Association:** *AIHA Mission Statement*. Fairfax, Va.: AIHA, 1994.
4. **World Health Organization (WHO):** Human Exposure Assessment. Environmental Health Criteria 214. Geneva, Switzerland: WHO, 2000.
5. **Woebkenberg, M.L:** Partnership in research: exposure assessment methods. *Chem. Health Safety* 1:24–26 (2000).

Outcome Competencies

After completing this chapter, the reader should be able to:

1. Define key terms used in this chapter.
2. Explain the purpose and objectives of risk assessment and discuss the increasing reliance on risk assessment in public policy and decision making.
3. Discuss the risk assessment process described in the Chapter
4. Recall sources of uncertainty in a risk assessment, the impact of uncertainty on outcome, and ways of expressing uncertainty in a risk assessment.
5. Describe how the dimensions of risk affect public perception and acceptance of risk.
6. Contrast the purposes and rationales of risk assessment and risk management, and list some of the "nonscientific" factors that may be incorporated into risk management.
7. Discuss the five general steps of the risk management process.
8. Describe the differences in levels of risk acceptability in environmental and occupational settings.
9. Describe the types of exposure criteria that may be used to address airborne exposure risks.
10. Describe the applications of emergency exposure levels.
11. Discuss a site conceptual model.

Prerequisite Knowledge

Prior to beginning this chapter, the reader should review the following chapters:

Chapter Number	Chapter Topic
History of Industrial Hygiene	
4	Occupational Exposure Limits
5	Occupational Toxicology
6	Occupational Epidemiology
7	Principles of Evaluating Worker Exposure
9	Comprehensive Exposure Assessment
10	Modeling Inhalation Exposure
34	Prevention and Mitigation of Accidental Chemical Releases
45	Risk Communication

Key Terms

acute effect • Acute Exposure Guideline Level (AEGL) • chronic effect •confidence level/limit • chronic daily intake • control banding • Emergency Response Planning Guideline (ERPG™) • hazard • hazard index • hazard quotient • Integrated Risk Information System (IRIS) • iterative risk assessment • lifetime cancer risk assessment • Military Exposure Guideline (MEG) • Monte Carlo analysis • reasonable maximum exposure • reference dose • risk • risk assessment • risk characterization • risk communication • risk estimate • risk management • screening risk assessment • toxic potential • toxicity assessment • toxicity value • uncertainty • variability

Key Topics

Occupational and Environmental Health Risk Assessment/ Risk Management

8

Gary M. Bratt, PhD, CIH, PE, BCEE; Deborah Imel Nelson, PhD, CIH; Andrew Maier, PhD, CIH, DABT; Susan D. Ripple, MS, CIH; David O. Anderson, PhD, CIH, CSP, QEP and Frank Mirer, PhD, CIH

Introduction

Purpose

In today's environment, occupational and environmental health (OEH) professionals will be involved in addressing a multitude of workplace, community, and public health risk issues. They will be employed in the private sector, as consultants, in federal, state, and local governments, in the military, and as private or federal contractors. They could be technical specialists such as occupational hygienists, environmental scientists, environmental engineers, or they could be managers, supervisors, researchers, or corporate executives. Depending on the job, they could be responsible for research and development, procurement, marketing, risk assessments, hazard analyses, risk communication, or risk management. Whatever their positions, they will need a sound background in risk assessment, risk management, and risk communication.

This chapter presents a basic overview of risk assessment and risk management processes, suggests useful tools, and provides numerous references.

- Section I presents introductory information, provides purpose and scope and objectives of the chapter.
- Section II includes background information on risk assessment/ management legislation, regulation, and policy.
- Section III discusses the risk management process.
- Section IV provides information on environmental risk assessment in the risk management process.
- Section V provides information on occupational hygiene and safety risk assessment in the risk management process.
- Section VI discusses uncertainty and variability in risk assessment.
- Section VII provides concluding remarks.

Additional references on risk assessment and risk management are available from AIHA®.[1,2]

Definitions

Relevant terms for this chapter (e.g., *risk, hazard, risk assessment, risk management* and *risk communication*) are used differently by laypersons, business people, and those in the various scientific disciplines. The following working definitions of risk-related terms provide a baseline for the discussions which follow.

- The definition of risk contains two components: the severity or impact of an adverse event, and the probability or likelihood of that event occurring. Therefore, with respect to chemical hazards, risk is a function of the toxicity of and exposure to a harmful substance.
- Hazard refers to the source of risk. In occupational and environmental hygiene, hazards may be chemical (the focus of this chapter), physical (e.g., ergonomic stressors, noise, temperature extremes), biological, and/or radiological (e.g., ionizing radiation) hazards.
- Toxic potential means the nature of the adverse effect, for example cancer,

caused by a chemical. Potency is measured by the fraction of a population affected by a specific dose, for example, the dose at which 50% of a population will develop cancer. Agents of increasing potency will achieve a population effect at a lower dose (level and duration of exposure). Increasing the exposure or the gravity of effect or potency of the chemical will result in increased risk.

- Risk assessment is the systematic process of determining the probability and magnitude of an undesired event and estimating the cost to human society or the environment in terms of morbidity, mortality, or economic impact, either quantitatively or qualitatively. Risk assessment is frequently described as a four-phase process: hazard identification, exposure response assessment, exposure assessment, and risk characterization. In the context of regulating environmental and occupational exposure to chemicals, risk assessment is the art and science of examining all relevant data about a chemical — its toxicity, environmental fate, routes of exposure, epidemiology, etc. — and characterizing its potential adverse effects on humans and/or the environment. For purposes of this chapter, risk assessment is the science-based evaluation of exposure to a chemical (or process or energy), followed by comparison with some measure of the known human health effects of exposure to that chemical; predicting the probability of health effects resulting from a given exposure. Risk assessment provides pertinent information to risk managers, policymakers, and regulators in helping set priorities and make decisions.[2]
- Risk management is the process of identifying, evaluating, selecting, and implementing actions to reduce risk to human health and to ecosystems. The goal of risk management is scientifically sound, cost-effective, integrated actions that reduce or prevent risks while taking into account social, cultural, ethical, political, and legal considerations. Risk management includes all activities undertaken to mitigate a hazard. These activities include the process of identifying, assessing, and controlling risks arising from operational factors and making decisions that may require balancing costs with benefits.[2]
- Risk communication is the exchange of information and opinions among interested parties about a hazard and the nature, magnitude, significance, and/or control of health risks. Risks and their management decisions must be credibly communicated to help ensure that messages are constructively formulated, transmitted, and received in a meaningful manner.[2] Effective risk communication is anchored by risk assessment and management decisions that are rational, defensible, and determined in an open and transparent manner, ultimately ensuring trust in the decision-making process.
- Scientific uncertainty about the effect, severity, or prevalence of a hazard tends to escalate unease.

Scope and Objectives

Risk assessment and management have always been integral to the OEH professions. IHs have long used risk assessment methods to assess risks in the workplace and in the environment, particularly to manage chemicals with no established exposure guidelines. Risk assessment methods are increasingly used to manage risks in federal government agency, military, and homeland security operations, and in emergency situations. Legislation and accepted state-of-the-art practices often specify risk assessment as an integral aid in managing risk; however, there is no universally acceptable model and no single risk assessment methodology is used by all organizations. In view of the broad diversity of work environments, the flexibility offered by in-depth knowledge of a variety of risk assessment methodologies is a professional strength.

The practice of risk assessment is distinctly different in the standard setting context (e.g., setting exposure limits) from that of the site-, process-, or product-specific contexts. In the standard setting context, underlying health information is analyzed to establish an exposure limit or guideline. Generally, occupational and environmental health professionals have limited involvement in governmental regulation setting. However, they may engage in such risk assessment when there is no established limit for a chemical, when their organization chooses to establish a limit, or when co-exposures show the established limit is inappropriate. For example, this could occur within the Department of Defense, especially where personnel are deployed in military operations in austere settings or involved with military-unique workplace, operations, equipment, and systems. It could occur with the development of a new drug, within the pharmaceutical industry. In addition, a hygienist may be involved in devising hazard communication warnings based on toxicological or epidemiological data. The more common context of risk assessment for OEH professionals is in site-specific evaluations, in which measured or estimated exposures are compared with established limits or guidelines. Both of these risk assessment roles — setting exposure limits and site-specific evaluations — are discussed in this chapter. Although conceptually related; risk assessments for noise, heat, radiation, ergonomics, acute traumatic injury, munitions-impacted areas, chemically-contaminated sites, infectious disease, and facility property damage, etc., use distinctly different data sets and analytical techniques, and are not addressed in this chapter.

Changes in the practice of industrial hygiene (and by extension, of risk assessment) have mirrored the technological advances and political events of the times.[3] Key events in the past century have included the shift from an agricultural to a manufacturing-based economy; the introduction of workers' compensation laws to assist victims and their families; founding of American Conference of Governmental Industrial Hygienist (ACGIH®) and the American Industrial Hygiene Association (AIHA®); and the enactment of the Williams-Steiger Occupational Safety and Health (OSH) Act of 1970.[3] In addition, the U.S. Environmental Protection Agency was established in 1970 to consolidate federal research, monitoring, standard-setting and enforcement activities to ensure environmental protection. Events such as the tragedy of Bhopal, India; economic pressures that have led to corporate downsizing; the reinvention of government; and the shift toward a service- and knowledge-based economy continued to affect the practice of occupational hygiene. In the 21st Century, events including the World Trade Center attacks and Hurricane Katrina have refocused national attention on emergency management in general and homeland security in particular. Corporate decision making continues to be concerned with enhancing profitability and avoiding liability, and increasingly, the need to respond to chemical management initiatives from the European Union. These changes call for constantly updated tools in the OEH professional's toolbox. Risk assessment is a powerful, value-added tool that can assist in decision making, priority setting, and protection of worker and community safety and health. The major goal of this chapter is to facilitate the integration of risk assessment into the practice of occupational and environmental hygiene. Specific objectives are to introduce risk and risk assessment, the broad application of risk assessment principles in OEH, and the role of risk assessment in risk management decision making.

This chapter does not cover the details of conducting risk assessments or making risk management decisions. An excellent resource for risk assessment principles and conduct of risk assessments is *Risk Assessment Principles for the Industrial Hygienist*.[4] Resources from the Environmental Protection Agency (EPA) for exposure scenarios and factors include: the EPA Exposure Factors Handbook[5,6], the Child-Specific Exposure Factors Handbook[7], Guidance for Selecting Age Groups for Monitoring and Assessing Childhood Exposures to Environmental Contaminants[8], Example Exposure Scenarios[9], and Sociodemographic Data Used for Identifying Potentially Highly Exposed Populations.[10]

EPA's Risk Assessment Guidelines were developed, based on recommendations from the National Academy of Science, to help guide EPA scientists in assessing the risks from chemicals or other agents in the environment. They also inform EPA decision makers and the general public about these procedures. The initial risk assessment guidelines related to cancer, mutagenic effects, developmental effects, exposure assessment, and chemical mixtures. Today EPA continues to develop new guidelines and also works to revise its original guidelines as experience and scientific knowledge improve.

Overview of Risk Assessment

Risk assessments are conducted to estimate how much damage or injury can be expected from exposures to a given hazard or harmful substance and to assist in judging whether these consequences are great enough to require increased management or guidance, or regulation. Depending on the type of hazard, the effects of primary concern might be workplace illness and injuries; reproductive and genetic abnormalities; diseases such as cancer, or other debilitating illnesses.

Risk assessment is frequently described as a phased process: identifying hazards; assessing hazards to determine risks; developing controls and making risk decisions; implementing controls; and supervising and evaluating. In the context of regulating environmental and occupational exposure to chemicals, risk assessment is the art and science of examining all relevant data about a chemical — its toxicity, environmental fate, routes of exposure, epidemiology, etc. — and characterizing its potential adverse effects on humans and/or the environment.

In the health, safety, and environmental fields, health risk is usually identified as the likelihood that individuals (or a population) will incur an increased incidence of adverse effects such as disabling injury, disease, or death. Risk frequently is expressed in quantitative probability terms—such as some number of additional cancer deaths over a lifetime in a population of 1 million exposed people. (A risk of 1 in 1,000 is often described as a "10^{-3} risk", 1 in 1 million as a "10^{-6} risk", and so on.) Historically, risks of less than 10^{-6} in magnitude have not been the object of concern. More qualitative characterizations are also used — such as low, medium, high, extremely high — where quantification is either infeasible or unnecessary.(11)

Development of the Art of Risk Assessment

Background

People have been exposed to hazards since the beginning of human history, so it is not surprising that risk assessment is not a new concept. Covello and Mumpower(12) described an early group of risk analysts who lived in the Tigris-Euphrates valley about 3200 B.C. These consultants would identify important dimensions of a problem, delineate alternatives, predict outcomes, and recommend the most favorable outcome — a process not dissimilar from modern risk assessment. Bernstein and Covello and Mumpower listed additional studies conducted during the sixteenth to the nineteenth centuries that established the basis for the analysis of environmental risk, including many familiar examples: Agricola's 1556 study linking health effects to mining and metallurgical practices; work by Ramazzini in the early 1700s identifying higher rates of breast cancer in nuns; Sir Percival Pott's study relating scrotal cancer to employment as a chimney sweep; John Snow's removal of the handle from the Broad Street pump in 1854 to prevent the spread of cholera.(12–14)

Paracelsus's (1493–1541) famous statement: "All substances are poisons; there is none which is not a poison. The right dose differentiates a poison and a remedy." has been long regarded as a fundamental concept in occupational health.(15) These early practitioners of the art of occupational and public health risk assessment paved the way for the formalization of risk assessment processes that were integrated into occupational and environmental regulation and health risk practice in the 20th century. The art of risk assessment continues to evolve to take advantage of developments in the fields of chemistry, biology, and biomathematics, and significant effort is being expended to look for new and more effective risk assessment approaches. For example, a report of the National Academy of Sciences (NAS) addressed trends for toxicity testing in the 21st Century that will better inform dose-response assessments for risk assessment.(16)

Federal Legislation on Environmental Risk in the United States

This section describes federal legislation to control environmental risks in the U.S.; agency-specific activities are discussed later. Federal regulation of environmental risks began very slowly in the U.S. with the River and Harbor Act of 1899, which prohibited the discharge of refuse into navigable waters.(17) In 1914, the railroad industry asked the U.S. Public Health Service to suggest their first drinking water standards to protect passengers from variable water quality along the routes. Although no laws or regulations were passed, it was understood that trains would not stop in towns that did not meet these standards.[18] In 1958, the Food, Drug, and Cosmetics Act was amended by the Delaney clause, which prohibited the intentional addition to food of any material found to cause cancer in humans or animals.

The late 1960s and early 1970s saw a virtual explosion in environmental legislation, such as the creation of the U.S. EPA and OSHA (via the passage of the Occupational Safety and Health Act), the Clean Air Act of 1970, and the Federal Water Pollution Control Act of 1971. These laws and the regulations promulgated under their authority addressed real and present problems: pollution of water and air, and hazards in the workplace. Many of these statutes (or subsequent amendments) contained language that implied but did not specifically require risk assessment: "toxic pollutants in toxic amounts;" "unreasonable risk to man or the environment" (see Table 8.1).

The second series of environmental laws, which included the Safe Drinking Water Act of 1974 and the Toxic Substances Control Act of 1976, addressed public concerns about pesticides and toxic chemicals.[19] Language became more risk oriented: "no known or anticipated adverse health effects;" "unreasonable risk of injury to health or the environment." Following events such as the hazardous waste disaster at Love Canal, N.Y., the third wave of legislation addressed hazardous waste handling practices and the cleanup of previously contaminated sites.[19] The Comprehensive Environmental Response, Compensation, and Liability Act (Superfund) of 1980 had a tremendous significance for modern environmental risk assessment through its requirement that EPA revise the National Contingency Plan, including addition of methods for evaluating and remedying releases from facilities that pose substantial danger to the public health or the environment. These revisions ultimately led to the frequently cited EPA series on risk assessment guidance for Superfund.[20–22] During this time period, the developing art of risk assessment was used increasingly as a means of bridging the gap between scientific study of the relationships between health effects of exposures to toxic chemicals, and the development of policies to protect the public and the environment from unreasonable risk. An increased reliance on quantification by policymakers was well evident by the early 1980s.[23] The acceptance of risk assessment in health, safety, and environmental policy was enhanced by the seminal report issued by the National Academy of Sciences (NAS) in 1983: *Risk Assessment in the Federal Government: Managing the Process*.[24] The report presented a logical approach to assessing environmental, health and safety risk that was widely accepted and used by government agencies.

Environmental legislation into the 1990s increasingly was directed at specific environmental risks (asbestos in schools, underground storage tanks, lead in drinking water, lead-based paint, etc.), leading indirectly to increased use of risk assessment.[19] The Clean Air Act Amendments (CAAA) of 1990 had a somewhat delayed impact on risk assessment. The amendments established a National Academy of Sciences study to review the risk assessment methodology used by EPA to determine carcinogenic risk associated with exposure to hazardous air pollutants and to suggest improvements in such methodology. Published as *Science and Judgment in Risk Assessment* in 1994, the document provided specific recommendations on the practice of risk assessment by EPA: the general retention of the conservative, default-based approach to screening analysis (subject to modifications), an iterative approach to risk assessment, and presentation of sources and magnitude of uncertainty along with point estimates of risk.[25]

The CAAA also established the President's Commission on Risk Assessment and Risk Management, which was charged with making a full investigation of the policy implications and appropriate uses of risk assessment and risk management in regulatory programs under various federal laws to prevent cancer and other chronic human health effects that may result from exposure to hazardous substances.[26,27]

An updated review of EPA Risk Assessment practices concluded that the basic use of the 1983 NAS paradigm should be retained, but suggested changes to the process to address needs for more timely and effective risk assessment decision-making.[28] Key recommendations of this report included:

Table 8.1 — Selected Major U.S. Statutes Involving Risk Assessment

Law	*Date*[A]	*Agency*	*Pertinent Language or Impact on Risk Assessment*
Delaney amendment to the Food, Drug and Cosmetic Act	1958	FDA	21 USC 348(c)(3): "That no additive shall be deemed to be safe it if is found to induce cancer when ingested by man or animal, or if it is found, after tests which are appropriate for the evaluation of the safety of food additives to induce cancer in man or animal"
Occupational Safety and Health Act	1970	OSHA	29 USC 655(b)(5): "no employee shall suffer material impairment of health or functional capacity"
Federal Water Pollution Control Act (Clean Water Act)	1971	EPA	33 USC 1251(a)(3): "It is the national policy that the discharge of toxic pollutants in toxic amounts be prohibited."
Federal Insecticide, Fungicide, and Rodenticide Act	1972	EPA	7 USC 136 (bb): "unreasonable adverse effect on the environment' means any unreasonable risk to man or the environment, taking into account the economic, social, and environmental costs and benefits of the use of any pesticide"
Safe Drinking Water Act	1974	EPA	42 USC 300 g-1(b)(4): "Each maximum contaminant level goal...shall be set at the level at which no known or anticipated adverse effects on the health of persons occur and which allows an adequate margin of safety"
Resource Conservation and Recovery Act	1976	EPA	42 USC 6903(5): "`hazardous waste' means . . . may cause, or significantly contribute to an increase in mortality or an increase in serious irreversible, or incapacitating reversible illness; or pose a substantial present or potential hazard to human health or the environment"
Toxic Substances Control Act	1976	EPA	15 USC 2601(a)(2): "Among the many chemical substances and mixtures...there are some whose manufacture, processing, distribution in commerce, use, or disposal may present an unreasonable risk of injury to heath or the environment... necessitates the regulation of intrastate commerce"
Comprehensive Environmental Response, Compensation and Liability Act (CERCLA, Superfund)	1980	EPA	Established a national program for responding to release of hazardous substances into the environment. Called for revision of the national contingency plan for the removal of oil and hazardous substances, originally required by 33 USC 1321, Federal Water Pollution Control Act. The revision was to include methods for evaluating and remedying releases from facilities that pose substantial danger to the public health or the environment.
Clean Air Act Amendments	1990	EPA	42 USC 7412(f)(1): "The Administrator shall investigate and report...methods of calculating the risk to public health remaining...after the application of standards, the public health significance of such estimated remaining risk"
			42 USC 7412(f)(2): "If standards . . . do not reduce lifetime excess cancer risks to the individual most exposed to emissions . . . to less than one in one million, the Administrator shall promulgate standards"
			Established the National Academy of Sciences to review risk assessment methodology used by EPA to determine carcinogenic risk associated with exposure to hazardous air pollutants and suggest improvements in methodology. Published as *Science and Judgment in Risk Assessment* by the National Research Council, 1994.
			Established the Risk Assessment and Management Commission, which was to investigate the policy implications and appropriate uses of risk assessment and risk management in regulatory programs under various federal laws to prevent cancer and other chronic human health effects that may result from exposure to hazardous substances. Published as *Risk Assessment and Risk Management in Regulatory Decision-Making—Draft Report for Public Review and Comment* on June 13, 1996.

[A]Most environmental legislation has been amended several times; EPA was not yet in existence when many of the major laws were first enacted.
Sources: Suggested by and adapted from Reference 77, Figure 3. Also, Superintendent of Documents' *Home Page*. Available: http://www.access.gpo.gov./su_docs/; *Selected Environmental Law Statutes*, 1994–95, educational ed. St. Paul, Minn.: West Publishing, 1994; and Reference 4.

- Increased focus should be placed on planning, scoping, and problem formulation to ensure that that the risk assessment is designed to address the identified concern.
- Guidelines should be developed for determining the degree to which variability and uncertainty analyses are needed to support decision-making for risk assessment applications.
- A unified approach should be developed for non-cancer and cancer effects that allows for determining risk probabilities for both.
- While continuing the use of defaults in risk assessment is appropriate, EPA should develop guidance on the level of evidence needed to justify use of chemical-specific data to move from defaults and should ensure current defaults embedded in existing methods are explicit.
- Methods (including prioritization and screening tools) are needed to increase the development of cumulative risk assessments (assessments that include combined risks posed by exposure to multiple agents or stressors; or aggregate exposure that includes all routes, pathways, and sources of exposure to a given chemical).
- A formal process is needed for stakeholder involvement in risk-based decision making.

Risk legislation can be divided into three main categories: (1) risk-based laws designed to reduce risks to zero; (2) balancing laws that balance cost and benefit and provide for some risk above zero, and (3) technology-based laws that require use of a specific technology or that force development of new technology.[29,30] Examples of risk-based regulations are the Safe Drinking Water Act provisions for maximum contaminant level goals established at a level to prevent adverse health effects, and the Delaney amendment to prohibit carcinogenic food additives. Examples of risk-benefit balancing include EPA's lead phase-down decision and proposed ban on asbestos-containing materials.[23]

The basis of the OSH Act is technology or balancing; that is, it "assures, to the extent feasible... that no employee will suffer material impairment of health or functional capacity."[30] The courts have agreed that OSHA can enforce a rule that will require development and/or distribution of new technologies.[23] Ironically, the cotton dust standard, which forced technological changes that industry feared would have negative impacts, resulted in improved competitiveness and productivity.[23] Similarly, the vinyl chloride standard resulted in lower industry costs and improved productivity.[3] Some laws may have two or three bases. For example, the stationary sources section of the Clean Air Act is risk-based, the vehicle section is technology-forcing, and the fuel section is risk-balancing.[29]

In the early 1980s "regulatory reform" legislation that would have required formal risk assessment and risk management (economic) analyses, as well as procedural mandates for consideration of these issues, began to be introduced in Congress.[31] Starting in 1994, many proposed comprehensive "regulatory reform" bills were introduced in Congress (although none have been passed). The Food Quality Protection Act of 1996 did contain several provisions regarding risk of pesticide chemical residues, and requires special consideration of children's health.[32] The Congressional Review Act (CRA) was passed along with the Small Business Regulatory and Fairness Act in 1996. This provided for Congressional veto of any regulation by majority vote of both houses of Congress. The CRA was used to disapprove OSHA's ergonomics standard in 2001.

Hazard Risk Assessment in the 1970s – Present

The most quoted framework for chemical hazard risk assessment is the paradigm advanced by the National Academy of Sciences Committee on Institutional Means for Risk Assessment in the Federal Government in 1983 (the "Red Book"). That Committee suggested four steps to risk assessment: hazard assessment; exposure-response assessment; exposure assessment; and, risk characterization.[24]

The most significant relationship to the occupational environment is seen in the evolving scheme being employed by OSHA. Evidence is required to show that a toxic substance is dangerous for workers and that adequate protection is essential in the occupational environment. Most central to providing hazard or toxicity information is the EPA scheme employed in the EPA Integrated Risk Information System (IRIS). Examples of numerous types of modeling that may be used including benchmark dose modeling approaches to replace traditional toxicology studies; physiologically-based pharmacokinetic modeling (PBPK) models to estimate organ or tissue doses, and inhalation dosimetry modeling to assess differences in respiratory tract distribution of inhaled chemicals.

U.S. Food and Drug Administration

Occupational and environmental health professionals within the U.S. Food and Drug Administration (FDA) perform duties to help protect the public health by assuring the safety, efficacy, and security of human and veterinary drugs, biological products, medical devices, the nation's food supply, cosmetics, and products that emit radiation. They may also help to prepare the U.S. for possible bioterrorism attacks by working with other federal agencies to ensure that adequate supplies of medicine and vaccines are available to the American public.

Historically the U.S. Food and Drug Administration (FDA) was the first agency to use quantitative risk assessment methods formally in the regulatory process.(33) Public health agencies generally face a problem for agents thought not to have a threshold such as carcinogens; any exposure to the agent carries an increase in risk, however small. Rather than simply ban the use of such a material, in a 1973 proposal on the regulation of food residues containing carcinogenic drugs, FDA suggested the "virtually safe dose" approach (corresponding to 10^{-8} risk) published by Mantel and Bryan in 1961.(34) Quantitative exposure response assessment was firmly established at FDA, which later adopted a maximally acceptable lifetime risk of 10^{-6}. From this point onward, the notion of extrapolating risk to levels not directly observable in a population in laboratory studies or epidemiological investigations, and choosing an acceptable level of risk in a population, became the dominant mode or risk assessment to support risk management decision making by federal public health agencies.(33)

U.S. Occupational Safety and Health Administration

Occupational and environmental health professionals within OSHA perform duties which could include industrial hygiene, health physics, environmental cleanup, ergonomics, and waste management. These duties support the varied operations within the OSHA which are primarily involved with preparing technical documents and legislation on occupational safety and health in the workplace. In addition, occupational safety and health professionals may be involved with workplace inspections or assistance.

Despite promulgation of new or updated Permissible Exposure Limits (PELs) for only 16 agents, the risk assessment scheme employed by OSHA provides evidence to show that the toxic substance is dangerous for workers and that adequate protection is essential in the occupational environment.(35) When OSHA was created in 1970, the enabling legislation directed it to adopt national consensus standards and existing federal standards. Thus, OSHA adopted some of the American National Standards Institute occupational exposure limits and the 1968 ACGIH® Threshold Limit Values® (TLVs®), which were legally enforceable for employers subject to the Walsh-Healey Public Contracts Act. The risk assessment methods for setting these legacy standards was not explicit, poorly documented, and likely inconsistently applied. Table 8.2 presents a chronology of OSHA's Permissible Exposure Limits (PELs), including the degree of reduction of permissible exposure. Highlights of important events are outlined in the following paragraphs; for simplicity, discussion of each specific risk issue, even those spanning decades, is contained in one paragraph.(3,29,33,36)

The framework for setting PELs was set by the Supreme Court 1980 decision siding with the American Petroleum Institute in overturning OSHA's first benzene standard, which had been promulgated in 1978. The critical terms are "material impairment of health or functional capacity" (language in the OSHA Act) and "significant risk" (created by the Supreme Court decision).

In July 1980 the Supreme Court, in a divided vote, invalidated OSHA's first attempt to set a benzene standard. The Court found that OSHA had failed to show that the standard would reduce a "significant risk in the workplace." Although hazard identification for benzene had been established by case reports and by an epidemiological study by NIOSH; neither data set was

Table 8.2 — Chronology of OSHA PELs

Substance	CFR 1910 Section	Date	Previous	Current	Reduction
Asbestos	1001	1971	12 f/cc	5 f/cc	2.4
13 Carcinogens	1003	1974	NA	na	
Vinyl Chloride	1017	1975	500 ppmM^3	1 ppm	500
Asbestos	1001	1976	5 f/cc	2 f/cc	2.5
Coke Oven Emissions	1029	1977	0.2 mg/M^3	0.15 mg/M^3	1.3
Inorganic Arsenic	1018	1978	0.5 mg/M^3	0.01 mg/M^3	50
Lead	1025	1978	200 µg/M^3	50 µg/M^3	4
DBCP	1044	1978	None	0.001 mg/M^3	na
Acrylonitrile	1045	1978	20 ppm	2 ppm	10
Cotton Dust	1043	1978	1 mg/M^3	0.2 mg/M^3	5
Asbestos		1984	2 f/cc	0.2 f/cc	10
Ethylene Oxide	1047	1986	50 ppm	1 ppm	50
Benzene	1028	1987	10 ppm	1 ppm	10
Formaldehyde	1048	1988	3 ppm	0.75 ppm	4
Cadmium	1027	1992	0.2 mg/M^3	0.005 mg/M^3	40
Methylenedianiline	1050	1992	None	0.01 ppm	na
Lead In Construction	1926.62	1993	200 µg/M^3	50 µg/ M^3	4
Asbestos	1001	1994	0.2 f/cc	0.1 f/cc	2*
Asbestos in Construction	1926.1101	1994		0.1 f/cc	na
Butadiene	1051	1996	1000 ppm	1 ppm	1000
Methylene Chloride	1052	1998	500 ppm	25 ppm	20
Chromium (VI)	1026	2006	52 µg/M^3	5 µg/M^3	10.4**

* The four PELs set for asbestos eventually mandated a 120-fold reduction from pre-OSHA PEL.
** Pre-existing PEL was in units of a different chemical form. Originally published as a "ceiling" level, OSHA reinterpreted the old PEL as a less protective time-weighted average.

associated with an exposure level. OSHA had declined to conduct a quantitative exposure-response assessment for benzene, instead arguing that identification of an agent as a carcinogen supported reducing exposure to the lowest feasible level. A quantitative exposure-response assessment had been advanced by the American Petroleum Institute. The Court ruled that some quantification of risk and the reduction of risk expected from the new standard were necessary for a standard to be upheld. In a footnote the Court suggested that a lifetime risk of occupational cancer of 1 in 1000 (10^{-3}) would "reasonably" be considered a significant risk, while 1 in 10,000,000 would not. The Court did not address how far below the 1 in 1000 level a significant risk could reasonably be thought to persist. Subsequently, OSHA in practice has used the 1 in 1000 risk as a benchmark of significance of risk in a population, but has stated the option of targeting a lower goal. Seven years later OSHA issued a new benzene standard of 1 ppm (8-hour) and 5-ppm short-term exposure limit based on quantitative risk assessments. The agency stated that this standard substantially reduced the significant risk to employees exposed at the existing level. The new benzene standard was effective December 1987.

The benzene decision was a landmark, both because the Court effectively established a requirement that the agency determine the existence of a "significant risk" before it initiated rulemaking and because it suggested a benchmark against which to judge occupational risk (i.e., 10^{-3}). It also affirmed the use of conservative assumptions that were supported by a body of reputable scientific thought, and the use of high-dose to low-dose extrapolation as a basis for human health risk assessment. Notably, all agents for which new chemical exposure standards were set after 1980 were considered to be carcinogens.

The legal tests for OSHA chemical exposure limits can be related to the stages in the NAS paradigm. The NAS hazard identification step is equivalent to OSHA's determination that an agent poses a threat to "material impairment of health or functional capacity." The NAS exposure-response relationship step is equivalent to OSHA's determination of "significant risk." Several case study summaries for establishment of chemical PELs are presented to highlight OSHA risk assessment approaches

- *Asbestos.* One of the very first actions taken by OSHA was to issue an Emergency Temporary Standard (ETS) for asbestos in May 1971, followed by a final standard of 5 fibers/cc in June 1972. In October 1975 rulemaking was initiated to reduce the PEL to 2 fibers/cc. These actions were based on OSHA's original approach that once the hazard identification step had found an agent had carcinogenic potential, a PEL at the lowest feasible level should be imposed. Following the 1980 benzene decision, OSHA adopted an approach including quantitative exposure-response analysis. In November 1983, based on its quantitative exposure-response assessment of asbestos exposure, OSHA issued an ETS lowering the PEL to 0.5 fibers/cc. As a result of an industry lawsuit, this ETS was overturned by the Fifth Circuit Court of Appeals, which stated that risk assessment of controversial issues requires public scrutiny through the notice-and-comment rulemaking procedure. In addition, the Court suggested that OSHA needed to identify a "significant risk" during the 6 months from ETS to permanent standard for an ETS to be valid. In June 1986 a final asbestos standard that lowered the PEL from 2.0 to 0.2 fibers/cc was issued. Although the Appeals Court for the District of Columbia upheld the standard, it was returned to OSHA for further study. In September 1988 OSHA promulgated a short term exposure limit of 1 fiber/cc for 30 minutes. In 1990 OSHA proposed to lower the PEL from 0.2 to 0.1 fiber/cc for all industries; this PEL was issued in August 1994. The standard was challenged in the Court of Appeals by both union and industry groups, but was upheld. OSHA's risk estimate for asbestos at 0.2 fibers/cc was 6.7 per 100 workers exposed over a 45-year working lifetime was based on developing asbestos related diseases including lung cancer.
- *Cancer policy.* Partly because of the benzene controversy and other matters regarding carcinogens, OSHA became an early player in carcinogenic risk assessment and regulation. There was considerable pressure for agencies to adopt formal, documented risk assessment guidelines. In 1977 the agency joined the Interagency Regulatory Liaison Group. OSHA also issued a draft cancer policy, the purpose of which was to provide a framework for the regulation of carcinogens. The cancer policy established criteria (decision rules) for deciding whether a material was carcinogenic, corresponding to the hazard identification step in risk assessment. OSHA found that quantitative exposure-response analysis was unreliable and would not be used. The policy also included a risk management element, stating that once a material was determined to be carcinogenic, the allowable exposure level would be the lowest feasible exposure, including banning the material. OSHA also committed to annual publication of a list of carcinogens. The policy thus included both risk assessment decision rules, risk communication and a risk management result. The risk assessment criteria are discussed later in this chapter. The final generic cancer policy was issued in 1980 and legally remains in effect. However, OSHA has stopped publishing the carcinogen list, and the "lowest feasible" risk management policy was essentially invalidated by the benzene decision.
- *Cotton dust.* The cost-benefit issue for occupational safety and health was decided with the cotton dust standard. After years of evidence linking cotton dust and byssinosis, OSHA published a proposed cotton dust standard in December 1976, followed by a final standard in June 1978. It was appealed and then affirmed by the Court of Appeals for the District of Columbia, which stated that the OSH Act prohibited the use of cost-benefit analysis to justify setting a higher exposure limit than indicated by health criteria in the statute. The Supreme Court upheld this decision. The Court stated that Congress itself had defined the cost-benefit relationship, placing the benefit of worker health above all considerations except those making this benefit unachievable. Cost-benefit analysis

could be used to adopt the least expensive means to achieve a given level of protection.

- *Ethylene oxide.* The ethylene oxide standard, which was based on quantitative risk assessment, was issued in June 1984. In ruling on the industry challenge to this standard, the Court of Appeals for the District of Columbia basically affirmed the OSHA PEL for ethylene oxide but remanded the issue to OSHA for further proceedings on the decision not to include a short term exposure limit. The ruling granted OSHA leeway in regulating on the frontiers of current knowledge, demanding no more than that OSHA "arrive at a reasonable conclusion based on all the evidence before it."[37] The Court also found that the no-threshold assumption was supported by substantial evidence. The Court of Appeals for the District of Columbia ordered OSHA to issue a final rule on the ethylene oxide short term exposure limit by March 1988; a 5-ppm short term exposure limit was issued in April 1988. OSHA estimates that the cancer risk at the new PEL is between 1.2 and 2.4 per thousand workers.
- *Formaldehyde.* Risk assessment also played a role in the formaldehyde standard, which was issued in 1987 (1-ppm PEL [8-hour], and 2-ppm short term exposure limit). Industry and union groups challenged it, and the Court of Appeals for the District of Columbia remanded the issue to OSHA, stipulating that (1) if a significant risk remained at 1 ppm, and it were feasible to do so, OSHA must promulgate a lower standard; and (2) the agency had failed to justify omitting medical removal protection. Concurring with a settlement of the lawsuit recommended by the labor and industry parties, OSHA issued a final rule on formaldehyde, dropping the PEL from 1 to 0.75 ppm and providing medical removal protection. Compared to other OSHA potency estimates, the risk assessment for formaldehyde is clearly an outlier. OSHA found that the so-called maximum likelihood estimate (MLE) at the old PEL of 3 ppm was 0.43 per 1000 [certainly within the range of "significant risk"] but the upper confidence interval (UCI) was 18 per 1000. The divergence between the MLE and the UCI implies that the potency estimate is indeterminate. The MLE model predicted a 77-fold reduction in risk for a 4-fold reduction in PEL, while the UCI prediction was only 7-fold.
- *The PEL Project.* Recognizing both the need to update the PELs and the difficulty of regulating substance-by-substance, in 1988 OSHA began the PEL Project, which was designed to revise and incorporate the TLVs as PELs. Shortly thereafter an article severely criticizing the TLV process was published in the *American Journal of Industrial Medicine* setting off a firestorm of comments and responses to the journal.[38] In 1989, hearings were held and the final revised air contaminants standard was issued. The standards were challenged by both management and labor groups, as well as being supported by some management groups. In July 1992 the Court of Appeals for the Eleventh Circuit ruled that OSHA's actions were invalid, even for substances for which limits were unchallenged either in the hearings or lawsuit. OSHA had failed to show, as required by the benzene decision, that each standard showed a significant risk in the workplace, and had made no calculation of the amount of risk that the new PEL reduced, or that the PELs were feasible. In March 1993 the agency announced that it would return to enforcement of the 1971 PELs. The agency did not attempt to articulate an exposure-response analysis policy for non-cancer endpoints.
- *Methylene Chloride.* In January 1997 OSHA issued a proposed standard for methylene chloride. The PEL, based on animal studies demonstrating lung and liver cancer in mice and mammary tumors in rats, was reduced to 25 ppm with no ceiling, and a short term exposure limit of 125 ppm for 15 min.[39] The rulemaking included two risk assessment related issues. First, evidence was presented that epidemiological studies which claimed to be null for lung cancer were too insensitive to find any increased risk at the exposure levels if

the risk were as predicted from the animal models. This was a first attempt to resolve an apparent divergence between laboratory and human studies by examining exposure-response effects. Secondly, OSHA was compelled to repeat its exposure response assessment using the industry model. OSHA demonstrated that competing assumptions generated the same result. According to OSHA's estimates, workers exposed at the new PEL suffer a 3.6 per thousand risk of cancer.

- *Chromium (VI)*. In February 2006, after a decade of litigation and nearly a decade after the methylene chloride standard was issued, OSHA promulgated a standard for chrome (VI) reducing allowable exposure from 52 μg/m³ to 5 μg/m³. This exposure response assessment was based on epidemiological studies of lung cancer in people. Several competing models were advanced by industry and other agencies. OSHA estimated that workers exposed at the new PEL will suffer an increased risk of 10 to 45 cancers per thousand.

U.S. Environmental Protection Agency (EPA)

EPA is involved in risk assessment for a variety of purposes to include regulation of new and existing chemicals under Toxic Substances Control Act (TSCA), registration/re-registration of pesticides and tolerance setting under Federal Insecticide, Fungicide, and Rodenticide Act (FIFRA), development of Maximum Contaminant Levels (MCLs) under Clean Water Act (CWA). It is also involved with cleanup of abandoned hazardous waste sites and dumps or compelling responsible parties to perform cleanups or reimburse the government for EPA-led site cleanups under Superfund. EPA also has had a substantial impact on risk assessment methodology. Because the legislation that the agency enforces is risk-balancing [FIFRA; Safe Drinking Water Act; TSCA; Clean Air Act (CAA)], risk-based [Resource Conservation and Recovery Act (RCRA), CAA], or technology-forcing [CAA], the agency has found itself right in the middle of the risk debate. Its risk assessment activities have been both program-specific and agency-wide, and have included development of risk assessment guidelines and methodologies and use of risk assessment in development of standards. Similar to OSHA, EPA often has found itself dealing with risk assessment in the courtroom, with results that have impacted risk assessment beyond the agency. For example, in 1976 the District of Columbia Circuit Court upheld EPA's order reducing lead in gasoline, ruling that actual injury was not required for endangerment to exist and that risk assessment could form the basis for health-related regulations under the CAA (*Ethyl Corp. v EPA*).[23] In 1976 EPA issued the first risk assessment guidelines.[29]

Occupational and environmental health professionals within EPA may perform duties which could include industrial hygiene, health physics, risk assessment, environmental protection, and environmental protection. These duties support the varied operations within the EPA which are primarily involved with preparing technical documents and legislation on environmental protection.

EPA has published extensively on risk assessment guidelines and methodologies. In 1984 EPA's *Risk Assessment and Management: Framework for Decision Making* appeared, followed in September 1986 by the Risk Assessment Guidelines.[40] These guidelines were partially in response to the National Academy of Sciences' recommendations and were designed to promote high technical quality and agency wide consistency.[41] Written by EPA scientists and receiving extensive peer-review, the guidelines covered carcinogenic risk assessment, estimating exposures, mutagenicity risk assessment, health assessment of suspect developmental toxicants, and health risk assessment of chemical mixtures. After decades of controversy, EPA published revised Guidelines for Carcinogen Risk Assessment and *Supplemental Guidance for Assessing Susceptibility from Early-Life Exposure to Carcinogens* in March 2005.[42,43]

In addition to use of risk assessment within the agency, in the mid-1980s EPA began issuing guidance for *Superfund risk assessors, including the Superfund Public Health Exposure Manual* (1986) and *Superfund Exposure Assessment Manual* (1988), followed by the *Risk Assessment Guidance for Superfund* series.[20–22] EPA Guidance on risk characterization was provided in the form of memoranda in 1992 and

1995.[44,45] In 2008, EPA Region III Toxicologist Jennifer Hubbard, published a Risk-Based Concentration (RBC) Table memorandum, that was originally developed to support the Superfund risk assessment screening process. Region III toxicologists have used RBCs to screen sites not yet on the National Priorities List, respond rapidly to citizen inquiries, and spot-check formal baseline risk assessments. The primary use of RBCs is for chemical screening during baseline risk assessment.[46] The Regional Screening table was developed with input from Regions III, VI, and IX, three Regions that have historically had their own versions of RBC Tables [also called Preliminary Remediation Goal (PRG) Tables], in an effort to improve consistency and incorporate updated guidance.[47]

EPA has also influenced health risk assessment and management with the establishment of acceptable risk levels. In 1981, EPA proposed worker radiation protection rules based on risk assessment (3 deaths per 1000) and comparison with death rates in the safest industries (2.7 per 1000).[29] NRC made a similar proposal in 1986. In 1982, the agency issued standards for pesticide residues in foods based on an acceptable risk level of 10^{-6}.

EPA compiles many hazard or toxicity assessments of chemicals of occupational and environmental importance under the heading of the Integrated Risk Information System (IRIS)[48], which is prepared and maintained by the EPA's National Center for Environmental Assessment (NCEA) within the Office of Research and Development (ORD). IRIS collects documents that describe in qualitative and in quantitative terms the health effects of individual substances (hazard identification and toxic potential). The hazard or toxicity assessments can be used in assessing risk. For noncancer effects, and for other effects known or assumed to be produced through a nonlinear (possibly threshold) mode of action, oral reference doses and inhalation reference concentrations (RfDs and RfCs, respectively) are generated using an extrapolation factor approach. For cancer effects, EPA characterizes the weight of evidence for human carcinogenicity, and presents oral and inhalation unit risks (exposure-response assessments) for carcinogenic effects. Where a nonlinear mode of action is established, references dose (RfD) and reference concentrations (RfC) values may be used. RfD and RfC values are calculated by an extrapolation factor method. First, a point of departure dose is identified. This may be a No Observed Adverse Effect Level (NOAEL) or a benchmark dose (a calculated NOAEL) for a specific adverse effect. If only the LOAEL is identified, an extrapolation factor of 10 is used to specify the point of departure. From there, uncertainty factors for human variability in resistance, animal to human, and acute to chronic, and a modifying factor for reliability of data are included, resulting in a reference concentration or dose as much as 1000-fold below the NOAEL.

Risk assessment was increasingly incorporated into environmental risk decision making in the 1990s. Following the Hazardous and Solid Waste Amendments of 1984, national interest in and limited resources for remediation of underground storage tank sites led to the introduction of risk assessment methodology for establishment of cleanup levels by the American Society for Testing and Materials (ASTM).[49] The Guide also established a framework for iterative risk assessment, described later in this chapter.

In recent years, EPA's risk assessment emphasis has shifted increasingly to a more broadly based approach characterized by greater consideration of multiple endpoints, sources, pathways and routes of exposure; community-based decision making; flexibility in achieving goals; case-specific responses; a focus on all of the environmental media; and significantly, holistic reduction of risk. This can be considered a cumulative risk assessment approach which covers a wide variety of risks. Currently, EPA assessments describe and where possible quantify the risks of adverse health and ecological effects from synthetic chemicals, radiation, and biological stressors.

Although much of EPA's activity has been in support of human health risk assessment, the agency also has developed guidance for ecological risk assessment.[50] EPA's involvement in risk assessment has been long and varied; only a few highlights have been presented. Additional information on risk assessment guidance and models and examples of chemical specific risk assessments are available on line at EPA's Risk Assessment Portal.[51,52]

U.S. Department of Defense

The provisions of the Occupational Safety and Health Act were implemented within the Federal sector with Executive Order 12196 — Occupational Safety and Health Programs for Federal Employees, February26, 1980.[53] The requirement to "Furnish to employees places and conditions of employment that are free from recognized hazards that are causing or are likely to cause death or serious physical harm" was thus extended to federal employees, including the Department of Defense (DoD) and the Department of Energy (DOE). Executive Order 13139, 30 September 1999 — Improving Health Protection of Military Personnel Participating in Particular Military Operations, (EO, 1999) provided additional health protection for military personnel.[54]

Within the DoD, a number of directives, instructions, and memoranda provide the basic policy to anticipate, recognize, evaluate, and control health hazards associated with occupational and environmental exposures to chemical, physical, and biological hazards in workplaces including military operations and deployments.[55–57]

Occupational and environmental health professionals within DoD perform duties involved with military or civilian workplaces or operations that are generally comparable to those of the private sector. Examples include facilities involved and work performed in the repair and overhaul of weapons, vessels, aircraft, or vehicles (except for equipment trials); construction; supply services; civil engineering or public works; medical services; and office work. In addition, they may perform duties associated with workplaces, operations, equipment, and systems unique to the national defense mission. These may include combat and operation, testing, and maintenance of military-unique equipment and systems such as military weapons, ordnance, and tactical vehicles. It also includes operations such as peacekeeping missions; field maneuvers; combat training; military-unique Research, Development, Test, and Evaluation activities; and actions required under national defense contingency conditions.

In the early 1980s, the US Army integrated the Manpower and Personnel Integration (MANPRINT) program into the development and procurement of major military systems, requiring consideration of human factors engineering, manpower, personnel, training, health hazards, system safety, and survivability throughout the Army materiel cycle.[58–60] In the 1990s, the Department of Defense (DoD) extended MANPRINT called "Human Systems Integration" within the DoD, to all military departments. It required System Program Managers to document acceptance of associated risks by the appropriate authorities before exposing people, equipment, or the environment to known system-related environmental, safety, and occupational health hazards.[61]

Risk management was formalized throughout DoD in the 1980s as a cyclical process involving anticipating and identifying hazards, assessing hazards to determine risks, developing controls and making risk decisions, implementing controls, and supervising, and evaluating.[62–64] Military public health personnel play a key role in the risk management process by identifying hazards, determining the significance of risk, determining appropriate control measures, and communicating risk information. Risk decisions within DoD are guided by the following risk management principles: accept no unnecessary risks, make risk decisions at the appropriate level, accept risks when benefits outweigh the costs, and anticipate and manage risk by planning.

The DoD organizations are involved with risk assessment and management, from traditional industrial hygiene, radiological and nuclear safety and health, environmental management and cleanup operations, to military-unique and chemical agent surety operations, and prevention of and preparation for emergencies from traditional and terrorist threats. The role of the military occupational and environmental hygienist in protecting the health and safety of military personnel whether they are in garrison or deployed wherever throughout the world is critical to military readiness, national defense, and the security of the U.S.

U.S. Department of Energy

The Department of Energy (DOE) as created in 1977 is responsible for energy policy and nuclear safety in the US, including the nuclear weapons program, energy conservation, energy-related research, radioactive waste disposal, and domestic energy production.

The nuclear technology and weapons development activities pursued by DOE and its predecessors (including the Atomic Energy Commission and Energy Research and Development Administration) dating back to the Manhattan Project of World War II have given rise to large quantities of radioactive and chemical wastes.(65) Since the end of the Cold War, DOE efforts have focused on environmental cleanup of the nuclear weapons complex, nonproliferation and stewardship of the nuclear stockpile, and technology transfer and industrial competitiveness.(66) Occupational and environmental health professionals within DOE may perform duties involved with traditional industrial hygiene, and with the proper qualifications or cross training, health physics, environmental protection, industrial safety, ergonomics and waste management. These duties support the varied operations within the DOE to include traditional industrial operations, nuclear operations, and environmental clean-up operations.

The principal goal of DOE's environmental management program is the control of risks to human health and the environment. As federal employees, the working conditions of DOE employees in general are covered by Executive Order 12196 of 1980.(53) Specific non-radiological OSH issues are regulated under 10 CFR 851, "Worker Safety and Health Program."(67) DOE's environmental management activities are controlled by numerous laws, regulations, and agreements.(68) The principal environmental laws specifying how cleanup is to be performed at weapons sites are the Resource Conservation and Recovery Act (RCRA) as amended(69); the Atomic Energy Act of 1954 as amended(70); the Federal Facility Compliance Act of 1992(71); and the Comprehensive Environmental Response, Compensation, and Liability Act (CERCLA) as amended(72) which mandates that applicable or relevant and appropriate requirements (ARARs) of federal and state environmental laws must be taken into account. In addition, for sites undergoing CERCLA cleanup, DOE is required to enter into agreements with EPA on how the cleanup is to be carried out. States have joined in such agreements as well, making them tripartite compliance agreements. Activities at such sites are also subject to DOE's own rules, the requirements of the Clean Water Act, OSHA standards, recommendations from the Defense Nuclear Facility Safety Board, as well as recommendations from the Environmental Management Advisory Board, the National Research Council, and other agencies. DOE's facilities for the disposal of high-level radioactive waste and spent nuclear fuel are regulated by the Nuclear Regulatory Commission, under regulations implementing standards promulgated by EPA.(65,73)

DOE's risk assessment approaches continue to evolve, and now include the Environmental Restoration Priority System (ERPS), the Risk Data Sheet (RDS), and Project Baseline Summaries. The ERPS differs from previous approaches in that it includes activity screening, information analysis, and criteria regarding socioeconomics; it is not limited to the facilities within DOE Defense Programs; and it is designed for use as an external tool, with outside involvement.(65,73)

The RDS advanced DOE's risk-based approach for prioritizing its environmental management activities by explicitly linking risk with program planning and budget formulation.(65,73) The RDS is a standardized form used to rate environmental management activities in addressing public health and safety, site personnel health and safety, environmental protection, compliance with pertinent laws and regulations, mission impact, mortgage reduction, and avoidance of adverse social, cultural, and economic impacts.

Since the fall of 1997, each DOE Operations/Field Office has been required to submit to DOE Headquarters a Project Baseline Summary (PBS) for each of its approved projects. The PBS generally includes a detailed summary of the project's scope, schedule and cost baseline, life-cycle metrics, annual performance targets, financial history, budget, and data on risk, safety, and health. A project risk evaluation addresses the concerns of regulators, stakeholders, and Tribal Nations. For each applicable risk category (public, worker, environment), the level of risk is defined by the intersection of two qualitatively assessed parameters (i.e., impact and likelihood), and the risk is classified as Urgent (U), High (H), Medium (M), Low (L), or Not Applicable (NA).(65,73)

DOE is currently examining standardized risk assessment methods that would improve creditability and reproducibility throughout the department. A risk-based approach for prioritizing DOE's environmental management activities has been endorsed by a National Research Council study, which concluded that its use would be feasible and successful, provided that its purposes and limitations were clearly defined, the public was involved in the process sufficiently early and fully, and that the approach gave adequate consideration to the full range of cultural, socioeconomic, historical, religious, and political concerns of interested stakeholders.[73]

U.S. Department of Homeland Security

Following terrorist attacks on September 11, 2001, President George W. Bush created the White House Office of Homeland Security. Soon after, Congress passed the Homeland Security Act of 2002 (PL 107-296) which created the Department of Homeland Security (DHS) resulting in the largest reorganization of the federal government since the U.S. Department of Defense was created in 1947.[74,75] DHS focuses primarily on security of the U.S., e.g., issuing advisories to alert travelers of security risks, or levels of national security risk.

Within DHS, the Office of Risk Management and Analysis is responsible for synchronizing, integrating, and coordinating risk management and risk analysis approaches, with a focus on homeland security risk doctrine and policy, integrated risk management, and integrated risk performance. Their strategic objectives include:

- Serving as the DHS's executive agent for national-level risk management analysis standards and metrics;
- Developing and embedding a consistent, standardized approach to risk;
- Developing a coordinated, collaborative approach to risk management;
- Assessing DHS-level risk performance; and
- Communicating the DHS's "risk story" in a manner that reinforces the value of the risk-informed approach.

The DHS Risk Lexicon, developed by the DHS Risk Steering Committee, provides a comprehensive list of terms and meanings relevant to the practice of homeland security risk management and analysis.[76] Industrial hygienists working in the area of homeland security risk assessment should familiarize themselves with specific usages contained in this document, which may differ slightly from those used in our profession. For example, risk assessment is defined as a "product or process which collects information and assigns values to risks for the purpose of informing priorities, developing or comparing courses of action, and informing decision making".

Risk for Chemical Facility Anti-Terrorism Standards (CFATS)

In Section 550 of the Homeland Security Act, Congress directed DHS to identify and secure those chemical facilities that present the greatest security risk, as determined by the consequence of a successful attack on a facility (consequence), the likelihood that an attack on a facility will be successful (vulnerability), and the intent and capability of an adversary in respect to attacking a facility (threat). DHS's interim final rule implementing this mandate imposes comprehensive federal security regulations for high-risk chemical facilities and establishes risk-based performance standards. It creates a risk-based tier structure which allows DHS to focus its resources on high-risk chemical facilities. To that end, facilities are assigned to one of four risk-based tiers ranging from high (Tier 1) to low (Tier 4) risk. Assignment of tiers is based on an assessment of the potential consequences of a successful attack on assets associated with chemicals of interest. DHS uses information submitted by facilities through a two-stage process to identify a facility's risk, which is a function of consequences, vulnerabilities, and threat. Based on information submitted in the Chemical Security Assessment Tool (CSAT) Top Screen, a facility may be required to submit the more detailed Security Vulnerability Assessment (SVA) and to develop and implement Site Security Plans, which include measures that satisfy the risk-based performance standards. DHS considers a variety of factors in determining the appropriate tier for each high-risk facility, including information about the public health and safety risk and the presence of chemicals with a critical impact on the governance mission and the economy. Occupational and environmental hygienists play a key role in facility information submissions.

Other DHS programs of interest to industrial hygienists include the National Incident Management System (NIMS)[77] and the National Infrastructure Protection Plan (NIPP).[78] Industrial hygienists who are involved in a health and safety advisory role in emergency management should be familiar with NIMS, specifically the Incident Command System (ICS). Within the NIPP, Sector-Specific Plans (SSPs) are required.[78] The SSPs detail the application of the NIPP risk management framework to the unique characteristics and risk landscape of each sector and provide the means by which the NIPP is implemented across all critical infrastructure and key resources (CIKR) sectors. Specifically, there are SSPs available for industrial groups including agriculture and food, banking and finance, communications, defense industrial base, energy, and information technology. Industrial hygienists in these industries may be involved sector-specific risk assessments.

All agencies within the Department of Homeland Security are involved with risk assessment and management, from border, port, and sky protection, to prevention of and preparation for emergencies, and responding to and recovering from disasters. The role of the occupational and environmental hygienist in protecting the health and safety of the public in general and of workers in specific is critical to our national preparedness efforts.

The Risk Management Process

Background of Risk Management

Risk management assists decision makers in reducing or offsetting unnecessary risk by systematically identifying, assessing, and controlling risk arising from operational factors, and by making decisions that weigh risks against mission benefits. An unnecessary risk is any risk that, if taken, will not contribute meaningfully to production or operation accomplishment or will needlessly endanger lives or resources. Risk management should be integrated into planning, preparation, and execution of business at all levels.[4,62–64] Leaders should ensure that adequate time and resources are dedicated to apply risk management early in the planning process for example, a new production line, industrial operation, waste treatment or disposal operation, when risks can be more readily assessed and managed.

The basic principles that provide a framework for implementing the risk management process include accepting no unnecessary risk, making risk decisions at the appropriate level, accepting risk when benefits outweigh the cost, and anticipating and managing risk by planning. The acceptable risk level developed using these principles will vary depending on the circumstances. For example, an acceptable health risk in a military-unique workplace operation may be comparable to a similar workplace operation in the continental U.S. However the health risk associated with a military unique operation is balanced with other operational risks and may not be the most important risk when determining how to accomplish the job. Similar assessments may be required by non-military organizations to assess risks for specific workplace situations and scenarios. For example, the selection of control measures may be based on the risks associated with them. Management would make the selection of the appropriate control measure which would result in the least risk to employees. For a variety of reasons, the level of risk considered acceptable in the workplace is typically higher than for the environment.

In industry, risk decisions should be made at the appropriate level of leadership, authority, and accountability. The individual or group making risk decisions must be able to eliminate or minimize the hazard, implement controls to reduce the risk, or accept the risk. The risk management process should include those accountable for production, the mission, or the task. If the supervisor, leader, or individual responsible for executing the production, mission, or task determines that available controls will not reduce risk to an acceptable level, decisions should be elevated to the next higher supervisor/leader. The process of weighing risks against opportunities and benefits helps to maximize the development and success of a new production line or operation. Balancing costs and benefits is a subjective process and should be an organizational leader's decision; however, these decisions must take into account the perspectives and needs of all stakeholders, in particular those who will be exposed to the hazard in question. If at all possible, stakeholders should be included in risk management decision making.

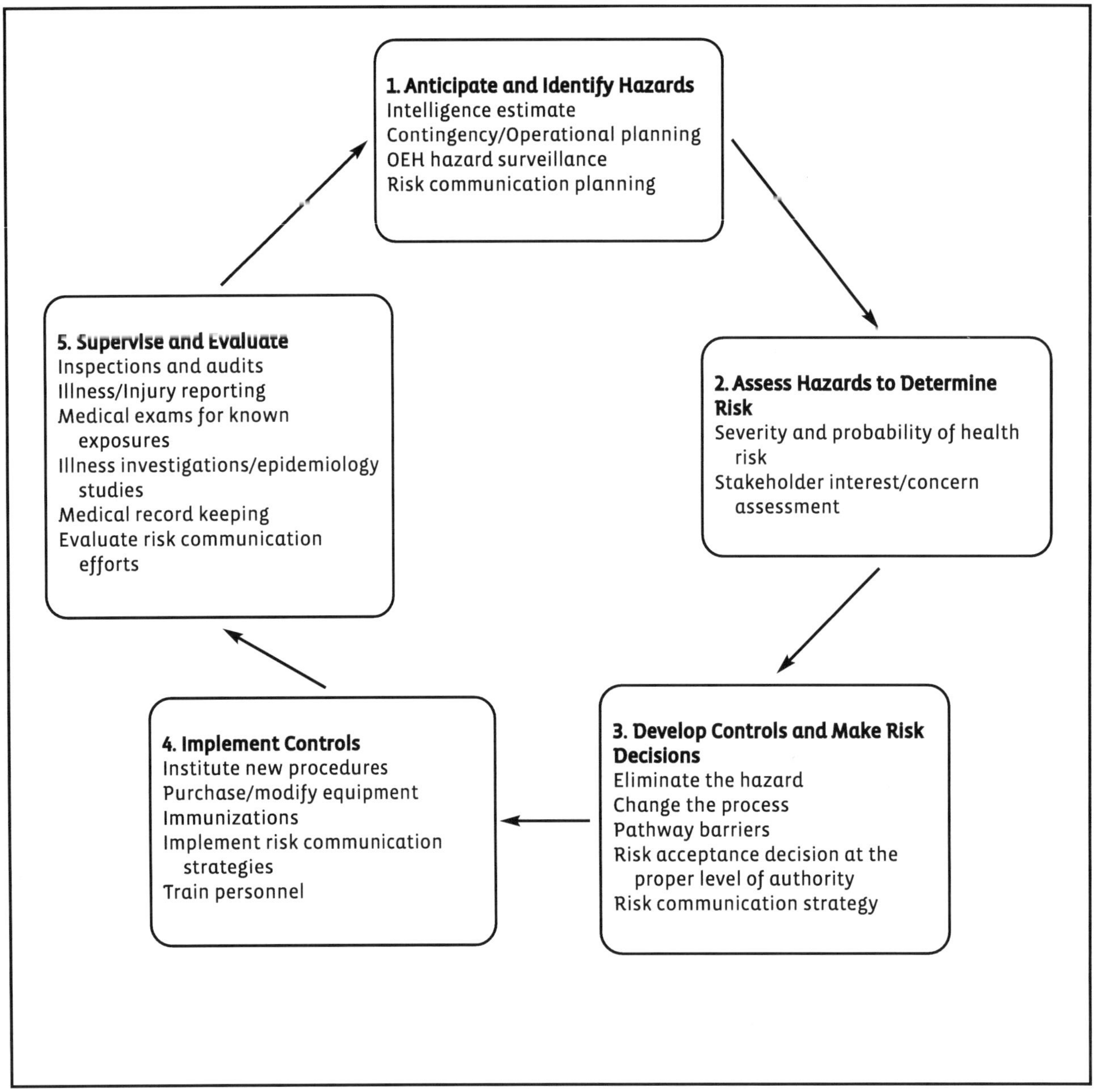

Figure 8.1 — Notional Risk Management Process.

The risk management process steps may vary, however the following steps are usually addressed[4,61]:

1. Identifying hazards.
2. Assessing hazards to determine risks.
3. Developing controls and making risk decisions.
4. Implementing controls.
5. Supervising and evaluating.

The process is cyclic. Figure 8.1 depicts a notional risk management process that could be employed by any type of organization (e.g., universities, industries, etc.) The figure shows some notional examples of tasks within this process.

Risk Assessment, Acceptable Risk, and Risk Management

This section briefly examines the role of risk assessment in the selection of risk management goals and techniques. In 1983, the National Research Council envisioned a clear line between risk assessment and risk management:

> "We recommend that regulatory agencies take steps to establish and maintain a clear conceptual distinction between assessment of risks and consideration of risk management alternatives; that is, the scientific findings and policy judgments embodied in risk assessments should be explicitly distinguished from the political, economic, and technical considerations that influence the design and choice of regulatory strategies."[41]

Risk assessment was to be composed of hazard identification, dose-response assessment, exposure assessment, and risk characterization. Risk management was to consist of development of regulatory options; evaluation of public health and technical considerations; and the economic, social, and political consequences of regulatory options. In other words, risk assessment was to be a value-neutral scientific process, whereas risk management could be influenced by nonscientific concerns. Most people agree that the most accurate risk assessment possible is the basis for a good decision, which may also take into account non-risk factors. But however good this sounds in theory, it is very difficult to put it into actual practice. The reader should be aware of the many points in the risk assessment/management process where there are uncertainty and variability in the data and a conservative decision is rendered to protect the health of the population or individual: use of more stringent exposure criteria, toxicological data from the most sensitive species, high-end exposure calculations, selection of the linear multistage model, and so forth. It needs to be recognized up front that there is no clear separation between the processes of risk assessment and risk management. The EPA has recommended that in the ecological risk assessment process, the risk assessor should meet frequently with the risk manager, so that risk can be evaluated in policy-relevant terms.[79] Within the DoD, risk assessment and risk management are institutionalized and are an inherent part of all military operations to address safety and occupational and environmental health risks. Risk analysis, as defined by Cohrssen and Covello[80], goes beyond the scientific process and includes decisions that should be guided by social, cultural, moral, economic, and political factors (i.e., determination of the significance of a risk and the communication of risk information to affected publics). This definition embraces risk assessment, risk management, and risk communication, which actually are difficult to separate. With these cautions in mind, several terms can be defined:

- R_T — true risk, the actual level of risk
- R_E — estimated risk, the risk assessor's best estimate of risk
- R_A — acceptable risk, the level of risk the public is willing to accept

An understanding of the relationship between risk (i.e., estimated risk, because true risk is not known) and acceptable risk is critical to this discussion because if the risk in a situation exceeds acceptable risk, then risk management efforts must be started. The decision about how much hazard mitigation (risk reduction) is adequate is based on the gap between the estimated risk and acceptable risk; if R_E greatly exceeds R_A, then risk mitigation efforts probably will be significant and immediate. The OEH professional estimates the level of risk based on hazard exposure severity and probability of health effects per exposure, using the risk assessment principles outlined. He or she knows that R_T does not equal zero, however, its true value might never be known. Therefore, R_E is selected from what is believed to be the top of the confidence interval about R_T, for example, the 95% upper confidence level, because if a mistake is to be made, the bias is toward protection of the population or individual. The OEH professional determines whether R_E is acceptable based on social, political, economic, public health, and technical considerations. In those areas where compliance with legislation is involved, society may also determine whether R_E is acceptable.
Sometimes society decides that R_A is too low and can be raised. An excellent example was provided when highway speed limits were raised, and experts predicted an increase in traffic deaths. Despite the fact that this prediction proved true, society did not protest the higher speed limits. In contrast, it has been decided that there are too many deaths from environmental tobacco smoke, as

evidenced by the successful efforts to gradually eliminate public smoking.

Although it seems that society would prefer zero risk, even demanding it at times, zero risk is not attainable unless the hazard in an operation is eliminated. There are different levels of risk that are acceptable in different situations. The reduction of a hazard exposure to a negligible risk is usually desirable. However, it may be necessary to accept a risk that is not negligible. For example, a moderate risk in an operation in a combat situation may not be acceptable for a similar operation in the continental U.S. For some manufacturing or research development situations, the exposure risk may be higher because using traditional hazard control methods may not be feasible, and if they were imposed, the product development task may be adversely affected. If this occurs it may be necessary to institute health surveillance measures.

Some levels of risk acceptability have been formalized. In establishing appropriate risk levels for Superfund sites, EPA works in the range of 10^{-6} to 10^{-4}; this is interpreted as 'one case per million persons exposed' up to 'one case per 10,000 persons exposed.' In contrast, OSHA accepts higher risk levels, in the range of 10^{-4} to 10^{-3}. There are reasonable arguments in favor of this differential: Workers are generally the healthiest members of society, they are trained in occupational hazards and have some degree of control over their exposure, they are financially compensated for their exposure to risk, and exposures are usually limited to 40 hours per week. The public comprises the young and the old, the healthy and the sick, and persons who may have occupational or environmental exposures to other chemicals. They may not be aware of these exposures, generally have no control over them, and receive no financial compensation. In the case of air contamination, exposures may be more or less continuous. In some situations the level of acceptable risk has been captured in acceptable exposure levels: Workplace Environmental Exposure Levels (WEELs™), TLVs® and PELs in the occupational setting, National Ambient Air Quality Standards for community air, and certain regional soil cleanup levels for hazardous waste sites. Thus, whether institutionalized or determined individually by leadership or management, the selection of R_A allows determination of corresponding exposure levels to contaminants in air, water, and soil.

Determination of Appropriate Exposure Levels

The acceptable risk level, along with economic, social, political, and technical considerations, is one of the inputs used in selection of acceptable exposure limits and the methods used to achieve these limits. Selection of risk management methods in occupational hygiene also is influenced by the hierarchy of controls: engineering, administrative, and personal protective equipment. If available, knowledge of exposure to other chemicals on the same or different jobs, presence of sensitive subpopulations, and exposures in the home environment might also influence the acceptable level of occupational exposure. Given all these factors, how does the risk manager or occupational hygienist make an appropriate selection? To some extent the determination of acceptable exposure limits for occupational and environmental settings seems to have followed two different trends. As described by Corn[3], the approach to establishing TLVs® was to determine the concentration of material that caused injury and to set threshold values based on the concentrations measured. The risk would then be negligible if exposure levels were kept below certain acceptable levels. (Note that the majority of alterations in TLVs® and PELs have been downward, reflecting increasing concern about chronic health effects.) Establishment of acceptable environmental exposures seems to have come from the other direction, as exemplified by the 1958 Delaney clause, which prohibited the use in food of any food additive shown to cause cancer in animals or humans at any oral dose.[17,81] The many food additives in use at that time were exempted from the rigorous testing requirements and were listed as GRAS (generally regarded as safe). It was later recognized that long-term use was no guarantee of safety, and several substances, including cyclamates and coal-tar dyes, have been taken off the list. FDA now has four regulatory categories: food additives, GRAS substances, prior-sanctioned substances, and color additives. The Delaney clause was later subject to legislative change (e.g., saccharin) and interpretation through the GRAS list (e.g., the use of methylene chloride to decaffeinate coffee).

Because site-specific cleanup levels for hazardous waste sites also have been based on findings of chronic toxicological or epidemiological studies, there has been a similar upward trend from zero or background levels to risk-based, or in some cases, technology-based levels. This so-called risk-based approach to establishing cleanup levels has been formalized in the EPA documentation[21], as well as the ASTM *Standard Guide for Risk-Based Corrective Action Applied at Petroleum Release Sites*.[49] These approaches are based on equations used to calculate risk with the target risk (lifetime cancer risk estimate for carcinogens, or hazard index for noncarcinogens) in this case as a known quantity, and the concentration of the chemical in the media of concern as the dependent variable. Risk equations allow calculations to be made to determine acceptable risk-based concentrations of contaminants in food, soil, or air.[82] If there is exposure to more than one chemical, or if exposure occurs by more than one route or pathway, the acceptable concentration must be reduced accordingly.

The importance of restricting risk assessment, when possible, to scientific concerns while allowing value judgments to enter into risk management decisions has been stressed. This is a distinction that may cause discomfort to some scientists and engineers, who may execute technically accurate risk assessments and risk management analyses only to see political and social preferences sway decisions to, in their opinions, less appropriate risk management techniques. It is useful to remember that, whenever possible, risk management decisions should benefit all stakeholders, for many of whom the economic, social, and political factors are of more immediate importance than the accuracy of the risk assessment itself.

Exposure Criteria Continuum

There are many types of exposure scenarios which OEH professionals may encounter and there is a wide array of exposure criteria used to address risks to airborne exposures.[83] No single value is appropriate for all applications. Figure 8.2 generically shows a range of the types of published airborne exposure criteria developed by various organizations for different applications. Examples from the workplace include ACGIH® TLVs®, AIHA® WEELs™, and OSHA PELs. Protective action criteria for chemical release events include Acute Exposure Guideline Level (AEGL) values published by EPA.[84,85] and Temporary Emergency Exposure Limit (TEEL) values developed by the Subcommittee on Consequence Assessment and Protective Actions (SCAPA).[86] For additional information see Protective Action Criteria for Chemicals — Including AEGLs, ERPGs™, & TEELs; Occupational safety and health standards for PELs and TWAs; American Conference of Governmental Industrial Hygienists® (ACGIH®) Policy Statement on the Uses of TLVs® and BEIs®; and Documentation for Immediately Dangerous to Life or Health Concentrations (IDLH).[87–89]

The OEH professionals working in any sector should become familiar with the different exposure guidelines in Figure 8.2, because they may find them applicable in addressing specific occupational and environmental health scenarios. In addition, all OEH professionals should be aware of the Department of Defense military exposure guidelines (MEGs). A MEG is a chemical concentration which represents a safe-sided estimate of the level above which certain types of health effects may begin to occur in individuals within the exposed population after an exposure of the specified duration. MEGs are established from multiple exposure criteria. MEGs are designed to assess a variety of military exposure scenarios, such as a single release of large amounts of a chemical, temporary exposure conditions lasting hours to days, or for continuous ambient environmental conditions, such as a regional pollution. The quantity and quality of the health effects and toxicological data upon which the MEGs are based varies substantially across the chemicals. Since existing toxicological databases and health criteria were utilized to develop the MEGs, the quality and extensiveness of toxicological and epidemiological information underlying these guidelines is comparable, and as variable as that used by federal agencies for worker and civilian applications. The appropriate application of MEGs for military deployment exposures provides a defensible, logical and consistent decision-making framework, however, it requires a basic

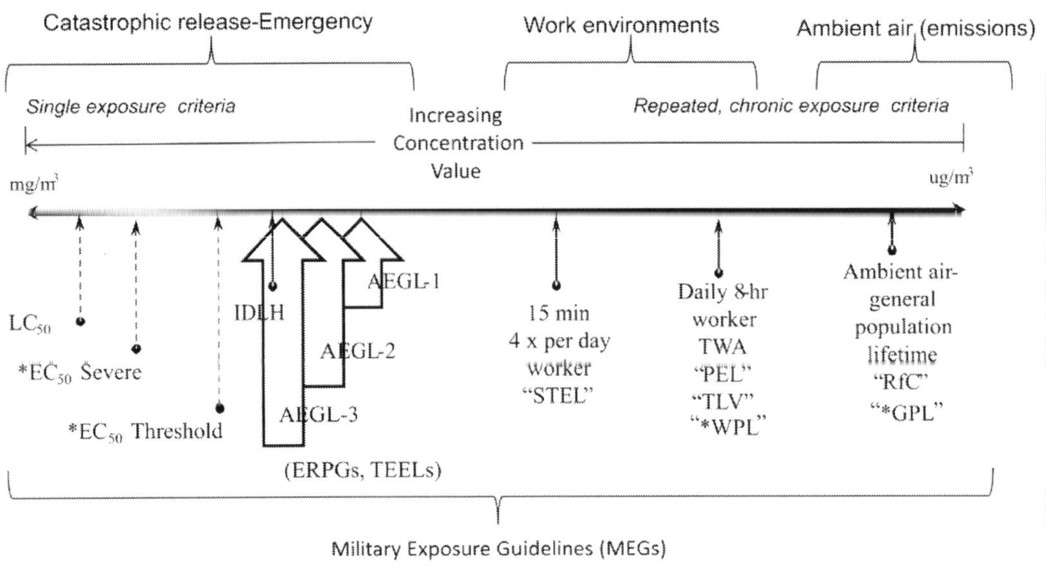

Notes: Source-USACHPPM, Presentation, "The C in CBRN – From Critical Exposure Levels to Clean-up Levels, We Know More Than You Might Think," US Army Force Health Protection Conference, August 2009.
*military unique terms for chemical warfare agents.

Legend:

µg/m³ — micrograms per cubic meter.

mg/m³ — milligrams per cubic meter.

LC_{50} — lethal concentration 50%, military casualty prediction, concentration fatal to ½ of exposed group

*EC_{50} — effective concentration-50%, military casualty prediction, for severe or mild/threshold effects: concentration at which ½ of an exposed group would be expected to have symptoms of designated severity.

IDLH — Immediately Dangerous to Life or Health, occupational use, 30 minute standard used as criteria for donning full protective gear.

AEGL — acute exposure guidelines level - for civilian emergencies, multiple durations (10 minutes, 30 minutes, 1 hour, 4 hour, 8 hour), published by National Academy of Sciences.
- AEGL-1 is initial level above which discomfort (minor transient effects) may be noted.
- AEGL-2 is level above which more significant effects may impair normal activities.
- AEGL-3 is level above which effects may begin to be very severe.

ERPG® — Emergency Response Planning Guideline, developed by American Industrial Hygiene Association, air concentration guidelines for single exposures to agents.

TEEL — Temporary Emergency Exposure Level, chemical exposure guidelines to use for emergency planning (if no AEGL or ERPG is available).

STEL — Short-Term Exposure Limit, occupational use, time-weighted average exposure limit for 15 minute period.

TWA — time-weighted average, average exposure to a contaminant workers may be exposed without adverse effect over a period such as in an 8-hour day or 40-hour week.

PEL — permissible exposure limit, acceptable exposure level as specified in regulatory standards; generally expressed as 8-hour time-weighted average concentration.

TLV® — threshold limit value (TLV® is a registered trademark of the American Conference of Governmental Industrial Hygienists), 8-hour time weighted average developed by ACGIH®, used in occupational settings to ensure most people can work for 8 hours a day, daily, with no harmful effects.

*WPL — worker population limit, military, used for chemical warfare agents, represents standards similar to TLV®.

RfC — reference concentration, estimated concentration that could be breathed continuously every day for a lifetime without adverse effects (developed by EPA, primarily used in environmental health risk assessments).

*GPL — general population limit, term used for chronic protection levels developed by Centers for Disease Control and Prevention for Army for chemical warfare agents, represents criteria similar to adjusted reference concentration.

Figure 8.2 — Chemical airborne exposure criteria continuum[83]

understanding of health risk assessment concepts and models (e.g., exposure assessment) and of key scientific limitations associated with the MEGs (e.g., dose- response and toxicology).[90]

Workplace

An occupational exposure limit (OEL) is considered a level that should protect a typical worker for 8 hours per day, 5 days per week for 40 years. The only occupational exposure limits that are mandatory for regulatory compliance in the U.S. are the Permissible Exposure Limits (PELs) established by the Occupational Safety and Health Administration.

There are a number of types of occupational exposure limits that are guidelines developed by non regulatory bodies. These include recommended exposure limit (RELs) developed by the National Institute for Occupational Safety and Health (NIOSH); threshold limit values (TLVs®) developed by the American Conference of Governmental Industrial Hygienists (ACGIH®); and WEELs™ developed by the American Industrial Hygiene Association (AIHA®),

Europe's most significant catalyst in setting health-based occupational exposure limits is the European Regulation on Registration, Evaluation, Authorisation and Restriction of Chemical substances (REACH), which was passed by the European Parliament on December 13, 2006 and entered into force in June 2007. Not least among the changes was the creation of Derived No-Effect Levels (DNELs) and Derived Minimum Effect Levels (DMELs) that represent levels above which humans (inclusive of consumers, workers, etc) should not be exposed. These levels are determined based on exposure scenarios that describe how a substance is manufactured or used during its life-cycle and how the manufacturer or importer or downstream user controls or recommends controlling exposure of humans and the environment. Manufacturers and importers are required to calculate DNELs and DMELs as part of their Chemical Safety Assessment (CSA) for any chemicals used in quantities of 10 tons or more per year or imported into the European Union in quantities of one ton or more per year. The DNEL is to be published in the manufacturer's Chemical Safety Report and, for hazard communication purposes, in an extended Safety Data Sheet (SDS).

It is assumed that the major manufacturers and suppliers have a very broad range of technical resources and expertise to do expansive hazard assessments to develop DNELs and to perform the exposure risk assessments leading to registration of their products. It is likely that small manufacturers will not have the toxicological resources to perform the required animal studies and thus may default to use the algorithm-based calculations to derive the DNELs.

DNELs and DMELs are based solely on animal toxicology data and have very conservative uncertainty factors applied to extrapolate to human physiological responses. DNELs are generally more conservative than conventional OELs. The calculation of DNELs follows a rule-based approach in which a series of standardized assessment factors is applied to the toxicological endpoints to allow for uncertainties and inter- and intra -species differences. This can result in a very conservative figure, perhaps two or three orders of magnitude lower than that from the traditional OEL setting process. The DNELs and DMELs are not set in the same manner as the existing health-based OELs set on a weight of evidence basis utilizing professional experience and expertise. DNELs and DMELs will not be consensus recommendations, but rather calculated reference concentration values determined by the manufacturer or supplier of the material.

The DNEL is used in the risk characterization section of the CSA as a benchmark to determine adequate control for specified exposure scenarios in both the consumer market and the worker segments. Risk to humans can be considered to be adequately controlled if the exposure levels estimated do not exceed the appropriate DNEL. REACH specifies that DNELs shall reflect the likely routes, duration and frequency of exposure. If more than one route of exposure is likely to occur (oral, dermal or inhalation), then a DNEL must be established for each route of exposure and for the exposure from all routes combined. It may also be necessary to identify different DNELs for each relevant human population (e.g., workers, consumers or humans subject to exposure indirectly via the ambient environment) and possibly for certain vulnerable sub-populations (e.g., children, pregnant women). The DNEL methodology is intended to harmonize the approach to occupational health risk assessment with those used for other types of risk such as environmental exposure. This is important under REACH, as manufacturers must assess not only human health risks but environmental and physical safety risks as well.

DNELs calculated by individual manufacturers and importers are not subject to any requirement for consultation or opportunity for input by interested parties. In contrast, the European process for setting Indicative OELs has been well established, involving experts from member countries on the Scientific Committee on Occupational Exposure Limits (SCOEL) and providing an opportunity for stakeholders in industry and government to comment on the proposals. These inputs are not included in the REACH process.

Debate is also underway to decide what to do when a DNEL cannot be established, although the current proposal is to set a DMEL based on a concept of acceptable or negligible risk, (such as the "Threshold of Toxicological Concern") rather than banning such materials automatically because they cannot be adequately controlled. Under REACH, the DNELs must be completed by 2010 for the 'grandfathered' substances registered for commerce and all products must be registered for commerce and use in member states by 2018. It is likely that the European Agency for Chemicals (ECHA) will set up a strategy to look at the validity and coherence of DNELs (even if it is on small samples randomly selected).

The REACh regulations will change the playing field in risk assessment for workers since all substances must be registered to be a part of the EU commerce, and to do so requires that an adequate chemical profile be made available for assessment of all uses and associated risks to the workers and consumers. With regard to the quality and availability of REACH hazard assessment input data:

- The reliability of a study which becomes part of the OEL toxicological data set needs to be understood and evaluated using a verified scoring system (i.e., Klimisch scoring) to rate the validity of a study for use as a pivotal endpoint in setting an OEL. There is precedence for this in the U.S. in that the Office of Management & Budget (OMB) requires this for some EPA work and the EU REACH and Biocidal Products Directive (BPD) protocols require Klemisch scoring.[91]
- It is difficult to capture all pertinent data for setting OELs because most company data has not been made public. The result is often incomplete data sets, resulting in final endpoints which are not accurate. Efforts to encourage companies to share their scientific data should be considered beyond the REACH submissions which may remain proprietary or business confidential. However, all endpoints selected as a point of departure for the derivation of a DNEL must be published on the internet by ECHA for the public access.
- REACH legislation requires ECHA to publish a database on the internet of the DNELs that are officially accepted for various substances.

Community

Community health risks include exposures from ambient air emissions from industry, hazardous material exposures from accidental chemical releases, and possible terrorist threats involving the intentional release of chemical, biological, or physical agents. The Emergency Planning and Community Right-to-Know Act (EPCRA) was passed in response to health risk concerns regarding the environmental and safety hazards posed by the storage and handling of toxic chemicals.[92] EPCRA establishes requirements for emergency planning and "Community Right-to-Know" reporting on hazardous and toxic chemicals. The Community Right-to-Know provisions help increase the public's knowledge and access to information on chemicals at individual facilities, their uses, and releases into the environment. States and communities, working with facilities, can use the information to reduce potential health risks to improve chemical safety and protect public health and the environment.

Accidental Release Prevention

Requirements: Risk Management Programs Under Clean Air Act Section 112(r)(7) requires companies that use certain flammable and toxic substances to develop a Risk Management Program, which includes a hazard assessment, a prevention program, and an emergency response program with procedures for informing the public and response agencies (e.g., the fire department) should an accident occur.[93] The Risk Management Program (RMP) is about reducing health risk at the local level. This information helps local fire, police, and emergency response personnel (who must prepare for and respond to chemical accidents), and is useful to citizens in understanding the chemical hazards and potential health risks in their communities. Making the RMPs available to the public stimulates communication between industry and the public and helps to improve accident prevention and emergency response practices at the local level.

Emergency Exposure Guidelines

The accidental release of methyl isocyanate in Bhopal, India, in December 1984 resulted in approximately 2,000 deaths and 20,000 injuries and had a global impact on chemical management. One result of this tragedy was the founding of the AIHA® Emergency Response Planning Committee in 1987 for the purpose of developing guidance levels that would define safe, toxic, and potentially lethal levels of chemical exposures which might be predicted to occur in the event of an accidental chemical release.[94] It was envisioned that these values could be used by emergency planners to anticipate and put controls in place to prevent or reduce the impact from chemical spills or accidents, and provide guidance in the event of chemical accident or terrorist action. The founders of the ERP Committee, which arose from the WEEL™ Committee, recognized that such guidance levels needed to be developed with a uniform process, relying on the input and expertise of many people to achieve consensus. Through the years, the committee has increasingly involved experts from a variety of organizations and companies. As of 2009, the ERP Committee has developed over 130 guidance documents and ERPG™ values.[95,96]

Another outcome of the Bhopal tragedy was the passage of the Superfund Amendments and Reauthorization Act (SARA) of 1986, which required EPA to identify extremely hazardous substances (EHSs) and provide guidance for Local Emergency Planning Committees in conducting health-hazard assessments for emergency response plans for sites where EHSs are produced, stored, transported, or used. EPA supported the work of the AIHA® ERP Committee, and in 1988 held a workshop to introduce the ERP program to interested federal and state regulators and the public.

Because of its extensive experience in this area, the National Research Council (NRC) Committee on Toxicology was asked by EPA and the Agency for Toxic Substances and Disease Registry (ATSDR) in 1991 to develop a methodology for establishing emergency exposure guidelines levels for EHSs for the general population. Since 1995, the National Advisory Committee for Acute Exposure Guideline Levels for Hazardous Substances (NAC/AEGL) has been tasked with developing Acute Exposure Guideline Levels (AEGLs) for high-priority, acutely toxic chemicals in a wide range of settings, including the community, the workplace, transportation, and the military.[98] These guidelines find application in emergency planning, notification, response, and training for chemical spills and other catastrophic incidents. The NAC/AEGL includes representatives from federal and state agencies, academia, corporations, and non-governmental organizations. Currently there are final, interim, and proposed AEGLs for more than 190 chemicals (SCAPA).[99]

ERPGs™[100] and AEGLs[97] are similar in concept but have important differences. ERPGs™ are "maximum airborne concentration below which it is believed that nearly all individuals could be exposed for up to 1 hour without experiencing" various health effects. They are established primarily with chemical accidents or terrorist activities in mind. AEGLs represent airborne concentrations above which it is believed that the general population would begin to experience various health effects. Since AEGLs are established for a broader purpose, including hazardous waste activities, they are determined for five different time periods: 10 minutes, 30 minutes, 1 hour, 4 hours, and 8 hours.[97]

The exacting processes in place to develop both ERPGs™ and AEGLs involve primary scientific literature review, initial proposed limits, extensive peer review, and subsequent revisions before final limits are

Table 8.3 — Selected Emergency Exposure Levels[89,94,97,101,102]

Emergency Exposure Value	*Emergency Response Planning Guides (ERPGs™)*	*Acute Exposure Guideline Levels (AEGLs)*	*Temporary Emergency Exposure Limits (TEELs)*	*Immediately Dangerous to Life or Health (IDLH)*
Owners	Emergency Response Planning Committee, American Industrial Hygiene Association (AIHA®)	Environmental Protection Agency (EPA), National Academy of Sciences, and a public / private partnership. Method developed with the National Academy of Sciences	Department of Energy (DOE) Subcommittee on Consequence Assessment and protective Actions (SCAPA), Chemical Exposures Working Group	National Institute for Occupational Safety and Health (NIOSH), USDOL Occupational Safety and Health Administration (OSHA)
Philosophy	Intended to be used as planning tools in accident prevention and emergency response, including transportation and community emergency response plans. Estimate concentrations at which most people will begin to experience health effects. May be used to help protect the public during short-term chemical releases when there is no AEGL available.	Represent level above which certain health effects are expected from once-in-a-lifetime, or rare, exposure to airborne chemicals.	TEELs are approximations to ERPGs™, and are temporary guidance to be used only until AEGLs or ERPGs™ are developed.	IDLHs were originally established for 387 substances in the mid-1970s for use in selecting respiratory protection equipment.
Levels	Up to 3 levels, developed for 1-hour exposures. ERPG-3: "the maximum airborne concentration below which it is believed that nearly all individuals could be exposed for up to 1 hour without experiencing or developing life-threatening health effects." ERPG-2: "the maximum airborne concentration below which it is believed that nearly all individuals could be exposed for up to 1 hour without experiencing or developing irreversible or other serious health effects or symptoms which could impair an individual's ability to take protective action." ERPG-1: "the maximum airborne concentration below which it is believed that nearly all individuals could be exposed for up to 1 hour without experiencing other than mild transient adverse health effects or perceiving a clearly defined, objectionable odor."	Developed for 5 time periods: 10 minutes, 30 minutes, 1 hour, 4 hours, 8 hours. AEGL-1: airborne concentration "above which it is predicted that the general population, including susceptible individuals, could experience notable discomfort, irritation, or certain asymptomatic nonsensory effects. However, the effects are not disabling and are transient and reversible upon cessation of exposure." AEGL-2: is the airborne concentration "above which it is predicted that the general population, including susceptible individuals, could experience irreversible or other serious, long-lasting adverse health effects or an impaired ability to escape." AEGL-3: airborne concentration "above which it is predicted that the general population, including susceptible individuals, could experience life-threatening health effects or death."	Original method was based on hierarchies of published concentrations limits; expanded method incorporates published toxicity data. TEEL-0 is the "threshold concentration below which most people will experience no appreciable risk of health effects. Definitions for TEEL-1, TEEL-2, and TEEL-3 match those for the ERPGs™, with the exception that TEELs are recommended as peak 15-minute time-weighted concentrations at the receptor point.	Based on 30 CFR 11.3(t): a concentration from which a worker could escape without injury or without irreversible health effects in the event of respiratory protection equipment failure. In determining IDLHs, "the ability of a worker to escape without loss of life or irreversible health effects was considered.
Protected Population	Nearly all members of the public but not sensitive individuals.	General population, including infants and children, susceptible individuals.	Workers and the general public.	Workers, in emergency situation only, for 30 minutes or less.

established. These processes have resulted in highly-respected emergency exposure values, but because of the degree of rigor required, only a few hundred chemicals have been evaluated.[99] In contrast, there are thousands of chemicals in use by industry, academia, and governmental organizations. The SCAPA has developed a methodology to advise the U.S. Department of Energy (DOE) and the National Nuclear Security Administration (NNSA) on Protective Action Criteria (PAC) for chemicals without AEGLs or ERPGs™. The PAC data set is maintained by the Chemical Exposures Working Group and includes AEGLs, ERPGs™, and Temporary Emergency Exposure Limits (TEELs). The TEELs are determined using a SCAPA developed methodology. The original method was based on hierarchies of published concentrations limits (e.g., IDLH, PEL-Ceiling values, etc.).[101,102] The expanded method incorporates published toxicity data with a preference for human data, resulting in TEELS for over 3000 chemicals.[99,103]

Industrial hygienists who will be conducting risk assessments for emergency planning should be familiar with the use of these emergency exposure values, as well as the OSHA Permissible Exposure Limit and ACGIH® Threshold Limit Value® short-term exposure and ceiling limit values. (See Table 8.3 for a comparison of selected emergency exposure levels.)

Environmental Risk Assessment in the Risk Management Process

As noted in the description of EPA, environmental risk assessment activities impact diverse regulatory programs. EPA risk assessment activities have been both program-specific and agency-wide, and have included development of risk assessment guidelines and methodologies described in the various sections of this chapter and use of risk assessment in development of standards. These uses include risk assessments related to new chemicals introduced to commerce, pollutants released into the air or water, pesticides, and hazardous and solid waste streams. In general, risk assessment activities associated with these diverse activities can be found on the respective EPA Program Office web pages; general methodologies are found on the web pages for the Office of Research and Development.

The NRC Risk Assessment Paradigm

In the National Research Council's Red Book, a widely quoted four-step paradigm of risk assessment was outlined, along with the recommendation that insofar as possible, these steps were to be guided by the best scientific information available. (In contrast, it would be appropriate for risk management decisions to include political, economic, and social/cultural factors.) These steps, and the questions they ask, are as follows:

1. **Hazard identification** — Is there a causal link between this chemical and potential human health effects at any exposure level? This corresponds to the statement in the OSHA law that standards assure to the extent feasible that "no employee will suffer material impairment of health or functional capacity even if such employee has regular exposure to the hazard".[104]
2. **Dose-response assessment** — What is the relationship between levels of exposure and the fraction of the population affected? This corresponds to the legal determination that a level of exposure poses a "significant risk," that is, a high enough risk rate.
3. **Exposure assessment** — What is the level of exposure to the chemical either currently in the workplace or at the levels to be found following promulgation of a standard? Following the PEL decision, OSHA must determine there are exposures above the level at which the agency intends to set the PEL, so that the rule will have benefit.
4. **Risk characterization** — What is the overall level of risk?

These four questions have been memorably rephrased: Is this stuff toxic? How toxic is it? Who is exposed to this stuff, how long, how often? So what?[105]

This paradigm, which has had broad use, has served to crystallize thinking about scientific data and inferences (default assumptions). It has provided a structure and a vocabulary for the risk assessment process. Its limitations include the fact that it is a single-chemical rather than holistic approach to risk assessment, and it cannot address adversity of effects, such as cancer versus teratogenic effects.[105] Despite these limitations the paradigm provides a useful model for discussing risk assessment. Each of these steps, along with some of the most important issues surrounding them, is discussed below. It should be noted that there are some differences between the approaches typically taken by occupational hygiene and environmental risk assessors. Also, the various steps of risk assessment may be conducted by different analysts.

The eventual level of risk is implicit rather than explicit in risk assessment for agents not regulated for carcinogenicity. For most of the history of industrial hygiene, and still for most groups that establish OELs, an approach based on the presumption of some threshold in the development of adverse effects is applied. This approach is based on selecting a concentration from a critical epidemiology or toxicology study which determined no adverse effect levels (i.e., No Observable Adverse Effect Level or NOAEL), the lowest dose that caused effects (i.e., Lowest Observed Adverse Effect Level or LOAEL), or a dose-response modeled estimate of the effect boundary (i.e., a benchmark dose or BMD). This effect level or point of departure is adjusted for data uncertainties with the application of uncertainty factors. Many OEL groups have traditionally applied this approach for all agents, including carcinogens. Other OEL-establishing groups, such as NIOSH and German MAK, have not traditionally established quantitative OELs for genotoxic carcinogens (which are assumed not to have a threshold). The approach based on adverse effect levels with adjustments for areas of uncertainty is more formally presented in the methods for reference doses and reference concentrations established by EPA.[106] Newer cancer assessment methods use mode of action understanding to apply alternative approaches based on risk probability or developing sub-threshold doses for tumors.[107] Thus, the reference dose approach is a more formal version of the traditional OEL approach, starting from a NOAEL, then reducing an allowable dose by uncertainty factors for population variability, acute to chronic, and laboratory to human extrapolation. These uncertainty factors are often misnamed safety factors.

This approach of developing sub-threshold estimates can be translated into the risk probability perspective of the National Academy of Science (NAS) paradigm. At the Lowest Observed Adverse Effect (LOAEL), the effect rate achieves statistical significance in a population or is otherwise recognized. This observation accomplishes the hazard identification step and starts the exposure-response assessment. At a robust NOAEL below a LOAEL, the population risk rate is likely 10 percent, which is typically the border of statistical significance in feasible laboratory or clinical studies. Thus an exposure limit at the NOAEL (below a LOAEL) subjects a population to a significant risk. The NOAEL is less protective if derived from a smaller study population, a higher background rate for the health effect targeted, and/or a lower quality of the study. The "benchmark dose" is a statistically robust NOAEL and is typically a 10 percent population risk.

Therefore, to reach equivalence with the practice for carcinogens, the allowable exposure must be set below the NOAEL. An extrapolation factor of 10 below the NOAEL, merely reflecting the expected exposure-response relationship in the range just below feasible observation, still leaves behind an approximate 1 percent risk if one assumes linearity in the dose-response curve.

EPA Superfund Risk Assessment

Methodology

The EPA has had a significant impact on the development of environmental risk assessment methodology due to the inclusion of risk assessment as an integral part of the Superfund remediation process, as well as in many other EPA programs. The Superfund methodology is straightforward, although it relies heavily on default assumptions, and allows comparison of dissimilar hazardous waste sites across the nation. The baseline risk assessment process for Superfund sites was based on the National Research Council's four-step paradigm of data collection and evaluation, the simultaneous steps of exposure assessment and toxicity assessment, and the final process of risk characterization, which combines data from the first three steps to develop risk predictions.[24] This section briefly examines each of these four steps.

Data Collection and Evaluation

The purpose of the EPA baseline risk assessment process is to develop sufficient information to support an informed risk management decision. The outcome of this step is highly site specific and consists of developing three interconnected parts:

(1) a list of chemicals of potential concern that may be present at the site;
(2) reliable data on concentrations of these chemicals in site media; and
(3) a site conceptual model (i.e., a source-path-receiver model of the site that hypothesizes ways in which humans may contact the chemicals).

Site Conceptual Model

A site conceptual model is used to plan the risk assessment and associated data collection activities and is often revised periodically as data become available at a site. A conceptual site model is a schematic diagram that:

- Identifies the primary source of contamination in the environment (e.g., releases from a leaking storage tank, waste material poured on the ground)
- Shows how chemicals at the original point of release might move in the environment (e.g., a chemical in soil might penetrate down into groundwater or might volatilize into air)
- Identifies the different types of human populations (e.g., resident, workers, recreational visitors) who might come into contact with contaminated media
- Lists the potential exposure pathways (e.g., ingestion of contaminated water, inhalation of chemicals in air, dermal contact with contaminated soil) that may occur for each population

Figure 8.3 provides a notional example of a conceptual site model based on the approach by the EPA.

Exposure Assessment

The product of the exposure assessment is identification of the nature of the exposed populations (e.g., workers, residents, children, etc.), and estimates of the magnitude, duration, and frequency of exposures. This process requires the risk assessor to characterize the physical setting, identify potentially exposed populations, identify potential exposure pathways, estimate exposure concentrations, and then estimate chemical intakes, usually in terms of milligrams per kilogram per day. Because age, activities, relationship to the site, and media intake all influence the expected exposure, the characteristics of potentially exposed persons play an important role in evaluation of exposure. The general population can be divided into subpopulations characterized by different demographic, geographic, and activity patterns. Exposure

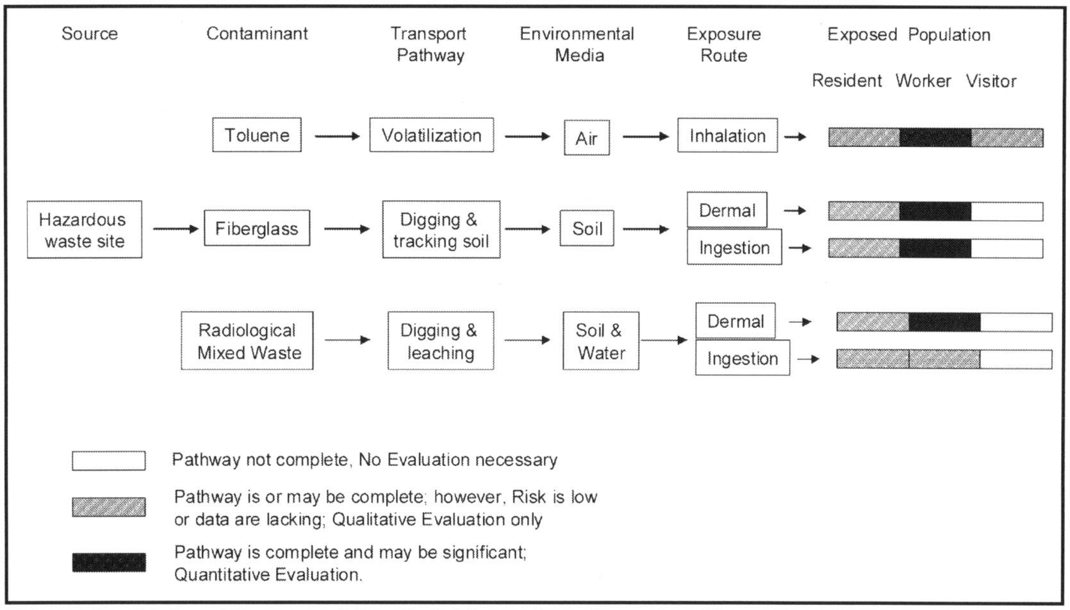

Figure 8.3 — Notional Conceptual Site Model Example — Hazardous Waste Site.

assessments usually are conducted for subpopulations that share similar characteristics, such as children with residential exposure or adults with occupational exposure.

The product of the exposure assessment is average daily exposure to the contaminants through all relevant media: air, water, soil, or biota. Equation 8.1 is generic and must be adapted to calculate exposures for each route of entry: ingestion, inhalation, or dermal absorption.

Calculation of Chronic Daily Intake

$$CDI = \frac{C_m \times I_m \times EF \times ED}{BW \times AT} \qquad (8.1)$$

where:

CDI = chronic daily intake (mg/kg/day)
C_m = concentration in affected media (e.g., mg/L)
I_m = intake of affected media (e.g., L/day)
EF = exposure frequency, days/year
ED = exposure duration, years
BW = body weight, kg
AT = averaging time, days

In most cases the specific information required in this calculation is not available, so generic assumptions or default values usually are substituted (see Table 8.4).

These values are based on upper bound estimates of probability distributions of

Table 8.4 — Selected Standard Default Exposure Factors

Hazard Identification Issues	*Toxicological Assessment Issues*	*Exposure Assessment*	*Risk Characterization*
Key toxicological studies • quality of data • laboratory versus field studies • single or multiple species • single or multiple tumor sites • benign or malignant tumors • endpoints other than carcinogenicity • other supporting studies • conflicting studies • significant data gaps	Data used to develop dose-response curve • animal species (most sensitive, average) • epidemiological data	Sources of environmental exposure • data from different media • significant pathways	Overall picture of risk
Clinical or epidemiological studies • type of study • exposure assessment • confounding factors • other causal factors	Model used to develop dose-response curve • rationale • noncarcinogenic hazards — calculation of RfD/RfCA — assumptions, uncertainty factors — confidence • carcinogenic hazards — dose-response model — basis for its selection — other valid models	Populations • general • highly exposed • highly susceptible	Major conclusions and strengths
Toxicological mechanisms • relevant studies • implications for health effects	Exposure • route, level • same as expected human exposure • impact of exposure extrapolations	Basis for exposure assessment • monitoring • modeling • exposure distributions	Major limitations and uncertainties
Nonpositive data • humans • animals (laboratory or wildlife)	Adverse effects in wildlife species	Key descriptors • average, high end, susceptible populations • central tendency • high-end estimate • highly exposed subgroups	Science policy options
Summaries of • confidence in conclusions • alternative conclusions • significant data gaps • major assumptions		Cumulative exposures • ethnic, socioeconomic	Qualitative characteristics of risk • voluntary versus involuntary, etc. • impact of risk perception
		Wildlife species	Alternatives to hazard
		Conclusions • different approaches • limitations • confidence	Risks of hazard alternative(s) • comparison to similar risks • comparison to similar decisions • limitations of comparisons
			Community concerns • public perception of risk
			Other risk assessments on this chemical
			Any other useful information

ARfC = reference concentration
Source: Reference 24.

typical exposures.[108,109] For example, the reasonable maximum exposure (RME) of residents to contaminants in drinking water is based on consumption of 2 L of water each day, for 350 days/year at a home that is occupied for 30 years by a "standard man" who weighs 70 kg. Chronic daily intakes (CDI) calculated from Equation 8.1 will be in terms of milligrams of contaminant per kilogram of body weight per day, or mg/kg/day, for appropriate comparison with toxicity values developed in the next stage. Note that the averaging time is different for carcinogens and non-carcinogens. The latency period for carcinogens is frequently measured in decades, so the carcinogenic risk is estimated on a per lifetime basis. In contrast, toxicity testing of non-carcinogens is more concerned with health effects occurring during real time (i.e., during the actual exposure time). Therefore, calculation of the CDI for noncarcinogens is averaged over the actual exposure time, which for RME calculations is taken to be 30 years.

Toxicity Assessment

In conducting a Superfund site risk assessment, the toxicity assessment is the least site-dependent of all the stages of risk assessment; therefore, the results should be consistent from site to site. The information needed includes the kinds of health effects (cancer or non-cancer effects) that could occur from exposure and the toxicity values of the chemicals:

- Slope factors for oral or dermal exposures carcinogens, expressed in terms of risk/(mg/kg-day) or unit risks for inhalation exposures, expressed in terms of risk/μg/m³ based on the slope of the dose-response curve; and
- RfDs for oral or dermal exposures to non-carcinogens, expressed in terms of mg/kg-day or RfC's for inhalation exposure expressed in terms of μg/m³.

Rather than conducting toxicological or epidemiological studies, the risk assessor typically searches the published literature and databases, beginning with EPA's IRIS database and other databases of risk assessment values or toxicity data as described elsewhere in this chapter such as the International Toxicity Estimates for Risk (ITER) database or the database of minimal risk level (MRL) values derived by the Agency for Toxic Substances or Disease Registry. Most available cancer risk values are based on ingestion, but some are available for inhalation exposure. Fewer still have been determined for dermal absorption. EPA has developed additional guidance on evaluating dermal[110] and inhalation[111] exposures. Moreover, separate toxicity values may be available for carcinogenic and non-carcinogenic effects, oral or inhalation exposure, and for different exposure periods. Extrapolation of values outside of their initial intent should be done only with the advice and consent of a toxicologist.

Risk Characterization

The actual calculation of risk estimates for a Superfund risk assessment is a fairly straightforward spreadsheet operation, given that correct exposure levels and toxicity values are available and appropriately matched. The type of health effect, the route of exposure, and the length of the exposure period must all be considered. Table 8.5 presents a sample spreadsheet that calculates the carcinogenic risk of adult residential ingestion of arsenic-contaminated soil. The dimensionless risk resulting from exposure to a carcinogen is calculated by multiplying the exposure, in terms of mg/kg-day, by the slope factor in risk/(mg/kg-day) and canceling the units (see Equation 8.2.1).

Lifetime Cancer Risk Estimate (low risk, < 0.01)

$$\text{Risk} = \text{CDI} \times \text{SF} \qquad (8.2.1)$$

where

CDI = chronic daily intake, mg/kg/day
SF = slope factor, 1/(mg/kg/day)

Note: CDI and SF must be expressed in reciprocal units and must represent the same route of entry (ingestion, inhalation, dermal absorption).

Noncancer Hazard Quotient

$$\text{HQ} = \text{CDI} / \text{RfD} \qquad (8.2.2)$$

where

HQ = hazard quotient, dimensionless
CDI = chronic daily intake, mg/kg/day
RfD = reference dose, mg/kg/day

Table 8.5 — Example of Spreadsheet Calculations for Risk Characterization

Carcinogenic Risk Calculations for Ingestion of Arsenic in Soil, Residential AdultExposure

2	(A)	(B)	(C)	
3	Factor	Value	Units	
4	Intake rate	100	mg/day	
5	Conversion factor	1.00E-06	kg/mg	
6	Exposure frequency	350	days/year	
7	Exposure duration	30	years	
8	Body weight	70	kg	
9	Averaging time	25550	days	
10	Slope factor	1.75	mg/kg/day	
11				
12	*Risk Based on Mean of Arsenic-in-Soil Sample Values*			
13	Area	Mean, mg/kg	Intake, mg/kg/day	Risk (unitless)
14	Area A	13.31	7.82E-06[A]	1.37E-05[B]
15	Area B	41.96	2.46E-05	4.31E-05
16				
17	*Risk Based on 95% Upper Confidence Limit (UCL) of Arsenic-in-Soil Sample Values*			
18	Area	95% UCL, mg/kg	Intake, mg/kg/day	Risk (unitless)
19	Area A	13.94	8.18E-06	1.43E-05
20	Area B	60.04	3.52E-05	6.17E-05

[A]Intake = (B14*B4*B5*B6*B7)/(B8*B9)
[B]Risk = (C14*B10)

Note: CDI and RfD are expressed in the same units and must represent the same exposure period (chronic, subchronic, or shorter-term) and the same route of entry (ingestion, inhalation, or dermal absorption).

This product is a true probabilistic estimate of risk and can be used to predict the upper bound on the number of cases of cancer per exposed population.

For non-carcinogens or carcinogens that have risk values based on non-linear dose-response techniques the CDI, expressed as , is simply compared with the appropriate RfD derived from the modified NOAEL (or LOAEL) or benchmark dose and expressed in terms of mg/kg-day (Equation 8.2.2). The resulting ratio of CDI and RfD, which is dimensionless, is the Hazard Quotient (HQ). Unlike the calculations for carcinogens, the HQ is not a true probabilistic estimate of risk of occurrence of adverse health effects and cannot be used to predict the rate of occurrence in a population, the risk of an individual experiencing the adverse health effects, or even the seriousness of any resulting health effects. However, as noted above there is ongoing development of methods as recommended by the NAS to present non-cancer effects as risk probabilities.[112]

Exposure to multiple chemicals, from a variety of pathways, often occurs at Superfund sites. Guidelines for assessing cumulative risk (exposure to several chemicals or other stressors) or aggregate risk (exposure to a chemical via multiple pathways) are addressed in the current guidance, but new approaches are actively being developed in response to the recognition of the importance of these combined exposures.[112] Although it is not currently practical to sum carcinogenic and non-carcinogenic risks, it may be appropriate to aggregate risks within each category. In the absence of specific toxicological information on the effects of multiple chemical exposures, it is usually assumed that the doses (and by extension, the lifetime cancer risk estimate or HQ) are additive. However, the addition of carcinogenic risk estimates or hazards may be excessively conservative. Kodell, et al have suggested a procedure to reduce conservatism in risk estimation for mixtures of carcinogens and EPA has developed additional guidance on assessing risk to chemicals mixtures that moves beyond the simplified hazard index or cancer risk addition approaches.[113,114]

The final step is to prepare a risk assessment report that is understandable to all stakeholders. EPA guidance stresses that risk characterization should be based on reliable scientific information from many different sources, and that documentation should be clear, transparent, reasonable, and consistent. The risk assessment report should discuss key scientific concepts, data, and methods from each stage of the process. It also should include acknowledgment and analysis of uncertainties and an estimate of confidence in the risk characterization. The risk assessment should present several types of risk information. A range of exposure scenarios and multiple risk descriptors (central tendency, high end of individual risk, population risk, important subgroups) should be included. The numbers must be supported by documentation of data, concepts, assumptions, models, and conclusions.[44,45]

Tiered Approach to Risk Assessment

An important objective of this chapter is to emphasize that risk assessment efforts must be appropriately matched to the situation at hand. In a deregulated environment the occupational hygienist is under even greater pressure to recommend risk management decisions that appropriately balance the costs of risk assessment and risk management with the potential impacts of unmitigated risks. The most effective protection of worker health and safety will result from a tiered or iterative approach which matches the level of evaluation and control with the risk at hand. Often this approach translates to the intent to apply health protective assumptions to drive risk management decisions when faced with lack of data (i.e., when uncertainties are high and data confidence is low). If the implications of such a health protective approach are undesirable, additional resources can be devoted to gathering more data, perhaps justifying the use of assumptions that better reflect the actual situation under investigation as opposed to worst-case scenarios, which can yield assessments that are more than adequately protective. Risk assessment efforts continue until there is acceptable balance among the cost of the risk assessment, the costs of the risk management, and the cost of the unmitigated risk. Additional inputs to selecting the level of risk assessment effort also include legal requirements, complexity of the situation, time available for analysis, the technical expertise of the analyst, and risk perceptions of workers, management, and the public. Occupational hygienists apply this full continuum of approaches from qualitative to quantitative methods as described below.

One approach to tiered risk assessments is similar in concept to that developed by ASTM in *Risk-Based Corrective Action Applied at Petroleum Release Sites*[49], abbreviated here as ASTM–RBCA. The purpose of this framework is the determination of cleanup levels (i.e., goals for remediation efforts) for sites such as those contaminated by leaking underground storage tanks. The first step is to determine whether there are any obvious safety hazards that should be corrected before analysis proceeds to Tier I of ASTM–RBCA. Tier I requires a low level of effort and resources, primarily involving the collection and analysis of site samples. The results are compared with lookup tables that contain suggested concentrations of contaminants in soil, water, and air. These lookup tables are based on EPA CDI equations and do not take into account any physical, chemical, or biological degradation or transfer. If the cost of achieving Tier I cleanup levels is deemed unnecessary or unfeasible, and continued risk assessment resources are available, the analyst may continue to Tier II. This requires a moderate level of resources, including site-specific data for input to (1) the same risk-based equations used to develop the lookup tables in Tier I or (2) screening-level models. If degradation or transfer processes are considered, these cleanup levels probably will be higher than those suggested by the lookup tables in Tier I. If, however, these cleanup levels also are deemed to be unnecessary or infeasible and sufficient risk assessment resources exist, the analyst may continue to Tier III. A significant increase in site-specific data and the use of complex modeling characterize this level, but the extra effort may be justified by even higher cleanup levels. Whether or not Tier III cleanup levels are higher, this is considered the last step in the risk assessment. The goal of this tiered approach is not to justify less protection to the public; each tier should achieve a similar level of

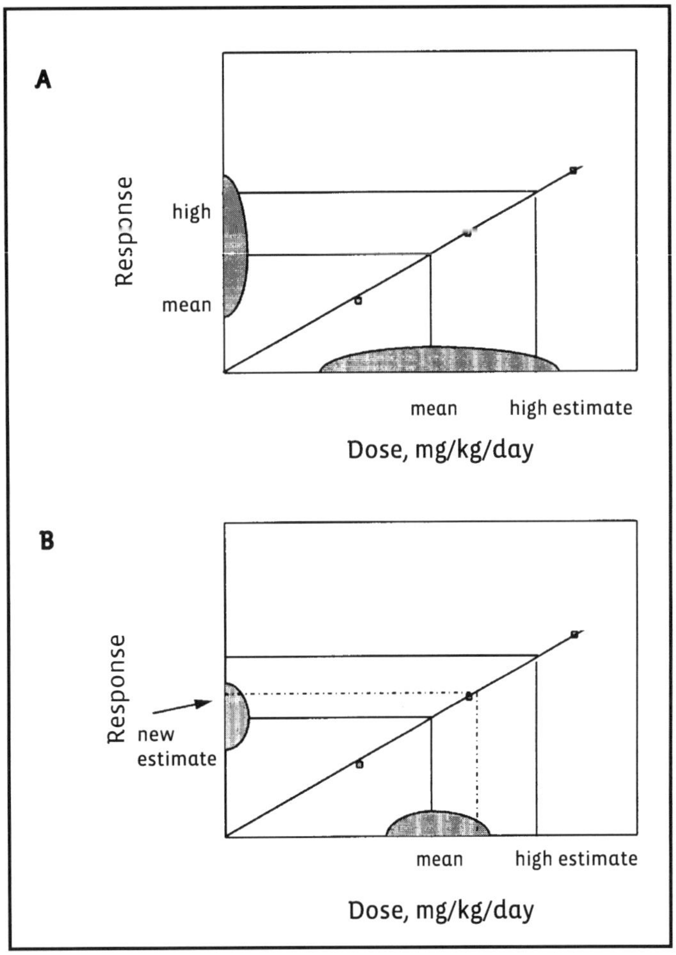

Figure 8.4 — Improved exposure assessment shrinks error bands. A: Dose and risk estimates are conservative; B: shrinking the error bands around the exposure estimate reduces the risk estimate.

protection. Rather, the goal of the higher tiers is to allow development of more realistic site-specific cleanup levels.

Collecting additional information or conducting a higher tier of risk assessment may have the effect of shrinking the error bands around the exposure assessment or of shifting the risk estimate to lower (or higher) values. As shown in Figure 8.4, this may allow a more accurate risk estimate and allows for making risk management decisions with greater confidence. Errors in risk assessment can be of two types: over- or underestimation of risk. In this case the Type I error can be defined as selecting more risk management than is actually needed; the impact is mainly financial. The Type II error is selecting less risk management than is actually needed; the potential impact is more significant, as it involves human health. Higher tier risk assessments should reduce the probability of making either the Type I or Type II error and allow more efficient allocation of risk management resources.

Occupational Hygiene and Safety Risk Assessment in the Risk Management Process

Risk Assessment Types

This section will discuss a number of risk assessment types, including quantitative, semi-quantitative, qualitative, control banding, and hazard/process hazard analyses.

Quantitative Risk Assessment

Quantitative risk assessment is practiced by occupational hygienists in the field whenever exposure measurements are compared with occupational exposure limits. The risk assessment process as practiced by occupational hygienists follows the basic steps laid out in the NRC (1983) report and *Patty's Industrial Hygiene and Toxicology*.[41,115] Hazard identification and dose –response assessments are employed as the basis for deriving OELs. The outcome of a quantitative exposure assessment is then compared to the OEL to support judgments about risk (i.e., risk characterization). The comparison of the quantitative estimate of exposure to the OEL is often called a hazard quotient (HQ). The outcome of this type of risk assessment will be a determination that the exposure is less than, equal to, or greater than acceptable levels. Occupational exposure limits are not typically based on linear dose-response models. Therefore, the degree to which the actual exposure is greater or less than the OEL is not a linear estimate of risk. Although reducing the actual exposure level by half would reduce the risk, one could not say that the resulting risk would be reduced by half. Advanced techniques have been proposed for use in developing probabilistic estimates for non-cancer health effect risk characterizations, but have not been formally adopted by most agencies that develop OELs.[116,117]

Table 8.6 — A chronology of selected events impacting occupational hygiene risk assessment

Date	*Event*	*Reference*
1930s	Industrial hygiene and occupational medicine professionals developed concept of dose-response relationship	1
1938	Founding of the organization now known as the American Conference of Governmental Industrial Hygienists	1
1938	First suggested guidelines for asbestos, Dreessen et al., 1938	1
1939	Founding of the American Industrial Hygiene Association (AIHA)	
1940	Bowditch et al. article on occupational exposure limits	1
1940s	ACGIH began to develop guidelines for occupational exposure limits, now known as threshold limit values	1
1947	Enactment of Federal Insecticide, Fungicide, and Rodenticide Act (FIFRA)	10
1958	Passage of Delaney amendment to the Pure Food, Drug, and Cosmetic Act	14
1961	Mantel and Bryan article on virtually safe doses published in the Journal of the National Cancer Institute	18
1970	Creation of OSHA, NIOSH, and EPA	
1971	*(May)* OSHA adopted 1968 ACGIH TLVs as permissible exposure limits	1
1973	Early FDA regulatory decision utilizing risk assessment based on Mantel and Bryan (1961)	18
1975	Eighth Circuit Court's decision on Reserve Mining Co. v. EPA	10
1976	EPA proposed the 1976 interim guidelines, the first risk assessment guidelines	14
1976	In Ethyl Corp v. EPA, the District of Columbia Circuit Court upheld EPA's order reducing lead in gasoline, ruling that actual injury was not required for endangerment to exist, and that risk assessment could form the basis for health-related regulations under the Clean Air Act.	10
1976	Enactment of the Toxic Substances Control Act. Regulation of toxic substances became a major theme of federal environmental statutes, which are characterized by unwillingness to wait for definitive proof.	10
1977	Formation of the Interagency Regulatory Liaison Group (abolished in 1981)	14
1977	OSHA Draft Cancer Policy issued	14
1977	FDA regulatory decisions used 10^{-6} guideline	18
1977	*(April)* OSHA issued ETS for benzene	20
1977	*(May)* Court of Appeals for the Fifth Circuit issued a temporary restraining order against the ETS for benzene	10
1978	OSHA issued new permanent standard for benzene	1, 20
1978	Congress required publication of annual list of known or suspected carcinogens to which a significant number of people are exposed. National Toxicology Program created to coordinate federal government toxicity testing.	10, 14
1978	*(October)* Benzene standard vacated by the Court of Appeals for the Fifth Circuit	20
1979	Scientific Bases for Identification of Potential Carcinogens and Estimation of Risks published by the Interagency Regulatory Liaison Group	1, 14
1979	Court of Appeals for the District of Columbia affirmed the cotton dust standard	10
1980	Comprehensive Environmental Response, Compensation and Liability Act (also known as Superfund) enacted	
1980	OSHA issued the Final Generic Cancer Policy	14, 20
1980	*(July)* U.S. Supreme Court invalidated the benzene standard	10, 18, 20
1981	Executive Order 12291 signed	1, 10, 20
1981	U.S. Supreme Court decision on OSHA cotton dust standard	10, 20
1982	EPA standards for pesticide residue in foods based on 10-6, FIFRA risk-benefit analysis	18
1983	The District of Columbia Circuit Court wrote that the correlation between declining blood lead levels and EPA-mandated reductions in lead-in-gasoline justified EPA's stricter lead limits imposed in 1982	10
1983	National Academy of Sciences published the "Red Book," *Risk Assessment in the Federal Government: Managing the Process*	
1984	Passage of the Hazardous and Solid Waste Amendments, eventually leading to increased use of risk assessment in management of leaking underground storage tanks	
1986	Passage of the Superfund Amendments and Reauthorization Act (SARA)	
1986	OSHA announced it would address "existing, significant risks" and that requirements would "significantly" reduce these risks	20
1986	*(November)* California voters approved Proposition 65	10
1986	EPA Cancer Guidelines, and the Superfund Public Health Exposure Manual	
1988	OSHA began the PEL Project, designed to revise and incorporate TLVs as standards	1, 20
1989	First volume in EPA Risk Assessment Guidance for Superfund published	7
1989	*(January)* OSHA published the final revised air contaminants standard	1, 20
1990	Enactment of CAAA, including certain requirements for risk assessments of hazardous air pollutants	
1992	*(February)* EPA issued Habicht Memorandum, "Guidance on Risk Characterization for Risk Managers and Risk Assessors"	
1992	*(July)* Court of Appeals for the Eleventh Circuit ruled that OSHA's actions under the PEL Program were invalid	20
1993	*(March)* OSHA announced it would enforce the 1971 PELs	20
1994	AIHA Risk Assessment Task Group completed the "AIHA Risk Assessment Position Paper" and "AIHA Risk Assessment White Paper"	
1994	As mandated by the CAAA, *Science and Judgment in Risk Assessment* published by the National Research Council	
1995	The American Society for Testing and Materials published Risk-Based Corrective Action Applied at Petroleum Release Sites, E 1739-95	
1995	*(January)* AIHA President Jerry Lynch testified at U.S. House of Representatives, Commerce Committee, hearings on H.R. 9, submitting the AIHA Risk Assessment Position Paper and White Paper into the record.	
1995	*(March)* EPA issued Browner Memorandum, "Policy for Risk Characterization at the U.S. Environmental Protection Agency"	
1997	U.S. Presidential/Congressional Commission on Risk Assessment and Risk Management (USPCCRARM): Framework for Environmental Health Risk Management, Final Report, vol. 1. Washington, D.C.: 1997.	
1997	U.S. Presidential/Congressional Commission on Risk Assessment and Risk Management (USPCCRARM): *Risk Assessment and Risk Management in Regulatory Decision-Making*, Final Report, Volume 2. Washington, D.C.: 1997	
1997	AIHA Risk Assessment Committee sponsored the first Risk Assessment Symposium for industrial hygienists, followed by symposia in 1999, 2000, and 2002	
2000	AIHA published *Risk Assessment Principles for Industrial Hygienists*, by Jayjock, Lynch, and Nelson	

Table 8.7 — Comparison of the classical occupational hygiene and environmental risk assessment models

Classical Occupational Hygiene	The Environmental Way
Anticipation/Recognition	Hazard identification (data collection/evaluation)
Evaluation	Exposure assessment Toxicity assessment Risk characterization
Control	Risk management
Hazard communication	Risk communication

The risk characterization is used in risk management decision making about the type and level of controls that may be necessary to protect worker health. Risk assessment has been an integral part of the development of OELs and its quantitative linkage with risk management was further developed through the benzene decision, in which the Supreme Court found that OSHA must first identify a significant risk of material health impairment and then show that the proposed standard would reduce that risk. As illustrated in Table 8.6, the standards that followed — the 1983 asbestos standard, ethylene oxide, formaldehyde, methylene dianiline, methylene chloride — were based on health risk assessments that when coupled with cost and technical feasibility data in the risk management process were used to arrive at the final PEL.

Thus, the basic concepts of risk assessment are not new to the occupational hygiene profession. Although the specific activities may vary between environmental and occupational risk assessment, the objectives of each stage remain the same. Evaluation of any exposure situation — environmental or occupational — requires knowledge of the pathways by which exposure may occur, quantification of the exposure and toxicity of the chemicals involved, and integration of this information (i.e., comparison of the level of exposure with the level of risk per unit of exposure). Table 8.7 compares the familiar model of occupational hygiene practice with the processes of environmental risk assessment, risk management, and risk communication. (It should be noted here that not all hygienists will agree with this mapping of risk assessment and occupational hygiene, maintaining that exposure evaluation is a risk management function.)

Although air sampling often is conducted by occupational hygienists, comparisons of airborne contaminant concentrations to PELs, TLVs®, WEELs™, or other OEL lists are not the only analytical tools available. A more thorough risk assessment could be performed by investing more resources in the exposure assessment processes, potentially resulting in a more accurate comparison of exposure to the OEL. Investing more resources in toxicity assessment processes might improve the OEL itself. A more complete exposure assessment might be performed by the addition of techniques that more fully characterize the actual "dose" received by the worker. Exposure assessments that characterize exposure to a chemical via multiple pathways (from multiple sources or multiple dose routes) are often called aggregate exposure assessments and can give a more accurate determination of the likelihood for adverse effects. Another refinement in the exposure assessment is to consider the ability of the chemical to be absorbed systemically and reach internal target tissues. Such assessments rely on evaluation of the total dose versus the external exposure and are compared to internal dose benchmarks (e.g., blood or urine levels of the chemical or its metabolite). The exposure assessment can also be enhanced by evaluating the distribution of exposures rather than characterizing exposure as a single value. Such techniques allow for the estimation of probabilities of exceeding an OEL under different scenarios. Examples of techniques include:

- Sampling and analysis of surface wipes for presence of heavy metals or pesticides and evaluation of dermal absorption to assess potential dermal contribution to the total dose;
- Collection and analysis of blood, urine, or breath samples from exposed workers for comparison to internal dose benchmarks;
- Evaluation of environmental (food, water, soil) as well as occupational exposures to the chemicals in question, along with determination of personal intake factors, such as quantity of contaminated food or water consumed daily, leading to estimation of chronic daily intake (CDI; mg/kg/day);

- Use of predictive models to estimate exposure to chemicals under varying conditions or to model exposure distributions.

When an expanded exposure assessment has been performed, incorporating data from personal and total environmental sampling, an expanded toxicity assessment may aid in full utilization of this data. Toxicity assessment for occupational hygiene typically begins with looking up the OEL and reading the associated documentation or other readily available reference on occupational and/or environmental toxicology to determine the target organs and types of adverse health effects to be expected. The toxicity assessment can be extended by updating the dose-response relationship that was used as the basis of the current OEL. The utility of taking this additional step will depend on the degree to which the current OEL reflects the current state of the science. A search of the literature may identify new epidemiology and toxicology data that ought to be considered. Moreover, dose-response analysis techniques used for deriving OELs have evolved over time and application of the newer methods to an existing data set might yield a revised OEL that can be developed with greater confidence. There are many enhancements in methodology that are increasingly being used to refine the determination of critical effects.(48) Some examples include:

- Benchmark dose modeling approaches to replace traditional toxicology study NOAEL/LOAEL values as the basis for identifying a critical effect level for such risk assessments.(118)
- Physiologically-based pharmacokinetic modeling (PBPK) models to estimate organ or tissue doses to extrapolate doses across exposure durations, species, or dose routes.(119,120)
- Inhalation dosimetry models assess differences in respiratory tract distribution of inhaled chemicals.(121)
- Advanced dose-response modeling tools to include the evaluation of biomarkers into the dose-response assessment.(122,123)
- Use of data on toxicokinetics or toxicodynamics (tissue response) to determine species differences in response or human variability in response to replace traditional uncertainty factors.(124)

Many of these techniques were applied initially in the field of environmental risk assessment, and are becoming more common in occupational risk assessments. Thus, an additional perspective may be gained by examining the traditional methods of environmental risk assessment. The individual worker's total exposure to the chemical in question, including primary and secondary occupational exposure, food, water, soil/dust, and other sources in the home, can be summed and compared with the slope factors or unit risks and/or RfD toxicity values, which were discussed in the section on environmental risk assessment. Many chemicals encountered in the workplace are included in EPA's Integrated Risk Information System (IRIS) file list and other free comprehensive resources such as the International Toxicity Estimates for Risk (ITER) system housed by the National Library of Medicine's TOXNET system. These and other resources provide extensive toxicological data and serve as an excellent starting point for further data searches, particularly for the many chemicals that are do not have published OELs.(125)

The application of environmental risk assessment methodologies to the practice of occupational hygiene, e.g., assessing worker exposure at a Superfund site, raises several issues, including (1) the use of averaging times and acute/chronic health effects; (2) situations in which there is a current OEL; and (3) toxicity values that have been developed for ingestion as opposed to inhalation as a route of entry. In addition, there are occupational hygiene risk assessment issues yet to be resolved: selection of mathematical models for low-dose extrapolation, assumptions made when adding risk across chemicals, pathways, populations, and so forth.

One of the first issues that must be addressed is that of averaging times in relation to regulatory requirements. When dealing with carcinogens, the practice in environmental risk assessment is to determine the reasonable maximum exposure (RME) over a 30-year period (that is, the 95% upper confidence level estimate of the length of a person's residency in a single home). The CDI over this 30-year period is averaged over the anticipated 70-year life span. For noncarcinogens the daily exposure is averaged over the actual exposure time, which will vary for comparison with RfDs based on short-term, subchronic, and chronic exposure periods. This differs from the usual practice in occupational hygiene, which is to measure actual exposure, typically averaged over an 8-hour day within the context of a 40-hour work week; some latitude is allowed in OELs to account for work schedules longer than 8 hours/day or 40 hours/week. The OSHA interpretation of its PELs is that any exposure above the 8-hour time-weighted average (after accounting for statistical variation) is a violation of the standards, regardless of whether the worker has any further exposure to the chemical that week or month. Although this "daily" approach is reasonable for chemicals that have acute health hazards, it does not make sense for those chemicals associated with chronic health effects and for which the appropriate quantity of concern is the long-term average body burden. A further contrast between occupational and environmental toxicity values is that the acceptable occupational exposure limits are based on intermittent exposures rather than continuous exposures; a higher exposure can be tolerated if frequent recovery periods are built in.

Another issue to be dealt with in application of the environmental risk levels (such as EPA RfDs) to occupational hygiene is the fact that many of them have been developed for ingestion rather than inhalation as the route of entry. Inhalation exposure is more complex due to the dynamics of the respiratory system and interactions with the physicochemical properties of chemicals. In many cases, lead for example, the route of entry is not as critical as is the actual dose absorbed. In the case of respiratory irritants or chemicals that are effectively metabolized by the liver, the route of entry can be critical. A toxicologist should be consulted prior to conversion of an oral slope factor or RfD to an inhalation or dermal toxicity value. For chemicals that have an established inhalation-based health benchmark, such as the U.S. EPA's RfC values, there is no issue related to route-to-route extrapolation. However, there are still uncertainties in application of such "environmental benchmarks." One issue is that of time averaging noted above. A second is that the EPA values are intended to be protective of the general population, including sensitive subpopulations. Thus, the uncertainty factors included to address human variability in sensitivity are often greater than those incorporated into risk assessments for workers.

Finally, assumptions made when adding risks across chemicals, pathways, and populations must be carefully examined. With respect to assumptions of linear additivity of health effects, it must be remembered that for noncarcinogens, the level of concern does not increase linearly as the RfD is approached or exceeded. Errors in risk estimation may result from the combination of HQs based on critical effects of varying toxicological significance or varying levels of confidence, uncertainty adjustments, and

Consequence					Increased Probability				
					A	B	C	D	E
Rating	People	Assets	Environment	Image	Never heard of in the world	Heard of incident in industry	Incident has occurred in our company	Happens several times/year in company	Happens several times/year in location
0	None	None	None	None	I	I	I	I	I
1	Slight	Slight	Slight	Slight	I	I	I	I	I
2	Minor	Minor	Minor	Minor	I	I	I	II	II
3	Major	Local	Localized	Considerable	I	I	II	II	III
4	1-3 Deaths	Major	Major	Major National	I	II	II	III	III
5	Many Deaths	Extensive	Massive	Major International	II	II	III	III	III

Figure 8.5 — Qualitative Risk Assessment Matrix.

modifying factors, and/or different health effects induced by different mechanisms of action. With respect to summation of carcinogenic risks, questions about linear additivity, weight of evidence in carcinogenic classification, and mechanisms of toxicological action also are relevant. The actual likelihood that any one individual would be exposed to all chemicals/pathways/scenarios also requires careful consideration.

Semiquantitative and Qualitative Risk Assessment

The emphasis in this chapter thus far has been on various quantitative approaches to determine the probability that a substance or situation will produce harm under specified conditions. In situations that must be assessed rapidly or that are not easily quantified, e.g., when there are inadequate data to support a quantitative risk assessment, semiquantitative or qualitative methods can be used. These methods often guide the user directly to a risk management option, skipping the intermediate step of estimating the degree of harm which may occur. Figure 8.5 Qualitative Risk Assessment Matrix presents an example of a risk assessment matrix that is similar to those used by many corporations to assess and manage risks to people, property, the environment, and public image. In this simplified assessment of severity and probability, the first step is to rate the potential consequence(s). Looking at potential human health consequences, the rating categories begin at none and slight, and progress to one or more fatalities. The next step is to determine the probability of the occurrence based on past history at the global, industry-wide, or company level. The recommended action is at the intersection of the severity row and the probability column. As an example, if the expected consequence is a major health effect that has already occurred several times at a specific location of the company, the situation would be judged to be intolerable, with immediate action required. A benefit of this approach is that resources are focused on risk management. Depending on the particular situation, however, the risk assessor may wish to follow up with a quantitative risk assessment (see previous discussion on iterative risk assessment).

Control Banding

Control banding (CB) is a qualitative and/or semi-quantitative approach to risk assessment and risk management which complements the more traditional quantitative methods, e.g., collection and analysis of air samples, followed by comparison to occupational exposure limits (OELs). Given the reality that appropriate occupational exposure limits cannot be established for every chemical in use, a chemical is assigned to a "band" for control measures, based on its hazard classification according to international criteria, the amount of chemical in use, and its volatility/dustiness. The outcome is a recommended control strategy. CB arose in the mid to late 1990s in response to the increasing number of chemicals posing a threat to worker health, legal challenges to the standards development process, lack of understanding of the traditional approach on the part of workers and of operators of small and medium size enterprises (SMEs), and the lack of resources to conduct toxicological and epidemiological research to establish the OELs and to collect and analyze samples.(126,127) CB has roots in a number of qualitative(128) and semiquantitative(129) risk assessment approaches that began to appear in the 1970s and evolved in the 1980s to assess the probability of catastrophic failure at large chemical facilities.(130) Active international collaboration and exchange of ideas among occupational hygienists in the chemical, biological, and pharmaceutical industries (where toxicity and exposure data were extremely limited in research and development applications)(131–133) culminated in 1998 in a series of papers from the United Kingdom describing COSHH Essentials(134–136) This approach is likely the best known and most thoroughly evaluated of the various CB toolkits.

COSHH Essentials was developed by the Health and Safety Executive (HSE) in the United Kingdom to assist employers [particularly subject matter experts (SMEs)] in meeting the requirements of the 1988 Control of Substances Hazardous to Health (COSHH) regulations to conduct risk assessments of chemical exposures to workers. In COSHH Essentials, the hazard is combined with the exposure potential to determine a recommended level of control approach. European Union (EU) risk phrases (R-phrases) are used to rank the hazard of a chemical, and potential for exposure is estimated by the quantity in use and the volatility of liquids or dustiness of solids. This semiquantitative assessment of the hazard of a substance and the likelihood of exposure is meant to guide the user directly toward one of four risk management approaches: (1) general ventilation, which assumes good work practices are in place; (2) engineering controls, ranging from local exhaust ventilation to a ventilated partial enclosure; (3) containment, enclosure that allows limited breaches of containment; and (4) special controls, requiring expert advice. To assist non-expert users of COSHH Essentials in implementing the first three levels of control, over 300 control guidance sheets (CGS) have been developed to provide general and specific advice on a range of hazards (e.g., metalworking fluids, asbestos, silica), tasks (e.g., manufacturing, construction, agriculture), and worker protection topics (e.g., respiratory protection, engineering controls, containment).[137] In its continuing development of COSHH Essentials, HSE has also provided "direct advice" strategies which focus on the task performed to directly assign personal protective equipment (PPE) and control options without the interim step of assessing the potential of exposure. An interactive site designed to guide the user through the process is available online.[138]

Although COSHH Essentials is the best known and best studied example of CB, the reader should note that the terms *control banding* and *COSHH Essentials* are NOT synonymous. Other CB toolkits have been developed by corporations (e.g., Hallmark Cards, Inc.), by nations (including The Netherlands, Germany, France, Norway, Belgium, Singapore, and Korea), and by international organizations (International Chemical Control Toolkit, or ICCT, developed in collaboration by the International Labour Organization, HSE, and the International Occupational Hygiene Association).[139] In additional to chemical CB, applications are expanding rapidly, and now include for example safety[140], ergonomics[141], construction[142,143], and nanotechnology.[144]

Before CB strategies can be accepted, adapted, and implemented on a wider scale, however, a number of validation and verification issues must be addressed. Validation refers herein to the many components related to accuracy of the model itself, and verification refers to the correct installation, operation, and maintenance of controls. These issues are critical, as under-prescription of control can have serious consequences, while over-prescription could lead to significant unnecessary expense.[134,145] A framework to critique CB models includes toxicity measures, margins of safety, exposure issues, control issues, validation, verification, and miscellaneous issues.[127] For example, under the rubric of toxicity measures, questions remain about the process of assigning R-phrases to chemicals, and the availability and accuracy of R-phrases.[146,147] Margins of safety which have been calculated for COSHH Essentials differ than those for the ICCT.[148] An important component of any model is its ability to correctly predict exposure, which may require data in addition to volume in use and dustiness and/or volatility.[149] The need for exposure monitoring has been clearly expressed by many occupational hygienists, including developers of the various models.[134,145,146] Control issues include the accuracy and detail provided by CGSs, and the ability of the recommended control strategy to reduce concentrations to desired range.[150] User issues focus on the ability of the user to correctly interpret the model, including inputs and resulting advice.[150] Validation and verification both suffer from limited research with which to evaluate the various CB models.[128,130,136,145,151–153] Finally, questions remain as to the impact of CB approaches[130], the need to utilize CB in the context of a complete IH program utilizing a hierarchy of controls approach,[134] and protection of vulnerable populations.[154]

Major criticisms of CB are its oversimplification and reliance on limited data.[155] However, it must be remembered that CB was originally developed for application in situations with limited data available (e.g., pharmaceutical research) and refined for application in SMEs which had limited industrial hygiene resources. CB has also been promoted for application in developing countries, where millions of workers have extremely limited or no access to industrial hygiene expertise.[126,139,156,157] Properly understood and applied, CB approaches can leverage industrial hygiene resources in a variety of situations and provide improved working conditions for many of these underrepresented workers.

Subjective Risk Assessment

Risk assessment involves the use of judgment and intuition whether the assessment is quantitative or qualitative. OEH professionals frequently make intuitive decisions without attributing either quantitative or qualitative values to the risks involved. While intuition is often useful, it is usually preferable to employ more rigorous risk assessment techniques to more 'objectively' inform, aid, and document decision making. Risk assessment is often assumed to be objective, and its results — risk values and the decisions based on them — to be an estimate of what one would consider a "true" risk. However, the risk management process, including the techniques and methodologies used, involve subjectivity. The assessment process inherently has uncertainty, professional judgment is needed, individual perspectives and bias are involved, and the intrusion of inaccuracy or errors is present. Given the same data and information, the results obtained by OEH professionals will often differ. OEH professionals should use risk assessment techniques, methodologies, and procedures with an understanding of limitations and necessary assumptions. Once the risk assessment is done and results communicated to leaders, risk managers, and other stakeholders, subjectivity will enter into the equation in implementing recommendations provided. Training, experience, and use of standardized methods will minimize but not eliminate variation in results; therefore, documentation of risk assessment processes is critical in report preparation.

While subjectivity may be a vulnerability in the risk assessment process, it is also one of the principal strengths of the process. Identifying and analyzing hazards and making decisions about risks demand human thought and investigation. Automating the process may be considered in these types of situations; however, doing so would remove the benefit of the ability for a human to probe, to assess the situation, to apply judgment, and to account for non-quantifiable inputs. While automation and the use of artificial intelligence (AI) may prove beneficial in the future as automation technology advances, humans must still be involved. This means that something in an assessment is likely to be missed and some things may be wrongly judged.

It is important for OEH professionals to understand and allow for the subjective influences on the process. Individual bias and perceptions, subjectivity, uncertainty, and variability should be addressed in training and professional development.

Vulnerability Assessment (Food/Water/Infrastructure)

With the increased national attention on homeland security, vulnerability assessments are being conducted on information technology, energy supply, water supply, transportation, and communication systems to identify, quantify, and prioritize system vulnerabilities to events such as vandalism, sabotage, or terrorist attack. Although the process is similar to that of risk assessment as described in this chapter, the focus of vulnerability assessment is on the consequences of an adverse event on a system or structure, and the primary and secondary consequences for the surrounding environment. Vulnerability assessment can drive the risk management process by emphasizing mitigation, e.g., options for reducing consequences and managing future events.[158,159]

The Homeland Security Act (Chemical Facility Anti-Terrorism Standards, described above) and the Public Health Security and Bioterrorism Preparedness and Response Act of 2002 both contain legal requirements to conduct vulnerability assessments. The Bioterrorism Act requires drinking water utilities serving more than 3,300 persons to conduct vulnerability assessments and to update emergency response plans.[160] Examples of resources for conducting vulnerability assessments include EPA vulnerability assessment guidance[161], the National Oceanic and Atmospheric Administration (NOAA) Risk and Vulnerability Assessment Tool (RVAT)[162], and the Department of Homeland Security Chemical Security Assessment Tool.[163]

Hazard/Process Hazard Analyses

Many industrial processes contain inherent chemical or physical characteristics with the energy potential for damaging people, property, and/or the environment. The increased number and magnitude of catastrophic chemical, petrochemical, and oil industry incidents which have occurred since the 1970s as a result of process hazards has led to a legislative emphasis on developing effective safety programs, including the Emergency Planning and Community Right to-Know Act of 1986 (EPCRA), and provisions in the Clean Air Act Amendments (CAAA, 1990) to institute federal regulatory programs to prevent chemical accidents that harm workers, the public and the environment.[164]

Section 304 of the CAAA called for OSHA to develop chemical accident prevention and emergency response regulations to protect workers at hazardous chemical facilities. OSHA responded by developing the Process Safety Management (PSM) standard,[165] which places accident prevention and emergency response requirements on facilities having listed hazardous chemicals above certain threshold quantities. EPA was required by Section 112(r) of the CAAA to develop regulations to prevent and respond to chemical accidents that could affect the public and environment off-site. EPA met this obligation in 1996 by promulgating the Risk Manage-ment Program (RMP) regulations.[93] RMP is similar to OSHA's PSM standard, but also requires facilities to perform an Offsite Consequence Analysis (OCA), which is an analytical estimate of the potential consequences of hypothetical worst case and alternative accidental release on the public and environment around the facility.

In keeping with these legislative requirements, OSHA has delineated 137 "highly hazardous chemicals" plus flammables (as defined by HAZCOM standard — 1910.1200), and EPA has listed 77 toxic substances and 63 flammables.[93,165] Any facility that uses, stores, manufactures, handles, or moves any of the chemicals or flammables, at or above the threshold quantities, must have in place a program which includes Process Hazard Analysis and emergency planning and response. PHA is a methodology to identify and evaluate process hazards for the purpose of determining the adequacy of or need for control measures and will address:

a. Hazards of the process;
b. Identification of any previous incident which had a likely potential for catastrophic consequences in the workplace;
c. Engineering and administrative controls applicable to the hazards;
d. Consequences of failure of engineering and administrative controls;
e. Facility siting;
f. Human factors; and
g. A qualitative evaluation of a range of the effects of incidents on employees.

Checklists, hazard and operability studies (HAZOP), failure mode and effects analysis (FMEA), and fault tree analysis are among the methodologies which can be used to conduct process hazard analysis under the PSM and RMP requirements.

Beyond the Workplace

Exposures to toxic chemicals used in the workplace can also occur in workers' homes, in the community near known sources, during consumer use of manufactured products, and in the general environment, as for example, following improper waste disposal. In fact, a cradle-to-grave, lifecycle evaluation of a chemical must include all these settings. In addition, the home is a prime source of exposure to household hazards including chemicals, radon, and biologicals. OEH professionals can utilize their skills in evaluating potential problems within homes in their community and use their risk assessment knowledge to help homeowners prioritize the mitigation of the greatest household hazards.

In the past, effects to family members of chemicals carried home by workers on their clothes, skin, hair, tools, and vehicles have best been documented for materials with clear pathways and severe, specific health effects:

- In 1914, Oliver reported on lead poisoning in wives of house painters from laundering their husbands' overalls.[167]
- Asbestosis and mesothelioma have occurred in asbestos workers as a result of direct exposure and in family members from exposure to "take-home asbestos."[167–169]
- Family members of beryllium workers in the nuclear and aviation industries have suffered from chronic beryllium disease.[167]

Family members may include children, pregnant women, and elderly, ill, and disabled persons. The hand-to-mouth behavior of young children may result in greater exposure, and children may in fact absorb, distribute, and metabolize chemicals differently than do adults.[7] Recognizing the public health risks of take-home chemicals, the U.S. Congress passed the Workers' Family Protection Act in 1992.[170] This law directed NIOSH to study the potential for contamination of workers' homes with hazardous chemicals and substances carried home from work. The subsequent NIOSH report documented additional hazards associated with pesticides; caustic chemicals; chlorinated hydrocarbons; mercury; estrogenic substances; dusts; arsenic; fibrous glass; and infectious agents carried home by workers.[171] Socioeconomic conditions may compound the problem, as workers and their families often live in communities that have been built around sources of contamination, such as lead smelters, asbestos mills and mines, and so on, and access to health care may be limited. Additional exposures to family members also can occur from cottage industries such as battery breaking, or even from hobbies such as electronics (solder), stained glass work, casting of bullets and fishing weights, and pottery glazes.

The 2002 report of the Workers' Family Protection Task Force identified important gaps in knowledge of take-home exposures and their potential health consequences, and recommended the following research agenda.

- Characterization of the extent of home contamination with toxic workplace substances.
- Identification of populations at greatest risk of known and suspected take-home exposures.
- Assessment of the adverse health effects from take-home exposures.
- Identification of previously unrecognized toxic exposures that endanger the health of workers' families.
- Assessment of take-home exposure prevention (e.g., requirements in the OSHA Expanded Health Standards for separate lockers for street clothes and work clothes, and shower and change facilities) and remediation methods and evaluation of worker notification and training programs.

The Workers' Family Protection Task Force is thus recommending that a risk assessment be conducted of take-home chemicals. Meeting the goals of this research agenda will require the use of the risk assessment principles and practices described in this chapter.

Community Health Risk Assessment

Health risks also extend to the community environment, where the exposed populations and exposure conditions differ significantly from the workplace. Community members include the same sensitive subpopulations as workers' families, and they may be exposed to contaminants in air (indoor and outdoor) on a 24-hour basis, as well as in water (drinking and recreational contact), food, and soil. Although the level of exposures to contaminants may be lower in the community, there may be substantially more contaminants to which the community is exposed. For reasons including these, the acceptable level of risk for the workplace is usually much higher than the acceptable level of risk for community environmental exposures.

OEH professionals currently have numerous tools they may use in performing community risk assessments. One tool is the EPA Risk Assessment Portal containing the EPA Risk Assessment Guidelines discussed previously (e.g., *Risk Assessment Guidance for Superfund*).[172] These guidelines have been extremely useful over the years in advancing the practice of community environmental risk assessment. Another tool is the Green Media Toolshed "Scorecard". This "Scorecard" was transferred to Green Media Toolshed by the Environmental Defense Fund in November 2005.[173] Risk assessors can obtain information regarding but not limited to hazardous air pollutants, lead hazards, and toxic releases from industrial facilities. Information for use in developing risk assessments for radionuclides is available from EPA Health Effects Assessment Summary Tables — Radionuclide Table.[174] The Agency for Toxic Substances and Disease Registry (ATSDR) also provides information on Minimal Risk Levels (MRLs) for Hazardous Substances.[175] The ATSDR designed these MRLs as screening tools to allow OEH professionals and other public health professionals to identify hazardous waste sites that may not present an adverse risk. These tools provide the occupational and environmental hygienist with valuable information to assess community health risks from the environment.

These tools can also help OEH professionals to evaluate hazards in the home and to train community residents to evaluate hazards in the home. Household hazards include radon, environmental tobacco smoke, biological contaminants, stoves, heaters, fireplaces, and chimneys, household products, formaldehyde, pesticides, asbestos, and lead.[176,177]

Household chemicals are common ingredients in many products, including personal care products, such as hair sprays and spray deodorants; paints; hobby and home improvement supplies, such as glues and markers; aerosol sprays; cleaners and disinfectants; and automotive products. Household chemicals can irritate eyes, nose, and throat; cause headaches, visual disorders, and memory impairment; damage the central nervous system and kidneys; and possibly increase the risk of cancer.[176]

Radon is an odorless, colorless gas that comes from the breakdown of uranium that is in rocks and soil beneath the home. Radon is the second leading cause of lung cancer in the U.S. after smoking. About 15,000 people each year die from lung cancer caused by radon.[176]

Biological contaminants are or were living organisms and include bacteria, mold, mildew, animal dander, dust mites, cockroaches, and pollen. Two conditions are necessary to support biological contaminants: nutrients and moisture. Mold is a fungus (plant) that causes the disintegration of organic materials such as cloth, paint, and paper. Mildew is the coating and discoloring of the organic materials caused by the mold. Mold and mildew can irritate your eyes, nose, and throat; cause shortness of breath; dizziness; fever; digestive problems; and can trigger asthma.[176]

Public exposure standards and guidelines often are not readily available. There is very little basic hazard data available to support risk assessments for many chemicals that may find their way into the community environment. EPA developed the Chemical Right-to-Know initiative in 1998.[178] Due to the lack of basic hazard data, this has hindered risk assessment for many chemicals. Several efforts have been launched under this initiative.[178–180] For example, the voluntary High Production Volume Challenge program concerns the testing of chemicals produced or imported in quantities over one million pounds per year. There is also an initiative to develop a test rule for chemicals not tested under the voluntary HPV program. Finally, there is an initiative for a Voluntary Children's Chemical Evaluation program for selected chemicals of concern to the health of children. Although these programs will not generate immediate basic hazard data, in the future this data will support sound risk assessments by OEH professionals. The EPA Child-Specific Exposure Factors Handbook published in 2008 consolidates all child exposure data into one single document.[7] This handbook provides information on various physiological and behavioral factors commonly used in assessing children's exposure to environmental chemicals.

Emergency Management — An All-Hazards Approach

Emergency Management and Business Continuity Planning

It is often said that emergency management and business continuity planning are not new activities, having been included previously in such activities as civil defense, severe weather preparedness practiced by those on the Gulf Coast or in Tornado Alley, and good stewardship of business resources. However, events such as the Oklahoma City bombing (1995), Y2K (2000), 9-11 (2001), and Hurricane Katrina (2005) have focused national attention on emergency management and highlighted many areas for improvement. The Department of Homeland Security (DHS), and specifically FEMA have invested heavily in programs and initiatives to improve our national ability to manage disasters and catastrophes. National capacity has been upgraded by adoption of standard procedures such as the Incident Command System[182], and programs to assist local jurisdictions to purchase equipment and train staff.

The overarching philosophy of modern emergency management is prevention, mitigation, preparedness, response, and recovery from "all hazards," including human-caused, natural, and technological disasters. All-hazard management is based on the concept that proper preparation for hurricanes and terrorists, lead to better preparation for tornadoes and pandemic flu. In other words, the planning process is more valuable than the resulting plans. Public safety departments have traditionally been involved in response, but increasingly, environmental health and safety departments are involved in prevention / mitigation, preparedness, and recovery.

NFPA 1600 *Standard on Disaster/ Emergency Management and Business Continuity Programs*[183], which provides basic criteria for a comprehensive program, categorizes hazards as those caused by nature (geological, meteorological, and biological), by humans (accidental and intentional), and by technology. Geological hazards include earthquakes, floods, and volcanoes; meteorological hazards include storms, floods, and hurricanes; and diseases, epidemics, and infestations would be considered biological hazards. Fires, explosions, and fuel shortages would be considered accidental hazards caused by humans; while bomb threats, wars, riots, and sabotage would be considered intentional. Computer failures, equipment malfunctions, software bugs, and energy shortages are considered technological hazards.[184]

Even though the all-hazards approach is most effective in protecting an individual, organization, or community, emergency management efforts can be maximized by conducting risk assessments to evaluate the probability and impact of specific potential adverse events with respect to vulnerable populations, natural, and built resources. Potential roles for industrial hygiene risk assessors are illustrated in the following paragraphs.

1. Local Emergency Planning Committees, created under SARA, Title III, Emergency Planning Community Right to Know Act (EPCRA) regulations, must develop emergency plans for incidents involving the manufacture, storage, or transportation of hazardous materials.[185] Risk assessment skills are invaluable in weighing the probably and severity of various accident scenarios.
2. Since November 2004, FEMA has required cities, counties, and tribal governments to have approved disaster mitigation plans in place to be eligible for certain types of disaster-recovery aid following natural disasters. These plans must include a risk assessment and a description of mitigation measures.[186]
3. At the community level, homeland security threat and risk assessments are designed to further the national mission to prevent, protect, respond, and recover from enemy attack with CBRNE (chemical, biological, radiological, nuclear, and explosive) weapons. Local jurisdictions may conduct threat and vulnerability assessments, which are combined in the risk assessment. Individual vulnerability assessments may be conducted on potential targets, e.g., on hospitals, research facilities, or schools. The jurisdiction would then conduct a gap analysis to diagnose its resource needs by comparing desired capabilities with current capabilities.[187]
4. At the organizational level, a hazard vulnerability assessment is a comprehensive analysis of the potential for various hazards to impact an organization, and its ability to manage the situation and remain in business. Hazard identification and vulnerability assessment are combined in a risk analysis, which can then serve as the basis of an effective emergency preparedness, response, and recovery plan. In the first step, hazards are defined and described, taking into account physical characteristics, magnitude and severity, probability and frequency, causative factors, and locations/areas affected. The vulnerability of people and property are evaluated in the vulnerability assessment, which covers the extent of injury/illness and damage that might result from a hazardous event of a given intensity occurring over a certain geographic area. These two components are combined in the risk analysis, which compares the estimation of probability of the hazards with the vulnerability to damage and injury.[184] An example of a hazard vulnerability model is presented in Table 8.8, Hazard and Vulnerability Assessment Tool.
5. Other analyses conducted at the organizational level include business continuity and recovery (BCR) planning and continuity of operations planning (COOP). BCR planning asks what are the critical functions performed by a unit, who can perform those functions, what information, supplies, or equipment are needed to perform those functions, who is cross-trained to provide backup, and what alternate locations are available to conduct those functions.

The information technology department is normally involved in BCR planning. COOP planning is similar, but in common usage refers more to planning to maintain governmental operations in the face of catastrophic events.

6. The AIHA® White Paper on "Industrial Hygienists' Role and Responsibilities in

Table 8.8 — Hazard and Vulnerability Assessment Tool(184)

NATURALLY OCCURRING EVENTS								
		SEVERITY = (MAGNITUDE – MITIGATION)						
EVENT	PROBABILITY	HUMAN IMPACT	PROPERTY IMPACT	BUSINESS IMPACT	PREPARED-NESS	INTERNAL RESPONSE	EXTERNAL RESPONSE	RISK
	Likelihood this will occur	*Possibility of death or injury*	*Physical losses and damages*	*Interruption of services*	*Preplanning*	*Time, effectiveness, resources*	*Community/ Mutual Aid staff and supplies*	*Relative threat**
SCORE	*0 = N/A 1 = Low 2 = Moderate 3 = High*	*0 = N/A 1 = Low 2 = Moderate 3 = High*	*0 = N/A 1 = Low 2 = Moderate 3 = High*	*0 = N/A 1 = Low 2 = Moderate 3 = High*	*0 = N/A 1 = High 2 = Moderate 3 = Low or none*	*0 = N/A 1 = High 2 = Moderate 3 = Low or none*	*0 = N/A 1 = High 2 = Moderate 3 = Low or none*	*0 - 100%*
Hurricane								**0%**
Tornado								**0%**
Severe Thunderstorm								**0%**
Snow Fall								**0%**
Blizzard								**0%**
Ice Storm								**0%**
Earthquake								**0%**
Tidal Wave								**0%**
Temperature Extremes								**0%**
Drought								**0%**
Flood, External								**0%**
Wild Fire								**0%**
Landslide								**0%**
Dam Inundation								**0%**
Volcano								**0%**
Epidemic								**0%**
AVERAGE SCORE	**0.00**	**0.00**	**0.00**	**0.00**	**0.00**	**0.00**	**0.00**	**0%**
*Threat increases with percentage.								
		—	Risk=Probability x Severity					

Emergency Preparedness and Response"[188] is an excellent resource for IHs who wish to expand their professional horizons to include assessment and management of risks associated with natural disaster, hazardous material accidents, and terrorism events. Industrial hygiene training and experience are well suited to the incident management priority to save lives and protect the health and safety of the public, responders, and recovery workers.[189] Industrial hygienists skilled in risk assessment may be especially valuable in analyzing hazards and risks, both before and during incidents. They may participate in pre-planning for major incidents, specifically by defining the types of disasters likely to be encountered, identifying the specific hazards as a result of those disasters, identifying the immediate response, and the hazards associated with those response actions. Industrial hygienists may also conduct risk assessments of airborne chemical hazards during an incident such as a chemical spill, determining the risk to responders and to the public.

Emergency management as a profession has been promoted through continuing and professional education.[190,191] Academic programs are available ranging from bachelor to PhD degrees, and professional certifications. Professional associations of emergency managers include the International Association of Emergency Managers, which manages the Certified Emergency Manager® program, and the National Emergency Management Association. State-level associations such as the Colorado Emergency Managers Association provide local opportunities for training and networking. The industrial hygiene paradigm of "anticipation, recognition, evaluation, and control" and strong emphasis on prevention are very compatible with the emergency management model of mitigation / prevention, preparedness, response, and recovery. Combined with self-study or formal training programs, the traditional scientific and technical education and analytical experience of industrial hygienists are excellent preparation for work in emergency management.

Uncertainty and Variability in Risk Assessment

Uncertainty and Variability

Throughout the risk assessment process, the analyst is faced with variability and uncertainty. There is some inconsistency among authors in the use of these terms. The term *uncertainty* often includes both variability and lack of data. Variability is the result of heterogeneity or actual differences among members of a population. It may be more accurately characterized but not reduced with additional data. Uncertainty results from measurement limitations and may be related to study design and analytical techniques or application of data to unsampled populations. Further measurements ultimately will reduce uncertainty.[192,193] Pending additional data and complete understanding of the underlying physical and biological processes, uncertainty must be resolved through the use of expert judgment.[194] Evans, et al.[195] described a method that incorporates expert judgment, probability distributions, and probability trees in the uncertainty analysis of carcinogenic potency. The probability tree allows components of the risk analysis to be disaggregated, with the judgments of experts weighing more heavily in components related to their expertise. This method encourages differences of opinion and allows all relevant information to be considered in risk characterization.

In lieu of additional data or knowledge, however, risk assessors tend to make conservative assumptions to ensure that any errors in risk estimation are in the direction of public health protection. This may lead to risk estimates that are overly conservative. For example, using conservative estimates for all input factors (e.g., the 95th percentiles of the distributions for inputs that are positively correlated with risk and the 5th percentile of the inputs that are negatively correlated) may lead to risk estimates as high as the 99.99th percentile of the distribution of risk estimates.[196] The risk assessor thus has a responsibility to examine the risk assessment to delineate sources and approximate magnitudes of errors. This analysis has two important purposes: to acknowledge and inform the users of the risk assessment (expert and lay readers alike) of potential sources and directions of error, and to identify those data gaps that can be effectively narrowed through the collection of additional data.

Several methods are commonly used to analyze and present uncertainty and variability in risk assessment, ranging from qualitative to quantitative techniques. The appropriate level of uncertainty analysis depends largely on the level of effort devoted to the risk assessment itself (that is, screening, moderate, or complex). In many situations a qualitative uncertainty analysis will suffice. The risk assessor simply lists the possible sources of uncertainty and variability and indicates the likely direction and magnitude of impact that each source will have on the final risk estimates. If enough data is available, the risk assessor can calculate the risk using the mean of the exposure data (reasonable average exposure) and then compare that with risk associated with the reasonable maximum exposure (RME). The range in the risk values would represent the uncertainty in the estimates (i.e., a semi-quantitative uncertainty analysis). Another approach is the sensitivity analysis, in which an input variable is varied by ±10 or ±25% to determine impact on risk estimate.[197]

There are many ways to evaluate confidence in a risk assessment. The U.S. Army Public Health Command (Provisional) (formerly U.S. Army Center for Health Promotion and Preventive Medicine) developed a simple approach for helping to determining confidence in a risk assessment.[198] They selected and defined three confidence levels: High, Medium, and Low. They then provided some criteria (See Table 8.9) to determine a subjective risk confidence level. This determination might benefit risk communication since uncertainty in the risk estimate is further clarified.

- High Confidence. High confidence in a risk level implies significant understanding of all the variables used to determine the risk. It results from sampling data that is adequate to characterize typical exposures and the range of those types of exposures, as well as a good understanding of the exposure patterns of the population being characterized. Additionally, the endpoints indicated by the exposure guideline chosen should be plausible for the exposure of interest.
- Medium Confidence. Medium confidence in a risk level implies some understanding of most of the variables used to determine the risk. It results from sampling data that is plausibly adequate to characterize typical exposures and the range of those types of exposures. Additionally a reasonable assumption that the exposure patterns of the population being characterized will indicate a true lower risk could

Table 8.9 — Notional criteria for determining confidence in your risk assessment[197]

Confidence	*Criteria*
High	- Field Sampling data quality is very good — substantial samples over time/space. - Field activity patterns are well known. - True exposures are reasonably approximated. - Knowledge of the symptoms of hazard exposure relative to guideline is well known. - No important missing information. - The predicted health outcome is highly plausible (strong toxicological weight of evidence/human data) or already demonstrated.
Medium	- Field data quality is relatively good. - Estimates of field exposure are likely to be greater than true exposures due to incomplete data coverage relative to actual exposure durations. - Detailed information is lacking regarding true personnel activity patterns in the field. - Symptoms are well known for each individual hazard, but some scientific evidence suggests that the combined effects of all hazards may exacerbate symptoms. - Predicted health outcome is plausible but there is toxicological data but limited weight of evidence/ human data is lacking.
Low	- Important data gaps and/or inconsistencies exist. - Exposure conditions are not well defined. - Field personnel activity patterns are basically unknown. - Predicted health outcome is not plausible because it is not consistent with real-world events/experience.

also indicate this level of confidence. Toxicity endpoints indicated by the exposure guideline chosen should be plausible for the exposure of interest.

- Low Confidence. Low confidence is assigned when sampling data may not be adequate to characterize the situation, and when the assessor is making a best scientific assessment in the absence of complete information.

Quantitative uncertainty analysis, such as first-order Taylor series or Monte Carlo analysis requires the highest level of effect and amount of input data but also provides the greatest information about uncertainty in the risk assessment.

Monte Carlo Analysis

Monte Carlo analysis has been used for more than 50 years to compute difficult multidimensional integrals in physics, chemistry, and other technical disciplines.[193] Its ability to combine probability distributions for several input variables to generate probability distributions for output variables makes it an obvious selection for analysis of uncertainty in risk assessment. Readily available software for personal computers, such as spreadsheet packages (Excel for Windows™) and add-ons (CrystalBall™) has greatly simplified the computational aspects of Monte Carlo analysis.

In a deterministic risk assessment a point estimate for each input variable (concentration, intake, etc.) is used to calculate a point estimate of risk. The point estimate selected is usually a high-end estimate (high end of the distribution (e.g., 95th percentile), which might lead to overestimates of risk. In contrast, in Monte Carlo analysis a value for each input parameter is selected randomly from a probability distribution value, and risk is then calculated according to the model equation (see Figure 8.6). The process may be repeated thousands of times to produce a probability distribution for the risk estimate, allowing the risk assessor to determine the mean and upper bound of the risk estimate and identify the input variables contributing the most to uncertainty. A comparison conducted by Smith[199] indicated that at the site investigated, the deterministic RME cancer risk estimate was between the 95th percentile and the maximum estimate produced by Monte Carlo analysis, suggesting that the RME risk calculation was protective and the results of probabilistic and deterministic calculations were consistent.[198,199]

There are, however, limitations to this technique, including the requirement for knowledge of probability distributions and covariance (degree of dependence) for input parameters. Finley et al.[192] proposed age-specific distributions for a variety of exposure factors, including soil ingestion rates, tap water consumption, and soil-on-skin adherence). Exposure factors developed from short-term studies with large populations may not accurately represent long-term conditions in small populations. Also, the tails of Monte Carlo risk distributions, which are of greatest regulatory interest, are very sensitive to the shape of input distributions. For this reason, Burmaster and Anderson[193] suggested that the risk analyst should run enough iterations (usually 10,000) to demonstrate numerical stability of the tails of the outputs. Other principles of good practice for the use of Monte Carlo analysis developed by the authors include suggestions to show all formulae used, calculate and present estimates, restrict the use of probabilistic techniques to the pathways and compounds of regulatory interest, and to the extent possible, contrast variability and uncertainty. Whenever possible, use measurement data, present the name and statistical quality of the random number generator used, and discuss the limitations of the methods and interpretation of the results.

Occupational and environmental hygienists should familiarize themselves with the Monte Carlo technique. Its ability to provide a range of risk estimates in the form of a

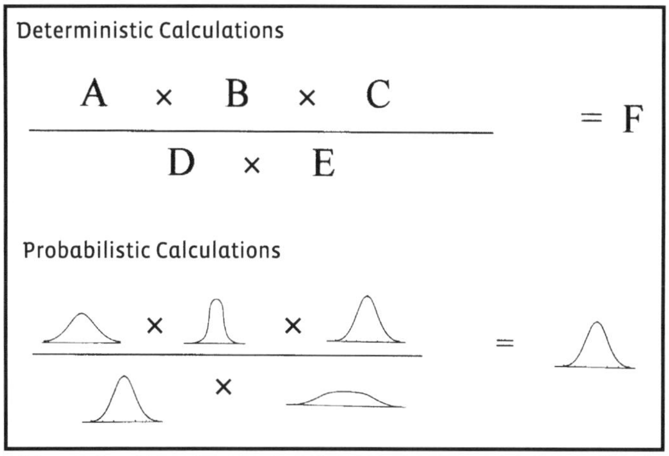

Figure 8.6 — Use of input distributions to generate output distributions in Monte Carlo analysis.

probability distribution makes it a potentially valuable tool in risk communication and in selection of risk management options. Several EPA regions have begun to accept Monte Carlo simulations submitted as uncertainty analysis given certain restrictions.[200] Many professional risk assessors have adopted Monte Carlo as a routine analytical technique and believe that it will continue to gain wider acceptance.

Conclusion

The purpose of this chapter has been to facilitate the integration of risk assessment into the practice of occupational hygiene. Toward that end, the basic concepts of risk assessment were introduced through discussions of risk, regulation of risk, and the risk assessment process. It has been suggested that political, economic, and technological changes force a new approach. Integration of risk assessment and occupational hygiene in an iterative framework can provide effective allocation of resources while minimizing errors, protecting worker and community health and safety, improving national security and emergency response, and meeting the traditional objectives of protecting the bottom line and avoiding liability.

Those who are responsible for worker health and safety, public health, emergency preparedness, environmental health, and the wider community must keep in mind the following points: first, there is a professional and ethical responsibility for the outcomes of evaluations and risk characterizations. Therefore, the recognition that OEH risk assessment extends beyond the collection of airborne concentration data and comparison with the occupational exposure limits is essential. New approaches and methods will continue to be developed independently or adapted from the companion OEH, safety, and security disciplines. Second, workers and the public need to be protected from occupational, environmental, and nontraditional hazards in a manner that is effective and cost efficient. As the experts in risk assessment for occupational and environmental scenarios, OEH professionals must continue to explore and develop new methodologies of practicing the profession, especially in the face of economic challenges, a deregulated environment, and nontraditional hazards.

Risk assessment, with all its diversity and flexibility, is a proven tool in the risk management process that belongs in the OEH professional's toolbox.

Key Terms and Definitions:

Acute effect: An adverse effect (usually) arising from a short exposure (minutes to hours) to a chemical.

Acute exposure: Large dose/short time.

Acute toxicity: The adverse effects resulting from a single dose or single exposure to a substance. Ordinarily refers to effects occurring within a short time following administration. Terminology and units used for different descriptive categories of toxicity vary. Examples of toxicity classifications as defined by different organizations are:

Acute Exposure Guideline Levels (AEGLs): Developed by the EPA, these guidelines represent threshold exposure limits for the general public and are applicable to emergency exposure periods ranging from 10 minutes to 8 hours. AEGL-2 and AEGL-3, and AEGL-1 values as appropriate, will be developed for each of five exposure periods (10 and 30 minutes, 1 hour, 4 hours, and 8 hours) and will be distinguished by varying degrees of severity of toxic effects. It is believed that the recommended exposure levels are applicable to the general population including infants and children, and other individuals who may be susceptible.

Benchmark Dose (BMD): An exposure due to a dose of a substance associated with a specified low incidence of risk, generally in the range of 1% to 10%, of a health effect; or the dose associated with a specified measure or change of a biological effect.

Catastrophe: an adverse event which involves multiple communities, with long-term severe impacts to the population, built environment, and normal operations

Cancer Slope Factor: The slope of the curve representing the relationship between dose and cancer risk. When estimated with the linearized multistage model, the slope factor is the upper 95 percent confidence limit of the slope (upper-bound estimate of risk). Also called cancer potency factor. Expressed as risk (mg/kg-day)$^{-1}$ **or** risk per mg/kg-day.

Chronic daily intake: Intake averaged over a long period of time (seven years to lifetime).

Chronic effect: Disease symptom or process of long duration, usually frequent in occurrence, and almost always debilitating.

Chronic exposure: Small dose/long time.

Chronic toxicity: Adverse health effects that can occur from prolonged, repeated exposure to relatively low levels of a substance; might have a chronic effect from an acute exposure.

Confidence Limit: An estimated value below (or above) which the true value of an estimated parameter is expected to lie for a specified percentage of such estimated limits.

Control banding: A complementary approach to protecting worker health by utilizing finite resources to identify and implement exposure controls. Given the reality that appropriate occupational exposure limits cannot be established for every chemical in use, a chemical is assigned to a "band" for control measures, for example, based on its hazard classification according to international criteria, the amount of chemical in use, and its volatility/dustiness. The outcome is a recommended control strategy.

Disaster: an adverse event whose management requires external resources, e.g., mutual aid

Effective concentration "X" (ECX): The concentration of a material that has caused a biological effect to X percent of the test animals.

Emergency: an adverse event which can be managed with standard operating procedures and local resources

Emergency Response Planning Guidelines (ERPGs™): Values above which one could reasonably anticipate observing adverse health effects (see ERPG-1; ERPG-2; ERPG-3). The term also refers to the documentation that summarizes the basis for those values. The documentation is contained in a series of guides produced by the Emergency Response Planning Committee™ of AIHA®.

Exposure: (1) As it pertains to air contaminants, it is the state of being exposed to a concentration of a contaminant. (2) Subjection of an employee in the course of employment to a chemical that is a physical or health hazard, and includes potential (e.g., accidental or possible) exposure. "Subjected" in terms of health hazards includes any route of entry (e.g., inhalation, ingestion, skin contact, or absorption). (3) Contact of an organism with a chemical or physical agent, quantified as the amount of chemical available at the exchange boundaries of the organism and available for absorption. Usually calculated as the mean exposure and some measure of maximum exposure. (4) The amount of an environmental agent that has reached the individual (external dose) or has been absorbed into the individual(internal dose or absorbed dose).

Exposure route: The way an organism comes into contact with a chemical or physical agent (e.g., ingestion, inhalation, dermal contact, etc.).

Hazard: Source of risk. A condition with the potential to cause injury, illness, or death of personnel; damage to or loss of equipment or property; or mission degradation.

Hazard index: Sum of more than one hazard quotient for multiple substances and/or multiple exposure pathways. Calculated separately for chronic, subchronic, and shorter-duration exposures.

Hazard quotient: Ratio of a single substance exposure level over a specified period to a reference dose (RfD) for that substance derived from a similar exposure period.

Immediately Dangerous to Life and Health (IDLH): Any atmosphere that poses an immediate hazard to life or poses immediate irreversible debilitating effects on health.

Integrated Risk Information System (IRIS): U.S. EPA database containing verified reference doses (RfDs), cancer slope factors, and current health and regulatory information. It is the EPA's preferred source of toxicity information for Superfund.

Iterative risk assessment: A process in which increasingly complex and data-rich risk assessments are conducted

Lifetime cancer risk estimate: The result of the exposure and toxicity assessments of a carcinogen. Represents the upper bound of the probability of an individual developing cancer as a result of lifetime exposure to the chemical.

LC_{50}: The airborne concentration of a given substance that when inhaled over a period of time will kill 50% of the animals under test.

Lowest Observed Adverse Effect Level (LOAEL): The lowest dose or exposure level of a chemical in a study at which there is a statistically or biologically significant increase in the frequency or severity of an adverse effect in the exposed population as compared with an appropriate, unexposed control group.

Military exposure guideline (MEG): MEGs are concentrations for chemicals in air, water, and soil that can be used to assist in assessing the significance of exposures to occupational and environmental chemical hazards during deployments. They are designed to assess a variety of military exposure scenarios, such as a single release of large amounts of a chemical, temporary exposure conditions lasting hours to days, or for continuous ambient environmental conditions, such as a regional pollution.

Military-unique workplace, operations, equipment, and systems: A DA military and civilian operation and workplace that is unique to the national defense mission. This includes combat and operation, testing, and maintenance of military-unique equipment and systems such as military weapons, ordnance, and tactical vehicles. It also includes operations such as peacekeeping missions; field maneuvers; combat training; military-unique Research, Development, Test, and Evaluation activities; and actions required under national defense contingency conditions.

Monte Carlo analysis: A method that obtains a probabilistic approximation to the solution of a problem by using statistical sampling techniques.

No Observed Adverse Effect Level (NOAEL): An exposure level at which there are no statistically or biologically significant increases in the frequency or severity of adverse effects between the exposed population and its appropriate control; some effects may be produced at this level, but they are not considered as adverse or precursors to adverse effects. In an experiment with several NOAELs, the regulatory focus is primarily on the highest one, leading to the common usage of the term NOAEL as the highest exposure without adverse effect.

Nonmilitary-unique workplace or operation: A DA military or civilian workplace or operation that is comparable generally to those of the private sector. Examples include facilities involved and work performed in the repair and overhaul of weapons, vessels, aircraft, or vehicles (except for equipment trials); construction; supply services; civil engineer or public works; medical services; and office work.

Occupational Exposure Limit (OEL): A health-based workplace standard to protect workers from adverse exposure (e.g., PELs, TLVs®, RELs, WEELs, etc.).

Permissible Exposure Limit (PEL): Established by OSHA (see 29 CFR 1910.1000, Subpart Z). The permissible concentration in air of a substance to which nearly all workers may be repeatedly exposed 8 hours a day, 40 hours a week, for 30 years without adverse effects.

Potency: Potency is measured by the fraction of a population affected by a specific dose, for example, the dose at which 50% of a population will develop cancer. Agents of increasing potency will achieve a population effect at a lower dose (level and duration of exposure). Increasing the exposure or the gravity of effect or potency of the chemical will result in increased risk.

Reasonable Maximum Exposure: (RME): Used in conservative exposure assessment calculations. Based not on worstcase scenario, but on 90% or 95% upper confidence limits on input parameters.

Reference Concentration (RfC): An estimate (with uncertainty spanning perhaps an order of magnitude) of a continuous inhalation exposure to the human population (including sensitive subgroups) that is likely to be without an appreciable risk of deleterious non-cancer effects during a lifetime.

Reference dose: (RfD): U.S. EPA toxicity value for evaluating noncarcinogenic effects resulting from exposures at Superfund sites. An estimate (with uncertainty spanning an order of magnitude or greater) of daily exposure level for humans, including sensitive subpopulations, that is likely to be without an appreciable risk or deleterious effects during a lifetime.

Risk: Contains two components: the severity or impact of an adverse event, and the probability or likelihood of that event occurring. With respect to chemical hazards, risk is thus a function of the toxicity of and exposure to a harmful substance.

Risk assessment: The systematic process of determining the probability and magnitude of an undesired event and estimating the cost to human society or the environment in terms of morbidity, mortality, or economic impact, either quantitatively or qualitatively.

Risk characterization: The risk assessment step that characterizes the potential for adverse health effects and evaluates the uncertainty involved.

Risk communication: the exchange of information and opinions among interested parties about a hazard and the nature, magnitude, significance, and/or control of health risks.

Risk estimate: Different expressions of risk may have different implications: (1) individual lifetime risk — the risk of an individual developing the adverse health effect sometime during the remaining lifespan; (2) population or societal risk - the integration of the individual lifetime risk over the exposed population; (3) relative risk -the probability of developing a specific adverse health effect given exposure to a risk agent compared with the same probability given no exposure to the agent; (4)standardized mortality ratio (SMR) - death rate due to a specific cause in an exposed population compared with the death rate in the general population; used often in occupational epidemiology studies; 5) loss of life expectancy — individual lifetime risk multiplied by 36 years equals the average remaining lifetime.

Risk management: the process of identifying, evaluating, selecting, and implementing actions to reduce risk to human health and to ecosystems. The goal of risk management is scientifically sound, cost-effective, integrated actions that reduce or prevent risks while taking into account social, cultural, ethical, political, and legal considerations. Risk management includes all activities undertaken to mitigate a hazard. These activities include the process of identifying, assessing, and controlling risks arising from operational factors and making decisions that may require balancing costs with benefits.

Screening Risk Assessment: A risk assessment performed with few data and many assumptions to identify exposures that should be evaluated more carefully for potential risk.

Short-Term Exposure Limit (STEL): (1) Maximum concentration for continuous 15-minute period. Allowed four times a day, with at least 60 minutes between exposures. (2) Used in reference to the OSHA PEL–STEL and ACGIH's TLV–STEL. The STEL represents a time weighted average (TWA) exposure that should not be exceeded for any 15-minute period. (3) STELs are recommended when exposures of even short duration to high concentrations of a chemical are known to produce acute toxicity. It is the concentration to which workers can be exposed continuously for a short period of time without suffering from 1) irritation; 2)chronic or irreversible tissue damage; or 3) narcosis of sufficient degree to increase the likelihood of accidental injury, impaired self-rescue, or reduced work efficiency. A STEL is defined as a 15-minute TWA exposure that should not be exceeded at any time during a workday, even if the overall 8-hour TWA is within limits, and it should not occur more than four times per day. There should be at least 60 minutes between successive exposures in this range. If warranted, an averaging period other than 15 minutes can also be used.

Temporary Emergency Exposure Limits (TEELs): Values intended to provide estimates of concentration ranges above which one could reasonably anticipate observing adverse health effects. The term also refers to the documentation that summarizes the basis for those values. The four levels of TEEL values are based on a 15-minute time-weighted average (similar to a short-term exposure limit) for a total of four values.

Threshold Limit Value (TLV®): Used by the American Conference of Governmental Industrial Hygienists (ACGIH®) to designate degree of exposure to contaminants and expressed as parts of vapor or gas per million parts of air by volume at 25°C and 760 mmHg pressure, or as approximate milligrams of particulate per cubic meter of air (mg/m^3). (See also permissible concentration.) An exposure level under which most people can work consistently for 8 hours a day, daily, with no harmful effects. TLVs® are listed as either an 8-hour TWA or a 15-minute STEL.

Threshold Limit Value–Time-Weighted Average (TLV®–TWA): The time-weighted average concentration for a normal 8-hour workday and a 40-hour workweek to which nearly all workers may be exposed repeatedly, day after day, without adverse effects.

Toxicity assessment: Both qualitative and quantitative data are developed in a toxicity assessment: 1) a description of the types of health effects that might be expected to occur in humans; and 2) some estimate of toxicity, such as the dose required to cause these health effects. Conceptually, this estimate of toxicity is based on a dose-response curve. The outcome of the toxicity assessment may be a slope factor or an exposure limit. Slope factors are based on the slope of the dose response curve and can be used to develop a probabilistic risk estimate.

Toxicity value: Numerical expression of a substance's dose response relationship. The most common values used in Superfund risk assessments are reference doses (RfDs) for noncarcinogenic effects and slope factors for carcinogenic effects.

Uncertainty: The unknown effects of parameters (e.g., effect, severity, or prevalence of a hazard), variables, or relationships that cannot or have not been verified or estimated by measurement or experimentation.

Variability: Observable diversity in biological sensitivity or response, and in exposure parameters (such as breathing rates, food consumption, etc.) These differences can be better understood, but generally not reduced by further research.

Workplace Environmental Exposure Level (WEEL™) guides: Exposure guidelines developed by AIHA intended to protect the health and safety of workers exposed to hazardous substances or conditions.

Worker Population Limit (WPL): Maximum allowable 8-hour time-weighted average concentration of chemical agent that an unmasked worker could be exposed to for an 8-hour workday and 40-hour week for 30 years without adverse effect.

References

1. **Harris, M.K. (ed.):** *Essential Resources for Industrial Hygiene: A Compendium of Current Practice Standards and Guidelines.* AIHA Standards Practice and Guidelines Committee, Fairfax, VA: AIHA Press, 2000.
2. **Bratt, G.M., C. Laszcz-Davis, and M.A. Jayjock:** *Risk Assessment, Management and Communication*, Chapter 7, Industrial Hygiene Compendium of Current Practice Standards and Guidelines. Fairfax, VA: AIHA Press, 2007.
3. **Corn, J.K.:** *Response to Occupational Health Hazards: A Historical Perspective.* New York: Van Nostrand Reinhold, 1992.
4. **Jayjock, M.A., J.R. Lynch, and D.L. Nelson:** *Fundamentals of Risk Assessment for the Industrial Hygienist,* Fairfax, VA: AIHA Press, 2000.
5. **U.S. Environmental Protection Agency (EPA):** *Exposure Factors Handbook* (EPA/600/P-95/002); Washington, D.C.: EPA, 1997.
6. **U.S. Environmental Protection Agency (EPA):** *Exposure Factors Handbook* (EPA/600/8-89/043). Washington, D.C.: EPA, 1990.
7. **U.S. Environmental Protection Agency (EPA):** *Child-Specific Exposure Factors Handbook.* Washington, DC.: EPA, 2008.

8. **U.S. Environmental Protection Agency (EPA):** Guidance on selecting age groups for monitoring and assessing childhood exposures to environmental contaminants. National Center for Environmental Assessment, Washington, D.C.: EPA/630/P-03/003F, 2005. Available from: National Technical Information Service, Springfield, VA, and online at http://epa.gov/ncea.
9. **U.S. Environmental Protection Agency (EPA):** Example Exposure Scenarios. National Center for Environmental Assessment, Washington, D.C.: EPA/600/R-03/036, 2003. Available from: National Information Service, Springfield, VA; PB2003-103280 and at http://www.epa.gov/ncea
10. **U.S. Environmental Protection Agency (EPA):** Sociodemographic Data Used for Identifying Potentially Highly Exposed Populations. U.S. Environmental Protection Agency, Washington, D.C.: EPA/600/R-99/060, 1999.
11. **American Chemical Society:** Understanding Risk Analysis, A Short Guide for Health, Safety, and Environmental Policy Making. Washington, D.C.: American Chemical Society, 1998.
12. **Covello, V.T. and J. Mumpower:** Risk analysis and risk management: An historical perspective. *Risk Anal. 5*:103–120 (1985).
13. **Bernstein, P.L.:** *Against the Gods: The Remarkable Story of Risk.* Hoboken, NJ: John Wiley & Sons, 1996.
14. **Hempel, S.:** *The Strange Case of the Broad Street Pump: John Snow and the Mystery of Cholera* . Berkeley, CA: University of California Press, 2007.
15. **Williams, P.L., and J.L. Burson:** *Industrial Toxicology: Safety and Health Applications in the Workplace.* New York: Van Nostrand Reinhold, 1985.
16. **National Academy of Sciences:** *Toxicity Testing in the Twenty-first Century: A Vision and a Strategy.* Washington, D.C.: National Academies Press, 2007.
17. **Salvato, J.A.:** *Environmental Engineering and Sanitation*, 4th edition. New York: John Wiley ə Sons, Inc., 1992.
18. **Vesilind, P.A., J.J. Peirce, and R.F. Weiner:** *Environmental Pollution and Control*, 3rd edition. Boston, MA: Butterworth-Heinemann, 1990.
19. **Andrews, R.N.:** Reform or Reaction: EPA at a crossroads. *Environ. Sci. Tech. 29*:505A–510A (1995).
20. **U.S. Environmental Protection Agency (EPA):** *Risk Assessment Guidance for Superfund*, vol. I, part A (EPA/540/1-89/002). Washington, DC: EPA, 1989.
21. **U.S. Environmental Protection Agency (EPA):** *Risk Assessment Guidance for Superfund*, vol. I, part B (Pub. 9285.7-01B). Washington, DC: EPA, 1991.
22. **U.S. Environmental Protection Agency (EPA):** *Risk Assessment Guidance for Superfund*, vol. I, part C (Pub. 9285.7-01C). Washington, DC: EPA, 1991.
23. **Percival, R.V., A.S. Miller, C.H. Schroeder, and J.P. Leape:** *Environmental Regulation: Law, Science, and Policy.* Boston, MA: Little, Brown and Co., 1992.
24. **National Research Council, Committee on the Institutional Means for Assessment of Risks to Public Health, Commission on Life Sciences:** *Risk Assessment in the Federal Government: Managing the Process.* Washington, D.C.: National Academy Press, 1983.
25. **National Academy of Sciences:** *Science and Judgment in Risk Assessment.* Washington, D.C.: National Academy of Sciences, 1994.
26. **U.S. Presidential/Congressional Commission on Risk Assessment and Risk Management (USPCCRARM):** *Framework for Environmental Health Risk Management*, Final Report, vol. 1. Washington, D.C.: USPCCRARM, 1997.
27. **U.S. Presidential/Congressional Commission on Risk Assessment and Risk Management (USPCCRARM):** *Risk Assessment and Risk Management in Regulatory Decision-Making*, Final Report, vol. 2. Washington, D.C.: USPCCRARM, 1997
28. **National Academy of Sciences:** *Science and Decisions: Advancing Risk Assessment.* National Academies Press, Washington, D.C. 2008.
29. **Rushefsky, M.E.:** *Making Cancer Policy.* Albany, NY: State University of New York Press, 1986.
30. **United States Code**, Title 29, Chapter 15 *Occupational Safety and Health*, Section 655(b)(5), page 157, Washington DC, 2001. "Occupational Safety and Health Act," Pub. Law 91-596, Section 2193. 91st Congress, Dec. 29, 1970; as amended, Pub. Law 101-552, Section 3101, Nov. 5, 1990.
31. **Congressional Information System, Inc. (CIS):** *Abstracts of Congressional Publications and Legislative History Citations* (Quadrennial series, including 1974, 1978, 1982, 1986, 1990, and 1994). Washington, D.C.: CIS.
32. **U.S. Environmental Protection Agency (EPA):** *Food Quality Protection Act of 1996.* [Online] Available: http://www.epa.gov/pesticides/regulating/laws/fqpa/fqpahigh.htm. Published 31 January 2001. (Accessed 31 March 2009).
33. **Rodricks, J.V., S.M. Brett, and G.C. Wrenn:** Significant risk decisions in federal regulatory agencies. *Reg. Toxicol. Pharmacol. 7*: 307–320 (1987).

34. **Mantel, N., and W.R. Bryan:** Safety testing of carcinogens. *J. Nat. Cancer Inst. 27*:455–460 (1961).
35. **Laborers' Health &. Safety Fund of North America:** Memorandum to U.S. Department of Labor, Office of the Assistant Secretary for Policy, Subject: *Risk Assessment Policy*, Available: http://www.defendingscience.org/case_studies/upload/Laborers-on-DOL-RA-Sept-2008.pdf, September 29,2008
36. **Mintz, B.:** *History of the Federal Occupational Safety and Health Administration.* In B.A. Plog, J. Niland, and P.B. Quinlan, editors, *Fundamentals of Industrial Hygiene*, 4th ed., Itasca, Ill.: National Safety Council, 1996.
37. **Public Citizen Health Research Group v. Tyson,** 796 F2d 1479 (D.C. Cir. 1986).
38. **Castleman, B.I., and G.E. Ziem:** Corporate influence on threshold limit values. *Am. J. Ind. Med. 13*:531–559 (1988).
39. **Federal Register 62:** *Methylene chloride..* p. 1493. 10 January 1997
40. **U.S. Environmental Protection Agency (EPA):** *The Risk Assessment Guidelines of 1986* (EPA/600/8-87/045). Washington, D.C.: EPA, 1987.
41. **National Research Council, Committee on the Institutional Means for Assessment of Risks to Public Health, Commission on Life Sciences:** *Risk Assessment in the Federal Government: Managing the Process.* Washington, D.C.: National Academy Press, 1983.
42. **U.S. Environmental Protection Agency (EPA):** Guidelines for Carcinogen Risk Assessment ((PDF) EPA/630/P-03/001F), March 2005.
43. **U.S. Environmental Protection Agency (EPA):** *Supplemental Guidance for Assessing Susceptibility from Early-Life Exposure to Carcinogens.* Washington, D.C.: U.S. EPA, March 2005.
44. **Habicht, F.H.:** "Guidance on Risk Characterization for Risk Managers and Risk Assessors." [Memo] Washington, D.C.: U.S. Environmental Protection Agency, 1992.
45. **Browner, C.:** "Policy for Risk Characterization at the U.S. Environmental Protection Agency." [Memo] Washington, D.C.: U.S. Environmental Protection Agency, 1995.
46. **U.S. Environmental Protection Agency (EPA):** Regional Guidance EPA/903/R-93-001, "Selecting Exposure Routes and Contaminants of Concern by Risk-Based Screening." Washington, D.C.: U.S. EPA, 1993.
47. **U.S. Environmental Protection Agency (EPA):** Memorandum, SUBJECT: Risk-Based Concentration Table, J. Hubbard, US EPA September 11, 2008. http://www.epa.gov/reg3hwmd/risk/human/pdf/covsep08.pdf. [Accessed August 3,2009.
48. **U.S. Environmental Protection Agency (EPA):** *Integrated Risk Information System.* Available: http://cfpub.epa.gov/ncea/iris/index.cfm. Updated February 6, 2009. [Accessed March 31, 2009.]
49. **American Society for Testing and Materials (ASTM):** *Standard Guide for Risk-Based Corrective Action Applied at Petroleum Release Sites (ASTM E 1739-95).* West Conshohocken, PA: ASTM, 1995.
50. **U.S. Environmental Protection Agency (EPA):** *Ecological Risk Guidance.* Available at http://www.epa.gov/risk/ecological-risk.htm. Updated March 18, 2008. [Accessed March 31, 2009.]
51. **U.S. Environmental Protection Agency (EPA):** *Risk Assessment Portal.* Available: http://www.epa.gov/risk/. Updated March 17, 2009. [Accessed March 31, 2009.]
52. **U.S. Environmental Protection Agency (EPA):** *Basic Information.* Available: http://www.epa.gov/risk/basicinformation.htm#g. Updated December 9, 2008. [Accessed March 31, 2009.]
53. **Executive Order 12196:** *Occupational safety and health programs for Federal employees*, 26 February 1980.
54. **Executive Order 13139:** *Improving Health Protection of Military Personnel Participating in Particular Military Operations*, 30 September 1999.
55. **U.S. Department of Defense:** DoD Instruction 6490.03, *Deployment Health*, August 11, 2006
56. **Office of the Chairman of the Joint Chiefs of Staff:** Memorandum, MCM 0028-07, "Updated Procedures for Deployment Health Surveillance and Readiness," November 2, 2007.
57. **U.S. Department of Defense:** DoD Instruction 6055.05, *Occupational and Environmental Health (OEH)*, November 11, 2008.
58. **Booher, H.R. (ed.):** *MANPRINT—An Approach to Systems Integration.* New York: Van Nostrand Reinhold, 1990.
59. **U.S. Army, Army Regulation 40–10, Medical Services:** *Health Hazard Assessment Program in Support of the Army Acquisition Process.* July 27, 2007.
60. **U.S. Army, Army Regulation 602-2:** *Manpower and Personnel Integration (MANPRINT) in the System Acquisition Process.* June 1, 2001.
61. **U.S. Department of Defense:** DoDI 5000.02, *Operation of the Defense Acquisition System*, December 8, 2008.
62. **U.S. Department of Defense:** DoD Directive 4715.1E, *Environment, Safety, and Occupational Health (ESOH)*, March 19, 2005.

63. **U.S. Department of Defense:** DoD Instruction 6055.1, *DoD Safety and Occupational Health (SOH) Program*, August 19, 1998.
64. **U.S. Army:** Field Manual 3-100.12/MCRP 5-12.1C/NTTP 5-03.5/AFTTP(I) 3-2.34, *Risk Management Multiservice Tactics, Techniques, and Procedures for Risk Management*, February 15, 2001.
65. **Consortium for Risk Evaluation with Stakeholder Participation (CRESP):** *Peer Review of the U.S. Department of Energy's Use of Risk in its Prioritization Process*, December 15, 1999.
66. **U.S. Department of Energy:**, DOE HR-0098, *US Department of Energy 1977-1994, a Summary History*, November 1994.
67. **Title 10, Code of Federal Regulations (CFR):** Part 851, *Worker Safety and Health Program*, February 9, 2006
68. **U.S. Department of Energy:** *DOE Safety Management System Policy*, DOE P 450.4, October 15, 1996.
69. **40 Code of Federal Regulations (CFR):** Parts 239-282, *Resource Conservation and Recovery Act (RCRA) of 1976*
70. *Atomic Energy Act of 1954*, available at http://www.nrc.gov/reading-rm/doc-collections/nuregs/staff/sr0980/, 30 August 1954. Accessed 31 March 2009.
71. *Federal Facility Compliance Act of 1992*, Public Law 102-386 (106 Statute 1505).
72. **Title 42, Chapter 103:**—*Comprehensive Environmental Response, Compensation, and Liability Act*, 1980.
73. **National Academy of Sciences/National Research Council (NAS):** *Building Consensus Through Risk Assessment and Risk Management in the Department of Energy's Environmental Remediation Program.* Washington, D.C.: National Academy Press, 1994.
74. **Department of Homeland Security (DHS):** *Homepage.* Available: www.dhs.gov. Updated February 13, 2009. [Accessed February 14, 2009.]
75. *Homeland Security Act of 2002.* [Online] Available at http://frwebgate.access.gpo.gov/cgi-bin/getdoc.cgi?dbname=107_cong_public_laws@docid=f:publ296.107.pdf (Accessed 15 February 2008).
76. **U.S. Department of Homeland Security:** DHS Risk Lexicon. September 2008. [Online] Available at http://www.dhs.gov/xprevprot/publications/gc_1232717001850.shtm (Accessed February 15, 2009).
77. **FEMA 2009:** *NIMS Resource Center.* [Online] Available at http://www.fema.gov/emergency/nims/ (Accessed 15 February 2009).
78. **U.S. Department of Homeland Security (DHS):** *National Infrastructure Protection Plan. 2009b.* [Online] Available at http://www.dhs.gov/xprevprot/programs/editorial_0827.shtm (Accessed 15 February 2009).
79. **U.S. Environmental Protection Agency (EPA):** *Guidelines for Ecological Risk Assessment. U.S. Environmental Protection Agency,* Risk Assessment Forum, Washington, DC, EPA/630/R095/002F, 1998..
80. **Cohrssen, J.J. and V.T. Covello:** *Risk Analysis: A Guide to Principles and Methods for Analyzing Health and Environmental Risks.* Washington, D.C.: U.S. Council on Environmental Quality, 1989.
81. **Nadakavukaren, A.:** *Man and Environment: A Health Perspective*, 4th edition. Prospect Heights, IL: Waveland Press, 1995.
82. **Smith, R.L.:** "Risk-Based Concentration Table, January-June 1995." [Memo], U.S. Environmental Protection Agency, Region III, Philadelphia, PA, March 1995.
83. **Hauschild, V., A. Watson, and G. Bratt:** The C in CBRN — From Critical Exposure Levels to Clean-up Levels, We Know More Than You Might Think. USACHPPM Presentation. U.S. Army Force Health Protection Conference, August 2009.
84. **National Academy of Sciences Committee on Toxicology, Subcommittee on Acute Exposure Guidelines Levels:** *Acute Exposure Guidelines Levels for Selected Airborne Chemicals,* Volume 3. Washington, DC: National Academy Press. 2003.
85. **American Industrial Hygiene Association® (AIHA®):** *ERPGs™ for 2007*, available at: (http://www.aiha.org/1documents/Committees/ERP-erpglevels.pdf). Accessed April 1, 2009.
86. **Subcommittee on Consequence Assessment and Protective Actions (SCAPA),** *Protective Action Criteria for Chemicals—Including AEGLs, ERPGs™, and TEELs*, Available at: (http://orise.orau.gov/emi/scapa/teels.htm) [Accessed April 1, 2009.]
87. **Occupational Safety and Health Administration (OSHA):** 29 CFR Part 1910, Occupational Safety and Health Standards.
88. **American Conference of Governmental Industrial Hygienists® (ACGIH®):** *Policy Statement on the Uses of TLVs® and BEIs®*, [Threshold Limit Values® (TLVs®) and Biological Exposure Indices (BEIs®). Cincinnati, OH: ACGIH®, 2007. Available: http://www.acgih.org/Products/tlv_bei_intro.htm. [Accessed April 1, 2009.]

89. **National Institute for Occupational Safety and Health (NIOSH):**, *Documentation for Immediately Dangerous to Life or Health Concentrations (IDLH): Introduction.* NTIS Publication No. PB-94-195047. Available online at http://www.cdc.gov/niosh/idlh/idlhintr.html#BKD May 1994. [Accessed February 27, 2009.]
90. **U.S. Army Center for Health Promotion and Preventive Medicine,** Technical Guide 230, Version 1.3 – Updated May 2003, With January 2004 Addendum. Chemical Exposure Guidelines for Deployed Military Personnel.
91. **Klimisch, H.J., M. Andreae, and U. Tillman:** A systemic approach for evaluating the quality of experimental toxicological and ecotoxicological data. *Reg.Toxicol. Pharmacol. 25*: 1–5 (1997).
92. **Public Law 99-499, Superfund Amendments and Reauthorization Act of 1986, Emergency Planning and Community Right-to-Know Act (EPCRA) 40 CFR Parts 355 and 370,** *Amendments to Emergency Planning and Notification; Emergency Release Notification and Hazardous Chemical Reporting* (http://www.epa.gov/fedrgstr/EPA-WASTE/2008/November/Day-03/f25329.htm), November 2008. Accessed 1 April 2009.
93. **U.S. Environmental Protection Agency (EPA): 40 CFR Part 68:** *Accidental Release Prevention Requirements: Risk Management Programs Under the Clean Air Act, Section 112(r)(7); List of Regulated Substances and Thresholds for Accidental Release Prevention, Stay of Effectiveness; and Accidental Release Prevention Requirements: Risk Management Programs Under Section 112(r)(7) of the Clean Air Act as Amended,* Guidelines; Final Rules and Notice, (http://www.epa.gov/emergencies/content/lawsregs/rmpover.htm) 61 FR 31668, June 20, 1996. Accessed 1 April 2009.
94. **American Industrial Hygiene Association® (AIHA®)ERP Committee:** "Procedures and Responsibilities." Fairfax, VA: AIHA, November 2006.
95. **Ripple, S.D.:** *Personal communication regarding ERPGs™.* March 2009.
96. **Rusch, G.M.:** *Personal communication regarding ERPGs™ and AEGLs.* March 2009.
97. **U.S. Environmental Protection Agency (EPA):** *AEGL Program.* Available at http://www.epa.gov/oppt/aegl/. December 11, 2008. [Accessed February 27, 2009.]
98. **National Research Council Subcommittee on Acute Exposure Guideline Levels, Committee on Toxicology, Board on Environmental Studies and Toxicology, Commission on Life Sciences:** *Standing Operating Procedures for Developing Acute Exposure Guideline Levels for Hazardous Chemicals.* National Academy Press, Washington, D.C. Available at http://www.nap.edu/openbook.php?record_id=10122&page=4. 2001. (Accessed 28 February 2009).
99. **Subcommittee on Consequence Assessment and Protective Actions (SCAPA):** *Protective Action Criteria for Chemicals — Including AEGLs, ERPGs, & TEELs* http://orise.orau.gov/emi/scapa/teels.htm (Accessed 7 March 2009)
100. **American Industrial Hygiene Association® (AIHA®):** *Emergency Response Planning Committee.* http://www.aiha.org/Content/InsideAIHA/Volunteer%2bGroups/ERPcomm.htm. February 23, 2009. [Accessed February 27, 2009.]
101. **Craig, D.K., J.S. Davis, R. DeVore, D.J. Hansen, A.J. Petrocchi, and T.J. Powell:** Alternative Guideline Limits for Chemicals without Emergency Response Planning Guidelines. *Am. Ind. Hyg. Assoc. J. 56*:919–925 (1995).
102. **Craig, D.K., J.S. Davis, D.J. Hansen, A.J. Petrocchi, T.J. Powell, and T.E. Tuccinardi:** Derivation of Temporary Emergency Exposure Limits (TEELs). *J. Appl. Toxicol. 20*:11–20 (2000).
103. Occupational Safety and Health Act, 29 US Code 15 Part 655 (b) (5), 2001]
104. **Barnes, D.G.:** Times are tough—brother, can you paradigm? *Risk Anal. 14*:219–223 (1994).
105. **Emergency Management Issues Special Interest Group (EMI SIG) (undated).** Subcommittee on Consequence Assessment and Protective Actions (SCAPA) (undated). Available at http://orise.orau.gov/emi/scapa/default.htm (Accessed 28 February 2009).
106. **U.S. Environmental Protection Agency (EPA):** *Methods for Derivation of Inhalation Reference Concentrations and Application of Inhalation Dosimetry.* EPA/600/8-90/066F. October 1994.
107. **U.S. Environmental Protection Agency (EPA):** *Guidelines for Carcinogen Risk Assessment.* EPA/630/P-03/001B. March 2005.
108. **U.S. Environmental Protection Agency (EPA):** *Exposure Factors Handbook* (EPA/600/8-89/043). Washington, D.C.: EPA, 1990.
109. **U.S. Environmental Protection Agency (EPA):** *Exposure Factors Handbook* (EPA/600/P-95/002); Washington, D.C.: EPA, 1997.
110. **U.S. Environmental Protection Agency (EPA):** *Guidance for Superfund Volume I: Human Health Evaluation Manual (Part E, Supplemental Guidance for Dermal Risk Assessment).* EPA/540/R/99/005). 2004.
111. **U.S. Environmental Protection Agency (EPA):** *Guidance for Superfund Volume I: Human Health Evaluation Manual (Part F, Supplemental Guidance for Inhalation Risk Assessment).* EPA-540-R-070-002). 2009.

112. **NAS:** *Science and Decisions: Advancing Risk Assessment.* The National Academy of Sciences. National Academies Press, Washington, D.C. 2008.
113. **Kodell, R.L., and J.J. Chen:** Reducing conservatism in risk estimation for mixtures of carcinogens. *Risk Anal. 14(3)*:327–332. 1994.
114. **U.S. Environmental Protection Agency (EPA):** *Guidelines for the Health Risk Assessment of Chemical Mixtures. 1986, Federal Register 51(185):34014-34025.] EPA 2001) [Supplementary Guidance for Conducting Health Risk Assessment of Chemical Mixtures (PDF)* EPA630-R-00-002. August, 2001.
115. **Haber L., J. Dollarhide, A. Maier, M. Dourson:** Noncancer Risk Assessment: Principles and Practice in Environmental and Occupational Settings. In *Patty's Industrial Hygiene and Toxicology.* New York: John Wiley and Sons, 2000.
116. **Dourson, M.L., L.K. Teuschler, P.R. Durkin, and W.M. Stiteler:** Categorical Regression of Toxicity Data: A Case Study Using Aldicarb. *Reg. Toxicol. Pharmacol. 25*:121–129 (1997).
117. **Swartout J.C., P.S. Price, M.L. Dourson, H.L. Carlson-Lynch and R.E. Keenan:** A Probabilistic Framework for the Reference Dose (Probabilistic RfD). *Risk Anal. 18(3)*:271–282 (1998).
118. **U.S. Environmental Protection Agency (EPA):** *Benchmark dose technical guidance document.. External Review Draft.* EPA/630/R-00/001. Additional documentation and software available at: http://www.epa.gov/ncea/bmds/. October 2000. Accessed April 1, 2009.
119. **U.S. Environmental Protection Agency (EPA) National Center for Environmental Assessment (NCEA):** *Approaches for the Application of Physiologically Based Pharmacokinetic (PBPK) Models and Supporting Data in Risk Assessment (Final Report).* U.S. Environmental Protection Agency, Washington, D.C., EPA/600/R-05/043F. http://cfpub.epa.gov/ncea/cfm/recordisplay.cfm?deid=157668. 2006. Accessed 1 April 2009.
120. **The International Programme on Chemical Safety (IPCS):** *Harmonization project to promote best practice in PBPK modeling — draft guidance.* 2008. http://www.who.int/ipcs/methods/harmonization/areas/pbpk_guidance/en/index.html. [Accessed April 1, 2009.]
121. **Jarabek, A.** Inhalation RfC methodology: Dosimetric adjustments and dose-response estimation of noncancer toxicity in the upper respiratory tract. *Inhal. Toxicol. 6*:301–325 (1994).
122. **Schulte, P.A.** A conceptual framework for the validation and use of biologic markers. *Environ. Res. 48*:129–144 (1989).
123. **Maier, A., R.E. Savage Jr., L.T. Haber:** Assessing biomarker use in risk assessment – A survey of practitioners. *J. Toxicol. Environ. Health Part A. 67*:687–695 (2004).
124. **The International Programme on Chemical Safety (IPCS): Harmonization Project Document; No. 2:** *Chemical-specific adjustment factors for interspecies differences and human variability: guidance document for use of data in dose/concentration–response assessment.* (http://whqlibdoc.who.int/publications/2005/9241546786_eng.pdf). (2005). [Accessed April 1, 2009.]
125. **Maier, A.:** *Occupational Health Resources. Information Resources in Toxicology.* Wexler, P. and B. Hakkinen (eds.). San Diego, CA: Academic Press, 2009.
126. **Zalk, D.M. and D.I. Nelson:** History and evolution of control banding: A review. *J. Occup. Environ. Hyg. 5(4)*:330–346 (2008).
127. **Nelson, D.I., and D.M. Zalk:** Control Banding: Background, Critique, and Evolution. In *Patty's Industrial Hygiene and Toxicology,* 6th edition. In Review. 2009.
128. **Swuste, P., A. Hale, and S. Pantry:** Solbase: A databank of solutions for occupational hazards and risks. *Ann. Occup. Hyg. 47(7)*: 541–547 (2003).
129. **Balsat, A., J. de Graeve, and P. Mairiaux:** A structured strategy for assessing chemical risks, suitable for small and medium-sized enterprises. *Ann. Occup. Hyg. 47(7)*:549–556. (2003).
130. **Money, C. D.:** European experiences in the development of approaches for the successful control of workplace health risks. *Ann. Occup. Hyg. 47(7)*:533–540(2003).
131. **Chemical Industries Association (CIA):** *Safe Handling of Colourants 2: Hazard Classification and Selection of Occupational Hygiene Strategies.* London: CIA, 1993.
132. **Association of the British Pharmaceutical Industry (ABPI):** *Guidance on Setting In-house Occupational Exposure Limits for Airborne Therapeutic Substances and Their Intermediates.* London: ABPI, 1995.
133. **Naumann, B.D., E.V. Sargent, B.S. Starkman, W.J. Fraser, G.T. Becker, and G.D. Kirk:** Performance-based exposure control limits for pharmaceutical active ingredients. *Am. Ind. Hyg. Assoc. J. 57(1)*:33–42(1996).
134. **Russell, R.M., S.C. Maidment, I. Brooke, and M.D. Topping:** An introduction to a UK scheme to help small firms control health risks from chemicals. *Ann. Occup. Hyg. 42(6)*:367–76(1998).
135. **Brooke, I.M.:** A UK scheme to help small firms control health risks from chemicals: Toxicological considerations. *Ann. Occup. Hyg. 42(6)*:377–90(1998).

136. **Maidment, S.C.:** Occupational hygiene considerations in the development of a structured approach to select chemical control strategies. *Ann. Occup. Hyg. 42(6)*: 391–400(1998).
137. **Health & Safety Executive (HSE):** *Control of Substances Hazardous to Health (COSHH) Essentials Guidance Publications.* Updated September 22, 2008. [Online] Available at http://www.hse.gov.uk/pubns/guidance/index.htm [Accessed February 23, 2008.]
138. **Health and Safety Executive (Great Britain):** *COSHH ESSENTIALS Easy steps to control health risks from chemicals.* 2009. [Online] Available at http://www.coshh-essentials.org.uk [Accessed February 15, 2009.]
139. **Nelson, D.I., S.V. Chiusano, A.L. Bracker, L.A. Erickson, C.L. Geraci, M. Harper, C. Harvey, A.A. Havics, M. D. Hoover, T.J. Lentz, R.W. Niemeier, S.D. Ripple, E.J. Stewart, E.A. Sullivan, and D.M. Zalk:** *Guidance for Conducting Control Banding Analyses.* Fairfax, VA: AIHA®, 2007.
140. **Zalk, D.M.:** Practical prevention in safety: from control banding to barrier banding. In Proceedings of the International Working on Safety Conference. The Eemhof, The Netherlands, September 15, 2006.
141. **Zalk, D.M.:** *Control banding principles to reduce musculoskeletal disorders: the ergonomics toolkit.* V5 (p. 327). In Proceedings of the International Ergonomics Association XVth Triennial Congress. IEA: South Korea, 24–29 August 2003.
142. **Spee, T.:** *Risk assessment from toxic substances and control measures in the Dutch construction industry.* Presented at Third International Control Banding Workshop. Pilanesberg, South Africa, 21 September 2005.
143. **Center to Protect Workers' Rights (CPWR):** *Construction Solutions.* 2007. [Online] Available at http://www.cpwr.com/rp-constructionsolutions.html. [Accessed February 24, 2008.]
144. **Maynard, A.D.:** Nanotechnology: the next big thing, or much ado about nothing? *Ann. Occup. Hyg. 51(1)*:1–12(2007).
145. **Jones, J. and M. Nicas:** *Evaluation of the ILO Toolkit with regards to hazard classification and control effectiveness.* Presented at Second International Control Banding Workshop. Cincinnati, OH, March 1–2, 2004.
146. **Guest, I.:** The Chemical Industries Association Guidance on Allocating Occupational Exposure Bands. *Ann. Occup. Hyg. 42(6)*:407–411(1998).
147. **Ruden, C. and S.O. Hansson:** How accurate are the European Union's classifications of *chemical substances. Toxicol. Lett. 144(2)*:159–72(2003).
148. **Jones, R.M. and M. Nicas:** Margins of safety provided by COSHH Essentials and the ILO Chemical Control Toolkit. *Ann. Occup. Hyg. 50(2)*:149–56(2006).
149. **Kromhout, H.:** Design of measurement strategies for workplace exposures. *Occup. Environ. Med. 59(5)*:349–54(2002).
150. **Topping, M.:** *COSHH Essentials: from concept to one-stop system.* Presented at First International Control Banding Workshop. London, November 4–5, 2002.
151. **Kromhout, H.:** Design of measurement strategies for workplace exposures: Author's reply. *Occup. Environ. Med. 59*:788–89(2002).
152. **Tischer, M., S. Bredendiek-Kamper, and U. Poppek:** Evaluation of the HSE COSHH Essentials exposure predictive model on the basis of BAuA field studies and existing substances exposure data. *Ann. Occup. Hyg. 47(7)*:557–69(2003).
153. **Jones, R.M. and M. Nicas:** Evaluation of COSHH Essentials for vapor degreasing and bag filling operations. *Ann. Occup. Hyg. 50(2)*:137–47(2006).
154. **Obadia, I.:** *ILO and control banding: the way forward.* Presented at First International Control Banding Workshop. London, November 4–5,2002.
155. **American Conference of Governmental Industrial Hygienists (ACGIH®):** Control *Banding: Issues and Opportunities: A Report of the ACGIH® Exposure/ Control Banding Task Force.* Publication #08-001. Cincinnati: ACGIH®, 2008.
156. **Tischer, M. and S. Scholaen:** Chemical management and control strategies: experiences from the GTZ pilot project on chemical safety in Indonesian small and medium-sized enterprises. *Ann. Occup. Hyg. 47(7)*:571–75(2003).
157. **Howard, J.:** *Navigating uncharted territory in occupational safety and health research: 21st century challenges.* Presented at American Industrial Hygiene Conference and Exposition. Dallas, TX, May 13, 2003.
158. **U.S. Environmental Protection Agency, Office of Water:** *Vulnerability Assessment Fact Sheet*, EPA 816-F-02-025, November 2002. Available at http://www.epa.gov/ogwdw/security/index.html. [Accessed February 27, 2009.]
159. **Lövkvist-Andersen, A.-L., R. Olsson, T. Ritchey, M. Stenström:** *Modeling Society's Capacity to Manage Extraordinary Events—Developing a Generic Design Basis (GDB) Model for Extraordinary Societal Events using Computer-Aided Morphological Analysis,* Adaption of paper at Society for Risk Analysis Conference, November 15–17, 2004. Available at http://www.swemorph.com/pdf/sra.pdf. [Accessed February 27, 2009.]

160. **Bioterrorism Act, Public Law 107–188:** *Title IV—Drinking Water Security and Safety, Section. 401. Terrorist and Other Intentional Acts, Section. 1433. Terrorist and Other Intentional Acts.* June 12, 2002,
161. **U.S. Environmental Protection Agency (EPA):** *Water Security Vulnerability Assessments* [Online] [http://cfpub.epa.gov/safewater/watersecurity/home.cfm?program_id=11. [Accessed February 27, 2009.]
162. **National Oceanic and Atmospheric Administration (NOAA):** *Risk and Vulnerability Assessment Tool (RVAT)* [Online] [http://www.csc.noaa.gov/rvat/. Accessed February 27, 2009.
163. **Department of Homeland Security:** *Chemical Security Assessment Tool* [Online] [http://www.dhs.gov/xprevprot/programs/gc_1169501486197.shtm]. Accessed February 27, 2009.
164. **Public Law 101-549:** *Clean Air Act Amendments of 1990,* Title III, Sections 304, 301, November 15, 1990.
165. **Occupational Safety and Health Administration (OSHA):** 29 CFR Part 1910,: *Process Safety Management of Highly Hazardous Chemicals; Explosives and Blasting Agents,* Final Rule, 57 FR 6356, February 24, 1992.
166. **U.S. Department of Energy Handbook Chemical,** DOE-HDBK-1100-2004, Process Hazards Analysis, Available at http://www.hss.doe.gov/nuclearsafety/ns/techstds/standard/hdbk1100/hdbk1100.pdf. August 2004. [Accessed February 27, 2009.]
167. **National Institute for Occupational Safety and Health (NIOSH):** *Report to Congress on Workers' Home Contamination Study Conducted under the Workers' Family Protection Act (29 U.S.C 671a).* September 1995. Available: http://www.cdc.gov/niosh/contamin.html. [Accessed February 27, 2009.]
168. **Newhouse, M.L., and H. Thompson:** Mesothelioma of pleura and peritoneum following exposure to asbestos in the London area. *Br. J. Ind. Med. 22*:261–269 (1965).
169. **Anderson, H.A., R. Lillis, S.M. Daum, and I.J. Selikoff:** Asbestosis among household contacts of asbestos factory workers. *Ann. NY Acad. Sci. 330*:387–399 (1979).
170. **Workers' Family Protection Act of 1992:** (Public Law 102-522, 29 U.S.C. 671a, 1992
171. **National Institute for Occupational Safety and Health (NIOSH):** *Protecting Workers' Families: A Research Agenda. Report of the Workers' Family Protection Task Force.* May 2002. Available: http://www.cdc.gov/niosh/pdfs/2002-113.pdf. [Accessed February 27, 2009.]
172. **U.S. Environmental Protection Agency (EPA):** *Risk Assessment Guidance for Superfund), volume. I, Human Health Evaluation Manual (Part D, Standardized Planning, Reporting and Review of Superfund Risk Assessments).* Publication 9285.7-47. December 2001. Available: http://www. epa.gov/superfund/programs/reforms/docs/vv_RAGsD.pdf. [Accessed February 25, 2009.]
173. **Green Media Toolshed:** *Scorecard, The Pollution Information Site.* Available: http://www.scorecard.org. [Accessed February 25, 2009.]
174. **U.S. Environmental Protection Agency (EPA):** *EPA Health Effects Assessment Summary Tables (HEAST).* Available: http://www.epa.gov/radiation/heast/index.html#index. Updated April 2, 2009. [Accessed April 2, 2009.]
175. **Agency for Toxic Substances and Disease Registry (ATSDR):** *Minimal Risk Levels (MRLs) for Hazardous Substances.* Available: http://www.atsdr.cdc.gov/mrls.html. December 2001. Updated January 14, 2009. [Accessed February 25, 2009.]
176. **U.S Environmental Protection Agency (EPA):** The Inside Story: A Guide to Indoor Air Quality, http://www.epa.gov/iaq/pubs/insidest.html. Updated April 1, 2009. [Accessed April 2, 2009.
177. **National Safety Council (NSC):** Safety and Health Policy Center, Washington D.C. http://nsc.org/ehc.aspx
178. **U.S. Environmental Protection Agency (EPA):** *Chemical Right-to-Know Initiative.* Available: http://www.epa.gov/chemrtk . Updated April 2, 2009.
179. "Data Collection and Development on High Production Volume (HPV) Chemicals." Federal Register 65:248 (26 December 2000) pp. 81686–81698.
180. "Proposed Rule: Testing of Certain High Production Volume Chemicals." Federal Register 65:248 (26 December 2000). pp. 81657–81685.
181. "Notice: Voluntary Children's Chemical Evaluation Program." Federal Register 65:248 (26 December 2000). pp. 81699–81718.
182. **Federal Emergency Management Agency (FEMA):** NIMS Resource Center. Available at http://www.fema.gov/emergency/nims/ (undated) (Accessed February 25, 2009).
183. **National Fire Protection Association (NFPA):** *NFPA 1600, Standard on Disaster/Emergency Management and Business Continuity Programs,* 2007 Edition. Quincy, MA: NFPA, 2007.
184. **Laszcz-Davis, C., R.R. McHaney,S.P. Pereira, K.J. Nardi, L.M. Gibbs, D. Akers, J. Jabara, M.D. Buckalew, F. Lebourgeois:** Emergency & Disaster Preparedness, Response &Recovery. In *Patty's Industrial Hygiene and Toxicology,* 6th edition. Hoboken, NJ: John Wiley &Sons, Inc., 2009.

185. **U.S. Environmental Protection Agency (EPA):** *Emergency Planning and Community Right-to-Know Act (EPCRA) Requirements.* Available at http://www.epa.gov/emergencies/content/epcra/index.htm. February 12, 2009. [Accessed February 26, 2009.]
186. **Federal Emergency Management Agency (FEMA):** *Hazard Mitigation Planning,* updated 11 February 2009. http://www.fema.gov/plan/mitplanning/index.shtm.
187. **Texas A&M University System, Texas Engineering Extension Service, National Emergency Response and Rescue Training Center:** *Homeland Security Threat and Risk Assessment, Participant Manual,* MGT310. College Station, TX. 2006.
188. **American Industrial Hygiene Association (AIHA®):** *White Paper: Industrial Hygienists' Role and Responsibilities in Emergency Preparedness and Response.* Fairfax, VA. (undated). Available at http://www.aiha.org/1documents/governmentaffairs/eprwhitepaper_final.pdf. [Accessed February 26, 2009.]
189. **Department of Homeland Security (DHS):** *National Response Framework.* P. 11. (2008 January). Available at http://www.fema.gov/pdf/emergency/nrf/nrf-core.pdf [Accessed February 26, 2009.]
190. **Waugh, W.L. and K. Tierney:** *Emergency Management: Principles and Practice for Local Government,* 2nd edition. Washington, D.C.: International City/County Management, 2007. p. 321.
191. **Federal Emergency Management Agency (FEMA):** *FEMA Training Resources* (updated 5 February 2009). Available at http://training.fema.gov/ (Accessed 25 February 2009).
192. **Finley, B., D. Proctor, P. Scott, N. Harrington, D. Paustenbach, and P. Price:** Recommended distributions for exposure factors frequently used in health risk assessment. *Risk Anal. 14*:533–553 (1994).
193. **Burmaster, D.E., and P.D. Anderson:** Principles of good practice for the use of Monte Carlo techniques in human health and ecological risk assessments. *Risk Anal. 14*:477–481 (1994).
194. **Lipton, J., and J.W. Gillett:** Uncertainty in risk assessment: Exceedence frequencies, acceptable risk, and risk-based decision making. *Reg. Toxicol. Pharmacol. 15*:51–61 (1992).
195. **Evans, J.S., G.M. Gray, R.L. Sielken, A.E. Smith, C. Valdez-Flores, and J.D. Graham:** Use of probabilistic expert judgment in uncertainty analysis of carcinogenic potency. *Reg. Toxicol. Pharmacol. 20*:15–36 (1994).
196. **Cullen, A.C.:** Measures of compounding conservatism in probabilistic risk assessment. *Risk Anal. 14*:389–393 (1994).
197. **Thompson, K.M., D.E. Burmaster, and E.A.C. Crouch:** Monte Carlo techniques for quantitative uncertainty analysis in public health risk assessments. *Risk Anal. 12*:53–63 (1992).
198. **U.S. Army Center for Health Promotion and Preventive Medicine**, Technical Guide 230, Version 1.3 - Updated May 2003, With January 2004 Addendum. Chemical Exposure Guidelines for Deployed Military Personnel.
199. **Smith, R.L.:** Use of Monte Carlo simulation for human exposure assessment at a Superfund site. *Risk Anal. 14*:433–439 (1994).
200. **U.S. Environmental Protection Agency (EPA):** *Use of Monte Carlo Simulation in Risk Assessments* (EPA903-F-94-001). Philadelphia: EPA, 1994.

Outcome Competencies

After completing this chapter, the reader should be able to:

1. Define underlined terms used in this chapter.
2. Describe the advantages of a comprehensive exposure assessment strategy.
3. Discuss the goals of comprehensive exposure assessment.
4. Outline the major steps in a comprehensive exposure assessment strategy.

Key Terms

authoritative OELs • basic characterization • compliance strategy • comprehensive exposure assessment• comprehensive strategy • exposure profile • exposure rating • internal OELs • occupational exposure limit (OEL) • regulatory OELs • similar exposure groups (SEGs) • working OELs

Prerequisite Knowledge

Prior to beginning this chapter, the user should review the following chapters:

Chapter Number	Chapter Topic
4	Occupational Exposure Limits
5	Occupational Toxicology
7	Principles of Evaluating Worker Exposure
8	Occuaptional and Environmental Health Risk Assessment/Risk Management
10	Modeling Inhalation Exposure
11	Sampling of Gases and Vapors
12	Analysis of Gases and Vapors
14	Sampling and Sizing of Airborne Particles

Key Topics

I. Introduction
   A. Growing Variety of Present and Future Risks
   B. Efficient and Effective Programs

II. Shifting State-of-the-Art: Compliance Monitoring to Comprehensive Exposure Assessment

III. Overview of Exposure Assessment Strategy
   A. Start — Establish the Exposure Assessment Strategy
   B. Basic Characterization
   C. Exposure Assessment
   D. Further Information Gathering
   E. Health Hazard Controls
   F. Reassessment
   G. Communications and Documentation

Comprehensive Exposure Assessment

9

John R. Mulhausen, PhD, CIH and Joseph Damiano, MS, CIH, CSP

Introduction

Occupational hygienists must anticipate, recognize, evaluate, and control health hazards and related risks in the workplace. Central to this effort is the assessment of occupational exposures. Comprehensive exposure assessment is the systematic review of the processes, practices, materials, and division of labor present in a workplace that is used to define and judge all exposures for all workers on all days. Such a rational and methodical approach to exposure recognition and evaluation helps ensure that all health risks are managed, that all related risks are considered, that all organization stakeholders are involved, and that occupational hygiene programs and resources are focused on the most important risks. It also positions the occupational hygiene program to better anticipate and manage future risks.

Increasing Challenges in Exposure Assessment

Modern workplaces are becoming more complex. The variety of risks associated with workplace exposure to chemical, physical, and biological agents is increasing. While the first priority of the occupational hygienist is to protect the health of workers, health risk is not the only risk he or she is asked to manage. Other risks include the risks posed by noncompliance with regulations, legal risks such as those associated with potential lawsuits or third-party liability, and risks related to the anxiety associated with many people's response to potential exposures.

Occupational hygienists must consider the fact that organizations today are accountable to many more -and more varied- stakeholders than organizations in the past. These new stakeholders include the customers, labor unions, regulators, stockholders, the press, and the communities in which the organization operates. Organizations rely on occupational hygienists to satisfy the concerns of these stakeholders on matters related to workplace exposures.

When evaluating risks to employees and the organization, occupational hygienists must also remember that today's programs will be held accountable not only for today's state-of-the-art, but tomorrow's as well. It is not sufficient to limit the question to "Are employee exposures below established exposure limits?" Instead, occupational hygienists must ensure that exposures are characterized well enough, and controlled well enough, to keep present risks within acceptable limits and to position the organization to manage future risks. Questions that must be considered include the following:

- How might this exposure affect the health of employees?
- How good is the exposure limit?
- What additional risks does this exposure present to the organization?

Compliance with current limits is just the start. The majority of chemicals do not have an occupational exposure limit (OEL), and the information used to set existing limits is often incomplete. Also, the limits that are set are not always designed to protect all workers or might be out of date.

New toxicological and epidemiological information is gathered each day. That means that new exposure limits will be generated for environmental agents that formerly had none, and that many of the limits currently in place will change. Experience has shown that most exposure limits are lowered when they are changed, and there is no reason to believe that trend will not continue.

Unfortunately, when new limits are set, or old limits are changed, there may be a population of workers who have been exposed to the chemical for some time at concentrations above the new limit. The occupational hygienist today must think about how he or she should position the current occupational hygiene program so it is best able to manage those changes and minimize the future risks they will pose. Having a historical database for all exposures will often allow identification of employees who were exposed above the lowered exposure limit and enable estimation of the extent of their past exposure. This then allows the formation of a strategy for medical management of the health of those employees.

Efficient and Effective Programs

At the same time that occupational hygienists are being asked to manage a growing variety of risks, their programs are being more carefully scrutinized for efficacy, efficiency, and cost-effectiveness. Economic factors demand that each organizational unit demonstrate its worth and its ability to operate waste-free. Occupational hygiene programs are no exception. The ability to efficiently understand, prioritize, and manage exposures and risks requires a more systematic, better documented approach to occupational hygiene than has typically been practiced in the past.

Occupational Hygiene Program Management

The better the occupational hygienist understands exposures, the better he or she is able to direct and prioritize the occupational hygiene program. This is true whether the goal of the exposure assessment process is regulatory compliance, a comprehensive description of all exposures, or a diagnostic evaluation of health hazard controls. The system for exposure assessment must be integrated with other systems for defining, prioritizing, and managing worker health protection. Assessment results are used to determine the needs and priority for health hazard controls, build exposure histories, and demonstrate regulatory compliance.

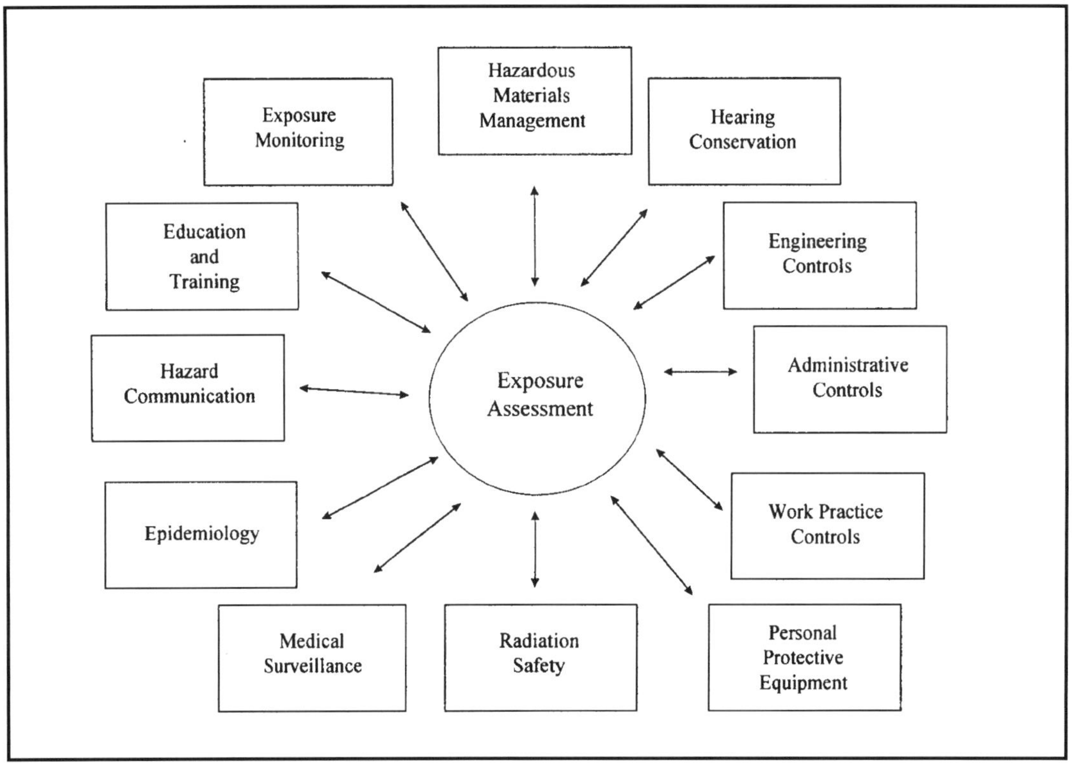

Figure 9.1 — Occupational hygiene program management.

Exposure assessment is at the heart of an occupational hygiene program as it supports all of its functional elements (see Figure 9.1). A well-rationalized program relies on a thorough understanding of what is known and not known about exposures. For example, to understand where best to spend precious resources on a monitoring program, the occupational hygienist must have an understanding of potential exposures that need better characterization or careful routine tracking. A thorough characterization of exposures allows the occupational hygienist to focus worker training programs, better target medical surveillance programs, and define specific requirements for personal protective equipment (PPE).

Better Prioritization of Control Efforts and Expenditures

The better the understanding of exposures and the risks they pose, the more assurance there is that the most important (highest risk) exposures are being controlled first. Control efforts, whether engineering, work practice, or PPE programs, are usually costly to implement and maintain. Therefore, it is critical that those efforts be appropriately prioritized, deployed, and managed.

A thorough understanding of exposures allows prioritization of control efforts to use limited funds wisely. The right combination of control efforts-including short-term, long-term, temporary, and permanent controls-can be implemented based on the prioritized exposure assessments. Plans can be made for improving controls and moving from short-term solutions such as PPE to long-term solutions such as local exhaust ventilation. Management will be assured that money is being spent on the most needed controls first and not wasted on unnecessary control efforts.

Better Understanding of Worker Exposures

A full understanding of exposures, combined with work history, allows better characterization of individual worker exposures and better management of employee medical concerns. Exposure histories, along with health effects information, can indicate the risk that workers have of developing occupational illness and disease. An understanding of exposures allows medical practitioners to target clinical examinations, medical surveillance, or other diagnostic techniques better to detect health effects early. The management of issues related to public health in the community in which the organization operates may be enhanced if there is a well-developed understanding of occupational exposures. When combined with morbidity or mortality data, the comprehensive characterization of exposures greatly improves the power of epidemiologic studies and better positions health care providers to answer questions about an individual's exposures and how they may have affected his or her health.

Shifting State-of-the-Art: Compliance Monitoring to Comprehensive Exposure Assessment

During the past decade, the characterization of exposures has received the attention of occupational hygiene professionals and regulatory agencies worldwide.[1–5] The state-of-the-art approach has shifted from compliance monitoring, which focuses on the maximum risk employee to determine whether exposures are above or below established limits, to comprehensive exposure assessment, which emphasizes the characterization of all exposures for all workers on all days.

Regulations in many countries now mandate some periodic review of exposures throughout an organization.[6–8] While current regulations are highly variable in scope and enforcement, the trend is clear, and the reasoning behind the trend indisputable: A comprehensive approach to assessing occupational exposures better positions an organization to understand the risks associated with the exposures and better positions the organization to manage those risks.

No longer is a compliance-based approach to occupational hygiene sufficient. If a broadened definition of risk is accepted, and it is agreed that the customers-workers and the organizations that employ occupational hygienists-are looking to occupational hygiene to help them manage those risks, one comes to the conclusion that the practice of occupational hygiene must progress to embrace a comprehensive and systematic approach to the evaluation of exposures and the risks they pose. Such an approach will include logical systems and strategies for evaluating all exposures, interpreting and assessing the many present and future risks those exposures might pose, and efficiently managing those exposures that present unacceptable risks.

Overview of Exposure Assessment Strategy

An overview of the comprehensive exposure assessment strategy is shown in Figure 9.2. The strategy is cyclic in nature and is most effectively used in an iterative manner that strives for continuous improvement. Early cycles will begin by collecting available information that is relatively easy to obtain. The results of initial exposure assessments based on that information will be used to prioritize follow-up control and information-gathering efforts. Resources should be focused on those exposures that have the highest priority based on the potential health risk they present. As those exposures are better understood and controlled, they will drop in priority and the next cycles through the strategy will focus on the next tier priority exposures.

The major steps in the strategy follow.

1. Start-establish the exposure assessment strategy.
2. Basic characterization-gather information to characterize the workplace, work force, and environmental agents.
3. Exposure assessment-assess exposures in the workplace in view of the information available on the workplace, work force, and environmental agents. The assessment outcomes include groupings of workers having similar exposures, a defined exposure profile for each group of similarly exposed workers, and a judgment about the acceptability of each exposure profile.
4. Further information gathering-implement prioritized exposure monitoring or the collection of more information on health effects so that uncertain exposure judgments can be resolved with higher confidence.
5. Health hazard control-implement prioritized control strategies for unacceptable exposures.
6. Reassessment-periodically perform a comprehensive re-evaluation of exposures. Determine whether routine monitoring is required to verify that acceptable exposures remain so.
7. Communication and documentation-although there is no element in Figure 9.2 for communication and documentation, the communication of exposure assessment findings and the maintenance of exposure assessment data are underlying and essential features in each step of the process.

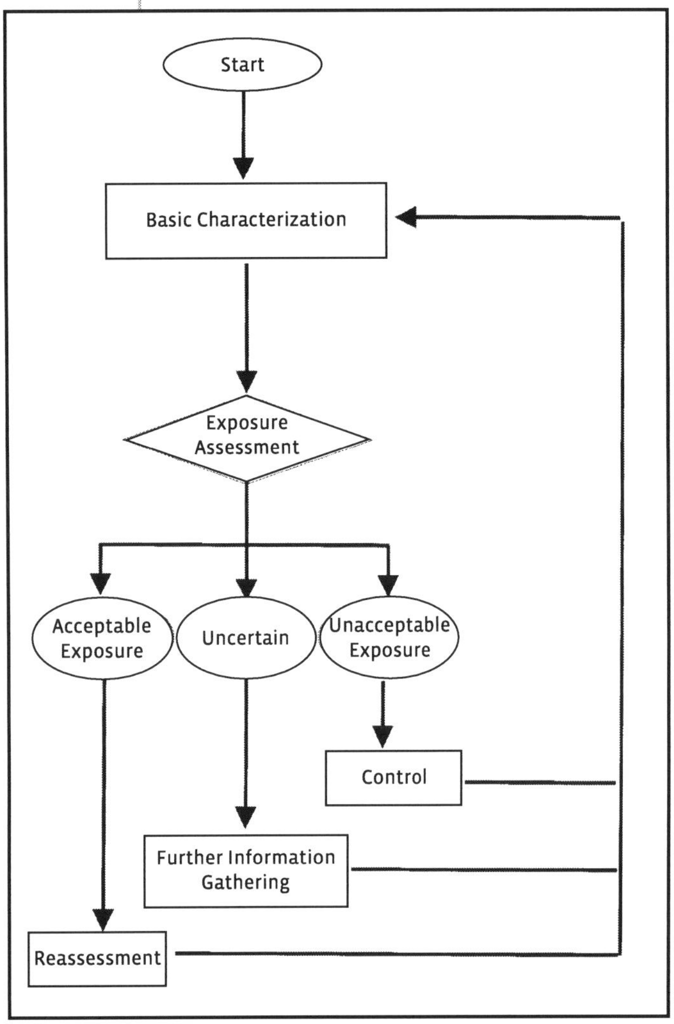

Figure 9.2 — A strategy for assessing and managing occupational exposures.

Start-Establish the Exposure Assessment Strategy

In establishing an organization's exposure assessment strategy, several issues should be carefully addressed, including the role of the occupational hygienist, the exposure assessment goals, and the written exposure assessment program.

Role of the Occupational Hygienist

Exposure assessments should be done by or under the direction of an occupational hygienist. Occupational hygienists have training and experience that make them uniquely qualified to form judgments about exposure profiles and their acceptability. They are best able to define information gathering needs and strategies. They have an understanding of the control options that would be most effective for a particular situation. They are best equipped to direct program modifications and identify prioritizations that take advantage of the results of the exposure assessment.

The participation of other technically knowledgeable professionals such as engineers, environmental scientists, toxicologists, safety professionals, physicians, nurses, and epidemiologists will facilitate exposure assessment programs and improve the quality of assessments. The interaction of occupational hygienists with colleagues in the occupational health professions will enhance worker protection and help ensure the effective implementation of the exposure assessment and management strategy.

Exposure Assessment Goals

Each organization must define goals for its own exposure assessment program. The goals may include (1) the identification and characterization of actual or potential health hazards; and (2) the development and maintenance of an occupational exposure database. The goals should be clearly articulated and lead to one of two general exposure assessment strategies: compliance strategy or comprehensive strategy.

The compliance strategy usually uses worst-case monitoring with a focus on exposures during the time of the survey. An attempt is made to identify the maximum-exposed workers in a group. One or a few measurements are then taken and simply compared with the occupational exposure limit. If the exposures of the maximum-exposed workers are sufficiently below the OEL, then the situation is acceptable. This strategy provides little insight into the day-to-day variation in exposures levels and is not amenable to the development of exposure histories that accurately reflect exposures and health risk. However, in many organizations with more limited funding, the compliance strategy may be an appropriate first step.

The comprehensive strategy is directed at characterizing and assessing exposure profiles (exposure average and variability) that cover all workers, workdays, and environmental agents. These exposure profiles are used to picture exposures on unmeasured days and for unmeasured workers in the similarly exposed group. In addition to ensuring compliance with OELs, this strategy provides an understanding of the day-to-day distribution of exposures. Exposure assessment findings can be used to address present-day health risks and construct exposure histories. If a historical database is maintained, the exposure assessment data may be used to address future health issues for individual workers and/or groups of workers. In the latter case, the data may be used to support epidemiological studies.

The goals of a system for comprehensive exposure assessment include the following:

- Characterize exposures to all potentially hazardous chemical, physical, and biological agents, including those without formal occupational exposure limits.
- Characterize the exposure intensity and temporal variability faced by all workers.
- Assess the potential risks (e.g., risk of potential harm to employee health, risk of noncompliance with governmental regulations, etc.).
- Prioritize and control exposures that present unacceptable risks.
- Identify exposures that need additional information gathering (e.g., baseline monitoring).
- Document exposures and control efforts, and communicate exposure assessment findings to all affected workers and others who are involved in worker health protection (e.g., management, labor representatives, medical staff, engineering staff, etc.).
- Maintain a historical record of exposures for all workers, so that future health issues can be addressed and managed in view of actual exposure information.
- Accomplish the above with efficient and effective allocation of time and resources.

Because a comprehensive approach to exposure assessment provides a more complete understanding of exposures than the compliance approach, it enables better management of occupational hygiene-related risks. It helps provide assurance to an organization's management, customers, employees, and the communities in which the organization operates that occupational health risks are understood and that the proper steps are being taken to manage the risks.

Written Exposure Assessment Program

A written exposure assessment program is an important reference tool for documenting how an organization will administer occupational exposure assessments. It specifies the strategies, methods, and criteria used in performing the assessments. The written program should address the following:

- Goals of the occupational exposure assessment program.
- Role and responsibilities of the occupational hygienist and other technical support staff.
- Methods for systematized information gathering to form a basic characterization of the workplace, work force, and environmental agents.
- Methods for defining groups of similarly exposed workers and the exposure profile for each group.
- Criteria for making a judgment as to whether the exposure profile for a group is acceptable, unacceptable, or uncertain. Decisions surrounding the selection and application of OELs are crucial, as are decisions regarding the appropriate decision statistic (e.g. 95-percent confident that the 95th percentile exposure is less-than the OEL).
- Systems for prioritizing and gathering the additional information needed to better characterize uncertain exposure assessments and make a more confident judgment about their acceptability, whether exposure monitoring data or health effects information.
- Exposure thresholds and criteria for conducting exposure monitoring (e.g., baseline monitoring if the initial exposure estimate is greater than 10% of the OEL).
- A system for ensuring that unacceptable exposures are prioritized and controlled.
- Systems for communicating and documenting exposure assessment findings and health hazard control recommendations.
- Systems and criteria for periodic reassessment of workplace exposures, including routine monitoring programs to ensure that acceptable exposures remain acceptable.

Basic Characterization

At the start of the exposure assessment process is the collection and organization of basic information needed to characterize the workplace, work force, and environmental agents. Information is gathered that will be used to understand the tasks being performed, the materials being used, the processes being run, and the controls in place so that a picture of exposure conditions can be made. At a minimum, the information gathered by the occupational hygienist should include an understanding of the operations, processes, and facilities, including:

1. Work force, tasks, and division of labor;
2. Potentially hazardous chemical, physical, and biological agents in the workplace;
3. How and when workers are exposed to the hazardous environmental agents;
4. Exposure controls present in the workplace, including engineering, administrative, and work practice controls and personal protective equipment;
5. Quantities of environmental agents;
6. Chemical and physical properties of the environmental agents; and
7. Potential health effects of the environmental agents, the mechanism of toxicity, and the OELs associated with each agent.

Health effect information about the environmental agents must be gathered, including OELs. Exposure assessments cannot be resolved without an OEL unless there is no exposure. These may be formal OELs such as regulatory OELs (set and enforced by governmental agencies), authoritative OELs (set and recommended by credible organizations, such as the American Conference of Governmental Industrial Hygienists or the American Industrial Hygiene Association), or internal OELs (formally set by an organization for its private use). Or they may be more

Control Banding

The exposure assessment process depends upon the identification an Occupational Exposure Limit (OEL). In the absence of a *governmental, authoritative* or *internal* OEL, the industrial hygienist can establish a working OEL to complete the exposure assessment. Control banding includes a hazard grouping or banding step that effectively establishes a working OEL for the agent of interest.

On the NIOSH website, control banding is defined as a process in which a single control technology (such as general ventilation or containment) is applied to one range or band of exposures to a chemical (such as 1–10 mg/m^3) that falls within a given hazard group (such as skin and eye irritants or severely irritating and corrosive). These target exposure bands can be used as working OELs in the exposure assessment process. Their expression as a range of exposure levels reflects the uncertainty in their derivation

Control banding originated in the pharmaceutical industry where it is it sometimes difficult to adequately characterize the toxicity of synthetic by-products in order to provide the basis for formal OELs. One system known as "Performance Based Exposure Control Limits" uses estimates of health risk to classify materials into hazard bands denoting ranges of OELs. Engineering control strategies are pre-assigned for each band and range from modest controls up to full containment with no human intervention.[13]

Perhaps the most substantial application of control banding is in the United Kingdom where a regulatory initiative known as COSHH, "Control of Substances Hazardous to Health", makes a control banding tool (COSHH Essentials) available for use by small and medium sized enterprises.[14]

COSHH Essentials utilizes various semiquantitative criteria to determine *working OELs* (hazard groups) and effective control strategies.[14] These criteria are a) "Hazard Groups" A, B, C, D, or E based upon a chemical's European Union R-Phrase prescribed for material safety data sheets -or an estimated range for the OEL, and b) "Exposure Predictor" levels 1 through 4 based upon chemical quantities, volatility and dustiness. The Hazard Groups and Exposure Predictors are used to determine the needed standard control strategies.

Hazard Group	*Target Airborne Concentration Range*	
A	>1–10 mg/m^3 dust;	>50–500 ppm vapor
B	>0.1–1 mg/m^3 dust;	>5–50 ppm vapor
C	>0.01–0.1 mg/m^3 dust;	>0.5–5 ppm vapor
D	<0.01 mg/m^3 dust;	<0.5 ppm vapor
E	Seek specialist advice	

Other applications of control banding can be found in laser safety and biosafety. The American National Standard for the Safe Use of Lasers defines hazard classifications for lasers and guidelines for controlling exposure to laser radiation based on those classifications. The hazard classes and control recommendations are designed to ensure compliance with the underlying OELs for laser radiation.[15]

The National Institutes of Health and the Center for Disease Control utilize a control banding strategy for managing exposure to biological agents in laboratories known as biosafety levels 1 through 4[16]:

BSL-1: Agents not associated with disease in healthy adults

BSL-2: Agents associated with disease, rarely serious and for which preventative interventions are available.

BSL-3: Agents associated with serious or lethal disease, interventions may be available; high individual risk and low community risk.

BSL-4: Agents likely to cause serious or lethal disease, interventions not usually available; high individual and community risk.

Standard practices, equipment and facilities are identified for each Biosafety Level.

informal working OELs that have been set by the occupational hygienist based on whatever information might be available to differentiate acceptable from unacceptable exposures. Working OELs are sometimes stated in ranges (e.g., 0.1–1.0 mg/m^3) or incorporate large safety factors to account for uncertainty.[12,13] Control banding approaches use hazard banding as a mechanism for defining working OELs for the purpose of determining targeted concentrations for control.

In assessing health effects data and reviewing existing OELs, the occupational hygienist should attempt to answer the following questions:

- Why was the existing OEL set at its particular level?
- What safety factor was used in deriving the OEL?
- What potentially important health effects were not considered?

- How adequate are the health data that support the OEL?
- Should the OEL be adjusted in the presence of a nontraditional work schedule?
- Is skin absorption a significant route of exposure?
- Are any concomitant exposures present in the workplace which pose additive or synergistic health risks?

The occupational hygienist must also consider the averaging time of the OEL. The averaging time refers to the time span for which an average exposure is estimated. The appropriate averaging time is set by the sponsor of the OEL and in principle can extend over any length of time from seconds or minutes, to a single shift, to multiple shifts, to months and years. To be in compliance with OELs, the occupational hygienist must follow the defined averaging time corresponding to the defined exposure level.

Choosing an appropriate averaging time for an OEL requires knowledge of the uptake, distribution, storage, elimination, and toxic action of the environmental agent. For substances that act quickly to elicit their toxic response, it is important to control the dose across a single shift (8-hour time-weighted average [TWA]) or shorter period of time (e.g., 15 minutes for short-term exposure limits [STELs] and instantaneous for ceiling limits).

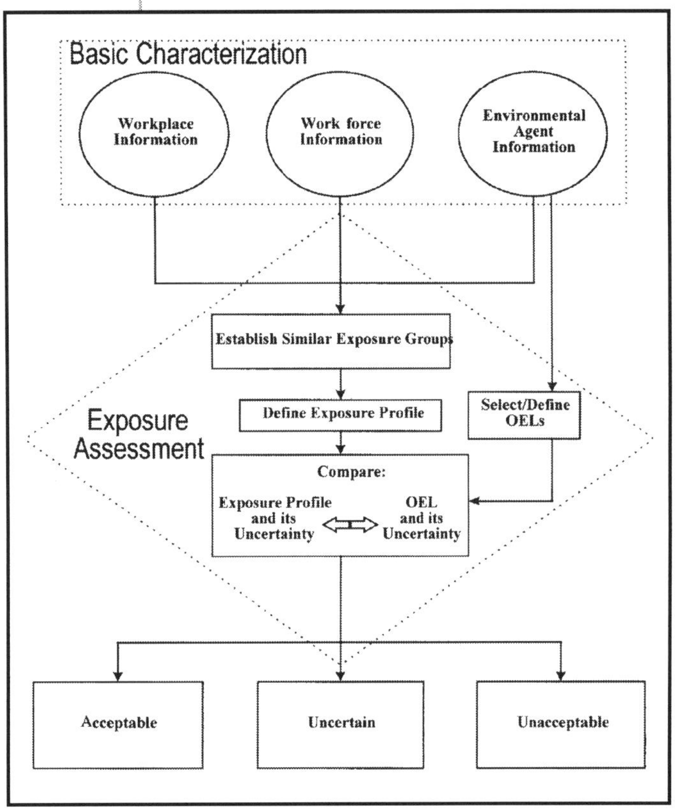

Figure 9.3 — Defining and judging exposure profiles.

Exposure Assessment

After the basic characterization has been performed, the occupational hygienist uses available data to assess exposures. The exposure assessment can be broken into several steps (see Figure 9.3), including establishing similar exposure groups (SEGs); defining the exposure profile, and comparing the exposure profile, with its uncertainty, to the OEL, with its uncertainty, to make a judgment that the exposure is acceptable, unacceptable, or uncertain.

Define SEGs

SEGs are groups of workers having the same general exposure profile for the agent(s) being studied because of the similarity and frequency of the tasks that they perform, the materials and processes with which they work, and the similarity of the way that they perform the tasks. SEGs are established using the information gathered during the basic characterization of the workplace, work force, and environmental agents. The occupational hygienist reviews this data and uses his or her training and experience to group employees believed to have similar exposures. SEGs are generally described by process, job, task, and environmental agent.

Define Exposure Profiles

An exposure profile is an estimate of the exposure intensity and how it varies over time for workers in an SEG. Information used for defining the exposure profile may include qualitative and/or quantitative data.

At the start of the exposure assessment process there may be very little quantitative data available, so most early exposure profiles will be based on qualitative information. As such, they may be accompanied by a great deal of uncertainty. As the information gathering and assessing cycle progresses, SEGs may be redefined and their exposure profiles modified and refined based on new information.

A useful tool for beginning to characterize the exposure profile is the exposure rating, particularly during the initial exposure assessments performed when monitoring data may be sparse or nonexistent.[1] An exposure rating is an estimate of exposure level relative to the OEL. Table 9.1 is an example of a categorization scheme for rating exposures. It is based on an estimate of the upper tail of the exposure profile (the 95th percentile) relative to the OEL.

Table 9.1 — Exposure Rating Categorization: Estimate of the Exposure Profile 95th Percentile Relative to the OEL

4	> 5% exceedance of the OEL (95th percentile > OEL)
3	> 5% exceedance of 0.5 × OEL (95th percentile between 0.5 × OEL and 1.0 × OEL)
2	> 5% exceedance of 0.1 × OEL (95th percentile between 0.1 × OEL and 0.5 × OEL)
1	Minimal to no exceedance of 0.1 × OEL (95th percentile < 0.1 × OEL)

The occupational hygienist's choice of exposure rating schemes will depend on how OELs are defined by regulatory and authoritative standards-setting organizations and on how they are applied in the exposure assessment. Exposure ratings are also useful for defining consistent exposure control follow-up and industrial hygiene program management (Table 9.2).

Table 9.2 — Recommended controls for exposure ratings

Exposure Rating Category	Recommended Control
0 (<1% of OEL)	No action
1 (<10% of OEL)	general HazCom
2 (10-50% of OEL)	+ chemical specific HazCom
3 (50-100% of OEL)	+ exposure surveillance, medical surveillance, work practices
4 (>100% of OEL)	+ respirators & engineering controls, work practice controls

In performing the initial exposure rating, there is value in assuming the absence of personal protective equipment used to control exposures. This will include respirators, hearing protectors, and chemically protective gloves. This approach will allow the occupational hygienist to determine precisely where and to what degree workers depend on personal protective equipment to control a health hazard.

Exposure ratings can be made on the basis of monitoring data (personal monitoring data; screening measurements with easy-to-use instruments such as sound level meters, detector tubes, or other direct reading devices); surrogate data (exposure data from another agent or another operation); and modeling (predictive modeling based on chemical and physical properties or process information).

Make Judgments about the Acceptability of the Exposure Profiles for Each SEG

Based on the SEG exposure profile and information collected about the toxicity of the agent, a judgment is made about the exposure. Specifically, the exposure profile (and the associated uncertainty in the exposure profile) is compared with the OEL (and the associated uncertainty in the OEL) and a judgment is made regarding the acceptability of the risk posed by the exposure. Possible judgments are that the exposure is acceptable, unacceptable, or uncertain.

Conceptually, uncertainty bands can be placed around the OEL and the exposure profile. If the uncertainty bands do not overlap, the occupational hygienist should be able to resolve the exposure assessment as acceptable or unacceptable regardless of the level of uncertainty associated with the OEL and the exposure profile.[9] On the other hand, if the uncertainty bands overlap, the occupational hygienist might not be able to judge whether the exposure is acceptable or unacceptable (see Figure 9.3). In that case he or she is forced to reduce the uncertainty associated with the OEL, the exposure profile, or both. The occupational hygienist must decide whether there is enough concern to classify the exposure as unacceptable and initiate a control program, or whether the existing exposure can continue while additional information is gathered.

The exposure judgment is used to prioritize control efforts or the collection of more information based on the environmental agent's estimated level of exposure, severity of potential health effects, and the uncertainty associated with the exposure profile and health effects information. In this system, unacceptable exposures are put on a prioritized list for control, uncertain exposures are put on a prioritized list for further information gathering, and acceptable

EXAMPLE — STATISTICAL ANALYSIS

Upper Tolerance Limit and Exceedance Fraction

Monitoring was performed in a furniture paint stripping operation to evaluate full-shift operator exposures to methylene chloride (OEL = 25 ppm). All results are eight-hour TWAs:

DATE	PPM	DESCRIPTIVE STATISTICS	
March 24	23	Number of Samples (n)	10
April 3	10	Maximum (max)	32
April 6	3	Minimum (min)	3
April 12	16	Range	29
April 17	6	Percent above OEL (%>OEL)	10
April 28	32	Mean	15.1
May 2	12	Median	14
May 5	24	Standard Deviation (s)	9.11
May 8	8	Geometric Mean (GM)	12.4
May 9	17	Geometric Standard Deviation (GSD)	2.1

Upper Tolerance Limit

The monitoring data was used to estimate the 95th percentile of the operator SEG exposure profile and calculate a 95%, 95% upper tolerance limit for comparison to the methylene chloride OEL of 25 ppm:

LOGNORMAL PARAMETRIC STATISTICS

95th Percentile:	40 ppm
Upper Tolerance Limit (95%, 95%):	100 ppm

Because the 95% upper tolerence limit of 100.4 ppm is far above 25 ppm, we are not 95% confident that the true 95th percentile is less than the 25 ppm OEL and may rate this exposure as "unacceptable."(1)

Exceedance Fraction

We can also use the exceedance fraction technique to evaluate the same monitoring data in order to estimate the percent of the operator SEG exposure profile that exceeds the methylene chloride OEL of 25 ppm(1):

LOGNORMAL PARAMETRIC STATISTICS

Percent Exceeding OEL (% > OEL)	16%
1,95% UCL % > OEL	38%

The exceedance fraction estimate is that 16 percent of the exposure profile is above the OEL. The one-sided 95% upper confidence limit (1,95% UCL) for that exceedence fraction tells us that we are 95 percent confident that 38 percent or less of the exposure profile is above the OEL. Based on those results we may conclude that such a high proportion of the exposure profile above the OEL is too risky and rate the SEG as "unacceptable."

exposures are documented as such and may be put on a list for periodic routine monitoring to verify that exposures continue to be acceptable.

At this point consideration is also given to refining worker membership in SEGs in view of the worker-to-worker variability in exposure that is sometimes associated with differences in work practices or other factors. Refining worker membership is particularly important in SEGs where exposure levels approach the OEL. If an individual worker in one of these critical SEGs has an exposure profile with significantly higher exposures than other workers in the SEG, then that individual worker may be exposed to an unacceptable health risk even though the SEG may have been judged acceptable. A monitoring

Improving Professional Judgment

Professional judgment is critical to efficient and effective exposure risk assessment and management and, indeed, to the successful practice of industrial hygiene. It is critical that judgments be accurate and free of bias. Recent studies indicate that industrial hygienists can improve the accuracy of their judgments through the introduction of some processes into their routine practice:

1) Use statistical analysis tools to evaluate monitoring results whenever data are available for an exposure assessment. Statistical tools inform the judgment by providing a robust characterization of exposure intensity, variability and data uncertainty. Statistical tools are particularly important for overcoming a common tendency to underestimate exposure risk when monitoring data are simply "eyeballed."[17]
2) Document key rationale for exposure judgments as part of the comprehensive exposure assessment. Numerous psychology studies of the accuracy of decisions indicate that accuracy is improved when people are forced to document the reasons for a particular decision.[18,19]
3) Incorporate a "feedback loop" into the exposure assessment process that requires comparison of initial exposure judgments made prior to the availability of monitoring data with judgments made using the statistical analysis of monitoring data when they become available. The Bayesian construct for integrating initial "prior" exposure decisions with data-based "likelihood" exposure decisions is particularly well suited for this purpose.[20]

Bayesian decision analysis provides an obvious feedback mechanism that can be used by an industrial hygienist to improve professional judgment. For example, if the likelihood decision distribution is inconsistent with the prior decision distribution then it is likely that either a significant process change has occurred or the industrial hygienist's initial judgment was incorrect. In either case, the industrial hygienist should readjust his judgment regarding this operation.

strategy may then be needed for these critical SEGs that incorporates ANOVA analysis of multiple measurements on multiple workers in the SEG in order to determine whether there is significant between-worker variability.[1,2]

Further Information Gathering

Exposure profiles that are not well understood, or for which acceptability judgments cannot be made with high confidence, must be further characterized by collecting additional information. Information-gathering efforts should be prioritized. Higher priority should be given to information needs associated with uncertain exposure assessments that involve high exposure rating estimates to highly toxic materials. In some cases, if exposure rating and toxicity estimates are high enough, consideration should be given to the use of personal protective equipment or other interim controls while the information is gathered or generated.

The occupational hygienist should also consider the installation of permanent controls in lieu of additional information gathering. It might, for example, be more cost-effective to implement additional controls than to spend resources attempting to characterize the exposure profile further.

The type of information needed may vary from one SEG to another. The exposure profile for one SEG may be very well understood but there may be little toxicity information available. In that case it will be important to collect, or even generate, toxicological or epidemiological data. Another SEG may have little data or prior knowledge available on which to base an estimate of the exposure profile. In that case it will be important to generate information to better characterize the exposure profile, either through exposure monitoring, modeling, or biological monitoring.

Exposure Monitoring. If an exposure profile is not well characterized, there may be a need for personal monitoring of worker exposures. This may include noise monitoring, air monitoring, skin exposure monitoring, or other environmental measurements.

Exposure Modeling. As tools for using mathematical modeling techniques to predict exposures based on workplace and worker parameters become more sophisticated, they will be used more and more to estimate exposure profiles. Exposure modeling is frequently used to estimate the potential

Bayesian Decision Analysis

A recently proposed approach to explicitly integrating qualitative judgments with the statistical analysis of monitoring data within a Bayesian statistical construct offers tremendous promise for improving the accuracy of exposure judgments and the effectiveness and efficiency of exposure management programs.[20]

The approach uses a common construct for depicting both qualitative exposure assessments and statistical analysis of quantitative data as decision probabilities that the 95th percentile of the SEG exposure distribution falls into a particular AIHA exposure category (e.g., 1%, 80%, 12%, 5%, and 2% probability that the exposure profile is a Category 0, 1, 2, 3, or 4 exposure). Bayesian statistical analysis is then used to combine the qualitative exposure characterization (prior) with the statistical analysis of the monitoring data (likelihood) to form an integrated depiction of the exposure (posterior).

Advantages of Bayesian decision analysis include: (a) decisions can be made with greater certainty; (b) prior data, professional judgment, or modeling information can be objectively incorporated into the decision-making process; (c) decision probabilities are easier to understand than the output of more traditional statistical analysis techniques; and (d) fewer measurements are necessary whenever the prior distribution is well defined and the process is fairly stable.[20]

exposures associated with new processes and products. Such models have the advantage of being less expensive and time-consuming than the actual measurement of environmental agents in the workplace.[21]

Biological Monitoring. Biological monitoring may be needed to assess the exposure profile if there are concerns about exposure through skin absorption or inadvertent ingestion. Due to the medical and ethical issues involved, the occupational hygienist should work closely with a physician whenever biological monitoring is considered.

Toxicological Data Generation. If the toxicity of the materials used in the workplace is not understood, then it is difficult to make a judgment about the acceptability of the exposure no matter how well that exposure profile is characterized. In those cases it may be necessary to obtain additional health effects information on the environmental agents of interest by eliciting the aid of toxicologists and other experts.

Epidemiological Data Generation. Epidemiological investigations are directed at evaluating the relationships between exposures and health. The results of epidemiological studies add to the available toxicological information for an environmental agent and enable better judgments about the acceptability or unacceptability of exposures. They can help determine whether adverse health conditions are associated with workplace exposures, and provide the basis for worker health management and workplace controls. Often one of the biggest weaknesses in epidemiological studies is the lack of useful exposure data.

Health Hazard Controls

SEG exposure profiles that are judged unacceptable should be put on a prioritized list for control. It is critical that occupational hygiene control programs be deployed and adjusted in view of exposure assessment findings. Control programs balance available resources with control needs to implement and maintain interim (e.g., respirator) or permanent (e.g., local exhaust ventilation) controls. Prioritization of resources for permanent controls can be performed based on the health risk posed by the exposure and the toxicity of the environmental agent. The prioritization factors may also include the uncertainty associated with the judgment, the number of workers exposed, and the frequency of exposure.

Exposure assessment findings can also be used to prioritize diagnostic monitoring, modeling, or other efforts to understand the important determinants of exposure so that effective control measures can be developed. Diagnostic monitoring is performed to identify the sources of exposure and to understand how the sources, tasks, and other variables (e.g., production rates) contribute to worker exposures. Modeling tools can help pinpoint the determinants that most influence exposure levels. They also offer a cost effective approach for exploring the effects of various control options. The results help the occupational hygienist devise the most appropriate and efficient control strategies for unacceptable exposures and determine whether the new or modified controls are effective.[21]

Reassessment

Exposures that are judged acceptable may need no further action, other than documentation, until the time comes for reassessment. Or there may be a need to collect further information, such as monitoring data, toxicology data, or epidemiological data to (1) validate the judgment of acceptability; and (2) ensure that the operation does not go out of control.

It is important that exposure profiles and SEGs be kept up-to-date as changes occur in the workplace that affect exposures. This will ensure that exposures continue to be well understood and that the organization's occupational hygiene program continues to respond to changing priorities.

The exposure assessment system should be linked to a management of change program that will help identify changes in the processes, materials, or work force that may significantly alter exposures or the allocation of employees to SEGs. These changes include (1) increased/decreased production rates; (2) increased/decreased production energy; (3) new or untrained workers introduced into the exposure group; (4) changed OELs; (5) new toxicity data; and (6) new or changed material (chemical or physical change).

There should also be a provision for required reassessment at some appropriate interval to account for the fact that many factors that influence changes in exposures are not readily foreseeable.

Communication and Documentation

The entire exposure assessment process, including all exposure assessment findings and follow-up, must be documented, whether or not monitoring data were collected. Moreover, the exposure assessment findings must be communicated in a timely and effective fashion to all workers in the SEG and others who are involved in worker health protection.

Lists of SEGs, their exposure profiles, and the judgments about their acceptability should be permanently stored so that individual exposure histories can be generated. Information on baseline and routine monitoring programs, as well as hazard control plans, must be kept along with evidence that the plans were implemented.

The data documentation efforts required by the comprehensive approach to exposure assessment in many organizations will be difficult to manage without the help of a computerized data management system. In planning an exposure assessment database, the occupational hygienist should carefully consider how exposure data will be used. Records should be established and maintained so that pertinent questions can be answered accurately and within a reasonable period of time. The occupational hygienist should recognize that other disciplines could have an interest in exposure data. This includes workers, management, and perhaps an organization's medical, engineering, and legal staff. Governmental agencies and industry associations may have an interest in occupational exposure data. Exposure records can also be a vitally important component of future epidemiological studies.[22,23]

Summary

Occupational hygienists throughout the world are recognizing that a systematic and comprehensive approach to exposure assessment is an effective mechanism for managing occupational hygiene programs. A thorough understanding of exposures allows the prioritization of the occupational hygiene program-including control efforts-to protect employees and manage exposure-related risks.

It also positions the occupational hygienist for better management of the unpredictable change that will occur both in knowledge of the health effects of environmental agents and in society's tolerance of workplace exposures. Coupled with good work-history information, comprehensive exposure assessments will enable better epidemiology and refinement of the understanding of the relationship between occupational exposures and disease.

The occupational hygienist is strongly encouraged to develop an exposure assessment program that is comprehensive in nature. Such a program will better position organizations to understand and manage ever-broadening occupational health-related risk.

References

1. **Mulhausen, J.R. and J. Damiano (eds.):** *A Strategy for Assessing and Managing Occupational Exposures,* 2nd edition. Fairfax, VA: AIHA Press, 1998.

2. **Ignacio, J. and W.H. Bullock (eds.):** *A Strategy for Assessing and Managing Occupational Exposures*, 3rd edition. Fairfax, VA: AIHA Press, 2006.
3. **American Industrial Hygiene Association (AIHA):** A Generic Exposure Assessment Standard. *Am. Ind. Hyg. Assoc. J. 55*:1009–1012.
4. **Organization Resources Counselors, Inc. (ORC):** "A Proposed Generic Workplace Exposure Assessment Standard." Washington, DC: ORC, 1992.
5. **Guest, I.G., J.W. Chessie, R.J. Gardner, and C.D. Money:** *Sampling Strategies for Airborne Contaminants in the Workplace* (British Occupational Hygiene Society Technical Guide 11). Leeds, UK: H and H Scientific Consultants Ltd., 1993.
6. **Health and Safety Executive (HSE):** The Control of Substances Hazardous to Health (Regulation 1657). London: Her Majesty's Stationery Office Publications Centre, 1988.
7. **Australia National Occupational Health and Safety Commission:** Control of Workplace Hazardous Substances. Canberra, Australia: Australian Government Publishing Service, 1993.
8. **Comité Européen de Normalisation (CEN):** Workplace Atmospheres-Guidance for the Assessment of Exposure by Inhalation of Chemical Agents for Comparison with Limit Values and Measurement Strategy (European Standard EN 689). London: CEN, 1995. [English version.]
9. **Jayjock, M.A., and N.C Hawkins:** A Proposal for Improving the Role of Exposure Modeling in Risk Assessment. *Am. Ind. Hyg. Assoc. J. 54*:733–741 (1993).
10. **Hawkins, N.C., M.A. Jayjock, and J. Lynch:** A Rationale and Framework for Establishing the Quality of Human Exposure Assessment. *Am. Ind. Hyg. Assoc. J. 53*:34–41 (1992).
11. **Claycamp, H.G.:** Industrial Health Risk Assessment: Industrial Hygiene for Technology Transition. *Am. Ind. Hyg. Assoc. J. 57*:423–427 (1996).
12. **Brooke, I.M.:** A UK Scheme to Help Small Firms Control Health Risks from Chemicals: Toxicological Considerations. *Ann. Occup. Hyg. 42*:377–390 (1998)
13. **Naumann, B.D., et al.:** Performance-Based Exposure Control Limits for Pharmaceutical Active Ingredients. *Am. Ind. Hyg. Assoc. J. 57*:33–42 (1996).
14. **Health and Safety Executive (HSE):** Control of Substances Hazardous to Health (Fifth Edition). Approved Code of Practice and Guidance. Health and Safety Executive, London. ISBN 0-7176-2981-3 2005
15. **Laser Institute of America (LIA):** ANSI Z136.1-2006 Safe Use of Lasers. Orlando, FL: LIA, 2007.
16. **Ryan, T.J.:** Biosafety Hazards in the Work Environment (Chapter 19). In *The Occupational Environment: Its Evaluation, Control and Management*, 2nd edition. DiNardi, S.R. (ed.). Fairfax, VA: AIHA Press, 2003.
17. **Logan, P.W. G. Ramachandran, J. R. Mulhausen, and P. Hewett:** Occupational exposure decisions: Can limited data interpretation training help improve accuracy? *Annals of Occ. Hyg.* 2009. [In Press].
18. **Kahneman, D., P. Slovic, and A. Tversky:** *Judgment Under Uncertainty: Heuristics and Biases.* New York: Cambridge University Press, 1982.
19. **Plous, S.:** *The Psychology of Judgment and Decision Making.* New York: McGraw-Hill, 1993.
20. **Hewett, P., P.W. Logan, J. Mulhausen, G. Ramachandran, and S. Banerjee:** Rating Exposure Control using Bayesian Decision Analysis. *J. Occup. Env. Health 3*:568–581, (2006).
21. **Keil, C.B. (ed.):** *Mathematical Models for Estimating Occupational Exposure to Chemicals.* Fairfax, VA: AIHA Press, 2000.
22. **Joint ACGIH-AIHA Task Group on Occupational Exposure Databases:** Data Elements for Occupational Exposure Databases: Guidelines and Recommendations for Airborne Hazards and Noise. *Appl. Occup. Environ. Hyg. 11*:1294–1311 (1996).
23. **Rajan, R., R. Alesbury, B. Carton, M. Gerin, et al.:** European Proposal for Core Information for the Storage and Exchange of Workplace Exposure Measurements on Chemical Agents. *Appl. Occup. Environ. Hyg. 12*:31–39 (1997).

Outcome Competencies

After completing this chapter, the reader should be able to:

1. Define underlined terms used in this chapter.
2. Define or recognize their options and responsibilities as occupational hygienists and practicing risk assessors.
3. Describe that true risk is never known but is typically overestimated vis-à-vis the Precautionary Principle.
4. Recall that the degree of risk overestimation is inversely proportional to the resources applied to the estimation.
5. Recognize that the occupational hygienist is a working technologist who uses science.
6. Recall that the heart and soul of this science is in the building, testing, and use of models.
7. Describe how expert judgment is legitimate and valued to the extent that the assumptions and data underlying it can be revealed and explained.
8. Recall that models that are overestimating can be useful, and that they are inexpensive in a tiered approach to risk assessment.
9. Apply equilibrium or steady-state vapor pressure models.
10. Apply the steady-state concentration single and two box model.
11. Apply the steady-state concentration dispersion model.
12. Recall that nonsteady-state concentration modeling is much more complicated.
13. Seek additional sources of information and guidance on exposure modeling.

Key Terms

box model • dispersion model • exposure limits • exposure modeling • exposure assessment • human health risk assessment • tiered approach • steady-state model • vapor pressure • zero ventilation model

Prerequisite Knowledge

Basic chemistry, physics, algebra.

Prior to beginning this chapter, the user should review the following chapters:

Chapter Number	Chapter Topic
8	Occupational and Environmental Health Risk Assessment/Risk Management
11	Sampling of Gases and Vapors
12	Analysis of Gases and Vapors
14	Sampling and Sizing of Airborne Particles
15	Principles and Instrumentation for Calibrating Air Sampling Equipment
17	Direct-Reading Instruments for Determining Gases, Vapors, and Aerosols Concentrations

Key Topics

Modeling Inhalation Exposure

10

Michael A. Jayjock, PhD, CIH

Introduction

Exposure modeling represents the essence of the science of exposure assessment and should be considered the primary stock in trade of the occupational hygienist. Before delving into the meaning and manner of exposure modeling, it is necessary to understand its context in the overall evaluation of potential impacts to worker health.

The primary function of occupational hygienists is to evaluate the potential risk of exposure to the health of workers. This is called human health risk assessment, and the subject is covered in much greater detail elsewhere in this book. However, for exposure modeling to make sense, it is necessary to present the following facts or touchstones of the process.

- Human Health Risk is driven equally by the exposure and the health effects per unit exposure.
- The essence of risk assessment in the context of industrial/occupational hygiene is the comparison of the estimated exposure to appropriate exposure limits.
- When faced with scientific uncertainty a precautionary approach[1] is typically applied which advises practitioners to err on the side of safety and thus overestimate risk or obtain more information to lower the uncertainty.
- Risk is estimated (typically overestimated) versus the true risk, and the true risk is never known.
- Risk assessment is typically a tiered approach starting with evaluations that generally overestimate risk but are inexpensive, and proceeding to more expensive but more accurate analytical tools.

It should be reasonably obvious from the information given above that occupational hygienists measure or otherwise estimate worker exposure, and this exposure has no contextual meaning without a valid exposure limit with which to compare it. The reader is encouraged to review the chapters in this book on risk assessment to understand the full meaning of these important concepts. Other references on this subject include various American Industrial Hygiene Association® (AIHA®) books and papers on risk assessment[2–4] and exposure assessment strategies.[5] Suffice it to say here that the following discussion of exposure modeling presents an approach that has as its end the comparison of an estimated exposure to a valid and appropriate exposure limit. Given that relationship it is necessary to understand the origin and basis of the exposure limits used. Anyone who has followed the downward trend in occupational exposure limits will understand that published exposure limits are never written in stone. The working limits, whether derived locally in working establishments or from the regulators or consensus groups such as the American Conference of Governmental Industrial Hygienists® (ACGIH®), should all be the subject of study, understanding, and judgment regarding their documentation and level of acceptable risk within societal norms.

This chapter is intended to introduce the general topic of exposure modeling. A general outline of the process and its importance will be presented along with a few operational tools. It will not get very deeply into the technical details of all of the models available or possible. Indeed, a full treatment of exposure modeling is not possible in a single chapter such as this. In fact, it is the subject of an entire book published by the AIHA®.[6] The second edition of *Mathematical Models for Estimating Occupational Exposure to Chemicals*[7] represents a significant addition to and enhancement of the first. Where it is appropriate, abstracted information from this second edition will be included in this chapter. These insights from the AIHA® modeling book are designed to inform the reader about the current state of the science and to encourage him or her to obtain this important text.

Why Do Exposure Modeling?

Indeed, why would one want to understand and use exposure models? The simple answer is that practicing occupational hygienists will never be able to monitor every situation everywhere. Also, as a technical expert, an occupational hygienist should have some objective and defensible rationale for why he or she did not do monitoring in the vast majority of exposure scenarios.

Consider a modern plant with hundreds of workers performing perhaps thousands of tasks within it. It is reasonably well established that the majority of tasks are never monitored because the occupational hygienist judges them to be safe.[8,9] That is, he or she has observed the situation and has concluded that the exposure limit is not exceeded. When asked how that determination was arrived at, the typical answer is that he or she applied "expert judgment"; the occupational hygienist uses his or her combined experience to make this call. When pressed further the hygienist may say that it is because the system or scenario under consideration is relatively "closed", that the vapor pressure is low, the exposure limit is relatively high, etc. These factors combine to tell an experienced occupational hygienist that overexposure will not occur. Some threshold must exist for these skilled estimators where conditions are such that predicted concentrations and exposures approach or exceed the exposure limit. At this point, the occupational hygienist typically moves to action and monitors the situation. The results of that monitoring determine whether controls are implemented.

Much of exposure assessment in general and industrial hygiene in particular, has been practiced using the reactive, reflective, qualitative, and undefined expert judgment as outlined above. Within the IH world, this manner and technique of working has generally protected many workers from overexposure and subsequent adverse health effects. However, it has a number of serious flaws, including:

(1) It is difficult or impossible to explain objectively.
(2) It is typically not supported by explicit quantified facts relating specific cause and effect.
(3) It is not amenable to technology transfer (i.e., those new to the field find it hard to learn).
(4) It is often insufficient to provide convincing evidence to affected workers or to defend against litigation or other legal challenges.

Thus, the standard method of direct measurement of selective scenarios is clearly not the best way to proceed. Indeed, sometimes measurements cannot be taken. Consider the following cases:

- You want to monitor exposures, but there is NO method available.
- You cannot measure exposures "right now" when they are occurring.
- You cannot measure exposures because you cannot be present, such as when they happen at another location, they happened previously (retrospective), or they have not happened yet (prospective).
- A small sample size of exposure monitoring events leads to a heavy bias toward concluding that unacceptable exposures are acceptable.[10]
- The financial burden associated with a technician's time to collect sample and analytical fees are real-world challenges that restrict monitoring efforts.

The stereotypical "old-time" occupational hygienist who is expert at determining which scenarios do not need monitoring is probably able to do so by running models subliminally or unconsciously in his or her mind while subconsciously comparing the results of this modeled exposure to the exposure limit. This chapter is designed to show how this process can be more open, conscious, objective, and most important, transferable to others. It strives to provide the practitioner with the basic rationale with the introduction of scientific tools and approaches for a technologist doing exposure assessment.

Practicing Occupational Hygienists are already Modelers

The reality is that every active occupational hygienist is already a modeler. It has already been established that a majority of potential exposures in the workplace are never monitored because the occupational hygienist judges them to be safe. How does he or she arrive at this conclusion? As discussed above, most occupational hygienists do it by applying a subliminal "model." This is done using the basic scientific method. To explain this further, consider the primary elements of the scientific method:

1. State the problem or premise
2. Form a hypothesis
3. Experiment and observe
4. Interpret the data
5. Draw conclusions and make predictions

In the course of evaluating the exposure/risk to workers, the occupational hygienist forwards a hypothesis or "model" of what he or she thinks is happening in the world relative to cause and effect. Their observations and interpretations in the vast majority of cases (or thought "experiments" in this example) support the hypothesis that exposures are below hazardous levels, and they conclude that the situation is safe.

As noted previously, when asked how they arrived at this conclusion for a majority of the scenarios under their responsibility, the usual answer is "expert judgment" which is operationally defined elsewhere[11] as:

> *"The application and appropriate use of knowledge gained from formal education, observation, experimentation, inference, and analogy."*

Clearly, the occupational hygienist has some model in mind when forming this hypothesis. A subliminal mathematical relationship or an algorithm was used to hypothesize, *"given the characteristics of all the causes of exposure in this situation, the resulting exposure will be less than the exposure limit."* Of course, much more often than not the hygienist is so sure of the hypothesis (the model) that he or she does not do the actual "experiment," namely; there is no physical measure of the exposure.

In some of the scenarios, and using the same subliminal model, the hygienist concludes that *overexposure* is possible. He or she is then compelled to test that hypothesis of relative safety. Thus, after observation, the occupational hygienist may conduct the experiment: someone measures the concentration and computes exposures. These monitoring data then provide direct and objective experimental evidence to accept or reject the hypothesis and to draw conclusions about the risk of this exposure. Perhaps more importantly, this process feeds the hygienist's internal database (*i.e.*, it increases experience) and allows for improvements in estimations and predictions about similar exposures in the future. That is, the use of data to evaluate the exposure hypothesis actually develops expert judgment. When the hypothesis that "exposures are low compared to the exposure limit" is rejected by monitoring data, it is imperative to learn what went wrong in judgment to not only improve expertise, but to ensure the health of the persons being served.

The occupational hygienist needs to realize that his or her expert judgment is an application of some "model," even if it has never been considered as such. Experienced occupational hygienists recall that as they were developing their technical skills, they improved with more experience, and they got better at understanding what they needed to know (the "inputs") to make better qualitative decisions on whether the scenario was "safe" or "let's monitor." This process is essentially the same as learning the technical details of mathematical modeling; however the latter process is infinitely more open and rational. As one progresses through the world of conscious modeling, he or she will learn what models gives when more complex algorithms and inputs are necessary to get better answers.

Some choose to call this typical subconscious hypothesis forming process of the occupational hygienist "qualitative exposure assessment," when in fact it involves the comparison of a quantitative estimate of the exposure (however unconsciously formulated) with a numerical exposure limit. The point of learning here is that there is clearly a quantitative model present and operating, if only subconsciously, and occupational hygienists need to have a more conscious understanding and explanation of the details of the decision-making process. This conscious understanding will help identify and fix a broken or defective model or understanding of reality. It will allow for the rational explanation to others as to how occupational hygienists operate professionally. Rather than simply invoking a claim of unsubstantiated professional judgment relative to their decisions, by using explicit mathematical modeling the occupational hygienist can understand and display the scientific rationale behind those decisions.

Model Elements

The primary element of a mathematical model is an algorithm. An algorithm in this context is simply an equation in which the predicted state, or exposure in this case, is on the left hand side and the inputs are on the right hand side of the equal sign. A general example is shown below:

$$\text{Predicted State} = f\,(\text{inputs}) \qquad (10\text{-}1)$$

The left-hand side of the equation (the predicted state in this case) is the dependent variable. The right hand side (inputs) represents the independent or predictor variables. The logic of the equation is that the inputs cause or drive the predicted state. The predicted state in exposure models is typically exposure or a concentration that leads to human exposure.

When exposure is measured directly the critical inputs or drivers that caused that exposure are typically not quantified. In the opinion of the authors this is a lost opportunity because understanding the predictors of exposure, should enable the prediction of exposures in many scenarios using models.

The reader will be exposed to some very explicit physical chemical models later in this chapter; however, they all have the basic form described above.

Below is a more concrete example of a relatively simple algebraic model commonly seen in mathematical or scientific training.

$$Y = (a)X_1 + (b)X_2 + (c)X_3 \ldots \qquad (10\text{-}2)$$

where:

Y = dependent variable (airborne concentration or breathing zone exposure)
X_1 = independent or predictor variable 1 (e.g., vapor pressure)
X_2 = independent or predictor variable 2 (e.g., evaporating surface area)
X_3 = independent for predictor variable 3 (e.g., ventilation rate)
a, b, c = predictor strength coefficients

In this model there are 3 inputs (vapor pressure, evaporating surface area and ventilation rate) all combining to cause the airborne concentration in the breathing zone of the exposed person. All of these inputs are independent of one another and all contribute to the airborne concentration. Vapor pressure and evaporating surface area are said to be source factors while ventilation rate is a control factor which limits the exposure. The predictor strength coefficients quantitatively describe the relative weight of their respective contributions within this model.

If such a model was reasonably developed and validated, it would be a valuable aid to anyone seeking to advance their understanding of what specifically might be causing the airborne concentrations to occur from passively evaporating sources.

Indeed, workers' exposures can be fully understood only to the extent that the physical world and the entities within it that cause exposures (i.e., the independent or predictor variables) are known and explicated. Even given a rich database of monitored airborne concentrations (i.e., dependent variable data), one must relate those results to the determinants (i.e., predictors) in the world that produced those exposures.[12] This is necessary to assure the continued validity of the predicted exposures in the future and allow for prediction of different scenarios.

The construction and use of these models is not mysterious, it is simply science. In the context of modeling inhalation exposure for occupational hygiene, this effort can be thought of as investigating and seeking to understand the determinants of airborne contaminant source generation and control. As the critical variables governing the generation and control of airborne toxicants are discerned, the tools are formed that will build one's experience, knowledge-base, and confidence to predict actual concentrations and exposures in the real world with simulated scenarios. As discussed above, model development consists of formulating hypotheses about the predictors of exposure and then testing them with data from experiments examining cause and effect. It is simply the scientific method as described above.

As understanding of why and how physical-chemical models are developed grows, it also becomes clear that the models represent a principal structural basis for the science of exposure assessment. These models, along with the statistical modeling of monitoring data, form the scientific foundation for characterizing worker exposure. Comparing the exposure to the toxicity or the health effect/exposure provides the basis for risk assessment.

Physical-chemical inhalation models are not limited to predicting present exposures. They can be used to estimate historical exposures that cannot easily be re-created and possible future exposures in hypothetical situations or scenarios. By employing a model, an occupational hygienist's insight about possible exposures is enhanced, even if the model is not perfectly accurate. A noted statistician, G.W.E. Box, has been credited with the profound observation that "all models are wrong, but some are useful."

What Box knew and others should keep in mind is that all scientific models, including occupational exposure models, are more or less generalized (and therefore relatively crude) representations of reality. Even remarkably elegant and presumably complete and correct basic scientific models such as those devised by Sir Isaac Newton to describe the laws of motion are wrong under certain conditions as described by Einstein. Thus, predictions from physical-chemical inhalation models can be extremely valuable; however, at this point these models are far from being considered elegant or complete. As such, they should be interpreted with caution and the usual judgment and intelligence that an occupational hygienist brings to his or her craft.

Submodels and Assumptions in Exposure Modeling

Many human exposure models do not estimate human exposure directly. In the case of inhalation models, they estimate the concentration of toxicant in the air and assume that the person is breathing the same air with this concentration. As such the model estimating the airborne concentration can be considered a submodel to a more general model which includes the concentration, contact and inhaling the contaminated air. Indeed, certain elements of the air concentration model may be composed of specific submodels. A prime example would be a model to estimate the vapor pressure of a component in a mixture which would then be feed into model to estimate airborne concentration levels.

With regard to dermal exposure some models simply estimate the amount of the toxicant that goes onto the surface of the skin and then assume either all or some specific portion of it penetrates into the systemic circulation of the body. This could be part of a submodel to estimate systemic or adsorbed dose.

The use of the above and various other assumptions are obviously important and necessary in exposure assessment. However, they can also clearly be problematic. In order for those who view and are affected by occupational hygiene to understand it, they need to be able to review the assumptions of the occupational hygienist. Indeed, it is vital to the integrity of the process to sort out and identify each and every assumption used in the modeling and subsequent estimation of exposure.

Tiered Approach to Modeling Exposure

There is a natural and appropriate tendency within any human endeavor to be efficient and cost-effective in accomplishing any goal or end product.

As such, it is typical to start with relatively simple models that not require much in the way of resources and thus are simple, easy and quick to run. The inputs to these simple models are purposely designed to be relatively easy to attain and use. For example, one can assume complete airborne saturation of vapors from an evaporating source which is easily done simply by knowing the vapor pressure. The downside is that this simple model could indeed dramatically overestimate the exposure potential of the scenario under investigation. Thus, depending on the conclusions of the predicted level of exposure compared with the exposure limit (i.e., the hazard index or exposure/exposure limit ratio), it may be necessary to apply more sophisticated modeling tools. These more complicated models cost more time, effort, and money but they render answers that are less overestimating.

During the tiered process it is not unusual to run out of modeling resource before gaining a definitive answer, and in this case either a better model (or model inputs) needs to be developed or representative air monitoring is performed. Unfortunately, for the general development of physical-chemical models the second solution (monitoring) has historically been chosen almost invariably because it is relatively inexpensive and answers the question at hand expeditiously.[12] Thus, exposure models in general have not been reasonably validated or developed to provide more precisely accurate portrayals of reality. Instead they exist as somewhat underdeveloped (albeit still useful) tools for the overestimation of airborne concentration, exposure and risk. It has been the authors long-lasting belief and assertion that the true promise of exposure assessment as a science will not be realized until resources are allocated to appropriately evaluate (validate) and develop these models in a standard development cycle.[13]

Hierarchy of Modeling Estimation Techniques

Below is a somewhat consolidated discussion and presentation of inhalation exposure modeling techniques. It is provided to introduce these tools. Much of the fine details are left out, and the reader is encouraged to go to the references for more information, including *Mathematical Models for Estimating Occupation Exposure to Chemicals*, 2nd edition.

Exposure modeling can become technically complicated very quickly. Indeed, one could easily spend an entire career in this field (although few have). However, the purpose here is to introduce the topic and thus only a few of the most generally used and useful models are discussed, these being the saturation or zero ventilation model, the box model, and the dispersion model. They are presented here in the form of an example.

For the case study the inhalation exposure potential to toluene from an aqueous solution containing 1 ppm w/w (one weight part per million weight parts, or w/w) of toluene will be considered. In this example the models are shown in order of tiers with increasing sophistication and level of information needed to use them appropriately and successfully. Thus, the first model one should think of using is the simple saturation model, followed by the box and dispersion models. More sophistication is brought into the investigation only if the overestimation cannot be tolerated in the evaluation of the risk.

Given minimal information about the use scenario and physical properties of a material, one can estimate the saturation concentration as an estimation of worst case airborne exposure to vapors in a Tier 1 analysis.[14,15]

Tier 1: Saturation or Zero Ventilation Model

This very basic and typically very conservative inhalation exposure model calculates the maximum possible concentration of vapor (i.e., saturation) in air. It is best used for gases and vapors emitted without mist formation when there is no information on ventilation or the details of use.

For any liquid, saturation will eventually occur in the air above a liquid surface if there is no ventilation and enough liquid is present for its saturated vapors to fill the available volume. In this case, the evaporation rate ultimately overwhelms any removal mechanism such as absorption, adsorption, or chemical transformation.

Figure 10.1 illustrates this phenomenon.

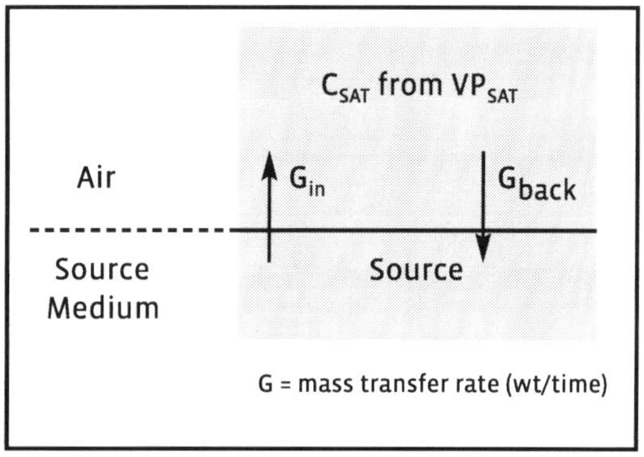

Figure 10.1 — Zero Ventilation or Saturation Model.

The equilibrium saturation concentration (C_{sat}) in volume parts of contaminant per million volume parts of air (ppm v/v) can be readily calculated using the following algorithm:

$$C_{sat} = \frac{VP_{sat}}{760}(1{,}000{,}000) \quad (10\text{-}3)$$

C_{sat} = airborne concentration in ppm v/v
VP_{sat} = saturation vapor pressure in Torr or mmHg

Vapor pressure (VP_{sat}) at any ambient temperature is an experimentally determined quantity; however, it can also be estimated from boiling point data for any class of liquids either at atmospheric pressure or under vacuum.[16] The estimation of the vapor pressure of components within mixtures is significantly more complicated but can also be estimated using established procedures.[17] This saturation model is usually conservative for the prediction of workroom air concentrations. It has been the authors' experience that it overestimates workroom air concentrations of vapor (i.e., non-particulate) in all but worst case scenarios (e.g., large spills indoors with poor ventilation) by a factor ranging over four orders of magnitude (10–10,000X). This observation is the result of comparing scores of measured concentrations of organic air contaminants in occupational settings with their saturation concentrations calculated from vapor pressure or boiling point data. Worst case scenarios include those in which significant aerosol is released or there is a relatively large area (greater than a few square meters) of evaporating liquid. In these situations the saturation model is often not very overestimating.

This model's value lies in its simplicity as a screen with only a few basic physicochemical properties required as input. As a typically very conservative estimate it represents a good first step in a tiered risk assessment. If exposure levels determined by the model are below the compound's ascribed toxic exposure level (e.g., an occupational exposure limit), a high degree of confidence exists that actual vapor concentrations do not pose an unacceptable risk to worker health via inhalation exposure. Of course, other routes of potential exposure (e.g., dermal or oral) and aerosol generation are not considered in this method.

If one knows very little about the details of the actual exposure scenario, then it can be said that he or she is highly uncertain about the actual level of exposure. However, it is very unlikely that the airborne concentration of toluene in this example in most reasonably conceived scenarios with this product will be higher than its predicted saturation concentration (C_{sat}).

In this evaluation one literally assumes that the person breathes the equivalent of headspace concentration of vapors all day. This mythical person would not have the benefit of general dilution ventilation; thus, this is sometimes called the zero ventilation model.

Tier 1 assessment can be done with very little information and at relatively low cost. In the example, the unitless Henry's law constant (H_A) is used, which is defined as

$$H_A = \frac{C_A\text{ (air), in mg/m}^3\text{ air}}{C_A\text{ (aq), in mg/m}^3\text{ water}} \quad (10\text{-}4)$$

where:

C_A (air) = equilibrium concentration of toxicant in the air above the liquid (i.e., headspace)
C_A (aq) = bulk concentration of toxicant in the liquid (typically water) in weight/volume of liquid

Technically H_A is not dimensionless; it has the units of "volume water to volume air." That is, m^3 water/m^3 air.

For this example, HA is estimated[18] to be 0.23.

The example product with 1 ppm (w/w) of toluene in aqueous solution has 1000 mg of toluene per cubic meter of water.

$$\left[\frac{1}{10^6}\right]\left[\frac{10^9\text{ mgH}_2\text{O}}{1\text{ m}^3\text{ H}_2\text{O}}\right] = \frac{1000\text{ mg}}{\text{m}^3} \quad (10\text{-}5)$$

It follows from Equation 10-5 that the predicted saturation airborne concentration of toluene over the solution is the product of the HA (which is 0.23) and 1000 mg/m^3 or

230 mg/m³ (61 ppm v/v). See conversion equation 10.6 for mg/m³ to ppm v/v below.

Thus, the estimate of the exposure using this relatively crude model is 61 ppm v/v toluene, which is above the 2010 ACGIH® Threshold Limit Value® exposure limit of 50 ppm (v/v). In this example the exposure determined in Tier 1 exceeds the exposure limit, and one needs to go to Tier 2. However, please note that if the product had contained 0.1 ppm (w/w) toluene, then the estimated Tier 1 exposure would have been 6.1 ppm (v/v) toluene, and there would have a fair degree of confidence that an exposure limit of 50 ppm (v/v) would not be exceeded.

Vapor Pressure, Partial Pressure, and Concentration

At this point the relationship between vapor pressure and airborne concentration of gases and vapors should be discussed. The Ideal Gas law from physical chemistry states that the volume of any ideal gas at any particular temperature and pressure is determined entirely by the number of gas molecules. Thus, a mole (6.02×10^{23} molecules) of hydrogen (H_2) at normal temperature and pressure has the same volume (24.4 L) as a mole of butane gas (C_4H_{10}). The Ideal Gas law allows us to express the concentration of a gas (or vapor) as volume parts of the gas (or vapor) per million volume parts of air (ppm v/v). The conversion between ppm v/v and milligrams of gas per cubic meter of air is given as:

$$\frac{mg}{m^3} = ppm \times \frac{MW}{24.4} \qquad (10\text{-}6)$$

MW = molecular weight of the gas in g/gmole.
24.4 = molar volume of any gas at 25C and 760mm Hg atmospheric pressure (liters)

An extension of the Ideal Gas law is Dalton's law, which states that in a mixture of gases the total pressure is equal to the sum of the partial pressures of the separate components. This means that at normal atmospheric pressure (or 1 atmosphere of pressure) all of the gases would add up to 1,000,000 ppm. In normal air this usually means that there is approximately 780,840 ppm v/v nitrogen; 209,476 ppm v/v oxygen; 9340 ppm v/v argon; 314 ppm v/v carbon dioxide; 18.2 ppm v/v neon; 8.7 ppm v/v xenon; 5.24 ppm v/v helium; 2 ppm v/v methane; 1.14 ppm v/v krypton; and 0.5 ppm v/v hydrogen.[19]

If any gas (including CO_2) or vapor is added to this typical air mass with the above concentrations, the partial pressures of all the constituents would reduce slightly so that they all still add up to 1 million volume parts per million parts and 1 atmosphere of pressure. For instance, if 61 ppm v/v of toluene from the example is added to this air mass, all of the above values would be proportionately readjusted slightly lower to allow for this partial pressure of toluene. However, the total pressure would remain at 1 atmosphere.

One meaning of Dalton's law is that one can convert directly between any airborne concentration of gas or vapor and its partial pressure. This is readily seen in Equation 10.3. In the case of the example with toluene, 61 ppm will exert a partial pressure of 61/1,000,000 atmospheres (6.1×10^{-5} atm). Since 1 atm is equal to 760 torr, the partial pressure of 61 ppm v/v is equal to (6.1×10^{-5} atm) (760 torr/atm) or 4.6×10^{-2} torr.

Tier 2: General Ventilation Box Model

One of the oldest and most used models in occupational hygiene is the box or general ventilation model. It relies very simply on the concept of the conservation of mass. The model is based on a "black box" of air, into which one cannot go or even look. But as an airborne contaminant is put into the box, any contaminant that subsequently comes out can be constantly measured. The average concentration in the box can be described as the amount that goes into the box minus the amount that leaves the box all divided by the volume of the box. This is expressed as an equation below:

$$\text{Concentration} = \frac{A_{in} - A_{out}}{V} \qquad (10\text{-}7)$$

A_{in} = amount that goes into the box (wt)
A_{out} = the amount that leaves the box (wt)
V = box volume

If the contaminant is going into the box at a steady rate and leaving with the outgoing air at the same rate, then the system is at steady state, and the average concentration in the box is constant.

If the concentration in the box is the same or homogeneous throughout the volume of the box, then the following assumptions need to be made: (1) the contaminant remains airborne (is not absorbed onto surfaces), (2) the contaminant does not change chemically within the box, and (3) the contaminant is instantly and completely mixed with the air inside upon entering the box. Using this simple steady-state model and assumptions, a general ventilation equation for this situation is

$$C_{eq} = \frac{G}{Q} \qquad (10\text{-}8)$$

C_{eq} = steady-state concentration, mg/m³
G = rate going into the box, mg/hr
Q = ventilation rate of air leaving the box, m³/hr

Of course, the real world is often much more complicated. The mixing of airborne contaminants is often not complete and instantaneous, and some substances are removed by non-ventilatory mechanisms such as adsorption, sedimentation or chemical reaction. Also, the nonsteady-state situation is significantly more complicated to describe mathematically. A differential equation that attempts to take all of these factors into account can be written for the pollutant concentration within the box for any time.[20]

$$VdC = Gdt - (C)(Q)(M)dt - (C)(k)dt \qquad (10\text{-}9)$$

V = the assumed volume of the box, m³
t = the time variable, hr
C = the concentration in the box at any given time, mg/m³
G = the rate of generation of pollutant within the box, mg/hr
Q = the volume flow rate of air exchange in the box, m³/hr
m = the dimensionless mixing efficiency of ventilation in the assumed box[21]
k = the removal rate by mechanisms other than ventilation and filtration, m³/hr

Typically, specific information is not available for the non-ventilatory loss rate (k), the mixing efficiency (m), or the time course of exposure. Thus, values for these factors and for the ventilation (Q) and generation rate (G) are assumed that render a reasonable upper bound estimate of C. Indeed, the steady-state condition is often the default for analysis. The following upper bound physico-chemical model assumptions are typically used for the estimation of airborne concentration (C) from evaporating sources.

Equilibrium Conditions (Time sufficiently long that dC = 0). Given a constant source, the maximum airborne concentration will occur at equilibrium. See the discussion on Time Element of Exposure.

G = Environmental Protection Agency (EPA) Algorithm[22]. This is presented in some detail below in the example; however, this algorithm is essentially driven by the mass transfer coefficient (Kt), which in turn is estimated with a relatively simple equation. In the instances where it has been compared with other techniques or measurements, it has significantly overestimated the rate of evaporation. It is used here only as an illustration, and the reader is encouraged to use more sophisticated less overestimating methods. A more sophisticated estimate of G from vaporizing sources (HBF model) is also presented later in this chapter.

Q = 0.1 Air Changes/Hour. Many, if not most, residences do not have specific provisions for the circulation of outdoor air. General ventilation often occurs via infiltration of outside air into the house via cracks. Recent data show the air change rates for fresh air in residences in the U.S.[23], Finland[24], and Denmark.[25] The U.S. and Finnish data indicate a median winter value around 0.5 to 0.6/hr. The Danish study reports a median air exchange rate of 0.3/hr. Over 75% of 140 homes in Baltimore, Md., in April had ventilation rates greater than 0.3 air changes/hr.

In the author's experience, typical indoor industrial ventilation rates are higher than 0.3 air changes per hour, and some are very much higher; thus, absent specific information, an assumption of 0.1 air change per hour appears to be a significant overestimating worst case.

m = 0.3. This is based on previous work[26] indoors without fans that reports m values in the range of 0.3 to 0.4. The concept and use of m has limitations. It has been found useful, even necessary, for estimating exposure; however, it violates the basic assumption of conservation of mass and thus has some severe qualifying factors. It might be better thought of as a safety or uncertainty factor associated with concentration hot spots associated with poor mixing around sources.

k = 0 (No non-ventilatory losses). Some, but relatively few, materials degrade in air quickly enough to significantly affect their airborne concentration.[27] Volatile and semi-volatile organic compounds can be deposited onto environmental surfaces where they can accumulate, degrade, or be re-emitted into the air. Short-term sources could have peak concentrations that are significantly lowered by these sink effects even in systems without degradation of the compound.[28] For long-term continuous sources, the equilibrium concentration is ultimately the same but delayed in systems with significant surface deposition. Also, the steady-state airborne concentration could be significantly lower in systems in which degradation is occurring after adsorption onto environmental surfaces.[29]

The following assumptions regarding human activity patterns will maximize the estimation of exposure (the product of airborne concentration × time): The worker is in this exposure field for the entire work shift, and a consumer is in the assumed exposure field for 24 hours/day.

Using these assumptions, the general ventilation model that incorporates the mixing factor and ignores k (i.e., set k = 0) is

$$C_{eq} = \frac{G}{(Q)(m) + k} = \frac{G}{(Q)(m)} \qquad (10\text{-}10)$$

Tier 2 Case Study-Modeling Toluene from an Aqueous Product

The calculation for this case study was started above with the Tier 1 zero ventilation model. In those calculation the headspace concentration and the worst case exposure potential associated with it has been estimated. This lower tier effort was done with only information on the concentration of toluene in the product and its Henry's law constant. To do a more detailed analysis (Tier 2 Box Model) in the case study, it is necessary to get more information about the actual exposure scenario. This aqueous product is typically used in light industrial settings in which the primary off-gassing and exposure comes from an open container of the product. The open surface area is 100 cm², and the workroom is maintained at 25°C. It is also determined that the workers are often in the room but very rarely immediately proximate to the open container. That is, average room concentrations are important rather than near-field concentrations or exposures very close to the open drum. The specific general ventilation rate has not been determined, and there is typically no local exhaust ventilation.

A physical-chemical model to estimate the source strength of an evaporating liquid has been presented by Fleischer[30] and has been used by the EPA.[31]

$$G = (10^3)\,\frac{(K_t)(MW)(AREA)(VPP - VPB)}{(R)(TL)} \qquad (10\text{-}11)$$

G = generation rate, mg/hr
K_t = mass transfer rate, m/hr
MW = molecular weight, g/mole
AREA = m^2
VP_P = vapor pressure of the substance, atm
VP_B = partial pressure of the toxicant in the room air, atm
R = gas constant (8.205×10^{-5} atm m^3/((mole)(K)))
TL = temperature of the evaporating liquid, K

For this exercise the mass transfer coefficient (K_t) estimated using the following relationship[22] will be used.

$$K_t = \sqrt[3]{\frac{18}{MW}} \qquad (10\text{-}12)$$

The use of algorithm in Equation 10.12 is done purely for clarity in the example, because this is a relatively simple relationship; however, because it has been found to overestimate exposure, other more detailed methods exist for this determination.[32–36]

In this example the input values found in Table 10.1 were used.

Table 10.1 — Values for Examples

Source	*Value*
K_t = 17.4 m/hr	Equation 10-12
MW = 92.1 g/mole	handbook
AREA = 0.01 m^2	100 cm^2 converted to m^2
VP_P = 61/1,000,000	61 ppm (v/v) from previous Henry's law calculation converted to atm
VP_B = 0	conservative assumption
R = (8.205 × 10^{-5} atm m^3/((mole)(deg K)))	Universal Gas Constant
T = 298 K	25°C converted to K
V = 50 m3 (room volume)	conservative assumption
m = 0.3	Ref: Drivas[14]
Air change/hr = 0.1	conservative assumption
G = 40 mg/hour	Using worst case 1984 algorithm[22]

One assumption in the above model is that the partial pressure of the contaminant in the box air (VP_B) is insignificant relative to the vapor pressure (VP_P) of the toxicant. This simplifying supposition overestimates the generation rate and thus the resulting concentration. It is useful and justified for relatively small evaporating sources (like the case study example), but it is not appropriate for large sources. The specifics of modeling large evaporating sources are covered elsewhere.[37]

Using these values in Equation 10-11 results in an estimated off-gassing rate of 40 mg/hour to the workroom.

The ventilation rate (Q) is equal to the room volume times the mixing air change rate per hour:

$$Q = (V)(\text{air change/hr})$$
$$Q = (50)(0.1) = 5\ m^3/hr$$

Assuming a mixing factor m = 0.3, Equation 10 predicts an average air concentration of toluene in the workroom of about 27 mg/m^3 (7 ppm v/v). This is below the current 188 mg/m^3 (50 ppm v/v) exposure limit. It should be noted that most of the predictors in the model have a linear effect on predicted concentration and less than a threefold increase in surface area and vapor pressure (from higher toluene concentration or higher temperatures) would have predicted exposure above this exposure limit. Thus, modeling a significantly larger, warmer, or more concentrated source would have resulted in a prediction of unacceptable upper bound estimate of risk.

Staying with the basic box model, a more sophisticated model to estimate the generation rate can also be used. This work was published and represents the method currently used by EPA to estimate inhalation exposures to new chemical substances.[34,35] The Hummel-Braun-Fehrenbacher (HBF) model describes the source rate as:

$$G = \frac{(7.2 \times 10^4)(MW)(VP_P)(AREA)}{(R)(TL)} \sqrt{\frac{(V_x)(D_{ab})}{(\pi)(\Delta x)}} \quad (10\text{-}13)$$

D_{ab} = diffusion coefficient, cm^2/sec of a through b (in this case b is air)
Δx = pool length along the direction of the airflow, cm
V_x = air velocity along the x-axis, cm/sec.

The diffusion coefficient (D_{ab}) is further defined as:

$$D_{ab} = \frac{4.09 \times 10^{-5}\,(TL)^{1.9}\left(\frac{1}{29} + \frac{1}{MW}\right)(MW)^{-0.333}}{P_t} \quad (10\text{-}14)$$

P_t = atmospheric pressure, atm.

This model has the added feature (and data requirements) of knowing or estimating the air velocity over the pool (V_x) and length of the pool in the direction of the air movement (Δx). If the pool is assumed to be essentially isometric, then the pool length is reasonably estimated as the square root of the AREA. It has been the author's experience that most indoor environments with reasonably calm air movement will have air moving in the range of 5–20 linear feet per minute in a rather random manner. If the example is continued with the square root of the AREA (converted to cm^2) for Δx and 5 ft/min (converted to cm/sec) for V_x, the estimated off-gassing rate is 15 mg/hr to the workroom. The predicted values are 21 and 30 mg/hr at indoor air velocities of 10 and 20 ft/min, respectively. The original estimate from the relatively crude mass transfer rate estimated using Equation 10.12 was 40 mg/hr. Thus, the use of this more sophisticated model allowed for a more refined estimate. Indeed, the HBF model predicts that the off-gassing rate will not reach 40 mg/m^3 from this pool until the airflow rate reaches around 50 linear feet per minute. This is a situation that is possible but not very likely in many indoor environments.

Tier 3: Two-Box Model

The general ventilation box assumes a well-mixed volume and can adequately estimate exposure intensity for individuals working at least a few meters from a contaminant emission source; however, this model usually underestimates airborne concentrations close to the source. It is intuitively obvious that the concentrations from the source will be higher close to the source than further from it in all but the most turbulently mixed environments. Thus, the general ventilation box model is good choice for estimating average concentrations within a room volume and could be reasonable for estimating the exposures from non-point sources or for persons that are distant a source in the same room. It is perhaps not the best choice for someone close to the source.

As previously discussed the mixing or "safety" factor **m** has been put forth to correct for this difference; however, it violates the basic assumption of conservation of mass and thus has some severe qualifying factors associated with its use. Also the assignment of the exact value of **m** as a positive finite value of >0 to 1 is problematic. Clearly it is close to 1 in small well-mixed volumes and much closer to 0 in large rooms with poor mixing. However, absent an extensive database one is simply guessing as to what value **m** should be.

A more technical and systematic approach has been to consider that the room volume is conceptually divided into two boxes. One box contains the emission source and is termed the "near field." Its dimensions are sized to include the breathing zone of the worker who is located near the source and whose exposure is to be estimated. The rest of the room is the conceptual second box and is termed the "far field." Figure 10.2 depicts this construct.

Nicas has taken this previously described concept[38] and derived the dynamic concentration equations that are presented below. These along with explicit steady state equations, also shown below, were published by Nicas in 1996.[39] The text below includes excerpted portions of Nicas' explanatory comments which appear in a full chapter on the 2-box model in the AIHA publication, *Mathematical Models for Estimating Occupational Exposure to Chemicals*, 2nd edition.[7]

It is assumed that air within each box of the 2 box model is perfectly mixed, but that there is limited air flow between the boxes. The inter-box air flow rate is denoted β in m^3/min; air simultaneously moves into and

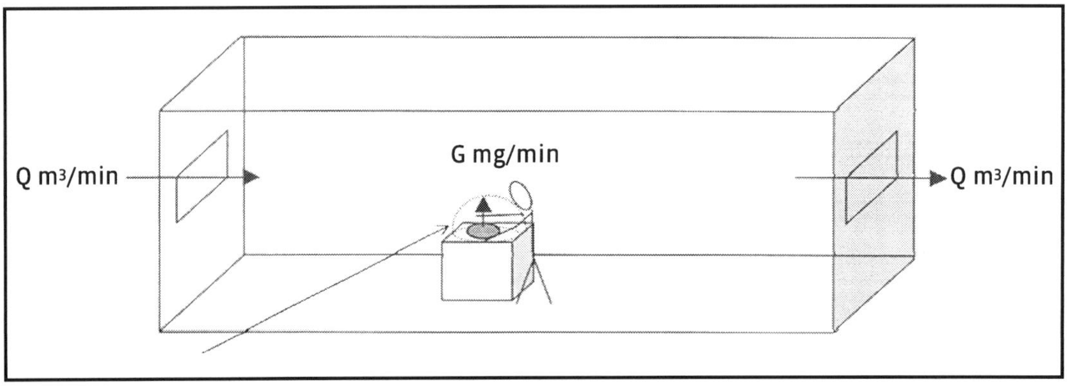

Figure 10.2 — Near field volume with the remaining room volume = far field.

out of the near field at rate β. Room mechanical supply air and/or infiltration air moves into and out of the far field at rate Q in m^3/min. Q is the same room supply air rate parameter used in the general ventilation single box model. In the two-box model described here, it is assumed that the contaminant mass emission rate is a constant value G in mg/min, and that the only way airborne chemical mass leaves a box is via air flow.

This description leads to the following coupled mass balance equations:

Near Field $$V_N dC_N = Gdt + \beta C_F dt - \beta C_N dt \quad (10\text{-}15)$$

Far Field $$V_F dC_F = \beta C_N dt - (\beta + Q)C_F dt \quad (10\text{-}16)$$

V_N and V_F = the near-field and far-field volumes, respectively (m^3)
C_N and C_F = the near-field and far-field concentrations, respectively (mg/m^3)
G = constant mass emission rate (mg/min)
β = air flow rate (m^3/min) between the near and far fields
Q = room supply air rate (m^3/min)
dt = an infinitesimal time interval (min)

In Equation 10-15, the left-hand side is the change in mass in the near field in the interval dt. Mass enters the near field in two ways: (1) it is emitted from the source (the G term), and (2) it is carried in from the far field by the inter-box air flow β. Mass leaves the near field in the same inter-box air flow. Next, consider Equation 10-16. The left-hand side is the change in mass in the far field in the interval dt. The only mass entering the far field is that carried in from the near field by the inter-box air flow β. However, mass leaves the far field in two ways: (1) it is carried back into the near field by the inter-box air flow, and (2) it exits the room altogether in the exhaust air flow Q.

If the initial contaminant concentration in each box is zero, the general solutions for the time-varying concentrations in the near field, $C_N(t)$, and in the far field, $C_F(t)$, are the following:

$$C_N(t) = \frac{G}{\left[\frac{\beta}{\beta + Q}\right] Q} + G\left[\frac{\beta Q + \lambda_2 V_N(\beta + Q)}{\beta Q V_N(\lambda_1 - \lambda_2)}\right] e^{\lambda_1 t} \times G\left[\frac{\beta Q + \lambda_2 V_N(\beta + Q)}{\beta Q V_N(\lambda_1 - \lambda_2)}\right] e^{\lambda_2 t} \quad (10\text{-}17)$$

$$C_F(t) = \frac{G}{Q} + G\left[\frac{\lambda_1 V_N + \beta}{\beta}\right]\left[\frac{\beta Q + \lambda_2 V_N(\beta + Q)}{\beta Q V_N(\lambda_1 - \lambda_2)}\right] e^{\lambda_1 t} - G\left[\frac{\lambda_2 V_N + \beta}{\beta}\right]\left[\frac{\beta Q + \lambda_1 V_N(\beta + Q)}{\beta Q V_N(\lambda_1 - \lambda_2)}\right] e^{\lambda_2 t} \quad (10\text{-}18)$$

where

$$\lambda_1 = 0.5\left[-\left[\frac{\beta V_F + V_N(\beta + Q)}{V_N V_F}\right] + \sqrt{\left[\frac{\beta V_F + V_N(\beta + Q)}{V_N V_F}\right]^2 - 4\left[\frac{\beta Q}{V_N V_F}\right]}\right]$$

$$\lambda_2 = 0.5\left[-\left[\frac{\beta V_F + V_N(\beta + Q)}{V_N V_F}\right] + \sqrt{\left[\frac{\beta V_F + V_N(\beta + Q)}{V_N V_F}\right]^2 - 4\left[\frac{\beta Q}{V_N V_F}\right]}\right]$$

The general solutions are complicated, but once numerical values are inserted for the various parameters, the resulting equations are relatively simple. The model parameters λ_1 and λ_2 correspond to air turnover rates (in units of min^{-1}) and do not depend on the contaminant emission rate. The absolute value of λ_1 is approximately equal to the air turnover or exchange rate in the far field (general room), or $|\lambda_1| \cong Q \div V_F$. The absolute value of λ_2 is approximately equal to the air turnover rate in the near field, or $|\lambda_2|$ $\beta \div V_N$. Because the parameters λ_1 and λ_2 are real, distinct, negative numbers for nearly all realistic scenarios, the terms $\exp(\lambda_1 \times t)$ and $\exp(\lambda_2 \times t)$ go to zero as t gets large, in which case the steady-state contaminant concentrations in the near field, $C_{N,SS}$, and in the far field, $C_{F,SS}$, are as follows:

$$C_{N,SS} = \frac{G}{Q} + \frac{G}{\beta} \qquad (10\text{-}19)$$

$$C_{F,SS} = \frac{G}{Q} \qquad (10\text{-}20)$$

If $\beta < Q$, then $C_{N,SS} > 2\, C_{F,SS}$, which signifies that exposure intensity is at least twice as high near the source as elsewhere in the room. On the other hand, if $\beta \gg Q$, then $C_{N,SS} \cong C_{F,SS}$, which signifies there is no difference in exposure intensity close to versus far from the source, which is to say that the room is essentially well-mixed. Therefore, for a given Q value, the difference between $C_{N,SS}$ and $C_{F,SS}$ depends on the value of β, which makes intuitive sense. If β is small, contaminant lingers near the source and can build up to a high concentration. If β is large, contaminant is quickly dispersed away from the source into the general room, so the concentration near the source does not build up to a high level.

The inter-box air flow rate β equals one-half the free surface area, FSA, of the near field zone times the average random air speed, S, which is assumed to be the same throughout the room, or:

$$\beta = \tfrac{1}{2} \times FSA \times S \qquad (10\text{-}21)$$

Please note that The right-hand side of Equation 10-19 for the steady-state near field concentration can be rearranged to yield the following expression for $C_{N,SS}$:

$$C_{N,SS} = C_{eq} = \frac{G}{\left[\dfrac{\beta}{\beta + Q}\right] Q} \qquad (10\text{-}22)$$

Following the running case study example we need to size the near-field volume and assign a value of β. The authors have found it useful to use a spherically shaped near-field volume assumed to be around the exposed person's breathing zone. For relatively near sources, a 1.24 m diameter (1 m^3) near-field volume typically is used. For source very near the head, a near-field diameter of less than 0.2 m Might be used. For this example, the near field volume is 1 m^3. Beta (β) is calculated from the near field volume and geometry and an estimated average room velocity rate of 0.167 m/s. This is approximately in the middle of the typical indoor air velocity in residences that reportedly[40] occurs within the range of 0.05 to 0.3 m/s.

Using these inputs along the previously estimated G = 40 mg/hour and Q of 5 m^3/hr the estimated equilibrium concentration is 8 mg/m^3. This should be a relatively conservative estimate since we used an estimated residential air velocity and velocities in industrial setting are expected to be higher. We also used a relatively low air exchange/ventilation rate. In short, we can reasonably, if tentatively (because of the uncertainty of the other inputs) predict, that actual exposure is quite likely to be less than this estimate.

Tier 3: Dispersion Model

The dispersion model is another advanced model that recognizes the above mentioned limitation of the general ventilation box. This model actually accounts for and mathematically describes the potentially sharp gradients of concentration for workers close to the emitting source. It is based on a diffusion model developed for heat flow[41] and applied to indoor air modeling.[42,43] A derivation of the equation for a continuous point source is presented in the references. It is designed to predict concentration at position r and time t for a spherically expanding source and is shown below.

$$C = \frac{G}{4(\pi)(D)(r)} \left[1 - \operatorname{erf} \frac{r}{\sqrt{4(t)(D)}}\right] \qquad (10\text{-}23)$$

erf = the error function[1]
C = airborne concentration, mass/volume, mg/m³
G = steady-state emission rate, mass/time, mg/hr
r = the distance from the source to the worker, m
D = the effective or eddy diffusivity coefficient, area/time, m²/hr
t = elapsed time, hr

Diffusion of contaminants in workroom air occurs primarily because of the turbulent motion of the air. In most industrial environments molecular diffusion is not a significant force in dispersing the contaminant between the emission source and the worker's breathing zone. Instead, the normal turbulence of typical indoor air causes eddys (or packet-like motions) that have the effect of breaking up the contaminant cloud and hastening its mixing with the workroom air. Therefore, applications of diffusion models in industrial environments use experimentally determined diffusion coefficients (D) called eddy or effective diffusivities. These eddy diffusivity coefficients are three to five orders of magnitude (1000 to 100,000 times) larger than molecular diffusivity.

The eddy diffusivity coefficient (D) can be based on experimental measurements at the site being modeled. Some eddy diffusivity values are also available in the literature.[44,45] Measurements of D in indoor industrial environments have ranged from 3–690 m²/hr with 12 m²/hr being a typical value.

Plotting the predicted airborne concentration (C) at one position r for many values of time t gives an increasing curve of concentration that approaches a steady-state level.

For sources (emitting into a hemisphere) on a surface and at equilibrium, Equation 23 simplifies to

$$C_{eq} = \frac{G}{2(\pi)(D)(r)} \qquad (10\text{-}24)$$

Note that the term in the denominator goes to 2 for hemispherical diffusion in Equation 24, while it is 4 in Equation 10.23 which described spherical diffusion.

Consider the previous example with G = 40 mg/hr and a person working within 1 m of the source (r = 1 m). It is known that the lowest D measured in a very limited database was 3 m²/hr. If this value is used, the estimated equilibrium airborne concentration of toluene is about 2 mg/m³. This is less than one-tenth of the amount predicted with the box model. However, the worst case ventilation could be very low, and this could result in very little mixing and a true D value that is much lower than 3 m²/hr. The fact is that there simply is not enough data to use this model with much confidence. It is useful in that it allows estimation of the effect of distance from the source on worker exposure. It predicts that it is a straight inverse relationship with the exposure going down twofold for every doubling of distance from it from a theoretic point source.

There is little doubt that the eddy diffusivity model could be a very valuable tool that can potentially provide near- and far-field exposure estimations; however, this approach in general suffers because it lacks the reasonable characterization of the primary predictor variable, eddy diffusivity.

Despite the lack of information needed to effectively invoke Tier 3 models and their resulting uncertainty it is interesting to see the progression of estimates from the various models in Table 10.2 below:

---

[1] The error function is related to the normal or Gaussian distribution. This is a bell-shaped curve described by the function $\phi(x) = \frac{1}{\sqrt{2(\pi)}} e^{-\frac{x^2}{2}}$. This curve is called the Normal Curve of Error and the area under this curve represents a probably integrals such that $\int_2^x \phi(x)dx = \frac{1}{2} \operatorname{erf} \frac{x}{\sqrt{2}}$. For example to evaluate erf(2.3) proceed as follows: Since $\frac{x}{\sqrt{2}} = 2.3$ one finds $x = (2.3)\sqrt{2} = 3.25$. In the normal table entry for the areas opposite x = 3.25, the value of 0.4994 is given. Thus erf(2.3) = 2(0.4494) = 0.9988. Modern PCs and software (e.g., EXCEL and Mathcad) can evaluate the erf without effort or table lookup.

Table 10.2 — Estimates from the various models

Model	*Prediction Concentration (mg/m³)*	*Confidence that Prediction is an overestimation*
Zero Ventilation	230	High
General Ventilation Single Box	27	High
2-Box	8	Moderate - High
Diffusion	2	Low

Determining or Estimating Generation Rates in Other Situations

This chapter has concentrated on the estimation of generation rate of vapors from evaporation. This was done because vaporizing sources are often important, and the subject readily allows the illustration of physical-chemical modeling. It should be mentioned that there are other sources and other ways of estimating these rates. If it is known or measured that a certain amount of gas is released from a vessel, and the time of release is also known, an average source term or G can be calculated by simply dividing the released mass by the time of release. Sometimes measuring G directly is the best and most expeditious way to attain it for use in a model. For example, painting a glass slide or piece of wood and measuring its loss of weight over time could provide very valuable information for this emission rate. Another example would be to weigh a can of a gaseous product (e.g., refrigerant gas) before and after a measured period of discharge to the air.

Airborne particle concentrations can also be estimated in this manner, but this situation is much more complicated in that relatively large aerodynamic particles will rapidly settle out of the air column. Also, some sprayed aerosol particles are constantly changing their diameter and mass while in the air because of vaporization. Modeling of this situation using indoor-sprayed pesticide as the example has been accomplished with a complicated and very detailed model.[46]

Finally, simulated scenarios can be run to estimate the particulate emission rate. Conducting simulations in a purposely well-mixed and well-characterized box will allow for back calculation of the generation rate (G). This rate can then be used in a generalized model for predicting real world exposure.

Indeed, this empirical approach was used by the authors to estimate the short term constant emission rate for particulates associated with machining a product during construction activities. A chamber environment was used to control the main determinants of exposure other than G; filtered air was moved through the chamber at a constant rate whose volume V was known. A typical machining rate was pre-determined and also held constant. Air samples were collected at multiple locations within the chamber to ensure airborne concentrations were relatively consistent, verifying well-mixed room conditions. This allowed the Well-Mixed box model to be used. The particulate measurements gave a measure of the airborne concentration averaged over the trial time period — giving C_{avg}. Knowing the value of the other variables in the time-integrated equation for C_{avg}, the equation was simply rearranged it to solve for G:

$$G = \frac{C_{avg}Q^2}{Q + \frac{V}{t}\left(e^{-Qt/V} - 1\right)} \qquad (10\text{-}25)$$

Where volume V= 15 m³ in which fresh, filtered air was directed through at Q = 75 m³/hr (5 ACH). The product was machined at a constant rate for time = 10 minutes. The air samples yielded an average concentration of 0.5 mg/m³, so G (mg/hr) calculated from C_{avg} was equal to 114.9 mg/hr.

This generation rate is portable; it can be inserted into any model chosen to represent a defined scenario facilitating 'what if' exercises. The predicted outcome is likely to reflect a much more realistic estimate of the true concentration than those whose generation rate is derived from conservative theoretical approaches. This is a particularly useful method when dealing with particulate exposures because G for particles cannot be derived from first principles. A more detailed explanation of the algorithms and application thereof has been presented elsewhere.[47,48]

Linked Monitoring and Modeling

The relationship between modeling and monitoring workplace airborne concentrations becomes particularly important when one has some monitoring data to add to the estimates being made by modeling. One can estimate or refine purely model-estimated exposures for an agent by combining the information from monitoring with the theoretical construct of and result from a model.

Simple examples include the predictions of workplace concentrations given some monitoring data and a change in source or ventilation rate or distance from a point source. Using the above box or eddy diffusivity models it can be predicted that reducing the source by half or doubling the ventilation rate will result in a concentration reduced by half. Also, doubling the distance from a true point source in a random dispersion field will also halve the concentration. These predictions will work for relatively simple situations. However, the more that is known about modeling, the better the understanding of where they might not work. Large evaporating sources, for example, will not render half the concentration when the ventilation rate is doubled. The reason and working model for this is presented elsewhere.[37]

Another more detailed example of linking monitoring and modeling is to first run a model on a mixture that predicts a relative exposure to a number of components of that mixture. If there happens to be monitoring data on one of the components in the modeled scenario, the estimates of actual exposure potential can be checked and refined. That is, the monitoring data on the substance can be used to predict the airborne levels of the other components. Using the ratios predicted by the model and multiplying the monitored data by these ratios allows prediction of the concentrations of the other components.

As a tangible illustration of this, assume there is exposure data on substance A (X ppm v/v), but the exposure for substance B (Y ppm v/v) needs to be estimated. Both are components of the same mixture in a process stream. Their percentages in the stream (%X and %Y) and their vapor pressures (VP_A and VP_B) are known. Assuming their molecular weights are similar, the percentage concentration can be used in place of their mole fractions.

$$Y_{ppm} = \left(\frac{\%Y}{\%X}\right)\left(\frac{VP_y}{VP_x}\right)(X_{ppm}) \qquad (10\text{-}26)$$

This modeling approach assumes that the mixture acts as an ideal solution, which may not be true. In any event, the point is that modeled ratios can be combined with monitored data to give more refined estimates of exposure for species that are being monitored.

A more formal process using a hybrid approach to blending modeling and monitoring data is presented through the use of Bayesian hierarchal modeling. This statistical framework allows us to incorporate different kinds of information yielding a more robust and transparent exposure assessment. This technique has only recently been applied to industrial hygiene[49] and dose reconstruction[50] and still more recently to modeling.[51,52] By incorporating different types of information stemming from different sources, it is reasonable to expect the output resulting from consideration of all the information to be more reliable and robust.

To illustrate, consider the following example:

An occupational hygiene survey was conducted to evaluate a workplace exposure. Three air samples were collected and yielded concentrations that were between 15% and 30% of the OEL. In and of themselves, these data are insufficient to make any firm conclusions regarding the acceptability of this exposure.

Additional information is available regarding the workplace and process and tasks: the room dimensions are known and the airflow has been qualitatively described. A review of the literature for airflow rates in similar processes and environments helped to define a reasonable universe of values for Q and the inter-zonal airflow, β (see above discussion on two-box model). The agent of concern is a volatile solvent that becomes airborne as it evaporates from an open tank. Using first principles, the generation rate can be estimated using one of several algorithms such as those discussed earlier in this chapter. The worker conducts tasks that require him to be in close proximity to the source for 30 minutes of every hour. With this information a screening level model can be used to estimate exposure, recognizing that there will be a relatively high degree of uncertainty associated with the predicted exposure.

While it is beyond the scope of this chapter to provide specific details of the analysis, these different types of information (monitoring and modeling) can be integrated to derive a more robust, objective and transparent estimate of the exposure using a Bayesian hierarchal model. Modern computing power and readily available software such as WINBUGS(53) have contributed to the popularity of this statistical approach. While there is still a great need for further research in this area, Bayesian hierarchal modeling has already been proven to be a remarkably valuable and potentially powerful tool in the exposure sciences.(54–56)

Time Element of Exposure

Figure 10.3 shows the time course of concentration for nonsteady-state and steady-state models in the case study.

The solid line is the point in time concentration assuming that the source (G) started at t=0. Note that under these conditions and assumptions over 10 hours are required for the space to approach the equilibrium concentration (C_{eq}) denoted by the dotted line at 27 mg/m^3.

The steady-state Equations 10-8, 10-10, and 10-24 are independent of the room volume (V), and the only thing required about time t is that it be long enough to have attained steady state. The models shown in these equations is thus appropriately applied only to situations that have come to apparent equilibrium. That is, an equilibrium

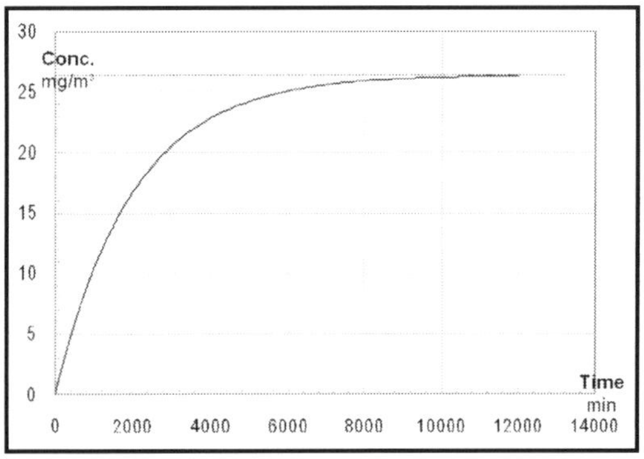

Figure 10.3 — Case Study Non-steady state concentration buildup.

or steady-state model will render some ultimate and unvarying steady-state concentration. However, it says nothing about the time course of the exposure. A steady-state model also says nothing about the actual exposure that occurred at the beginning of the exposure period. This question becomes critical if this is the only time a person might be exposed, such as in a batch job that is done at the beginning of an exposure and completed quickly.

The thoughtful reader might ask:

1. How long must a typical operation run before a steady-state concentration is established?
2. How can an exposure that occurs before this apparent equilibrium is established from a source that starts at t=0 be estimated?
3. How can an exposure be estimated that occurs after steady state is established from a source that is then turned off?

Since theoretical steady state is approached but rarely achieved, a practical solution to the problem of gauging the time scale of concentration buildup is to calculate the time required to achieve some percentage of this ultimate concentration. Solving Equation 10-9 for time (with C=0 @ t=0) yields

$$t = \frac{-V}{(Q)(m) + k} \, 1n[G - ((Q)(m) + k)(C)/G] \qquad (10\text{-}27)$$

At 90% of equilibrium Equation 10 becomes

$$C = \frac{0.90(G)}{(Q)(m) + k} \qquad (10\text{-}28)$$

Combining Equations 18 and 19 gives

$$t\,(@\ 90\%\ \text{of equilibrium}) = 2.303 \frac{V}{(Q)(m) + k} \qquad (10\text{-}29)$$

Equation 10-29 shows that large volumes with low ventilation rates and poor mixing take a relatively long time to reach a substantial portion of equilibrium. In the running example, this time (time to attain 90% of equilibrium) is 2.303(50)/((5)(0.3)) or 77 hours. The practical lesson from this is that if one is modeling essentially batch processes where C=0 @ t=0, and the length of time for the exposure is of relatively short duration (less than 1–2 hours), one needs to consider the time-weighted average concentration the worker may be exposed to under non-steady-state conditions.

Ignoring m and k Equation 10-29 reduces to approximately 2.3 (V/Q). As previously mentioned most residences have about a 50% mixing air exchange every hour because of infiltration. Thus Q/V = 0.5/hr and V/Q = 2 hr. Thus, the normal house attains 90% of C_{eq} from a beginning source in 4–5 hrs.

In the converse situation, there is an occupied air volume containing a concentration of toxicant in which the source has been turned off or removed. Under the same conditions (i.e., large volume, low ventilation rate, poor mixing) it will take a relatively long time to clear this concentration. This scenario is examined and presented below in more detail.

The above analysis and equations of the time variation of airborne concentration assumes that the initial concentration is nil (i.e., C=0 @ t=0), which is a common situation; however, in many industrial situations the initial concentration should not be neglected. If the operation has been ongoing and relatively steady for many hours one cannot make this assumption and using C_{eq} as the starting concentration may be warranted.

Also, in a situation where worker exposure is modeled in the morning and afternoon, and the source is turned off at lunch time (when workers take a 30-minute break), then it might be important for the afternoon estimate to include an initial concentration term based on the decay calculated for the lunch period.

With the source turned off (G=0):

$$C = C_0 e^{-\frac{(Q)(m)(t)}{V}} \qquad (10\text{-}30)$$

C_0 = concentration just before lunch and just before source was turned off

C = concentration immediately after the lunch period

t = elapsed time for lunch period

After the lunch break one may need to model the situation as the source is again turned on. This is done by setting k to 0 (unless you have some data on k) and solving Equation 10.9 for C (with C=C_0 @ t=0).

$$C = \frac{G}{(Q)(m)} + C_0 - \frac{G}{(Q)(m)} e^{-\frac{(Q)(m)(t)}{V}} \qquad (10\text{-}31)$$

In this situation C_0 in Equation 10-22 should be set equal to C from Equation 10-21; that is, the final airborne concentration after the lunch break becomes the initial concentration for the beginning of the afternoon work session.

Please note, if one is modeling a scenario in steady state (i.e., one at apparent equilibrium relative to the airborne concentration of contaminant), initial concentrations need not be accounted for or kept track of, and Equations 10-10 and 10-16 should be used.

The question of whether an equilibrium or nonequilibrium model should be used is probably best answered by looking at the scenario of interest and using a reasonable worst case approach. The product of (C_{eq})(time) will always render the highest estimate of exposure for any reasonably constant and long-lived source. However, if this typically overestimated value is not satisfactory for the evaluation of exposure, one may need to do the more sophisticated analysis of integrating nonequilibrium conditions. Relatively long exposure times and a steady source rate will render essentially the same estimates of exposure regardless of whether one uses a steady-state or nonsteady-state model.

Future of Occupational Hygiene Exposure Modeling

As can be seen, the above analyses usually render significantly lower estimates of exposure as they become more sophisticated. These values often remain significant overestimates of the actual exposure. This is because lack of knowledge of basic model details is appropriately dealt with by using overestimating, conservative assumptions.

Unfortunately, one can often run out of resources at a relatively low level in Tier 2 and not be able to progress with the modeling approach. If the estimated exposure still exceeds the exposure limit, the assessor needs to go beyond this point to the next stage (Tier 3). He or she has a choice of

(1) reducing the uncertainty of the model with research (typically run well controlled simulations) or (2) doing direct monitoring measures of the exposure scenario. The second choice has almost invariably been taken because the first choice is very expensive in the short term. Because direct monitoring databases only look at and provide data on the outcomes of exposure (i.e., the resulting airborne concentrations) and not the determinants that caused the exposure to happen, they have not been useful for model development and validation.

An example of reducing model uncertainty with its concomitant overestimation would be gathering better data on the ventilation rates and conditions extant in different classes of buildings and workplaces. If, for example, one had a probability distribution function of air change rates and eddy diffusivities for rooms in light industrial buildings, he or she could do a Monte Carlo simulation[57,58] showing the range of the predicted exposure in this environment by repeatedly sampling these distributions and using Equation 10-23 or 10-24. Of course, this analysis would have to be combined with best estimates of toxicant generation rates (G) to render an over estimate of airborne concentration and exposure potential.

Because the topic is essentially generic, research in the area of exposure modeling will benefit everyone who does exposure assessment and would be in the best interest of the profession.

More Information

As mentioned a few times in this chapter, there is an entire book on this specific subject.[7] The book contains complete chapters on the following subjects in much greater detail than presented in this chapter:

- General Principles
- Generation Rates
- Well Mixed Single Box Model
- Well Mixed Single Box Model with Changing Conditions
- Two-Box Model
- Diffusion Model
- Computerized Fluid Dynamics Models
- Knowledge Based Models
- Statistical Models
- Model Uncertainty Analysis
- Bayesian Decision Analysis
- Dermal Exposure Modeling
- Model Selection
- 21st Century Regulatory Initiatives Requiring Models

The authors believe it represents the single most comprehensive source of information on this topic available.

References

1. **United Nations:** United Nations Conference on the Environment and Development (UNCED). Rio de Janeiro: United Nations, 1992.
2. **Jayjock, M., J. Lynch, and D. Nelson:** *Risk Assessment Principles for the Industrial Hygienist.* Fairfax, VA: AIHA Press, 2000.
3. **Jayjock, M.A. and N.C. Hawkins:** A proposal for improving the role of exposure modeling in risk assessment. *Am. Ind. Hyg. Assoc. J. 54*:733–741 (1993).
4. **Jayjock, M.A., P.G. Lewis and J.R. Lynch:** Quantitative Level of Protection Offered to Workers by ACGIH Threshold Limit Values Occupational Exposure Limits. *Am. Ind. Hyg. Assoc. J. 62*:4–11 (2001).
5. **Ignacio, J.S., and W.H. Bullock (eds.):** A *Strategy for Assessing and Managing Occupational Exposures*, 3rd edition. Fairfax, VA: AIHA Press, 2006.
6. **Keil, C.B. (ed.):** *Mathematical Models for Estimating Occupational Exposure to Chemicals.* Fairfax, VA, AIHA Press, 2000.
7. **Keil, C.B., C. Simmons, and T.R. Anthony (eds.):** *Mathematical Models for Estimating Occupational Exposure to Chemicals*, 2nd edition. Fairfax, VA, AIHA Press, 2009.
8. **Mulhausen, J.R:** "Interpreting Monitoring Data: Are We Making the Right Judgments?" presented at the Professional Conference of Industrial Hygiene. Denver, CO. Oct. 25, 2005.
9. **Mulhausen, J.R.:** "Exposure Judgments: Continuously Improving Accuracy Using the AIHA Strategy with its Exposure Control Banding Approach" in Roundtable RT 233 at the AIHce. Chicago, IL. May 18, 2006.
10. **Damiano, J and J.R. Mulhausen:** *A Strategy for Assessing and Managing Occupational Exposures*, 3rd edition. Fairfax, VA: AIHA Press, 1998.
11. **Damiano, J and J.R. Mulhausen:** A Strategy for Assessing and Managing Occupational Exposures, 2nd edition. Fairfax, VA: AIHA Press, 1998. p. 16.
12. **Jayjock, M.A. and N.C. Hawkins:** Exposure database improvements for indoor air model validation. *Appl. Occup. Environ. Hyg. 10*:379–382 (1995).
13. **Jayjock, M.A., C.F. Chaisson, S. Arnold, and E.J. Dederick:** Modeling Framework for Human Exposure Assessment. *J. Exp. Sci. Env. Epidemiol. 17*:S81–89 (2007)

14. **Jayjock, M.A.:** Assessment of inhalation exposure potential from vapors in the workplace. *Am. Ind. Hyg. Assoc. J. 49*:380–385 (1988).
15. **Hawkins, N.C.:** "Uncertainly and Residual Risk." Presentation on behalf of the Chemical Manufacturers Association to the National Research Council/National Academy of Science Committee on Risk Assessment of Hazardous Air Pollutants, Washington, DC, November 1991.
16. **Haas, H.B. and R.F. Newton:** Correction of boiling points to standard pressure. In *CRC Handbook of Chemistry and Physics,* 59th edition. Boca Raton, FL: CRC Press, 1978. p. D-228.
17. **Lyman, W.J., W.F. Reehl, and D.H. Rosenblat:** *Handbook of Chemical Property Estimation Methods.* New York: McGraw Hill, 1982. Chapters 11, 14, 15.
18. **Meylan, W.M. and P.H. Howard:** Bond contribution method for estimating Henry's law constants. *Environ. Toxicol. Chem. 10*:1283–1293 (1991).
19. **Lide, D.R.:** *Handbook of Chemistry and Physics,* 76th edition. New York: CRC Press, 1996. Sec. 14, p. 14.
20. **Tichenor, B.A., Z. Guo, J.E. Dunn, L.E. Sparks, et al.:** The interaction of vapor phase organic compounds with indoor sinks. *Indoor Air 1*:1–23 (1991).
21. **Brief, R.S.:** A simple way to determine air contaminants. *Air Eng. 2*:39–41 (1960).
22. **U.S. Environmental Protection Agency (EPA):** A Manual for the Preparation of Engineering Assessment. Washington, DC: EPA, September 1984. [Unpublished draft]
23. **Wallace, L.A.:** "EPA/ORD/Monitor-ing Program." Presentation before the Science Advisory Board Panel on Indoor Air Quality and Total Human Exposure Committee, Washington, DC, March 29, 1989.
24. **Ruotsalainen, R., R. Ronnberg, J. Sateri, A. Majanen, et al.:** Indoor climate and the performance of ventilation in Finnish residences. *Indoor Air 2*:137–145 (1992).
25. **Harving, H., R. Dahl, J. Korsgaard, and S.A. Linde:** The indoor air environment in dwellings: a study of air-exchange, humidity and pollutants in 115 Danish residences. *Indoor Air 2*:121–126 (1992).
26. **Drivas, P.J., P.G. Simmonds, and F.H. Shair:** Experimental characterization of ventilation systems in buildings. *Environ. Sci. Technol. 6*:609–614 (1972).
27. **Tou, J.C. and G.J. Kallos:** Kinetic study of the stabilities of chloromethyl methyl ether and bis(chloromethyl) ether in humid air. *Anal. Chem. 46*:1866–1869 (1974).
28. **Sparks, L.E.:** Modeling indoor concentrations and exposure. *Ann. N.Y. Acad. Sci. 641*: 102–111 (1992).
29. **Jayjock, M.A, D.R. Doshi, E.H. Nungesser, and W.D. Shade:** Development and evaluation of a source/sink model of indoor air concentrations from isothiazolone treated wood used indoors. *Am. Ind. Hyg. Assoc. J. 56*:546–557 (1995).
30. **Fleischer, M.T.:** "An Evaporation/ Air Dispersion Model for Chemical Spills On Land." Shell Development Center, Westhollow Research Center, P.O. Box 1380, Houston, Texas, 1980. [Pamphlet]
31. **U.S. Environmental Protection Agency (EPA):** A Manual for the Preparation of Engineering Assessment. Washington, DC: EPA, September 1984. [Unpublished draft]
32. **Schroy, J.M. and J.M. Wu:** Emission from spills. In *Proceedings on Control of Specific Toxic Pollutants.* Gainesville, FL: Air Pollution Control Association, 1979.
33. **Chemical Manufacturers Association (CMA):** PAVE-Program to Assess Volatile Emissions, Version 2.0. Washington, DC: CMA, 1992.
34. **Braun, K.O. and K.J. Caplan:** Evaporation Rate of Volatile Liquids [EPA/744-R-92-001; NTIS PB 92-232305]. Washington, DC: U.S. Environmental Protection Agency, Office of Pollution Prevention and Toxics, 1989.
35. **Hummel, A.A., K.O. Braum, and M.C. Fehrenbacher:** Evaporation of a liquid in a flowing airstream. *Am. Ind. Hyg. Assoc. J. 57*:519-525 (1996).
36. **Fehrenbacher, M.C. and A.A. Hummel:** Evaluation of the mass balance model used by the Environmental Protection Agency for estimating inhalation exposure to new chemical substances. *Am. Ind. Hyg. Assoc. J. 57*:526-536 (1996).
37. **Jayjock, M.A.:** Back pressure modeling of indoor air concentration from volatilizing sources. *Am. Ind. Hyg. Assoc. J. 55*:230-235 (1994).
38. **Hemeon, W.C.:** *Plant and Process Ventilation,* 2nd edition. New York: Industrial Press, 1963.
39. **Nicas, M.:** Estimating exposure intensity in an imperfectly mixed room, *Am. Ind. Hyg. Assoc. J. 57*:542–550 (1996).
40. **National Academy of Sciences (NAS):** *Clearing the Air: Asthma and Indoor Air Exposures.* Committee on the Assessment of Asthma and Indoor Air, Division of Health Promotion and Disease Prevention, Institute of Medicine, National Academy Press ISBN: 978-0-309-06496-5, Wash. D.C. (2000). p. 410.
41. **Carslaw, H.S. and J.C. Jaeger:** *Conduction of Heat in Solids,* 2nd edition. London: Oxford University Press, 1959. pp. 260–261.
42. **Roach, S.A.:** On the role of turbulent diffusion in ventilation. *Ann. Occup. Hyg. 24*:105–132 (1981).

43. **Wadden, R.A., J.L. Hawkins, P.A. Scheff, and J.E. Franke:** Characterization of emission factors related to source activity for trichloroethylene degreasing and chrome plating processes. *Am. Ind. Hyg. Assoc. J. 52*:349–356 (1991).
44. **Wadden, R.A., P.A. Scheff, and J.E. Franke:** Emission factors from trichloroethylene vapor degreasers. *Am. Ind. Hyg. Assoc. J. 50*:496–500 (1989).
45. **Scheff, P.A., R.L. Friedman, J.E. Franke, L.M. Conroy, et al.:** Source activity modeling of Freon emissions from open-top vapor degreasers. *Appl. Occup. Environ. Hyg. 7*:127–134 (1992).
46. **Matoba, Y., J. Ohnishi, and M. Matsuo:** A simulation of insecticides in indoor aerosol space spraying. *Chemosphere 26*:1167–1186 (1993).
47. **Arnold, S. and M. Jayjock:** Calculating Average Airborne Concentrations from and Generation Rates for Emissions for Constant Short-Lived Sources. AIHce Podium Session 129. Philadelphia, PA, 2007.
48. **Arnold, S. and M. Jayjock:** Applying Emission Source Data to Determine Average Airborne Concentrations from and Generation Rates for Emissions for Constant Short-Lived Sources. AIHce Podium Session 126. Toronto, Ont., 2009.
49. **Hewett, P., P. Logan, J. Mulhausen, G. Ramachandran, and S. Banerjee:** Rating Exposure Control Using Bayesian Decision Analysis. *J. Occ. Env. Hyg. 3(10)*:568–581 (2006).
50. **Ramachandran, G. and J. Vincent:** A Bayesian approach to retrospective exposure assessment. *App. Occup. and Env. Hyg. 14(8)*: 547–557 (1999)
51. **Zhang, Y., S. Banerjee, R. Yang, C. Lungu, and G. Ramachandran:** Bayesian Modeling of Exposure and Air Flow Using Two-zone Models. *Ann. Occ. Hyg. 53(4)*:409–424 (2009).
52. **Sottas, P.E., J. Lavoué, R. Bruzzi, D. Vernez, N. Charrière, and P.O. Droz:** An empirical hierarchical Bayesian unification of occupational exposure assessment methods. *Stat. Med. 28(1)*:75–93 (2009)
53. **WINBUGS:** www.mrc-bsu.cam.ac.uk/bugs/welcome.shtml. [Accessed on September 24, 2009].
54. **Ferrari, P., R. Carroll, P. Gustafson, and E. Riboli:** A Bayesian multilevel model for estimating the diet/disease relationship in a multicenter study with exposures measured with error: The EPIC Study. *Stat. Med. 27*:6037–6054 (2008).
55. **Chatterjee, A., G. Horgan, and C. Theobald:** Exposure Assessment in Pesticide Intake from Multiple Food Products: A Bayesian Latent-Variable Approach. *Risk Anal. 28(6)*:1727–1736 (2008).
56. **Elliott, P. and D. Savitz:** Design Issues in Small-Area Studies of Environment and Health. *Env. Health Persp. 116(8)*:1098–1104 (2008).
57. **Hawkins, N.C.:** Evaluating conservatism in maximally exposed individual (MEI) predictive exposure assessments: a first-cut analysis. *Reg. Toxicol. Pharmacol. 14*:107–117 (1991).
58. **Evans, J.S., D.W. Cooper, and P.L. Kinney:** On the propagation of error in air pollution measurements. *Env. Mon. Assess. 4*:139 (1984).

Outcome Competencies

After completing this chapter, the reader should be able to:

1. Define underlined terms used in this chapter.
2. Explain sample collection principles to practicing professionals and the public.
3. Select sampling methods for gases and vapors that satisfy occupational hygiene objectives
4. Select sampling parameters for gases and vapors that satisfy the requirements of the method and the occupational hygiene objectives.
5. Evaluate the applicability of specific media and methods for sampling gases and vapors in defined situations.
6. Perform necessary calculations to ensure the collection of reliable data when sampling gases and vapors.
7. Interpret air sampling data collected.

Key Terms

absorbing medium • active sampling • adsorbing medium • analytical methods • back pressures • backup layer • breakthrough volume • cold traps • constant flow • desorption efficiency • diffusive samplers • electromagnetic susceptibility • fritted glass bubblers • gas • gas washing bottles • grab sampling • impinger • integrated sampling • intrinsically safe • limit of detection (LOD) • limit of quantitation (LOQ) • lower boundary of working range • passive sampling • personal sampling • pressure drop • primary standards • sampler capacity • sampling media • sampling strategy • secondary standards • solvent extraction • sorbent tube • stainless steel canister • target concentration • thermal desorption • treated filter • upper measurement limit • vapor • whole air sampling • working range

Prerequisite Knowledge

Basic understanding of chemistry and occupational hygiene sampling.

Prior to beginning this chapter, the user should review the following chapters:

Chapter Number	Chapter Topic
15	Principles and Instrumentation for Calibrating Air Sampling Equipment
17	Direct-Reading Instruments for Determining Concentrations of Gases, Vapors & Aerosols

Key Topics

I. Sample Collection Principles
   A. Integrated Samples
   B. Grab Samples
   C. Operational Limitations of Sampling and Analysis
II. Sampling Media for Gases and Vapors
   A. Solid Sorbents
   B. Chemically-Treated Filters
   C. Liquid Absorbers
   D. Sampling Bags/Partially-Evacuated Rigid Containers
   E. Cold Traps
III. Calculations and Interpretation of Air Sampling Data

Sampling of Gases and Vapors

11

Deborah F. Dietrich, CIH

Introduction

This chapter introduces the techniques available to the occupational hygienist for evaluating exposures to gases and vapors arising in or from the workplace. Occupational hygienists in the twenty-first century face new responsibilities in light of the shift from an industrial to a service-based economy in the U.S. and other developed countries and a heightened awareness of environmental issues in the general community. Therefore, current practitioners must be aware of technology available to assess gases and vapors in the traditional industrial environment as well as in indoor and ambient air. It is also important that occupational hygienists recognize the capabilities and limitations of various methodologies for specific applications. In this chapter, the applications and limitations of a variety of sampling media and techniques are reviewed.

When developing a particular sampling strategy, the reader should review sampling and analytical methods available for the contaminants of interest for specific applications. Several governmental and consensus organizations have compiled and published manuals of sampling and analytical methods for gases and vapors. Addresses and websites of these organizations are provided in Table 11.1.

The occupational hygienist should carefully select the sampling and analytical methods most suitable for the specific application. If air sampling is being done for the purposes of OSHA compliance, the choice of a NIOSH or OSHA method may be most appropriate. Note, however, that OSHA does not mandate the sampling method. OSHA standards for individual chemicals will typically list the methods that have been tested by OSHA or NIOSH, but this does not preclude the use of alternative equivalent methods. The employer has the obligation of selecting a method that meets the sampling and analytical accuracy and precision requirements of the standard under its unique field conditions. These requirements typically stipulate measurement at the permissible exposure limit (PEL) within ±25% of the "true" value at a 95% confidence level.[1] The U.S. EPA publishes methods for pollutants in indoor air and for toxic compounds in ambient air. These methods are designed to measure the lower levels typically found in these environments.

Before beginning a sampling program, it is important to select and consult with a qualified analytical laboratory. The American Industrial Hygiene Association (AIHA®) maintains a list of laboratories that have been accredited under the Industrial Hygiene Laboratory Accreditation Program. A qualified laboratory can assist in choosing sampling and analytical methods that meet the sensitivity and specificity criteria appropriate to the environment being evaluated. The laboratory can also help choose a sampling medium and strategy that are compatible with the analytical method selected and can advise on any special handling procedures not included in the published method. Two key factors necessary for the selection of the most appropriate method are (1) knowledge of the occupational environment and (2) an overall perspective of the limitation of the chemistry of the sampling and analysis.

Caution should be exercised when using a traditional workplace sampling method for measuring contaminants in indoor or ambient air as the expected concentrations may be below the working range of the method. NIOSH offers some specific recommendations for circumstances when industrial hygienists must "push a method to the limit." To obtain the sensitivity required for measurement of low levels, NIOSH recommends that practitioners exceed the recommended air volume, while observing the recommended maximum

Table 11.1 — Available Publications on Sampling and Analytical Methods for Gases and Vapors

U.S. Government Agency Methods

National Institute for Occupational Safety and Health (NIOSH)
NIOSH Manual of Analytical Methods, Fourth Edition
National Institute for Occupational Safety and Health
4676 Columbia Parkway
Cincinnati, OH 45226-1998
http://www.cdc.gov/niosh/nmam/

Occupational Safety and Health Administration (OSHA)
OSHA analytical Methods Manual
OSHA Salt Lake Technical Center
8660 South Sandy Parkway
Sandy, UT 84070
http://www.osha.gov/dts/sltc/methods/toc.html

OSHA Chemical Sampling Information
http://www.osha.gov/dts/chemicalsampling/toc/toc_chemsamp.html

Environmental Protection Agency (EPA)
Compendium of Methods for the Determination of Toxic Organic Compounds in Ambient Air
Atmospheric Research and Exposure Assessment Laboratory
Office of Research and Development
Research Triangle Park, NC 27711
http://www.epa.gov/ttn/amtic/airtox.html

Compendium of Methods for the Determination of Air Pollutants in Indoor Air
Atmospheric Research and Exposure Assessment Laboratory
Office of Research and Development
Research Triangle Park, NC 27711
http://www.arb.ca.gov/research/indoor/methods.htm

International Government Agency Methods

UK Health and Safety Executive
Methods for the Determination of Hazardous Substances
Health and Safety Laboratory
Sheffield, UK
http://www.hse.gov.uk/pubns/mdhs/index.htm

Consensus Organization Methods

ASTM International
Annual Book of ASTM Standards
100 Barr Harbor Dr.
West Conshohocken, PA 19428

ASTM Committee D22 publishes standards related to sampling of gases and vapors in different environments.
http://www.astm.org

American National Standards Institute (ANSI)
1819 L St. NW
Suite 600
Washington, DC 20036

ANSI publishes test protocols and performance standards for air sampling devices.
http://www.ansi.org

flow rate.[2] This is because the recommended air volume is generally a conservative value so as to protect against breakthrough under worst-case conditions of high humidity and high concentrations. While considerable leeway exists for the air volume, breakthrough should be monitored by observing the amount of contaminants on the primary and backup sections of the sampler.

For industrial hygiene purposes, a substance is considered a gas if this is its normal physical state at room temperature (25°C) and one-atmosphere pressure. Examples of gases are carbon monoxide, chlorine, oxygen, and nitrogen. If, however, the substance is normally a liquid (or solid) at normal temperature and pressure, then the gaseous component in equilibrium with its liquid (or solid) state is called a vapor. Carbon tetrachloride, formaldehyde, and benzene are examples of compounds that are present in the vapor state.

Sample Collection Principles

There are a number of considerations when designing a sampling plan such as the location of samples, the number of workers to be sampled, and the duration of samples. Such considerations are reviewed in the exposure assessment chapters of this publication. Practitioners should also consider non-chemical factors when choosing sampling options in various environments. Equipment noise is an important consideration when doing indoor air sampling in occupied public buildings and residences. Similarly, equipment size and flow rate should be suitable for the space requirements and should not disturb normal ventilation. Security of sampling equipment must also be addressed to avoid sample tampering and theft.

This discussion will focus on the means of collecting valid samples of gases and vapors. Two basic types of samples are used to evaluate employees' exposures to gases and vapors in the workplace: integrated and grab. Sampling using continuous monitors will be considered in the chapter on direct-reading instrumental methods.

Integrated sampling for gases and vapors involves the passage of a known volume of air through an absorbing or adsorbing medium to remove the desired contaminants from the air during a specified period of time. With this technique, the contaminants of interest are collected and concentrated over a period of time to obtain the average exposure levels during the entire sampling period. Grab sampling techniques involve the direct collection of an air-contaminant mixture into a device such as a sampling bag, syringe, or evacuated flask over a short interval of a few seconds or minutes. Thus, grab samples represent the atmospheric concentrations at the sampling site at a given point in time.[3]

Occupational hygienists may also encounter the term, whole air sampling. Whole air sampling involves the collection of air into a sealable container such as a stainless steel canister or sampling bag for subsequent analysis. Whole air samples can be collected in canisters over a short period of time as grab samples or integrated over a longer period of time to obtain time-weighted average (TWA) concentrations.

Integrated Samples

Integrated sampling, covering the entire period of exposure, is required because airborne contaminant concentrations during a typical work shift vary with time and activity. Instantaneous measurements (grab samples) taken at any given period, therefore, do not reflect the average exposure of the worker for the entire shift and may not capture intermittent high or low exposures. Most integrated sampling is done to determine the 8-hour TWA exposure and results are compared with the OSHA PELs, the threshold limit values (TLVs®) of the American Conference of Governmental Industrial Hygienists (ACGIH®), or other applicable limits or guidelines such as the NIOSH recommended exposure limits. Integrated sampling is also required for determining compliance with short-term exposure limits performed over a 15-minute period.

When collecting an integrated sample, it is important that the appropriate sample duration and flow rate are chosen relative to the purpose of sampling, the sensitivity of the analytical method, and the expected concentration of the contaminant of interest. It is also essential that the flow rate and time be accurately measured. The accuracy of any industrial hygiene measurement depends on the precise determination of the mass of contaminant collected as well as the volume of air sampled.

Active Sampling

Most integrated sampling methods published by OSHA or NIOSH use active sampling techniques. Active sampling is a means of collecting an airborne substance that employs a mechanical device such as an air sampling pump to draw the air/contaminant mixture into or through the sampling device such as a sorbent tube, treated filter, or impinger containing a liquid medium. A key element when using active sampling techniques is calibration that reliably measures the pump's flow rate, thus allowing for an accurate determination of air volume.

Air Sampling Pumps. An integrated air sampling method requires a relatively constant source of suction as an air-moving device that can be calibrated to the recommended flow rate. OSHA Analytical Methods specify that personal sampling pumps be calibrated to within ±5% of the recommended flow rate with the collection media in line.[4] There are a number of lightweight, battery operated pumps available that can be used with a variety of collection devices. Most utilize a rechargeable battery pack that allows for extended sampling over the 8-hour workday or longer. They can be attached to the wearer's belt for personal sampling in the worker's breathing zone or they can be used as area samplers.

Sampling pumps are available with a variety of flow ranges and automatic features including timers, fault shutdown, constant flow capabilities, and computer compatibility. Most recently developed pumps weigh no more than two pounds and are intrinsically safe allowing safe operation even in potentially explosive environments. Many pumps now also include a mechanism to address electromagnetic susceptibility, as it has been found that degraded instrument performance can result from radio frequency interference or electromagnetic interference from devices such as walkie-talkies, high voltage equipment, and electric motors.[5]

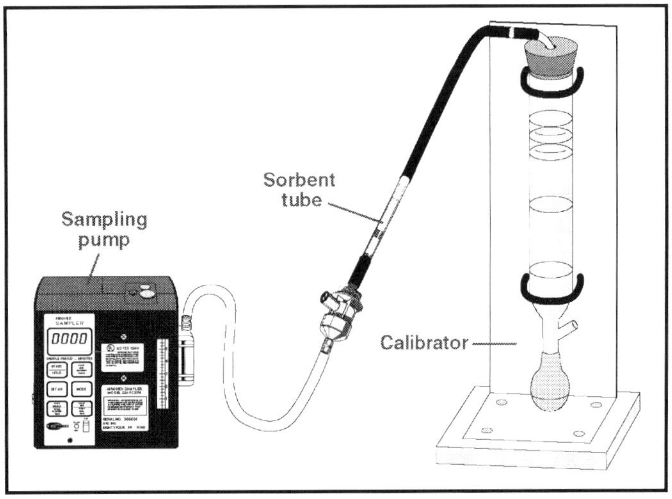

Figure 11.1 — Sampling train connected to calibrator.

Pumps must be capable of maintaining the desired flow rate over the entire sampling period with the sample collection device in line. This is not normally a problem when sampling gases and vapors with solid sorbent tubes. However, when the sorbent material is of a fine mesh size or when sorbent tubes with a relatively high pressure drop are being used to collect short-term samples at flow rates of 1 L/min or greater, some pumps may not be able to handle the pressure drop.[2] Most recently designed personal samplers have a constant flow feature to continuously compensate for varying back pressures. Others have a constant pressure feature to allow for sampling with multiple sorbent tubes each with an independently set flow rate.

Calibration. Pump flow rate must be calibrated with the entire sampling train assembled, as it will be used in the field. (See Figure 11.1). Good industrial hygiene practice dictates that pumps be calibrated before and after sampling on the same day under pressure and temperature conditions similar to those at the sampling site. Calibration should not be done using built-in rotameters found on many sampling pumps. These are not precision devices and will not give a quantitative measure of the rate of airflow. Some newly released sampling pumps incorporate an internal flow sensor that indicates the flow rate digitally on the pump display. Like built-in rotameters, these flow sensors are secondary standards that require calibration and verification using an external primary standard. Users are cautioned to read closely the instructions from the manufacturer regarding the accuracy of the readout and the frequency of calibration using a primary standard.

A wide variety of devices are currently available to measure airflow accurately; these are covered in greater detail in another chapter of this book. Flowmeters that are termed primary standards are based on direct and measurable linear dimensions, such as the length and diameter of a cylinder.

These include spirometers, bubble meters, and Mariotte bottles. Manufacturers of electronic bubble meters and near-frictionless piston meters report that their devices are also primary standards. Like manual bubble meters, electronic bubble meters operate by measuring the flow rate of gases over a fixed volume per unit time. The fixed volume is that of the flow cell. The time for the soap film to travel from the first infrared sensor to the second sensor is measured with a microprocessor, calculated as volume per unit time and displayed as the flow rate. With near-frictionless piston meters, the pump or flow source evacuates or pressurizes air in a flow cell causing a piston to rise. The piston breaks the light beam as it passes. When a second beam is broken a clock measures the time between the two breaks and the flow measurement is displayed. Since the volume of the flow cell and the timer are NIST traceable, the manufacturer reports that this device is a true primary standard.[6] Secondary standards are flowmeters that trace their calibration to primary standards and maintain their accuracy with reasonable care and handling in operation.[7] Secondary standards include precision rotameters, wet test meters, and dry gas meters.

Sample Collection Media. Occupational hygienists should consult air sampling methods developed by NIOSH, OSHA, or other recognized testing organizations to determine the appropriate collection media for a specific chemical contaminant. (A more complete discussion of sample collection media is given later in the chapter.) These published methods have been extensively researched and collaboratively tested, and deviations from the requirements are not recommended.

It is important, however, for the occupational hygienist to review the method to determine its applicability relative to the field conditions. ASTM International has published a *Standard Guide for Selection of Methods for Active, Integrative Sampling of Volatile Organic Compounds in Air*.[8] This document provides critical parameters that can be used to determine appropriate sampling methods for designated compounds including vapor pressure, boiling point, and reactivity in air. Target analytes are listed for various sampling media along with advantages and limitations for each. Particular attention should be paid to interfering compounds, humidity and temperature effects, and appropriate measuring range. The physical state of the contaminant(s) being sampled is also an important consideration. Air contaminants may often simultaneously exist in multiple-phases, e.g., particulate and vapor phase. It is important to choose the proper sample media to collect all phases of the contaminant of interest.[2]

Advantages and Disadvantages of Active Sampling. Active sampling techniques offer considerable advantages for the measurement of airborne contaminants. Since most methods published by OSHA and NIOSH are active methods, there has been extensive testing and documentation of reliability. If the purpose of sampling is for OSHA compliance, it is possible to select the same active sampling method that would be used by compliance personnel during an inspection.

From a technical standpoint, active sampling methods offer the advantage of a calibrated, measured airflow for assurance in accuracy of sample volume. Also, most solid sorbent tubes have a secondary layer of sorbent that serves as a backup layer for the indication of sample breakthrough. (See Figure 11.2). If contaminants exist in multiple phases, it is possible to use a series of samplers, such as a pre-filter with a sorbent tube, or a specialty tube with internal filters to effectively collect both phases simultaneously from one air sample with one pump.

A disadvantage of active sampling is that the equipment is often cumbersome and may interfere with the job if workers have to wear a pump and sample media throughout the entire workday. Pump calibration can

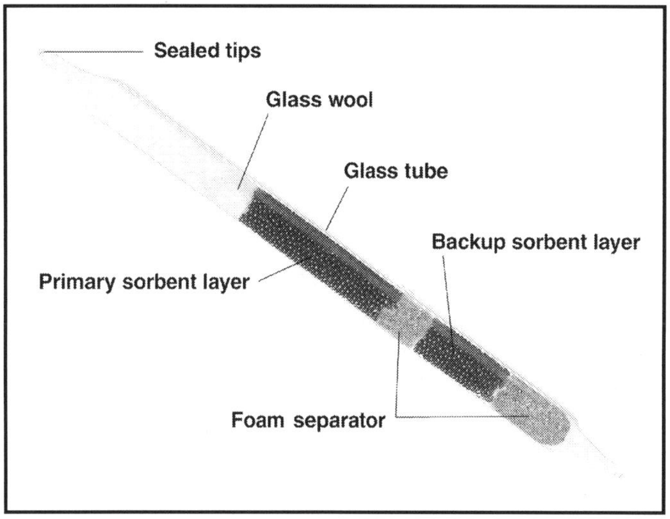

Figure 11.2 — Sorbent sample tube with backup sorbent layer.

also be time consuming, and technical training is required to perform the necessary tasks. As pumps age, they may become less reliable at maintaining constant flow over the entire sampling period, and more frequent calibration may be necessary.

Passive Samplers

Among the most important developments in air sampling technology in recent years is the development of passive sampling devices. This technology was first introduced to the occupational hygiene profession in a 1973 article by Palmes and Gunnison.[9] Passive sampling is the collection of airborne gases and vapors at a rate controlled by a physical process such as diffusion through a static air layer or permeation through a membrane without the active movement of air through an air sampler. Most passive samplers that are commercially available operate on the principle of diffusion. Diffusive samplers rely on the movement of contaminant molecules across a concentration gradient, which for steady-state conditions can be defined by Fick's First Law of Diffusion.[10]

The following equation gives the steady-state relationship for the rate of mass transfer:

$$W = \left[\frac{DA}{L}\right](C_1 - C_0) \qquad (11\text{-}1)$$

where:

W = mass transfer rate, ng/sec
D = diffusion coefficient, cm^2/sec
A = cross-sectional area of diffusion path, cm^2
L = length of diffusion path, cm
C_1 = ambient concentration of contaminant, ng/cm^3
C_0 = concentration of contaminant at collection surface, ng/m^3

Diffusive samplers consist of a diffusion gap between the external air and a sorbing medium. The sorbing medium serves not only to collect the chemicals of interest, but also to maintain the concentration of these chemicals as close to zero as possible at the end of the diffusion path.[11] If this occurs throughout the sampling period, Fick's First Law reduces to:

$$Q = \left[\frac{DA}{L}\right](CT) \qquad (11\text{-}2)$$

where:

Q = amount collected (ng)
D = diffusion coefficient (cm^2/min)
A = cross-sectional area of the diffusion path (cm^2)
L = diffusive path length (cm)
C = airborne concentration (mg/m^3)
T = sampling time (min)

Note that the units of D (A/L) are volume per unit time, the same as for active air-moving devices such as personal sampling pumps.

Each gas or vapor being sampled has a specific diffusion coefficient (D). Therefore, a passive sampler will probably have a different sampling rate for each analyte in the mixture. Diffusion coefficients for various compounds of interest can be determined experimentally or they may be estimated using one of several equations.[12] The diffusion coefficient and the sampler geometry can be used to determine a theoretical uptake rate. In practice, however, uptake rates may vary under various field conditions.[13] To more reliably assess the overall accuracy and precision of a passive sampler, a validation of its performance characteristics can be done using validation protocols published by NIOSH or other testing agencies.[14, 15] These protocols stipulate the testing of those aspects unique to passive sampling, as well as those aspects common to both active and passive sampling (see Table 11.2).

In recent years, there have been a variety of publications related to evaluating the performance characteristics of diffusive samplers:

1. European Standard EN 838 for evaluating the performance of diffusive samplers.[16]
2. U.K. Health and Safety Executive Method for the Determination of Hazardous Substances 88 for volatile organic compounds in air using diffusive samplers.[17]
3. ASTM Standard Practice for Evaluating the Performance of Diffusive Samplers Designation: D 6246-08.[18]

Table 11.2 — Performance Characteristics Evaluated in the NIOSH Validation Protocol for Passive Samplers.

Analytical recovery	Relative humidity
Sampling rate and capacity	Interferents
Reverse diffusion	Monitor orientation
Storage stability	Temperature
Analyte concentration	Accuracy and precision
Exposure time	Shelf life
Face velocity	Behavior in the field

Note: Data from Cassinelli et al.[14]

4. American National Standard for Air Sampling Devices—Diffusive Type for Gases and Vapors in Working Environments (ANSI/ISEA 104-1998 R2009).[19]

In 1998, the OSHA Salt Lake Technical Center released a research report that attempted to determine sampling rate variation for specific passive sampler designs.[20] The concept of passive sampling rate variation was equated to active sampling pump error (which is typically assumed to be ±5%). This was significant in that the use of the sampling rate variation for a particular passive sampler along with the analytical error component allowed the calculation of the overall sampling and analytical error (SAE). OSHA inspectors must use SAEs along with the sample results to determine if an OSHA PEL has been exceeded. This research report paved the way for the development and use of passive sampling methods by OSHA. Within a few years of this research report, OSHA passive sampling methods were validated and published for toluene, tetrachloroethylene, trichloroethylene, xylenes, ethyl benzene, methyl ethyl ketone, methyl isobutyl ketone, benzene, formaldehyde, and butyl acetates.[4]

Types of Passive Samplers. To meet the wide range of sampling needs, many different types of passive samplers are now commercially available. Direct-reading passive samplers provide users an inexpensive option for chemical screening or for alerting wearers to the presence of highly toxic substances. Direct-reading passive samplers typically employ colorimetric techniques. The length of the color band or the intensity of the color change is read on a scale or compared with a chart for determination of concentration levels.

For example, with passive color tubes, users break open one end and insert the color tube into a holder that is clipped in the breathing zone or fixed-point location. Target chemicals diffuse into the tube, chemically react with the tube ingredients, and the resultant color band is compared to the tube's printed scale to determine chemical levels as ppm-hrs. Dividing by the number of hours sampled provides ppm concentrations in air. Direct-reading passive samplers offer convenience and immediate results for field applications. But they have sources of error that limit their accuracy for compliance sampling.

Passive samplers that require laboratory analysis are a better option for applications requiring high accuracy, as they do not have the sources of error found with colorimetric samplers. In addition, users can reference published sampling methods or research reports to document sampling reliability. In many cases, validated passive samplers provide accuracy and precision levels comparable to those found with active samplers.

Passive samplers that require laboratory analysis typically use solid sorbents or chemically treated paper to collect the contaminant of interest. Both types have grown in their application and level of sophistication in recent years. Organic vapor samplers with solid sorbents are now commercially available for ppm-level determinations using solvent extraction and GC analysis or ppb-level determinations using thermal desorption and GC analysis. (See a discussion on Desorption of Contaminants later in this chapter.) Passive samplers for ppm-level measurements are suitable for routine occupational hygiene applications including 8-hour TWA and 15-minute STEL determinations. (See Figure 11.3) Samplers for ppb-level determinations are useful for indoor and ambient air measurements.

Specific design modifications are used by passive sampler manufacturers to allow the determinations of lower exposure levels found in ambient and indoor air. For example, the patented Radiello® diffusive sampling system uses a radial design with a 360° sampling surface instead of the axial design of traditional diffusive samplers. The manufacturer reports that the radial design provides contaminant uptake rates at least three times higher than axial diffusive samplers with the same dimensions.[21] The patented ULTRA® passive sampling system

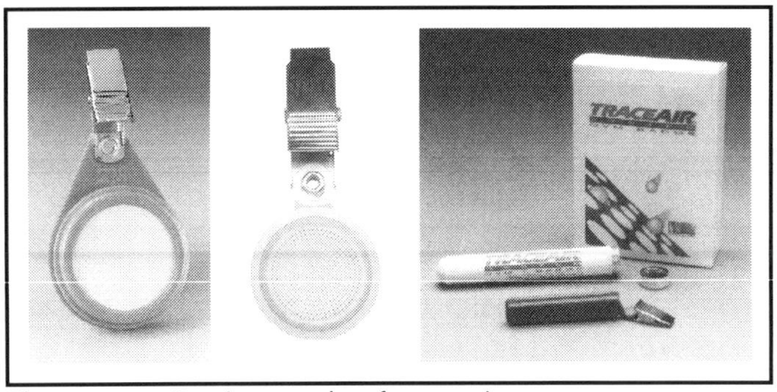

Figure 11.3 — Passive samplers for organic vapors.

allows direct transfer of the solid sorbent from the sampler to a thermal desorption tube in the laboratory to achieve lower detection limits.[22] (See Figure 11.4).

In addition to organic vapor samplers designed to collect a broad range of compounds, specialty passive samplers are available to preferentially collect specific compounds. Three diffusive samplers that employ dinitrophenylhydrazine (DNPH) chemistry are specified in OSHA Method 1007 for the sampling and analysis of formaldehyde. OSHA Method ID-140 specifies the use of a specialty solid sorbent for the collection of inorganic mercury vapor in both a passive sampler and in a sorbent tube.[4] For more information on different sorbent materials, see the section on Types of Sorbent Materials or Table 11.3 later in this chapter.

Advantages and Disadvantages of Passive Samplers. Passive samplers offer many advantages to the occupational hygienist. They are very easy to use, allowing samples to be collected by personnel with less technical training. Passive samplers are also

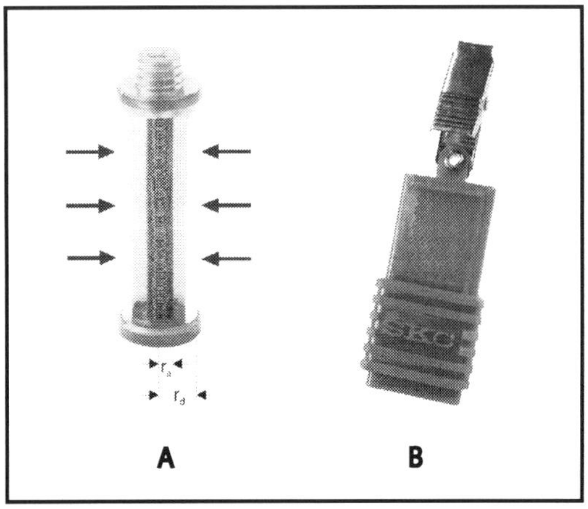

Figure 11.4 — Passive samplers designed for low-level measurements. (A) Radiello® sampler with radial design of (B) ULTRA® III sampler with sample and blank in one sampler.

less expensive than active sampling when compared to the costs of pumps and flowmeters, and they are less obtrusive to the wearer. Finally, for most occupational hygiene applications the mass of contaminant collected by passive samplers is not significantly affected by temperature or pressure.[23]

Users should weigh these advantages against the possible disadvantages of these devices. In many cases, there are no OSHA or NIOSH methods to reference to ensure the reliability of data when using passive samplers. The sampling rate, if theoretically calculated, may not prove to be valid under field conditions. Reverse diffusion may also be a factor whereby some chemicals diffuse onto the sorbent, but are not adequately retained. Reverse diffusion can be a particular concern if transient peaks of vapor occur in the workplace air. Molecules entering the sampler may not have enough time to reach the sorbing medium before the concentration drops disrupting the diffusive process. This is more of a concern in tube-type diffusive samplers than in badge-type samplers.[10]

Environmental parameters may influence the collection efficiency of passive samplers. Stagnant air (i.e., face velocities less than 25 ft/min) will cause "starvation" of the sampler. As the diffusion zone (L) is lengthened due to the lack of fresh contaminant molecules outside the sampler, the sampling rate is decreased causing a low measurement of the actual concentration. Alternatively, high face velocities can cause turbulence to occur in the air gap affecting sampling.[24] (This effect is minimized, however, as most manufacturers use a windscreen to dampen the effect of turbulent air.)

Interfering compounds can affect the ability of passive samplers to collect the target contaminant. For example, two possible interferences are reported in OSHA Method 1007 when using passive samplers for formaldehyde. Ozone is a known interferent for samplers using DNPH to derivatize formaldehyde. Ozone can react with DNPH decreasing the amount available to react, or it can decrease the amount of formaldehyde-DNPH already formed. OSHA advises users not to use DNPH-based passive samplers for formaldehyde if the ozone levels are greater than 0.5 ppm. OSHA also noted an interfering effect on passive sampler performance when formalin is the source of formaldehyde exposures. The methyl alcohol in the formalin solutions chemically reacts with formaldehyde to form methoxymethanol and dimethoxymethane which have different diffusive sampling rates than formaldehyde.[4]

Users are advised to exercise caution when using passive samplers for indoor air quality investigations or ambient area sampling. The low uptake rates of passive samplers may not provide the sensitivity required for low level determinations, and extended sampling times of 24 hours or more may enhance reverse diffusion effects. When sampling in unoccupied buildings, stagnant air may affect the performance of the sampler as described above. ASTM International has issued standard guidelines on the use of diffusive samplers for gaseous pollutants in indoor air to assist practitioners working in this environment.[24]

Grab Samples

Grab samples are collected to measure gas and vapor concentrations at a point in time and are used, therefore, to evaluate "peak" exposures for comparison to "ceiling" limits. Grab samples can be used to identify unknown contaminants, to evaluate contaminant sources, or to measure contaminant levels from intermittent processes or other sources. Grab or instantaneous samples of air to be analyzed for gaseous components are collected using rigid containers, such as syringes, partially evacuated flasks or canisters, or in nonrigid containers, such as sampling bags. See a complete discussion of these devices later in this chapter.

Instantaneous (as well as integrated) measurements of gases and vapors may also be performed using detector tubes or direct-reading instruments. These methods are described in another chapter of this book.

An advantage of collecting an air-contaminant mixture directly into a rigid or nonrigid container is that frequently it can be analyzed immediately by direct injection into a gas chromatograph (GC) or by using direct-reading instruments. Thus, quick decisions can be made in the field, such as choosing personal protective equipment, determining the source of leaks, or permitting entry into a vessel. The samples can also be retained for more thorough laboratory analysis at a later time.

A disadvantage of this technique is that for most applications contaminants are collected but not integrated over time. Only some containers such as stainless steel canisters will allow for the placement of a metering device, such as a critical orifice on the inlet, that will enable the collection of a sample at near constant flow over a period of time to provide a TWA concentration. While grab samples provide information relative to peak exposures, using multiple grab samples to assess full-shift exposures is time consuming and subject to error. This technique requires statistical analysis and will not be discussed in this book.

Operational Limits of Sampling and Analysis

When using any sampling technique, consideration must be given to the inherent limitations of the method, including sampler capacity, limit of detection (LOD), limit of quantitation (LOQ), and the upper measurement limit, which define the useful range for the method.[25] In a given application one or more of these factors will determine the minimum, maximum, or optimum volume of air to be sampled and may determine the confidence that can be placed in the results.

Sampler capacity (W_{max}) is a predetermined conservative estimate of the total mass of contaminant that can be collected on the sampling medium without loss or overloading. For gases and vapors, researchers at NIOSH have defined W_{max} as two-thirds of the experimental breakthrough capacity of the solid sorbent, i.e., 67% of the mass of contaminant on the sorbent at the breakthrough volume.[25] Breakthrough volume is defined as that volume of an atmosphere containing two times the PEL for the contaminant that can be sampled at the recommended flow rate before the efficiency of the sampler degrades to 95%.

The American Chemical Society (ACS) Committee on Environmental Analytical Chemistry defines the LOD as the lowest concentration level than can be determined to be statistically different from a blank sample. The recommended value of the LOD is the amount of analyte that will give rise to a signal that is three times the standard deviation of the signal derived from the media blank. The LOQ is the concentration level above which quantitative results may be obtained with a certain degree of confidence. The recommended value of the LOQ is the amount of analyte that will give rise to a signal that is 10 times the standard deviation of the signal from a series of media blanks. This corresponds to a relative uncertainty in the measurement of ±30% at the 99% confidence level.[26]

The OSHA Salt Lake Technical Center, in their *Method Evaluation Guidelines for Organic Compounds* of June 1993, describe detection limit in terms of both the detection limit of the analytical procedure and the detection limit of the overall procedure.[27] OSHA reports that in general, detection limits are defined as the amount of analyte that gives a response that is significantly different (three standard deviations) from the background response. If the amount of analyte was derived from an analytical standard, it would represent the detection limit of the analytical procedure. If the amount of analyte was derived from media spikes, it would represent the detection limit of the overall procedure.

The upper measurement limit (W_u) is the useful limit (mg of analyte per sample) of the analytical instrument. If the sample is above the upper measurement limit of the analytical instrument, it can on most occasions be re-diluted and re-analyzed. The values of LOD, LOQ, and Wu for a given contaminant and analytical procedure should be obtained from and/or discussed with the analytical laboratory before sampling.

The target concentration (C_t) is a preliminary estimate of the airborne concentration of the contaminant of interest relative to the purpose of testing. This parameter can be used to determine minimum and maximum air volumes. The target concentration may be estimated by using previous sampling data, by using direct-reading instruments, or by relying on the professional judgment of the occupational hygienist.

A minimum sample volume for a quantitative determination (Vmin) at the target concentration may be calculated as follows:

$$V_{min}\,(L) = \frac{LOQ(mg) \times 10^3\,(L/m^3)}{C_t\,(mg/m^3)} \qquad (11\text{-}3)$$

Example: It is desired to collect valid samples of acetaldehyde given the following information: method, NIOSH 3507; range given in method, 2 to 60 mg per sample; target concentration, 200 ppm (360.2 mg/m³). What is the minimum air volume required?

$$V_{min}\,(L) = \frac{2\text{ mg} \times 10^3\text{ L/m}^3}{360.2\text{ mg/m}^3} = 6\text{ L} \qquad (11\text{-}4)$$

The maximum sample volume that may be collected with minimum risk of bias due to Breakthrough or sampler overloading may be calculated as follows:

$$V_{max}\,(L) = \frac{W_{max}(mg) \times 10^3\,(L/m^3)}{C_t\,(mg/m^3)} \qquad (11\text{-}5)$$

The working range of a method is the range of contaminant concentration (mg/m³) that may be quantitated at a specified air volume (liters) expressed as mg/m³ or ppm. The lower boundary of the working range is defined by a sample that has a mass of contaminant equal to the LOQ. The upper boundary is defined by sampler capacity. Therefore, the working range may be calculated as follows:

$$\text{Lower Boundary}\,(mg/m^3) = \frac{LOQ(mg) \times 10^3\,(L/m^3)}{V\,(L)} \qquad (11\text{-}6)$$

$$\text{Upper Boundary}\,(mg/m^3) = \frac{W_{max}(mg) \times 10^3\,(L/m^3)}{V\,(L)} \qquad (11\text{-}7)$$

Sampling Media for Gases and Vapors

Solid Sorbents

The most widely used sampling media for gases and vapors are solid sorbents that adsorb the contaminant onto the surface of the sorbent material. Solid sorbents typically consist of either small granules or beads. To be effective, a sorbent should:

1. Trap and retain all or nearly all of the contaminant from an air stream;
2. Be amenable to desorption of the trapped contaminants from the sorbent;
3. Have sufficient capacity to retain a large enough amount of the contaminant to facilitate analysis without creating too large a pressure drop across the sampling media;
4. Not cause a chemical change of the contaminant except when the analytical method is based on derivitization of the contaminant; and

5. Adsorb the contaminant of interest even in the presence of other contaminants, possibly in higher concentrations than the contaminant of interest.[28]

Properties of commonly used solid sorbents are shown in Table 11.3.

Collection Efficiency of Solid Sorbents

Validated air sampling methods will specify a sorbent material that will effectively trap the contaminant(s) of interest. But several factors may affect the collection efficiency of solid sorbents[31]:

Temperature. Because the adsorption process is exothermic, adsorption efficiency is limited at higher temperatures. In addition, reactivity increases with rising temperatures.

Humidity. As water vapor is adsorbed by a sorbent, the sorbent's adsorption capacity for the contaminant of interest may decrease. This effect is most pronounced for sorbents such as charcoal.

Sampling Rate. Higher flow rates lower the sampling efficiency of solid sorbents. For sorbents whose capacity is significantly reduced by high humidity, reducing the sample flow rate may improve the collection efficiency.

Other Contaminants. The presence of significant concentrations of air contaminants (other than the contaminant of interest) may also reduce the collection efficiency of the sorbent for the target compound. This effect is most pronounced for contaminants within the same chemical family. Some classes of compounds can displace other less tightly adsorbed analytes in mixed atmospheres and cause breakthrough or losses.

Sample Breakthrough. Most commercially available sampling tubes consist of two sections of sorbent separated by glass wool or polyurethane foam. In charcoal tubes, the second or backup section is usually one-third of the total weight of the charcoal. These two

Table 11.3 — Properties of Solid Sorbents Commonly Used in Industrial Hygiene Sampling.

Sorbent	*Type*	*Specific Sorbent Surface Area (m^2/g)*	*Pore Type*[A]	*Upper Temperature Limit (°C)*	*Composition*
Activated charcoal	elemental carbon	>1000	I	>400[B]	coconut shell or petroleum-based charcoal
Silica gel	inorganic	300–800	I–II	n/a[B]	amorphous silica
Tenax® GC	organic polymer	20	III	350–400	polymer of 2,6-diphenyl-p-phenylene oxide
Chromosorb®					
102	organic polymer	300–400	II	250	copolymer of styrene and divinyl benzene
104	organic polymer	100–200	III	250	copolymer of acrylonitrile and divinyl benzene
106	organic polymer	700–800	II	250	cross-linked polystyrene
Amberlite®					
XAD-2	organic polymer	300–400	II	200–250	copolymer of styrene and divinyl benzene
XAD-4	organic polymer	500–850	I–II	200–250	copolymer of styrene and divinyl benzene
XAD-7	organic polymer	325–450	I–II	200–250	acrylate polymer

Note: Data from Crisp,[28] Harper and Purnell,[29] and Stanetzek et al.[30]
[A]Pore type: I is <2 nm; II is 2–50 nm; III is >50 nm.
[B]Not normally used for thermal desorption.

sections are desorbed and analyzed separately in the laboratory. As a guideline, if 25% or less of the amount of contaminant collected on the front section is found on the backup section, significant loss of the compound (breakthrough) has probably not occurred. If greater than 25% is detected, breakthrough is evident and results should be reported as "breakthrough, possible sample loss." More specific information can be obtained by a detailed study of the breakthrough profiles for each specific sorbent and chemical.[32]

In some cases, a false indication of breakthrough may be caused by diffusion (migration) of the compounds collected on the front section to the backup section over an extended storage period. Sample migration can be reduced by refrigerating or freezing samples as soon as possible, or it can be eliminated by separating the front and backup sections immediately after sampling. Several methods specify the use of two tubes in series rather than a double-layer tube to avoid this problem (e.g., NIOSH Method 1024 for 1,3-Butadiene). In some cases, field desorption is recommended before transport or storage of the samples.

Desorption of Contaminants

Air contaminants are desorbed from solid sorbents using solvent extraction or thermal desorption techniques. With solvent extraction, a few milliliters of a specific solvent are used to extract the contaminants of interest from the adsorbent material. Desorption efficiency is a measure of how much analyte can be recovered from the sorbent tube. It is determined typically at 0.1, 0.5, 1, and 2 times the target concentration based on the recommended air volume and expressed as a percent of analyte spiked on the sorbent tube.[4] Desorption efficiency should be determined for each lot number of solid sorbent used for sampling and should be done in the concentration range of interest. Solvent desorption, the most frequently used technique, is specified by NIOSH for most occupational hygiene analyses. The most common desorption solvent is carbon disulfide because it has a high desorption efficiency for many organic compounds and produces minimum interference in GC analysis using flame ionization detection.

In some cases, however, the recoveries are poor when using carbon disulfide. For example, higher desorption efficiencies can be attained with mixtures such as methanol and methylene chloride when analyzing for Cellosolves®. For specific alcohols, better desorption efficiencies are obtained with a mixture of carbon disulfide and another alcohol.

Thermal desorption works by driving the contaminant off the sorbent by subjecting it to a high temperature. The desorbed contaminant is carried in an inert gas stream such as nitrogen, argon, or helium directly into the analytical instrument, typically a GC or gas chromatograph/mass spectrometer (GC/MS). Because the contaminant is not diluted by a desorption solvent, the entire mass of contaminant collected can be introduced directly into the analytical instrument (rather than an aliquot of a solution).

As a result, thermal desorption can be used to measure very low airborne concentrations, often subparts per billion. Indeed, thermal desorption is specified in U.S. EPA methods for measurement of low level volatile organic compounds in indoor and ambient air following collection with sorbent tubes.[33,34] Even in general industry, however, thermal desorption may prove to be the trend of the future for measuring contaminants with low exposure limits, such as benzene. Researchers report that thermal desorption combined with capillary gas chromatography can increase the sensitivity over 500 times that achieved with solvent desorption.[35] At the present time, most published methods specifying thermal desorption are for samples collected with sorbent tubes. The future will undoubtedly see an increase in the use of thermal desorption techniques following sample collection with diffusive sorbent samplers.

Types of Sorbent Material

There are four general categories of sorbent materials for air sampling: inorganic, elemental carbon, graphitized carbon, and organic polymers.[36]

Inorganic Sorbents. Inorganic sorbents including silica gel and alumina are typically used to collect polar organic compounds such as alcohols, amines, and phenols followed by solvent extraction. Silica gel is less reactive than charcoal, and it allows for effective analytical recoveries when using nonpolar desorbing solvents such as carbon disulfide.[37] A significant disadvantage of silica gel, however, is that it shows a sharp decrease in capacity with increasing humidity. In fact, silica gel is so hydrophilic that it will preferentially bond water molecules at any humidity causing displacement of less strongly held compounds.[38] Furthermore, it can be difficult to separate co-collected water from the contaminant of interest in the gas chromatographic analysis.[36] Silica gel has been specified in OSHA and NIOSH methods for the collection of aliphatic and aromatic amines, aminoethanols, and nitrobenzenes. Several inorganic acids can also be collected using a special prewashed silica gel tube with a glass fiber prefilter inside the tube. Alumina is not widely used for air sampling at this time.

Elemental carbon. Activated charcoal is the most widely used solid sorbent for occupational hygiene sampling as many of the OSHA and NIOSH sampling procedures for organic vapors specify this material. Charcoal can be obtained from a variety of sources, including coconut shells, coal, wood, peat, and petroleum.[28] Each form has its own characteristics and uses. At this time, the only form used for occupational hygiene sampling is derived from coconut shells. Petroleum based charcoal used in the past is no longer available commercially. Activated charcoal has a high adsorptive capacity due to its microporous structure and its high surface area-to-weight ratio. This high adsorptive capacity makes activated charcoal an ideal sorbent for sampling chemically stable compounds over a wide concentration range. High humidity, however, has an adverse effect on the adsorptive capacity of charcoal.[39] If high humidity or other factors that might limit capacity are present in the sampling environment, it may be necessary to use a sampling tube with a larger amount of sorbent material than the one specified in the method.

Despite its wide application, charcoal has some limitations. It is not an efficient collector for very volatile low molecular weight hydrocarbons such as methane and ethane.[40] Nor is it effective for low boiling compounds such as ammonia, ethylene, and hydrogen chloride. Due to its oxidizing surface, charcoal is not suitable for the collection of reactive compounds such as mercaptans or aldehydes.[2] Coconut charcoal in particular has been found to be a poor collector for ketones. When ketones are adsorbed, they break down by reactions involving water that are catalyzed by the charcoal surface. Hence, desorption efficiency and storage stability are poor.[41]

A beaded activated charcoal, Anasorb® 747, has been specified in a variety of new government agency methods. This beaded carbon has a high surface area and is an effective collector of both polar and nonpolar organic compounds. It offers the additional advantages of a uniform mesh size, more uniform recovery characteristics and it is more hydrophobic than coconut shell charcoal. Therefore, the collection capacity is less affected by humidity. Anasorb 747 (with and without chemical treatment) is specified in OSHA methods for several compounds including sulfur dioxide, anesthetic gases, ethylene oxide, propylene oxide, methanol, ethanol, and isopropanol.

Carbonized or Graphitized Sorbents. Graphitized carbons such as Anasorb GCB1 and Carbotrap® B offer a low to moderate surface area, but are suitable for sampling compounds of intermediate to high volatility. They offer the advantage of being hydrophobic and thermally stable, which allows for thermal desorption. Other sorbents in this group are carbon molecular sieves such as Carbosieve®. They have a high surface area and small pore sizes, which make them effective collectors of very volatile organic compounds.[36]

Organic Polymers. Organic porous polymers are used extensively in both occupational hygiene and environmental sampling. The wide variety of these materials allows for selectivity to particular applications, and the stability of some polymers at high temperatures enables them to be thermally desorbed.[28] Commercially available porous polymers include Tenax®, Porapaks®, Chromosorbs®, and Amberlite® XAD resins.

Tenax is a polymer of 2,6 diphenyl-p-phenylene oxide. It is the sorbent of choice for sampling for low-level contaminants due to its high thermal limit of 375°C, which is amenable to thermal desorption. At very low concentrations, such as those found in environmental samples, the relatively small surface area of Tenax is not as significant a concern. Tenax can be used to collect a broad range of organic compounds, particularly volatile, nonpolar organics having boiling points in the range of 80 to 200°C.[33] It is also used as the sorbent for some explosives, such as trinitrotoluene (TNT) and dinitrotoluene (DNT).

Porapaks comprise a group of porous polymers with a wide range of polarity. The least polar member of the group, Porapak P, has chromatographic properties that facilitate the separation of compounds such as ketones, aldehydes, alcohols, and glycols.[28] Porapak P is specified by NIOSH for the collection of dimethyl sulfate. At the other end of the spectrum, Porapak T is sufficiently polar to separate water and formaldehyde and is useful for the collection of hexachlorocyclopentadiene. Porapaks offer a range of sorbents, but the most polar members have disadvantages because of strong water retention and the greater energy required to remove contaminants for analysis.

Chromosorbs have properties similar to those of the Porapaks. Chromosorb 101 is the least polar member of this sorbent group, while Chromosorb 104 is the most polar. Chromosorb 102 is particularly useful as a sorbent for air contaminants because of its large specific surface area. NIOSH methods specify this sorbent for the collection of pesticides including chlordane and endrin. In a 1995 interlaboratory study, Chromosorb 106 was found to be the most desirable sorbent for occupational hygiene applications in Europe using thermal desorption as the method of analysis.[42]

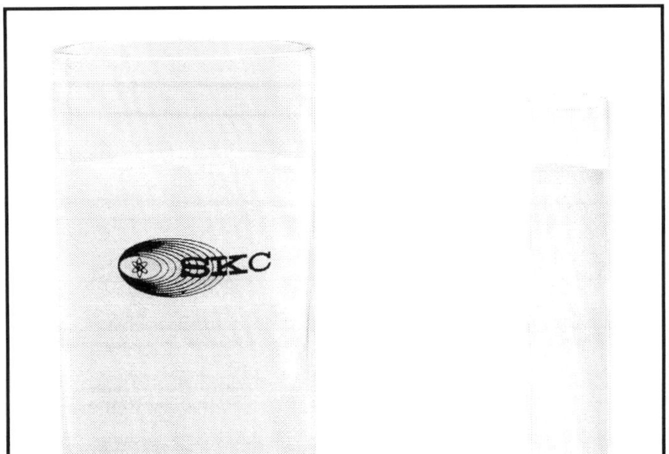

Figure 11.5 — Glass sorbent cartridges with polyurethane foam.

Amberlite XAD resins include a number of different types, but most air sampling methods using these materials specify XAD-2. NIOSH and OSHA specify XAD-2 for the collection of a wide variety of organophosphorus pesticides, and both agencies have also developed methods for collecting formaldehyde using XAD-2 coated with 2-(hydroxymethyl) piperidine. XAD-7, 8, 9, and 12 are most suitable for polar compounds and XAD-1, 2, and 4 for nonpolar compounds.

Other Sorbent Material. Glass sorbent cartridges containing polyurethane foam (PUF) or PUF in combination with other solid sorbents such as XAD are specified in methods for sampling and analysis of organochlorine pesticides and polychlorinated biphenyls in indoor and ambient air.[43,44] Low volume and high volume PUF tubes are available for different applications and expected concentrations (see Figure 11.5).

Sorbent Combinations. In some situations, such as at hazardous waste cleanup sites, occupational hygienists are called on to evaluate employee or community exposures to complex mixtures of organic contaminants. In recent years, sorbent tubes containing multiple layers of different sorbents have been used for such applications. Typically, three sorbents of increasing retentivity are used and air is drawn first through the weakest sorbent to collect less volatile substances and last through the strongest sorbent to collect the more volatile substances.[36] Analysis and compound identification involves thermal desorption, gas chromatography/mass spectrometry, and computerized analytical library searches.

Sorbent/Filter Combinations. Sorbent tubes are also used in combination with filter cassettes to effectively trap multiphase contaminants. For example, the NIOSH method for sampling PNAs (Method 5506) uses a PTFE (polytetrafluoroethylene) filter to collect the particulate fraction, followed by an XAD-2 sorbent tube to collect vapors. Another example is measurement of organotin compounds (NIOSH Method 5504) using a glass fiber filter followed by an XAD-2 sorbent tube.

Some recent NIOSH and OSHA methods specify sampling tubes with one or more filters contained within the tube itself. These internal filters serve one of two purposes: to trap the aerosol phase of the target compound or to scrub out interfering compounds. The OSHA Versatile Sampler (OVS) is a specially designed glass tube that contains either a glass fiber or quartz filter to trap the aerosol phase and a two-section sorbent bed to adsorb vapors. OVS tubes are currently specified for the collection of organophosphorus pesticides, TNT, DNT, phthalate esters, and glycols (See Figure 11.6). A 2006 OSHA method for hydrogen sulfide specifies the use of glass tubes containing an uncoated glass fiber filter, a sodium carbonate/glycerol coated glass fiber filter, and silver nitrate coated silica gel sorbent. The uncoated filter scrubs out particulates, the coated filter scrubs out sulfur dioxide, and the target compound is trapped in the sorbent.[4]

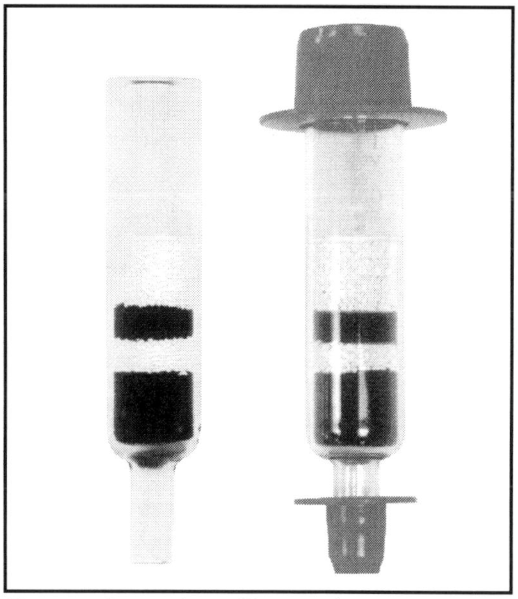

Figure 11.6 — Sorbent/filter combination tubes.

Chemically Treated Filters

Filters have proven to be an effective substrate for various liquid media that can trap a variety of airborne contaminants. Most liquid media used to treat filters chemically derivatize the contaminant(s) of interest producing a more stable compound for storage and analysis. To further enhance the stability of samples, some methods stipulate that filters should be transferred a short time after sampling to glass vials containing a specified liquid.

When compared to wet chemistry methods using bubblers, chemically treated filters are less cumbersome, safer to use in the field, and can provide improved collection efficiency for some compounds (e.g., methyl mercaptan). In addition, a front and a back filter can be used in one cassette to determine if sample breakthrough has occurred. Chemically treated filters are specified by OSHA or NIOSH for the collection of a variety of compounds including phosphine, glutaraldehyde, diisocyanates, and fluorides.

Liquid Absorbers

Sampling techniques that use liquid sampling media either include absorption based on solubility or may involve a reaction of the contaminant with the sampling solution. Four basic types of sampling devices have been used in conjunction with liquid absorbers: gas washing bottles, spiral and helical absorbers, fritted bubblers, and glass-bead columns. Of these, only the gas washing bottles and fritted bubblers are now used routinely in occupational hygiene sampling (see Figure 11.7).

Gas Washing Bottles

Gas washing bottles include Drechsel types, standard Greenburg-Smith devices, and midget impingers. The air is bubbled through the liquid absorber to secure intimate mixing of air and liquid, and the length of travel of the gas through the collecting medium is equivalent to the height of the absorbing liquid. These scrubbers are suitable for gases and vapors that are readily

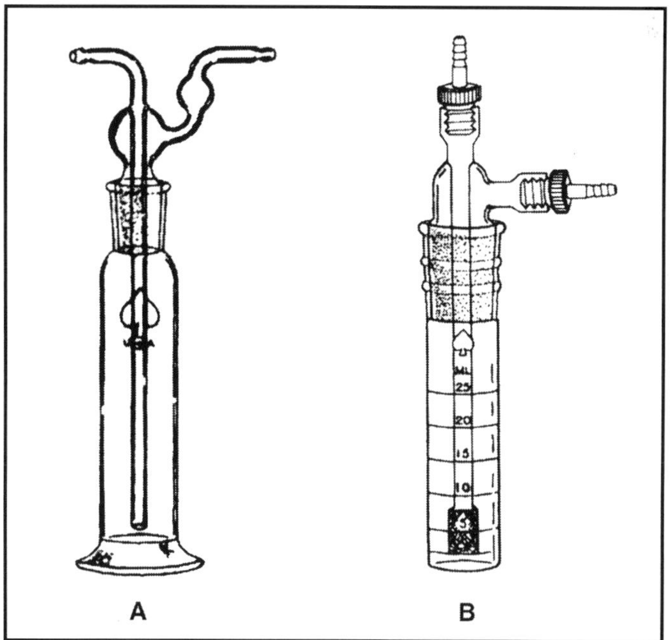

Figure 11.7 — Liquid absorbers: (A) gas washing bottles (B) fritted bubblers.

soluble in the absorbing liquid or react with it. One unit or two units in series may be enough for efficient collection; however, in some cases, several in series may be needed to attain the efficiency of a single fritted glass bubbler. The advantages of these devices include simple construction; ease of rinsing; and, with the exception of Greenburg-Smith impingers, small liquid volume requirements.

Fritted Glass Bubblers

With fritted glass bubblers, air passes through formed porous glass plates and enters the liquid in the form of small bubbles. The size of the air bubbles depends on the liquid and the diameter of the orifices from which the bubbles emerge. Frits are classified as fine (25–50 μm), coarse (70–100 μm), or extra coarse (145–175 μm) depending on the pore size. The extra-coarse frit is used when a higher flow rate is desired. The heavier froth generated by some liquids increases the time of contact of gas with liquid. Fritted glass bubblers are more efficient collectors than gas washing bottles and can be used for the majority of gases and vapors that are soluble in the reagent or react rapidly with it. Flow rates between 0.5 and 1.0 L/min are commonly used. Fritted glass is not suitable for sampling contaminants that form a precipitate during sampling that could clog the fritted glass or inhibit quantitative recovery of the sample. In this case, a gas washing bottle should be used. To prevent clogging, it may also be necessary to include a prefilter at the bubbler inlet when sampling air with a high particulate content.

Glass sampling devices are cumbersome, especially for on-worker sampling. Many liquid absorbers contain corrosive or toxic substances, including strong acids, bases, or toxic organics and pose safety and exposure problems for the users. In addition, the evaporation of liquid media poses problems of sample loss and worker exposure. Thus, the use of liquid absorbers has declined in favor of solid sorbent samplers or chemically treated filters.

Sampling Bags/Partially Evacuated Rigid Containers

In certain applications, users may prefer to collect an air sample into a vessel for subsequent analysis. This type of sample is referred to as a whole air sample and typically involves the use of flexible sampling bags or partially evacuated rigid containers. Whole air samples are frequently collected in the following applications:

- Low level measurements of organic vapors in ambient or indoor air
- Soil vapor sampling and other field applications where samples will be analyzed on site using portable, direct-reading instruments
- Leak, spill, or other emergency situations requiring quick sample collection and analysis so that appropriate control measures can be taken
- Measurements of peak concentrations of contaminants from specific plant processes or worker tasks
- Collection of gases or highly volatile compounds for which adsorption methods are not available or are not efficient

Commercially available sampling bags are listed in Table 11.4. The major advantage to collection of air samples with bags is that most volatile organic compounds are collected and retained for analysis. A major disadvantage, however, is the limited storage time, typically 24–48 hours in Tedlar or similar materials. In addition, loss of contaminant from a sampling bag may occur through reaction of the contaminant, adsorption of the contaminant onto the bag material, diffusion of the contaminant through the bag material, leakage around the valve stem and seams, and rupture during transport and handling. Despite these drawbacks, flexible sampling bags are widely used. To minimize errors, the following precautions should be taken:

1. Bags should be purged several times with an inert gas such as nitrogen to remove any trace contaminants before sampling.
2. Sampling bags selected should be relatively impermeable to the contaminant being sampled.
3. Storage of the sample in the bag should not be extended beyond the recommended time for the specific air contaminant and bag material.
4. Bags should not be completely filled, especially if they will be transported by airplane. Changes in pressure or temperature can cause the bag to rupture.
5. If bags are being used in a heavily contaminated area, it may be desirable to

Table 11.4 — Commercially Available Sampling Bags

Type	*Chemical Composition*
Five-layer aluminized	inner layer-polyethylene
Halar	copolymer of ethylene and trifluoroethylene
Saran®	polyvinylidene chloride
Tedlar®	polyvinyl fluoride
Teflon®	FEP (fluorinated ethylene, propylene)

Note: Data from Posner and Woodfin[45]

place the bags into an evacuation chamber and fill by negative pressure to avoid contamination of the pump or a degradation of analyte concentration by interaction with the pump (see Figure 11.8.)

A major question facing practitioners is the reusability of air sampling bags. Researchers have evaluated whether Tedlar bags could be flushed and reused after an extended holding time without carryover caused by the previous sample.[46] Their results indicated that long-term storage of compounds into Tedlar bags is not recommended as chemicals can adsorb onto the bag surface, and this can lead to significant off-gassing of contaminants into subsequent samples. If bags are to be reused, these researchers suggest that bags be cleaned immediately after their initial use with a rigorous flushing and heating procedure, then stored in an evacuated state.

Evacuated flasks include heavy-walled glass containers (Figure 11.9) and other plastic or metal containers in which 99.97% or more of the air has been removed by a heavy-duty vacuum pump. Sampling is conducted by breaking the seal to permit the air to enter the flask. Commercially available evacuated flasks include glass bulbs and flasks provided by most laboratory supply houses.

Pre-evacuated stainless steel canisters have been widely used as an air collection vessel for contaminants found at extremely low levels for environmental assessments. To prevent reaction of the sample with the canister, the interior of the canister is either treated with an electropolishing process to remove or cover reactive metal sites (i.e., SUMMA® process) or is deactivated by a fused silica coating process (i.e., Silcosteel®). Canisters are available in both subatmospheric and pressurized sampling models. Subatmospheric sampling involves the use of a flow controller with a critical orifice to regulate the rate and duration of sampling into the canister without a pump. Pressurized sampling requires a pump to provide positive pressure to the sample canister. After sample collection, 100–500 mL of air is withdrawn; the contaminants are concentrated onto a cryogenically cooled trap and analyzed by GC coupled to one or more appropriate GC detectors.[47] Laboratory equipment is commercially available to clean the canisters for reuse.

Canister sampling in ambient air has typically been done using canisters with a volume of 6L. This large volume is required to measure concentrations down to parts per trillion. Measurements in the ppm range, however, require a much smaller volume of air. Therefore, smaller canisters with an overall volume of 400 ml have been introduced for sampling gases and vapors in typical workplace environments (see Figure 11.10). For personal sampling, the small canisters

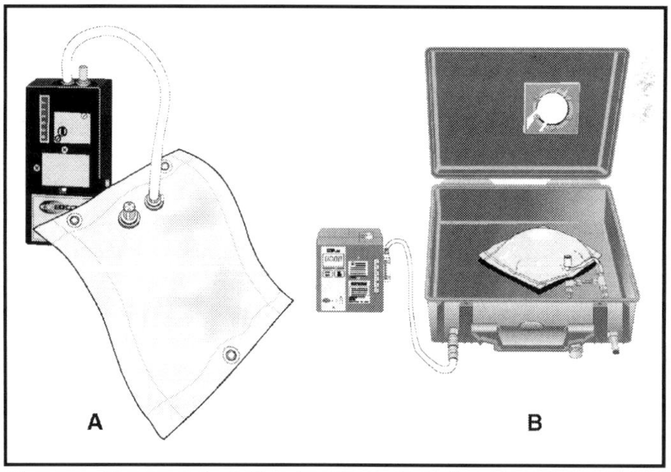

Figure 11.8 — Sample Collection Using Sampling Bags: (A) positive pressure collection (B) negative pressure collection.

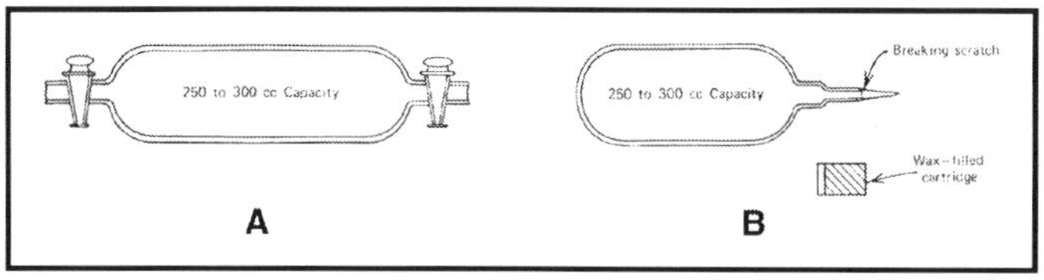

Figure 11.9 — Grab Sample Bottles: (A) gas or liquid displacement (B) evacuated flask.

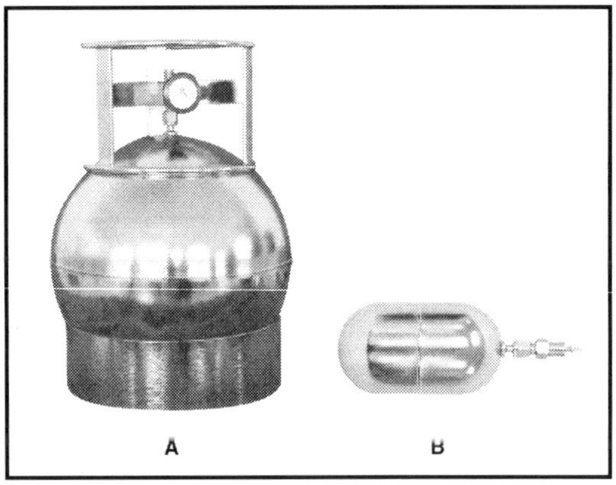

Figure 11.10 — Stainless Steel Canisters: (A) 6L canister (B) 400 ml canister.

can be mounted onto a belt with a Teflon sample line extending to the breathing zone. They can also be used for area sampling for applications such as indoor air quality investigations, emergency response, and fence-line sampling.

A new technology has recently been introduced for personal diffusive sampling with canisters using the principle of helium diffusion. The HDS Personal Monitor is a collection vessel that is vacuum cleaned and filled with helium prior to use. The sampler is then positioned onto the individual and the external valve is removed which exposes a diffusion capillary tube to the surrounding air.(48) The helium diffuses out and ambient air diffuses in at predictable uptake rates. After sampling 4 to 8 hours, the external valve is replaced and the sampler is shipped to the laboratory for GC analysis.

Canisters offer the advantages of longer storage times than bags, no breakthrough problems, and sample durations ranging from a quick grab sample to an integrated sample over several days. Disadvantages include the expense of the equipment and analysis, the inability to perform analysis in the field, and analytical problems caused by water vapor.

Cold Traps

Cold traps have been used to collect analytes from a sampled air stream when the compounds are too unstable or reactive to be collected efficiently by other techniques. Cold traps have also been used to collect unknown contaminants in liquid or solid form for identification purposes. With this technique, vapor is separated from air by passing it through a coil or other vessel that has been immersed in a cooling system such as dry ice, liquid air, or liquid nitrogen.

A variety of traps are available, including the U-tube design. The most efficient traps for field use, however, are the reverse gas washing bottle-type in which the analytes are frozen from the air stream by first contacting the cold outer walls of the vessel. The air stream is drawn through the sampling vessels by a constant flow pump. The cold trap technique can also be combined with stainless steel canister sampling in which the sample air is metered into a chilled canister. Sample vapors are transferred from the trap to the analytical instruments by warming, followed by vacuum trapping or selective temperature gas flows using inert gas streams. Cold trap techniques cannot be conveniently used for personal sampling, but apply well to area sampling of indoor or ambient air.

Calculations and Interpretation of Air Sampling Data

The analytical laboratory will determine the total amount of analyte collected on the sampling device and will normally report the results in total mass of the specified contaminant and air concentration based upon the sample volume supplied by the sample submitter. To determine the airborne concentration, it will be necessary to divide the mass of contaminant by the volume of air sampled. The air volume is calculated by multiplying the average flow rate of the sampler by the sampling time. To more easily convert to ppm, the results will typically need to be calculated in mg/m. It may be necessary to first convert the analytical results from micrograms to milligrams and the air volume from liters to cubic meters (micrograms × 10^{-3} = milligrams; mg/liter × 10^3 = mg/m^3).

If sampling was conducted near normal temperature and pressure, the following simplified formula can be used to convert the measured analyte concentration from mg/m^3 to ppm:

$$\text{ppm} = \frac{\text{mg/m}^3 \times 24.45}{\text{Molecular Weight}} \qquad (11\text{-}8)$$

Once airborne concentrations have been determined, it is necessary to compare those levels to appropriate exposure standards. To determine compliance with full-shift occupational exposure limits, 8-hour TWAs will need to be calculated:

$$\text{8-hr TWA} = \frac{C_1T_1 + C_2T_2 + C_3T_3 + \dots + C_nT_n}{8} \quad (11\text{-}9)$$

where:

C_n = concentration of an individual sample
T_n = sample time of an individual sample

The number eight is used in the denominator as most standards are based on an 8-hour exposure followed by 16 hours of rest.

Example: If three benzene samples collected on a refinery worker over an 8-hour workday revealed the following exposures — 0.5 ppm for a 4.5 hour sample; 1.5 ppm for a 1.0 hour sample; and 0.8 ppm for a 2.5 hour sample — what would be the 8-hour TWA?

$$\text{8-hr TWA} = \frac{(0.5)(4.5)+(1.5)(1)+(0.8)(2.5)}{8} = 0.7\ \text{ppm}$$

If individuals are working extended or unusual shifts in which the exposure time is lengthened or the recovery time is lessened, occupational exposure limits may need to be adjusted. Brief and Scala have developed one such model that has been used to make adjustments to workplace exposure standards for extended or unusual work shifts.[49] This model reduces the allowable limit for both increased exposure time and reduced recovery time. A complete review of literature relating to the adjustment of occupational exposure limits for unusual work schedules has been published.[50] This article provides valuable information on the options available to health and safety professionals faced with this situation.

Additional Sources

- Air sampling method manuals by OSHA and NIOSH (Listed in Table 11.1).
- **Cohen, Beverly S. and C.S. McCammon (eds.):** *Air Sampling Instruments for Evaluation of Atmospheric Contaminants*, 9th edition. Cincinnati, OH: ACGIH, 2001.
- **Yocum, J.E. and S. McCarthy:** *Measuring Indoor Air Quality.* Cincinnati, OH: ACGIH®, 1991.
- **Wright, G.D.:** *Fundamentals of Air Sampling.* Boca Raton, FL: Lewis Publishers/CRC Press, 1994.
- **Greulich, K.A. and C.E. Gray (eds.):** *Manual of Analytical Methods for the Industrial Hygiene Chemistry Laboratory.* Springfield, VA: NTIS, 1991.

References

1. *Code of Federal Regulations,* Title 29, Part 1910. 1995. (See standards on individual chemicals, e.g., 1910.1047, 1910.1048, and 1910.1028.)
2. **McCammon, C.S. and M.L. Woebkenberg:** General considerations for sampling airborne contaminants. In *NIOSH Manual of Analytical Methods,* 4th edition. Cincinnati, Ohio: U.S. Department of Health and Human Services. 1994, Second Supplement 1/15/98. pp. 17–35.
3. **Soule, R.D.:** Industrial hygiene sampling and analysis. In *Patty's Industrial Hygiene and Toxicology,* Vol. 1. New York: John Wiley & Sons, 1991. pp. 73–135.
4. **U.S. Department of Labor:** OSHA *Analytical Methods Manual.* Salt Lake City, Utah: U.S. Department of Labor, Occupational Safety and Health Division Directorate for Technical Support, 1990. See also http://www.osha.gov/dts/sltc/methods/toc.html.
5. **Feldman, R.F.:** Degraded instrument performance due to radio interference: criteria and standards. *Appl. Occup. Environ. Hyg. 8*:351–355 (1993).
6. **Bios International Corporation:** *Defender 500 Series Instruction Manual.* Butler, NJ, 2006.
7. **Lippmann, M.:** Calibration. In *Patty's Industrial Hygiene and Toxicology,* Vol. 1. New York: John Wiley & Sons, 1991. pp. 461–530.
8. **ASTM International:** ASTM Standard D6345-98 (2004): Standard Guide for Selection of Methods for Active, Integrative Sampling of Volatile Organic Compounds in Air. West Conshohocken, PA: ASTM, 2004.
9. **Palmes, E.D. and A.F. Gunnison:** Personal Monitoring Devices for Gaseous Contaminants. *Am. Ind. Hyg. Assoc. J. 34*:78–81 (1973).

10. **Rose, V.E. and J.L. Perkins:** Passive dosimetry-state of the art review. *Am. Ind. Hyg. Assoc. J. 43*:605–621 (1982).
11. **Harper, M.:** Diffusive Sampling. *Appl. Occup. Environ. Hyg. 13(11)*:759–763 (1998).
12. **Lugg, G.A.:** Diffusion coefficients of some organic and other vapors in air. *Anal. Chem. 40*:1072–1077 (1968).
13. **Hickey, J.L.S. and C.C. Bishop:** Field comparison of charcoal tubes and passive vapor monitors with mixed organic vapors. *Am. Ind. Hyg. Assoc. J. 42*:264–267 (1981).
14. **Cassinelli, M.E., R.D. Hull, J.V. Crable, and A.W. Teass:** Protocol for the evaluation of passive monitors. In *Diffusive Sampling: An Alternative Approach to Workplace Air Monitoring*. London: Royal Society of Chemistry, Burlington House, 1987. pp. 190–202.
15. **Brown, R.H., R.P. Harvey, C.J. Purnell, and K.J. Saunders:** A diffusive sampler evaluation protocol. *Am. Ind. Hyg. Assoc. J. 45*:67–75 (1984).
16. **EN 838 Workplace Atmospheres:** Diffusive Samplers for the Determination of Gases and Vapors—Requirements and Tests Methods, Comité Européen de Normalisation, Brussels, Belgium (1995).
17. **Health and Safety Executive:** *Methods for the Determination of Hazardous Substances*. Sheffield, UK: Health and Safety Laboratory, Health and Safety Executive, (1997). Method 88.
18. **ASTM International:** ASTM Standard D6246-98: Standard Practice for Evaluating the Performance of Diffusive Samplers. West Conshohocken, PA: ASTM, 2008.
19. **American National Standards Institute:** ANSI/ISEA Standard 104-1998 R2009: Air Sampling Devices—Diffusive Types for Gases and Vapors in Working Environments, New York, (2009).
20. **Hendricks, W.:** Determination of Sampling Rate Variation for SKC 575 Series Passive Samplers, OSHA Salt Lake Technical Center In-house file, Salt Lake City, UT (1998). See http://www.osha.gov/dts/sltc/methods/studies/skc575.html.
21. **Sigma-Aldrich:** *Supelco Edition Radiello Manual*. Bellefonte, PA. See www.sigma-aldrich.com/radiello.
22. **SKC, Inc.:** *ULTRA Sampler Operating Instructions*. Eighty Four, PA. See www.skcinc.com.
23. **Lautenbeger, W.J., E.V. Kring, and J.A. Morello:** Theory of Passive Monitors. *Ann. of Am. Conf. Gov. Ind. Hyg. 1*:91–99 (1981).
24. **ASTM International:** ASTM Standard D6306-98: Standard Guide for Placement and Use of Diffusion Controlled Passive Monitors for Gaseous Pollutants in Indoor Air. West Conshohocken, PA: ASTM, 1998.
25. **Eller, P.M.:** Operational limits of air analysis methods. *Appl. Ind. Hyg. 2*:91–94 (1986).
26. **Keith, L.H., W. Crummett, J. Deegan, R.A. Libby, J.K. Taylor, and G. Wentler:** Principals of environmental analysis. *Anal. Chem. 55*:2210–2218 (1983).
27. **U.S. Department of Labor:** *Method Evaluation Guidelines*. Salt Lake City, Utah: U.S. Department of Labor, Occupational Safety and Health Division Directorate for Technical Support, 1993. See http://www.osha.gov/dts/sltc/methods/index.html.
28. **Crisp, S.:** Solid sorbent gas samplers. *Ann. Occup. Hyg. 23*:47–76 (1980).
29. **Harper, M. and C.J. Purnell:** Alkylammonium montmorillonites as adsorbents for organic vapors from air. *Environ. Sci. Technol. 24*:55–62 (1990).
30. **Stanetzek, I., U. Giese, R.H. Schuster, and G. Wunsch:** Chromatographic characterization of adsorbents for selective sampling of organic air pollutants. *Am. Ind. Hyg. J. 57*:128–133 (1996).
31. **Melcher, R.G.:** Laboratory and field validation of solid sorbent samplers. In *Sampling and Calibration for Atmospheric Measurements*, ASTM STP 957. Philadelphia: American Society for Testing and Materials, 1987. pp. 149–165.
32. **Harper, M.:** Evaluation of solid sorbent sampling methods by breakthrough volume studies. *Ann. Occ. Hyg. 37*:65–88 (1993).
33. **U.S. Environmental Protection Agency (EPA):** *Compendium of Methods for the Determination of Toxic Organic Compounds in Ambient Air* by W.T. Winberrry, N.T. Murphy and R.J. Riggan (EPA/600/4-89/017), Research Triangle Park, NC: US EPA/Office of Research and Development, 1988. Methods TO-1, TO-2, TO-17.
34. **U.S. Environmental Protection Agency (EPA):** *Compendium of Methods for the Determination of Air Pollutants in Indoor Air* by W.T. Winberry, L. Forehand, N.T. Murphy, A. Ceroli, B. Phinney and A. Evans (EPA/600/4-90/010), Research Triangle Park, NC: US EPA/Office of Research and Development, 1990. Method IP-1B.
35. **Verma, D.K. and K. des Tombe:** Measurement of Benzene in the Workplace and its Evolution Process, Part II: Present Methods and Future Trends. *Am. Ind. Hyg. J. 60*:48–56 (1999).
36. **ASTM International:** ASTM Standard D6345-98: Standard Guide for Selection of Methods for Active, Integrative Sampling of Volatile Organic Compounds in Air. West Conshohocken, PA: ASTM, 1998.

37. **Guenier, J.P., F. Lhuillier, and J. Muller:** Sampling of gaseous pollutants on silica gel with 2400 mg tubes. *Ann. Occup. Hyg. 30*:103–114 (1986).
38. **Harper, M.:** Novel sorbents for sampling organic vapours. *Analyst 119*:65–69 (1994).
39. **Rudling, J. and E. Bjorkholm:** Effect of adsorbed water on solvent desorption of organic vapors collected on activated carbon. *Am. Ind. Hyg. Assoc. J. 47*:615–620 (1986).
40. **Tang, Y.Z., W.K. Cheng, P. Fellin, Q. Tran, and I. Drummond:** Laboratory Evaluation of Sampling Method for C1-C4 Hydrocarbons. *Am. Ind. Hyg. Assoc. J. 57*:245–250 (1996).
41. **Harper, M. and M.L. Kimberland, R.J. Orr, and L.V. Guild:** An evaluation of sorbents for sampling ketones in workplace air. *Appl. Occup. Environ. Hyg. 8*:293–304 (1993).
42. **European Commission:** Study of Sorbing Agents for the Sampling of Volatile Compounds from Air (EC Contract MAT1-CT92-0038). Measurements and Testing Programme of the European Commission. Sheffield, UK: Health and Safety Laboratory, Health and Safety Executive, 1995.
43. **ASTM International:** ASTM Standard D4861-94a, Standard Practice for Sampling and Selection of Analytical Techniques for Pesticides and Polychlorinated Biphenyls in Air. West Conshohocken, PA: ASTM, 1994.
44. **U.S. Environmental Protection Agency (EPA):** *Compendium of Methods for the Determination of Toxic Organic Compounds in Ambient Air*, by W. T. Winberry, N.T. Murphy, and R.J. Riggan (EPA/600/4-89/017). Research Triangle Park, NC: U.S. Environmental Protection Agency/Office of Research and Development, 1988. Method TO-10 and TO-13.
45. **Posner, J.C. and W.J. Woodfin:** Sampling with gas bags I: Losses of analyte with time. *Appl. Ind. Hyg. 1*:163–168 (1986).
46. **McGarvey, L.J. and C.V. Shorten:** The Effects of Adsorption on the Reusability of Tedlar Air Sampling Bags. *Am. Ind. Hyg. Assoc. J. 61*:375–380 (2000).
47. **U.S. Environmental Protection Agency:** *Compendium of Methods for the Determination of Toxic Organic Compounds in Ambient Air*, by W. T. Winberry, N.T. Murphy, and R.J. Riggan (EPA/600/4-89/017). Research Triangle Park, NC: U.S. Environmental Protection Agency/Office of Research and Development, 1988. Method TO-14.
48. **Entech Instruments, Inc.:** *HDS Personal Monitor Brochure*, Simi Valley, CA. See www.entechinst.com.
49. **Brief, R.S. and R.A. Scala:** Occupational Exposure Limits for Novel Work Schedules. *Am. Ind. Hyg. Assoc. J. 36*:467–469 (1975).
50. **Verma, D.K.:** Adjustment of Occupational Exposure Limits for Unusual Work Schedules. *Am. Ind. Hyg. Assoc. J. 61*:367–374 (2000).

Outcome Competencies

After completing this chapter, the reader should be able to:

1. Understand the fundamental concepts of a chromatographic separation as used in the analysis of vapors and gases.
2. Distinguish between the three chromatographic techniques (GC, HPLC, & IC) used in the analysis of vapors and gases.
3. Describe detectors commonly used with each of the chromatographic techniques.
4. Describe the types of hazardous substance commonly analyzed by each of the three chromatographic techniques.
5. Locate primary sources of analytical methodology used in occupational exposure assessment.
6. Identify analytical procedures that may not be state of the art for analysis of gases and vapors.

Key Terms

Beer-Lambert law • conductivity detector (CD) • diode array detector (DAD) • discharge ionization detector • electrochemical detector • electron capture detector (ECD) • flame ionization detector (FID) • flame photometric detector (FPD) • fluorescence detector • gas chromatography (GC) • gas chromatography/mass spectrometry (GC/MS) • high-performance liquid chromatography (HPLC) • ion chromatography (IC) • nitrogen chemiluminescence detector (NCD) • nitrogen-phosphorus detector (NPD)• photoionization detector (PID) • retention time • spectrophotometry • sulfur chemiluminescence detector (SCD) • thermal conductivity detector (TCD) • UV-vis absorbance detector (UV-vis)

Prerequisite Knowledge

General chemistry

Prior to beginning this chapter, the reader should review the following chapters:

Chapter Number	Chapter Topic
11	Sampling of Gases and Vapors
13	Quality Control for Sampling and Laboratory Analysis
16	Preparation of Known Concentrations of Air Contaminants

Key Topics

I. Chromatographic Techniques
   A. Gas Chromatography
   B. Gas Chromatography/Mass Spectrometry
   C. High-Performance Liquid Chromatography
   D. Ion Chromatography
II. Volumetric Methods
III. Spectrophotometric Methods

Analysis of Gases and Vapors

12

By Gerald R. Schultz, CIH and Warren D. Hendricks

Introduction

This chapter introduces the practicing occupational hygienist to the range of analytical techniques used to quantify gases and vapors in the environment. These analytical chemistry techniques allow the occupational hygienist to determine employee exposure to a large variety of hazardous workplace contaminants.

Unlike their predecessors, modern occupational hygienists rarely conduct the chemical analyses of samples they collect. Due to a general increase in specialization, and specifically due to the accreditation requirements for laboratories analyzing occupational hygiene samples, virtually all occupational hygiene samples are now analyzed by a relatively small number of regional and national laboratories served by overnight delivery services. Based on a large volume of analyses, these laboratories have the resources to maintain a high degree of analytical proficiency for a wide variety of substances along with rigorous quality control programs that are simply not economically feasible in a laboratory conducting a small number of analyses.

Despite these changes it is still crucially important for the occupational hygienist to have at least a working understanding of analytical methods and procedures. The most prominent example of the need for such knowledge comes in the selection of a sampling and associated analytical method. The occupational hygienist must be fully cognizant of the requirements and limitations of the analytical method prior to conducting any air sampling survey. This includes working closely with the laboratory.

It is important to be aware of possible interferences that may be present that may complicate or invalidate analysis. An example of this problem is in the collection and analysis of formaldehyde using National Institute for Occupational Safety and Health (NIOSH) Method 3500.[1] Using this analytical methodology, the presence of phenol in the sample results in an apparent reduction in the amount of formaldehyde present, a phenomenon called "negative interference." If the occupational hygienist is not aware of this methodological limitation, the resulting estimate of worker exposure will be significantly reduced, with possible health and/or regulatory implications. However, a thorough occupational hygienist will be mindful of these limitations and select another sampling and analytical method, such as NIOSH Method 2541[2] or Occupational Safety and Health Administration (OSHA) Method 52[3] (which are not subject to this problem) or will inform the laboratory to take steps to eliminate the phenol interference. Compensation for the presence of analytical interferences in the laboratory is not always possible, however, and it is important for the occupational hygienist to maintain communication with the laboratory to prevent such occurrences.

The occupational hygienist also must be very cognizant of the detection limits of the analytical method selected. Sampling and analytical efforts can be wasted if the detection limit of the analysis exceeds the analyte's regulatory or consensus exposure standard. With a knowledge of the detection limit and a defined sampling goal, such as being able to detect a concentration 10% of an exposure standard, a sample volume can be calculated, that when used will assure the occupational hygienist that if the substance was not detected, the concentration is low and not of concern.

Analytical methods typically are associated with a particular sampling procedure and are generally presented in the context of a combined sampling and analytical method. To the extent possible, it is important to use reference sampling and analytical methods. These are procedures that have been thoroughly evaluated or are considered valid through a broad consensus. Of particular importance for workplace exposure evaluation are the sampling and analytical methods recommended by NIOSH[(4)], OSHA[(5)], and to a lesser extent the U.S. Environmental Protection Agency (EPA).[(6)] The AIHA Industrial Hygiene Methods Exchange Network (IHMEN) Data-base website also provides resources for analytical methods[(7)] and a source of consensus methods would be ASTM.[(8)] Many laboratories may also have in-house methods that have been thoroughly evaluated.

As noted previously, it is important to select and consult with a qualified laboratory prior to undertaking any sampling activity. Laboratories accredited by the Industrial Hygiene Laboratory Accreditation Program (IHLAP) of the AIHA® Laboratory Accreditation Programs, LLC meet this qualification.

A wide range of analytical techniques is available for the quantification of gases and vapors. A list of analytical techniques with examples of analytes based on the NIOSH and OSHA methods websites is presented as Table 12.1. The generic layout of a front page for current NIOSH methods is presented as Figure 12.1 and for current OSHA methods as in Figure 12.2. For discussion purposes, analytical techniques for gases and vapors are grouped into chromatographic, volumetric, and spectrophotometric methods.

Table 12.1 — List of Analytical Techniques and Examples of Common Analytes

Analytical Technique	*Examples of Analyte Compounds*
GC/flame ionization detector	PNAs or PAHs, ketones, halogenated hydrocarbons, alcohols, ethers, aliphatic hydrocarbons, aromatic hydrocarbons
GC/nitrogen phosphorus detector	acrolein, nicotine, acetone cyanohydrin, organophosphate pesticides
GC/flame photometric detector	mercaptans, carbon disulfide, tributylphosphate, pesticides containing a sulfur or phosphorous atom
GC/electron capture detector	butadienes, pentadienes, chlordane, polychlorinated benzenes, PCBs, ethylene oxide
GC/thermal conductivity detector	carbon dioxide, oxygen, nitrogen
GC/photoionization detector	ethylene oxide, tetraethyl lead, tetramethyl lead
GC/discharge ionization detector	carbon monoxide, carbon dioxide, methane, hydrogen
GC/nitrogen chemiluminscence detector	nitrosoamines, nitrogen containing pesticides
GC/sulfur chemiluminscence detector	sulfur containing pesticides
GC/mass spectometry	aldehyde screening, identification of unknowns
HPLC/UV-vis detector	acetaldehyde, anisidine, p-chlorophenol, diethylenetriamine, ethylenediamine, maleic anhydride, p-nitroaniline, PNAs
HPLC/fluorescence detector	isocyanates, PNAs or PAHs
HPLC/electrochemical detector	isocyanates, peroxides
IC/conductivity detector	aminoethanol compounds, ammonia hydrogen sulfide, inorganic acids, iodine, hydrogen sulfide, sulfur dioxide
IC/electrochemical detector	Iodine, cyanides
IC/UV-vis detector	hexavalent chromium, ozone
Visible absorption spectrophotometry	acetic anhydride, formaldehyde, hydrazine, nitrogen dioxide, phosphine

Source: National Institute for Occupational Safety and Health (NIOSH) website http://www.cdc.gov/niosh, and Occupational Safety and Health (OSHA) website http://www.osha.gov.

NAME OF SUBSTANCE METHOD #

FORMULA Molecular Weight Chemical Abstracts Service # RTECS #

Method numbers are followed by the issue number. In the middle is the type of evaluation (Full, partial, or unrated). On the right is the first issue date and this method's issue date if the method has more than one issue date.

OSHA: These exposure limit values are
NIOSH: those in effect at the time of
ACGIH®: printing of the method

PROPERTIES: Boiling/melting points, density, equilibrium vapor pressure, and molecular weight determine the sample aerosol/vapor composition

SYNONYMS: Common synonyms for the substance, including Chemical Abstract Service (CAS) numbers

SAMPLING	MEASURMENT
SAMPLER: Brief description of sampling equipment **FLOW RATE:** acceptable sampling range, L/min **VOL –MIN:** Minimum sample volume (L) corresponds to Limit of Quantitation (LOQ) at OSHA PEL **-MAX:** Maximum sample volume (L) to avoid analyte breakthrough or overloading **BLANKS:** Each set should have at least 2 field blanks, up to 10% of samples, plus 6 or more media blanks in the case of coated sorbents, impingers solutions, or other media which may have a background of analyte **ACCURACY** Data are for experiments in which known atmospheres of substance were generated and analyzed according to the method. Target accuracy is less than 25% difference from actual concentration at or above the OSHA PEL	**TECHNIQUE:** The measurement technique used. **ANALYTE:** The chemical species actually measured A summary of the measurement EQUIPMENT, SAMPLE PREPARATION, and MEASUREMENT steps appearing on the second page of the method is given here **CALIBRATION:** Summary of type of standards used **RANGE:** Range of calibration standards to be used; from LOQ to upper limit of measurement (Note: More concentrated samples may be diluted in most cases to fall within the calibration range.) **ESTIMATED LOD:** limit of detection (background + 3 σ) **PRECISION:** Experimental precision of spiked samplers

APPLICABILITY: The conditions under which the method is useful, including the working range in mg/m (from LOQ to the maximum sampler loading) for a stated air volume are given here.

INTERFERENCES: Compounds or conditions which are known to interfere in either sampling or measurement are listed here.

OTHER METHODS: Other NIOSH or OSHA methods which are related to this one, along with literature methods are listed here and keyed to **REFERENCES.**

Figure 12.1 — Layout of cover page for NIOSH sampling and analytical methods.

Chromatographic Methods

Chromatographic methods are powerful tools for the separation of gaseous contaminants and their subsequent individual analysis.

Chromatographic techniques were developed in the early 1900s and were followed in the mid-1940s by the development of modern gas chromatography (GC) elements.(10) The word "chromatography" is taken from the Greek for "colorwriting" because early efforts involved separating plant pigments. In general, chromatography is the process of separating the components of a mixture by using a mobile phase and a stationary phase. A diagram of the chromatographic process is presented in Figure 12.3. The chromatographic techniques routinely used in an industrial hygiene laboratory are defined by the nature of the mobile phase used. If the mobile phase is a gas, the separation process is called gas chromatography; if the mobile phase is a liquid or liquid solution of desired polarity, it is

Analyte(s) Name(s)	
Method no.:	This is the method number
Target Concentration: OSHA PEL: ACGIH® TLV®:	The Target Concentration is the concentration at which the method was validated.
Procedure:	The sampling media, sample extraction, and analytical technique are described.
Recommended sampling time and sampling rate:	Recommended sampling time and rate for active samplers or range of sampling times for passive samplers.
Reliable quantitation limit:	This is the lowest amount that can be reliably quantitated. This is similar to the limit of quantitation (LOQ) found in NIOSH methods.
Standard error of estimate at the target concentration:	This is the combined error associated with the analytical method and the sampling method.
Special requirements:	Any special requirements in sampling or shipping are placed here, such as samples need to be refrigerated, or samples need to be protected from light.
Status of Method:	The method will be listed as Evaluated or Validated, and Partially Evaluated or Partially Validated. OSHA Evaluated is the same as Validated, and partially evaluated is the same as partially validated.
Chemist:	Date:
Methods Development Team Industrial Hygiene Chemistry Division OSHA Salt Lake Technical Center Sandy UT 84070-6406	

Figure 12.2 — Layout of cover page for OSHA sampling and analytical methods.

liquid chromatography; and if it is a liquid solution with a desired ionic composition, it is ion chromatography. The stationary phase is a solid that reversibly adsorbs the sample components, or a liquid on a solid substrate into which the sample components reversibly dissolve. The stationary phase is contained in a chromatography column.

Samples are introduced onto the chromatographic column that has a low flow of mobile phase passing through it. The repeated interaction between the solutes (sample) in the mobile phase and the stationary phase differentially retards the passage of individual solutes in a mixture, providing separation. Once separated, the individual analytes can be detected using nonselective detectors to quantify the amount of analyte present.

The output signal of a chromatographic detector normally is plotted against time. This plot is called a chromatogram, an example of which is shown in Figure 12.4. The response of the detector to carrier gas produces a constant signal referred to as the baseline. The baseline, therefore, represents a detector signal of zero (i.e., when the

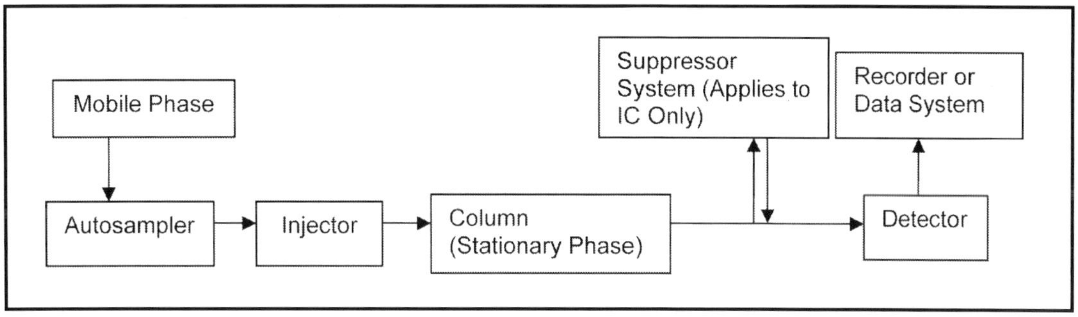

Figure 12.3 — Schematic of a chromatographic system.

detector does not detect anything eluting from the column). A peak is a rise in the plot when one or more chemicals are detected as they elute from the column. The length of time between sample injection and the maximum height of a peak is called the retention time. Retention time is constant for an analyte under a constant set of analytical conditions. Note, however, that retention time does not in and of itself provide definitive identification of a peak; some chemicals may have identical or nearly identical retention times.

The size (area) of the chromatographic peak corresponding to a given analyte is directly proportional to the mass of the analyte injected. The area of the peak is usually determined by electronic integration using various algorithms. With proper calibration the analyst can determine the mass of analyte in an unknown sample. Note, however, that chromatographic detectors do not respond identically to all substances; identical masses of two different contaminants may result in hugely different chromatographic peak areas. The ratio of mass to its response is known as the response factor and is unique for each analyte. The uniqueness of each contaminant's response factor, when coupled with the factors that influence retention time, requires individual calibrations for each analyte of interest under the standard analytical conditions selected for analysis. Also, the response factor may vary over a range of analyte mass, therefore calibrations must be performed over a range of concentrations that would bracket the sample concentrations that are anticipated to be found.

Chromatographic detectors are based on a variety of detection concepts, most with wide linear ranges. The linear range is the range of detected analyte mass for which the response factor remains constant, thus resulting in a calibration curve consisting of a straight line with a slope equal to the response factor. Linear responses offer the analyst a much more efficient instrument calibration than nonlinear responses. Detectors that must be used in their nonlinear ranges require a more detailed calibration to accurately determine the calibration curve. A calibration curve is produced by graphing a set of detector responses against the concentrations of the corresponding analytical reference standards that produced those responses. The production of calibration curves and their use in determining the amount of analyte present in a sample, based on sample detector responses, is nowadays usually performed by electronic means.

The following sections discuss the types of chromatography commonly used for the

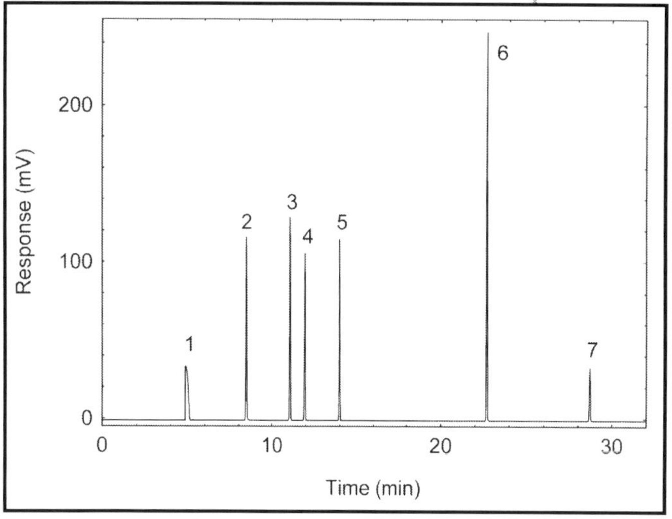

Figure 12.4 — GC chromatogram using a capillary column and a flame ionization detector. The extraction solvent is carbon disulfide with *n*-hexyl benzene as internal standard. The peaks are: (1) carbon disulfide, (2) *tert*-butyl acetate, (3) *sec*-butyl acetate, (4) isobutyl acetate, (5) *n*-butyl acetate, (6) *N,N*-dimethyl formamide, and (7) *n*-hexyl benzene.

analysis of gases and vapors in air samples (i.e., GC, high-performance liquid chromatography [HPLC], ion chromatography [IC], and GC/mass spectrometry).

Gas Chromatography

The major analytical technique for gases and vapors listed in Table 12.1 is gas chromatography, employing different detectors. GC provides a powerful tool for the analysis of low-concentration air contaminants. GC analysis is applicable to compounds with sufficient vapor pressure and thermal stability to dissolve in the mobile phase and pass through the chromatographic column in sufficient quantity to be detectable. Air samples to be analyzed by GC typically are collected on sorbent tubes and desorbed into a liquid for analysis (see Chapter 11).

There are numerous methods that use GC for air sample analysis. NIOSH Method 1500 for hydrocarbons with boiling points between 36 and 126°C is an example of such a method. This method (which applies to a range of compounds including benzene, toluene, n-hexane, and n-octane) specifies GC/flame ionization detector (FID) analysis.[11]

The basic components of a gas chromatograph are a carrier gas system, a sample injector system, a column, a detector, and a recording system. In GC the mobile phase is a gas and is referred to as the carrier gas. The carrier gas system is usually a pressure-regulated compressed nonreactive gas (e.g., hydrogen, helium, or nitrogen), chosen because it does not interact with the stationary phase.

Samples can be injected onto a GC column as a volatile liquid or as a gas. Injection volumes typically range from 0.1 to 10 µL for volatile liquids and from 0.05 to 100 mL for gas samples. The sample must be injected rapidly and evenly to optimize chromatographic separation as it passes through the column. The injector is maintained at a higher temperature than the column to prevent condensation of the solvent and/or analyte. Gas or liquid samples can be injected into the column using a syringe with the hypodermic needle inserted through a self-sealing septum contained in the injection port. Laboratories that analyze large numbers of samples use automated sample injection systems that provide for rapid analysis and more precise injection. Gas samples can also be injected onto the column using gas sampling valves, although this is not common for routine occupational hygiene analyses performed by GC. A GC gas sampling valve involves the use of a fixed-volume sample loop that can be flushed onto the column with mobile phase (similar to the common HPLC injection system described later).

Injection systems are available that involve the use of thermal desorption from sorbent tubes and subsequent gas phase injection of the entire sample. In thermal desorption systems the contaminant is driven from the sorbent at a high temperature into a carrier gas. Because the analytes are not diluted in a desorption solvent, a much larger portion of analyte can be introduced directly into the gas chromatograph. Using this procedure it is possible to determine lower concentrations of contaminants, often in the sub-parts per billion (ppb) range. A limitation of thermal desorption is that there normally is only one chance for successful analysis because the entire sample is consumed in the injection process. Although there are thermal desorbers which allow the sample to be split, and part of the sample reabsorbed onto a resin bed for reanalysis after a second thermal desorption, this injection technique, in general, lacks the efficiency of the commonly used sample desorption with a solvent and liquid injection.

After a sample is injected onto the head of a chromatographic column, each component in the sample repeatedly sorbs onto the stationary phase and desorbs into the mobile phase. The stationary phase exhibits a different affinity for each component of the sample mixture. Chemical compounds that are more strongly attracted to the stationary phase take longer to be swept through the column by the mobile phase. The end result is that individual compounds elute from the column at different times. Accurate quantification, therefore, depends on the combined abilities of the chromatographic column, carrier gas flow rate, and temperature conditions to separate analytes from other sample components prior to reaching the detector.

GC analysis of samples collected from workplace atmospheres uses either packed or capillary columns. Packed columns are typically 0.5- to 2-m long metal or glass tubes in straight, bent, or coiled form, usually filled with a liquid-coated solid support material. The purpose of the solid support, typically diatomaceous earth, is to provide a large uniform and inert surface area for distributing the liquid coating with which the analytes interact. The versatility of GC as an analytical tool derives from the wide variety of substances that can be used as stationary phase coatings in GC columns. The stationary phase polarity, chemical composition, surface area, and amount of liquid coating are the major factors influencing the separation process. In general, the composition of the stationary phase chosen will depend on the composition of the analyte. For the most efficient separation the liquid phase should be chemically similar to the sample being analyzed. For example, non-polar hydrocarbons are best separated using long chain hydrocarbons, such as paraffin or squalene as the stationary liquid phase. Polar compounds are better separated using alcohol or amide liquid phases.

In contrast to packed columns, capillary columns are long (15–150 m) open tubes of small diameter (0.20–0.75 mm) with the inside of the tubing containing a coated or bonded liquid phase. Capillary columns provide better peak resolution because their low resistance to flow allows for longer columns. The tradeoff, however, is that because of their small internal volume, smaller injection volumes must be used. Most gas chromatographic sample analyses for occupational hygiene are nowadays performed with capillary column technology.

The column of a GC is maintained in a temperature controlled environment (the GC oven) where the column temperature can be rigidly controlled. This temperature control allows chromatographic separations to occur isothermally or with the use of programmed temperature changes. Column temperature is adjusted so that it is high enough for the analysis to be accomplished in a reasonable amount of time and low enough that the desired separation is obtained. A rule of thumb is that the retention time of an analyte in a column will double for every 30°C decrease in temperature.[12] When there are multiple analytes with a wide range of physical properties in a single sample, temperature programming may be needed to achieve separation in a reasonable time. Temperature programming allows for the separation of analytes with a wide range of boiling points. When a sample is injected onto a relatively cool column, the early peaks result from low boiling compounds that move quickly through the column. Higher boiling compounds, however, are more strongly retained by the stationary phase and will elute very slowly, resulting in long broad peaks. If the temperature in the column is caused to rise through a programmed temperature increase at a set time-interval from the time of sample injection, the high boiling point compounds will move more quickly through the column resulting in sharper peaks.

Selection of the appropriate detector for the analyte of interest is essential to realize the full potential of GC analysis. The following detection systems are available to maximize analytical sensitivity and selectivity.

Flame Ionization Detector (FID)

The FID is very sensitive to most organic compounds, including aliphatic and aromatic hydrocarbons, ketones, alcohols, ethers, and halogenated hydrocarbons. It is one of the most widely used gas chromatographic detectors because it has high sensitivity and exhibits a linear response over a wide dynamic range. The FID has a linear range of six to seven orders of magnitude. FIDs respond only to compounds with oxidizable carbon atoms and therefore will not respond to water vapor; elemental gases; carbon monoxide; carbon dioxide; hydrogen cyanide; formaldehyde; formic acid; water; or to most other inorganic compounds. Importantly, FIDs show little response to carbon disulfide. For this reason carbon disulfide frequently is used as a charcoal tube desorption solvent for methods using an FID. (Often GC-FID methods may specify that a small amount of another solvent be added to the carbon disulfide to modify the polarity of the solution for the purpose of increasing sample desorption efficiency.) In an FID, effluent from the GC column is mixed with hydrogen in excess air prior to passing through a small opening or jet, where it is burned. Ionized combustion products are attracted to a metal "collector" around the flame. The collector is electrically charged at about +200 volts relative to the jet, attracting ions produced by the flame to the collector. Ions reaching the collector create an electrical current, which is amplified and recorded.

The methanizer flame ionization detector is a special FID detector used to detect low levels of carbon monoxide and carbon dioxide. The detector assembly contains a removable jet that is packed with a nickel catalyst and heated to 380°C. The GC column effluent is mixed with hydrogen before it passes through the jet where carbon monoxide and carbon dioxide are catalytically converted to methane which is detected by the FID. The reaction occurs after the compounds have passed through the GC column; therefore, their retention times are not changed. Hydrocarbons are not affected as they pass through the jet.

Nitrogen-Phosphorus Detector (NPD)

The NPD, also called a thermionic or alkali flame detector, is highly sensitive and selective for nitrogen and phosphorous compounds, including amines and organophosphates. The detector is similar in principle to the FID, except that ionization occurs on the surface of an alkali metal salt, such as cesium bromide, rubidium silicate, or potassium chloride. The older version of this detector, the alkali flame detector, uses a flame to heat the alkali metal salt. Newer detector designs electrically heat the alkali metal salt to improve stability and reduce response to hydrocarbon interferences.

Flame Photometric Detector (FPD)

The FPD is used to measure phosphorus-containing and sulfur-containing compounds such as organophosphate pesticides and mercaptans. The FPD measures phosphorus-containing or sulfur-containing compounds by burning the column effluent in a hydrogen-air flame with an excess of hydrogen. Sulfur and phosphorus compounds emit light above the flame; a filter optimized to pass light at 393 nm is used to detect sulfur compounds; a filter optimized to pass light at 535 nm is used to detect phosphorus compounds. A photomultiplier tube is then used to quantify the amount of light passing through the selective filter.

Electron Capture Detector (ECD)

The ECD is selective and highly sensitive for halogenated hydrocarbons, nitriles, nitrates, ozone, organo-metallics, sulfur compounds, and many other electron-capturing compounds. Selectivity is based on the absorption of electrons by compounds that have an affinity for free electrons because their molecules have an electronegative group or center. In an ECD, electrons are generated using radioactive beta-emitting isotopes, such as nickel-63 or tritium, and captured at a positively charged collector. This electron flux produces a steady current amplified by an electrometer. When an electron-capturing compound is present in the gas chromatograph column effluent, fewer electrons reach the collector. The resulting decrease in current is amplified and inverted so that the output signal from the detector increases as compounds are detected. The loss of current is a measure of the electron affinity of the analytes passing through the detector. Non-halogenated hydrocarbons have little electron affinity and therefore are not detected using an ECD. Selective sensitivity for halides makes this detector particularly useful for halogenated pesticides and other halogenated hydrocarbons such as polychlorinated biphenyls. A limitation of the ECD is its narrow linear range, which necessitates careful calibration in the range of interest.

Thermal Conductivity Detector (TCD)

The TCD is the most universal gas chromatographic detector because it can measure most gases and vapors. It has low sensitivity compared with the other detectors, however, and is used primarily for analysis of low molecular weight gases such as carbon dioxide, nitrogen, and oxygen. This detector measures the differences in thermal conductivity between the column effluent, and a reference gas consisting of uncontaminated carrier gas. The most common carrier gas with this detector is helium. The detector has two flow through sensor cells, one through which pure carrier gas flows as a reference and the other through which the column effluent flows. Each cell contains an identical fine filament of platinum or tungsten that is heated by an electric current. The thermal conductivity (and heat capacity to some extent) of the gas passing through the column effluent cell changes slightly as sample components elute. This change in thermal properties of the gas will change the temperature of the filament and thus its electrical resistance. The difference in resistance between the filaments of column effluent cell and the reference cell is electronically measured, amplified and recorded as a detector response. This detector is also known as a hotwire detector.

Photoionization Detector (PID)

The PID is sensitive to compounds with low ionization potentials that can be ionized by ultraviolet light. PIDs can be used to selectively detect a wide range of compounds including aromatics, alkenes, ketones, or amines in the presence of aliphatic chromatographic interferences. This detector is similar in principle to the FID except that, instead of using a flame, it uses ultraviolet light to ionize the analyte molecules. Absorption of a photon by a molecule can cause the molecule to lose an electron if the energy of the photon is greater than the ionization potential of the molecule. Different PID lamps are available to provide different photon energy levels. The lamp photon energy is chosen for selectivity of the analyte over the chromatographic interferences present in the sample. For example, benzene has an ionization potential of 9.2 electron volts (eV), and hexane has an ionization potential of 10.2 eV. A lamp that emits photons with an energy of 11 eV will ionize both, although it may be more sensitive to benzene. With a 10 eV lamp, the PID will detect only the benzene, even with a large amount of hexane present.

Discharge Ionization Detector (DID)

The DID has high sensitivity to permanent gases and low molecular compounds (carbon monoxide, carbon dioxide, nitrogen, oxygen, argon, hydrogen, methane). High-voltage electricity is used to energize a stream of helium probably producing photons, electrons and metastable helium. This excited helium stream is mixed with the column effluent where energy is transferred to the effluent components and result in their ionization. Ionized analyte creates an electrical current to a charged collector. This current which will be proportional to the amount of analyte in the effluent is amplified and recorded. The DID is useful in industrial hygiene laboratories that analyze gas bag samples for determining the quality of breathing air.

Nitrogen & Sulfur Chemiluminescence Detectors (NCD) & (SCD)

These detectors when configured appropriately can be highly sensitive and selective towards nitrogen or sulfur containing compounds. The NCD is based on the reaction of ozone with nitrogen oxide (and other species) produced when column effluent is combusted in an electrical furnace. Photons emitted from the ozone-nitrogen oxide reaction are detected and amplified with a photomultiplier tube and recorded. This detector can have unique utility in an industrial hygiene laboratory for trace-level analysis of nitrosamines and nitrogen-containing pesticides. The SCD operates similarly except the detected photons are produced by the reaction of ozone with sulfur oxide, hydrogen sulfide and other reaction species produced inside the electrical furnace.

GC/Mass Spectrometry (GC/MS)

A gas chromatograph interfaced with a mass spectrometer can be used to both quantitate and conclusively identify analytes. Its unique capabilities for conclusive qualitative identification make it a powerful tool in identifying or confirming the presence of hazardous substances. Today, small bench-top mass spectrometers are available that are specifically designed for use a GC.

GC column effluent is introduced into the mass spectrometer and ionized, producing parent ions and ion fragments that are accelerated and separated by their mass-to-charge ratio. The mass spectrum is the record of the numbers of each kind of ion. The relative numbers of each ion are characteristic for every compound, including isomers.

The basic parts of a mass spectrometer are the (1) inlet system; (2) ion source, where the sample is ionized; (3) accelerating system, which separates the ions by their mass; and (4) detector system, which measures the number of ions emerging from the accelerating system. The spectrometer is maintained at a high vacuum. Because GCs operate at atmospheric pressures, specialized devices have been developed to inject extremely small samples of the GC effluent into the mass spectrometer to maintain the vacuum.

Ion sources are the primary component of a mass spectrometer. They produce ions without mass discrimination, which are accelerated and passed into the mass analyzer. The most common type of ionization source produces ions by electron impact. As the column effluent from the gas chromatograph enters the mass spectrometer, the low molecular weight carrier gas is removed, and the rest of the column effluent travels through a beam of electrons in a high vacuum. Some of the molecules are fragmented by the electron beam into numerous ions and neutral fragments. The positively charged ions then enter the accelerating system, where rapidly changing electrical and magnetic radiation fields separate the ions according to their mass, allowing ions with each selected mass to pass sequentially through to the detector system. The detector system consists of an ion-multiplier, which measures the number of ions passing through the mass analyzer. As ions strike a collector, the ion-multiplier causes the emission of electrons, which are collected and amplified by an electron multiplier.

A computer is used to store information on the abundance and associated mass of ions detected by the ion-multiplier. For each scan of the mass analyzer, the set of mass and abundance data pairs is called a mass spectrum, typically displayed as a bar graph or a table showing the abundance of positively charged ions at each mass. The mass spectrum pattern provides information about the structure of the original chemical compound and in many cases is sufficient for identification. An example of a mass spectrum is presented in Figure 12.5. Some common applications of GC/MS are:

- Evaluation of complex mixtures, such as mixtures of polynuclear aromatic hydrocarbons (PAHs), or identification of individual component vapors from photocopier and other office machine emissions; GC alone is not capable of positive identification;
- Identification of pyrolysis and combustion products from fires;
- Analysis of insecticides and herbicides— conventional analytical methods frequently cannot resolve or identify the wide variety of industrial pesticides currently in use, but GC/MS can both identify and quantify these compounds.

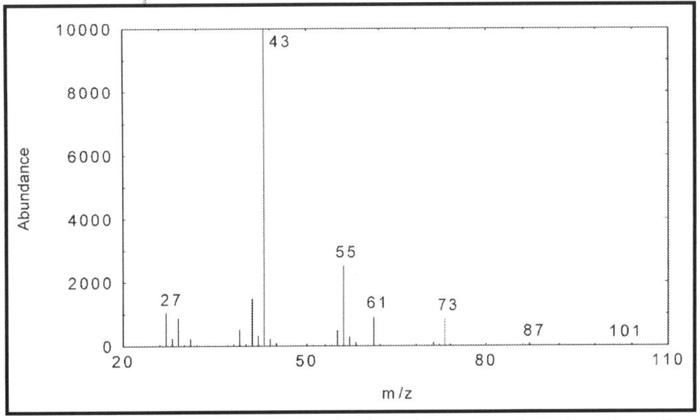

Figure 12.5 — Mass spectrum of *n*-butyl acetate showing the relative abundance of each mass fragment.

A specific example of a GC/MS method is NIOSH Method 2539 for aldehyde screening.[13] This method is designed to identify individual aldehydes in an air sample or in a bulk liquid. Another GC/MS method is EPA Method TO-17, which is designed for the determination of volatile organic compounds (VOCs) in indoor air.[14] This method is based on the collection of VOCs on Tenax® sorbent tubes followed by thermal desorption and capillary GC/MS analysis.

High-Performance Liquid Chromatography (HPLC)

Although GC is used to analyze the vast majority of airborne organic compounds, it is not suitable for compounds that may be unstable at elevated temperatures or have very high boiling points (low vapor pressures). For these substances, HPLC is usually a viable alternative for measuring occupational concentration levels. Certain compounds from the following chemical types are commonly analyzed by HPLC: isocyanates (through analysis of a stable chemical derivative, i.e. reaction product), pesticides, and substances associated with carcinogenicity such as polynuclear aromatics hydrocarbons (PNAs or PAHs) and nitrosamines.

Examples of a specific HPLC methods are NIOSH Method 5506[15], and OSHA Method 58[16] for polynuclear aromatics and coke oven emissions These methods are designed for a range of PAHs including benz[a]anthracene, and benzo[a]pyrene.

Whereas in GC the chromatography of an analysis is optimized by altering the column (stationary phase) used and the column temperature, in HPLC it is usually optimized by altering the column used and the polarity of the liquid mobile phase. HPLC analyses are usually performed with the column at ambient temperature or slightly above, and the polar nature of the mobile phase is controlled by use of the appropriate liquid or solution of liquids. One of the most commonly used solutions is a 50/50 water / acetonitrile solution.

The injection system for HPLC is similar in design to the gas sampling valve that is sometimes used in GC, and can be automated. The injector has a plumbing configuration that allows a small isolated sampling loop of known volume to be filled with sample solution. After being filled with sample, this loop of tubing is switched into the pressurized plumbing of the instrument where mobile phase flushes the sample from the loop to the head of the column. HPLC columns are made of rigid metal tubing 2.5 to 25 cm in length and, as with GC, the stationary phase can be a solid material or a solid substrate with a bonded phase usually in the form of 5 to 10 µm particles. The flow rate of mobile phase through the column is usually in the range of 0.5 to 2 mL/min.

A new variation of HPLC is emerging on the scene which uses higher pressure than the traditional HPLC, usually ranging from 3,000–10,000 psi, with small columns containing 1 to 3 µm particle sized packing. The result is sharper peaks and shorter retention times.

Commonly used HPLC detectors used in industrial hygiene laboratories include UV-Visible detector, fluorescence detector, and to a lesser extent the electrochemical detector. Also liquid chromatography/ mass spectrometry (LC/MS) technology is available, but not presently in wide use for measuring occupational exposures. An HPLC chromatogram is presented in Figure 12.6.

UV-vis Absorbance Detector

The UV-vis detector measures the ultraviolet (UV) or visible light absorbance of the column effluent. Compounds highly sensitive to detection must be strong absorbers of the wavelength used by the detector. The basic components of the UV-vis detector are a UV lamp, a visible lamp, a flow-through cell with windows that are transparent to UV and visible light, and a photodiode or other light-measuring device. Some UV detectors can be operated at only one wavelength, typically 254 nm, whereas most can also operate at additional wavelengths. This detector was originally developed to measure in the UV range only, typically to measure compounds with benzene rings which absorb at 254 nm. In the 1980s, the addition of visible lamps became common, which extended the detector's usefulness into the visible wavelength range. A variable UV-vis detector can be tuned to any wavelength within its operating range. A diode array detector (DAD) is a UV-vis detector that can simultaneously measure the absorbance of a substance at selected wavelengths in the UV-vis spectrum. This allows the analyst to quantify and confirm the presence of a given analyte by its unique absorbance fingerprint across the spectrum. Spectral libraries can be developed to aid in the confirmation of samples and identification of unknown peaks.

Fluorescence Detector

The fluorescence detector measures the emission of light produced by fluorescing analytes and is extremely sensitive to highly conjugated aromatic compounds such as PAHs. Some analytical methods use derivatization reagents to react with the analyte to form a fluorescent derivative. In these methods a light source raises the fluorescent analyte to an unstable higher energy level, which quickly decays in two or more steps, emitting light at longer wavelengths. The basic detector components are a lamp, a flow cell with transparent windows, filters or diffraction gratings to select the excitation and emission wavelengths, and a photomultiplier tube or other light-measuring device.

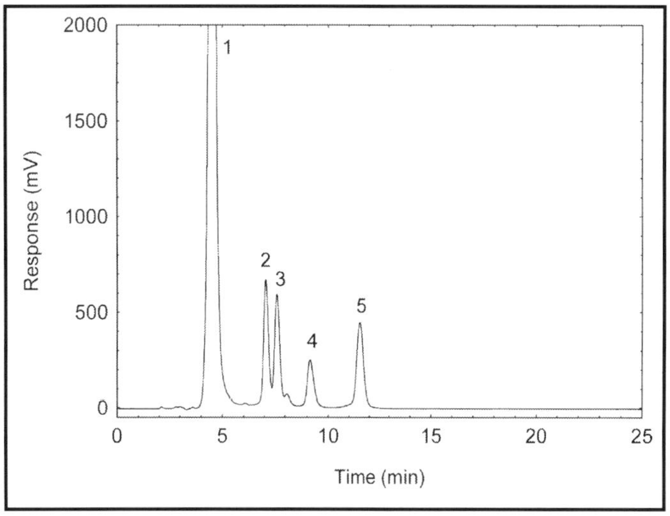

Figure 12.6 — HPLC chromatogram using a UV-vis detector. The peaks are: 1) DMSO, 2) toluene-2,6-diisocyante, 3) toluene-2,4-diisocyanate, 4) 1,6-hexamethylene diisocyanate, and 5) methylene bisphenyl isocyanate.

Fluorescence detectors vary in sensitivity and selectivity. Some use a collection of lamps, wave-plates, and filters to provide a range of excitation and emission wavelengths. Most fluorescence detectors can be tuned to any wavelength within their range. Most automated models can rapidly change the wavelengths during chromatographic analysis of one sample to optimize the detector for different analytes that elute at different retention times.

Electrochemical Detector

An electrochemical detector responds to compounds (such as phenols, aromatic amines, ketones, aldehydes, peroxides, and mercaptans) that can be readily oxidized or reduced. Electrode systems use working and reference electrodes to quantify analytes over a range of six orders of magnitude.

Ion Chromatography (IC)

IC is used for the separation and detection of analytes that can dissociate into ionic species. The mechanisms of separation differ from those of HPLC, but IC could be considered an element of HPLC because of the similarities. Both require the basic components of a chromatographic system (Figure 12.3), use a liquid mobile phase, and operate at similar internal pressures. The main differences are that IC operates with an ionic mobile phase, requires a column containing stationary phase that is appropriate for ionic separations, and the chromatographic components must be made of inert materials not necessary in HPLC. IC is useful in an industrial hygiene laboratory for the analysis of a variety of substances that include mineral acids and hexavalent chromium.

Examples of IC methods are NIOSH Method 7903 for inorganic acids[17] and OSHA Method ID165SG[18] for acid mist. Both of these methods use IC to analyze for mineral acids by their respective anion, such as nitrate for nitric acid and sulfate for sulfuric acid.

An IC analysis is optimized by altering the column (stationary phase) used and ionic nature of the mobile phase, which is known as the eluent. IC analyses are usually performed with the column at ambient temperature, and the ionic nature of the eluent (which is mainly water) typically controlled with the addition small amounts of a weak acid or base. For example, both of the methods mentioned in the previous paragraph use millimolar solutions of sodium carbonate and sodium bicarbonate as the eluents.

The injection system for IC is similar to that described for HPLC but all plumbing and surfaces that may be exposed to eluent must be constructed of a material that is inert to acidic or basic solutions. Metal surfaces must be avoided because they are subject to corrosion from exposure to eluent, or may interact with the analyte's ionic species. Internal tubing and surfaces are typically made of organic polymeric materials. IC columns, also made of organic polymeric materials, consist of tubing 2.5 to 25 cm in length. The stationary phase is usually composed of an appropriate ion exchange resin in the form of 5 to 10 μm particles. Ion exchange resins are available as anionic exchangers and cationic exchangers. Some of the anions most suitable for anion exchange IC analysis include bromide; sulfate; nitrate; phosphate; chromate; chloride; cyanamide; sulfite; and thiocyanate. Cation exchange IC can be used for the analysis of alkali and alkaline earth metals, inorganic ammonium salts, and salts of various amines. Cation exchange has been used for the analysis of carcinogens such as beta-naphthylamine, benzidine, hydrazines, azoarenes, and aziridines. The flow rate of the mobile phase through the column is in the range of 0.5 to 2 mL/min.

An additional component commonly used in IC is the suppressor system, which is placed inline between the column and the detector. The function of the suppressor system is to suppress the ionic nature of the eluent and enhance that of the analyte for conductivity detection. This reduces the eluent background signal and increases sensitivity of the analyte. Nowadays suppressor systems are usually membrane based and involve the use of small ion exchange screens and micro-membranes. This suppressor system has mostly replaced the suppressor columns once used in IC, which contained a strong cation exchange resin and had to be regenerated (as with the ion exchange resin in a household water softener). The suppressor system is required when a conductivity detector is used.

Most of the HPLC detectors, with appropriate adaptation, can be used with IC, but the most commonly used IC detector is the conductivity detector. An IC chromatogram is presented in Figure 12.7.

Conductivity Detector (CD)

The conductivity detector measures the conductivity of the total mobile phase. The electrical conductivity detector senses all the ions present, whether they come from the solute or from the mobile phase. Most IC instruments use ion suppressors which suppress the ions in the eluent so the analytes can be measured. The conductivity detector has a flow-through cell, a few micro-liters in volume containing two electrodes two or three millimeters apart. The electrodes are usually made of platinum, or some other noble metal, or occasionally stainless steel. The sensor monitors the resistance between the electrodes and the signal is modified to provide an output that is linearly related to the ion concentration. This detector is used for a large array of analyses which include many of those already described.

Electrochemical Detector (ED)

This detector has previously been described in the HPLC section. When adapted to IC, this detector can be used for the analysis of iodine and cyanide.

UV-vis Absorbance Detector and Fluorescence Detectors

When these detectors are used in IC, the analyte is either derivatized before analysis or derivatized after eluting from the column (post-column derivatization) to produce a reaction product that absorbs light in the UV-vis range or fluoresces. Most ionic species separated by IC are not strong absorbers in the UV-vis range nor exhibit fluorescence. These detectors have been used for the analysis of ozone as its nitrate derivative, and hexavalent chromium via post column derivatization.

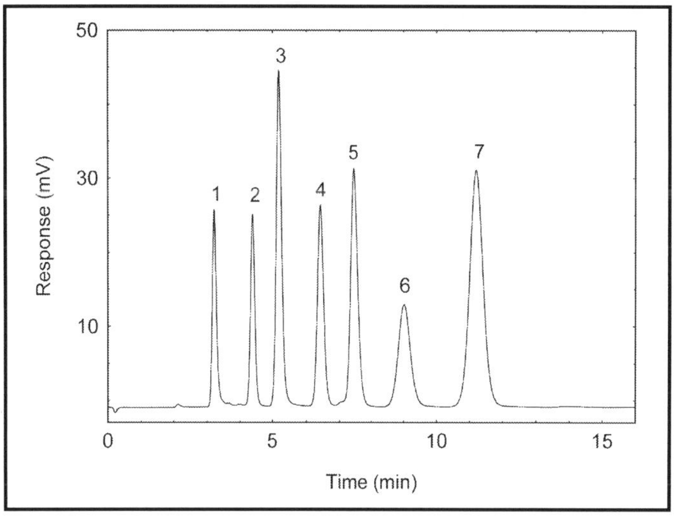

Figure 12.7 — IC chromatogram using a conductivity detector. The peaks are: 1) fluoride, 2) chloride, 3) nitrite, 4) nitrate, 5) bromide, 6) phosphate, and 7) sulfate.

Volumetric Methods

Analysis using volumetric methods, sometimes referred to as wet-chemical methods, is performed by measuring the volume of a solution of a known concentration required to react completely with the substance being determined. For the analysis of gases and vapors, titrimetric methods that involve measuring the quantity of a reagent required to react completely with the analyte that is dissolved in a solution are available. Detection of an endpoint is based on the observation of some property of the solution that undergoes a characteristic change near the equivalence point (endpoint). Changes in color, turbidity, electrical conductivity, electrical potential, refractive index, or temperature of the solution are the most commonly used properties to detect reaction endpoint.

For occupational hygiene applications, titrimetric techniques have been used historically to determine airborne concentrations of hydrogen chloride, nitric acid, caustic mist, sulfur dioxide, hydrogen sulfide, and ozone. Volumetric methods quantify all acids as an acid, making it impossible to quantify two acids separately, such as nitric acid and sulfuric acid. For the most part, these methods have been replaced by more specific analytical techniques, such as IC. Also, this has usually resulted more efficient sample collection procedures.

Spectrophotometric Methods

A common technique for many occupational hygiene analyses is the measurement of the absorption of light at a particular wavelength by a solution containing the analyte or a light absorbing derivative formed from the analyte. The process is termed "absorption spectrophotometry." (When visible light is used the process has been called colorimetry.) Spectrophotometric methods that use UV, visible, and infrared radiation also have been developed. The extent to which light is absorbed by the solution is related to the concentration of the analyte in solution and the length of the light beam passing through the absorbing solution.

Absorption photometry is described using the Beer-Lambert law, which relates the absorbance of light to the concentration of the absorbing material according to Equation 12.1.

$$A = \log\left[\frac{I_{in}}{I_{out}}\right] = \log\left[\frac{1}{T}\right] = a \times b \times c \qquad (12.1)$$

where:

- A = absorbance
- I_{in} = intensity of light entering the solution
- I_{out} = intensity of light leaving the solution
- T = transmittance
- a = molar absorptivity constant
- b = path length
- c = concentration of absorbing material

A plot of absorbance versus concentration of the absorbing material usually yields a straight line. This plot can be used to determine the concentration of that analyte in solution derived from an air sample. Changes in color intensity have been the basis of many occupational hygiene colorimetric methods. For example, a classic application is the use of Saltzman's reagent to determine the airborne concentration of nitrogen dioxide.

Spectrophotometric and colorimetric techniques have for the most part been replaced by more sensitive and convenient instrumental methods. For example, methods of analysis for many organic compounds by UV spectrophotometry have been replaced by GC and HPLC techniques. Chromatographic methods that use detectors such as the UV-vis detector are actually using spectrophotometry adapted to monitor separated sample components by use of a flow-through cell. Other than its adaptation to chromatography methods UV spectrophotometry used in occupational hygiene exposure monitoring is generally restricted to direct-reading field instruments, such as those used for measuring mercury vapors and real-time screening of organic compounds. Infrared spectrophotometric techniques are also used to quantify airborne organic compounds. One advantage of the infrared technique is that it can be adapted to direct-reading instruments to measure a variety of gases and vapors. This is discussed further in Chapter 17 on direct-reading instruments.

Summary

Chromatographic methods nowadays constitute the most common standard techniques for modern occupational hygiene gas and vapor sample analysis. Of these methods, GC methods are most prevalent, but HPLC and IC methods also are used for gases and vapors that are not well suited for GC analysis. HPLC is useful for heat labile substances and those with high boiling points, and the separation mechanisms used in IC are effective for substances that have an ionic nature, such as mineral acids. A variety of chromatographic mobile phases, chromatographic stationary phases, and detection concepts are used in chromatographic methods to optimize the separation of sample components, the removal of interferences, and the achievement of necessary levels of detection. Traditional volumetric and spectrophotometric methods have, by large, been replaced by instrumental chromatographic methods because of their advantages in specificity, sensitivity, and efficiency through automation.

Many laboratory methods for the analysis of specific gases and vapors have been established and are available through government agencies such as NIOSH and OSHA, and through AIHA's IHMEN. Additionally consensus organizations such as the American Society for Testing Materials (ASTM) can be useful sources of standardized analytical methodology.

The occupational hygienist must assure that analytical methodologies are available to meet his particular exposure monitoring needs. This can be accomplished by using a competent analytical laboratory and maintaining close contact with it, especially when novel exposure monitoring is going to be performed.

Acknowledgments

The authors wish to thank Michael A. Coffman, Jaswant Singh, Patrick N. Breysse, and Peter S. J. Lee, whose earlier work on this chapter provided the foundation of this version.

Additional Sources

Chapman, J.R.: *Practical Organic Mass Spectrometry*. New York: John Wiley & Sons, 1995.

Harris, D.C.: *Quantitative Chemical Analysis*. New York: W.H. Freeman, 2006.

Jennings, W.: *Analytical Gas Chromatography*. New York: Academic Press, 1997.

Meyer, V.: *Practical High-Performance Liquid Chromatography*. New York: John Wiley and Sons, 1993.

Willard, H., L. Merrit, J. Dean, and F. Settle: *Instrumental Methods of Analysis*, 7th edition. Belmont, CA: Wadsworth Publishing, 1988.

Weiss, J.: *Handbook of Ion Chromatography*. Weinheim, Germany: Wiley-VCH, 2004.

References

1. **National Institute for Occupational Safety and Health (NIOSH):** "Formaldehyde by Vis". [Online] Available at http://www.cdc.gov/niosh/nmam/pdfs/3500.pdf. [Accessed July 1, 2011].
2. **National Institute for Occupational Safety and Health (NIOSH):** "Formaldehyde by GC". [Online] Available at http://www.cdc.gov/niosh/nmam/pdfs/2541.pdf [Accessed July 1, 2011].
3. **Occupational Safety and Health Administration (OSHA):** "Acrolein and Formaldehyde." [Online] Available at http://www.osha.gov/dts/sltc/methods/organic/org052/org052.html. [Accessed July 1, 2011].
4. **National Institute for Occupational Safety and Health (NIOSH):** *NIOSH Manual of Analytical Methods* (NMAN). [Online] Available at http://www.cdc.gov/niosh/nmam/. [Accessed July 1, 2011].
5. **Occupational Safety and Health Administration (OSHA):** "Sampling and Analytical Methods". [Online] Available at http://www.osha.gov/dts/sltc/methods/index.html. [Accessed July 1, 2011].
6. **U.S. Environmental Protection Agency (EPA):** "Air Toxic Methods". [Online] Available at http://www.epa.gov/ttn/amtic/airtox.html. [Accessed July 1, 2011].
7. **American Industrial Hygiene Association® (AIHA®):** "WEEL Chemicals and the Industrial Hygiene Methods Exchange Network Database". [Online] Available at http://www.aiha.org/Content/InsideAIHA/Volunteer+Groups/IHMENdatabase.htm. [Accessed July 1, 2011].
8. **ASTM International:** "ASTM Standards." [Online] Available at http://www.astm.org/Standards/index/shmtl. [Accessed July 1, 2011].
9. **American Industrial Hygiene Association® (AIHA®):** "Proficiency Testing". [Online] Available at http://www.aiha.org/Content/LQAP/PT/pt.htm. [Accessed July 1, 2011].
10. **Santinder, A.:** *Chromatography and Separation Science*. Boston, MA: Academic Press, 2003.
11. **National Institute for Occupational Safety and Health (NIOSH):** "Hydrocarbons BP 36-216°C". [Online] Available at http://www.cdc.gov/niosh/nmam/pdfs/1500.pdf. [Accessed July 1, 2011].
12. **National Institute for Occupational Safety and Health (NIOSH):** "Aldehydes, Screening". [Online] Available at http://www.cdc.gov/niosh/nmam/pdfs/2539.pdf. [Accessed July 1, 2011].
13. "Method TO-17 Toxic Organic Compounds in Ambient Air". [Online] Available at http://www.epa.gov/ttn/amtic/files/ambient/airtox/to-17.pdf (Accessed July 1, 2011).
14. **Occupational Safety and Health Administration (OSHA):** "OSHA Method 42 1,6-Hexamethylene Diisocyanate (HDI), Toluene-2,4-Diisocyanate (2,4-TDI), and Toluene-2,6-Diisocyanate (2,6-TDI)" [Online] Available at http://www.osha.gov/dts/sltc/methods/organic/org042/org042.html and "OSHA Method 37 Methylene Bisphenyl Isocyanate (MDI)". [Online] Available at http://www.osha.gov/dts/sltc/methods/organic/org047/org047.html. [Accessed July 1, 2011].
15. **National Institute for Occupational Safety and Health (NIOSH):** "Polynuclear Aromatic Hydrocarbons by HPLC". [Online] Available at http://www.cdc.gov/niosh/nmam/pdfs/5506.pdf. [Accessed July 1, 2011].
16. **Occupational Safety and Health Administration (OSHA):** "OSHA Method 58 Coal Tar Pitch Volatiles (CTPV), Coke Oven Emissions (COE), and Selected Polynuclear Aromatic Hydrocarbons (PAHs)". [Online] Available at http://www.osha.gov/dts/sltc/methods/organic/org058/org058.html. [Accessed July 1, 2011].
17. **National Institute for Occupational Safety and Health (NIOSH):** "Acids, Inorganic" [Online] Available at http://www.cdc.gov/niosh/nmam/pdfs/7903.pdf. [Accessed July 1, 2011].
18. **Occupational Safety and Health Administration (OSHA):** "Acid Mist in Workplace Atmospheres". [Online] Available at http://www.osha.gov/dts/sltc/methods/inorganic/id165sg/id165sg.html. [Accessed July 1, 2011].

Outcome Competencies

After completing this chapter, the reader should be able to:

1. Define underlined terms used in this chapter.
2. Describe the function and organization of a laboratory quality management system.
3. Differentiate between quality assurance and quality control.
4. Differentiate between accuracy and precision, and between repeatability, replicability, and reproducibility.
5. Apply quality control concepts developed in this chapter to sampling and analysis activities.
6. Prepare an outline for a sampling project quality management plan.
7. Prepare an outline for a laboratory quality control plan.
8. Develop and evaluate the results of an intralaboratory quality control program, including the use of control charts and the evaluation of intra- and inter-analyst data.
9. Develop and evaluate the results of an interlaboratory quality control program.

Prerequisite Knowledge

College-level chemistry and algebra. Basic course in statistics recommended.

Prior to beginning this chapter, the reader should review the following chapters:

Chapter Number	Chapter Topic
7	Principles of Evaluating Worker Exposure
11	Sampling of Gases and Vapors
12	Analysis of Gases and Vapors
14	Sampling and Sizing of Airborne Particles
15	Principles and Instrumentation for Calibrating Air Sampling Equipment
16	Preparation of Known Concentrations of Air Contaminants
17	Direct-Reading Instruments for Determining Concentrations of Gases, Vapors & Aerosols
41	Program Management
42	Surveys and Audits

Key Terms

acceptance testing • accuracy • blank samples • calibration • control chart • corrective action • document control • duplicate samples • interlaboratory • management plan • management system • precision • preventive action • • quality • quality assurance • quality control • spiked samples • split samples • systems audit • Youden plot

Key Topics

I. Quality, Quality Control, Quality Assurance, and Quality Management
II. Field and Laboratory Quality Management Plan(s)
   A. Elements of a Quality Management Plan
III. Elements of Quality Control
   A. Accuracy, Bias, and Precision
IV. Quality Assurance for Sampling Activities
   A. Written Sampling Method
   B. Acceptable Sampling Materials
   C. Sampler Calibration
   D. Portable Instruments
V. Quality Assurance for Intralaboratory Operations
   A. Accreditation
   B. Other Types of Control Charts
   C. Evaluating Laboratory Methods
   D. Reporting Results
VI. Interlaboratory Quality Assurance
VII. Summary

Quality Control for Sampling and Laboratory Analysis

13

Keith R. Nicholson, MPH, CIH

Introduction

Goals and Objectives

Treatises on quality control have filled volumes in the literature. There are numerous approaches and viewpoints relating to the application of these to the control of processes. This particular chapter serves only as an introduction to this topic and provides some common applications of these to the collection of industrial hygiene samples and the analysis of the samples in the laboratory. The reader is encouraged to utilize the references included in this chapter and the myriad other references and resources available to further their knowledge of quality management, the associated statistical approaches, and how these can be applied in their particular application. It is not intended that the reader should require an in-depth understanding of statistics. As stated by Dr. W. J. Youden:[1]

> *There is an important reason for insisting on simple and intuitively acceptable statistical techniques. Presentation of evidence before a court, or to a producer whose product is rejected, will be more convincing if it is understandable.*

Quality, Quality Control, Quality Assurance, and Quality Management

Quality has many definitions. Even within the field, quality means different things to different people. Juran[2] defines quality as "freedom from deficiencies," thereby producing a product or service "meeting the needs of customers." Thus, Juran sees a quality product (or service) as one that is free of defects and performs those functions for which it was designed and constructed and produces client satisfaction. "Fitness for use" also describes such a product. Other definitions include the notion of conformance to specifications and/or standards, and client satisfaction at a competitive price. Producing a product that meets client needs is sometimes difficult because client needs are not always known, even by the client. Assistance may be needed to define the real needs of the client. Once these needs have been determined, they become the product specifications and, therefore, become the criteria by which the product will be evaluated.

Taylor[3] defines quality control (QC) as "a system of activities whose purpose is to control the quality of a product or service so that it meets the needs of users." Thus, a QC system is that system under which a product is tested to determine whether it meets specifications. This has been referred to as the quality function.

Suppose that some systematic error was being made in the use of the QC system. How would this error be discovered and then corrected? To ensure that the QC system is operating effectively, an additional QC system is implemented to assess the efficacy of the QC system monitoring the product. This additional control system is referred to as a quality assurance (QA) program. Thus, quality assurance could be defined as quality control on quality control.

Each sampling or laboratory organization is associated with a management system that

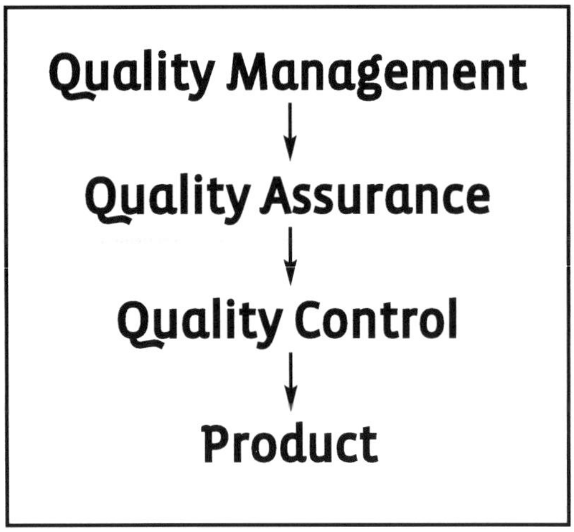

Figure 13.1 — The Quality Hierarchy.

defines the mission, goals, and values of the organization. In addition this management system provides financial systems, human resources, and administrative functions. The quality management system, a part of the overall management system, provides the policies, procedures, and organization that defines the quality assurance programs and how they interact with and are supported by the overall management system.

The quality hierarchy is pictured in Figure 13.1.

Field and Laboratory Quality Management Plan(s)

It has been said that if you don't know where you are going you will never get there. This is true of both sampling and analytical operations — there must be goals and objectives for each operation. In addition, the processes and procedures to be used, and the way these will be monitored and evaluated must be defined. The <u>management plan</u> is a written document that provides detailed policies and procedures. It may be formatted into a single document or, more often, into a manual of policies with separate standard operating procedures.

Elements of a Quality Management Plan

Following the ISO/IEC 17025:2005 Standard[4], there are 15 elements that are addressed in a management plan. These elements are:

1. Organization: This section describes how the organization is structured and how it relates to other parent or related organizations. Job descriptions and qualifications for positions within the organization are included.
2. Management System: This section outlines "top" management's commitment to the quality management system. A vital part of this section is a Quality Policy Statement that outlines management's goals, objectives, and vision for the quality management system. The policies pertinent to the system are organized in a quality (assurance) manual.
3. Document Control: An organization has many documents that describe its policies and procedures. The purpose of document control is to identify all of these documents, where they are located, how they are approved and modified, and how current they may be. Documents consist not only of the policies, procedures, forms, and so on that the organization creates but also texts, manuals, software, and similar items that have an impact on the quality of the product. It should be noted that documents and records are different. In general, documents describe how something is to be done, and records show that it was done
4. Review of Requests, Tenders, and Contracts: When a customer requests sampling or laboratory services, it is critical that the request be reviewed to ensure that the work is clearly defined, and that the organization is capable of providing the service in a manner that will meet the customer's requirements. Records of the request must be maintained as well as any subsequent clarifications or changes.
5. Subcontracting: If an organization subcontracts any activities that could impact the quality of its operations, it should be demonstrated that the subcontractor is capable of performing the work in accordance with specifications.
6. Service to the Customer: The adage "the customer is always right" is a foundation of customer service. This section of the management plan outlines the organizations commitment to the customer and their willingness to work with the customer.

7. Purchasing: Services and supplies used by the organization have a direct impact on the quality of the product. Vendors should be selected based on their ability to provide supplies and services that meet minimum quality requirements. This section describes record keeping of how vendors are selected, how supplies and services are ordered, how the quality of received supplies and services are verified, and how supplies are stored until use.
8. Control of Nonconformances: Nonconformances are events where the product or service does not meet operational or client specifications or where a process does not follow standard procedures. Nonconformances are often isolated events. This section describes how the organization should address these issues when they occur. If the investigation of a nonconformance identifies a systematic problem, then a corrective action is initiated.
9. Complaints: Complaints from customers are an indication that there may be a problem with the quality management system. Multiple, similar complaints or significant complaints may identify deficiencies in the system and should be elevated into the correction action system.
10. Improvement: The organization must be committed to continually improving its operations and have a plan for how this will be done.
11. <u>Corrective Action</u>: When significant or systematic problems are identified, the cause of the problem must be identified and a resolution put into place that will prevent the problem from occurring in the future. To find the cause of a problem, don't stop with the first answer, rather, dig into the problem and ask why several times. In some cases the cause may be obvious and, in others, obscure. The underlying cause of the problem is referred to as the "root" cause. Once the cause of a problem is identified it is easier to address and fix the problem.
12. <u>Preventive Action</u>: This is a proactive process to "fix" a problem before it occurs. It includes routine maintenance of equipment but also should include observing technical and administrative operations for potential problems and taking the steps necessary to prevent them from happening.
13. Control of Records: Records provide the history of how something was done. They need to be stored in a safe and organized manner. Records consist not only of paper forms and documents but electronic records (spreadsheets, word processing documents, email, data logs, etc.), photographs, recordings, and any other type of media.
14. Internal Audits: These provide an opportunity for the organization to evaluate their processes and procedures to ensure that they are meeting requirements (<u>systems audit</u>). They also include observation of sampling or laboratory processes to verify that they are in accordance with the approved procedures (process or procedural audit). A checklist of specific items and requirements prepared prior to the audit serves as the basis of the audit. Any deficiency identified is noted, and corrective actions are initiated to find the cause of the deficiency and make the needed corrections. All corrective actions should be entered into the organization's corrective action system. A systems audit should be conducted at least annually, whereas procedural audits may be conducted more often, if necessary, to ensure that procedures are being followed.
15. Management Reviews and Reports: At least annually, the organization's business management examines the quality management system and evaluates the effectiveness of the system in meeting the overall organizational goals. Based on this review, changes and improvements are made to the system. Regular reports to technical and business management provide short-term snapshots of how the system is operating.

In addition to the management plan, there are technical requirements that also must be met. These include:

1. Selection and Training of Personnel: The individuals performing work under the quality management plan must have been trained in all relevant aspects of the plan and in the performance of their job tasks. It is the

responsibility of the organization to ensure that personnel are able to perform their job functions correctly and effectively. Training requirements are determined based on job description, and training records are maintained.

2. Selection of Methods: The methods used for sampling or analysis must be based on sound scientific principles. Whenever possible the method selected should be one that has been published by national or international agencies and generally accepted or have been subjected to peer review. Methods should be validated to ensure acceptable performance.

   Often, an adopted standard method does not provide sufficient detail to ensure consistency in the way it is applied without further clarification and interpretation. In these instances, a standard operating procedure should be developed that describes the specific steps the organization takes to perform the method. The procedure should go through a validation process to ensure that it will work as anticipated and in accordance with the standard method.

3. Estimation of Uncertainty: Uncertainty is defined by ISO as the parameter associated with the result of a measurement that characterizes the dispersion of the values that could reasonably be attributed to the measurement.[5,6] In simpler terms, it can be regarded as how certain you are that the result is close to the true value. For example, if you measured a length of string with a ruler graduated at centimeter markings, how accurately could you report the length.

   Sources of the uncertainty should be identified and evaluated. In the ruler example, the source of uncertainty is the <u>accuracy</u> of the ruler graduations, and the uncertainty is the actual variations observed in the graduations and how well you can estimate a measurement between the graduations. In general, the sources of uncertainty in the sampling process are harder to estimate and are usually greater than those found in the laboratory.

4. Control of Data: Detailed records of all processes, observations, and measurements should be maintained. Examples include instrument adjustments, changes in supplies, sampling meteorological or environmental conditions, activities in the sampling area, details of laboratory analysis, and changes in the process being monitored.

   These records provide a history of the sampling/analysis event and allow reconstruction of the event. Records should be created at the time of the event and be maintained in an orderly manner and in a secure location. Bound notebooks, project files, and secure and backed up electronic files are examples of how these records may be maintained. All records should include the date the record was created and who created it.

   Calculations and data transfers should be verified. If possible, a second, qualified individual should perform this verification and ensure that calculations and data transfers were performed correctly. Computer programs developed by or for the user should be validated as performing properly and then secured from modification. Commercial software is normally considered validated as received from the developer; however, applications of the software may need to be validated. For example, spreadsheets should be validated, but the functions built into the program do not need to be validated.

5. Equipment and Instrumentation: The organization needs to have all of the sampling and analytical equipment and instrumentation necessary to complete the project. The equipment available must be capable of meeting all specifications and requirements of the project. <u>Calibration</u> programs should be established when output is vital to the sampling and analysis results. The calibration should be checked before and after each use.

   Personnel operating equipment should be thoroughly trained in its care, operation, and limitations. Pertinent manuals and instructions should be readily available.

6. Traceability: NIST defines traceability[7] as "the establishment of an unbroken chain of comparisons to stated references" and an unbroken chain of

comparisons to mean "the complete, explicitly described, and documented series of comparisons that successively link the value and uncertainty of a result of measurement with the values and uncertainties of each of the intermediate reference standards and the highest reference standard to which traceability for the result of measurement is claimed." The highest reference standard should be an internationally recognized standard.

7. Sampling: This is the detailed sampling plan for the organization doing the sampling. However, if laboratory personnel are involved in sampling or subsampling, the procedures they will use should be described and documented.
8. Handling of Test Items: Once samples are collected, they need to be transported to the laboratory. These requirements should also address requirements for storage of sampling media prior to sample collection, storage after sample collection, sample identification, shipping requirements (e.g., express shipping and refrigeration), and chain of custody requirements.

   At the laboratory, procedures need to be in place that address sample receipt, storage prior to analysis, identification, proper assignment to analytical groups, and retention and disposal.
9. Quality Assurance of Results: Results of tests and calibrations should be evaluated to assure compliance with requirements and specifications.
10. Reporting of Results: The results of sampling and laboratory analyses should be reported in a manner that is accurate, clear, unambiguous, and objective. Opinions and interpretations should be easily identified. The content and format of the report is dependent on the organization's normal procedures and the requirements of the customer.

The extent of elements that should be addressed may appear daunting at first. However, these can be scaled and adjusted to the size of the organization and the scope of the process(es) involved. Some elements may be eliminated, but all should be considered initially.

Elements of Quality Control

The purpose of quality control is to provide a level of assurance that the result of a process will meet specifications.

Accuracy, Bias, and Precision

The terms accuracy, bias, and precision are terms often used to describe how close a result is to the true or expected value.

According to NIST[8], *"accuracy is a qualitative term referring to whether there is agreement between a measurement made on an object and its true (target or reference) value"*, whereas, bias is a *"quantitative term describing the difference between the average of measurements made on the same object and its true value."* Bias is the difference between the average of observed results and the true value, and is determined over a period of time.

Precision is a quantitative measurement of the normal distribution of results due to the random error in the system. The term "standard error" is used to describe precision measurements. The smaller the standard error, the more precise are the measurements.

An example of these might be in the measurement of a mass. If one were to calibrate a balance against a NIST traceable weight and find that the balance reads 2% higher than the NIST traceable mass, one would say that the balance had a +2% bias. One could then correct for this bias. If they then took another mass and weighed it several times, they would have a series of readings clustered around an average. Precision is a measurement of the variability or standard error observed between the average value and the individual readings.

There are five related measures that are often used when evaluating precision. These are:

1. Range: The maximum value minus the minimum value of a measurement (often expressed as an absolute value). The relative range is the range divided by the average of the values.
2. Sample variance (s^2): Similar to range but based on the differences between the average of a series of measurements and the individual measurements. It is calculated as:

$$s^2 = \frac{\Sigma(\bar{x} - x)^2}{n - 1} \qquad (13\text{-}1)$$

Note that this is the "sample" variance calculated using $n - 1$, not the population variance (σ^2), which is calculated using n. When dealing with a series of measurements, the full population of possible measurements is seldom available. Instead, a subset, or sample, of the population is used.

3. Sample standard deviation (s): This is the square root of the variance.

$$s = \sqrt{\frac{\Sigma(\bar{x} - x)^2}{n - 1}} \qquad (13\text{-}2)$$

The standard deviation of this sampling is denoted by the symbol "s" and it is assumed that the properties (i.e., mean, median, and mode, of a normal, Gaussian, distribution) of the sample are good estimates of the properties of the population.

4. Coefficient of variation (CV): This is the standard deviation divided by the mean:

$$s = \frac{\sqrt{\dfrac{\Sigma(\bar{x} - x)^2}{n - 1}}}{\dfrac{\Sigma x}{n}} \qquad (13\text{-}3)$$

5. Standard error (SE): The estimate of expected error in the sample estimate of a population mean, or the sample standard deviation (s) divided by the square root of the sample size (n).

$$S_E = \frac{s}{\sqrt{n}} \qquad (13\text{-}4)$$

Both bias and precision are important values when evaluating a result. As illustrated in Figure 13.2, precise data may be biased and unbiased data may not be precise. The best data is data that is both unbiased and precise.

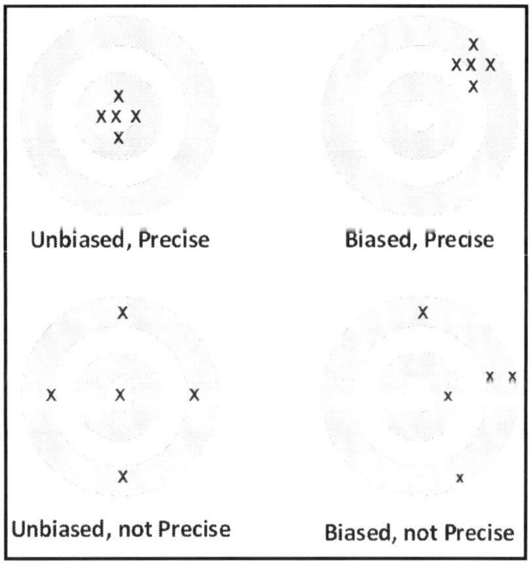

Figure 13.2 — Bias and Precision.

Quality Assurance for Sampling Activities

To be able to draw conclusions about airborne contaminant concentration, the extent to which workers have been exposed or may be exposed in the future, the efficacy of exposure controls, or for other reasons, samples must be collected properly and then analyzed properly. Since "you can't make a silk purse out of a sow's ear," the best laboratory can't improve a poorly collected sample. Sample collection and sample analysis are interrelated, and both are critical components of accurate data production.

The quality of collected samples is established by implementation of an effective management plan. Each of the items previously discussed should be carefully considered for inclusion in the plan. The management plan should be written in sufficient detail to fully describe each element and how it will be implemented.

Variability in many aspects of the sampling process is difficult to control, if even possible. Rigid adherence to written sampling methods can reduce this inherent variability. Materials used for sampling must be consistent in quality and use. Equipment and instruments used must be appropriate for the procedures employed. Some sampling equipment (e.g., sampling pumps) may lend themselves to statistical evaluations. However, due to the multitude of variables during sampling and the inability to control many of them, a full statistical evaluation becomes impractical to implement. One way to set up metrics for monitoring the sampling plan is through the use of samples that produce results that provide comparisons. These include duplicate samples, split samples, spiked samples, and blank samples.

Duplicate samples are used to evaluate the entire sampling/analysis method. Schlecht et al.[9] refers to duplicate samples as those samples collected "as close as possible to the same physical location, at identical time intervals, with approximately equal volumes sampled" as the actual samples. In other words, duplicate samples are collocated samples. Care must be taken that the duplicate samples are spatially located so that the collection of one of the duplicate samples does not affect the other. Care must be taken when evaluating the results of duplicate samples since wide variations can be observed even in closely controlled situations.[10]

Split samples, prepared by dividing a single sample into multiple portions, can be used but find limited application in industrial hygiene sampling. Bulk sampling methods (e.g., soil, water, paint), in general, lend themselves to the creation of split samples.

Spiked samples are among those most commonly used in occupational hygiene. To create a spiked sample, a known mass of contaminant is placed on the unused collection medium. A sample volume is devised to make the spike look like an actual sample. One disadvantage of this type of control sample is that there is no matrix effect (since no air is actually sampled, other compounds ordinarily collected while sampling will not be collected) like that found when analyzing an actual sample. Spiked samples must be stable under field conditions; otherwise, they are useless. The accuracy of the spiking of the samples is a factor in evaluating results from spiked samples. These samples should be prepared by an individual with extensive experience in the spiking of quality control samples.

There are several types of blank samples that can be used as controls: field blanks, transport blanks, and media blanks. A field blank is used to assess the extent to which an actual sample has been contaminated during the collection process. A field blank is treated as though it were an actual sample, that is, the field blank is handled as closely as possible to the way an actual sample is handled, except that it is not exposed to the contaminated atmosphere. The field blank should accompany the actual sample(s) through every stage of the sampling process, including transport to and from the sampling site. The mass of contaminant found on the field blank is subtracted from that found on the actual sample(s) before dividing by the air volume sampled in the determination of mass concentration of the contaminant. Each sampling method has a limit on the mass of contaminant permissible on the field blank. A contaminant mass above this limit makes the airborne concentration of contaminant found on actual samples questionable. A transport blank is similar to a field blank, but the sampler is not opened. It can be used to assess contamination of the actual sample(s) by the sample container, environmental conditions, and any preservative used during transport of the sample(s) back to the laboratory, as well as storage of the sample in the laboratory prior to analysis. A media blank is a sample of unexposed sampling media from the same lot as the samples. Often, the sampling media contain background levels of analyte or interferences. A media blank helps in the assessment of and correction for these background levels.

Written Sampling Method

Of the two processes, sampling and analysis, sampling generates the largest opportunity for variability. This is the result of several factors: the training, attitude, and attention of the person performing sampling; how representative the sample is; environmental factors, such as variability of temperature, relative humidity, barometric pressure; handling and transportation of samples from the field to the laboratory; and sample collection factors, such as variability in sampler volumetric flow, sampling time, collection efficiency, and variation in contaminant concentration during sampling.

Many organizations use methods published by national or international agencies for a designated contaminant. The method is printed out for use in the sampling project. However, methods are often not followed as written and are informally modified to suit the needs of the sampling organization; that is, these methods are modified, but no record is kept regarding the modifications made to the method. Sometimes parts of these methods are subject to interpretation, and these interpretations are usually left up to field personnel.

What is needed is a clearly written sampling method, or protocol, for use by field personnel. This usually entails taking an appropriate published method and modifying it for a specific sampling project. These modifications include specific instructions regarding assembly and use of sampling equipment (including sample labeling); conditions under which short-term and longer-term samples are collected, especially with regard to comparison of concentration data with an exposure standard, as well as personal vs. area samples; sample handling and transportation instructions; use and handling of "blank" samples; use of data forms and/or data recording devices and logbooks; decontamination processes; and data check sequences to ensure correct data transcription. This can be an involved process because every change to the published method must be reviewed for clarity, accuracy, and consistency. Opportunities for interpretation must be eliminated to the extent practicable.

Written sampling methods that are meticulously followed help to minimize this variability. Personnel performing sampling are trained to use the sampling method and are expected to understand the details of the procedure. Any necessary deviations from the written method are carefully recorded so these can be evaluated for impact on the results. Variables affecting the sampling process but which cannot be controlled during sampling are identified in the method and recorded during sampling. Procedures for equipment and instrument calibration and operation are specified and records generated at the time of performance.

Acceptable Sampling Materials

An important part of the written sampling method is the selection of sampling materials. Published methods identify the type of materials necessary for sample collection but do not generally specify the particular brands or lot numbers to be used. Whenever possible, materials should be obtained from recognized vendors who have implemented an effective quality assurance program.

It is the responsibility of the sampling organization to verify that the sampling materials are appropriate and meet the quality requirements. Materials obtained from vendors that have been approved by the sampling organization and have a proven track record are usually acceptable. Lot-specific certificates of analysis should be obtained for reagents. Sampling media should be subject to verification by lot and any available certifications obtained and maintained. If there is any question about the acceptability of the materials, they should be subjected to acceptance testing.

Sampler Calibration

A protocol for sampler calibration is an important part of the written sampling method. AIHA defines calibration as "a set of operations used to determine the accuracy of the reading of a test device to a stated uncertainty."[11] Applying this definition to flow calibration of a rotameter, for example, calibration is the process that associates the rotameter reading with a known flow rate within known limits.

Detailed records of each calibration performed include: date and time of the calibration, individual performing the calibration, model and serial numbers of all equipment involved, location, environmental conditions at the time, identification and calibration status of references, and details of calculations performed.

Together, the protocol and records provide complete traceability from the calibration, through any intermediate calibrations (e.g., calibration of an electronic bubble meter), to the appropriate international standard(s).

Portable Instruments

Portable instruments perform the same function as a laboratory. Their purpose is to provide a result that is used to make decisions. As such, they should be subject to many of the same quality assurance principles as a laboratory. Users need to be trained in the use of the instrument and be fully aware of the instrumentation capabilities and limitations. The instrument should be subject to appropriate calibrations before and after use. Maintenance intervals should be conscientiously followed. The accuracy and precision of the instrument should be determined and monitored on a regular basis. If practical, quality control samples should be analyzed regularly, and detailed records maintained.

Quality Assurance for Intralaboratory Operations

Accreditation

Accreditation is a formal recognition by a national or international authority of a laboratory's capability to perform certain testing and measurement activities. The purpose of accreditation is to provide information that will help in making informed decisions regarding laboratory selection. It demonstrates a laboratory's competence and capabilities. (AIHA Laboratory Accreditation Programs, LLC is a Full Member of the International Laboratory Accreditation Cooperation (ILAC) and a signatory (for testing) of the ILAC Mutual Recognition Arrangement (MRA).)

The AIHA® Laboratory Accreditation Program is a voluntary program. In general, the program requires a laboratory to operate a management system that is compliant with ISO/IEC Standard 17025:2005, participate in interlaboratory proficiency demonstration programs, and meet other technical requirements. Biennially, the laboratory submits an application for review and is subjected to an on-site evaluation by a qualified individual.

Laboratories that participate in this accreditation program have demonstrated an ability to perform industrial hygiene analyses. However, each sampling organization needs to perform their own evaluation of the laboratory to ascertain that the laboratory is capable of meeting the specific requirements of the sampling plan.

The Control Chart

A control chart is a graphical representation of data that is used to determine the state of a process. Walter A. Shewhart[12] is credited with having developed the technique most commonly used. The Shewhart chart is based on the normal distribution (Figure 13.3) — a symmetrical distribution in which the mean, median, and the mode all have the same value.

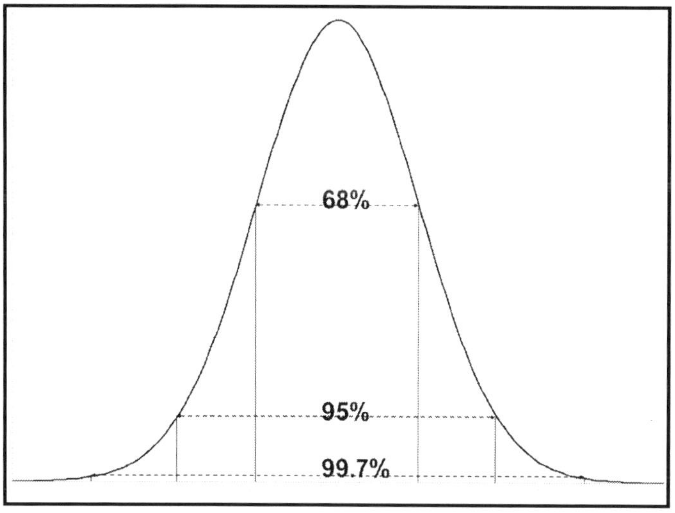

Figure 13.3 — The Normal Distribution.

Figure 13.3 shows that approximately 68% of the area under the normal distribution curve falls between the mean ±1 standard deviation (σ) approximately 95% of the area under the curve falls between the mean ±2 σ, and approximately 99.7% of the area under the curve falls between the mean ±3 σ.

The Central Limit theorem[8] declares that, for random samples of size n drawn from a population with mean μ and standard deviation σ, as n increases: (1) the mean of the sampling distribution of means approaches μ, the population mean; (2) the standard deviation of the sampling distribution of means approaches $\sigma / \sqrt{n}$, the standard error of the mean; and (3) the shape of the distribution of sampling means will approach the normal.

Referring once again to Figure 13.3, if the graph is rotated 90° and the lines that segment the distribution curve by standard deviation are extended, a control chart is formed (Figure 13.4).

The lines at $\bar{x} \pm 3s$ are called the upper control limit (UCL) and the lower control limit (LCL). The lines at $\bar{x} \pm 2s$ are the upper and lower warning limits. The line at $\bar{x}$ is called the Center Line. It is important to note here that QC data (like spike recoveries, check samples, and so on) are plotted on the control chart, not sample data.

It is not unusual for QC samples to be prepared at different values. To accommodate this, a common practice is to convert the found values for QC samples to recoveries (found divided by theoretical). The recovery value for each QC sample is then used to con-

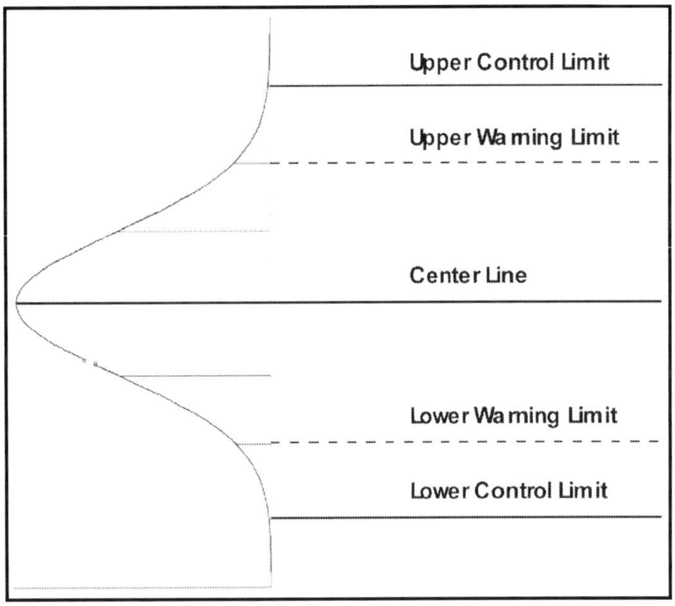

Figure 13.4 — Control Chart.

struct the control chart.

According to Shewhart:[8]

"It has also been observed that a person would seldom if ever be justified in concluding that a state of statistical control of a given repetitive operation or production process has been reached until he had obtained, under presumably the same essential conditions, a sequence of not less than twenty-five samples of size four that are in control."

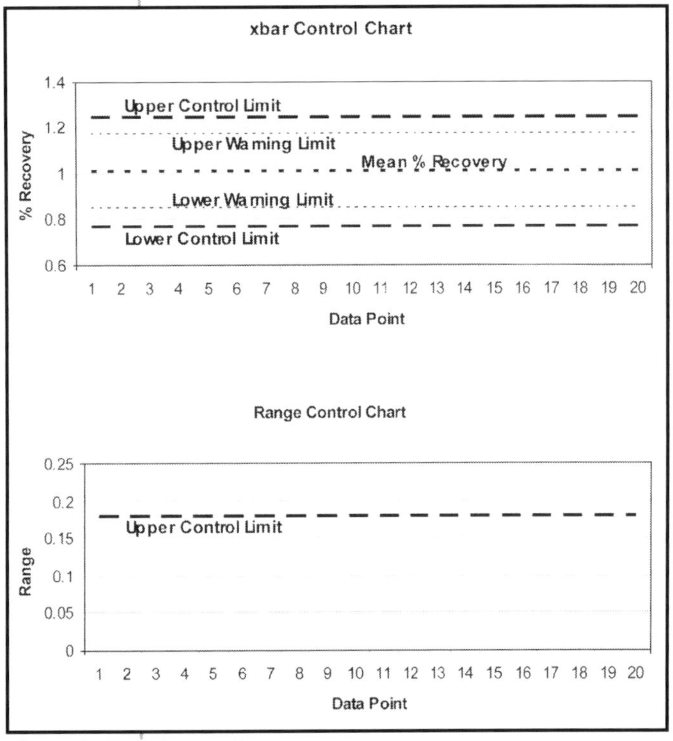

Figure 13.5 — xbar-R Chart.

Based on this rule of thumb, approximately 100 data points would need to be collected from a process that is in statistical control in order to calculate reliable control limits. In most situations, this would require a substantial amount of time to collect sufficient data. There needs to be a way to generate a control chart on significantly less data.

In a data-producing system there are two general types of variability: (1) that coming from assignable (or determinate) causes — systematic error, and (2) that coming from unassignable (indeterminate) causes — random error. A process is in a state of statistical control when all causes of systematic error have been minimized or eliminated, leaving only random error. Control chart data inform the user of the state of process quality with respect to systematic error over a specified time. For this reason, control charts should be updated regularly. The data used to calculate the control chart is then projected forward and is the basis for evaluation of future data points.

Two control charts are needed to evaluate the state of control of a particular analytical process. One control chart is needed to deal with bias, and another is needed to deal with precision. Since bias is related to central tendency, a common type of control chart for bias plots is a means ($\bar{x}$ or *x*bar) chart. Precision is a measure of variability, and it is commonly monitored by the use of a range ($\overline{R}$) chart. The combination of charts is referred to as an xbar-R chart (an *x*bar and R chart, Figure 13.5). Range has been used historically in statistical quality control because it is easy to calculate, and it can be related to the standard deviation; however, with computerized systems it is generally easy to calculate and use standard deviations when larger data sets are involved. Historically, control charts have been printed and examined visually. Databases now allow these evaluations to be performed by computer systems. Modern information management systems can automatically transfer data from instrumentation and perform these quality control evaluations without operator intervention. Visual presentations are still of great value, though, when evaluating out of control situations or process anomalies.

Evaluating Bias — The Control Chart

One way to calculate initial control limits is to use a limited data set and apply a factor to the data to account for the size of the data set. This approach relies on the mean of a data set (≤ 10 samples) as an estimator of the standard deviation adjusted with a multiplicative factor (d_2) that is a function of the number of data points in the set. To estimate a 3s control limit, the value of s is estimated to be $\overline{R} / d_2 \sqrt{n}$. To simplify the calculation of 3*s* the parameter A_2 is defined as $3 / d_2 \sqrt{n}$. Values for d_2 and A_2, and D_4 (which will be used later) are presented in Table 13.1.

Table 13.1 — Initial Control Chart Factors[8]

Number of Points in Data Set	d_2	A_2	D_4
2	1.128	1.880	3.267
3	1.693	1.023	2.575
4	2.059	0.729	2.282
5	2.326	0.577	2.115
6	2.534	0.483	2.004
7	2.704	0.419	1.924
8	2.847	0.373	1.864
9	2.970	0.337	1.816
10	3.078	0.308	1.777

Control limits are calculated using the following formulas:

$$UCL = \bar{x} + A_2 \times \overline{R} \quad (13\text{-}5)$$

$$LCL = \bar{x} - A_2 \times \overline{R} \quad (13\text{-}6)$$

where $\bar{x}$ is the mean recovery for the data, and is the range of the recoveries.

As an example, initial analysis of spiked samples for hexavalent chromium (Cr^{+6}) by OSHA method ID-215 yielded the data in Table 13.2.

Table 13.2 — Initial Spike Data

Sample	*Found (mg)*	*Theoretical (mg)*	*Recovery*
1	8.4250	8.9654	0.9397
2	6.2790	6.7477	0.9305
3	4.1980	4.4732	0.9385
4	8.1890	8.7947	0.9311
5	6.1100	6.5771	0.9290
6	4.0200	4.2458	0.9468
Average Recovery			0.9359
Range of Recovery			0.0178

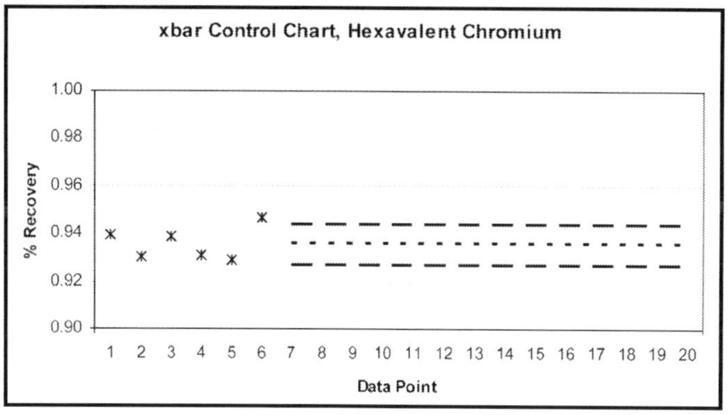

Figure 13.6 — Initial xbar Control Chart.

Since we have six data points (two groups of three), the value of A_2 from Table 13.1 is 0.483. The calculations then become:

$$UCL = 0.9359 + 0.483 \times 0.0178 = 0.944$$

$$LCL = 0.9359 - 0.483 \times 0.0178 = 0.927$$

Figure 13.6 is the control chart generated from this data. Note that this chart demonstrates a known low bias in this method.

As data is collected, more than 10 points become available for the calculation (Table 13.3). At this point, the standard deviation of the data set can replace the range based estimate.

Table 13.3 — Additional Spike Data.

Sample	*Found (mg)*	*Theoretical (mg)*	*Recovery*
1	8.4250	8.9654	0.9397
2	6.2790	6.7477	0.9305
3	4.1980	4.4732	0.9385
4	8.1890	8.7947	0.9311
5	6.1100	6.5771	0.9290
6	4.0200	4.2458	0.9468
7	7.0670	8.5484	0.8267
8	5.9840	6.4824	0.9231
9	4.1110	4.2079	0.9770
10	7.7620	8.2641	0.9392
11	6.1130	6.4824	0.9430
12	3.8900	4.0751	0.9546
Average Recovery			0.9316
Standard Deviation(s) of Recovery			0.0359

The control limits are now calculated using the formula $\bar{x} \pm 3s$ to give the following:

$$UCL = 0.9316 + 3 \times 0.0359 = 1.0393$$

$$LCL = 0.9316 - 3 \times 0.0359 = 0.8239$$

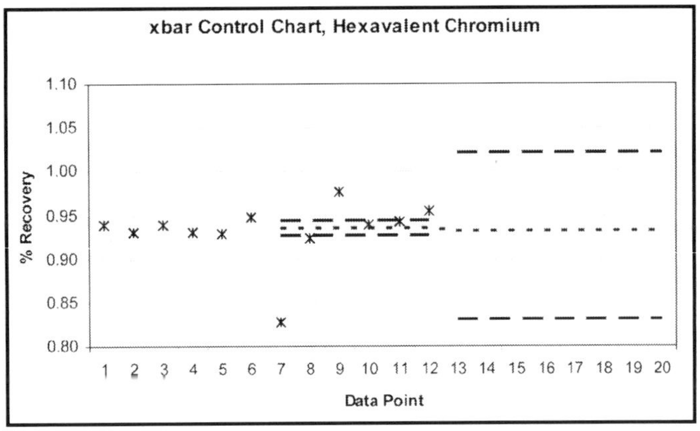

Figure 13.7 — *x*bar Control Chart with 12 Data Points.

Note the recovery for several of the samples above the UCL or below the LCL initially calculated, in particular, the recovery for Sample 7. This point could have been discarded for being significantly outside the control limits. However, since there is very limited data at this point, it should be included unless a substantial reason for the low value is available (e.g., the sample had been spilled during preparation). As more data is collected, the impact of individual points on the full data set will be minimized.

After a total of 24 data points have been collected, the control limits become:

$$UCL = 0.9283 + 3 \times 0.0324 = 1.0255$$

$$LCL = 0.9283 - 3 \times 0.0324 = 0.8311$$

This process is continued until 100 spiked samples have been analyzed.

Evaluating Precision — The $\overline{R}$ or s Control Chart

An $\overline{R}$ or *s* control chart is used to evaluate the precision of a process. Control limits are calculated using the range or *s* of the spiked samples data collected each time the process is run. In industrial hygiene, there are usually only two spiked samples analyzed per run with a single analysis of each sample. The spiked samples are prepared at similar theoretical values. The range (R) of the analysis becomes $recovery_1 - recovery_2$. Table 13.4 shows an example.

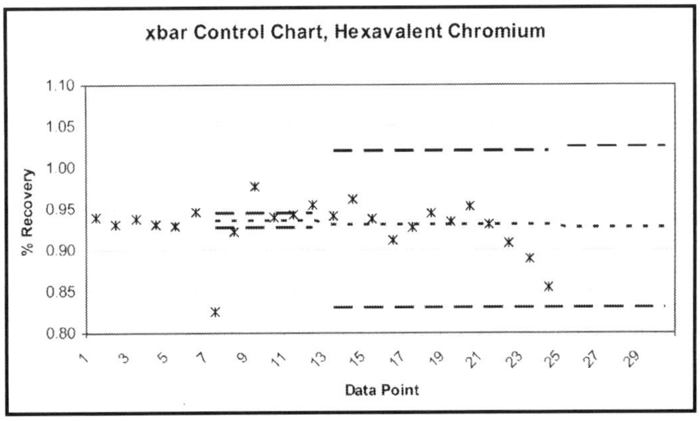

Figure 13.8 — *x*bar Control Chart with 24 Data Points.

Table 13.4 — Initial Precision Data.

Run	*Recovery$_1$*	*Recovery$_2$*	*Range*
1	0.9397	0.9311	0.0086
2	0.9305	0.9290	0.0015
3	0.9385	0.9468	-0.0083
Average Range			0.0006
Range of the Range			0.0169

Using the factor in Table 13.1 for three data points the control limits can be calculated as:

$$UCL = 0.0006 + 0.729 \times 0.0169 = 0.013$$

$$LCL = 0.0006 - 0.729 \times 0.0169 = -0.012$$

When more than 10 sets of data are obtained, the range based estimate can be replaced with the sample standard deviation (*s*).

Table 13.5 — Additional Precision Data.

Run	*Recovery$_1$*	*Recovery$_2$*	*Range*
1	0.9397	0.9311	0.0086
2	0.9305	0.9290	0.0015
3	0.9385	0.9468	-0.0083
4	0.8267	0.9421	-0.1154
5	0.9231	0.9623	-0.0392
6	0.9770	0.9375	0.0395
7	0.9392	0.9118	0.0274
8	0.9430	0.9280	0.0150
9	0.9546	0.9454	0.0092
10	0.9349	0.9083	0.0266
11	0.9527	0.8904	0.0623
12	0.9316	0.8557	0.0759
Average Range			0.0086
Standard Deviation of the Range			0.0496

$$UCL = 0.0086 + 3 \times 0.0496 = 0.1574$$

$$LCL = 0.0086 + 3 \times 0.0496 = -0.1402$$

It can be argued that, for industrial hygiene, the order of the recoveries carries little meaning, unlike a manufacturing process where the order may be meaningful. This lends itself to an approach using the absolute value of the range instead of maintaining the sign. With this approach there is no center line or lower control limit, the base line for the control chart is zero, and the upper control limit is calculated using the absolute value of the range. Table 6 shows this approach using the data from Table 13.5.

Table 13.6 — Additional Precision Data — Absolute Value of Range.

Run	*Recovery*$_1$	*Recovery*$_2$	*/Range/*
1	0.9397	0.9311	0.0086
2	0.9305	0.9290	0.0015
3	0.9385	0.9468	0.0083
4	0.8267	0.9421	0.1154
5	0.9231	0.9623	0.0392
6	0.9770	0.9375	0.0395
7	0.9392	0.9118	0.0274
8	0.9430	0.9280	0.0150
9	0.9546	0.9454	0.0092
10	0.9349	0.9083	0.0266
11	0.9527	0.8904	0.0623
12	0.9316	0.8557	0.0759
Average Range			0.0357
Standard Deviation of the Range			0.0339

The upper control limit becomes:

$$UCL = 0 + 3 \times 0.0339 = 0.1017$$

Evaluating Control Charts

Laboratories have an ethical and often legal obligation to produce data that are unbiased and precise. This requires the laboratory to be in a known state of statistical control. The control chart simplifies the evaluation of a process.

In 1956, Western Electric Company published a quality control handbook that has become a basis for statistical process control. This handbook provided a series of statistically derived rules (WECO Rules) that may be used to evaluate a control chart for an "out of control" situation. To apply these rules, additional limits need to be added to a control chart at ±1*s* and ±2*s*, in addition to the ±3*s* control limits. The rules define an out of control situation as any of the following[8]:

1. Any point that is more than ±3*s* from the mean.
2. Any two of three consecutive points are more than ±2*s* from the mean.
3. Any four out of five consecutive points are more than ±1*s* from the mean.
4. Any eight consecutive points that are on the same side of the mean.

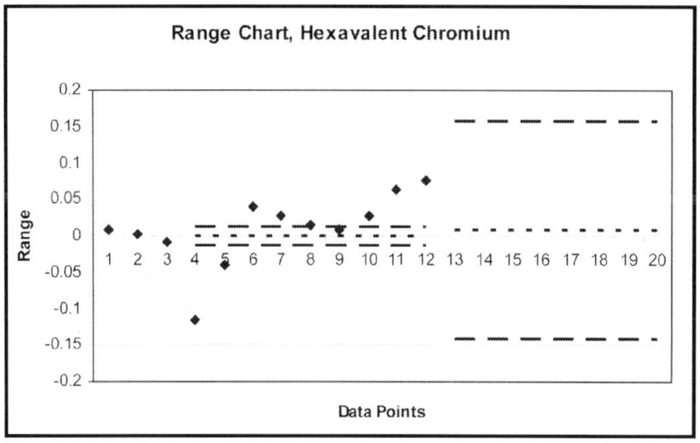

Figure 13.9 — Range Control Chart.

Two additional "trend rules" are also included:

5. Six consecutive points in a row that trend up or down.
6. Fourteen consecutive points in a row that alternate up and down.

An out of control situation, as defined by rules, does not necessarily mean that the process is out of statistical control. Since the rules are based on probability, there is always a possibility of a "false alarm." Based on WECO Rule #1, there is a probability, on the average, of a false alarm every 371 points. Adding all of the WECO rules increases this probability to once every 91.75 points.[8] Whenever an out of control is flagged, the situation needs to receive further evaluation. Often these situations include non-statistical errors that should be excluded from the data set.

In addition to established rules, simple visual evaluation of a control chart can also

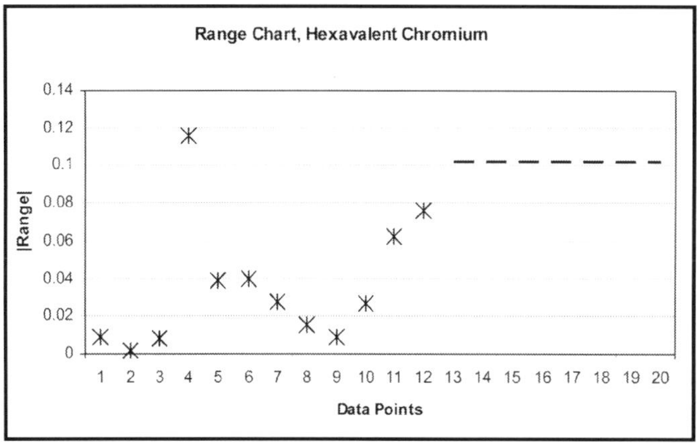

Figure 13.10 — Range Control Chart Using Absolute Value of Range.

provide information that may be missed by automated systems. These include long-term cycles, such as seasonal changes, and long-term drift that causes a mean to slowly increase or decrease.

Outliers are data points that do not appear to conform to the normal distribution. In referring to outliers, the following quotation expresses concisely the nature of, and concerns about, these data.

> *In almost every true series of observations, some are found, which differ so much from the others as to indicate some abnormal source of error not contemplated in the theoretical discussions, and the introduction of which into the investigations can only serve . . . to perplex and mislead the inquirer.*[13]

It is interesting that this quotation was made almost 150 years ago, and seemingly, outlier data was a concern even then. Now, it is recognized that outliers do not necessarily "perplex" or "mislead," nor are they necessarily "bad" or "erroneous." In some instances researchers may not reject them; they may even welcome them as unexpectedly useful.

An outlier is defined as a data point that "appears to be markedly different from other members of the sample in which it occurs."[14] Notice the use of the word "appears." One should be very careful in deciding that a piece of data may be an outlier. For one reason, the data in question could be an extreme value in the distribution. It could be also that the data results from some gross deviation from the analytical method used, or a mathematical blunder. So, before assuming that some questionable data is outlying, one may wish to investigate the process and the calculations first. If there is no apparent deviation from the method, and if the calculations were completed correctly, it may be that the data in question are outlying. Outlier data are neither discarded nor deleted. These data are flagged in some appropriate manner then not used in calculations.

Three ways to handle outlier data are the Dixon Ration test, the Grubbs test, and Huber's method. Statistical texts include numerous other approaches that also may be appropriate.

The Dixon Ratio test[15] is one that can be used to detect a single outlying datum. It is easy to use and the calculations are simple. It is only used to remove a single data point from the data set, it is not repeated. The Dixon Ratio test assumes an underlying normal distribution of data. To perform the test (1) rank the data in ascending order, X_1 (lowest) to X_n (highest); (2) select the significance level for rejection; (3) calculate the Dixon Ratio (Tables 13.10 and 13.11 show Dixon Ratio information and calculations); (4) look up the critical value for the appropriate r-value in the Dixon Ratio table (Table 13.12); and (5) if the $r_{calculated} > r_{table}$ for the confidence level selected in Step 2 above, conclude that the suspect point is an outlier; otherwise, retain the data point.

Table 13.7 — Dixon Ratio Information.

Number of Data Points	*Ratio to be Calculated*
3 to 7	r_{10}
8 to 10	r_{11}
11 to 13	r_{21}
14 to 25	r_{22}

Table 13.8 — Dixon Ratio Calculations.

r	*If X_n is Suspect*	*If X_1 is Suspect*
r_{10}	$(X_n - X_{n-1})/(X_n - X_1)$	$(X_2 - X_1)/(X_n - X_1)$
r_{11}	$(X_n - X_{n-1})/(X_n - X_2)$	$(X_2 - X_1)/(X_{n-1} - X_1)$
r_{21}	$(X_n - X_{n-2})/(X_n - X_2)$	$(X_3 - X_1)/(X_{n-1} - X_1)$
r_{22}	$(Xn - X_{n-2})/(X_n - X_3)$	$(X_3 - X_1)/(X_{n-2} - X_1)$

The Grubb's test is another method to delete outlier data. This test can be repeated on the data set after removing a data point. Due to the complexity of the calculations, this test is usually performed using a statistical software package.

The mean ($\bar{x}$) and standard deviation (*s*) of the data set are first calculated. The test statistic, G, is calculated for a single point (*x*) using the equation:

$$G = \frac{|x - \bar{x}|}{s} \qquad (13\text{-}7)$$

The test statistic is calculated based on the number of points in the data set (*N*) and the significance (α) of the test (a value of 0.1 is often used) using the equation:

Table 13.9 — Values for Use in the Dixon Ratio Test.

Statistic	*Number of Observations*	*Risk of False Rejection* 0.5%	1%	5%	10%
r10	3	0.994	0.988	0.941	0.886
	4	0.926	0.889	0.765	0.679
	5	0.821	0.780	0.642	0.557
	6	0.740	0.698	0.560	0.482
	7	0.680	0.637	0.507	0.434
r11	8	0.725	0.683	0.554	0.479
	9	0.677	0.635	0.512	0.441
	10	0.639	0.597	0.477	0.409
r21	11	0.713	0.679	0.576	0.517
	12	0.675	0.642	0.546	0.490
	13	0.649	0.615	0.521	0.467
r22	14	0.674	0.641	0.546	0.492
	15	0.647	0.616	0.525	0.472
	16	0.624	0.595	0.507	0.454
	17	0.605	0.577	0.490	0.438
	18	0.589	0.561	0.475	0.424
	19	0.575	0.547	0.462	0.412
	20	0.562	0.535	0.450	0.401

$$G_{test} = \frac{(N-1)}{\sqrt{N}} \sqrt{\frac{t^2(\alpha / 2N, N-2)}{N-2+t^2(\alpha / 2N, N-2)}} \quad (13\text{-}8)$$

where $t(\alpha/2N, N-2)$ is the critical value of the *t*-distribution with N–2 degrees of freedom and a significance level of α / 2N.

If $G > G_{test}$, the point may be excluded from further calculations.

The test is started using the point with the greatest deviation from the mean of the data set. It is then repeated for the point with the next greatest deviation until a point is not discarded. On small data sets (<10) it is possible to eliminate points that should be included.

Huber's method[16] utilizes a process called winsorization to estimate the mean ($\bar{x}$) and standard deviation (s) of the data set. For this method, the $\bar{x}$ and s of the data set are calculated. Any value that is greater than $\bar{x} + 1.5s$ is replaced with $\bar{x} + 1.5s$. Likewise, a value smaller than $\bar{x} - 1.5s$ is replaced with $\bar{x} - 1.5s$. The $\bar{x}$ and standard deviation s of the data set of the winsorized data set is then calculated. This process is repeated until it converges to an acceptable degree of accuracy, and the Huber mean ($\bar{x}_{Hub}$) and standard deviation (s_{Hub}) are obtained.

Other Types of Control Charts

The Shewhart *x*bar-R control chart has become a standard in the industrial hygiene laboratory. It is easy to understand; trends can be often be seen visually, and the chart can be constructed using readily available software or spreadsheets or even by hand. However, it does have limitations and may not be the best chart for all applications. In these instances, other types of control charts may be more applicable. For example, an Individuals and Moving Range (ImR or XmR) chart may be used to monitor precision when only a single quality control sample is included in each run, for example, a control chart that monitors the results of an initial calibration verification standard.

An ImR chart monitors the mean recovery of the QC parameter as an xbar chart. The precision is then monitored on a moving range (mR) chart. This is done by calculating the moving range: for each point in the chart the moving range is the absolute value of the difference between the point and the immediately preceding point, as in Table 6. The mean of the ranges and the mean of the individuals are calculated. The control limit is calculated as:

$$UCL = \overline{R} \times D_4 \quad (13\text{-}9)$$

Since the range is calculated from two points, the value of D_4 is selected from Table 13.1, Initial Control Chart Factors, for n=2 (2.575). Using the data in Table 10, the following can be calculated and charted (Figure 13.10):

	$s = 3.57$	$\bar{x} = 100.4$
For Recovery:	UCL = 104.0	
	LCL = 96.8	
For Moving Range:	$\overline{R} = 4.1$	
	UCL = 10.6	

Table 13.10 — Moving Range.

Recovery	*Moving Range*
99.2	—
98.4	0.8
99.2	0.8
102.9	3.7
97.9	5.0
96.4	1.5
101.8	5.4
109.4	7.6
98.6	10.8
98.0	0.6
101.2	3.2
107.6	6.4
96.9	10.7
100.7	3.8
101.9	1.2
98.9	3.0
97.8	1.1

Care must be taken when interpreting this chart, since an out of control situation can be caused by the point, the previous point, or a combination of the two. In addition, the WECO rules cannot be applied to this type of chart.

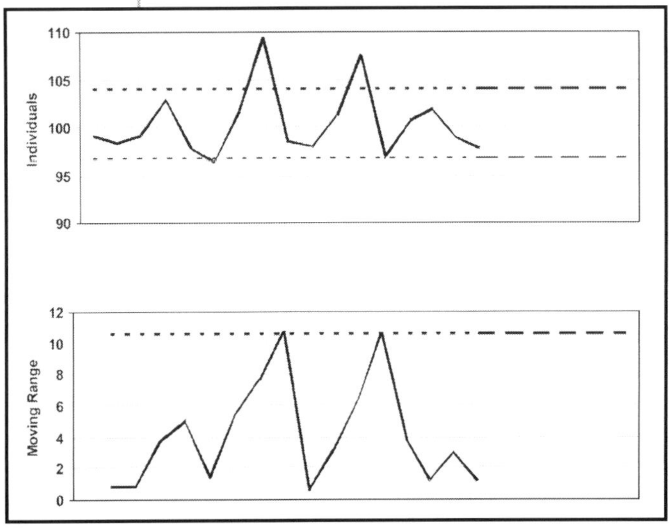

Figure 13.11 — ImR Control Chart.

Evaluating Laboratory Methods

Most methods used in industrial hygiene include instructions for both sampling and laboratory analysis. These methods have been subjected to various validation protocols prior to being published. Few organizations have the resources to subject a sampling method to a full validation, since this involves collecting samples from simulated workplace atmospheres. Thus, the sampling part of the method is often accepted as published and then evaluated further based on field studies and comparison with other methods. The laboratory portion of the method should be validated for the analytes, instrumentation, and procedures involved. In particular, it should be demonstrated that each laboratory is capable of performing the method and achieving results that are comparable with the criteria specified in the method. This is generally done through preparation of spiked samples followed by processing in accordance with the laboratory's standard operating procedures.

The instrumentation, equipment, and supplies available in a given laboratory are usually different from those used to develop and validate a method. As laboratory science advances, new equipment and instrumentation is adopted by laboratories. These and other factors result in a laboratory modifying a published method. Whenever a method is modified, the impact of the modification should be evaluated.

Assume that a laboratory has modified a method for the analysis of toluene by gas chromatography by using a new type of column. Does the modified method produce accurate (unbiased) data when compared with the original method? One rigorous approach to this uses the following steps. This approach may also be used when a laboratory implements a standard method and validates their procedure against the published data.

Step 1. Make the following decisions.

- What is α? (α is the Type I error; in this case, the risk of concluding the method is biased when it is not. A typical value for α is 0.05.)

- What is β? (β is the Type II error; in this case, the risk of concluding the method is accurate when it is not. A typical value for β is 0.10.)
- What is the MDB? (MDB is the minimum detectable bias; if the method produces data equal to or greater than the MDB, it should be detected with (1–β) probability. The value used for MDB is typically 0.5 to 2 times the standard deviation.)
- What is σ_{TEST}? (σ_{TEST} is the standard deviation of the unmodified method. If a laboratory is implementing a standard method, the value of σ_{TEST} is the published standard deviation for the analytical portion of the method.)
- What is the standard concentration to be used to determine method accuracy?

Step 2. Determine how many tests must be performed.

$$MDB = \frac{z \bullet \sigma_{TEST}}{\sqrt{N}} \qquad (13\text{-}10)$$

Where $z = (z\alpha/2 + z\beta)$. (Note: z is a z-score found in z tables in any statistics text.)

Rearranging, $n = \dfrac{z^2 \cdot \sigma^2_{TEST}}{MDB^2}$

If n is not an integer, round it up.

Step 3. Perform the calculated number of tests.

Step 4. Determine $\bar{x}$, the average of the n tests.

Step 5. Determine the method precision for n tests, $\sigma x = \sigma_{TEST} / \sqrt{n}$

Step 6. Compare x with the standard concentration. If x is within units of the standard concentration, conclude that the method is accurate. If not, then conclude the method is biased.

For example, consider the following: α = 0.05, β = 0.10, σ_{TEST} = 4 ppb, MDB = 2 ppb (0.5 σ_{TEST}), standard concentration = 10 ppb. Determine the (1–α)% confidence interval on the mean: $\bar{x} \pm t_{(\alpha/2,n-1)}\, s / \sqrt{n}$. If the interval contains the known value and is not "too wide," assume the test is accurate.

$$n = \frac{z^2 \bullet \sigma^2_{TEST}}{MDB^2} = \frac{(1.96 + 1.282)^2 \bullet 4^2}{2^2} = 42.04$$

So, 43 tests of the 10 ppb standard should be made. Assume that 43 analyses were performed on the 10 ppb standard, and that the mean concentration reported for those 43 tests was 9.62 ppb.

$$\sigma_x = \sigma_{TEST} / \sqrt{n} = 4 \text{ ppb} / \sqrt{43} = 0.61 \text{ ppb}$$

$$\bar{x} \pm z_{a/2} \bullet \sigma_{\bar{x}} = 9.63 \pm 1.96 \bullet 0.61 = 9.62 \pm 1.20 = 8.42 \text{ to } 10.82 \text{ ppb}$$

Since the range 8.42 ppb to 10.82 ppb contains the standard concentration (10 ppb), the method is not biased.

If the laboratory was implementing NIOSH method 1501 for toluene, the value for σ_{TEST} from the method is 0.022, and the calculation becomes:

$$\sigma_{\bar{x}} = 9.62 \pm (1.96)(0.022) = 9.62 \pm 0.04 = 9.42 \text{ to } 10.02 \text{ ppb}$$

As in the previous example, the standard concentration is within the range; therefore the conclusion is that the laboratory implementation of the method is not biased.

Reporting Results

The laboratory test report must provide the customer with the information necessary to make informed decisions. The report must clearly identify both the laboratory and the customer. Pertinent observations must be noted. The results must represent both the validity and accuracy of the analysis.

Reporting Limits

AIHA® defines the reporting limit as "the lowest concentration of analyte in a sample that can be reported with a defined, reproducible level of certainty." There are many approaches to the determination of a reporting limit, and there are also many related terms that may be confused with a reporting limit.

Environmental chemistry utilizes three "limits" that may clarify (or add confusion to) the definition of a reporting limit.[17]

- Critical Limit: This is the lowest measured concentration above which one can confidently assert that the analyte has been detected.

- Detection Limit: The lowest concentration at or above which an analyte can confidently be distinguished from zero. Thus, the detection limit defines the lowest concentration at which the measurement signal consistently emerges from the noise.
- Quantitation Limit: The lowest concentration at which there is some confidence that the reported measurement is relatively close to the true value.

A method detection limit (MDL)[(18)] is commonly determined as 3.14*s*, where *s* is the standard deviation of seven samples spiked near the expected MDL. This limit can be considered a critical limit or, possibly, a detection limit.

In industrial hygiene laboratories, the reporting limit is often similar to a quantitation limit. However, in many instances, the analyte concentrations that are of concern in a workplace are substantially higher than the instrument is capable of quantifying. Therefore, it is common for a laboratory to adopt a reporting limit that is higher than a quantitation limit they could achieve. One approach to demonstrating that the laboratory's reporting limit can be supported is:

- Review the regulatory or other exposure limits and the customer's requirements and select a tentative reporting limit.
- Determine an acceptable recovery range for the reporting limit (e.g., ±25%).
- Prepare multiple spiked samples at or below this reporting limit.
- Analyze the samples using the specified laboratory procedure.
- Evaluate the results against the acceptance criteria.

If the sample results are within the acceptance criteria, the laboratory has demonstrated that they are able to achieve the reporting limit. If they are not within criteria, the analytical process must be examined and adjusted, or it may be necessary to raise the desired reporting limit to a level where the acceptance criteria can be met.

Once a reporting limit has been established, the laboratory should verify that it can be achieved by analysis of a calibration sample in each run that represents a value at or below the reporting limit.

Significant Figures

It is the responsibility of a laboratory to report results that reflect the "true" value. The number of significant figures presented in a reported value implies the precision that can be attributed to the result. The following are general rules that apply to the determination of the number of significant figures in a result:

- In a calculation, the least precise measurement determines the number of significant figures.
- All digits are retained during the calculation and the final result is rounded to the appropriate number of significant digits.
- In a result: (all examples have four significant figures)
  - All non-zero digits are significant (1234, 1.234).
  - Leading zeros are not significant. (001234, 0.01234).
  - Zeros between non-zero digits are significant (1002, 1.002).
  - Trailing zeros to the right of a decimal are significant (0.01230).
  - Trailing zeros in a number without a decimal may or may not be significant (12300 may have three, four, or five significant figures).
  - Scientific notation eliminates potential confusion (1.230×10^4 has four significant figures).

When considering the measurements that go into a laboratory analysis, it may be difficult to justify more than two or possibly three significant figures in a result.

Uncertainty

There are two types of error that contribute to uncertainty: random errors and biases. Biases are usually the result of contributors than can be corrected or minimized. These include errors in calibration of standards and references by other laboratories, reproducible errors in the preparation of calibration materials and samples, environmental conditions, and incorrect procedures. The contribution of these is often observed as an overall average deviation on the process control charts from the theoretical midline. Random errors are the result of contributors that cannot be corrected. These include errors due to normal instrument variability, inability to precisely repeat a process, uncontrollable environmental contributors, unknown contributors, and human variability.

Theoretically, biases are corrected during the analytical process. For instance, a purchased standard material with a nominal 1000 ppm value may have a certified value of 990 ppm. The laboratory calculations can be adjusted to account for this -1% bias. The summation of any uncorrected bias in a controlled system will usually appear as a shift from the control chart mid-line.

Random error is the prominent contributor to the precision control chart. It can be measured but cannot be corrected.

Laboratory analytical error is a combination of both random error and uncorrected bias. In the approach used by OSHA,[19] the $\bar{x}$ control chart provides a basis for estimating the analytical error. The chart is generated from spiked samples analyzed concurrently with the field samples. Ideally, the spiked samples are prepared from known sources of the analyte that are independent of the calibration materials, have a known bias, and have been corrected for the bias. The data is calculated as the value reported by the analysis divided by the theoretical value for the spike. Thus, this recovery value (found/theoretical) incorporates both the random error of the analysis and the uncorrected biases.

The focus of many industrial hygiene projects is to determine if a specified contaminant concentration has exceeded the exposure limit. Because of this focus, the lower control limit is of little concern, and our attention is on the upper control limit. This allows us to only consider the upper part (>$\bar{x}$) of the normal distribution (Figure 13.12). The formula for the calculation of the analytical error is:

$$\text{Analytical Error} = 1.645\sqrt{(SD / \bar{x})^2}$$

In the sampling process, the calibration check of a sampling pump's flow is usually required to be within ±5% of the initial calibration. This error can be added to the analytical error to arrive at a sampling analytical error (SAE) calculated using the formula:

$$SAE = 1.645\sqrt{(SD / \bar{x})^2 + 0.050^2}$$

This SAE is expressed in terms of a coefficient of variation (CV) and may be used to construct control limits when applied to a value that is expressed in similar terms. When comparing to an exposure limit the needed ratio can be obtained by dividing the analytical result by the exposure limit. The SAE is then added to the ratio to obtain the upper control limit or subtracted to obtain the lower control limit.

$$UCL = \frac{result}{limit} + SAE$$

$$LCL = \frac{result}{limit} - SAE$$

The question becomes: Has the exposure limit been exceeded? There are three possible answers to this question:

1. The reported value is above the UCL, therefore it has been exceeded.
2. The reported value is below the LCL, therefore it has not been exceeded.
3. The reported value is between the LCL and the UCL, and it is not possible to say definitely it has either been exceeded or not exceeded. Therefore, it must be assumed that the exposure limit may not have been exceeded.

Interlaboratory Quality Assurance

Ideally the result from the analysis of a sample would be the same regardless of the laboratory where the sample was analyzed. However, just as there is variability within a laboratory, there is variability between

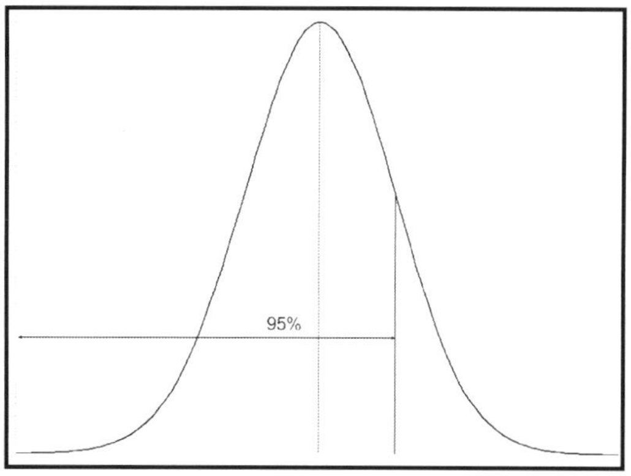

Figure 13.12 — One-sided Confidence Limit.

laboratories. The determination of this variability is an expensive task, both financially and in other resources. Fortunately there are approaches to evaluating interlaboratory analytical performance that can reduce these costs.

One of the benefits of a laboratory accreditation program is that the costs associated with conducting an interlaboratory quality assurance program are diffused throughout the customer base of the participating laboratories. AIHA® has operated an industrial hygiene laboratory accreditation program since 1974. Though it does not guarantee absolute consistency, it does require that participating laboratories perform in accordance with internationally recognized standards. Laboratories participate in interlaboratory testing programs to demonstrate general competency. AIHA® operates proficiency testing programs for laboratories analyzing organics (gas chromatography); metals (spectroscopy); silica (X-ray diffraction, infrared, or colorimetric); fibers (phase contrast microscopy); and asbestos (polarized light microscopy). Participation in these programs is not limited to accredited laboratories. Laboratories that are not able to maintain a proficient rating in a program should closely examine their internal policies and procedures, since this is indicative of a systematic problem.

There are several schemes for the evaluation of small groups of laboratories. One common approach is the establishment of a round-robin between the laboratories. The details of how such a program is operated should be outlined in a written procedure available to and accepted by all of the participants. This procedure should include:

- How samples are prepared and distributed to the participants, including a schedule.
- Number of samples prepared (four or more for each analyte/matrix combination are recommended).
- Any limitations on analytical methodology.
- The statistical treatment of the data.
- How the results of the round-robin are reported to the participants.

Data from the round-robin can be evaluated using techniques similar to those employed in a laboratory's internal quality assurance program.

One method that can be used to assess laboratory-to-laboratory variability is what has come to be known as the Youden test.[20] In this test, participating laboratories are sent several of the same samples for analysis. Each laboratory reports the data to the coordinating laboratory for statistical analysis. Each laboratory is ranked for each sample. If seven labs participate in a round-robin, the laboratory with the lowest reported concentration for a given sample is given a "1" and the highest is given a "7." Ranking is performed for each sample. When ranking is complete, scores are totaled and compared with Youden's table. This table produces a score range: lab scores lower than the lower limit of this range are biased low; labs with scores higher than the upper limit are biased high. Examine the data set in Table 13.14 for three labs and seven samples.

Table 13.11 — Example Data Set — Three Labs, Seven Samples

	Lab 1	*Lab 2*	*Lab 3*
Raw Data			
Sample 1	11.6	15.3	21.1
Sample 2	11.0	14.8	20.8
Sample 3	21.0	10.8	15.0
Sample 4	15.0	10.8	20.6
Sample 5	14.9	11.2	20.7
Sample 6	21.3	24.9	24.9
Sample 7	18.8	20.2	25.5
Ranked Data			
Sample 1	1	2	3
Sample 2	1	2	3
Sample 3	1	2	3
Sample 4	2	1	3
Sample 5	2	1	3
Sample 6	1	2	3
Sample 7	1	2	3
Total	9	12	21

The Youden table[15] shown in Table 13.12 gives the approximate 5% two-tailed limits for ranking scores.

The approximate 5% limits for three laboratories analyzing seven samples are 8 and 20. Laboratories scoring between 8 and 20 are not significantly different. A laboratory scoring lower than 8 is biased low, and one scoring greater than 20 is biased high. Based on the data in Table 13.11, Labs 1 and 2 are not significantly different; Lab 3 is biased high.

Large variations in results reported from different laboratories analyzing the same samples might be explained by random

Table 13.12 — 5% Two-tailed Limits on Ranked Scores

Number of Laboratories	*Number of Samples Analyzed Upper Limit/Lower Limit*							
	3	*4*	*5*	*6*	*7*	*8*	*9*	*10*
3		4 12	5 15	7 17	8 20	10 22	12 24	13 27
4		4 16	6 19	8 22	10 25	12 28	14 31	16 24
5		5 19	7 23	9 27	11 31	13 35	16 38	18 42
6	3 18	5 23	7 28	10 32	12 37	15 41	18 45	21 49
7	3 21	5 27	8 32	11 37	14 42	17 47	20 52	23 57

errors in the measurements or by systematic errors in the different laboratories. Practically speaking, it is highly probable that systematic errors made by the participating laboratories are the cause for these wide variations. This can be evaluated using another technique for analyzing interlaboratory variability, the "two-sample" or Youden plot.[21] In this graphical technique, each participating laboratory is sent two slightly dissimilar samples (A and B, where B is within ±10% of the value of A) and asked to perform one analysis on each sample. When Sample A results are returned, they should be plotted with respect to the results obtained by the same laboratory for Sample B. Median lines are drawn, and outliers are identified and discarded from the data set. If there was no bias in the results, the plotted points should be randomly distributed around the intersection of the two median lines drawn. It is rare that this is observed. Generally what is observed is that the plotted points fall around a line drawn at 45° from the intersection of the two median lines, indicating that each participating laboratory has its own technique (an internal consistency) for analyzing the samples. Laboratories that report one sample high are more likely to report the second sample high. The converse is true also. Through the use of two samples similar in concentration, an estimate of precision can be made. This is done by constructing a perpendicular line from the plotted point to the 45° line.

Table 13.13[22] shows the data for nine laboratories that analyzed two samples, A and B. The averages for A and B were calculated as was the difference (A–B) and the average difference. In the last column, the average difference was subtracted from the absolute value of (A–B), and this difference was then averaged. The data are plotted as shown in Figure 13.13.

Table 13.13 — Example Data — Nine Labs, Two Samples

Lab Number	*A*	*B*	*A–B*	*|(A–B)| -0.24*
1	35.1	33.0	2.10	1.86
2	23.0	23.2	-0.20	0.44
3	23.8	22.3	1.50	1.26
4	25.6	24.1	1.50	1.26
5	23.7	23.6	0.10	0.14
6	21.0	23.1	-2.10	2.34
7	23.0	21.0	2.00	1.76
8	26.5	25.6	0.90	0.66
9	21.4	25.0	-3.60	3.84
Avg	24.8	24.5	0.24	1.51

The average of the absolute values of (A–B) - 0.24, when multiplied by 0.886, gives an estimate of the standard deviation: 1.51 × 0.886 = 1.34. The estimate of the standard deviation for precision allows the construction of a circle centered on the intersection of the median lines within which any given percentage of points can be expected to fall, given that the participating laboratories can eliminate all bias or constant errors. For 95% of points to be within the circle, the multiple of the standard deviation is 2.448. Therefore, 2.448 × 1.34 = 3.28 is the radius of the circle. Once the circle is constructed, points falling outside the circle represent laboratories with substantial systematic errors incorporated into their analytical technique.

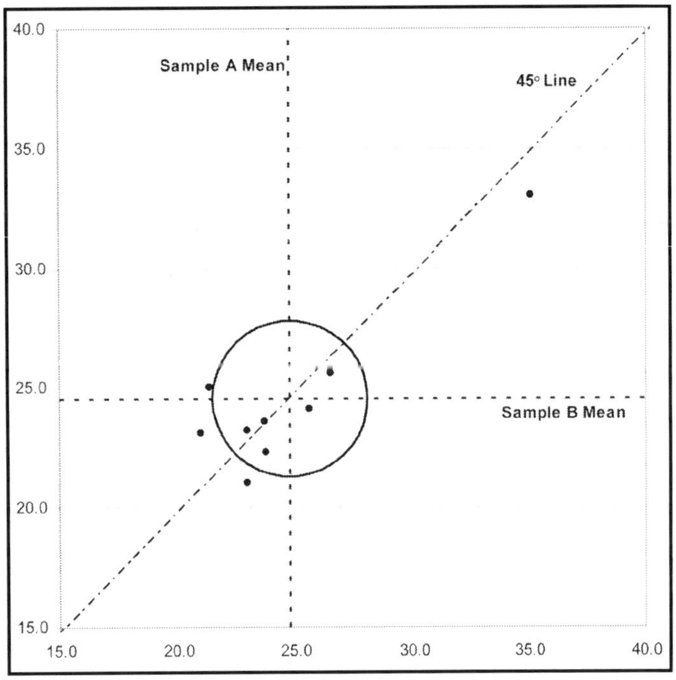

Figure 13.13 — Youden Plot.

Summary

The accuracy of the results of a workplace sampling project is dependent on many factors. By having the sampling and the analysis processes "in control," process variation and associated errors can be reduced and estimated. The amount of control necessary in any given project is dependent on the standards and requirements against which the results will be evaluated. By examining the factors that may affect the performance of the project, suitable controls can be put in place. Written plans, procedures, and records provide the basis for establishing and documenting the controls and, ultimately, the accuracy of the project results.

In most projects, the sampling process provides the greatest opportunity for errors and variability. This process is best controlled through the use of clearly and strictly defined sampling procedures. These procedures should be rigorously followed. Instruments and equipment used during sample collection must be carefully calibrated and operated. Controls applied during analysis cannot compensate for a poorly collected sample.

The laboratory is generally a more controlled environment than the sampling environment. Whenever possible, the laboratory analysis come from a process that is determined to be stable and in statistical control. Since the laboratory provides a place where the greatest control can be exerted, its contribution to the overall inaccuracy of the project must be minimized.

Acknowledgements

Reginald C. Jordan, Ph.D., CIH (previous Author)

Donna LaGarde (Chemist, OSHA Salt Lake Technical Center)

References

1. **Cornell, J.A.:** W.J. Youden — The man and his methodology. In *Statistics Division Newsletter.* Milwaukee, WI.: American Society for Quality Control *13(2)*:9–18 (1993).
2. **Juran, J.M. (ed.):** *Juran's Quality Control Handbook*, 4th edition. New York: McGraw-Hill, 1999.
3. **Taylor, J.K.:** *Quality Assurance for Chemical Measurements.* Chelsea, MI: Lewis Publishers, 1987.
4. **ASTM International (ASTM):** *General Requirements for the Competence of Testing and Calibration Laboratories* (ANS/ISO/IEC 17025:2005 (E)). West Conshohocken, PA: ASTM International, 2005.
5. **AIHA®:** *Guidelines for Uncertainty Estimation.* [Online] http://www.aihaaccreditedlabs.org/PolicyModules/Documents/GuidanceEstimationUncertaintyMeasurement.pdf [Accessed October 2010].
6. **International Organization for Standardization (ISO):** *International Vocabulary of Metrology — Basic and General Concepts and Associated Terms (VIM)* (ISO/IEC Guide 99:2007). Geneva, Switzerland: ISO, 2007.
7. **National Institute for Standards and Technology (NIST):** *NIST Policy on Traceability.* [Online] http://ts.nist.gov/Traceability/Policy/nist_traceability_policy-external.cfm [Accessed October 2010].
8. **Croarkin, C., and P. Tobias:** *NIST/SEMATECH e-Handbook of Statistical Methods.* [Online] http://www.itl.nist.gov/div898/handbook/ [Accessed October 2010].
9. **Schlecht, P.C., J.V. Crable, and W.D. Kelley:** Industrial hygiene. In *Quality Assurance Practices for Health Laboratories.* Washington, DC: American Public Health Association, 1978. p. 801.
10. **Reut, S., R. Stadnichenko, D. Hillis, and P. Pityn:** Factors affecting the accuracy of airborne quartz determination. *J. Occup. Environ. Hyg. 4(2)*:80-86 (2007).

11. **AIHA®:** *Laboratory Accreditation Policies.* [Online] http://www.aiha.org/Content/LQAP/documents/2008LabAccredPolicyRevision.htm [Accessed October 2010].
12. **Shewhart, W.A.:** *Economic Control of the Quality of Manufactured Product.* Princeton, NJ: Van Nostrand Reinhold, 1931.
13. **Peirce, B.:** Criterion for the rejection of doubtful observations. *Astr. J. 2*:161–163. [Online] http://articles.adsabs.harvard.edu/full/1852AJ......2..161P.1852 [Accessed October 2010].
14. **American Society for Testing and Materials (ASTM):** *Standard Practice for Dealing with Outlying Observations* (E 178-80). West Conshohocken, PA: ASTM, 1980.
15. **Taylor, J.K.:** *Statistical Techniques for Data Analysis.* Chelsea, MI: Lewis Publishers, 2004.
16. **Analytical Methods Committee:** Robust statistics: A method of coping with outliers. *AMC Technical Briefs.* London, UK: Royal Society of Chemistry. No. 6. April 2001.
17. **Gibbons, R.D., and Coleman, D.E.:** *Statisticals Method for Detection and Quantification of Environmental Contamination.* New York: John Wiley & Sons, 2001.
18. **U.S. Government Printing Office:** *Title 40 Code of Federal Regulations Part 136 Appendix B.* [Online] http://www.gpoaccess.gov/cfr/index.html [Accessed October 2010].
19. **U.S. Department of Labor, Occupational Safety and Health Administration:** *Personal sampling for air contaminants. OSHA Technical Manual.* [Online] http://www.osha.gov/dts/osta/otm/otm_ii/otm_ii_1.html [Accessed October 2010].
20. **Youden, W.J.:** Measurement agreement comparisons. In *Proceedings of the 1962 Standards Laboratory Conference* (NBS misc. pub. 248). Washington, DC: Government Printing Office, 1962.
21. **Youden, W.J.:** Collection of papers on statistical treatment of data. *J. Qual. Technol. 4*:1–67 (1972).
22. **Linch, A.L.:** Quality control for sampling and laboratory analysis. In *The Industrial Environment—Its Evaluation and Control.* Washington, DC: U.S. Government Printing Office, 1973.

Other Useful References

Arthur, J.: *Lean Six Sigma Demystified.* New York: McGraw-Hill, 2007.

Burkart, J.A., L.M. Eggenberger, J.H. Nelson, and P.R. Nicholson: A practical statistical quality control scheme for the industrial hygiene chemistry laboratory. *Am. Ind. Hyg. Assoc. J. 45*:386–392 (1984).

Ellison, S.L.R., M. Rosslein, and A. Williams: *Quantifying Uncertainty in Analytical Measurement.* EURACHEM/CITAC Guide GC 4. 2000.

Ratliff, T.A.: *The Laboratory Quality Assurance System: A Manual of Quality Procedures and Forms.* New York: Van Nostrand Reinhold, 2003.

Smith, L.D., Bolyard, M.L, and Eller, P.M.: Quality Assurance. In *NIOSH Manual of Analytical Methods.* [Online] http://www.cdc.gov/niosh/nmam/pdfs/chapter-c.pdf [Accessed October 2010].

U.S. Environmental Protection Agency (EPA): *Quality Assurance Handbook for Air Pollution Measurement Systems,* Vol. I (EPA/600/R-94/038a). [Online] http://www.epa.gov/ttn/amtic/files/ambient/qaqc/r94-038a.pdf [Accessed October 2010].

Outcome Competencies

After completing this chapter, the reader should be able to:

1. Define underlined terms used in this chapter.
2. Identify the importance of mass, particle count, and surface area in risk assessment.
3. Describe basic aerosol morphology and descriptive classifications.
4. Identify the primary mechanisms of aerosol particle movement and deposition.
5. Describe commonly used techniques for aerosol sampling and size analysis.
6. Calculate critical descriptors of aerosol particle size distribution.

Key Terms

50% cut point size • aerosol • diffusion • dose • dust • fiber • fog • fume • gravimetric analysis • hygroscopicity • impaction • inhalable fraction • interception • mist • nasopharyngeal region • particle aerodynamic diameter • pulmonary (or alveolar) region • respirable fraction • sedimentation • smoke • Stokes diameter • terminal settling velocity • thoracic fraction • tracheobronchial region

Prerequisite Knowledge

Prior to beginning this chapter, the reader should have an understanding of basic Newtonian physics and mathematics through college algebra. In addition, the reader should review the related chapters:

Chapter Number	Chapter Topic
5	Occupational Toxicology
7	Principles of Evaluating Worker Exposure
17	Direct-Reading Instruments for Determining Concentrations of Gases, Vapors, and Aerosols

Key Topics

I. Definitions

II. Aerosol Morphology

III. Motion of Airborne Particles
   A. Sedimentation
   B. Inertial Motion and Deposition
   C. Diffusion
   D. Interception
   E. Other Particle Transport Mechanisms
   F. Particle Retention on Surfaces

IV. Deposition of Inhaled Particles

V. Aerosol Sampling and Analysis in Industrial Environments
   A. Sampling Theory Exposure
   B. Particle Size-Selective Sampling
   C. Filtration-Based Techniques
   D. Sedimentation-Based Techniques for Collecting Finer Particle Fractions
   E. Impaction-Based Techniques
   F. Optical Techniques
   G. Microscopy Techniques

VI. Aerosol Size Distribution Analysis

Sampling and Sizing of Airborne Particles

14

Mary E. Eide and Dean R. Lillquist, PhD, CIH, CHMM

Introduction

For common use, the term aerosol often refers to the spray produced from an "aerosol can" containing a liquid and a compressed gas used as a propellant (e.g., spray paints, spray lubricants, spray adhesives, etc.). However, for technical discussions, an aerosol is described as solid and/or liquid particles dispersed in a gaseous medium. In the context of occupational hygiene, were the primary focus is on worker exposure assessment, the gaseous medium is almost always air. Aerosols range in size from visible dust "floating" in air (> 50 µm in diameter), to microscopic particles invisible to the naked eye. In fact, the particles of most concern are generally those which can't be seen.

There are many aerosol-producing workplace activities which may lead to worker exposures. Some traditional examples include the "dusty trades" such as hard rock and coal mining which produce dust aerosols. High-temperature metal work including welding, cutting, and smelting which can produce very fine metal fume aerosols; liquid based cleaning activities which can produce liquid sprays and mists; biological aerosol from various sources including droplet aerosols from blood and body fluids potentially containing pathogenic organisms and biologically contaminated machining fluids, agricultural products. Recently, there has extensive interest and research in ultra-fine particles, including nanometer sized particles from both environmental and engineered (commercial) sources.

Regarding worker risk assessment, inhaled particles have adverse health affects by being deposited and damaging tissue locally or being dissolved and distributed systemically. Depending on the size and chemical properties of aerosols; the airborne concentration and time of exposure; and many other factors; health effects of exposure may range from simple temporary irritation, to chronic illness, to terminal disease. Occupational aerosol hazards have been recognized since at least the first century A.D., when Pliny described how boat painters covered their heads with hoods to prevent the inhalation of lead dust.(1) A crude form of respiratory protection also was worn by miners at the beginning of the Renaissance, as described by Agricola (1494–1555) in his treatise on European mining practices of the time.(2)

In the 300 years since Bernardino Ramazzini initiated the formal study of occupational diseases, work-related aerosol exposures have been shown to cause numerous diseases of the respiratory tract and other tissues. In the past 100 years, specific toxicological mechanisms been identified to explain how these diseases develop and progress. And during this time, advances in aerosol science and inhalation toxicology have extended our understanding of the relationship between aerosol exposure, uptake, and fate. This improved understanding has in turn promoted the development of refined techniques for aerosol exposure characterization.

Although still important in the developed and expanding economies around the world, it would be a mistake to limit our thinking about aerosol-related illness to such historically important occupational lung diseases as silicosis, black lung (coal miners' pneumoconiosis), and asbestos-related lung cancer. This is because other aerosol-related health effects continue to gain more attention. For example, ultra fine and nano-sized aerosols (both environmental and engineered), diesel combustion aerosol, radon progeny aerosol, environmental tobacco smoke, man-made fibers, and infectious and allergenic bioaerosols are of increasing interest in occupational hygiene work. Research continues to reveal more on the health effects of exposure to many of these aerosols. The occupational hygienist plays a critical role in the identification of exposure, characterization and quantitation, epidemiological study, standards development, and hazard prevention. Techniques for aerosol sampling and characterization continue to evolve in a dynamic process driven by advances in technology and our understanding of disease etiology.

Evaluating aerosols can be theoretical research exercises using extremely sophisticated instruments. However, practicing occupational hygienists are often called upon to characterize worker aerosol exposures. Therefore, it is important for the occupational hygienist to be familiar with the properties of aerosols in occupational environments and the techniques available for their assessment. Although no single sampling and analysis technique is appropriate for all needs, standard sampling and analytical techniques should be used whenever they exist.

This chapter focuses on the sampling and analytical methods and equipment commonly used in assessing aerosols of occupational health concern. It does not address many other areas of aerosol science interest such as ambient atmospheric aerosols, ultrafine particles in cleanroom environments, or pharmaceutical aerosol preparations. It only incidentally addresses bioaerosols (see Chapter 22 for a detailed discussion of biohazards). Neither does it address techniques and instrumentation not suited to use in the occupational hygiene field. For a discussion of these and other topics related to aerosol generation and measurement the reader is referred to the excellent texts by Baron and Willeke(3), Cox and Wathes(4), and Vincent.(5)

Definitions

Aerosols are encountered in several forms in occupational hygiene practice.(6)

Dusts are comprised of particulate aerosols produced by mechanical processes such as breaking, grinding, and pulverizing. They are encountered in most mining activities (excavation, conveyor transport, pulverizing), materials handling operations (loading, unloading, transport), and dry material preparation and packaging processes (ball milling, sieving, bagging). Dusts particles are chemically unchanged from the original parent material, except that their smaller size and higher specific surface area (surface area per unit mass or volume of material) may enhance their ability to become (and remain) airborne, their ability to be inhaled and penetrate into the respiratory tract, their toxicity, rate of solubility, or their explosion potential. As shown in Figure 14.1, dust particles range in size from less than 1 μm (or 10^{-6} m; e.g., ground talc) to as large as 1 mm (e.g., fertilizer and ground limestone). Individual dust particles are very often regular in shape (in the sense that they have no preferred dimension). Crystalline material fractures along structural lines and may be columnar or cubic in shape with relatively sharp edges or flat surfaces. However, the ratio of length to width or diameter is less than 3:1. But there are some notable exceptions to this, including dusts comprised of fibrous particles (e.g., asbestos) and platelet-like particles (e.g., talc, anthracite coal).

Fumes as defined for occupational health purposes are not noxious vapors, as they are often described in the vernacular, but are in fact fine solid aerosol particles produced from the re-condensation of vaporized solid material. Material that is normally solid at standard conditions is melted and vaporized (as, for example, during welding or the smelting of ores). Condensation and the formation of very small primary particles (of the order of 0.01 μm in size) occurs during the cooling of the hot vapor in a process known as nucleation. Such particles come together in collisions by the process of coagulation, thus leading to the formation of agglomerates that are of the order of about 1 μm in diameter. Typically these agglomerates are nearly spherical in configuration. It is the aerosol made of such agglomerates that is usually known as fume. Fumes from welding and smelting processes are usually in the form metal oxides or a mixture of the metal and metal oxide. They are small enough to penetrate readily to the deep lung. They also may be chemically quite reactive and may pose a significant hazard to workers. Zinc oxide fume produced during welding or cutting on galvanized (zinc-coated) metal may cause welders to become nauseous. Fresh cadmium oxide fume, which is produced when cadmium-bearing silver solder is used to braze together low-melting-point metals (e.g., when joining copper radiator components) is extremely hazardous and can cause potentially fatal pulmonary edema. Anticorrosion cadmium coatings on metal bolts are another source of cadmium oxide fume if fasteners are cut using an oxy-acetylene torch. Metalizing operations, in which worn metal parts such as shafts are "built up" prior to re-machining, involves spraying molten metal onto the worn surface. Fume can cause a flu-like immunologic reaction called "metal fume fever." Plastics can also be melted, vaporized, and re-condense into fumes and worker exposures have been associated with a polymer fume fever response.

Mists are spherical droplet aerosols produced from bulk liquid by mechanical processes such as splashing, bubbling, or spraying. The droplets are chemically unchanged from the parent liquid and range in size from perhaps a few microns to over 100 µm. The upper end of this size range is limited by the ability of a droplet to remain physically intact when the force of gravity (that distorts the droplet) is significantly greater than the force of surface tension (that is holding the droplet together). Any vigorous process involving liquids has the potential to produce a mist aerosol. Indeed, processes such as spray painting and some types of crop spraying operations are designed specifically to produce mists. In the health care setting the mist droplet aerosols produced by the coughing or treatment of infected patients have received increased attention in recent years due to concerns about occupational exposure of health care workers to multidrug resistant tuberculosis and other pathogens.

Fogs are also droplet aerosols, but are produced by physical condensation from the vapor phase. Fog droplets are typically smaller than mechanically generated mist droplets, and are of the order of 1 to 10 µm. Whereas mists may visibly settle toward the ground, fogs appear to remain suspended in the air.

Smokes are complex mixtures of solid and liquid aerosol particles, gases, and vapors resulting from incomplete combustion of carbonaceous materials and are formed by complex combinations of physical nucleation-type mechanisms and chemical reactions. Tobacco smoke, for example, contains thousands of chemical species, many of which are toxic or carcinogenic.[7,8] Smokes from burning plastics, synthetic fabrics, and other petrochemical products may be extremely toxic and are often more widespread and hazardous than the actual flame in a building or aircraft fire. Primary smoke particles are on the order of 0.01 to 1 µm in diameter; but just like fumes, agglomerates containing many particles may be much larger.

Fibers are elongated particles with length much greater than width. Fibers may be naturally occurring, for example, in materials such as plant fibers and asbestiform silicate minerals, or synthetic, such as vitreous or graphite fibers. In the context of occupational health, asbestos is highly studied and regulated, and it the convention to define a "fiber" as a particle with a ratio of length to width greater than 3:1. It is well known that asbestos is very hazardous to health if significant amount of small fibers become airborne and are inhaled. Asbestos-related lung diseases include asbestosis (a chronic fibrosis of the lung), mesothelioma (cancer of the lining of the lung cavity), and bronchial carcinoma (cancer of the conducting airways of the lung). These diseases have been associated with heavy asbestos exposure in ship builders, pipe fitters, and insulation installers.

Increasing use of refractory ceramic fibers, mineral wools, spun glass, and composite materials incorporating reinforcing synthetic fibers has fueled concerns that these fibers may have unsuspected toxic potential.[9,10] One theory is that if a particle has the shape, appearance, durability of asbestos fibers, it should be treated with the same caution. In terms of their physical and biological behaviors fibrous aerosols display aerodynamic and health effects behaviors that differ in many respects from spherical or near-spherical particles of the same material and mass, so that aerosol characterization is typically more complex for fibers than for other aerosols.

Aerosol distribution in virtually all occupational environments are not one size, exhibit a range of particle sizes, and are

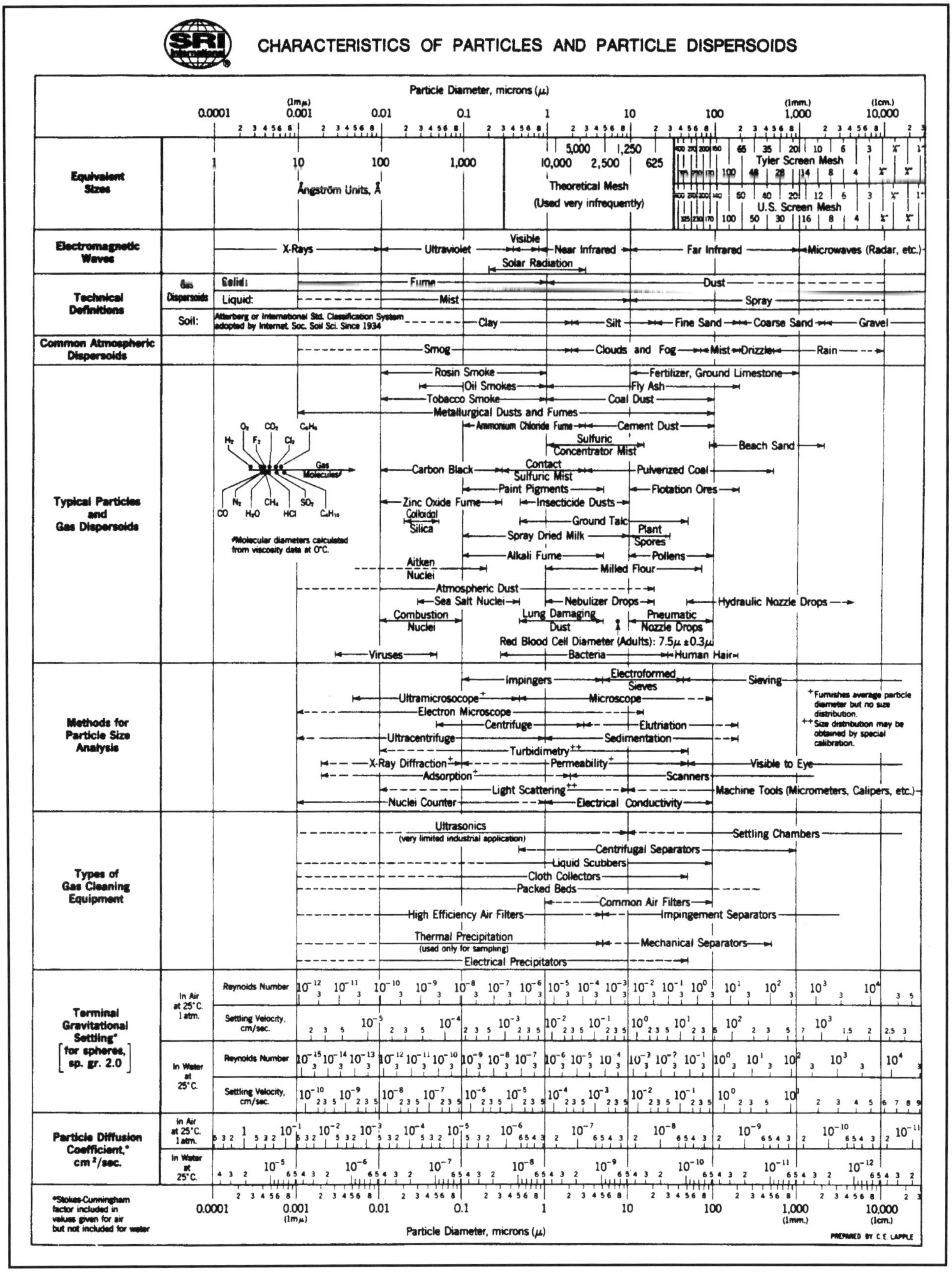

Figure 14.1 — Characteristics of particles and particle dispersoids (Source: C.E. Lappler, SRI Journal 5:94 [1961].)

described as a polydispersed aerosol. By contrast, aerosols that do contain only a single size particle are termed monodispersed. Monodispersed aerosols are difficult to generate and maintain and are usually only encountered in research and calibration activities. It is common to express the "particle size distribution" in terms of the lognormal distribution, with a "tail" in the distribution that extends out to large particles.

Traditionally, aerosols concentrations in air are often assessed by mass per unit volume (mg/m^3). Because volume is a cubic function to diameter, when using mass, large particles have the most significant impact on total mass. Small particles do not contribute significantly to the total mass of aerosols. Just how much do "small" particles contribute to total mass?

mass = volume × density

volume of a sphere = $4/3\pi r^3$

Example for unit density particles (density = 1 gm/cm^3) with diameters = 1 µm and 10µm

for 1.0 micron size, $4/3\pi(1\ \mu m)^3 = 0.52\ \mu m^3$
$0.52\ \mu m^3 \times 1\ gm/cm^3 \times 1 cm^3/1{,}000{,}000{,}000{,}000\ \mu m^3$
$= 5.2 \times 10^{-13} gm$

for 10 micron size, $4/3\pi(10\ \mu m)^3 = 524\ \mu m^3$
$524\ \mu m^3 \times 1\ gm/cm^3 \times 1 cm^3/1{,}000{,}000{,}000{,}000\ \mu m^3$
$= 5.2 \times 10^{-10} gm$

It takes 1000 particles with 1 µm diameter to equal the mass of one 10 µm particle.

Similarly, it takes one million 0.1 µm diameter to equal the mass of one 10 µm particle.

Other methods used to assess aerosols include particle counting (historical units - millions of particles per cubic foot or mppcf) and total surface area.[9] These evaluations tools can account for the contribution of reactive surfaces and give considerations to smaller particles. They are good evaluation tools for assessing risk of ultrafine and nanomaterials.

Table 14.1 — Comparison of properties for unit density spheres with different diameters

Diameter (µm)	*Mass of particle (gm)*	*# of particles per gram*	*Surface area (m²) per gram*
0.1	5.2×10^{-16}	1.9×10^{15}	60
1.0	5.2×10^{-13}	1.9×10^{12}	6
10	5.2×10^{-10}	1.9×10^{9}	0.6

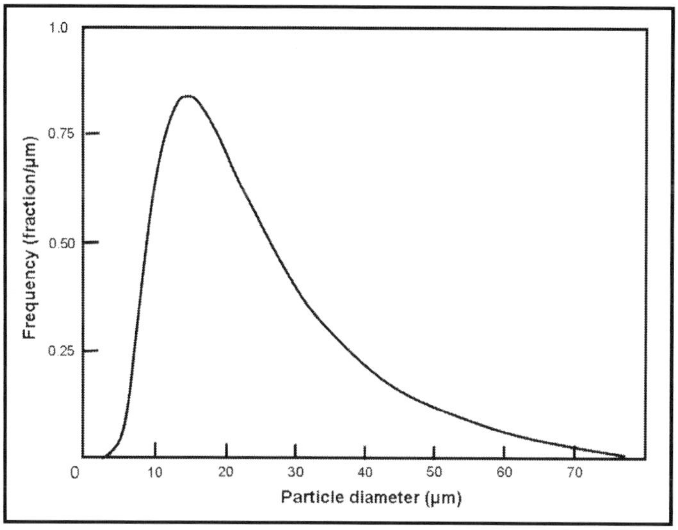

Figure 14.2 — Example of size distribution of polydispersed aerosol.

Aerosol Morphology

Airborne particles may also be described in terms of their morphology, or shape and appearance. Particles with a characteristic length dimension independent of particle orientation are known as "isometric." Some aerosol scientists refer to such particles also as "compact" or "regular." For such particles, it is possible to describe the shape by a single dimension. For the case of a spherical particle this dimension is simply its diameter. Metal fumes and liquid droplets are spherical due to liquid surface tension (during the molten phase for the fumes), except when they are large enough that the forces of gravity become comparable to the forces of surface tension and so the droplet can become distorted. Many bioaerosol particles are also spherical or essentially so, including allergenic pollens and dust mite fecal pellets.

Some aerosol particles are not spherical but are essentially isometric. Examples of such particles are dusts produced from grinding or pulverizing processes and some crystalline particles. For the dynamic behavior of such particles, it is suitable to treat them as isometric or having a single dimension. One may assume, for simplicity, that such particles are spherical; to be more precise (as might be desired in some specific case, or in some types of aerosol research) a "dynamic correction factor" may be applied to account for the effects of nonsphericity on particle aerodynamic behavior.[12]

Other particles are clearly nonisometric and are treated as ellipsoids of revolution. If the axis of rotation is the major axis of the ellipse, the resulting particle is known as a prolate spheroid. A fiber is the limiting case of such a particle in which the length exceeds the diameter. As mentioned previously, the conventional definition of a fiber is an elongated particle with a length-to-diameter ratio greater than 3:1. Some rod-shaped bacilli and chain aggregates of these and other microorganisms may have an aspect ratio of greater than 3:1. Conversely, if the axis of rotation is the minor axis of the ellipse, the particle is an oblate spheroid. A plate-like particle is the limiting case of such a particle in which the particle diameter exceeds its thickness. Fiber particles occur frequently in industrial aerosols. Examples include asbestos, metal whiskers, carbon fibers, and other fiber particles used in composite materials. Examples of plate-like particles include paint pigments, insect parts, mica, and crystalline particles.

The particles just discussed are "singlet particles." That is, they are formed as single discrete particles and remain so for their entire lifetimes in the airborne state. But when the initial concentration of particles is high (greater than 106 particles/cm^3) particles may coagulate or flocculate to form aggregate particles. This is most commonly the case when the initial particles are in the ultrafine size range (0.001 to 0.1 µm). Such aggregate particles may contain hundreds of primary particles. It is very difficult to analyze the dynamic behavior of such particles as the gross dimensional structure of the aggregates varies widely from one particle to another. The relationship between the primary and secondary structure of aggregates has been investigated by considering the particles as "fractal" structures. This general approach was pioneered by Mandelbrot[13] and has been applied to aerosol aggregates by several investigators.[14]

Soot particles, produced by the incomplete combustion of hydrocarbon fuels, are a prime example of aggregates. Compared to primary particles, aggregates display certain important characteristics, chief among which is the very large surface area per unit mass of particle. This large specific surface area may enhance surface condensation of vapors and catalytic reaction of simple vapors to produce new gaseous species.

The most common approach to the determination of particle morphology is by optical or electron microscopy. When one observes a particle by optical microscopy, a two-dimensional object is seen. For a particle that is not actually spherical, a number of ways have been proposed to determine an appropriate dimension. The simplest method of delineating the dimension is with the equivalent diameter based on equivalent projected area (i.e., the diameter of a spherical particle which, when viewed under the microscope, would have the same projected area as the particle of interest). To infer the three-dimensional structure of the particle, it is necessary to make some assumptions regarding the third dimension. An additional problem is the possibility that particles collected on a substrate for microscopy may suffer deformation due to attractive (or other) forces between the particle and the substrate. Electron microscopy, because it requires a high vacuum, is not feasible for liquids or other volatile substances, so this limits the type of particles that may be morphologically analyzed by this method.[15]

Motion of Airborne Particles

Airborne particles may exert their toxic effects only after contact with body tissues. Dose depends on the exposure history of the subject over time, particle deposition efficiency, pharmacokinetics including clearance processes, and the intrinsic toxicity of the substance. Bioaccumulation will change over time as the result of ongoing exposure, biologic defense and clearance, or both. Possible negative responses including irritation, localized tissue damage, systemic absorption, progressive disease, etc. It is perhaps more helpful to think in terms of the "dose rate," because this can be directly related to what is measured by an occupational hygienist: airborne concentration in the workplace to estimate worker exposure.

For aerosols, worker exposure and dose is influenced to a large extent by the aerosol's physical properties that govern how the particles may follow the motion of the air itself, be inhaled through the nose and or mouth, and penetrate into and deposit in the respiratory tract. Aerosol particle size, shape, density, and hygroscopicity (tendency to absorb water vapor) determine to a large extent how the particles behave in the air and how efficiently they are inhaled and deposited in the respiratory tract.

This section describes the basic particle descriptors and primary particle transport mechanisms of inertial motion, sedimentation, diffusion, and interception. Also discussed briefly are the mechanisms of particle transport under electrostatic and thermophoretic forces. Following sections discuss the influence of these forces on aerosol inhalation and deposition in the body and in turn how they are applied in various aerosol sampling and sizing techniques.

Sedimentation

Sedimentation refers to movement of an aerosol particle through a gaseous medium under the influence of gravity. The rate of settling depends on the particle's size, shape, mass, and orientation (for nonspherical particles) and on the air density and viscosity. An airborne particle is subject to a gravitational force and falls vertically according to Newton's second law. The accelerating force is given by the product of the particle mass and the gravitational constant, g, which for a sphere of diameter d_p and density ρ is:

$$F_g = \frac{\pi d_p^3}{6} \rho g \qquad (14\text{-}1)$$

Opposing this force is the drag force on the particle due to gas viscosity. The drag force on a spherical particle moving with velocity U through a medium having a viscosity η is given, for practical purposes for most aerosols of interest in occupational hygiene, to a fair approximation by Stokes' law:

$$F_D = 3\pi\eta d_p U \qquad (14\text{-}2)$$

where $\eta = 1.84 \times 10^{-4}$ g/cm/sec at normal temperature and pressure (NTP) (1 atm, 25°C). Because the particle displaces its own volume of air even at rest, there is also a small buoyant force acting opposite the gravity force, namely:

$$F_b = \frac{\pi d_p^3}{6} \rho f g \qquad (14\text{-}3)$$

where ρ_f is the density of the fluid medium (for air, $\rho_f = 1.29 \times 10^{-3}$ g/cm³ at NTP). The gravitational and buoyant forces are constant, but the drag force increases linearly with particle velocity, so that at some point the sum of the buoyant and fluid drag forces exactly equals the gravitational force, the acceleration becomes zero, and the particle attains a constant velocity (Figure 14.3a). This terminal settling velocity is obtained by setting the sum of the forces equal to zero. Normally the buoyant force is negligible compared with the gravitational force. Making this assumption, one obtains an expression for the terminal settling velocity:

$$U_t = \frac{d_p^2 \rho}{18\eta} g = \tau g \qquad (14\text{-}4)$$

where τ is the particle's "relaxation time" and has units in seconds. When the particle diameter is of the order of the gas mean free path, an additional factor must be included in Stokes' law to take account of the "slip" of the particle, when the particle interacts with the surrounding gas medium as a series of individual discrete collisions. This factor is known as the Cunningham slip correction and is given by the expression

$$C_c = \frac{0.166}{d_p} \qquad (14\text{-}5)$$

where d_p is the particle diameter in micrometers. This expression is appropriate for air at NTP for particles down to approximately 0.1 μm.[16]

A particle reaches terminal velocity when the downward force of gravity (F_g) equals the upward force of drag (F_d) and buoyancy. The net force is zero and the result is that the velocity of the object remains constant. Terminal settling velocities range from approximately 10^{-4} to 10^{-1} cm/sec for 0.1 to 10 μm diameter particles, respectively. The time required for a particle initially at rest to reach terminal settling velocity U_t is approximately 7_t, which ranges from 10^{-6} to 10^{-3} sec for particles in the range of 0.1 to 10 μm, respectively. The effect of gravitational forces is greater for larger particles.

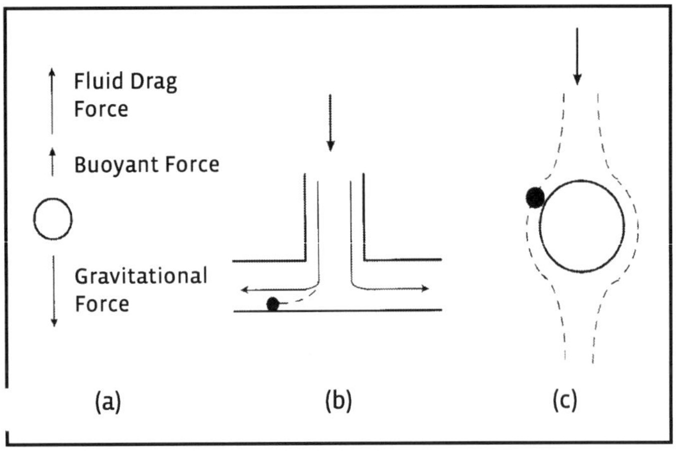

Figure 14.3 — Aerosol Particle collection mechanisms: (a) sedimentation at terminal settling velocity; (b) inertial impaction; and (c) interception.

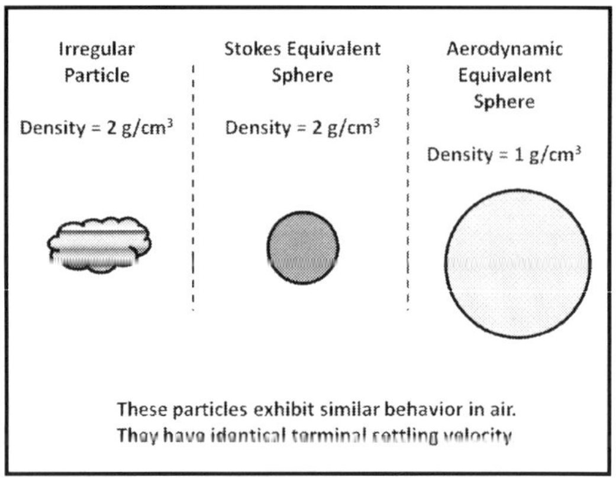

Figure 14.4 — Comparison of irregular, Stokes, and Aerodynamic Equivalent spheres.

When the particles are not spherical, the right side of Equation 14.2 may be multiplied by a "shape factor" with a characteristic particle dimension substituted for sphere diameter. Discussion of such an equation is beyond the scope of this chapter, but may be explored in aerosol science texts including Hinds[12], Vincent[14], and Mercer.[17]

For spherical particles between 1 and 100 μm (i.e, negligible slip), the equation for terminal settling velocity becomes:

$$V_{grav} \cong 3 \times 10^{-8} \rho_p d^2_p \tag{14-6}$$

Stokes and Aerodynamic Diameter

In considering particle sedimentation the shape, size, and density of particles is often unknown. It is convenient to discuss particle size in terms of the diameter of a spherical particle of the same density that would exhibit the same behavior as the particle in question; this value is termed the Stokes diameter, d_{St}. The d_{St} may be calculated from Equation 14-4 for a measured U_τ and known ρ; however, the usual practice is to extend this analogy to the concept of aerodynamic equivalent diameter, d_{ae}, which is the diameter of a unit density sphere (density = 1 g/cm³) that would exhibit the same settling velocity as the particle in question. For unit density aerosols, $d_{St} = d_{ae}$. The advantage of using aerodynamic equivalent diameter rather than Stokes diameter is that aerodynamic equivalent diameter "normalizes" different aerosols to a common basis so that their behaviors may be directly compared.

Particle Stokes and aerodynamic diameters are important for inertial and gravitational deposition, collector design, and data interpretation. As discussed previously, most particles are irregularly shaped. Deposition and collection efficiency are often expressed using particle aerodynamic diameter.

Inertial Motion and Deposition

A particle's inertia, defined as its tendency to resist a change in its motion, provides an important deposition mechanism both for human inhalation/deposition and also for aerosol sampling. A particle in motion through a fluid moves in a straight line unless acted on by a net external force, as described by Newton's first law of motion. When the airflow is forced to change direction suddenly (for example, at a lung bifurcation, in a duct of changing cross-section, or around a blunt obstacle), the particle's inertia carries it across flow streamlines some distance before its forward motion in that direction is dissipated by fluid mechanical drag forces such as those already mentioned. If a surface is within the distance traveled, the particle may be captured by impaction on the surface (Figure 14.3b). In general, the likelihood of impaction increases with the mass and velocity of the particle and with the sharpness of the change in direction. These particle- and system-specific factors are reflected in the Stokes number, St, given by

$$St = \tau \frac{U}{D} C_C \tag{14-7}$$

where τ and C_c are as previously defined, and U and D are characteristic velocity and dimension values for the system. For example, for a spherical particle in air flowing around a much larger spherical body, D might be the diameter of the larger sphere and U the velocity of the airstream approaching the sphere. Here, therefore, St is the ratio of the relaxation time of the particle (i.e., the time it takes for it to come into equilibrium with its fluid surroundings) and the time scale associated with the flow change in question. The latter is approximated by D/U. The Stokes number may take various values depending on the characteristics of the flow system, but for a given system the efficiency of impaction increases with increasing St. As for gravitational forces, the preceding discussion shows that inertial forces are greater for larger particles.

Diffusion

Aerosol particles in a gaseous medium are bombarded by collisions with individual gas molecules that are in random Brownian motion associated with their fundamental microscopic thermal behavior. This in turn causes the particles to undergo random displacement that is known as "diffusion" and, unlike for gravitational or inertial-controlled motion, this effect is more prominent for small particles than for large ones. The particle parameter that describes this process is the particle diffusivity (or diffusion coefficient), D_B, and this is given by the Stokes-Einstein equation:

$$D_B = \frac{k_B T}{3\pi\eta d_p} C_C \qquad (14.8)$$

where k_B is Boltzmann's constant (1.38×10^{-23} J/ degrees K), and T is absolute temperature. The diffusion coefficient is inversely proportional to the particle's geometric size and is independent of particle density. The units of D_B are centimeters squared per second. Net motion by diffusion occurs when a particle concentration gradient exists and acts in the direction such that there is a net flux of particles from regions of high number concentration to regions of lower concentration. Fick's law of diffusion states that the flux of particles, J (particles per unit cross sectional area per unit time), is the product of the diffusivity, D_B, and the concentration gradient, dc/dx. Diffusive transport is favored by small particle diameter, large concentration differences, and short distances over which diffusion occurs.

Interception

Flow of an aerosol past a surface may produce particle deposition by the process of interception (Figure 14.3c). This deposition process does not depend on particle motion across fluid streamlines, as is the case for inertial impaction. Instead, it depends on the particle coming close enough to a flow boundary (by any means) that it may be collected by virtue of its own physical size. That is, for particle trajectories that carry a particle to a distance equal to or less than one-half the particle diameter, the particle will be captured by touching the surface. For a collecting object whose characteristic dimension is X_I, the probability of collection by interception is related to the ratio d_p/X_I. The collection mechanism is particularly significant for the case of elongated particles (e.g., fibers) for which d_p is replaced by the particle length, d_l. Fibers are therefore much more likely to be captured by interception than are spherical or near-spherical particles of equivalent mass.

Other Particle Transport Mechanisms

Other particle transport mechanisms that are relevant to aerosols in the occupational hygiene context, either in terms of deposition in the respiratory tract or sampling, include centrifugation, electrical, and thermophoretic motions. In centrifugal motion, particles in a body of air that is rapidly rotated (e.g., in a centrifuge) experience a centrifugal force that is directly analogous to the force of gravity in the vertical direction. The difference here, however, is that the magnitude of the acceleration (and hence the force) is controllable by changing the rate of rotation of the air and the size of the containing surfaces. In electrical motion a particle that is electrically charged experiences a force if an external electric field is applied and migrates accordingly, in a direction depending on the relative charge on the particle and the polarity of the electric field.

Thermophoretic particle motion occurs for a particle in air when there is a temperature gradient such that the particle experiences collisions from gas molecules that are more energetic on one side than the other. In that way, greater momentum is transferred to the particle from the "hot" side than from the "cold" side, such that the particle moves through the temperature gradient toward cooler air. Of these three transport mechanisms, centrifugal and electrical forces are more effective for larger particles. On the other hand, thermophoretic forces are more effective for small particles. All three of these mechanisms have been applied in aerosol sampling devices at one time or another.

Particle Retention on Surfaces

Particles coming into contact with surfaces may be acted on by various forces, some of which cause particles to be retained on the surface and some of which may tend to cause the particle's release, or resuspension, from the media. Forces governing retention include short-range van der Waals forces (arising form molecular interactions between the surfaces of the particle and the collection surface respectively), electrostatic attraction due to electrical charge differences between the particle and surface, and capillary forces arising from the adsorption of a water (or other liquid) film between the particle and the surface.[12,18] The forces that tend to prevent particles from being retained on contact mainly relate to particle bounce (governed by the coefficient of restitution that influences particle and surface elastic deformation when they come into contact at a finite velocity). Forces that influence the ability of the particle to be retained after it has been deposited relate to the fluid mechanical drag forces that may overcome the retaining forces and cause "blow-off." The physics of adhesion and resuspension are complex, but in general it is sufficient to say that smaller particles are more difficult to dislodge than larger ones.

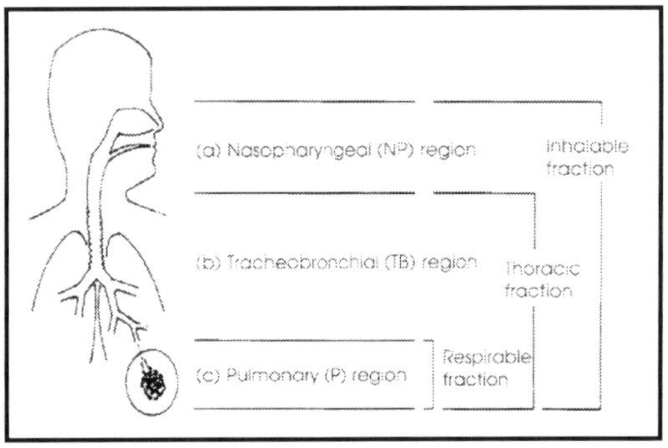

Figure 14.4 — Regions of the respiratory tract.

Deposition of Inhaled Particles

Aerosolized materials can directly affect the skin and eyes and can be systemically absorbed via these routes. However, inhaled aerosols are usually of primary occupational health concern. For a given exposure situation the amount of aerosolized material actually inhaled, the fraction of inhaled aerosol depositing in the different regions of the respiratory tract, and the fate of the deposited material are functions of many factors. These factors include the physical and chemical nature of the aerosol (e.g., particle size distribution, hygroscopicity, shape, solubility in water and lipids, chemical reactivity), the exposure conditions (e.g., airborne concentration, temperature, relative humidity, air velocity, physiologic demands on the worker), and characteristics of the individual (e.g., gender, body size, age, overall health, work practices, smoking status). This section discusses respiratory tract morphology and its effect on particle deposition in general terms. Detailed discussion of the fate of deposited aerosol particles and the diseases associated with them are found, for example, in Vincent[14], Phalen[19], or Rosenstock and Cullen.[20]

During breathing, a volume of air is drawn into the nose (or mouth) from the immediate region of the face. This frequently is referred to as the "breathing zone" and is where occupational hygienists position personal samplers to assess inhalation risk. Aerosol particles in this zone can experience forces described above, and due to the sharply varying air velocity in this region can be drawn toward the nose. As a result, some particles in the inspired air volume are inhaled into the nose and/or mouth,whereas others, particularly the larger ones, may fail to be inhaled. Experimental studies have shown that only half of all particles greater than approximately 50 μm in aerodynamic diameter are inspired from still air.[21] Particles in the inspired fraction actually entering the respiratory tract (i.e., the inhaled fraction) must first traverse the moist and convoluted passageways of the nasal turbinates of the nasopharynx (Figure 14.4). Larger particles, on the order of 10 μm and bigger, have difficulty negotiating the sharp turns at the high velocities in the nasal passages and deposit by impaction on the nasal mucosa. Further, particles made up of or coated with hygroscopic materials may absorb a significant mass of water in this warm and humid nasopharyngeal (NP) region of the respiratory tract, thereby increasing the likelihood that they will be captured by inertial deposition. Inertial impaction is by far the most significant deposition mechanism in the NP region.

Particles not captured in the NP region are respired into the tracheobronchial (TB) region consisting of the trachea and conducting airways (bronchi and bronchioles). This thoracic fraction contains particles generally smaller than 10 μm in aerodynamic diameter. Although various models of lung morphology exist,[22] for discussion purposes the TB region may be described as having a branched structure consisting of 16 generations lined with a mucus-covered, ciliated epithelium.[23] The airways branch at angles of up to 45 degrees[24,25], with the individual airways inclined from the vertical (in an upright person) at angles of from 0 (trachea) to 60 degrees.[25] The conducting airways are not involved in the gas exchange of respiration; their function is to distribute the inhaled air quickly and evenly to the deeper portions of the lung. Airway diameters become progressively smaller with each generation, but the number of airways increases geometrically. The net effect is that air velocities through the conducting airways decrease from approximately 200 cm/sec in the trachea and main bronchi to only a few centimeters per second in the terminal bronchioles, and the time of transit through an airway segment (its residence time in the segment) increases from approximately 0.01 sec in some of the larger bronchi to 0.1 sec in the terminal bronchioles.[26] Higher velocities favor inertial impaction, whereas lower velocities and higher residence times favor sedimentation and diffusion. Thus, the relative influence of inertial impaction decreases and the influence of sedimentation and diffusion increase from the top to the bottom of the TB region. However, diffusion is not considered a significant deposition mechanism in the conducting airways due to the large diffusion distances involved.

Particles not captured in the TB region can penetrate to the pulmonary (P) region containing the respiratory bronchioles, alveolar ducts, and alveolar sacs across which gas exchange occurs. Particles capable of migrating to this region of the lung comprise the respirable fraction of the aerosol. Air velocities in the P region drop from approximately 1 cm/sec in the highest respiratory bronchioles to less than 0.1 cm/sec in the alveolar ducts and sacs, whereas residence times increase to over 1 sec.[26] Inertial deposition is unimportant at these velocities. Depending on the particle size, either sedimentation or diffusion is the dominant deposition mechanism in the P region. Particles less than 0.1 μm exhibit significant diffusion and may deposit in large numbers on delicate pulmonary tissues. Although they may represent a small total mass, these particles may cause severe injury and disease. For some types of particles, if they are carrying sufficient electric charge, they may be deposited by attractive electrostatic image forces. Animal studies have suggested that this may be particularly significant for long thin fibers such as asbestos.[27]

Mouth breathing, due to nasal obstruction or heavy physiologic demand, causes air to bypass the nasal passages and can significantly alter the fraction of inhaled aerosol penetrating to the thoracic region. Individual aerosol deposition patterns are determined by respiratory tract morphology, breathing rate, minute volume, nose versus mouth breathing practices, and numerous other factors.[28] In addition, fiber deposition behavior may be significantly different from that of compact particles of equivalent mass; for example, fibers are more likely to be captured by interception simply due to their shape. Accurate prediction of respiratory tract aerosol deposition patterns continues to be a major area of research.

Aerosol Sampling and Analysis in Industrial Environments

Sampling Theory

The general objective of aerosol sampling is to obtain information about aerosol concentrations and properties over a specified length of time. To achieve this, a sample of the air containing the aerosol of interest is aspirated by suction (by means of a pump) into the body of a sampler through an entry orifice and either deposited on a filter for subsequent analysis, or conveyed to a sensing zone for real-time detection. The former is historically the most common approach in routine occupational hygiene aerosol sampling and often involves both gravimetric and chemical analysis. In systems such as this, the nature of the airflow and particle motion in the vicinity outside and inside the sampling device becomes a critical issue in assessing the performance characteristics of the device.

Of the many aerosol properties that can be assessed, the most common is the aerosol mass per unit air volume (mass concentration) for particles falling within specific particle size fractions relating to how they might penetrate into the human respiratory tract after inhalation. This measure is the basis of most current standards for aerosol exposures. A traditional approach to aerosol sampling, one that is still widely applied in the United States and many other countries, involves sampling for what is commonly referred to as "total dust." The intention here is that all particles in the air should be collected with equal efficiency, so that the sample is collected without respect to any particular particle size fraction. Whether this is true has been the subject of much research (see, for example, the summary of Hinds[29]). By contrast, particle size-selective sampling is intended to separate the aerosol into size fractions based on based on health rationale. A complete review of sampling theory is given by Vincent[30], to which the interested reader is referred. Several important conclusions can be drawn from this review of theory: (1) All aerosol sampling in reality is size-selective (i.e., common samplers do not collect all the aerosol that exists in situ); (2) numerous losses occur in the process of sampling, both external and internal to the sampler; (3) the particle size-selective efficiency of a sampler is a complex function of sampler geometry, sampling rate, flow external to the sampler, and sampler orientation with respect to the direction of external flow; and (4) sampler theory is still quite rudimentary, but is sufficient to be useful in helping an industrial hygienist choose a sampler for a specific application and for assessing losses during sampling to identify "correction factors."

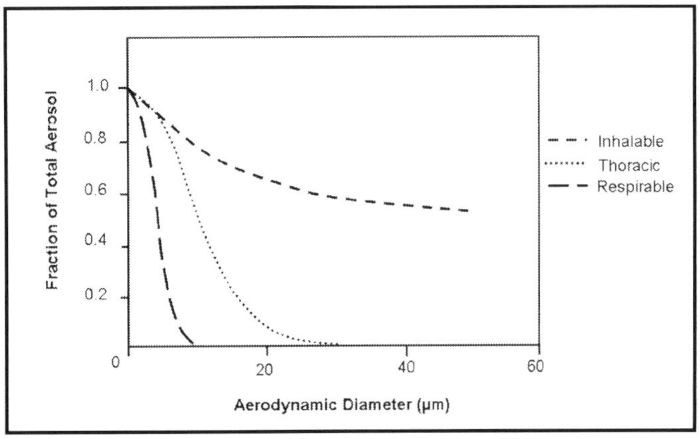

Figure 14.5 — Collection efficiency as a fraction of total aerosol of samplers performing according to the ACGIH/ISO/CEN size-selective sampling criteria.

Under certain conditions, it is possible for the efficiency of an aerosol sampler to be greater than 100% (because the nature of the particle motion near the sampler entry might be such as to actually increase the particle concentration.) One important fact that arises from considerations of sampler theory is that aerosol sampler performance is very complicated, and that the performances of individual samplers intended nominally for collecting the same fraction (e.g., total dust) may in fact be quite different. Here, therefore, the industrial hygienist must exercise caution in choosing an aerosol sampler to do a specific job and make sure that the chosen sampler does indeed collect the particle size fraction of interest. When available, the use of standard sampling and analytical methods allow for reproducible and comparable results.

No single aerosol sampling and analysis technique is suited to all possible information needs concerning aerosol exposure and control. Methods and devices are developed to answer specific questions, within the limits of available technology. Advances in both technology and our understanding of aerosol behavior and health effects are continual drivers for further development. This section describes aerosol sampling and analysis techniques in common use for workplace evaluation. Techniques designed for laboratory or research use, or for characterizing aerosols in ducts, stacks, and so forth are not discussed; these techniques are reviewed in detail by others (see, for example, Cohen and McCammon[31]).

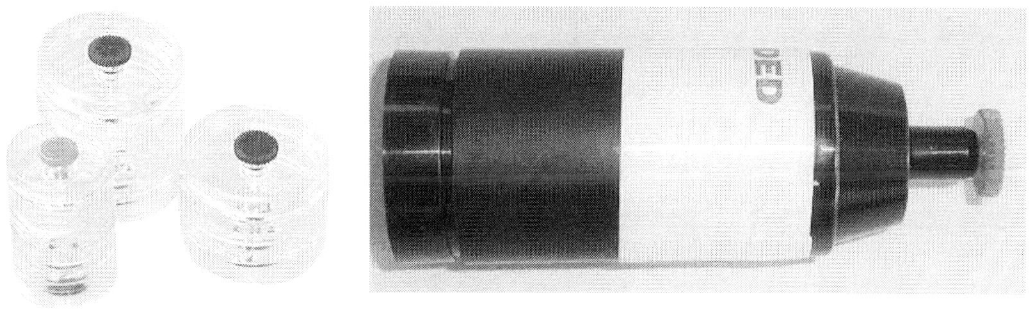

(a) (b)

Figure 14.6 — Examples of filter cassettes. (a) acrylonitrile cassettes, (b) polypropylene 25-mm cassette with cowl.

Particle Size-Selective Sampling

Aerosol particle size greatly influences where deposition occurs in the respiratory tract, and the site of deposition often determines the degree of hazard represented by the exposure. Aerosol sampling techniques have been developed to measure aerosol as inhalable, thoracic, or respirable fractions. This strategy assesses particle size fractions that penetrate progressively further into the respiratory tract, are very useful in assessing the hazard potential of occupational aerosol exposures. In recent years international agreement has been reached on how such criteria should be defined for the purposes of aerosol standards. Sampler performance exactly matching the criteria would collect particles of various sizes with the efficiencies shown in Figure 14.6. In practice, samplers with performances falling within prescribed tolerance bands are acceptable. Size-selective samplers for inhalable, thoracic, and respirable sampling are discussed in detail elsewhere (see, for example, Vincent[30] and Lippmann[32]) and Several of these are illustrated in the following sections.

Filtration-Based Techniques

Filters have been used for aerosol collection since the ancients first covered their faces with cloth veils to avoid breathing dust and they are still used in numerous air cleaning applications including respiratory protection, pollution control, and recovery of valuable fugitive materials. In exposure characterization, filtration-based techniques allow the study of aerosol mass concentration, number concentration, particle morphology, radioactivity, chemical content, and biohazard potential. Many types of filter media are available, and the choice of media depends on the aerosol characteristics and the analytical technique to be used. A brief overview of these topics is provided here; for more detailed information the reader is referred to the summaries of filtration theory and methods, filter media, and filter holders by Lee and Mukland[33] and Lippmann.[34]

Gravimetric analysis involves drawing a known volume of aerosol-laden air through a filter of known initial weight, then reweighing the filter to determine the mass captured. The average aerosol concentration is this mass divided by the volume of sampled air, typically expressed in terms of milligrams of aerosol per cubic meter of air sampled. In personal (breathing zone) sampling, conventional practice is to use a 25-, 37-, or 47-mm diameter filter cassette containing a filter supported by a screen or backing pad, orientated at a 45 degree angle down from horizontal. The cassettes may be used open-faced (with or without an extension hood) or closed-faced. Examples include the three-piece 25-mm cassette with extension cowl used for asbestos sampling, and the three-piece 37-mm polystyrene and two-piece 47-mm stainless steel cassettes used with the intention of collecting "total" aerosol (Figure 14.7). Here total is used in the sense defined earlier. However, research has shown that these samplers significantly and consistently under-sample even with respect to the inhalable fraction of larger particle sizes in typical workplace conditions.[35]

Studies and analysis of the results by researchers at the U.K. Health and Safety

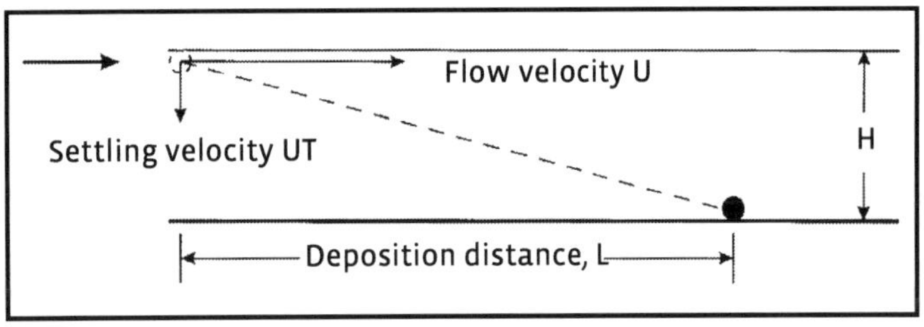

Figure 14.7 — Idealized horizontal elutriator.

Laboratory and the National Institute of Occupational Safety and Health (NIOSH) were carried out to examine the performances of a number of candidate samplers for the inhalable fraction. These showed that the currently available sampler that best collects the inhalable fraction is the so-called Institute of Occupational Medicine (IOM) sampler (SKC Ltd., Blandford Forum, Hants, U.K.).[36–38] This 2 L/min sampling device features a 25-mm filter in a removable capsule and a 15-mm circular inlet and has been shown to accurately sample the inhalable fraction of ambient aerosol for particles up to at least 80 μm in aerodynamic diameter and for wind speeds up to 2.6 m/sec.[14]

Filter media of the types most widely used are classified as fiber, porous membrane, or straight-through (capillary) membrane filters.[33] Fiber filters commonly are composed of cellulose, glass, or quartz fibers. They exhibit a low pressure drop at high sampling flow rates, have a high loading capacity, and are relatively inexpensive; however, they may not be adequately efficient for submicron particle sizes, and water absorption may present problems in gravimetric analyses. Because filters must be removed from cassettes for reweighing, the high mechanical strength of fiber filters can be a distinct advantage over other filter types.

Porous membrane filters are produced from gels of cellulose ester, polyvinyl chloride, and other materials that set in a highly porous mesh microstructure leaving convoluted flow paths. Membrane filter efficiency is reflected in a pore size rating that ranges from approximately 0.1 to 10 μm, but pore size rating can be a misleading indicator. For example, mixed cellulose ester (MCE) membrane filters of 5-μm pore size are typically greater than 98% efficient even for 1-μm and smaller particles, and 8-μm MCE filters are greater than 92% efficient for these particles.[33,39] These filters, like fiber filters, are considered to be "depth filters," because deposition is throughout the filter matrix, but porous membrane filters have generally higher flow resistance and lower loading capacity than fiber filters.

Straight-through, or capillary, membrane filters are made of polycarbonate or polyester film perforated with straight-through pores of nearly uniform size and distribution. The holes result from neutron bombardment followed by chemical etching to the desired size. Straight-through filters have a high pressure drop and low loading capacity compared to other filters and are susceptible to static charge buildup that can affect particle capture and retention. However, they have distinct advantages for optical or electron microscopic particle analysis. Here, viewing is excellent because particles larger than the pore size are captured at the filter surface, which is extremely flat and smooth.

Polyester foam media may represent a filtration technology suited to simultaneous sampling of multiple aerosol fractions in a single sampler. A sampler designed by Vincent et al.[40] utilizes two foam plugs in series with a final high efficiency filter to separate the inhalable, thoracic-less-respirable, and respirable fractions of sampled aerosol. The advantages of such a device are obvious; however there are unresolved questions about its usefulness for other analytical needs and about the feasibility of large-scale manufacture of uniform and well-characterized foams.

Major suppliers market numerous varieties and sizes of fiber filters, membrane filters, and straight-through membrane filters[34], so choice of the appropriate media for a particular application can be a challenge. When standard methods do not specify the sampling media and method, supplier technical representatives or the supporting analytical laboratory may provide useful guidance.

In any type of filter sampling there is a risk of losing volatile material during collection and of suffering unplanned chemical reactions between collected material and the filter media. Volatiles may be captured on sorbent media placed in series with and downstream of the filter media, and in some cases chemically treated filters are available that react with and retain the contaminant. Careful choice of sampling media may prevent undesirable species-media reactions.

Sedimentation-Based Techniques for Collecting Finer Particle Fractions

Sedimentation-based aerosol sampling techniques are conceptually simple. The horizontal elutriator first emerged in the 1950s. The theory of horizontal elutriation formed the basis of the first definition for the respirable fraction (i.e., the British Medical Research Council definition, later referred to as the "Johannesburg curve" after it was accepted as an international definition at a 1959 conference in Johannesburg on pneumoconiosis). The aspirated aerosol passes in the laminar airflow between two narrowly spaced horizontal plates as shown in Figure 14.7. An aerosol particle in this flow settles under gravity at its terminal settling velocity UT, so that in a sufficiently long elutriator the particle eventually reaches the bottom plate and is captured. It may be shown that for a particle entering at the top plate of the elutriator, its deposition distance L from the elutriator entrance is

$$L = H \frac{U}{U_T} \tag{14-9}$$

where H is the height of the channel. The actual path traveled by the particle is not linear, as suggested by this equation; rather, it follows a curved path due to the parabolic velocity profile of the laminar airflow between the plates.[14] Although simple to design and build, horizontal elutriators are not suited to personal sampling and do not provide good resolution of particle sizes. However, they are effective as preselectors in area samplers for respirable aerosol. For example, the British MRE type 113A area sampler incorporates a multichannel horizontal elutriator preseparator to remove nonrespirable particles from sampled aerosol prior to filtration. This device is still used in the British and some European coal mining industries.

Cyclones

Cyclone separators utilize centrifugal forces to effect particle capture. Cyclones cause the sampled air to be spun in a tapering tube, as shown conceptually in Figure 14.8. In the complicated flow inside the body of the cyclone, particles migrate toward the tube walls and are removed. The remaining suspended particles pass out of the device with the airstream and are collected on a filter. The so-called cut size of the device indicates the aerodynamic diameter of particles for which penetration through the cyclone is 50%, that is, the d_{50}. Cyclones are most efficient for large particle sizes and are used in occupational hygiene primarily as preseparators. Because they can be made very compact, they have been developed as miniature versions for personal sampling. The d50 for a cyclone is controlled by the configuration of the cyclone and the flow conditions and decreases with decreasing cyclone diameter and increasing flow rate. Common examples in use as preselectors for the respirable fraction for the purpose of occupational hygiene sampling are the Dorr-Oliver nylon cyclone preclassifier operating at 1.7 L/min (Zefon International, St. Petersburg, Fla.), the Casella cyclone sampler operating at 1.9 L/min (Casella CEL, Amherst, N.H.), and the SKC GS-3 conductive plastic cyclone sampler (SKC Inc., Eighty Four, Pa.) (Figure 14.9). The SKC Spiral Sampler provides an alternative method of collecting respirable samples in a compact configuration. In each device the respirable aerosol fraction passes through the cyclone to be captured on a filter for subsequent analysis. Collection efficiency performance criteria adopted by the

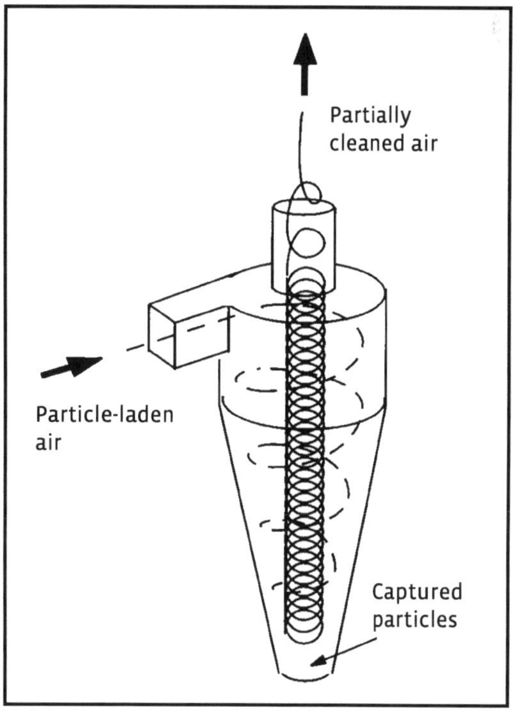

Figure 14.8 — Cyclone separator.

American Conference of Governmental Industrial Hygienists and the International Standards Organization/European Standardization Committee specify that cyclones and other respirable aerosol sampling devices should exhibit a d_{50} of 4 µm for the respirable fraction.[41]

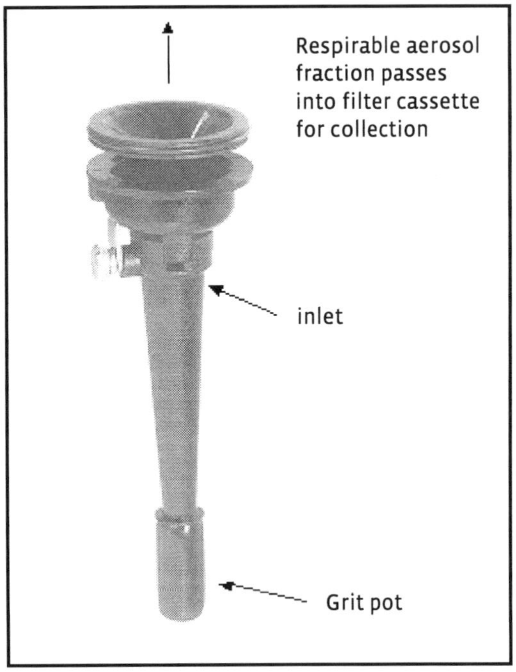

Figure 14.9 — Personal cyclone. Exploded view of a personal respirable dust sampling assembly incorporating an SKC aluminum cyclone and 37-mm three-piece filter cassette. Nonrespirable particles are collected in the grit pot at the base of the cyclone, and the respirable fraction is collected on the filter for subsequent weighing or chemical analysis (graphic courtesy SKC, Inc.).

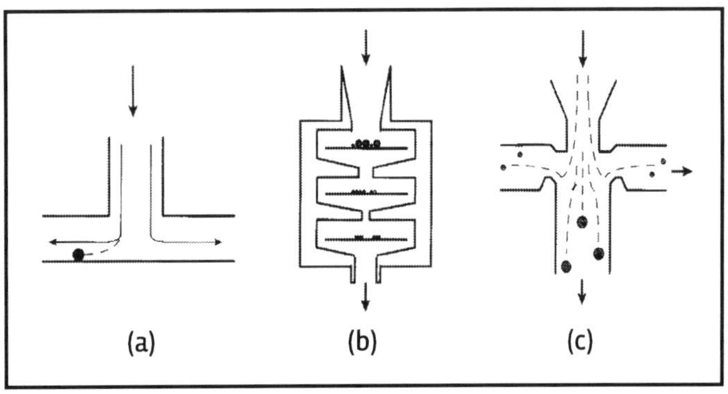

Figure 14.10 — Inertial impactors: (a) conventional jet-to-plate; (b) multi-stage or cascade impactor; and (c) virtual impactor or dichotomous sampler.

Impaction-Based Techniques

Impaction-based sampling devices are commonly used for aerosol characterization in relation to particle size. In essence, an impactor relies on a particle's inertia to carry it onto a collection surface on which the sample airstream impinges (Figure 14.10a). Jet-and-plate impactors direct a high-velocity jet against a collection surface such that the air is forced to make an abrupt 90 degree turn. Depending on its mass and position in the jet, an entrained particle may or may not strike the plate and be captured. The likelihood of capture increases with increasing Stokes' number as shown in Equation 14-6, where the characteristic velocity and dimensions of the system are the jet's average velocity and the slot half-width for a rectangular slot impactor or throat radius for a circular jet impactor. The parameter often used to characterize impactor performance is again the 50% cut point size, d_{50}, which is the particle size captured by the impactor with 50% efficiency.

Single-stage impactors often are used as preseparators for other sampling devices, as in samplers designed to measure only particulate matter less than a specified size. For example, the diesel particulate matter (DPM) personal sampler (SKC, Inc.), which was

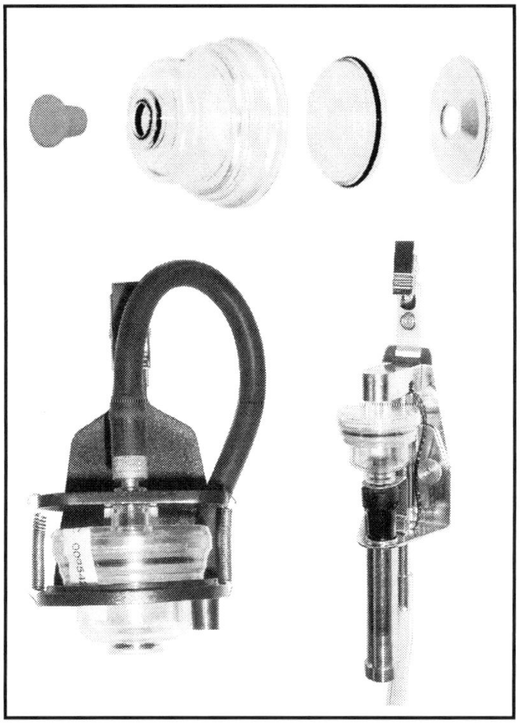

Figure 14.11 — Diesel particulate matter (DPM) personal sampler.

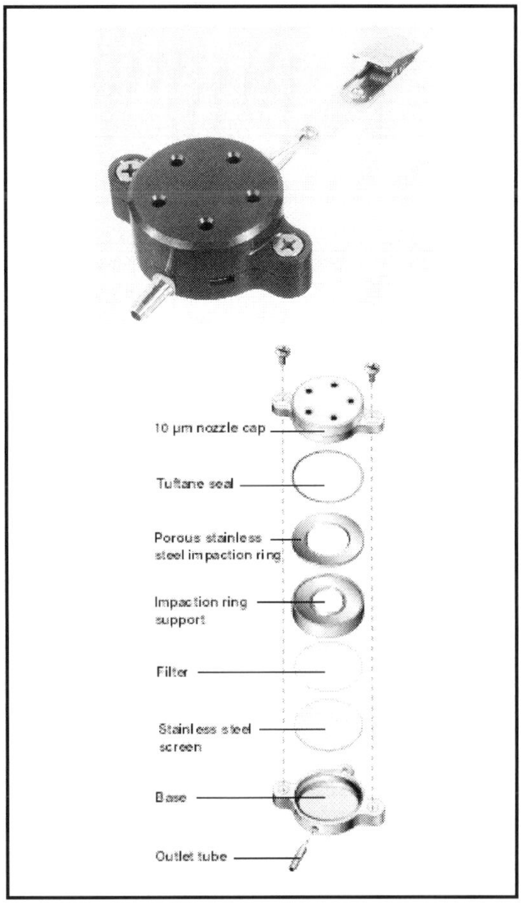

Figure 14.12 — Personal environmental monitor (PEM) sampler.

designed to separate diesel particulate aerosol from coarser dusts in mines, employs a four-nozzle precision-jeweled impactor with a 0.9 µm cut size at a 1.7 L/min flow rate (Figure 14.11). Particles smaller than this size, which are taken to represent the aerosol fraction associated with diesel exhaust particulate, pass through the impactor and are captured on a filter for analysis (for a discussion of mining aerosols see Cantrell and Volkwein[42]). The sampler may be preceded by a respirable cyclone preseparator to avoid overloading the impactor. A similar device is the personal environmental monitor (PEM) sampler (SKC, Inc.) (Figure 14.12). The PEM features five nozzles in an interchangeable cap, with nozzle sizes allowing cut points of either 2.5 or 10 µm at a flow rate of 2, 4, or 10 L/min (i.e., six-cap models are available). Particulate matter smaller than the cut point size again is collected on a filter for analysis. The device may be used by itself as shown in the exploded view at Figure 14.11 or may be preceded by a respirable cyclone preseparator (graphics courtesy SKC, Inc.).

When the impactor itself is the primary instrument, multistage designs usually are used in a cascade configuration as shown in Figure 14.10b. Cascade impactors place impactors of descending cut size in series so that the largest particles are removed in the first stage, and serially smaller particles are removed in the subsequent stages. In a well-designed device each stage collects a narrow range of particle sizes, so that the sampled aerosol is separated into distinct and, ideally, nonoverlapping size fractions (in practice there is always some overlap). In the simplest approach the mass of particulate material collected on each stage is used to generate a cumulative mass distribution that may then be plotted against a characteristic particle size for each stage. Such data for aerosols with log-normally distributed particle sizes plots as a straight line on log-probability paper, so that the distribution's geometric mean particle size and geometric standard deviation may be graphically determined (see, for example, Lodge and Chan[43]). It is recognized, however, that this approach is highly simplistic, because it is mathematically impossible to infer a continuous particle size distribution from just a small number of discrete pieces of information. With the advent of computers and modern spreadsheet software, a range of mathematical inversion methods has been developed that can provide more accurate results from the original raw data.[44]

Well-known cascade impactors are the Andersen 8-stage area sampler operated at 28.3 L/min and the Marple personal cascade impactor operated at 2 L/min.[45] The IOM 2-L/min personal inhalable dust spectrometer (PIDS) is similar to the Marple personal cascade impactor sampler except that the PIDS uses circular rather than slot jets. In addition, use of the PIDS allows inclusion in the analysis of particulate material collected in the inlet of the sampler above the first impactor stage, and so—when used with an appropriate mathematical algorithm—can accurately provide particle size information over the whole inhalable range of particle aerodynamic diameter up to 100 µm.

Material collected by cascade impaction may be analyzed in various ways. Gravimetric analysis of the total mass collected on each plate, chemical or radiometric analysis to determine the distribution of species across particle size, and extraction and mutagenic evaluation of different size fractions are some options. These data may be extremely useful in hazard evaluation because more will be known about what potentially hazardous materials are present and where they might deposit in the respiratory tract. Specially designed samplers that hold growth media (agar) are available for microbiological sampling.

An interesting variation on the conventional plate-type impactor is the virtual impactor (Figure 14.10c). In this device there is no collection surface. Rather, the aerosol jet exiting the nozzle impinges on the surface of lower-velocity "minor flow" in the collection probe. As the major portion of the flow is forced to reverse direction and exit the device, larger particles fail to negotiate the turn and penetrate into the body of the minor flow. The minor flow thus contains the larger size fraction and the major flow contains the smaller size fraction, and both flows are available for further use or analysis. Such "dichotomous" samplers have been designed specifically to separate the $PM_{2.5}$ fraction from the PM_{10} fraction in ambient air samples to distinguish between the "fine" and "coarse" fractions of PM_{10}.[46] $PM_{2.5}$ and PM_{10} refer to the subfractions of airborne particulate matter (PM) that are smaller than 2.5 µm or 10 µm, respectively.

Another variation of the impactor is the liquid impinger. Liquid impingers project an aerosol jet against a wetted surface (May Multistage Liquid Impinger, Figure 14.13a), a submerged surface (AGI-4 All Glass Impinger), or a liquid surface (AGI-30 impinger, Figure 14.13b). These devices are especially useful when sampling mist aerosols that might evaporate on a dry collection plate or when it is otherwise desirable to react either the collected aerosol or a gas phase component with the collection liquid. The collection liquid may be examined in various ways, including particle counting. Particle counting was used in the past to characterize dust exposure from impinger samples, with dust concentrations expressed in units of millions of particles per cubic foot (mppcf).[47] Epidemiologists conducting retrospective exposure assessments of the dusty trades must often wrestle with the difficulties of converting data in millions of particles per cubic foot to equivalent exposures in milligrams per cubic meter.

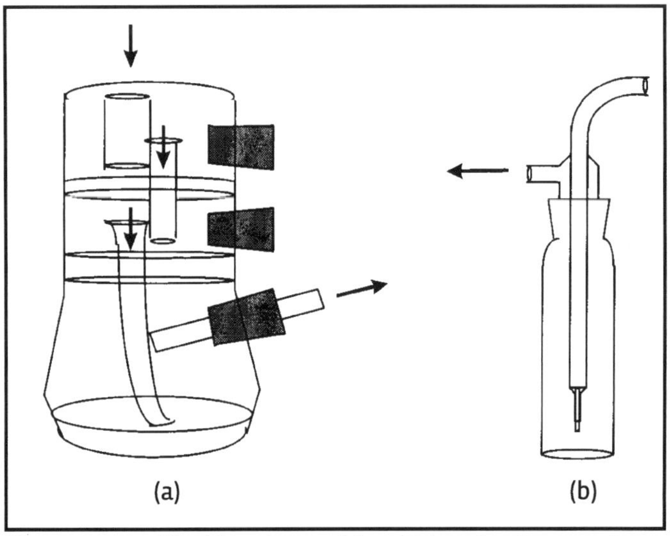

Figure 14.13 — Liquid impingers: (a) multistage impinger; and (b) common all glass impinger.

Optical Techniques

Optical aerosol measurement methods employ scattered light to characterize the concentration and/or particle size distribution of aerosols. This technology is applicable for particles from 0.05–20 µm. Some devices simply count the number of particles present in a sample to provide a count concentration; some both count the particles and individually measure their size to provide count concentration and count size distribution information (the number of particles in each discrete particle size range); and some estimate the aerosol mass concentration of a cloud of aerosol particles. These methods historically required large and often complex instrumentation and were limited to research applications or area monitoring. Recently, laser diode illumination sources and the availability of miniaturized solid state electronics with on-board data logging have promoted the recent development of miniaturized aerosol monitors that may be used as personal samplers. These devices provide near real-time aerosol measurement with high temporal resolution, downloadable time-stamped data sets, and both on-board and remote data processing, analysis, and display. However, like all instruments they have their limitations, and it is important to understand these limitations to avoid systematic measurement errors and be able to interpret result.

Light incident on an aerosol particle may be absorbed by the particle or scattered by it. The combined effect of absorption and scattering is extinction. Scattered light is light that is reflected, refracted, or diffracted by the particle so that it deviates from its original path. The interaction of light and a particle is related to both light factors and particle factors, namely the wavelength of the light (λ), the particle size (d), the particle shape, and particle material refractive index (m). The wavelength and particle size are related by the size parameter, $\alpha = \lambda$. For $a \ll 1$, say for visible light with $\lambda \sim 0.5$ µm and $d < 0.05$ µm, that is, $\alpha \sim 0.3$, the interaction is described by Rayleigh's theory, which indicates that light incident on a particle of arbitrary shape will be radiated symmetrically in the direction of the incident beam (forward scattering) and opposite to the beam direction (backward scattering). The intensity of scattered light at any angle q from the beam direction is a function of beam wavelength, particle size, and particle refractive index. Rayleigh scattering is important primarily for small particles. For $\alpha \gg 1$, say for visible light and $d > 50$ µm, that is, α on the order of 100–1000, the light is treated as rays and behaves according to the laws of classical optics. The amount of diffraction is of special interest because diffraction is dependent on particle size (the parameter of interest) but independent of refractive index (a parameter typically not known for an industrial aerosol). Further, diffraction effects dominate the scattered light at low scattering angles, so aerosol particle measurement devices are often forward-scattering devices that measure the amount of light scattered at a small angle from the incident beam direction.

Most of the particles of inhalation concern fall in the size range between the Rayleigh and ray optics regions. The more complex Lorenz-Mie theory (which encompasses Rayleigh theory and classical ray optics) is required to mathematically describe their extinction behavior. For particle sizes on the order of the wavelength of incident light, for example, 0.1–1 µm (100–1000 nm), multiple particle sizes may produce the same scattering intensity, so that a measured signal may represent any of several particle sizes. Further, in this region the scattering signal is also strongly influenced by the particle refractive index. Therefore, optical instruments that characterize particle size from scattered light must be calibrated for the aerosol being measured.

Measurements may be of individual particles or of the aerosol as an ensemble of many particles. In a single-particle optical particle counter/sizer photometer, aerosol particles are passed individually through a sensing zone and illuminated by a light source. The pulse of scattered light is collected over some scattering angle, focused with a lens onto a photodetector, and the photodetector output signal is then amplified and analyzed for peak height or area as an indication of particle geometric size. Current instruments automatically log the counts in size intervals or "bins" and process the data into displays or summary statistics. Different instruments are distinguished primarily by the scattering angle used. Forward-scattering instruments collect diffracted light at a low scattering angle. These devices have difficulty in accurately distinguishing particle sizes over the 0.7–1.2 µm range due to the problem of multivalued scattering signals, as discussed previously. Other instruments collect scattered light over a larger angle and may be termed "near forward scattering," and are therefore affected by the refractive index and shape of the measured particles.

An occupational hygiene application of single-particle optical counters is the condensation nucleus counter (CNC) which measures particles in the range of 0.005 – 1.0 µm. An example is the CNC component of respirator quantitative fit-test systems such as the Portacount Plus (TSI Inc., St. Paul, Minn.). Naturally occurring airborne particles that are normally too small to be detected by an optical instrument are passed through an alcohol vapor chamber in which the alcohol condenses around the particle to form a liquid droplet. The droplets are large enough to produce a detectable scattered light pulse when passed through the instrument's beam, so that a count concentration of condensation nuclei is obtained from the number of counts and the sampling flow rate. The ratio of condensation nuclei concentrations measured outside and inside the respirator facepiece provide a quantitative measure of leakage through the face-to-facepiece seal—the higher the ratio, or fit factor, the better the seal. It should be noted that CNC and other single-particle optical counting instruments provide count concentration but not size distribution information.

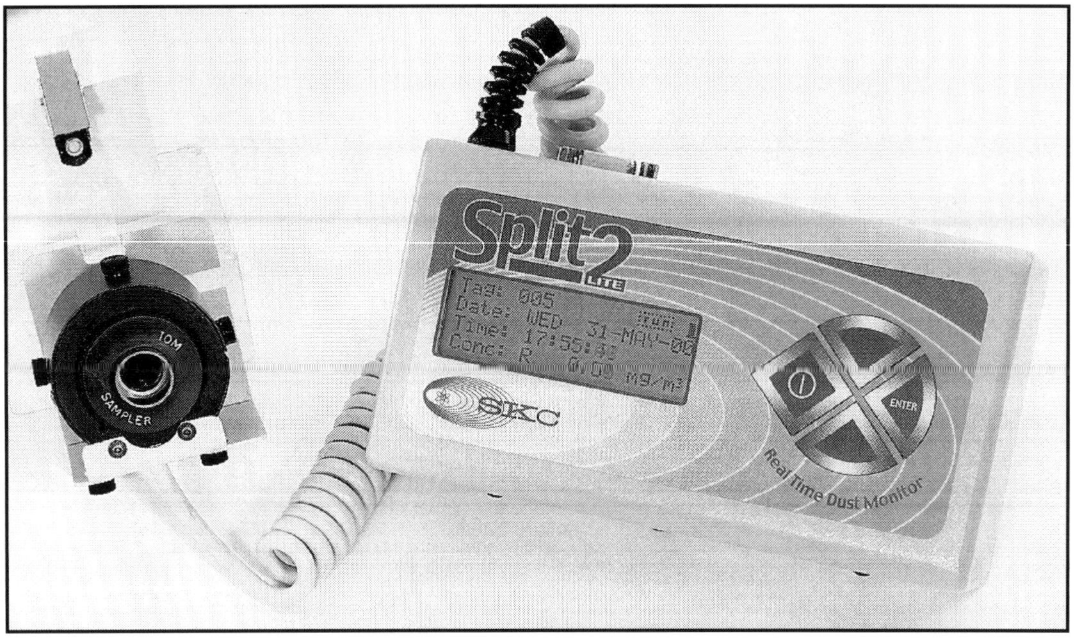

Figure 14.14 — Personal ensemble aerosol photometer (nephelometer).

In an "ensemble-sensing" device, also termed a nephelometer, the light beam passes through a cloud of particles and the cumulative amount of light scattered into a given solid angle is collected by a photodetector. The photodetector signal is a function of the beam wavelength as well as the aerosol particle size distribution, refractive index distribution, and concentration, as well as the angle at which the light is scattered. For aerosol of a given material and particle size distribution the photometer signal varies linearly with aerosol concentration over wide ranges of concentrations. When the concentration of the particle cloud is high, light scattered from one particle may subsequently be rescattered by other particles. This multiple-scattering situation reduces the instrument's sensitivity to concentration changes, and the instrument is said to be "overloaded." When such concentrated aerosols are measured it may be necessary to dilute the sample before introducing it into the instrument's sensing volume. Ensemble data-logging aerosol photometers suitable for personal sampling include the MIE Personal DataRAM (Realtime Aerosol Monitor) (MIE, Billerica, Mass.) and the SKC Split2 Real-time Personal Dust Sampler (SKC Inc.), Figure 14.14. Neither instrument requires an air pump, relying instead on normal air currents to move aerosol into the sensing zone; however, both devices have battery-operated pump add-on accessories that allow air to be drawn through the sensing zone and subsequently onto a collection filter, as well as preseparator add-ons to allow size-selective aerosol measurement. The addition of these accessories substantially increases the size and weight of the samplers and reduces their ease of use for breathing-zone or personal sampling. Active sampling particulate monitors incorporating an internal pump and battery may also be fitted with size-selective sampling heads. All of these instruments provide output in mass concentration units (mg/m^3), but they are factory calibrated against a standard fine dust test aerosol (e.g., Arizona road dust), and the indicated values may be inaccurate for a different aerosol. So it is important to calibrate the devices for the aerosol of interest if reliable concentration estimates are needed. The air pump and filter accessories may be used in calibrating the instruments for the aerosol of interest in actual sampling conditions.

Microscopy Techniques

Aerosol analysis by microscopy involves examination of the aerosol particles after they have been deposited on a suitable substrate, such as a filter or an electron microscope grid.[48] Commonly used techniques include phase contrast microscopy, polarized light microscopy, scanning electron microscopy, and transmission electron microscopy. As with other sampling methods the aerosol particle size characteristics are an important determinant of the method chosen. Of primary importance is the particle size with respect to the resolving power of the microscope. In the case of an optical microscope, the resolving power is a function of the wavelength of the light, which varies from 0.4 μm (violet) to 0.7 μm (red). Under ideal conditions the resolving power is approximately 0.2 μm, which is to say that smaller particles cannot be sized by optical microscopy. The primary current application of optical microscopy is to obtain information about the aerosol count concentration (such as fiber concentration of asbestos aerosol samples) or about the aerosol count size distribution. Maximum optical magnification, using an oil immersion objective, is limited to approximately 1000×.

Electron microscopy requires a special collecting substrate, such as carbon film, and a film support structure that will fit the microscope sample holder. The two commonly used electron microscopy (EM) methods are transmission EM and scanning EM. In transmission EM the support structure is a thin metal grid having a diameter of 2 mm. The electron beam is directed perpendicular to the sample grid, and particles are detected by the differing electron transmission of the particles and the substrate. Transmission EM resolving power is of the order of 10 ηm. In its simplest form transmission EM yields a two-dimensional image of the particles. It is common to "shadow" the sample by evaporating a metal under vacuum conditions to produce a thin metal film onto the particles and substrate; by orienting the metal vapor source oblique to the sample, a shadow is produced behind each particle that yields some information about the third dimension.

In scanning EM the electron beam itself is oriented oblique to the sample, and the scattered electrons are detected to yield images. This approach is somewhat similar to the shadowing of transmission EM samples in that some three-dimensional information is obtained. However, scanning EM differs in that the scattering of electrons by particles is fundamentally different from electron transmission. The contrast between particles and substrate is generally greater for transmission EM. Some particles are difficult to detect in scanning EM because of their low scattering efficiency. Additionally, the resolving power of scanning EM is substantially less than that for transmission. Resolution is approximately 0.01 μm for scanning EM compared with 0.001 μm for transmission EM. Therefore, the choice between these two methods depends on both the particle composition and size.

A major problem with both EM methods is the question of a representative sample. The area of the collecting substrate for both methods is very small, and it is not feasible to collect an entire sample onto a grid or substrate. Only an extremely small fraction of the total aerosol is collected onto the substrate, and the surface density of particles is quite low. It is thus difficult to obtain a number or mass concentration of an aerosol from an EM analysis. Rather, it is more common to consider the particles as representative of the size distribution and use the results for this purpose.

For additional information on optical and EM microscopy techniques relevant to occupational hygiene practice, please see the detailed discussions provided by Silverman et al.[48] and Cradle.[49]

Other Samplers

Significant research into new technologies and applications for aerosol analysis continues. Interest in ultrafine and nanometer sized particulates is increasing. Engineered nanoparticles (particles with at least one dimension less than 100 ηm) may have designed physical, chemical, or biological properties.

The Tapered-Element Oscillating Microbalance (TEOM) air sampler provides a real-time measurement of particulate by measuring the rate of vibration of a quartz crystal. Although this technique has been used primarily for measuring outdoor samples, it is readily adaptable to industrial applications for continuous monitoring within a plant site.

Electrical Aerosol Detectors (EAD) work by imparting a charge to particles and measuring the charge with an electrometer.

Denuder systems and diffusion batteries collect gases, vapors, and ultra-fines by differential diffusion mobility and can be used in conjunction with aerosol samplers to separate these materials from larger particulates.[50, 51] These are research tools used to collect ultrafine or nano-particles between 1 m–0.1 µm.

Aerosol Size Distribution Analysis

Natural and industrial aerosols are virtually always polydisperse—that is, they are made up of particles that are not all of the same size. Indeed, for most aerosols encountered in the occupational hygiene setting, the range of particle sizes found may be very wide. The simplest case might be that of a mist aerosol, such as might be mechanically generated in an industrial process through splashing, spraying, or agitation. Here the particles are morphologically and chemically similar in that they are spherical droplets of the parent material, with the only real difference between particles being in their diameter. As is the case for many quantities occurring in nature, particle sizes in such an aerosol are often approximately lognormally distributed; that is, the logarithms of the particles sizes follow a Gaussian, or normal, frequency distribution. This is fortunate because it allows the entire distribution to be characterized with two descriptors or "statistics": geometric mean (or median) size and geometric standard deviation (GSD). The distribution is likely to be expressed using either the count median diameter (CMD) and GSD, or the mass median aerodynamic diameter (MMAD) and GSD, depending on how the measurement data were obtained. Count-based frequency distributions result from such measurement devices as optical particle counters/sizers, which determine the geometric size of a particle from the amount of incident light scattered by the particle at a specified angle as previously discussed (see also, for example, Chen and Pui and[52]). Particle counts are grouped in size intervals, and the CMD and GSD may be calculated as:

$$\log \text{CMD} = \frac{\sum_{i=l}^{N} n_i \log d_i}{\sum_{i=l}^{N} n_i - 1} \qquad (14\text{-}10)$$

$$\log \text{GSD} = \sqrt{\frac{\sum_{i=l}^{N} N_i (\log \text{CMD} - \log d_i)^2}{\sum_{i=l}^{N} n_i - 1}} \qquad (14\text{-}11)$$

where n_i is the number of particles in a given interval, d_i is the midpoint size for the interval, and N is the total number of intervals collected. These calculations, which are tedious to perform, may give a misleading impression of mathematical certainty, because measurement data may be only approximately lognormally distributed. Fortunately, a simple graphical technique is available that is useful for both checking the lognormality of the data and obtaining the CMD and GSD. As shown in Table 14.1, the fraction of the total count in each size interval is as reported by the measurement instrument, the cumulative fraction less than a stated size (e.g., the interval midpoint) is calculated, and the data are graphed as a cumulative frequency distribution in a log-probability plot as shown in Figure 14.15. Note that the top-most data point (that corresponding to 100%) is not plotted. If the data are lognormally distributed, then a straight line may be fitted to the data points—the general practice among hygienists is to perform an "eyeball regression." CMD is taken as the particle size corresponding to the 50% probability of occurrence, and the GSD is calculated as either the ratio of CMD to the 15.87% particle size or the ratio of the 84.13% particle size to the CMD (both will give the same GSD value). If a single straight line cannot be fitted to the data, then the distribution is not lognormal, as might be the case for mixtures of aerosols originating from different sources. For example, coal mine aerosols may be made up of aerosols from diesel engine exhausts, which are largely fine soot particles, mixed with much coarser carbon based mine dust. The aerosols taken individually are likely to exhibit lognormally distributed particle sizes but with much different median diameters and GSDs. The combined aerosol will then be multimodal, with multiple modes, or peaks, instead of only one. Measurement data for the aerosol would not fall in a straight line on a log-probability plot. Thus, log-probability plots provide more interpretive information than the calculated values from Equations 14.10 and 14.11.

Cascade impactors are examples of mass-based measurement instruments that characterize the mass fraction rather than count fraction in specified particle size intervals. In this case the size intervals represent aerodynamic particle size and are usually reported in terms of aerodynamic equivalent diameter, d_{ae}. The data analysis is similar to that performed in Table 14.3 in that the fraction of total collected mass represented by each size interval (collection stage) is calculated, the cumulative mass frequency distribution is determined, a log-probability plot is prepared, and the MMAD and GSD are obtained. Note that for a given lognormally distributed aerosol the MMAD will be larger than the CMD.[12] As mentioned earlier, this approach is quite crude, although it may be sufficient for many practical occupational hygiene applications. But for more accurate results, the application of an appropriate mathematical inversion algorithm may be used.[44]

Occupational hygienists and epidemiologists may find it necessary to compare occupational exposure data obtained using different measurement techniques. For example, it might be desirable to combine data from cascade impactor sampling with data from optical particle counting when classifying worker exposures. This is by no means a simple task, because such factors as particle shape, density, and refractive index must be well understood if data of one type are to be mathematically converted to another type.

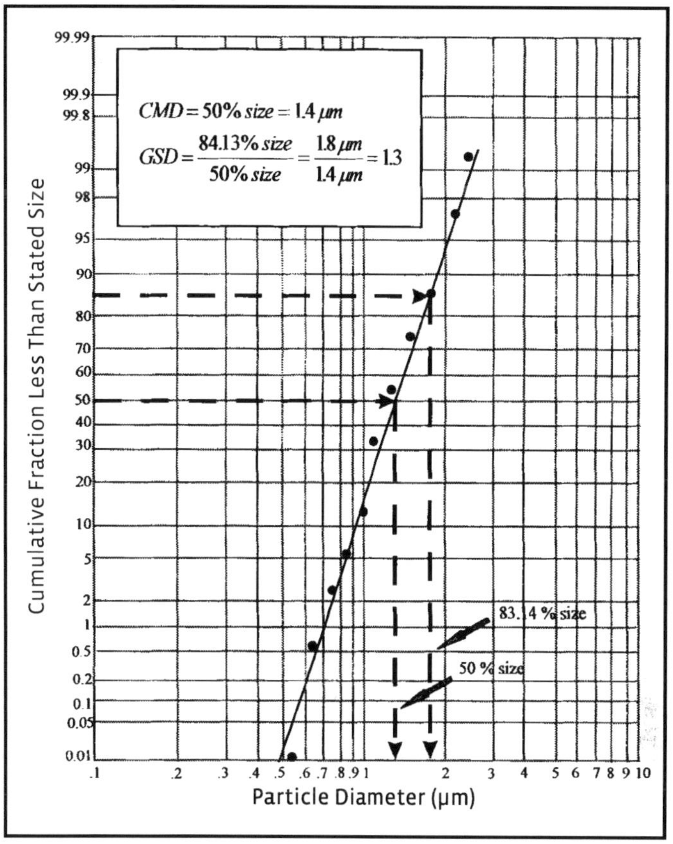

Figure 14.15 — Aerosol size distribution cumulative probability plot. The aerosol particle sizes are approximately log normally distributed if a straight line provides a good fit to the measurement data. CMD and GSD are determined from the plotted line. Count-based distributions result from optical measurement instruments that estimate particulate size by examining particle light scattering behavior.

Table 14.2 — Analysis of Particle Count Data

Lower Interval Size (μm)	*Upper Interval Size (μm)*	*Midpoint Interval Size d_i (μm)*	*Number in Interval n_i*	*Fraction Interval (%)*	*Cumulative Fraction less Than d_i (%)*
0.46	0.54	0.50	3770	0.74	0.74
0.54	0.63	0.585	13,000	2.56	3.30
0.66	0.74	0.685	55,100	10.84	14.14
0.74	0.86	0.80	62,900	12.38	26.52
0.86	1.0	0.93	98,800	19.44	45.96
1.0	1.2	1.1	109,000	21.45	67.41
1.2	1.4	1.3	98,800	19.44	86.85
1.4	1.6	1.5	37,200	7.32	94.17
1.6	1.8	1.7	17,000	3.35	97.52
1.8	2.2	2.0	9710	1.91	99.43
2.2	2.5	2.35	2850	0.56	99.99
2.5	2.9	2.7	52	0.01	100
			508,182		

Summary

Numerous sampling and analysis techniques are available to characterize potentially hazardous aerosol exposures in occupational environments. Selection of the appropriate technique is a matter of recognizing the potential hazard based on an understanding of process variables and aerosol behavior, defining the information needs required for hazard evaluation, then identifying a sampling and analytical method that will satisfy those needs. No single method can address all possible questions about a given aerosol, nor can any single method answer a given question for all possible aerosols. The choice of which instrument or media to use, or which analysis to perform, may be based on regulatory requirements, current accepted practice, or individual judgment. In all cases an understanding of the capabilities and limitations of the technique used is critical to effective data interpretation and accurate exposure characterization.

References

1. **Hunter, D.:** *The Diseases of Occupations*, 6th edition. London: Hodder and Stroughton, 1978.
2. **Agricola, G.:** De Re Metallica. Basel: 1556. Trans. C.C. Hoover and L.H. Hoover. New York: Dover Publications, 1950.
3. **Baron, P.A., and K. Willeke (eds.):** *Aerosol Measurement: Principles, Techniques and Applications*, 2nd edition. New York: John Wiley & Sons, 2001.
4. **Cox, C.S., and C.M. Wathes (eds.):** *Bioaerosols Handbook*. Boca Raton, Fla.: Lewis Publishers, 1995.
5. **Vincent, J.H.:** *Aerosol Sampling: Science, Standards, Instrumentation and Application*. Chichester, U.K.: John Wiley & Sons, 2007.
6. **Reist, P.C.:** *Aerosol Science and Technology*, 2nd edition. New York: McGraw-Hill, 1993.
7. **U.S. Department of Health, Education and Welfare (DHEW):** Smoking and Health: A Report of the Surgeon General (Publication no. DHEW [PHS] 79050066). Washington, D.C.: U.S. Government Printing Office, 1979.
8. **U.S. Department of Health and Human Services (DHHS):** The Health Consequences of Smoking: Chronic Obstructive Lung Disease. A Report of the Surgeon General (Publication no. DHHS [PHS] 84-50205). Washington, D.C.: U.S. Government Printing Office, 1984.
9. **U.S. Environmental Protection Agency (EPA):** Workshop Report on Chronic Inhalation Toxicity and Carcinogenicity Testing of Respirable Fibrous Particles (Publication no. EPA-748-R-96-001). Washington, D.C.: U.S. Government Printing Office, 1996.
10. **Donaldson, K., R.C. Brown, and G.M. Brown:** Respirable industrial fibers: Mechanisms of pathogenicity. *Brit. Assoc. Lung Res. 48*:390–393 (1993).
11. **Ruzer, L.S. and N.H. Harley (eds.):** *Aerosols Handbook: Measurement, Dosimetery, and Health Effects*. Boca Raton, Fla.: CRC Press 2000.
12. **Hinds, W.C.:** *Aerosol Technology-Properties, Behavior, and Measurement of Airborne Particles*, 2nd edition. New York: John Wiley & Sons, 1999.
13. **Mandelbrot, B.B.:** *The Fractal Geometry of Nature*. New York: Freeman, 1983.
14. **Vincent, J.H.:** *Aerosol Science for Industrial Hygienists*. New York: Elsevier Science, 1995.
15. **Miller, A.L., et al.:** *Microscopic Analysis of Airborne Particles and Fibers*. Cincinnati, Ohio: ACGIH®, 2008.
16. **Cunningham, E.:** On the velocity of steady fall of spherical particles through fluid medium. *Proc. Royal Soc. A83*:357–365 (1910).
17. **Mercer, T.T.:** *Aerosol Technology in Hazard Evaluation*. New York: Academic Press, 1973.
18. **Esmen, N.A.:** Adhesion and aerodynamic resuspension of fibrous particles. *J. Environ. Eng. 122*:379–383 (1996).
19. **Phalen, R.F.:** Airway anatomy and physiology. In *Particle Size-Selective Air Sampling for Particulate Air Contaminants*. Vincent, J.H. (ed.). Cincinnati, Ohio: ACGIH®, 1999. pp. 29–50.
20. **Rosenstock, L. and M.R. Cullen:** *Textbook of Clinical Occupational and Environmental Medicine*. Philadelphia: W.B. Saunders, 1994.
21. **Vincent, J. and L. Armbruster:** On the quantitative inhalability of airborne dust. *Ann. Occup. Hyg. 24*:245–248 (1981).
22. **Yu, C.P., and C.K. Diu:** A comparative study of aerosol deposition in different lung models. *Am. Ind. Hyg. Assoc. J. 43*:54–65 (1980).
23. **Weibel, E.R.:** *Morphometry of the Human Lung*. New York: Academic Press, 1963.
24. **Hansen, J.E., and E.P. Ampaya:** Human air space, shapes, sizes, areas and volumes. *J. Appl. Physiol. 38*:990–995 (1975).
25. **Yeh, H., and G.M. Schum:** Models of human lung airways and their application to inhaled particle deposition. *Bull. Math. Biol. 42*:461–480 (1980).
26. **Harris, R.L., and D.A. Fraser:** A model for deposition of fibers in the human respiratory system. *Am. Ind. Hyg. Assoc. J. 37*:73–89 (1976).

27. **Vincent, J.H.:** On the practical significance of electrostatic lung deposition of isometric and fibrous aerosols. *J. Aerosol. Sci. 16*:511–519 (1985).
28. **Rudolf, G., J. Gebhart, J. Heyder, C.F. Schiller, and W. Stahlhofen:** An empirical formula describing aerosol deposition in man for any particle size. *J. Aerosol Sci. 17*:350–355 (1986).
29. **Hinds, W.C.:** Sampling for inhalable aerosol. In *Particle Size-Selective Air Sampling for Particulate Air Contaminants.* Vincent, J.H. (ed.). Cincinnati, Ohio: ACGIH®, 1999. pp. 119–140.
30. **Vincent, J.H.:** *Particle Size Selective Sampling for Particulate Air Contaminants.* Cincinnati, Ohio: ACGIH®, 1999.
31. **Cohen, B.S., and C.S. McCammon, Jr. (eds.):** *Air Sampling Instruments for Evaluation of Atmospheric Contaminants,* 9th edition. Cincinnati, Ohio: ACGIH®, 2001.
32. **Lippmann, M.:** Size-selective health hazard sampling. In *Air Sampling Instruments for Evaluation of Atmospheric Contaminants,* 9th edition. Cohen, B.S. and C.S. McCammon, Jr. (eds.). Cincinnati, Ohio: ACGIH®, 2001. pp. 94–134.
33. **Lee, K.W. and R. Muklund:** Filter collection. In *Aerosol Measurement: Principles, Techniques and Applications,* 2nd edition. Baron, P.A. and K. Willeke (eds.). New York: John Wiley & Sons, 2001. pp. 197–228.
34. **Lippmann, M.:** Filters and filter holders. In *Air Sampling Instruments for Evaluation of Atmospheric Contaminants,* 9th edition. Cohen, B.S. and C.S. McCammon, Jr. (eds.). Cincinnati, Ohio: ACGIH®, 1995. pp. 281–314.
35. **Mark, D., C.P. Lyons, S.L. Upjohn, and L.C. Kenny:** Wind tunnel testing of the sampling efficiency of personable inhalable aerosol samplers. *J. Aerosol Sci. 25(suppl. 1)*: S339–S340 (1994).
36. **Mark, D. and J.H. Vincent:** A new personal sampler for airborne total dust in workplaces. *Ann. Occup. Hyg. 30*:89–102 (1986).
37. **Kenny, L.C., et al.:** A collaborative European study of personal inhalable aerosol sampler performance. *Ann. of Occup. Hyg. 41*:135–153 (1997).
38. **Bartley, D.L.:** Inhalable aerosol samplers. *Appl. Occup. and Environ. Hyg. 13*:274–278 (1998).
39. **Liu, B.Y.H., D.Y.H. Pui, and K.L. Rubow:** Characteristics of air sampling filter media. In *Aerosols in the Mining and Industrial Work Environments,* Vol. 3. Marple, V.A. and B.Y.H. Liu (eds.). Ann Arbor, Mich.: Ann Arbor Science, 1983. pp. 989–1038.
40. **Vincent, J.H., R.J. Aitken, and D. Mark:** Porous plastic foam media: Penetration characteristics and applications in particle size-selective sampling. *J. Aerosol Sci. 24*:929–944 (1993).
41. **ACGIH®:** Threshold Limit Values® for Chemical Substances and Physical Agents/Biological Exposure Indices®. Cincinnati, Ohio: ACGIH®, 2001.
42. **Cantrell, B.K., and J.C. Volkwein:** Mine aerosol measurement. In *Aerosol Measurement: Principles, Techniques and Applications,* 2nd edition. Baron, P.A. and K. Willeke (eds.). New York: John Wiley & Sons, 2001. pp. 801–820.
43. **Lodge, J.P., and T.L. Chan:** *Cascade Impactors: Sampling and Data Analysis.* Akron, Ohio: AIHA®, 1986.
44. **Ramachandran, G., and M. Kandlikar:** Inverse methods for analyzing aerosol spectrometer measurements: A review. *J. Aerosol Sci. 30*:413–437 (1999).
45. **Hering, S.V.:** Impactors, cyclones, and other inertial and gravitational collectors. In *Air Sampling Instruments for Evaluation of Atmospheric Contaminants,* 9th edition. Cohen, B.S. and C.S. McCammon, Jr. (eds.). Cincinnati, Ohio: ACGIH®, 2001. pp. 315–375.
46. **Watson, J.G. and J.C. Chow:** Ambient air sampling. In *Aerosol Measurement: Principles, Techniques and Applications,* 2nd edition. Baron, P.A. and K. Willeke (eds.). New York: John Wiley & Sons, 2001. pp. 821–844.
47. **Drinker, P., and T. Hatch:** *Industrial Dust: Hygienic Significance, Measurement and Control.* New York: McGraw-Hill, 1936.
48. **Silverman, L., C.E. Billings, and M.W. First:** *Particle Size Analysis in Industrial Hygiene.* New York: Academic Press, 1971.
49. **Cradle, R.D.:** *The Measurement of Airborne Particles.* New York: John Wiley & Sons, 1975.
50. **Y-S. Chen:** Denuder Systems and Diffusion Batteries. Cincinnati, Ohio: ACGIH®, 2008.
51. **Chen, D-R. and D.Y.H. Pui:** *Nanoparticles and Ultrafine Aerosol Measurements.* Cincinnati, Ohio: ACGIH®, 2008.
52. **Chen, D-R. and D.Y.H. Pui:** *Direct-Reading Instruments for Analyzing Airborne Particles.* Cincinnati, Ohio: ACGIH®, 2008.

Outcome Competencies

After completing this chapter, the reader should be able to:

1. Define underlined terms used in this chapter.
2. Explain the concept of traceability and calibration hierarchy.
3. Recognize the significance of the calibration process for IH measurement.
4. Describe the advantages and disadvantages of the various calibrators used in occupational air sampling.
5. Develop calibration procedures for specific air sampling equipment/methods.
6. Recognize what is needed to establish and maintain a laboratory calibration program.

Prerequisite Knowledge

General college physics
General college algebra

Prior to beginning this chapter, the user should review the following chapters:

Chapter Number	Chapter Topic
11	Sampling of Gases and Vapors
17	Direct-Reading Instruments for Determining Concentrations of Gases, Vapors, and Aerosols

Key Terms

bubble meter • by-pass rotameter • calibration • calibration curve • calibration program • critical flow orifices • critical orifices • displacement bottles • dry-gas meters • flask of Mariotte • flow rate standards • flow rate meters • frictionless piston meters • glass piston • graphite piston • heated element anemometer • hierarchical pathway • intermediate standards • laminar-flow meter • mass flowmeters • mercury-sealed piston • meter provers • orifice meters • precision rotameters • primary standards • prover bottle • rotameters • secondary standards • spirometers • strapping • thermal meter • traceability • variable-area meter • variable-head meters • velocity pressure • venturi meters • volume syringe • volume meters • wet test gas meter

Key Topics

I. Calibration Process
II. Flow Rate Standards
III. Calibration Hierarchy and Traceability
IV. Primary Standards (Volume Meters)
   A. Spirometers and Meter Provers
   B. Displacement Bottle
   C. Frictionless Piston Meters
V. Secondary Standards (Volume Meters)
   A. Wet Test Gas Meter
   B. Dry-Gas Meter
VI. Secondary Standards (Flow Rate Meters)
   A. Variable Head Meters
   B. Critical Flow Orifice
   C. Packed Plug Flowmeter
   D. Variable Area Meters
   E. Meters with Both Variable Head and Variable Area Elements
VII. Velocity Meters
   A. Mass Flow Meters
   B. Thermo-Anemometers
   C. Pitot Tubes
   D. Other Velocity Meters
VIII. Establishing and Maintaining a Calibration Program

Principles and Instrumentation for Calibrating Air Sampling Equipment

15

Glenn E. Lamson, CIH

Introduction

Air sampling is widely used in occupational hygiene to measure worker exposure and to characterize emission sources. It is frequently employed within the contexts of a general survey, investigation of a specific complaint, or for regulatory compliance. Regardless of the reason for air monitoring, the accuracy and precision of any air sampling procedure can be only as good as the sampling and analytical error that are associated with the sampling method. The difference between the air concentration reported for an air contaminant (on the basis of a meter reading or laboratory analysis) and the true concentration at that time and place represents the overall error of the measurement.

This overall error is a sum of all component errors rather than a single cause, and these smaller errors can add up to a high overall error if steps are not taken to minimize them. To minimize the overall error, it may be necessary to analyze each of the potential components and then concentrate one's efforts on reducing the largest component error. For example, it would not be productive to reduce the uncertainty in the analytical procedure from 10 to 1% when the error associated with the sample air volume measurement is as high as 15–20%. It is important to have the sampling error as small as possible by following proper calibration techniques to obtain the most accurate assessment of employee exposures.

In air sampling, the largest portion of the sampling error frequently is due to the flow rate of air and, ultimately, the underestimation or overestimation of the total volume of air that has passed through the sampling device. To define any exposure concentration, the quantity of the contaminant of interest per unit volume of air must be accurately measured. Therefore, to obtain the best estimate of the true concentration to which an employee has been exposed, one must have a thorough understanding of both the principles and instruments used for calibrating air sampling equipment.

The air sampling equipment may be calibrated with a primary calibration instrument or by a secondary calibration instrument. The air sampling equipment calibrated from a secondary calibration instrument should have traceability to a primary calibration instrument. The National Technology Transfer and Advancement Act of 1995 established a common testing strategy for commercial and federal agencies.[1] The U.S. Government published the National Standards Strategy for the U.S. in 2000, which made American National Standards Institute (ANSI) as the lead agency for establishing the testing methods.[2] Most ANSI and American Society for Testing Materials (ASTM) methods for calibrating instruments specify traceability to a National Institute of Standards and Technology (NIST) primary calibration instrument.

The Calibration Process

Before any air sampling device can be relied on as accurate, it must first be calibrated. <u>Calibration</u> is defined by ANSI as "the set of operations which establishes, under specified conditions, the relationship between values indicated by a measuring instrument or measuring system, and the corresponding standard or known values derived from the standard."[3] In perhaps somewhat simpler terms, the calibration process is a comparison of one instrument's response with that of a reference instrument of known response and known accuracy. Hence, the overall quality of the calibration process can be no better than the quality of the calibrator used or referenced.

Manufacturers have developed calibration procedures to address this need for reliable valid sampling equipment. Where possible, the primary or secondary calibration equipment is traceable to NIST following procedures by ANSI, ASTM, and Instrument Society of America (ISA). Global bodies for standardization and standards development are the International Electrotechnical Commission (IEC) and the International Organization for Standardization (ISO). The IEC provides technical specifications and publishes international standards for electrical, electronic, and related technologies. ISO provides procedural guidance and fills the need for standards outside of the electrical and electronic disciplines, and includes members from all over the world, including the United States. European standards development bodies also exist including the Comité Européen de Normalisation (CEN) and the Comité Européen de Normalisation Electrotechnique (CENELEC).

The calibrators most frequently used as primary or secondary calibration instruments for air sampling equipment can be divided into three basic groups, which are differentiated by the type of measurement that is to be checked. The first group is made up of volume meters, whereas the second group encompasses flow rate meters, both of which respond to the entire airflow of the sampler. The third group is referred to as velocity meters, which respond by measuring velocity at a particular point of the airflow cross-section. Several different devices within each of these categories have evolved over the years, primarily from the disciplines of engineering, chemistry, and medicine.

Volume meters include displacement bottles, spirometers/bell-type provers, frictionless meters, wet test meters, dry-gas meters, and positive displacement or roots meters. Flow rate meters are divided into two groups: (1) variable-head meters (which include orifice and venturi meters) and (2) variable-area meters (which include rotameters). Velocity meters, which are actually a type of flow rate meter, include mass flowmeters, thermoanemometers, and pitot tubes.

Flow Rate Standards

The calibrators used in flow rate measurements have in the past been classified as either primary, intermediate, or secondary. This classification system is based on the accuracy and ability to directly measure the internal dimensions of the calibrator. As a general rule most texts today limit classifications to either primary or secondary, with all previous intermediate standards now included in the secondary standards category. The following definitions for these classifications of calibrators are presented here.[4]

- Primary standards. Devices for which measuring volume can be accurately determined by measurement of internal dimensions alone; the accuracy of this type of meter is ±1% or better.
- Secondary standards. Devices for general use that are calibrated against primary or intermediate standards. Typically more portable, rugged, and versatile than devices in the other two categories, these devices generally have accuracies of ±5% or better. The need for recalibration depends on the amount of handling, frequency of use, and type of environment in which they are operated. For example, dust collection within a rotameter may require a recalibration as often as every 3 months.

The calibration of air sampling pumps is performed before and after each episode of sampling with the media in line, as the media provides resistance affecting the flow rate. Do not use the same individual media for the calibration and for sampling as the individual media may become contaminated during calibration from chemicals in the calibration room. ASTM D5337-04 Standard Practice for Flow Rate for Calibration of Personal Sampling Pumps provides a guide to the calibration of air sampling pumps.[5] Aerosol air sampling pumps should be calibrated following ASTM Standard D6061-01 (2007) Standard Practice for Evaluating the Performance of Respirable Aerosol Samplers.[6] OSHA sampling methods require the air sampling pumps perform within 5%, as a performance criteria of 5% is used in their calculation of the Sampling and

Analytical Error (SAE).[7] U.S. Environmental Protection Agency (EPA) has specific requirements for air quality monitoring found in 40 CFR Parts 50, 53, and 58. Part 50 is the National Primary and Secondary Ambient Air Quality Standards, Part 53 is the Ambient Air Monitoring Reference and Equivalent Methods, and Part 58 is the Ambient Air Quality Surveillance.[8,9] Records should be kept of the pre/post calibrations of each sampling episode. When post-calibration results differ from pre-calibration results by more than 5% the validity of the samples are in question and samples should be retaken. When post/pre-calibration results differ by less than 5% the flow rate used for total volume calculations will be determined by professional judgment. For most instances use the average of the pre and post calibrations.[10] By using the lower flow rate number the calculation errs on the side of increased worker protection. For enforcement purposes the larger flow rate must be used as it errs on the side of the employer.[7]

European Standard EN 1232 which has performance criteria for battery powered air sampling pumps with nominal volumetric flows of 5 mL/min to 5 L/min along with laboratory testing methods for pump performance tested under specific laboratory conditions.[10] The EN 12919:1999 has performance criteria for pumps with nominal flow rates over 5 L/min.[11]

Certification

Certification of air sampling equipment may be done by NIOSH, Mine Safety and Health Administration (MSHA), or by a contract testing laboratory such as Underwriters Laboratories (UL), or by a third party testing such as Safety Equipment Institute (SEI). These organizations may certify the equipment or oversee part or all of the assembly process. Outside of the U.S. third party certification is usually performed to see if the equipment conforms to the performance standards of that particular country, and may include an audit of the manufacturer's quality management system to ensure each piece of equipment conforms to that country's performance standards. In Europe the third party certifies the instrument and places the certification mark of Conformite' Européen (CE) on the instrument. Equipment can also be internationally certified by ISO.

Calibration Hierarchy and Traceability

The traditional concept of measurement traceability in the U.S. has focused on an unbroken hierarchical pathway of measurements that leads, ultimately, to a national standard.[13] For example, in industrial hygiene air sampling (or occupational hygiene air sampling) this hierarchical pathway might begin with the need to accurately set the flow rate of a personal air sampling pump at 2 L/min. In this scenario a precision rotameter (a secondary standard) is used to set this flow rate in the field. The accuracy of the rotameter has been maintained by means of a calibration curve that was generated in the laboratory using an electronic bubble meter (a primary standard). The laboratory checks the accuracy of its primary standard annually. This is done by either obtaining a transfer standard on site, which is directly traceable, or by sending the calibrator to an appropriate laboratory or agency for a direct comparison with a national standard. Virtually all calibration standards currently in use have at some time involved some form of traceability back to an acceptable reference standard of known accuracy. All too often, however, the evidence of traceability is either lost or simply not maintained. When dealing with low permissible exposure levels or low threshold limit values the true accuracy of the calibration must be a consideration. Even a small error in this accuracy when measuring low levels of contaminants may impact the results, leading to a potential overexposure.

It is important to note that many federally regulated organizations and their contractors are required to verify that the measurements they make are traceable and that they can support the claim of traceability by maintaining an audit record. This regulatory requirement implies the ability to relate individual measurement results through an unbroken chain of calibration to a common source, usually U.S. national standards as maintained by NIST.[14]

To adequately establish an audit trail for traceability, NIST recommends that a proper calibration result include (1) the assigned value, (2) a stated uncertainty, (3) identification of the standard used in the calibration, and (4) the specifications of any environmental conditions of the calibration when correction factors should be applied if the standard or equipment were to be used under different environmental conditions.[12] Records of the calibration of the secondary standards and its primary standard should be maintained together to provide the proper traceability of the equipment calibration. Most secondary calibration equipment, such as electronic flow rate calibrators, are secondary standards, and come from the manufacturer with a certification back to a NIST certified primary calibration. These certificates should be added to the audit trail of a particular piece of equipment. Most manufacturers of the secondary calibration equipment will provide a recommended recertification schedule. An audit trail of these records should be maintained for each piece of equipment with copies maintained with the equipment.

The primary and secondary standards which can be calibrated following ASTM D1071-83(2008) include: cubic-foot bottle, immersion type of moving-tank type; portable cubic-foot standard (Stillman-type); fractional cubic-foot bottle; burettes, flasks, and other volumetric measuring devices; calibrated gasometers (gas meter provers); gas meters (displacement type) liquid-sealed relating drums; gas meters (displacement type) diaphragm- or bellows-type meters, equipped with observation index; gas meters (displacement type) rotary displacement meters; gas meters (rate of flow) porous plug and capillary flowmeters; gas meter (rate of flow) float (variable area, constant head); orifice flow nozzle; and venturi-type flow meters.[15]

Primary Standards (Volume Meters)

Spirometers and Meter Provers

Spirometers and meter provers measure the total volume, V, of a gas that is passed through the meter while it is being operated. The time period, t, of operation and the temperature and pressure of the gas as it passes through the meter also are measured. The average flow rate, Q, is derived from the following equation.

$$Q = V/t \qquad (15\text{-}1)$$

The term "spirometer" was first applied by the English physician John Hutchinson in 1846 to describe an instrument that measured lung volume.[16] Hutchinson's spirometer required the patient to breathe into a delicately balanced receiver of known volume that was elevated in measurable increments with each expired breath. This work led to the first effective instrument for the detection of early or latent stages of consumption (tuberculosis) and was immediately put to use by the insurance industry.[17]

Today, spirometers include instruments that measure volume directly, as well as those that measure velocity or pressure differences and convert these indicators through the use of electronics to a volume reading. Only those spirometers referred to as water sealed, dry sealed, or dry rolling sealed actually measure volume directly and would therefore qualify as primary standards. Although spirometers were not originally designed to be calibrators, it is much easier to adapt the device for this purpose if it can be operated manually. Most dry seal or dry rolling sealed spirometers in use today are electronically operated, leaving the water sealed type as the most useful.

Traditionally, large water-sealed spirometers, also known as respirometers or gasometers, were manufactured with capacities of 100 to 600 L. The primary difference between these spirometers and Hutchinson's original design is the use of a liquid seal. A typical spirometer, for example, was made of two stainless steel cylinders, each with a sealed end. One cylinder or tank held water while the other, turned upside down like a bell, was suspended in the water by a chain and counterbalance. Volume was calculated by using a bell of known dimensions and measuring how far the bell was lifted when air entering the bell displaced the water. This was usually accomplished by fixing a volume scale to the side of the bell and attaching a pointer to the stationary tank. In this way the total volume entering the system over a given time was measured. Some models also had a built-in mixing fan mounted in the bell and a thermometer to facilitate the measurements needed for gas volume calculations. It was the size (volume) of these devices that made them attractive as calibrators; however, both the size and, therefore, weight of these measuring devices eventually made them impractical as lung function testers, and today they are no longer commercially available. What is commercially available is a somewhat more portable survey spirometer that uses guide rods instead of the traditional counter-weights and an internal bell that displaces most of the water in the tank, thereby reducing both volume and weight of the liquid (Figure 15.1). Although this smaller water-sealed spirometer has the advantage of availability, it also has the disadvantage of only a 10-L volume capacity.

Even though the large water-sealed spirometers are no longer commercially available, they may still be found in both commercial laboratories and university settings, where they function as primary standard calibrators or possibly training tools. For this instrument to be used as a calibrator, the bell is raised with the gas to be measured while ensuring that the water seal stays intact. At this point the bell can be considered fully charged. As the bell is lowered, the water acts as a piston that drives the gas out of the bell and through the flowmeter under test. The depth of immersion of the bell is a measure of the volume of the gas displaced and can be read off a calibrated scale. If large volumes are to be measured, the process has to be repeated several times, which can make the operation time consuming. Before this spirometer is used, it should be checked for corrosion on the internal surface of the bell and for damage to the shape of the bell that might affect the volume. Allow the water in the spirometer to come to room temperature and the air in the bell to equilibrate to the ambient pressure. The air volume can then be corrected to a standardized condition using the ideal gas laws:

$$V_{std} = V_{mes}\left(\frac{P_{mes}}{P_{std}}\right)\left(\frac{T_{std}}{T_{mes}}\right) \qquad (15\text{-}2)$$

where

V_{std} = volume at standard conditions (P_{std} = 760 mmHg at T_{std} = 298 K)
V_{mes} = volume measured at conditions P_{mes} and T_{mes}
T_{mes} = absolute temperature of V_{mes}
P_{mes} = measured pressure of V_{mes} (mmHg)

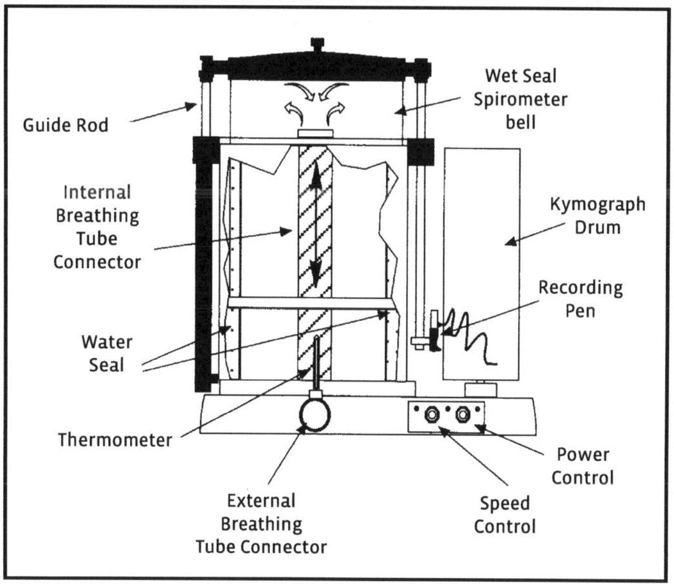

Figure 15.1 — Diagram of a portable survey water sealed spirometer referred to as a respirometer or pulmonary screener with a volume capacity of 10L (courtesy of Warren E. Collins, Inc., Braintree, Mass.).

Today, most portable dry sealed and water sealed spirometers are calibrated at the factory using a 1- to 3-L volume syringe (for examples see Figure 15.2) that is either certified by or traceable to NIST. Although it is possible to ship a large water-sealed spirometer to NIST for calibration, it would be more practical to use a NIST transfer standard and run the calibration on site. Another method that can be used to check the calibration would be a procedure known as "strapping," which consists of measuring the cylinder's dimensions with a steel tape and calculating the volume.[18] For this process to be part of an unbroken calibration hierarchy, the steel tape measure would have to be traceable to a recognized standard.

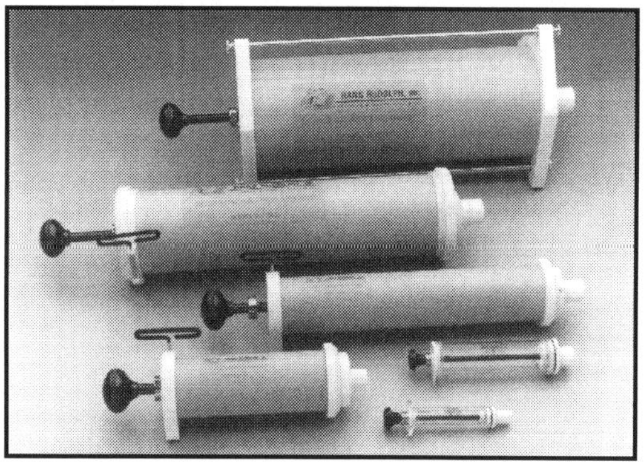

Figure 15.2 — Volume calibration syringes, 0.5 to 7 L (courtesy of Hans Rudolph, Inc., Kansas City, Mo.).

"Meter provers" refer to a proven tank capacity that is used to check the volumetric accuracy of a gas or liquid that is delivered by a positive-displacement meter. Meter provers, also known as bell provers, are primary volume standards that are actually very similar in both design and function to large water-sealed spirometers. However, unlike the traditional large water-sealed spirometers, bell provers are designed specifically to function as primary volume calibrators, are commercially available with internal volumes 0.18 m^3 (5 ft^3) to 0.71 m^3 (20 ft^3), and are currently in use by NIST. In addition, these instruments employ a low vapor pressure oil seal instead of a water seal and an internal bell or tank to reduce the overall volume of the liquid used to make the seal (refer to the diagram in Figure 15.1). As a gas flows through the device, it first enters the internal tank, and then the gas displaces the bell. The bell is counterbalanced throughout its travel by counterweights suspended on chains, just like a traditional spirometer. By attaching a small-gauge wire to the top of the bell and connecting a linear encoding system, the bell's location can be measured automatically as it is displaced by the gas flowing into the chamber. A computer can collect this information, as well as temperature and pressure measurements, and calculate an instantaneous reading of gas mass flow with an accuracy of 0.5%, according to the manufacturer (see Figure 15.3).

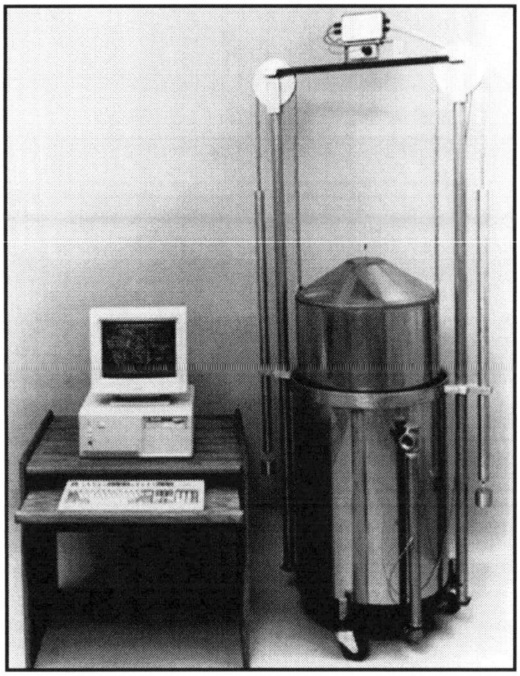

Figure 15.3 — The Sierra Automated Bell Prover was designed and built as a primary standard gas flow calibrator. It was constructed of 300-series stainless steel and fitted with inlet and outlet valving, two counterweights, an optical encoder for measuring bell travel, and automated inputs for both temperature and back pressure measurements (courtesy of Sierra Instruments, Inc., Monterey, Calif.).

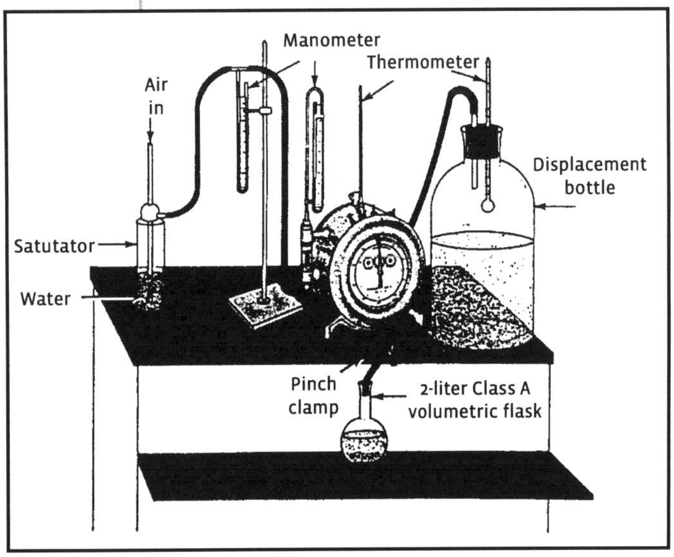

Figure 15.4 — Diagram of a displacement bottle used to calibraty a wet test meter (reprinted with permission from CRC Press, Inc.).[3]

Displacement Bottle

The displacement bottle, sometimes referred to as a prover bottle (see Figure 15.4), is a volume and flow rate calibrator that operates similarly to the bell prover, except that it measures displaced water instead of displaced gas. The operating principle of this instrument was first described in 1686 by the French hydraulician Edme Mariotte and has been referred to as the "flask of Mariotte."[19] Mariotte used a closed cylindrical container filled with water that had a bottom drain to let water out and an inlet tube to let air into the container. The instrument was used primarily to illustrate the weight of the atmosphere but is now commonly employed in the laboratory as a constant pressure head device.

Displacement bottles usually have a valve at the bottom of the bottle that allows the water to be drained out; this in turn draws air into the bottle in response to the lowered pressure. The volume of the air drawn in is equal to the change in water level multiplied by the cross-section at the water surface. A more accurate method used in the laboratory would be to collect the displaced water into a graduated cylinder or volumetric flask. By also measuring the time needed to displace a set volume of water, it is possible to calibrate low flowrate meters accurately in the range of 10 to 500 mL/min or less.[18] Measurements for temperature, pressure, and volume will need to be corrected to standard conditions. Wight suggests that when a displacement bottle is used to calibrate another device, there may be substantial negative pressure at the bottle inlet that will need to be a part of the correction process.[4]

"Frictionless" Piston Meters

Frictionless piston meters are cylindrical air displacement meters that use nearly frictionless pistons to measure flow rates as primary flow calibrators. The pistons in these instruments are designed to form gas-tight seals of negligible weight and friction and are made from a variety of materials including soap film, mercury, glass, and graphite. Variations in piston material have a direct effect on the meter's cost, accuracy, and portability.

Soap-Film Pistons or Bubble Meters

The bubble meter is arguably the most frequently used calibrator in occupational hygiene air sampling, primarily because it is both economical and relatively simple to operate. The first references to a bubble meter go back to the late 1800s, but it is difficult to know exactly to whom the honor of invention might belong. In its simplest form the bubble meter consists of a graduated tube, such as a laboratory glass burette, and a soap film. It is also possible to construct one of these meters by using an inverted plastic syringe with appropriate gradations (see Figure 15.5).

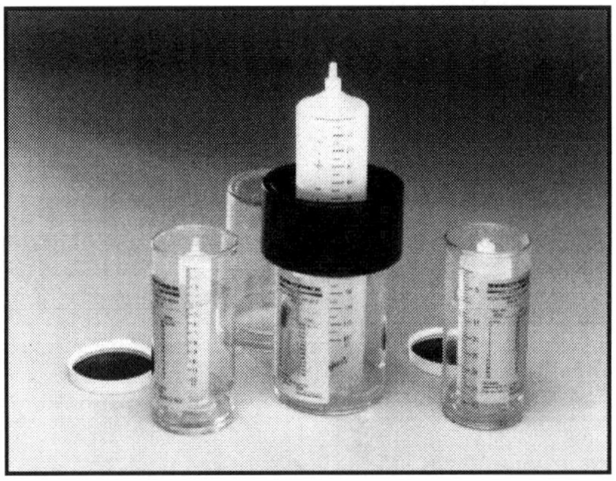

Figure 15.5 — Set of three bubble flowmeters, BFM-10, 40, and 100 (courtesy of Spectrex, Redwood City, Calif.).

A vacuum source, usually a personal sampling pump, is attached to the smaller end of the graduated tube or syringe while the other is immersed in a soap/water solution. This immersion should last only as long as it takes for a soap bubble to form and begin to rise in the wet tube. The volume displacement per unit time (i.e., flow rate) can then be determined by measuring the time required for the bubble to pass between two scale markings that enclose a known volume. These meters are generally accurate to within ±1%, although greater accuracy can be achieved under selected conditions.[20]

The simplicity of the soap bubble meter is not without some disadvantages. If the bubble meter is operated in the presence of relatively dry air (e.g., less than 50% relative humidity)[20] and at low flow rates, the air mass that passes over the soap film may become saturated with water vapor. When this occurs, the volume change being measured is due to the mixture of water vapor from the solution and the air being measured.[21] The percentage volume due to the water vapor can be obtained from tables of partial pressure of water versus temperature in references such as the *CRC Handbook of Chemistry and Physics*.[22] An appropriate correction factor can then be calculated and applied to any standard temperature and pressure corrections that might be needed (see Equation 15-3).[23]

$$V_{std} = V_{mes}\left[\frac{P_{mes} - P_{wv}}{P_{std}}\right]\left[\frac{T_{std}}{T_{mes}}\right] \qquad (15\text{-}3)$$

Where

V_{std} = volume at standard conditions (P_{std} = 760 mmHg at T_{std} = 298 K)
V_{mes} = volume measured at conditions P_{mes} and T_{mes}
T_{mes} = absolute temperature of Vmes
P_{mes} = measured pressure of V_{mes} (mmHg)
P_{wv} = partial pressure of water vapor at T_{mes} in mmHg.

Table 13.1 — Calculated Correction Factors for Water Vapor

Elevation (meters) of Sample Site	Air Temperature (°C) at Sample Site: 0	5	10	15	20	25	30	35
0	1.064	1.082	1.039	1.016	0.992	0.968	0.941	0.912
180	1.063	1.040	1.019	0.995	0.973	0.949	0.922	0.893
360	1.041	1.019	0.998	0.976	0.952	0.929	0.902	0.875
560	1.015	0.995	0.975	0.969	0.930	0.906	0.880	0.853
720	0.997	0.977	0.956	0.934	0.912	0.889	0.864	0.836
900	0.975	0.955	0.936	0.914	0.892	0.870	0.844	0.817
1080	0.953	0.933	0.915	0.893	0.872	0.850	0.824	0.798

Note: Correction factors for the error associated with the partial pressure of water vapor when using a soap bubble meter (assume low flow rates and dry air) at temperatures and elevations reasonable for a typical cold climate. Corrections are based on 760 mmHg and 25°C. The dashed lines separate increments of volume error by 5%.[14]

An alternative to the time involved in working out the above equation, but not the understanding, is a list of correction factors for reasonable temperatures and elevations that can be expected in a particular region. Such a list could be made for any number of regions, taking into account the uniqueness of both geography and climate.[24] Table 15.1 illustrates the water vapor correction factors that would be appropriate for the temperature

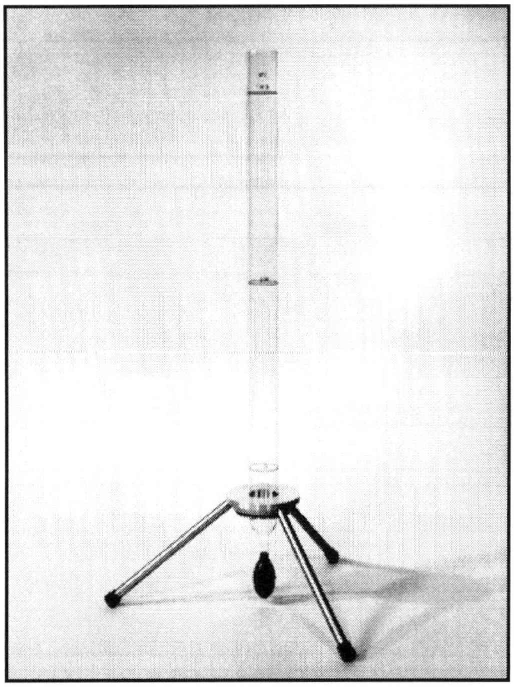

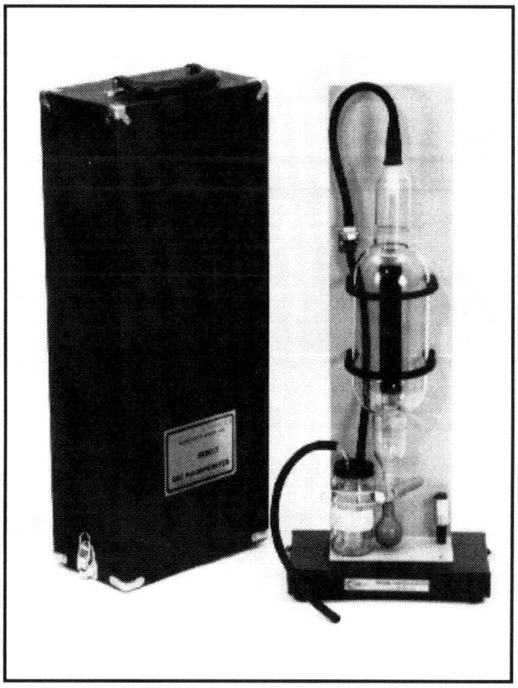

Figure 15.6 — (A) Manual laboratory film flowmeter series 211; (B) manual flowmeter kit model 302 with a range of 100 to 4000 mL/min (figures courtesy SKC, Inc., Eighty Four, Pa.).

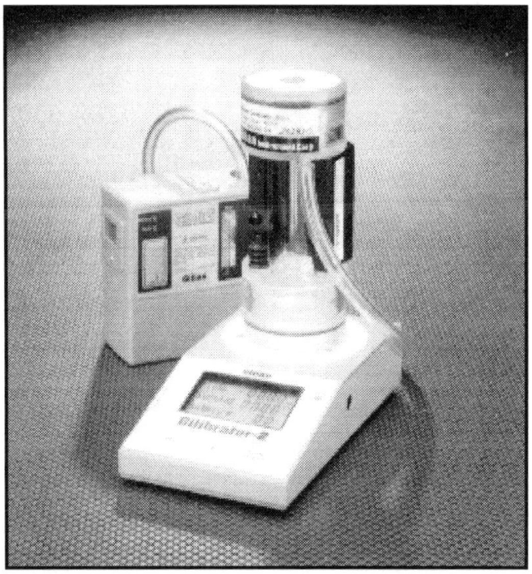

Figure 15.7 — An electronic soap bubble flowmeter, the Gilibrator-2, shown being used to calibrate a personal air sampling pump using one of three possible interchangeable cells (courtesy Sensidyne, Inc., Clearwater, Fla.).

and geographical diversity found in a typical cold climate in the United States.

Manufactured bubble meters are available from a variety of sources that offer both manual calculation of volume (Figures 15.6A and 15.6B) and electronically determined volumes (Figure 15.7). The electronically determined volumes use a pair of infrared optical triggers that measure the time it takes a piston to travel between two set points. Usually these meters are guaranteed to meet tolerances that are specified by NIST, or they can be certified for accuracy directly by NIST. Manufacturers usually certify electronic bubble meters for only one year, and the meters must be returned to the manufacturer for annual calibration. For non-electronic bubble meters the need eventually arises through use or misuse for some sort of calibration check of the tube volume. This can be accomplished gravimetrically by inverting the tube and filling it with distilled water between two graduated marks. The water is then drained from the tube, and the weight of the water is measured using a calibrated and traceable gravimetric scale. An accurate volume of the tube can then be determined after applying the appropriate temperature corrections to the liquid.

Mercury-Sealed Pistons

The mercury-sealed piston meter is another primary reference standard used by NIST. Although these meters are commercially available (see Figure 15.8A), they are extremely expensive and are usually designated for laboratory use only. The mercury-sealed piston meter consists of a precisely

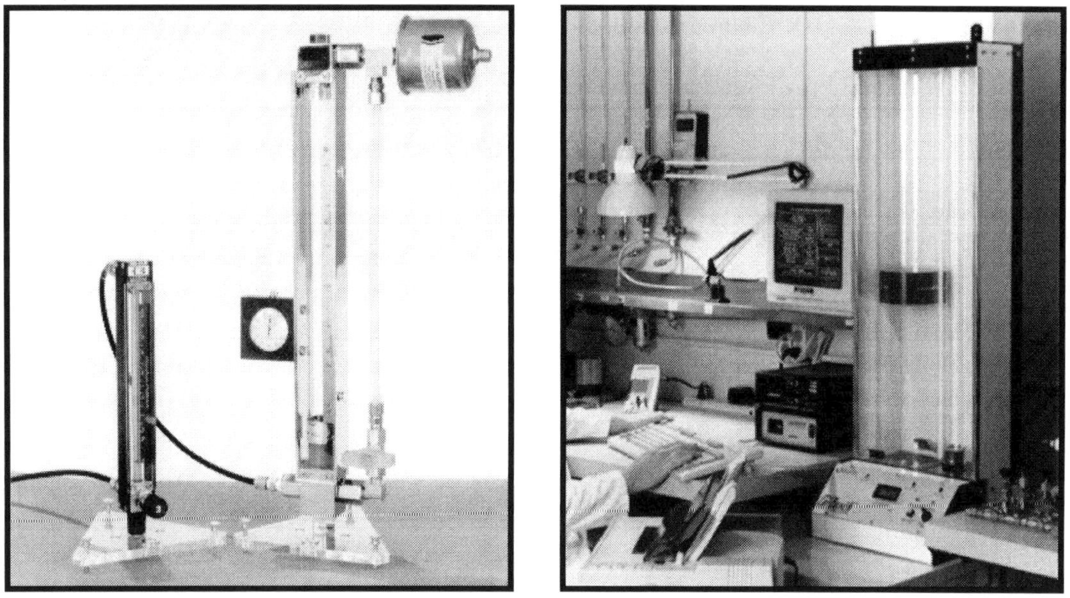

Figure 15.8 — (A) Brooks Vol-u-meter® (shown at right) calibrating a Brooks Sho-rate Purgemeter. Note the activated charcoal filter, designed to remove harmful mercury vapor (courtesy Brooks Instrument Division, Emerson Electric Division, Hatfield, Pa.); (B) the Cal-Bench® model 101, a completely automated primary standard (mercury sealed piston) calibration system (courtesy Sierra Instruments, Inc., Monterey, Calif.).

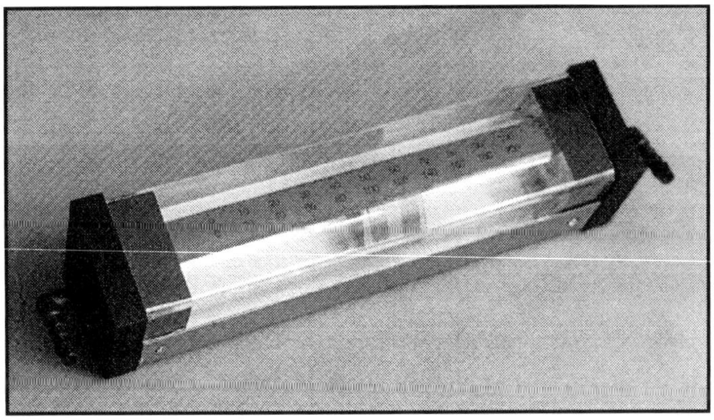

Figure 15.9 — Dry-Flow Flowmeter model 100a uses a glass piston instead of a soap-bubble film (courtesy Spectrex, Redwood City, Calif.).

bored borosilicate glass cylinder and a close-fitting plate of polyvinyl chloride. The plate is separated from the cylinder wall by an O-ring of liquid mercury that retains its toroidal shape through strong surface tension. The floating seal has a negligible friction loss, but the weight of the piston must be compensated for by calculations. With a manually operated timer the accuracy is said to be ±0.2% for timing intervals of 30 seconds or more.[18]

The mercury piston meter also can be designed as a completely automated system. The instrument pictured in Figure 15.8B is actually made up of three mercury-sealed piston meters. The tubes are sized to provide a 10:1 ratio in volumetric displacement between the tubes, which allows a calibration flow range of 1 to 50,000 standard cubic centimeters per minute. Instead of using infrared optical triggers, this system employs a specialized sonar transceiver at the top of each tube that emits a pulse of sound energy operating at approximately 50 kHz. As the pulse travels down the tube, it is reflected from the top of the piston and returns to the transceiver. A computer measures the transit time of the energy pulse and calculates the speed of sound based on ambient conditions of pressure, temperature, and relative humidity. By knowing the speed of sound and the transit time of the pulse, the position of the piston is said to be determined with a resolution of 0.152 mL (0.006 inches).

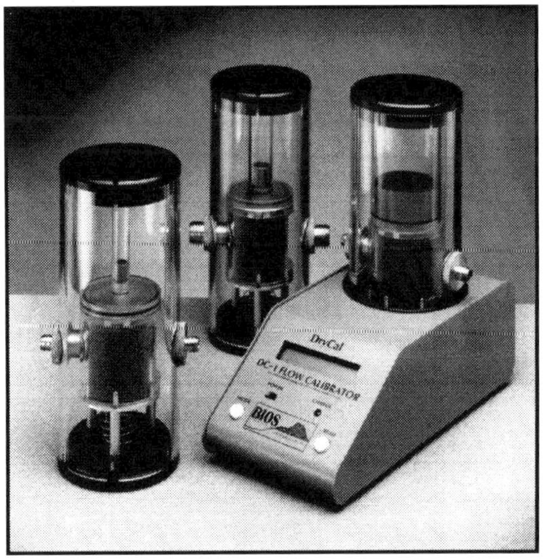

Figure 15.10 — Dry Cal® DC-1 flow calibrator, an example of a graphite piston flowmeter that is completely dry. Three interchangeable cells offer a wide volume range from 1 mL/min to 50 L/min (courtesy of Bois International, Pompton Plains, N.J.).

Glass and Graphite Pistons

Solid pistons offer some advantages over liquid seals made of either soap film or mercury. However, unlike the liquid pistons, air leakage can occur between the solid piston and the inside of the tube wall. Figure 15.9 is an example of a gas flowmeter that measures the displacement of a glass piston within the cylinder. The manufacturer suggests the use of flow rates that range from 10–200 mL/min with accuracy at 100% full scale of ±2%. By incorporating both electronics and a graphite piston into the flowmeter (Figure 15.10) many of the problems associated with soap bubble meters can be eliminated. The standard cell for this graphite piston meter covers a range of 10 mL to 9.999 L/m. Optional low- and high-flow cells extend the range from 1 mL to 50 L/m. Accuracy is reported by the manufacturer at ±1 to 2% depending on cell size. The variation is due to the clearance between the graphite piston and the cell wall, which creates a maximum leakage of approximately 0.005% of full scale.

One of the disadvantages of using a graphite piston, as pictured in Figure 15.10, is a phenomenon known as flow source pulsation. When using certain personal air sampling pumps, a high flow pulsation may develop when the flow is turned to the lower end of its range. This condition causes the piston to vibrate visibly during a measurement, resulting in a false or unstable reading.

This pulsation ceases with the insertion of an inline source pulsation damper (Figure 15.11).

Secondary Standards (Volume Meters)

Wet Test Gas Meter

It was not until 1816 that a practical attempt was made to measure commercial coal gas by an automatic and continuous instrument known as Crosley's drum or the wet meter drum.(25) The success of this instrument was in large part responsible for smoothing the way for the popularization of the commercial gas supply industry. The principles used in the Crosley drum are present today in the wet test gas meter (see Figure 15.12), which functions primarily as a laboratory calibrating standard. However, wet test gas meters are also frequently used to meter the flow of other gases directly.

The wet test gas meter is more commonly referred to as a wet test meter and consists of a partitioned drum half-submerged in a liquid (usually water) with openings at the center and periphery of each radial chamber. Air or gas enters at the center and flows into an individual compartment causing it to rise, thereby producing rotation. A dial on the face of the instrument indicates this rotation. The volume measured depends on the fluid level in the meter, because the liquid is displaced by air. A sight gauge for determining fluid height is provided, and leveling screws and a sight bubble are provided for this purpose. Correcting volume measurements to standard conditions is always required. There are several potential errors associated with the use of a wet test meter. The drum and moving parts are subject to corrosion from internal moisture and damage from misuse. There is friction in the bearings, and the mechanical counter and inertia must be overcome at low flows (<1 rpm). At high flows (>3 rpm), the internal liquid might surge and break the water seal at either the inlet or outlet. In spite of these factors the accuracy of the meter usually is within 1% when used as directed by the manufacturer.

Before the meter can be checked for accuracy, it must be leveled and filled with water to the calibration point. Then air is run through the meter for several hours to saturate the water and allow the meter to

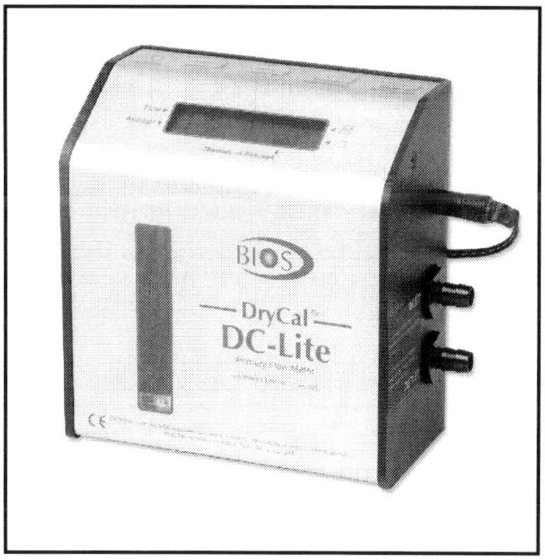

Figure 15.11 — DC-Lite® reported to be immune to flow source pulsation with a flow range of 1 mL/min to 30 L/min (courtesy of Bios International, Pumpton Plains, N.J.).

equilibrate.(26) At this point the meter is ready for calibration against a primary standard. Although it is possible to use a water sealed spirometer as a primary standard calibrator, it may be difficult to find one that has been properly maintained. Manufacturers of wet test meters use a NIST certified meter

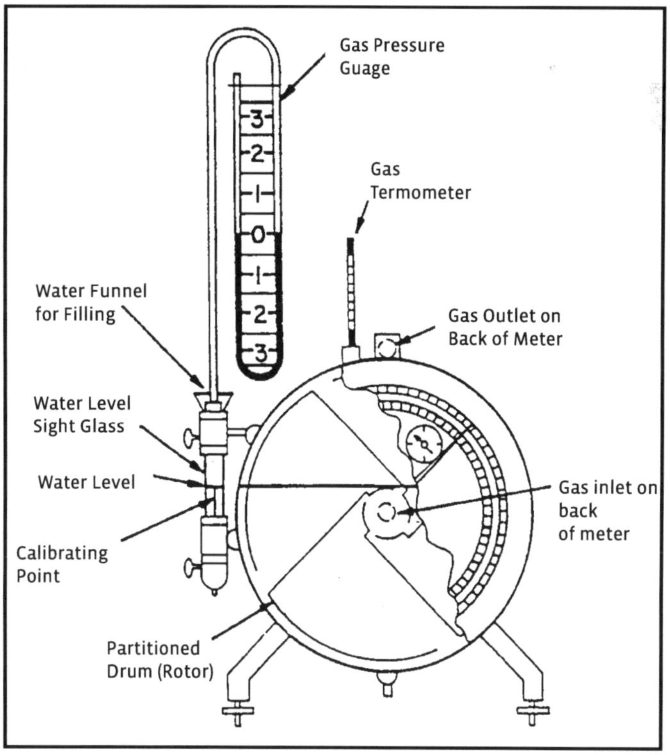

Figure 15.12 — Schematic of a wet test meter.

prover bottle as a primary standard that is capable of providing ±0.05% accuracy. The prover bottle is similar to the displacement bottle except the bottle is precisely manufactured to NIST tolerances. Calibration procedures using a prover bottle are described by ASTM D1071-83 (2008).[15]

Dry-Gas Meter

The Crosley drum was used as a consumer's meter from 1816 until the end of the century, by which time it had given way to a dry-gas meter that had come into practical use in 1844.[25] The dry-gas meter shown in Figures 15.13A and 15.13B is probably the second most widely used airflow calibrating device in the general field of air sampling. It consists of two bags interconnected by mechanical valves and a cycle-counting device. The air or gas fills one bag while the other bag empties itself; when the cycle is completed the valves are switched, and the second bag fills while the first one empties. The volume in cubic feet equivalents limits the maximum flow rate of these devices to a bagged capacity. Ness explains that a meter with a bag stamped DTM-200 is a dry-test meter that will safely pass a maximum of 200 dry feet per hour at a ½-inch water column differential.[26] Any such device has the disadvantage of mechanical drag, pressure drop, and leakage; however, the advantage of using the meter under rather high pressures and high volumes often outweighs these errors, which can be determined for a specific set of conditions. Although these meters are not normally used for occupational sampling, they are currently available with flow rates that average around 10–150 L/min (0.35–5.3 ft³/min). It is also possible to obtain the meter with either a digital or analog readout that measures flow in units of either cubic feet per hour or cubic meters per hour.

The dry-gas meter is calibrated against a primary standard, such as a bell prover, or a recently calibrated secondary standard, such as the wet test gas meter. In the absence of a suitable standard and to maintain a calibration hierarchy, the meter is returned to the manufacturer for annual calibration. Use of a displacement bottle or prover meter bottle is also a possibility following the same procedure employed when calibrating the wet test meter. Accuracy of the meter is corrected by adjusting the meter linkage. In practice, if the meter is within 1% of the known volume, a calibration factor is computed and used as a correction factor for meter readings.[4]

Secondary Standards (Flow Rate Meters)

Flow rate meters operate on the principle of the conservation of energy. More specifically, they use Bernoulli's theorem for the exchange of potential energy for kinetic

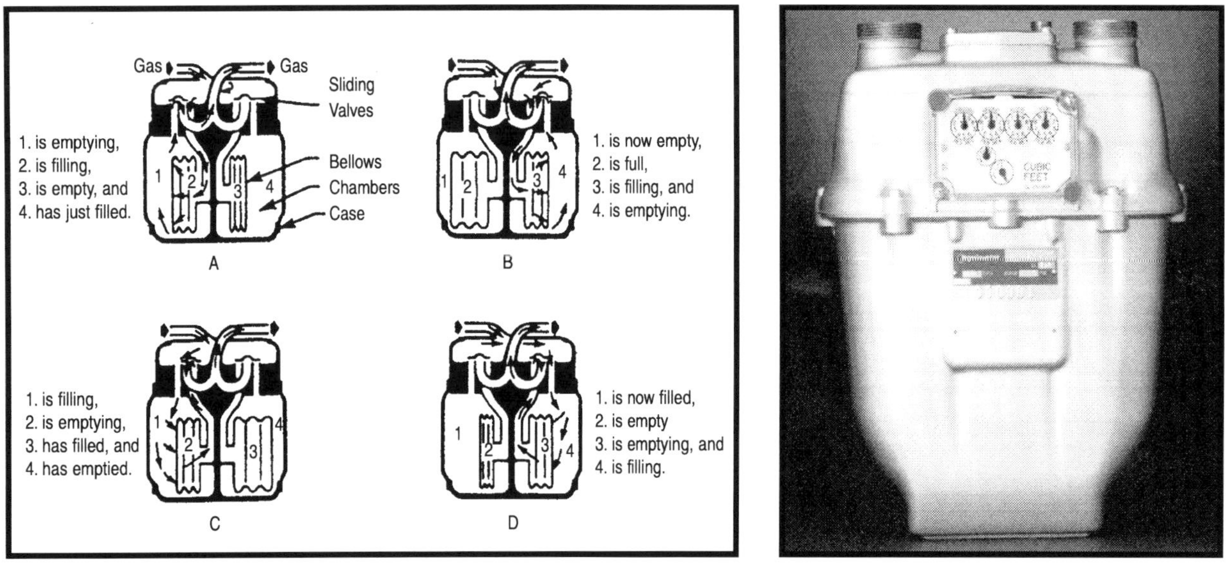

Figure 15.13 — (A) Internal mechanism of a dry-gas meter during operation (reprinted with permission from CRC Press(3)); (B) dry-gas meters are used extensively in stack sampling and pollution monitoring devices (courtesy of Equimeter, Inc., DuBois, Pa.).

energy and/or frictional heat. Each consists of a flow restriction within a closed conduit. The restriction causes an increase in the fluid velocity and therefore an increase in kinetic energy, which requires a corresponding decrease in potential energy, that is, static pressure. The flow rate can be calculated from knowledge of the pressure drop, the flow cross-section at the constriction, the density of the fluid, and the coefficient of discharge. This coefficient is the ratio of actual flow to the theoretical flow and makes allowances for stream contraction and frictional effects.

Flowmeters that operate on this principle are divided into two distinct groups. The first group includes orifice meters, venturi meters, and critical orifices. These have a fixed restriction and are known as variable-head meters because the differential pressure varies with flow. Flowmeters in the other group, which includes rotameters, are variable-area meters because a constant pressure differential is maintained by varying the cross-sectional area of the meter.

Variable-Head Meters

Venturi Meters

Variable-head meters, or head meters, are devices that produce a differential in pressure caused by a restriction in the airflow stream. This pressure difference was initially studied by Giovanni Battista Venturi in 1774, but it was not until 1894 that an engineer named Clemens Herschel invented the flowmeter, which he named in honor of Venturi.[28] Variations in these head meters include orifice meters, nozzles, and venturi tubes and are discussed in detail elsewhere.[29–31] These devices are used extensively in chemical processing and other industries but have little impact on occupational air sampling. One notable exception is a type of orifice meter known as a critical flow orifice that is used in the occupational environment to control airstreams in sampling equipment at predetermined constant flow rates.

Critical Flow Orifice

For a given set of upstream conditions the discharge of a gas from a restricted opening increases with a decrease in the ratio of absolute pressures P_2/P_1, where P_2 is the downstream pressure and P_1 the upstream pressure, until the velocity through the restriction reaches the velocity of sound. The value of P_2/P_1 at which the maximum velocity is just attained is known as the critical pressure ratio. The pressure in the throat will not fall below the pressure at the critical point, even if a much lower downstream pressure exists. For air, this condition is met when P_2 is less than 0.53 P_1, and the ratio of the upstream cross-sectional area (S_1) to the orifice area (S_2) is greater than 25.[32,33] Therefore, when the pressure ratio is below the critical value, the rate of flow usually depends on the upstream pressure. If there is a flow restriction (e.g., a filter) between the critical orifice and the room air, the upstream pressure (P_1) may be at less than ambient pressure.

For all differential-producing devices: when $P2<0.53\ P_1$, and $S_1/S_2>25$, the mass-flow rate W can be determined by the following equation.

$$W = \frac{C_v S_2 P_1 \text{ lbs / sec}}{T_1^{1/2}} \tag{15-5}$$

where

C_v = coefficient of discharge (normally ~ 1)
S_2 = orifice area in square inches
P_1 = upstream absolute pressure in pounds per square inch
T_1 = upstream temperature in degrees K

Critical flow orifices are widely used in occupational hygiene instruments such as the midget impinger pump for the maintaining and controlling of airstreams at constant flow rates. Systems using critical flow nozzles also have been used in place of bell provers for the calibration of gas meters. They can be purchased but need to be calibrated, or they can be constructed using a hypodermic needle. The flowmeter readings are then plotted against the critical flows to yield a calibration curve. The major limitation in their use is that only one critical flow rate is possible from each orifice, and the pressure differential is high. To a large degree this can be overcome by using several orifices in parallel downstream of the flowmeter under calibration. A second limitation is that these orifices are easily clogged and can erode over time and therefore require frequent examination and/or calibration against other reference meters as a part of a regular calibration program.

Variable-Area Meters

Rotameters

Rotameters are by far the most popular field instruments for flow rate measurements. The device consists of a float that is free to move up and down within a vertical tapered tube that is larger at the top than the bottom (Figure 15.14). Some of the shaped floats achieve stability by having slots that make them rotate. The term rotameter was first used to describe meters that used spinning floats, but now is generally used for all types of tapered metering tubes regardless of whether the float spins. As air flows upward, it causes the float to rise until the pressure drop across the annular area between the float and the tube wall is just sufficient to support the float. The tapered tube usually is made of glass or clear plastic and has a flow rate scale etched directly on one side. The height of the float indicates the flow rate. Floats of various configurations are used, as indicated in Figure 15.15. They are conventionally read at the highest point of maximum diameter, unless otherwise indicated.

Most rotameters have a range of 10:1 between their maximum and minimum flows. The range of a given tube can be extended by using heavier or lighter floats. Tubes are made in sizes from about 0.32 to 15 cm (0.125 to 6 inches) in diameter, covering ranges from a few milliliters per minute to over 28.3 m^3/min (1000 ft^3/min).

The most widely used material for construction is acrylic plastic. Because of space limitations, the scale lengths are generally small, ranging from 5 to 10 cm (2 to 4 inches). Unless they are individually calibrated, the accuracy is unlikely to be better than ±25%. When they are individually calibrated, ±5% accuracy can be achieved. It should be noted, however, that with relatively few scale markers on these rotameters, the accuracy of the readings may be a major limiting factor. Precision rotameters are usually larger, 30 cm (12 inches), made of glass, and have more accurate numerical scales. It is important to note that rotameters read correctly only at ambient pressure and temperature. Adding any restriction to the inlet, such as a filter or inlet valve, may produce significant errors in readings. In other words, the rotameter should never be placed between the sampling media and the pump.

Calibrations of rotameters are performed at an appropriate reference pressure and temperature, using either a primary standard or recently calibrated secondary standard such as the wet test meter following

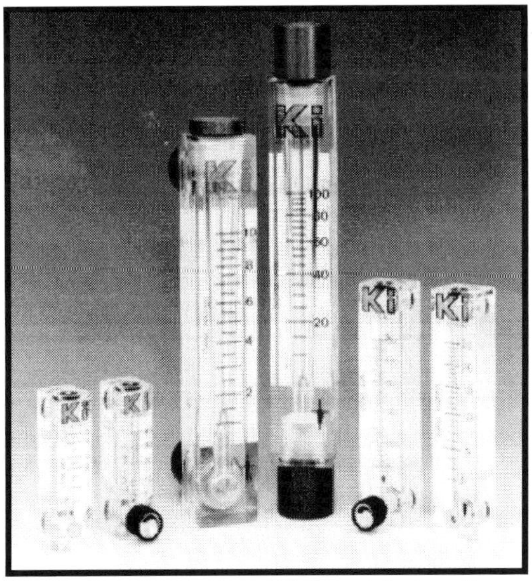

Figure 15.14 — A variety of lightweight (acrylic plastic) single float, field rotameters (courtesy Key Instruments, Trevose, Pa.).

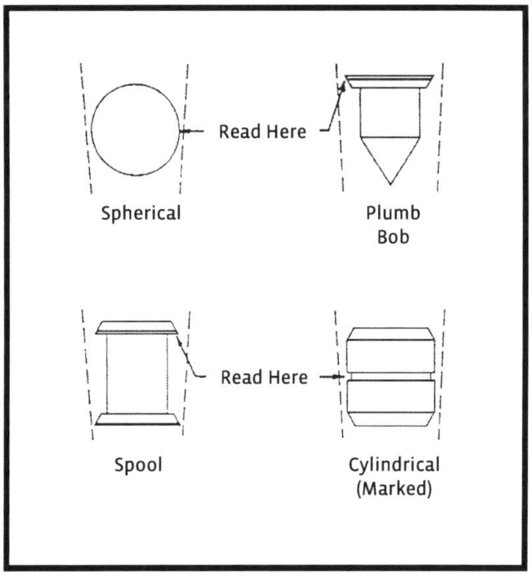

Figure 15.15 — Rotameter floats of various configurations showing reading point of highest maximum diameter for each.

ASTM D3195-90(2004).[34] The flow rate of a gas through a rotameter is seldom calculated from tube diameters and float dimensions, although the development and use of such equations are available.[35] Instead, curves are generated that relate meter readings to flow rates that are derived from a calibration by using a primary or accurate secondary standard. New rotameters usually are supplied with a vendor or manufacturer's generated calibration curve that should list the conditions of both temperature and pressure of the calibration. All rotameters should be recalibrated at or close to the conditions expected in the field or have appropriate corrections applied for the difference in calibrated and indicated flow rates.

For rotameters with linear flow rate scales, the actual sampling flow approximately equals the indicated flow rate times the square roots of the ratios of absolute temperatures to pressures of the calibration and field conditions.[28] The ratios increase when the field pressure is less than the pressure in the calibration laboratory or the field temperature is greater than that in the laboratory. Thus, if the flowmeter was accurate at ambient pressure, and the flow resistance of the sampling medium was relatively low (e.g., 30 mmHg), for a flow rate of 11 L/m the flow rate indicated on the rotameter would be $11 \times (730/760)^{0.5} = 10.8$ L/m, a difference of only 1.8%. On the other hand, for a 25 mm diameter AA Millipore with a 3.9 cm^2 filtering area and a sampling rate of 11 L/min, the flow resistance would be approximately 190 mmHg, and the indicated flow rate would be $11 \times (570/760)^{0.5} =$ 9.5 L/min, a difference of 14%. It should be noted that any other representative filter calibration should indicate a similar difference.

A similar correction is needed when sampling is done at atmospheric pressures and/or temperatures that differ substantially from those used for the calibration. For example, at an elevation of 1524 m (5000 ft) above sea level, the atmospheric pressure is only 83% of that at sea level. Thus, the standardized flow rate is 0.911 or 8.7% less than that indicated on a rotameter scale, based on the altitude correction alone. If the temperature in the field were 35°C while the meter was calibrated at 20°C, the standardized flow rate in the field would be 0.975 or 2.5% less than that indicated. For a summary of the corrections that would be used, refer to the following equation.[23]

$$Q_{std} = Q_{ind} \left[\frac{P_{amb}}{P_{std}} \times \frac{T_{std}}{T_{amb}} \right]^{0.5} \qquad (15\text{-}5)$$

Where

Q_{std} = standardized flow based on rotameter calibration at T_{std}
Q_{ind} = indicated rotameter reading at T_{amb} and P_{amb}
T_{amb} = ambient temperature in degrees K
P_{amb} = ambient pressure in mmHg
T_{std} = standardized temperature in degrees K
P_{std} = standardized pressure at 760 mmHg

When these kinds of corrections are needed for high altitude and high temperature, the overall correction for the preceding example would be 0.089 or 10.9%.

The correction in flow generated by the use of this equation is actually a function of the rotameter basic flow equation and not a simple gas-law correction.[36] Most of the terms in the rotameter basic flow equation can be considered constants, thereby allowing the fundamental equations of Boyle and Charles (referred to as the ideal gas law) to be in substitution for density, which will give a quick and reasonably accurate means of correcting flow.

In general, rotameter corrections should come into play only when a significant calibration shift has occurred between the calibration and field conditions. According to both the National Institute for Occupational Safety and Health (NIOSH) and the Occupational Safety and Health Administration (OSHA) a deviation of more than ±5% of the calibration value is considered to be a significant shift. In other words, a volume flow rate is corrected if measured conditions exceed calibration conditions by 5% or greater using Equation 15.4.

Once it is determined that a correction for flow is likely to be needed, the specific correction factor can be worked out by either measuring or calculating the sample site air pressure and temperature. When calculating air pressure from elevation information, use a conversion factor of 2.5 mmHg per 30 m elevation increase, or vice versa for an elevation decrease, using Environmental

Protection Agency Method 2A—Direct Measurement of Gas Volume Through Pipes and Small Ducts.[29] The actual flow correction would look like the following:

Conversion of elevation to equivalent pressure in mmHg:

$$\left[\frac{1080 \text{ meter}}{30 \text{ meters}}\right]\left[\frac{2.5 \text{ mmg}}{1}\right] = 670 \text{ mmHg}$$

Rotameter correction factor at occupational hygiene conditions at 760 mmHg and 25°C:

$$\left[\left[\frac{670 \text{ mmHg}}{760 \text{ mmHg}}\right]\left[\frac{298.15 \text{ K}}{303.15 \text{ K}}\right]\right]^{0.5} = 0.931$$

The preceding equation gives a correction factor value of 0.931, which indicates a 7% error in flow. To correct for this error, simply multiply 0.931 by the indicated flow rate from the rotameter calibration curve.

By applying a sufficient range of temperature corrections and pressure corrections (using elevation data), as could be generated by Equation 15.4, it is possible to demonstrate exactly under which field conditions a 5% or greater error in flow is likely to occur (see Figure 15.16).[24] If we use the same example as cited above, with an elevation of 1080 m (3543.3 ft) and a warm summer day of 30°C, Figure 15.16 can be used to show that the indicated rotameter flow would be in error by a value greater than 5%. After a detailed examination of Figure 15.16, it becomes evident that there is a rather significant range of temperatures and elevations that would not require a 5% error correction when using a rotameter that was originally calibrated at standard conditions. Whether one chooses to make a rotameter correction at 5% or greater in the long run depends on one's own professionalism and knowledge of the circumstances in which the error occurs.

Meters with Both Variable Head and Variable Area Elements

By-Pass Flow Indicators

In most high-volume samplers the flow rate is strongly dependent on the flow resistance, and flowmeters with a sufficiently low flow resistance are usually too bulky or expensive.

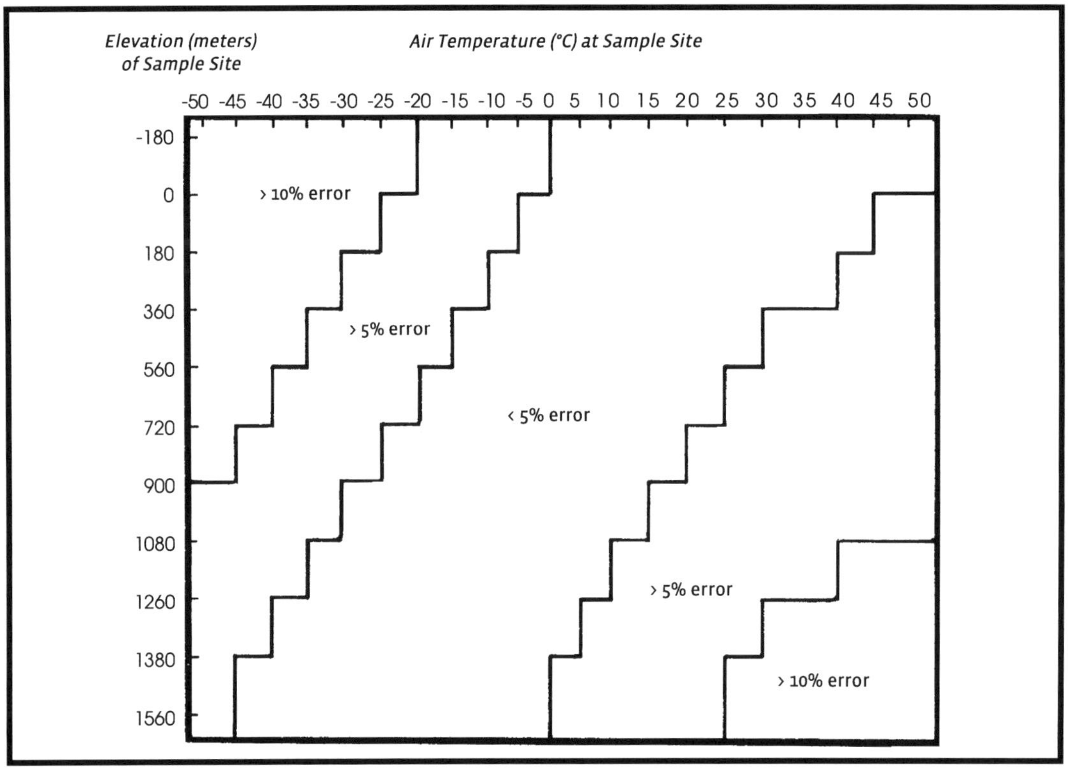

Figure 15.16 — Percent error of indicated flow when using a rotameter at temperatures and elevations that are different from a calibrated state of 760 mmHg and 25°C (normal conditions).[14]

A commonly used metering element for such samplers is the by-pass rotameter, which actually meters only a small fraction of the total flow that is proportional to the total flow. As shown schematically in Figure 15.17, a by-pass flowmeter contains both a variable-head element and a variable-area element. The pressure drop across the fixed orifice or flow restrictor creates a proportionate flow through the parallel path containing the small rotameter. The scale on the rotameter generally reads directly in cubic feet per minute or liters per minute of total flow. In the versions used on portable high-volume samplers, there is usually an adjustable bleed valve at the top of the rotameter that should be set initially and periodically readjusted in laboratory calibrations so that the scale markings can indicate overall flow. If the rotameter tube accumulates dirt, or the bleed valve adjustment drifts, the scale readings can depart greatly from the true flows.

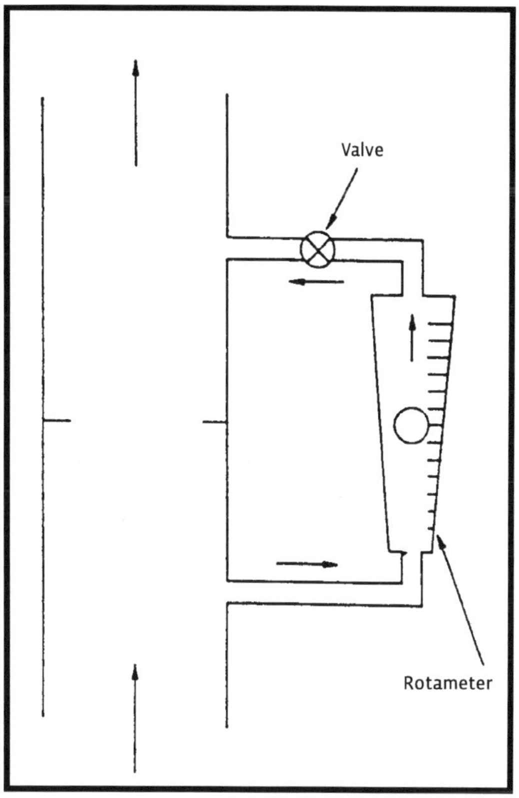

Figure 15.17 — Diagram of a by-pass flow indicator with both the variable-head element (valve) and the variable-area element (rotameter) labeled.

Velocity Meters

Because the flow profile is rarely uniform across the channel, the measured velocity invariably differs from the average velocity. Furthermore, because the shape of the flow profile usually changes with changes in flow rate, the ratio of point-to-average velocity also changes. Thus, when a point velocity is used as an index of flow rate, there is an additional potential source of error, which should be evaluated in laboratory calibrations that simulate the conditions of use. Despite their disadvantages, velocity sensors are sometimes the best indicators available, as, for example, in some electrostatic precipitators where the flow resistance of other types of meters cannot be tolerated.

Mass Flow Meters

A thermal meter measures mass airflow or gas flow rate with negligible pressure loss. Known as mass flow meters, these devices consist of a heating element in a duct section between two points at which the temperature of the airstream or gas stream is measured. The temperature difference between the two points depends on the mass rate of flow and the heat input. Ness stated that if these instruments are properly calibrated against a bubble burette their accuracy is within ±3%.[27] Figure 15.18 shows a mass flow meter that combines the primary standard calibrator capability of a frictionless piston meter with internal electronics that make corrections to standardized temperature and pressure. Accuracy of the unit is reported at ±1%.

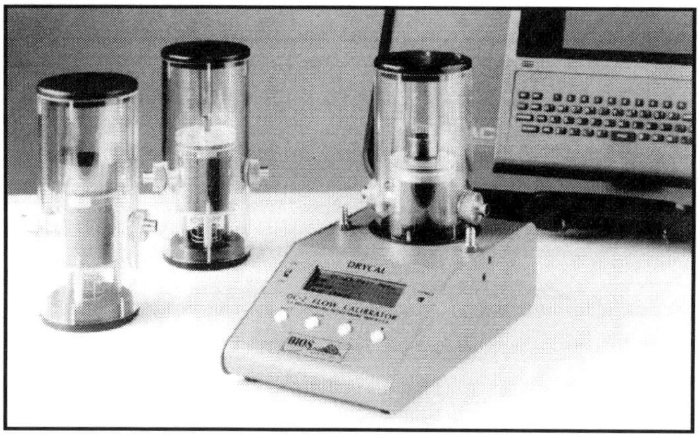

Figure 15.18 — Standardized mass flow calibrator, Dry Cal® DC-2M, in addition to giving true primary volume flow readings, the unit also contains internal barometric pressure and temperature sensors, which allows readings to be corrected to standard conditions (courtesy of Bois International, Pompton Plains, N.J.).

Thermo-Anemometers

Any instrument used to measure velocity can be referred to as an anemometer. In a heated element anemometer the flowing air cools the sensor in proportion to the velocity of the air. Instruments are available with various kinds of heated elements, such as heated thermometers, thermocouples, films, and wires. They are all essentially non-directional, that is, they have single element probes, measuring the airspeed but not its direction. They all can accurately measure steady-state airspeed, and those with low mass sensors and appropriate circuits also can accurately measure velocity fluctuations with frequencies above 100,000 Hz. Because the signals produced by the basic sensors depend on ambient temperature as well as air velocity, the probes are usually equipped with a reference element that provides an output that can be used to compensate or correct errors due to temperature variations. Some heated element anemometers can measure velocities as low as 0.05 m/sec (10 ft/min) and as high as 44 m/sec (8000 ft/min).

Pitot Tubes

The basic idea for an instrument that could be used as a reference for measuring the velocity of air was first published by Henri de Pitot in 1732.[19] A standard pitot tube, as it is known, consists of an impact tube with an opening facing axially into the flow and a concentric static pressure tube with eight holes spaced equally around it in a plane that is eight diameters from the impact opening. The difference between the static and impact pressures is the velocity pressure. Bernoulli's theorem applied to a pitot tube in an airstream simplifies to the dimensionless formula[37]:

$$V = 4005(h_v)0.5 \qquad (15\text{-}6)$$

where

h_v = velocity pressure in inches of water
V = velocity in feet per minute

If the pitot tube is carefully made it may function as a primary standard. Checking the calibration of a pitot tube, although rarely done, is a simple process that involves comparing the pitot tube with another velocity meter such as an anemometer or current meter that is traceable to a reference standard. There are several serious limitations to pitot tube measurements in most sampling flow calibrations. One is that it may be difficult to obtain or fabricate a small enough probe. Another is that the velocity pressue pressure may be too low to measure at the velocities encountered, even when using an inclined manometer or a low-range Magnehelic® gauge.

Other Velocity Meters

There are several other ways to use the kinetic energy of a flowing fluid to measure velocity. One way is to align a jeweled-bearing turbine wheel axially in the stream and count the number of rotations per unit time. Such devices generally are known as rotating vane anemometers. Some are very small and are used as velocity probes. Others are sized to fit the whole duct and become indicators of total flow rate and sometimes are called turbine flowmeters. These and other instruments such as the velometer or swinging vane anemometer are reviewed in *Industrial Ventilation: A Manual of Recommended Practice*.[37]

Establishing and Maintaining a Calibration Program

Each element of the sampling system should be calibrated accurately prior to initial field use. Protocols also should be established for periodic recalibration, because the performance of many transducers and meters changes with the accumulation of dirt, corrosion, leaks, and misalignment due to vibration or shocks in handling, and so on. The frequency of such recalibration checks initially should be high, until experience is accumulated to show that it can be reduced safely. The need for calibration and calibration frequency depends on several factors, as outlined by Wight[4]:

- Instrument characteristics: sensitivity and experience with its stability under similar use patterns
- Instrument use: rough handling, moving, heavy usage, and changing environments necessitate frequent calibration
- Instrument users: multiple users and users of various skill and experience

It is important to document the nature and frequency of calibrations and calibration checks to meet legal as well as scientific requirements. Measurements made to document the presence or absence of exposures are only as reliable as the calibrations on which they are based. Formalized calibration audit procedures established by federal agencies provide a basis for quality assurance where they apply. They also can provide a systematic framework for developing appropriate calibration procedures for situations not governed by specific reporting requirements. State and local air monitoring networks that are collecting data for compliance purposes must follow calibration procedures and external performance audits as outlined by the Environmental Protection Agency.(38) The OSHA instruction manual has forms to be followed when conducting equipment calibration and has specific requirements for field calibrations.(7) Another governmental source is NIOSH. The NIOSH *Manual of Analytical Methods*(39) recommends specific calibration procedures for both air sampling pumps and analytical equipment.

For any calibration program to be effective it must be performed under a definite, documented, and controlled procedure by a competent individual; in a repeatable manner; and under controlled conditions. It must be reported unambiguously and meet defined traceability requirements. For assurance of safety the calibrations should have an effective quality system. There also should be demonstrated competence in activities that affect reliability, safety, and performance.

The International Organization for Standardization (ISO) series 9000 standard requires that all measurements that affect quality shall be calibrated at prescribed intervals with certified equipment having a known valid relationship to nationally recognized standards. Certification to the ISO 9000 Quality System Standards is primarily in reference to the global business environment but also has an impact on calibration laboratories.(40) The ability to document equipment traceability will no doubt take on greater and greater significance as organizations develop international traceability standards.

The National Conference of Standards Laboratories, with the approval of the *American National Standards Institute, developed the American National Standard for Calibration-Calibration Laboratories and Measuring Test Equipment-General Requirements.*(14) The standard outlines the need for inventory, calibration history, location history, and maintenance history to be collected and used for calibration equipment. To satisfy this standard, five basic types of reports are necessary: (1) a calibration certificate or report that documents the calibration, (2) a due-for-calibration report, (3) an out-of-tolerance report, (4) a forward traceability report, and (5) a reverse traceability report.

Summary

In its simplest form the calibration process is a systematic comparison of one instrument's response to that of a standard reference of known response and known accuracy. Without this comparison the determination of an occupational exposure concentration cannot be relied on to be an accurate measure. Regardless of the method used for air sampling, one must have a through knowledge of both the principles and instrumentation used to perform, maintain, and document the calibration. The following comments summarize the guiding philosophy behind all air sampler calibrations.

- Determine in advance the type of calibrator needed. For example, decide whether a primary or secondary standard is necessary, what level of accuracy is needed, what range of flow will be used, and under what conditions the equipment and calibrator will be used (see Table 15.2).
- Always maintain the record of traceability for every calibration.
- Set up a calibration program. All standard instruments used as calibrators should have records available covering periodic calibration checks and annual comparisons with a known standard.
- Be sure to understand the operation of the instrument being calibrated as well as the calibrator before attempting the calibration procedure. Be sure that you are operating within the range of the instrument and standard.
- When in doubt about procedures or data, assure their validity before proceeding to the next operation.

Table 15.2 — Available Methods for the Calibration of Air Sampling Equipment

Standard Meters	*General Flow, Range, or Available Capacity*	*Reported Accuracy*	*Best Usage*
Primary standards			
Water sealed spirometers	100–600 L	±1%	laboratory
Bell provers or meter provers	0.14-0.57 m^3	±0.5%	laboratory
Volume calibration syringe	0.5–7 L	±0.25%	field or lab
Displacement or prover bottle	10-500 mL/min	±0.05 to 0.25%	laboratory
Soap film piston	<1 mL to 30 L/min	±1%	field or lab
Mercury sealed pistons	manual: 30–1200 cc automated: 1–50,000 standard cm^3/min	±0.2% ±0.2%	laboratory laboratory
Glass piston	10–200 mL/min	±2%	field or lab
Graphite piston (accuracy varies with cell size)	1 mL/min to 50 L/min	±1-2%	field or lab
Secondary standards			
Wet test meter	1–480 ft^3/hr (0.5–230 L/min)	±0.5%	laboratory
Dry-gas meter	20–325+ (10–150 L/min)	±1%	field
Rotameter (accuracy depends on calibration)	1 mL/min and up	±25 to 1%	field
Critical flow orifice	depends on orifice diameter	±0.5%	field or lab
Laminar-flow meter	use for very low flow rates	< ±1%	laboratory
Pitot tube traversing	velocities >50 ft/sec (15 m/sec)	±1%	field
Thermo-anemometer (accuracy depends on flow)	10 ft/min (0.05/sec) to 8000 ft/min (44 m/sec)	±0.1 to 0.2%	field
Electronic mass flow rate	0–10 mL/min to 0–3000 L/min	±3%	field or lab

Note: Adapted from M. Lippmann, Airflow Calibration.[22]

- To assure reliable calibration and sample collection in the field, it is essential that a battery maintenance program be developed when using personal sampling pumps with rechargeable batteries. Follow the manufacturer's recommendations for battery care and maintenance.
- All sampling and calibration train connections should be as short and free of constrictions and resistance as possible. Always check for leaks in both the sampling train and the pump.
- Allow sufficient time for equilibrium to be established, inertia to be overcome, and conditions to stabilize. The time needed for this may vary among equipment and be influenced by environmental conditions or frequency of use.
- Extreme care should be exercised to limit the potential for subjective responses that occur when reading scales, recording times, making adjustments, or even leveling equipment.
- Enough points or different rates of flow should be obtained on a calibration curve to give confidence in the plot obtained. Each point should be made up of more than one (minimum of three) reading whenever practical.
- Do not assume that temperature, pressure, and water vapor corrections do not apply to your particular calibration. First, prove what the correction would be mathematically, and then use professional judgment to determine whether to make the correction.
- Calibration curves should be properly identified as to conditions of calibration, device calibrated and what it was calibrated against, units involved,

range and precision of calibration, date, and who performed the actual procedure. Often it is convenient to indicate where the original data are filed and to attach a tag to the instrument indicating this information.

- A complete and permanent record of all calibration procedures, data, and results should be maintained and filed. This should include trial runs, known faulty data with appropriate comments, instrument identification, connection sizes, barometric pressure, temperatures, and so on.
- Once an instrument has been calibrated, it needs to be recalibrated whenever the device has been changed, repaired, received from a manufacturer, subjected to use, mishandled or damaged, and at any time when there is a question as to its accuracy.
- When a recalibration differs from previous records, the cause for this change in calibration should be determined before accepting the new data or repeating the procedure.

Acknowledgments

The author wishes to thank the previous authors of this chapter, Peter Waldron MS, MPH, CIH, and Morton Lippman, PhD, CIH, whose work provided the framework for this update as well as an expansion of the subject area. The author is also indebted to Mary Eide for her research assistance and editing skills.

References

1. **National Institute of Standards and Technology (NIST):** National Technology Transfer and Advancement Act of 1995 (Public Law 104-113). Available at http://www.nist.gov/director/ocla/Public_Laws/PL104-113.pdf. [Accessed March 2, 2009].
2. **ASTM International:** *National Standards Strategy for the United States.* Available at http://www.astm.org/NEWS/NSS_ANSI.htm. [Accessed March 2, 2009].
3. **NCSL International:** *American National Standard for Calibration—Calibration Laboratories and Measuring and Test Equipment—General Requirements* (ANSI/NCSL Z540-2-1997).Available at http://store.ncsli.org/ANSI_NCSL_Z540_2-1997_R2002__P118C35.cfm. [Accessed March 2, 2009].
4. **Wight, G.D.:** *Fundamentals of Air Sampling.* Boca Raton, Fla.: Lewis Publishers, 1994.
5. **ASTM International:** *Standard Practice for Flow Rate for Calibration of Personal Sampling* ASTM D5337-04. Available at http://www.astm.org/Standards/D5337.htm. [Accessed March 11, 2009].
6. **ASTM International:** *Standard Practice for Evaluating the Performance of Respirable Aerosol Samplers* ASTM D6061-01 (2007). Available at http://www.astm.org/Standards/D6061.htm. [Accessed March 11, 2009].
7. **Occupational Safety and Health Administration (OSHA):** *OSHA Technical Manual.* Available at www.osha.gov/dts/osta/otm/otm_toc.html. [Accessed November 3, 2008].
8. **Code of Federal Regulations:** National Primary and Secondary Ambient Air Quality Standards. *40 Code of Federal Regulations* Part 50. 2006. pp. 61144-61233.
9. **Code of Federal Regulations:** Ambient Air Monitoring Reference and Equivalent Methods *40 Code of Regulations Part 53 and 58.* 2006. pp 61236-61328.
10. **Biseli, M.S.:** *Industrial Hygiene Evaluation Methods.* Boca Raton, Fla.: Lewis Publishers, 2004.
11. **Comité Européan de Normalisation (CEN):** *Workplace Atmospheres — Pumps for Personal Sampling of Chemical Agents, Requirements and Test Methods* EN 1232:1997. Available at http://www.cen.eu/cenorm/homepage.htm. [Accessed March 3, 2009].
12. **Comité Européan de Normalisation (CEN):** *Workplace Atmospheres — Pumps for the Sampling of Chemical Agents with a Volume Flow Rate Over 5 L/min — Requirements and Test Methods* EN 12919:1999. Available at http://www.cen.eu/cenorm/homepage.htm. [Accessed March 3, 2009].
13. **Garner, E.L. and S.D. Rasberry:** What's New in Traceability. *J. Testing Eval. 21*:505–509 (1993).
14. **National Institute of Standards and Technology (NIST):** *NIST Calibration Services: Policies on Calibration and Traceability.* Available at http://ts.nist.gov/MeasurementServices/Calibrations/policy.cfm. [Accessed March 3, 2009).
15. **ASTM International:** *Standard Method for Volumetric Measurement of Gaseous Fuel Samples* D1071-2008. Available at http://www.astm.org/Standards/D1071.htm. [Accessed March 10, 2009].
16. **Reiser, S.J.:** *Medicine and the Reign of Technology.* Cambridge, U.K.: Cambridge University Press, 1978.
17. **Davis, A.B.:** *Medicine and Its Technology.* Westport, Conn.: Greenwood Press, 1981.

18. **Nelson, G.O.:** *Controlled Test Atmospheres: Principles and Techniques*. Ann Arbor, MI: Ann Arbor Science Publishers, 1971.
19. **Rouse, H. and S. Ince:** *History of Hydraulics*. Iowa City: Iowa Institute of Hydraulic Research, 1980.
20. **Levy, A.:** The accuracy of the bubble meter method for gas measurements. *J. Sci. Instrum. 41*:449–453 (1964).
21. **Baker, W.C., and J.F. Pouchot:** The measurement of gas flow. Part II. *Air Pollut. Control Assoc. J. 33*:156–162 (1983).
22. **Lide, D.R. (ed.):** *CRC Handbook of Chemistry and Physics*, 89th edition. Boca Raton, FL: CRC Press, 2008.
23. **DiNardi, S.R.:** *Calculation Methods for Industrial Hygiene*. New York: Van Nostrand Reinhold, 1995.
24. **Waldron, P.F.:** *Reducing Systematic Error Associated with Asbestos Air Sampling Through the Appropriate Use of Flowmeter Correction Factors*. MPH thesis, University of Massachusetts, Amherst, Mass., 1991.
25. **Parkinson, B.R:** The history and recent development of the wet gas meter, part 1: History. *Gas J. 252(8)*:104–106 (1947).
26. **Precision Scientific:** *Wet Test Gas Meters (catalog TS-63111 AT-8)*. Chicago: Precision Scientific, 1995.
27. **Ness, S.A.:** *Air Monitoring for Toxic Exposures: An Integrated Approach*. New York: Van Nostrand Reinhold, 1991.
28. **Leidel, N.A., Busch, K.A., and Lynch, J.R.:** "Occupational Exposure Sampling Strategy Manual" NIOSH Publication no. 77-173. Available at http://www.cdc.gov/niosh/docs/77-173. [Accessed November 3, 2008].
29. **Code of Federal Regulations:** Method 2A-Direct Measurement of Gas Volume Through Pipes and Small Ducts. *Code of Federal Regulations Title 40*, Part 60, App. A. 1999. pp. 580-583.
30. **Carvill, J.:** *Famous Names in Engineering*. London: Butterworth, 1981.
31. **Lippmann, M.:** *Airflow calibration. In Air Sampling Instruments*, 9th edition. Cohen, B.S. and S.V. Hering (eds.). Cincinnati, OH: ACGIH®, 2001. pp. 139–150.
32. **Cusick, C.F.:** *Flow Meter Engineering Handbook*, 3rd edition. Philadelphia: Minneapolis-Honeywell Regulator Co., Brown Instrument Division, 1961.
33. **Bradner, M., and L.P. Emerson:** Flow Measurement. In *Fluid Mechanics Source Book*. Parker, S.P. (ed.). New York: McGraw-Hill, 1987. pp. 203–207.
34. **ASTM International:** Standard Practice for Rotameter Calibration ASTM D3195-90 (2004). Available at http://www.astm.org/Standards/D3195.htm. [Accessed March 3, 2009].
35. **Fischer & Porter Co.:** *Variable Area Flowmeter Handbook Volume II: Rotameter Calculations*. [Pamphlet] Warminster, PA: Fisher & Porter Co., 1982.
36. **Caplan, K.S.:** Rotameter corrections for gas density. *Am. Ind. Hyg. Assoc. J. 46*:10–16 (1985).
37. **ACGIH®:** *Industrial Ventilation: A Manual of Recommended Practice*, 24th edition. Cincinnati, OH: ACGIH®, 2001.
38. **Code of Federal Regulations:** Standards of Performance of New Stationary Sources. *Code of Federal Regulations Title 40*, Part 60. 2000.
39. **National Institute for Occupational Safety and Health (NIOSH):** *NIOSH Manual of Analytical Methods*. Available at www.cdc.gov/niosh/nmam. [Accessed November 3, 2008].
40. **International Organization for Standardization (ISO):** *ISO 9000 Certification Standards*. Available at http://www.iso.org/iso/iso_catalogue.htm. [Accessed March 3, 2009].

Outcome Competencies

After completing this chapter, the reader should be able to:

1. Define underlined terms used in this chapter.
2. Recognize the needs for and uses of systems for preparing known concentrations of air contaminants.
3. Discuss state-of-the-art knowledge of available systems, their applications, advantages, and disadvantages.
4. Apply the calculations involved in the use of these systems.
5. Apply the appropriate system considering one's needs and available resources.
6. Discuss the operating principles of a permeation device.
7. Explain source devices to produce aerosols.

Prerequisite Knowledge

Prior to beginning this chapter, the reader should review *General Chemistry*[1] for general content and S.R. DiNardi, *Calculation Methods for Industrial Hygiene*, Van Nostrand Reinhold, 1995.

Prior to beginning this chapter, the user should review the following chapters:

Chapter Number	Chapter Topic
7	Principles of Evaluating Worker Exposure
11	Sampling of Gases and Vapors
12	Analysis of Gases and Vapors
14	Sampling and Sizing of Airborne Particles
15	Principles and Instrumentation for Calibrating Air Sampling Equipment
17	Direct-Reading Instruments for Determining Concentrations of Gases, Vapors, and Aerosols

Key Terms

bar • batch mixture • calibration • diffusion system • flow-dilution system • Ideal Gas law • molar gas volume • monodisperse aerosol • Pascal • permeation tube • SI metric units • validated sampling and analysis method

Key Topics

I. Preparation of Batch Mixtures of Gases and Vapors
   A. Sealed Chambers
   B. Bottles
   C. Plastic Bags
   D. Pressure Cylinders
   E. Calculations of Concentrations in Air
II. Flow-Dilution Systems
   A. Gas-Metering Devices
   B. Construction and Performance of Mixing Systems
III. Source Devices for Gases and Vapors
   A. Vapor Pressure Source Devices
   B. Motor Driven Syringes
   C. Diffusion Source Systems
   D. Porous Plug Source Devices
   E. Permeation Tube Source Devices
   F. Miscellaneous Generation Systems
   G. Illustrative Calculations for Flow-Dilution Systems
IV. Source Devices for Aerosols
   A. Dry Dust Feeders
   B. Nebulizers
   C. Spinning Disc Aerosol Generators
   D. Vaporization and Condensation of Liquids
   E. Miscellaneous Generation Systems
V. Multipurpose Calibration Components and Systems

Preparation of Known Concentrations of Air Contaminants

16

Bernard E. Saltzman, PhD, CIH, PE

Introduction

Known low concentrations of air contaminants are required for many purposes: for testing and validation of analytical methods, for calibrating instruments, and for scientific studies.

Because of legal and economic consequences of the measurements to determine regulatory compliance, each regulatory standard should include a validated sampling and analysis method. As part of the Standards Completion Program[2] the National Institute for Occupational Safety and Health validated methods for 386 compounds in 1976. Additional work was subsequently conducted to validate methods for 130 others.[3] An important part of these validation tests was the generation of known concentrations in air in the range of one half to two times the permissible exposure limit (PEL) against which to compare the test results. Many new methods are being developed utilizing charcoal tubes, passive samplers, and direct-reading devices and instruments that require validation.

Numerous electronic instruments are secondary measuring devices that require calibration with accurately known airborne concentrations. The Environmental Protection Agency's quality assurance procedures have been published.[4]

Another use for known concentrations is for toxicological and scientific investigations of the effects of these concentrations. Such work provides the basis for control standards.

Two general types of systems are used for generation of known concentrations. Preparation of a batch mixture has the advantages of simplicity and convenience in some cases. Alternatively a flow-dilution system may be employed. A flow-dilution system requires a metered flow of diluent air and a source for supplying known flows of gases, vapors, or aerosols; these flows are combined in a mixing device. This system has the advantages of compactness and of being capable of providing large volumes at known low concentrations, which can be rapidly changed if desired. Each of these techniques will be described in detail later in this chapter. Many articles have been published on the subject of making known concentrations. Broad coverage is given in articles.[5–18]

Preparation of Batch Mixtures of Gases and Vapors

These methods generally require relatively simple equipment and procedures. However, a serious disadvantage is the fact that only limited quantities of the mixture can be supplied. For reactive compounds erroneously low concentrations may result from appreciable adsorption losses of the test substance on the walls of the chamber. Losses in excess of 50% are common.[19,20] These methods may be used to prepare nominal concentrations of many substances that are not too reactive. They should not be used as primary standards without verification by chemical analyses.

Sealed Chambers

Known concentrations of gases and vapors were first prepared as batch mixtures by

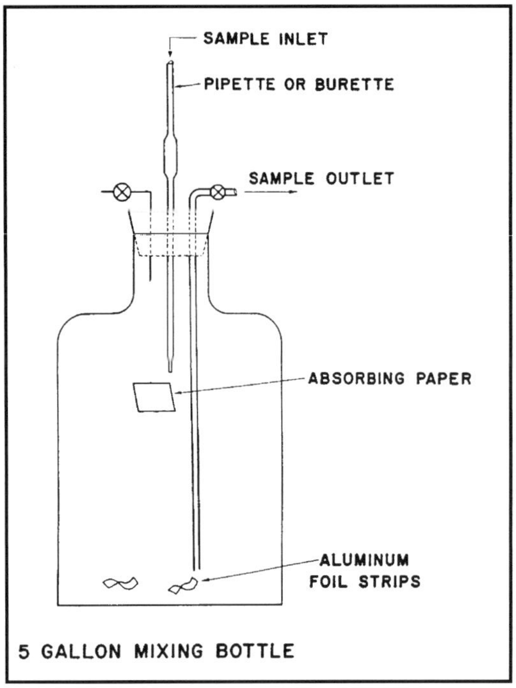

Figure 16.1 — Preparation of vapor mixtures in a glass bottle (Source: Reference 6).

introducing and dispersing accurately measured quantities of the test compound into a sealed chamber containing clean air with mixing provided by an electric fan. (Sparks from brushes may explode some mixtures. When air dilutions of solvents or other combustible materials are prepared, care must be taken to keep the concentrations outside of the explosive limits.) The mixture may be withdrawn from the center of the chamber through a tube. Leakage from sealed exposure chambers, most likely from deterioration of door gaskets, may be evaluated by pressurizing them (to 5 cm H_2O) and determining the rate of pressure drop with time.[21]

Bottles

Figure 16.1 illustrates a simple technique for preparation of vapor mixtures using a 5-gallon glass bottle. A quantity of volatile liquid is pipetted into the bottle onto a piece of paper to assist in its evaporation. The bottle may then be tumbled with aluminum foil inside to facilitate air and vapor mixing. The mixture is withdrawn through a glass tube from the bottom of the bottle rather than from the top to avoid leakage and losses occurring around the stopper.

As the mixture is withdrawn, air enters the top of the bottle to relieve the vacuum.

TABLE 16.1 — Decrease in Concentration Versus Fractional Volume Withdrawn from Chamber Mixture

W/V	0.05	0.10	0.25	0.50
C/C_0	0.951	0.905	0.779	0.607

It can be seen that the disadvantage of these techniques is that the concentration decreases during the withdrawal process as clean air enters. Assuming the worst possible case of complete turbulent mixing in the bottle or chamber, the change in concentration is given by Equation 1.

$$C/C_0 = e^{W/V} \qquad (16\text{-}1)$$

where

C = final concentration in bottle or chamber
C_0 = initial concentration
W = volume withdrawn, liters
V = original volume of mixture, liters

Some calculated values are shown in Table 16.1. This table shows the maximum depletion errors produced by withdrawal of the mixture. Smaller errors result if the incoming air does not mix completely with the exiting mixture. Up to 5% can be withdrawn without serious loss. These errors are avoided by use of plastic bags or pressure cylinders, as described below.

Figure 16.2 illustrates a simple commercial assembly for creating a known concentration of hydrocarbon for use in calibrating explosive-gas meters. A sealed glass ampule containing a hydrocarbon such as methane is placed inside a polyethylene bottle and broken by shaking against a steel ball. The mixture is then carefully squeezed into the instrument to be calibrated, taking care not to suck back air. Another commercial system for making a known concentration batch is comprised of a cartridge of isobutane, which is used to fill a small syringe. This is injected into a larger syringe that is then filled with air. The latter syringe serves as a gas holder for the mixture. These devices are relatively simple, convenient, and sufficiently accurate for calibrating explosive-gas meters.

Plastic Bags

A variety of plastic bags have been found to be very useful for preparing known mixtures in the laboratory. Among the materials used have been Mylar®, aluminized Mylar, Scotchpak, Saran®, polyvinyl chloride, Teflon®, Tedlar®, and Kel-F®. Tedlar, Teflon, and Kel-F are considerably more expensive materials preferred for use in photochemical smog studies involving ultraviolet irradiation. Surprisingly, for most applications the less expensive materials give superior performance. Mylar bags are popular because of their strength and inertness.

Bags are fabricated from plastic sheets by thermal sealing. Volatile contaminants are baked out of the plastic sheets by some fabricators by keeping them in an oven for a few days. A rigid plastic tube or a valve similar to the type used for tires may be sealed to a side or corner to serve as the inlet, as illustrated in Figure 16.3. The inlet tube to the bag may be closed with a rubber stopper, serum cap, cork, or a valve according to the substance being handled. Bags are available commercially from a number of vendors.[22] The 3 ft × 3 ft or 2 ft × 4 ft size contains over 100 L. Available sizes range from 0.5 L (6 inches × 6 inches) to 450 L (5 ft × 5 ft).

A simple arrangement may be used for preparing a known mixture in a plastic bag. The bag is alternately filled partly with clean air and then completely evacuated several times to flush it out. Then clean air is metered into it through a wet or dry test meter or using a rotameter and stopwatch. The test substance is added to this stream at a tee just above the entrance to the bag. If the test substance is a volatile liquid, it can be injected accurately by syringe through a septum. Sufficient air must subsequently be passed through the tee to completely transfer the injected material. When the desired air volume has been introduced, the bag is disconnected and plugged or capped. The contents may be mixed by gently kneading the bag with the hands.

The major advantage of using flexible bags is that no dilution occurs as the sample is withdrawn. These bags are transportable. Bags should be tested frequently for pinhole leaks. Initial screening tests may be done by filling them with clean air and sealing them. Usually leaks are large enough to produce detectable flattening within 24 hours.

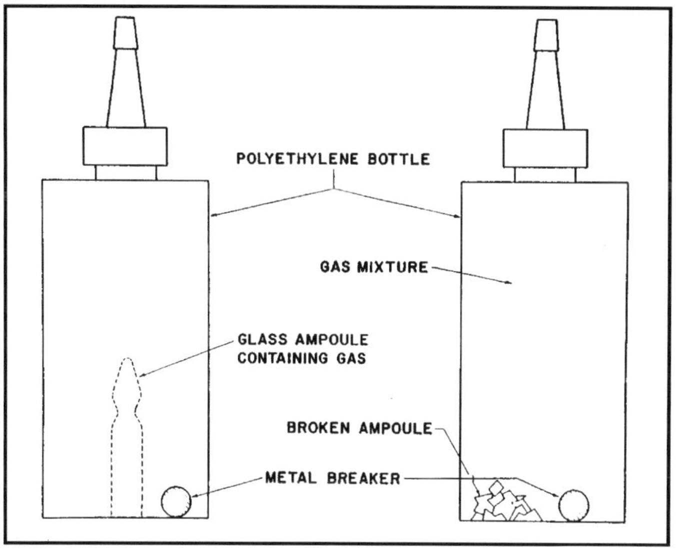

Figure 16.2 — Calibrator for explosive gas meters (Source: Reference 6).

Adsorption and reaction on the walls is no great problem for relatively high concentrations of inert materials such as halogenated solvents and hydrocarbons.[23] However, low concentrations of reactive materials such as sulfur dioxide, nitrogen dioxide, and ozone are partly lost, even after prior conditioning of the bags.[19,20,24,25] Larger bags are preferable to minimize the surface-to-volume ratio. Losses of 5 or 10% frequently occur during the first hour, after which the losses are a small percentage per day. Conditioning of the bags with similar mixtures is essential to reduce these losses. A similar or identical mixture is stored for at least 24 hours in the bag and then evacuated just before use. A tabulation[26] of the uses of these bags described in 12 articles lists the plastic material, the gas or vapor stored, their concentrations, and the researcher comments. Another

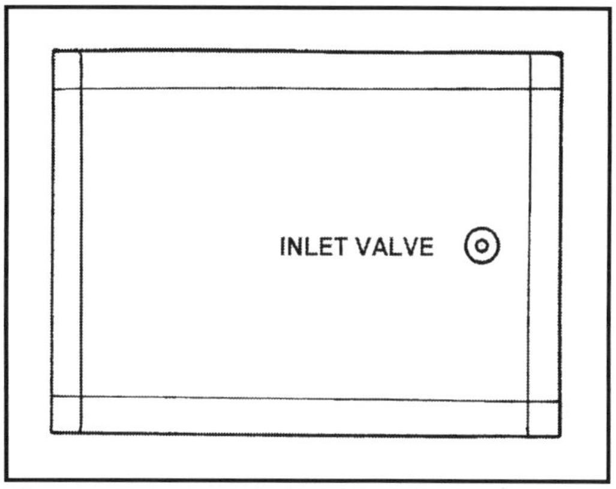

Figure 16.3 — Typical plastic bag for containing air samples.

study[27] focused on occupational hygiene applications of plastic bags. Good stability in Saran bags was found for mixtures containing benzene, dichloromethane, and methyl alcohol; and for Scotchpak bags containing benzene, dichloromethane, and methyl isobutyl ketone. Percentage losses were greater for lower concentrations (i.e., below 50 ppm). Losses greater than 20% were observed in the first 24 hours for Saran bags containing methyl isobutyl ketone vapors; however, concentrations stabilized after two to three days. Concentrations of batch mixtures calculated theoretically were compared with analyses by gas chromatography.[28] Although the theoretical slope was obtained, incorrect intercepts were observed for compounds of low vapor pressure (0.4–8 mm Hg at 25°C) because of significant wall adsorption in the instruments. Losses of carbon monoxide and hydrocarbons in sampling bags of various materials also have been studied.[29] Losses of occupational hygiene analytes with time have been reported.[30] If the mixture is stored for more than a day, permeation into as well as out of the bag must be considered, especially for thin plastic films. Permeation of outside pollutants (hydrocarbons and nitrogen oxides) into Teflon bags has been demonstrated.[31]

It is difficult to draw generalized conclusions from these reports, other than the need for caution in applying plastic bags for low concentrations. Losses should be determined for each material in each type of bag. Even the past history of each individual bag must be considered. For properly conducted laboratory applications, known mixtures can be prepared very conveniently in plastic bags.

Pressure Cylinders

Preparation of certain gas mixtures can be done conveniently in pressurized steel cylinders.[6] This is very useful for mixtures such as hydrocarbons or carbon monoxide in air, which can be stored for years without losses. With other substances, there are losses because of factors such as polymerization, adsorption, or reaction with the cylinder walls. In some cases, as the pressure decreases in the cylinder, material desorbs from the walls, yielding a higher final concentration in the cylinder than was initially present. Concentrations should be low enough to avoid condensation of any component at the high pressure in the cylinder, even at the lowest temperature expected during its use. Care must be taken to use clean regulators made with appropriate materials that will not adsorb or react with the contents of the cylinder. Specially coated aluminum cylinders rather than steel cylinders may be used to assure long-term stability of many reactive gases at ppm concentrations.

A serious safety hazard exists in preparation of compressed gas mixtures. As mentioned previously, there is a possibility of explosion of combustible substances. This may occur because of the heat of compression during a too rapid filling process. Excessive heat also may cause errors in the gas composition. Certain substances with high positive heats of formation, such as acetylene, can detonate even in the absence of oxygen. Also, explosive copper acetylid can be produced if copper is used in the manifolds and connections. Proper equipment, including armor-plate shielding, and experience are required for safe preparation. Because these and accurate pressure gauges are not ordinarily available, it is recommended that such mixtures be purchased from the compressed gas vendors who have professional experience and equipment for such work. These vendors can prepare mixtures either by using accurate pressure gauges to measure the proportions of the components or by actually weighing the cylinders as each component is added. They also can provide an analysis at a reasonable extra charge; however, these analyses are not always reliable.[32]

The Analytical Chemistry Division of the National Institute of Standards and Technology (NIST) supervises gas mixtures offered by certain specialty gas companies as NIST Traceable Reference Material. Mixtures in air include carbon dioxide, carbon monoxide, methane, propane, and nitrogen dioxide. Mixtures in nitrogen (or helium) include benzene, carbon monoxide, carbonyl sulfide, hydrogen sulfide, methyl mercaptan, nitric oxide, and propane.

Calculations of Concentrations in Air

When equations are used for calculations, values in appropriate units must be entered for each term. If there is a constant in the equation, its numerical value corresponds to the units required. Ambient pressures are commonly measured with a mercury barometer and expressed as mm of mercury. Air volumes are commonly measured in liters, and temperatures as degrees Celcuis. SI metric units have been agreed on internationally, including length: meter; mass: kg; temperature, °C; pressure: bar (= 10^6 dynes/cm^2), and Pascal (kg/m sec^2). Their relationships to commonly used units are as follows: 1 m^3 = 1000 L = 10^6 mL; 1 atmosphere = 760 mm Hg = 1.0133 bar = 1.0133×10^5 Pa.

The calculations for preparation of batch mixtures are based on close adherence to the Ideal Gas law[1] at low partial pressures. Calculations for dilute gas concentrations are based on the simple ratio of the volume of test gas to the volume of mixture, as shown in Equation 16-2.

$$\text{ppm} = 10^6\, v/V \qquad (16\text{-}2)$$

where

ppm = parts per million by volume (definition)
v = volume of test gas in the mixture, L
V = total volume of mixture, L

Changes in ambient temperature and pressure do not change the ppm value because both the numerator and denominator in this equation are changed by the same factor, which cancels out.

In the case of volatile liquids the calculation is based on the ratio of moles of test liquid to moles of gas mixture, Equation 3. The moles of liquid are determined in the numerator by dividing the weight injected by the molecular weight of the liquid compound. The moles of gas mixture are calculated in the denominator by dividing the total volume of mixture by the molar gas volume.

$$\text{ppm} = \left(\frac{10^6\, w/MW}{V/V_m} \right) \qquad (16\text{-}3)$$

where

w = weight of volatile test liquid introduced, g
MW = gram molecular weight of test liquid
V_m = gram molecular volume, L, of the mixture under ambient conditions

The molar gas volume is calculated from Equation 16-4 for the ambient temperature and pressure of the mixture.

$$V_m = 24.45 \left(\frac{760}{P} \right) \left(\frac{t + 273.15}{298.15} \right) \qquad (16\text{-}4)$$

where

24.45 = gram molecular volume, L, under standard conditions of 760 mm Hg, 25°C
P = ambient pressure, mm Hg
t = ambient temperature, °C

Calculations for batch mixtures in compressed gas tanks may be made on the basis of the ratio of the partial pressure of the test compound to the total pressure of the mixture, as shown in Equation 16-5.

$$\text{ppm} = 10^6\, p/P_T \qquad (16\text{-}5)$$

where

p = partial pressure of the test compound, and
P_T = total pressure of the mixture.

The same equation may be used for methods relying on the equilibrium vapor pressure of a volatile liquid as a source of a known concentration. In this case p is the equilibrium vapor pressure and P_T is the barometric pressure of the atmosphere.

A more common method of expressing concentrations is in terms of mg/m^3, defined simply as the weight of the test component divided by the volume of the mixture. In this case the ambient pressure and temperature affect the value only of the denominator and thus affect the value of the mg/m^3. For precise work the volume is corrected to standard conditions of 25°C, 760 mm Hg, using another form of Equation 16-4.

$$V_2 = V_1 \left(\frac{P_1}{P_2} \right) \left(\frac{t_2 + 273.15}{t_1 + 273.15} \right) \qquad (16\text{-}4a)$$

where

V_2 = corrected volume (desired at 25°C, 760 mm Hg)
V_1 = ambient volume
P_1 = ambient pressure
P_2 = desired corrected pressure (760 mm Hg)
t_2 = desired corrected temperature (25°C)
t_1 = ambient temperature °C

The standard conditions of 25°C and 760 mm Hg were selected to be close to usual ambient conditions so that the correction is small and is commonly ignored. Results of chemical analyses ordinarily are expressed in terms of milligrams (or micrograms). These may be divided by the sample volume in the same manner to yield mg/m³ (which is also µg/L).

The relationship under standard conditions between ppm and mg/m³ may be derived as follows. In a volume of 24.45 L containing 1 mole of mixture, the ppm is equal to the number of micromoles of the test component. Multiplying ppm by the molecular weight gives the number of micrograms for the numerator.

$$\frac{mg}{m^3} = \frac{\mu g}{L} = \frac{ppm \times MW}{24.45} \qquad (16\text{-}6)$$

$$ppm = \frac{24.45 \times mg/m^3}{MW} \qquad (16\text{-}6a)$$

In Equation 16-6a if the mg/m³ are at ambient temperature and pressure, the 24.45 L molar volume is replaced by the ambient value from Equation 16-4.

These calculations are illustrated by the following examples.

Example 1. A volume of 5 mL of pure carbon monoxide gas is slowly injected into a tube through which 105 L of air are being metered into a plastic bag. What is the concentration (ppm by volume) of the final carbon monoxide mixture?

Answer. Applying Equation 16-2: ppm = $10^6 \times 0.005$ L/105 L = 47.6 ppm.

Example 2. A dish containing 12.7 g of carbon tetrachloride is placed in a sealed cubical chamber with inside dimensions of 2.1 m for each edge. The final temperature is 22.5°C, and the barometer reading is 765 mm Hg. (a) What concentration (ppm) is achieved? (b) What is the concentration in mg/m³ under ambient conditions? (c) What is the concentration in mg/m³ under standard conditions?

Answers. (a) The ambient volume in liters is V = $(2.1)^3$ = 9.26 m³ × 1000 = 9260 L

Applying Equation 16-4,

$$V_m = 24.45 \times \left(\frac{760}{765}\right)\left(\frac{295.65}{298.15}\right) = 24.11L$$

Applying Equation 16-3,

$$ppm = \left(\frac{10^6 \times 12.7/153.84}{9260/24.11}\right) = 214.9 \text{ ppm}$$

(b) mg/m³ = 12,700 mg/9.26 m³ = 1371 mg/m³. (c) There are 1371 mg in a volume of 1 m³ under ambient conditions. Correcting this volume to standard conditions results in

$$\frac{mg}{m^3} = \frac{1371}{\frac{24.45}{24.11}} = 1351 \text{ mg/m}^3$$

Alternatively, Equation 16-6 could be applied to the ppm, which does not change with ambient pressure and temperature.

$$\frac{mg}{m^3} = \frac{214.9 \times 153.84}{24.45} = 1351 \text{ mg/m}^3$$

Flow-Dilution Systems

In flow-dilution systems air and test vapor, gas, or aerosol are continuously and accurately metered and combined in a mixing device. These systems offer the primary advantage of being very compact. Since it is possible to operate them continuously, very large volumes of gas mixture can be provided. In a properly designed system, concentrations also can be changed very rapidly. Because of the relatively small gas volume of this system, the explosive hazard is less than that of batch systems. Any losses by adsorption on surfaces occur only in the initial minutes of operation. After a brief period the surfaces are fully saturated and no further losses occur. Because of these advantages, flow-dilution systems are popular for accurate work with most substances.

Gas-Metering Devices

A variety of devices can be used to measure the air and test substance flows in a flow-dilution system. The accuracy of the final concentration, of course, depends on the accuracy of these measurements. Rotameters are commonly used. Mass flowmeters, orifice meters, and critical orifices are also frequently employed. The calibration equations and techniques for these devices are given in detail in Chapter 15 on instruments for calibration. Because rotameters are very commonly used, a few points of importance to their application in flow-dilution systems will be discussed.

The pulsating flows provided by some diaphragm pumps utilized in many flow-dilution systems may result in serious errors in interpreting meter readings on the basis of a steady flow calibration. The author has observed that rotameter readings may be high by a flow factor of as much as 2, depending on the wave form of the pulsating flow. It is, therefore, essential for accurate measurements to use a pump with a pulsation damper, or to damp out such pulsations by assembling a train comprised of the pump, a surge chamber, and a resistance, such as a partially closed valve or orifice. The error due to the pulsating flow can be determined as the flowmeter is recalibrated by running the pulsating flow through the rotameter and into a soap film meter or wet-test meter, and then comparing results with the steady flow calibration. The reason for this error is that although the mean flow rate of the pulsating flow is proportional to the mean of the first power of the gas velocity, the lifting force on the rotameter ball is proportional to the mean of the gas velocity raised to a power of between 1 and 2. For completely turbulent flows in the rotameter, which are common, the exponent is 2; in this case if the velocity fluctuates in a sine wave, the ball position will correspond to the root mean square value, which is 1.414 times the correct mean value. If the wave form is spiked, even greater deviations can occur. Similar relationships and errors may occur with other types of flowmeters. Wave forms have been measured[33] with small hot-wire anemometers for some popular air sampling pumps not provided with pulsation dampers.

There are two types of corrections of flowmeter calibrations made under standard conditions for readings made under a different ambient pressure and temperature. If the system has substantial pressure drops and the flowmeter is operating under pressure or vacuum, this is added to or subtracted from the barometric pressure to give the absolute pressure, which is used for the correction. The first is the correction because the calibration is dependent on the density, and in some cases the viscosity, of the gas flow, both of which are affected by ambient pressure and temperature. Applying this correction gives the correct ambient flow. The second correction may be applied to convert the actual gas flow rate under ambient conditions to that under standard conditions. The latter correction is made on the basis of the ideal gas relationship using Equation 16-4a. It should be kept clearly in mind that the first calibration correction depends on the specific device being employed. The two bases, ambient or standard conditions, should not be confused, and the proper one must be employed for the application. Corrections for high altitudes are related to atmospheric pressure.[34]

Construction and Performance of Mixing Systems

A flow-dilution system is comprised of a metered test substance source, a metered clean-air source, and a mixer to dilute the test substance to the low concentration required. The total flow of mixture must be equal to or greater than the flow needed. It is highly desirable to use only glass or Teflon parts for constructing the mixing system. Components preferably should be connected with ball or standard taper ground glass joints. Short lengths of plastic tubing may be used if not exposed in butt-to-butt connections of the glass parts. Some studies have shown that metal and plastic tubing must be conditioned with the dilute mixtures for periods of hours or days before they cease absorbing the test substances.[19,20,35]

Two other factors must be kept in mind in the construction of a mixing system. The first is that the pressure drops must be very small, and the system should preferably be operated at very close to atmospheric pressure. Otherwise, any changes in one part of the system will require troublesome readjustment of the flows of other components. The interactions may require several time-consuming reiterative adjustments. Also, if a monitoring instrument is being calibrated it may not draw the designed sample flow rate from a system not at atmospheric pressure, and the readings may be erroneous. The second factor to consider is that the dead volume of the system must be minimized to achieve a rapid response time. For example, assume that a flow of 0.1 mL/min is metered into a diluent airstream, and that the dead volume of the system to the dilution point is 1 mL. To accomplish one volume change will require 10 minutes. To be certain that this dead volume is completely flushed out, five volume changes are needed, corresponding to a time lag of 50 minutes before the full concentration of test gas reaches the dilution point.

Figure 16.4 illustrates a convenient all-glass system for making gas dilutions. The metered test gas is connected at the extreme right through a ball joint and capillary tube (1). The dilution air is metered into the side arm (2). A trap-like mixing device ensures complete mixing with very little pressure drop. The desired flow can be taken from the side arm (3) and the excess vented through the waste tube (4), which may be connected to a Tygon® tube long enough to prevent entrance of air into the flow system. If necessary, this vent tube should be run to a hood. By clamping down on the vent tube or submerging the outlet (4) in a beaker of water, any desired pressure can be obtained in the delivery system.

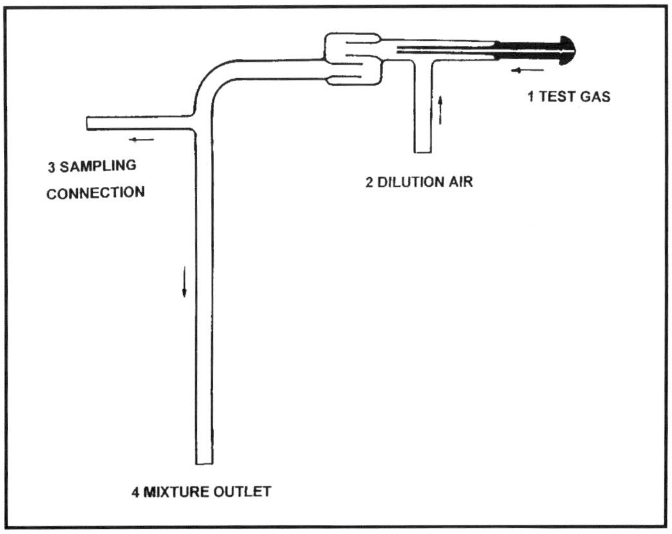

Figure 16.4 — All-glass flow-dilution mixer. 1: Inlet for metered gas; 2: inlet for meterd purified air; 3: samplong connection; 4: waste mixture outlet. (Source: Reference 5)

The dilution air must be purified according to the needs of the work. Air can be passed through an oil filter and then over a bed of carbon, silica gel, or Ascarite®, or bubbled through a scrubbing mixture of sodium dichromate in concentrated sulfuric acid if necessary. Organic compounds can be destroyed by passing the air over a hot platinum catalyst, or at a lower temperature over a Hopcalite® catalyst. Another convenient method of purification is to pass the air flow through a universal gas mask canister. The purification system must be designed according to the specific needs of the work.

Source Devices for Gases and Vapors

A variety of source devices are described below for providing high concentrations of gases and vapors that can be diluted with pure air to achieve the concentration desired. Each possesses specific advantages and disadvantages. Selection of a source device depends on the needs of the application and the equipment available to the user. Figure 16.5 shows a self-dilution device that can be generally applied to reduce the concentration provided by the source when necessary for work at very low concentrations. The flow of gas or vapor passes through the branches in proportions determined by restrictions R_1 and R_2. An appropriate absorbent such as carbon, soda lime, etc., in the lower branch completely removes the gas or vapor from the stream. Thus, the combined output of the two branches provides the delivered flow at a fractional concentration of the input depending on the relative values of the two flow restrictors. Furthermore, operation of the three-way stopcock also provides either the full concentration or zero concentration or completely cuts off the flow.

Vapor Pressure Source Devices

Figure 16.6 illustrates the method for providing a known concentration corresponding to the equilibrium vapor pressure of a volatile liquid. A flow of inert gas or purified air is bubbled through a container of the pure liquid (1) operated at ambient or elevated temperature. Liquid mixtures are less desirable because the more volatile components will evaporate first; thus, the vapor concentrations change as the evaporation proceeds. Because the output of the first bubbler may commonly be at only 50 to 90% of the saturation vapor pressure, equilibrium concentrations are obtained by then passing the vapor mixture through a second bubbler containing the same liquid, at an accurately controlled lower constant temperature. The excess vapor is condensed, and the final concentration is very close to equilibrium vapor pressure at the cooling bath temperature. A filter must be included to ensure that a liquid fog or mist does not escape. It is desirable to operate the constant temperature bath below ambient temperature so that liquid does not condense in the cool portions of the system downstream. The applications of this method to carbon tetrachloride[36] and mercury[37] have been described.

Another version of this arrangement is shown in Figure 16.7. This uses a wick feed from a small bottle containing the additive as a source of the vapor and an ice bath for the constant temperature.

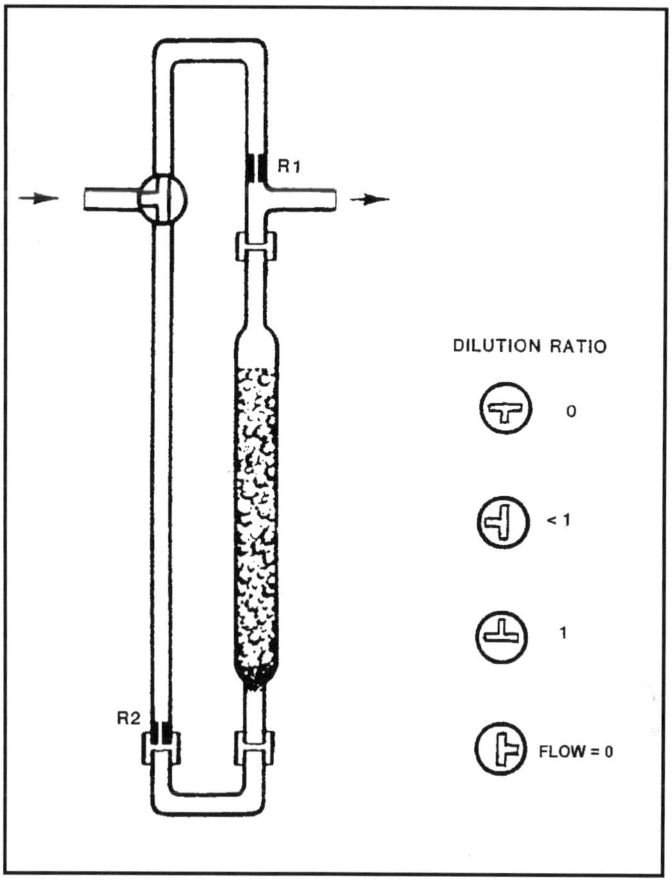

Figure 16.5 — Sel-dilution device. Dilution ratio is the ratio of the exiting to entering concentrations. (Source: Reference 7)

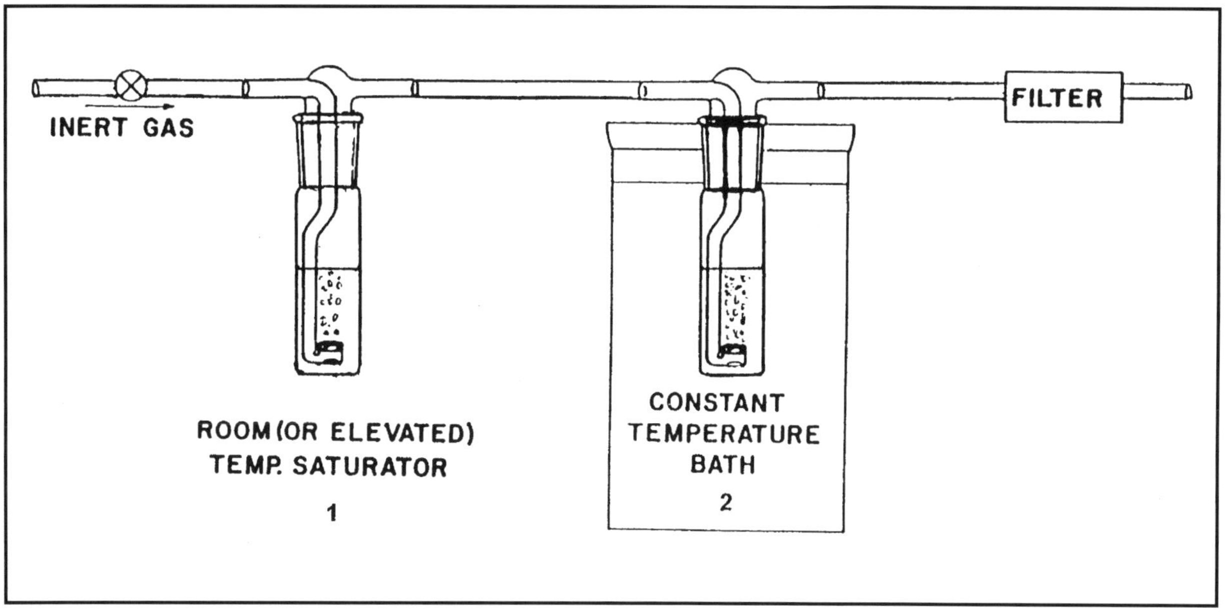

Figure 16.6 — Vapor saturator source system.

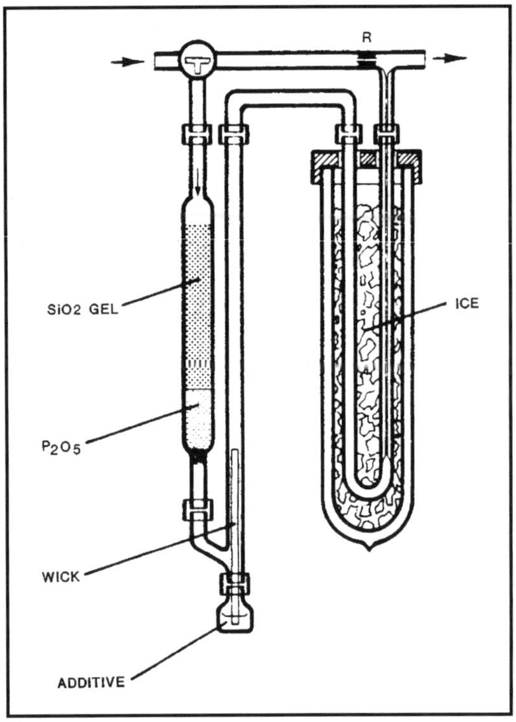

Figure 16.7 — Wick evaporator-condensor source system (Source: Reference 7).

Motor Driven Syringes

Figure 16.8 illustrates a source delivery system using a glass hypodermic syringe (4) that is driven by a motor drive at uniform rates that can be controlled to empty it in periods varying from a few minutes to an hour. A gas cylinder containing the pure test component or mixture is connected at the right side (1). The bubbler (2) is a safety device to protect the glass apparatus from excessive pressures if the tank needle valve is opened too wide. The tank valve is cautiously opened, and a slow stream of gas is vented from the outlet (3) of the bubbler. The syringe is manually filled and emptied several times to flush it with the gas. This is done by turning the three-way stopcock (5) so that on the intake stroke the syringe is connected to the cylinder at (1) and on the discharge stroke to the delivery end (6). After flushing, the syringe is filled from the cylinder and the motor drive is set to discharge it over the desired period of time. This motor drive should include a limit switch to shut off the motor before it breaks the syringe, and a revolution counter for measuring the displacement. From the known gear ratio, the screw pitch, and a measurement of the plunger diameter with a micrometer, the

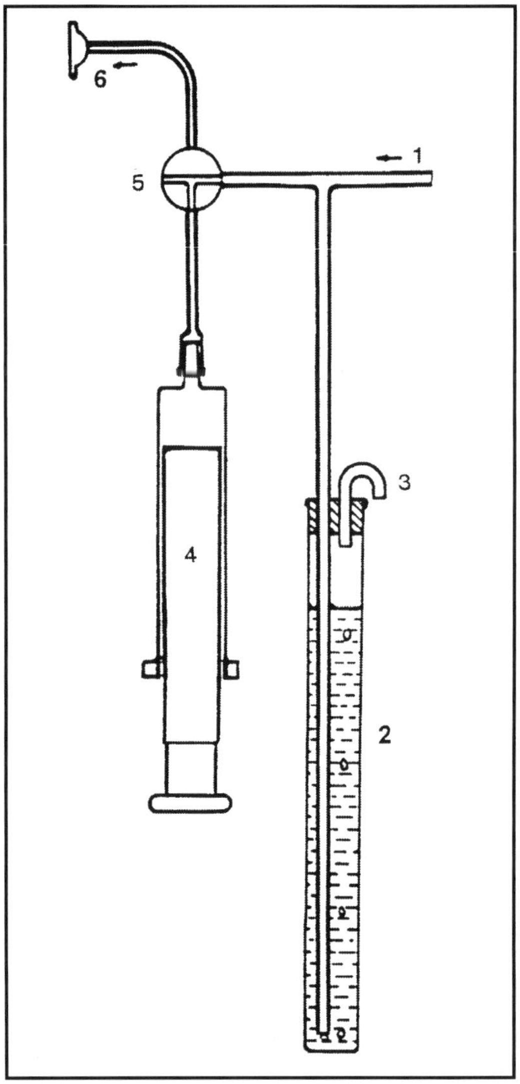

Figure 16.8 — Motor-driven syringe source system. 1: test gas inlet; 2: safety pressure release and flushing vent; 3: waste gas outlet; 4: motor-driven 50-mL glass syringe; 5: stopcock in syringe filling position; 6: metered gas outlet. (Source: Reference 5)

rate of feed can be calculated. An accuracy and reproducibility of parts per thousand can be achieved with an accurate screw and good bearings.

At low delivery rates the back diffusion of air into the syringe from the delivery tip may cause an error. Thus, if the syringe is set to empty over a 1-hour period, toward the end as much as half of the gas mixture contents could be air that has diffused in backward. This error is easily minimized by inserting a loose glass wool plug in the delivery system and using capillary tubing for the delivered flow. The device was designed to

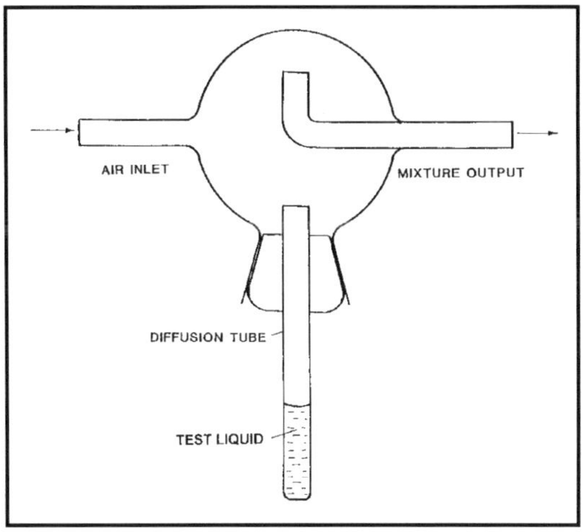

Figure 16.9 — Vapor diffusion source system.

connect to the dilution system illustrated in Figure 16.4. Syringes also may be used to meter a volatile liquid into an electrically heated vaporizer connected to an exposure chamber.[38,39] Concentrations can be routinely maintained within 10% of target levels. The possibilities of fire, explosion, or decomposition of a high-boiling compound must be considered.

Diffusion Source Systems

Figure 16.9 illustrates a diffusion system that can provide constant concentrations of a volatile liquid. The test liquid is contained in the bottom of a long thin tube and is kept at a known constant temperature. As the air flow is passed over the tip, vapor diffuses up through the length of the tube at a reproducible rate (assuming the temperature is closely controlled) and mixes with the stream. The rate is determined by the vapor pressure of the liquid, the dimensions of the tube, and the diffusion constants of the vapor and of air. If substantial amounts of a liquid are evaporated and the liquid level drops, the diffusion path length increases slightly. The quantity of liquid evaporated can be determined best from volume markings on the tube or by weighing the tube at the beginning and end of the period of use. It is possible to use a recording balance in some systems. Quantities calculated from the diffusion coefficient and the dimensions of the tube may be less accurate. Experimental values have been tabulated and the limitations of this method described.[40]

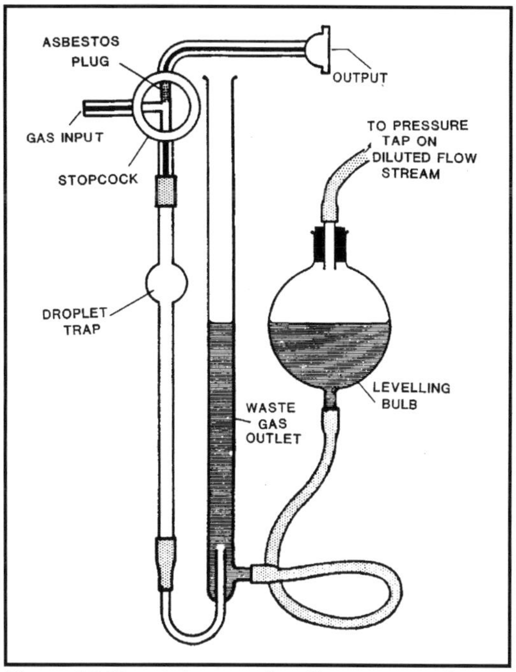

Figure 16.10 — Asbestos plug flowmeter and controller.

Porous Plug Source Devices

Figure 16.10 illustrates a micrometering system[5,41] that both measures and controls small flows of gas in the range of 0.02 to 10 mL/min. This is based on the principle of diffusion of test gas through an asbestos plug under a controlled pressure difference. The inlet is connected to a cylinder containing pure test gas or a mixture. An acid-washed asbestos plug is contained in one leg of the T bore of a three-way stopcock (which is never turned), as shown in the figure. Any similar inert material may be used if asbestos is not available. The degree of fiber tamping is determined by trial and error to provide the desired delivered flow range. The cylinder needle valve is opened cautiously to provide a few bubbles per minute from the waste outlet in the lower portion of the figure. The height of water or oil above the waste outlet determines the fixed pressure on the lower face of the asbestos plug, which produces a fixed rate of diffusion of the gas through the plug to the capillary delivery tip. The meter is calibrated by connecting the delivery end to a graduated 1-mL pipette with the tip cut off, containing a soap film or drop of water. The motion of the film or drop past the markings is timed with a stop watch. This is repeated for different heights of liquid obtained by adjustment of the leveling bulb. The calibration plot of flow rates in mL/min versus the heights of liquid over the waste outlet in cm is usually a straight line passing through the origin. After the gas cylinder is shut off it should never be disconnected before the liquid pressures equalize; otherwise, the liquid may surge up and wet the asbestos plug. If this occurs, it must be discarded, the bore dried and repacked, and the new plug calibrated.

This device is a very convenient and precise method for metering low flows in the indicated range. The output flow remains constant for weeks, but should be checked occasionally. The delivery tip is connected to the mixer shown in Figure 16.4. For low delivery rates, the dead volume is minimized by using capillary tubing.

The leveling bulb vent is connected to a tap on the diluted gas manifold. This provides a correction for back pressure of the system into which the flow is being delivered. An appreciable back pressure changes the pressure differential across the asbestos plug. The bulb vent connection causes the liquid level to rise in the vent tube. If the vent tube area is small compared with the area of the liquid surface in the bulb, this compensates almost exactly for the back pressure by increasing the upstream pressure on the plug enough to maintain a constant pressure differential.

Permeation Tube Source Devices

Permeation tubes[42, 43] are very useful sources for liquefiable gases and volatile liquids. Because of their potential precision they will be discussed in some detail here. NIST certifies sulfur dioxide and nitrogen dioxide permeation tubes. Each is individually calibrated at 25°C to within 1% of the stated permeation rate with 95% confidence. Thus, when maintained in a dry thermostated environment, they can serve as primary standards. Commercial sources[13,22] offer tubes for over 100 compounds and certify their permeation rates as a function of temperature to a precision of ±2%.

In these devices the liquid is sealed under pressure in inert plastic (commonly Teflon) tubes. The vapor pressure may be as high as 10 atmospheres. The gas or vapor permeates out through the walls of the tube at a constant rate (commonly of a few milligrams per day) for periods as long as a year. Figure 16.11 illustrates four commercial types of tubes. In the standard type (1) the liquified gas or volatile liquid is sealed in an inert plastic tube with solid plugs held in place by crimped bands. In some extended lifetime tubes a glass or stainless steel vial containing the liquified gas is attached to the Teflon tube (4). To slow the permeation rate, the low emission devices have thicker permeable walls (2) or wafers connected to an impermeable container (3) holding the liquid. In permeation tubes containing a liquid with a low vapor pressure, such as nitrogen dioxide (boiling point 21.3°C), a sufficiently tight seal may be obtained by pushing the Teflon tube onto the neck of a glass vial and by pushing a glass plug in at the top. For higher vapor pressures, such as in tubes containing propane (vapor pressure 10 atmospheres at 25°C), a stainless steel vial is used. Metals used for bottles or crimping bands must be selected for corrosion resistance, especially if the tubes are calibrated by weighing. In another type of seal, FEP (fluorinated ethylene propylene polymer), Teflon plugs are fused to an FEP Teflon tube by means of heat. Tubes are usually discarded when empty.

Figure 16.12 illustrates the typical use of a permeation tube in a commercial precision span gas standard generator for instrument calibration. A small constant flow is passed over the tube in an air oven thermostated to within ±0.05°C and then is diluted with a larger flow to produce the desired concentration and flow rate. In an alternative design that provides an extremely long-lived source, the liquid is contained in a sealed container in the oven. The air flows through the inside of a coiled Teflon tube immersed in the liquid in the container.

All tubes, especially if the contents are under pressure, should be handled with caution since they may present a toxic or explosive hazard. If they have been chilled in dry ice during filling, room for expansion of the liquid on warming to ordinary temperatures should be provided. Tubes should be protected from excessive heat. They should never be manually touched, scratched, bent, or mechanically abused. After a new tube has been prepared, several days or weeks are required before a steady permeation rate is achieved at a thermostated temperature. It

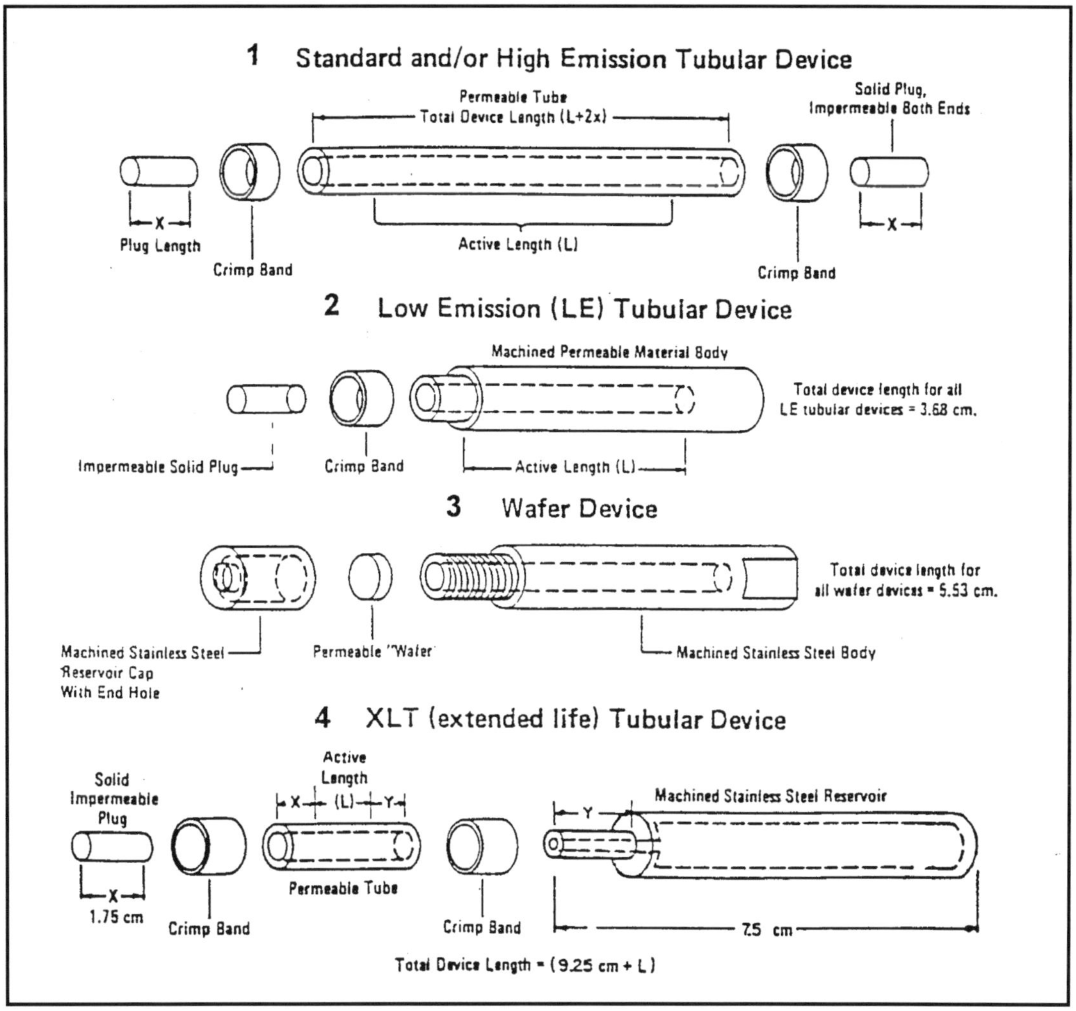

Figure 16.11 — Construction of some commercial permeation tubes (Courtesy of Dynacel® Permeation Devices, VICI Metronics Co.).

was reported[44] that tubes made of FEP Teflon should be annealed at 30°C for a period to relieve extrusion strains and equilibrate the Teflon to achieve a steady permeation rate. Otherwise, a pseudo-stable rate is achieved that is not reproduced after appreciable temperature fluctuations. Tubes made of TFE (tetrafluorinated ethylene polymer) Teflon are more porous than FEP Teflon and may be used to obtain 3 to 10 times higher permeation rates.

Gravimetric calibrations may be made by weighing the permeation tubes at intervals and plotting the weights against time. The slope of the line fitted by the method of least squares to the measured points is the permeation rate. This process may take as long as several weeks with an ordinary balance because of the necessity of waiting to

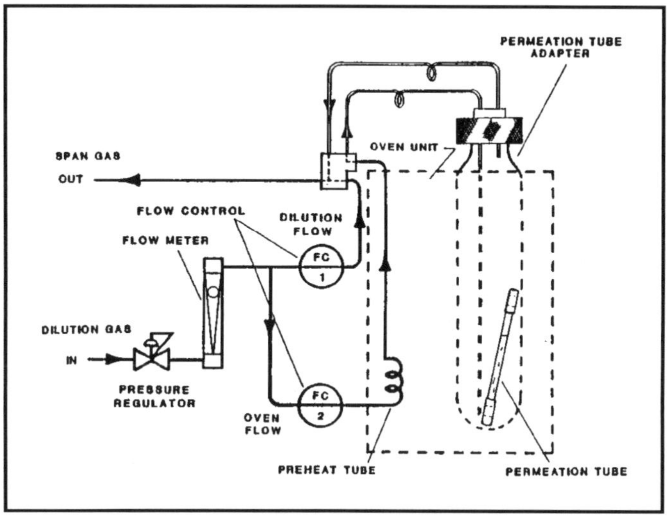

Figure 16.12 — A commercial calibration system using permeation tubes (Model 570C, Precision Gas Standards Generator, courtesy of Kin-Tek Laboratory Inc.).

obtain accurately measurable weight differences. However, if a good micro balance is available, the calibration can be shortened to a day. Static charges that develop on some permeation tubes can cause serious weighing errors unless discharged with a polonium strip static eliminator. For a corrosive gas, the balance may be protected from corrosion by inserting the permeation tubes into tared glass-stoppered weighing tubes. The weight history of a nitrogen dioxide tube over a 37-week period[44] is shown in Figure 16.13. The tube was alternately stored in a closed container over sodium hydroxide (to absorb the released gas) and in a container flushed with about 50 mL/min of air (from the laboratory system), with cylinder oxygen, and with cylinder nitrogen. The humidity affected the weights. The most reproducible results were obtained with the cylinder nitrogen.

The environment of some types of permeation tubes must be very carefully controlled. Materials can permeate into the tubes as well as out of them. Thus, nitrogen dioxide tubes exposed to high humidity develop blisters and long-term changes in permeation rates. Even the moisture content of the flowing gas passing over the tube affects the permeation rate. These effects are likely due to the formation of nitric acid within the Teflon walls and/or inside the tube in the liquid nitrogen dioxide. When shipped inside capped iron pipe nipples, the color of the contents changed from brown to green. This was caused by reduction of nitrogen dioxide gas by the iron to nitric oxide, which permeated backward into the tube to combine with nitrogen dioxide to form blue N_2O_3. Exposure to air (or oxygen) for a time restored the brown color by backward permeation of oxygen. A similar problem occurs with hydrogen sulfide tubes, which precipitate colloidal sulfur within the walls of the tube when exposed to oxygen. Depleted sulfur dioxide tubes sometimes contain liquid droplets that may be sulfuric acid from backward permeation of water vapor and oxygen. It is, therefore, desirable never to remove such tubes from their operating environments.

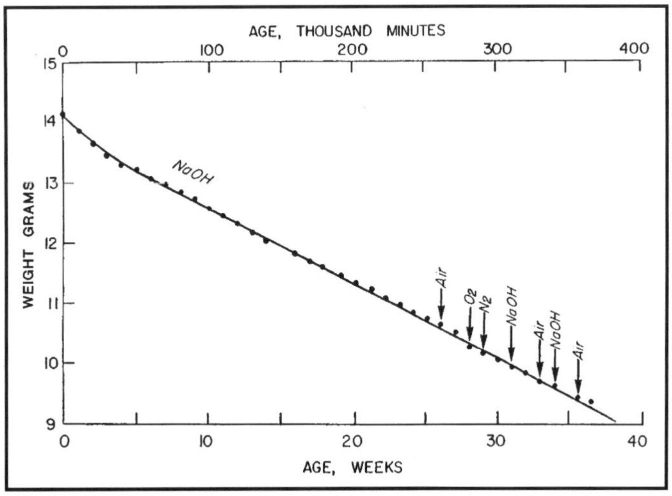

Figure 16.13 — Weight history of a nitrgen dioxide permeation bottle stored over NaOH or in flowing gas streams starting at indicated times (Source: Reference 44).

Figure 16.14 illustrates a system that maintains the tube in a constant environment during calibration, use, and storage. A slow stream (50 mL/min) of dry nitrogen (1) from a cylinder is passed through a coil in a thermostated water bath (2). The bath pump (3) circulates water through the coil (4) to maintain the same temperature in an insulated water bath (5), which is mixed by a stirrer (6). The nitrogen stream passes through the stopcock (7) and over the permeation tube (8) to flush away the permeated gases. This stream leaves through the outlet stopcock (9) to the inlet (10) and is blended with a metered pure air flow (11) entering the mixing device to provide known concentrations of the gas at the outlet (12).

The calibration can be made volumetrically[43,44] using a relatively inexpensive Gilmont Warburg compensated syringe manometer (9, 13, 14, 15, 16, 17) supported by a clamp (18). The gas flow from the nitrogen cylinder is temporarily shut down. Stopcock (7) is closed and stopcock (9) is turned to the position to connect the permeation tube chamber to the manometer inlet (13), and the manometer outlet (14) to the inlet of the mixer (10). The level of the manometer liquid is adjusted to the mark (15) by turning screw (16), and a stopwatch is started. The permeating gas causes the manometer liquid to move away from the mark (15). The pressure is relieved by withdrawing the plunger of the micrometer (17), on which the evolved volume after a timed interval can be read with a sensitivity of 0.2 µL. High precision has been obtained in less than an hour in this manner.

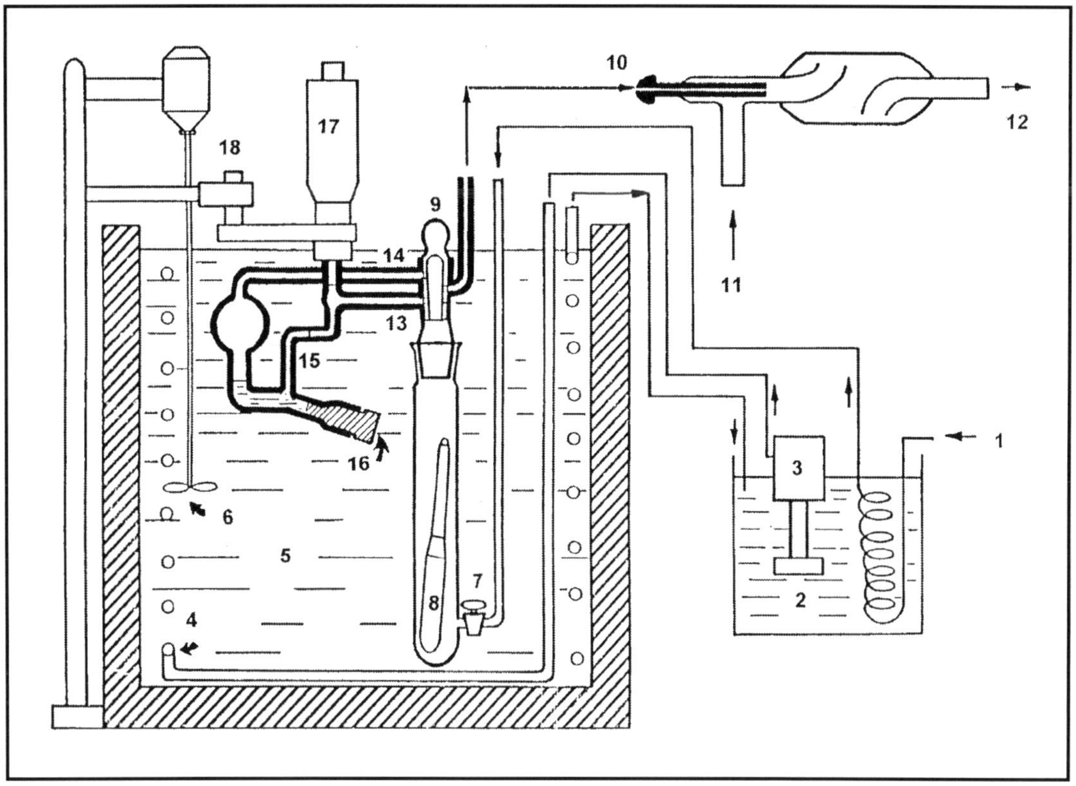

Figure 16.14 — Permeation tube flow system with in situ volumetric calibration. 1: connection for metered dry nitrogen from cylinder; 2: thermostated water bath; 3: circulating water pump; 4: thermostated water coil; 5: insulated water bath; 6: stirrer; 7: gas inlet stopcock; 8: permeation tube; 9: gas outlet stopcock; 10: connection for permeated gas flow; 11: connection for metered dilution air; 12: gas mixture outlet; 13: manometer inlet; 14: manometer outlet; 15: reference line; 16: adjusting screw; 17: 200-µL micrometer syringe; 18: clamp. (Source: Reference 44)

In other systems the permeation tube is suspended by a fiber from a microbalance so that it can be weighed at intervals without removal from a dry inert gas environment. Tubes containing corrosives such as chlorine, nitrogen dioxide, hydrogen fluoride, dimethyl sulfide, and ethyl nitrate should be purged with dry gas while stored.

The quantitative relationships for use of a permeation tube as a source for a flowing gas stream are given by Equation 16-7.

$$C = G\,L\,K\,/\,F \tag{16-7}$$

where

C = concentration in the flowing gas stream, ppm
F = flow rate, mL/min
G = permeation rate per cm of tube length, ng/min cm
L = permeation tube length, cm
K = gas reciprocal density, nL/ng (= V_m/MW)

Table 16.2 lists the values of G at 30 and 70°C for various compounds, for commercial tubes of 0.25-inch outside diameter and specified thicknesses. For tubes of other dimensions, the values of G_2 may be calculated from the table value G_1 as follows.

$$G_2 = G_1\left(\frac{\log(od/id)_1}{\log(od/id)_2}\right) \tag{16-8}$$

where

od = outside diameter of tube
id = inside diameter of tube subscripts 1 and 2 refer to values from the table and the new values, respectively

The tube lives listed in Table 16.2 are calculated on the assumption that the tubes are filled with liquid to 90% of their volume and are used at the calibration temperature until only 10% of their volume contains liquid.

Table 16.2 — Permeation Rates (ng/min cm) for Various Compounds

Material	*Temp (°C)*	*Wall Thickness (Inches)*	*G (Rate)*	*Life (Months)*
Acetaldahyde	30	.030TFE	235	11
Acetic acid	30	.030TFE	53	67
Acetic anhydride	70	.030TFE	239	15
Acetone	70	.030	270	10
Acrolein	30	.030TFE	164	17
Acrylonitrile	30	.030TFE	90	30
Allyl sulfide	70	.030TFE	48	62
Ammonia	30	.062	210	4.7
	35	.062	300	3.3
Aniline	70	.030TFE	35	99
Benzene	70	.030	260	11
	30	.030TFE	34	88
Bromomethane	30	.030	225	26
Bromine	30	.030TFE	240	42
Bromoform	70	.030TFE	127	77
Butadiene	30	.030	177	12
Butane	30	.030	24	82
1-Butene	30	.030	87	23
cis-Butene	30	.030	57	37
trans-Butene	30	.030	140	14
Butyl amine	70	.030TFE	326	7.7
n-Butyl mercaptan	70	.030TFE	242	11
tert-Butyl mercaptan	70	.030TFE	50	54
Carbon disulfide	30	.030	140	30
Carbon tetrachloride	70	.030	220	24
	30	.030TFE	150	14
Chlorine[A]	30	.062	1250	1.6
Chloroform	70	.030	713	7.1
	30	.030TFE	95	53
Chloroethane	30	.030	56	54
Chloromethane	30	.030	607	5.6
	30	.062	200	16
Cyclohexane	70	.030	20	132
1,2 Diaminoethane	70	.030TFE	448	10
1,2, Dibromoethane	70	.030	115	64
1,1, Dichloroethane	70	.030	265	15
1,2 Dichloroethane	30	.030TFE	69	60
	70	.030	260	16
1,1, Dichloroethene	30	.030	79	52
1,2 cis-Dichloroethene	30	.030TFE	270	16
1,2 trans-Dichloroethene	30	.030	145	29
Dichlorofluoromethane	30	.030	400	5.1
(F21)	30	.062TFE	101	45
Dichloromethane	70	.030	1600	2.8
	30	.030TFE	300	15
	30	.030	60	75
1,2 Dichlorotetra-fluoroethane (F114)	30	.062	670	2.6
Diethyl disulfide	70	.030TFE	58	58
Diethyl sulfide	30	.030TFE	14	202
	70	.030	51	56
Diisopropyl amine	70	.030TFE	157	30
m-Diisopropyl benzene	70	.030TFE	13	219
Dimethyl amine	30	.030TFE	240	9.6
N,N Dimethyl acetamide	70	.030TFE	48	66
Dimethyl disulfide	70	.030TFE	130	28
Dimethyl formamide	70	.030TFE	77	41
1,1 Dimethyl hydrazine	30	.030TFE	550	8.6
	70	.062	320	6.4
Dimethyl sulfate	70	.030TFE	60	75
Dimethyl sulfide	70	.030	300	9.5
	30	70	70	41
	70	.030TFE	1100	2.6
Ethanol	70	.030	49	54
Ethyl acetate	70	.030	296	10
Ethyl amine	30	.030TFE	77	31
Ethyl nitrate	30	.030TFE	224	20

(continued on next page.)

The permeation rates have high temperature coefficients. Equation 16-9 shows the usual relationship in the form of the Arrhenius equation:

$$\log\left(\frac{G_2}{G_1}\right) = \left(\frac{E}{2.303\,R}\right)\left(\frac{1}{T_1} - \frac{1}{T_2}\right) \qquad (16\text{-}9)$$

where

G_1, G_2 = permeation rates at different temperatures
T_1, T_2 = corresponding temperatures, °K (= °C + 273.15)
E = activation energy of permeation process, cal/g mol
R = gas constant, 1.9885 cal/g mol °K

Values of E have been reported[43] ranging from 10 to 16 Kcal/g mol. Thus, the value of the E fraction term on the right may range from 2184 to 3494. To obtain 1% accuracy the temperature must be controlled to at least 0.1°C.

Miscellaneous Generation Systems

Figure 16.15 illustrates an electrolytic generator that was developed[5] as a suitable source of arsine and stibine. The solution was electrolyzed by passing a DC current through the platinum wire electrodes. The lower electrode was the cathode at which hydrogen and small quantities of arsine or stibine were liberated. The stream of purified air bubbled through the fritted tube end near the cathode and flushed the gas mixture into the outlet. The generation of arsine or stibine was not proportional to the DC current but was substantially constant after an initial lag period.

Another system used successfully was an aerated chemical solution mixture.[5] Thus, a 30% w/v solution of potassium cyanide served as a source of hydrogen cyanide. A relatively constant concentration could be obtained for as long as 10 hours. The strength and pH of the solution affected the concentration of hydrogen cyanide produced. The air bubbled through the solution should be free from carbon dioxide, since carbonic acid can displace hydrogen cyanide. In other applications, hydrogen chloride was obtained by aeration of a 1:1 concentrated acid-water mixture, and

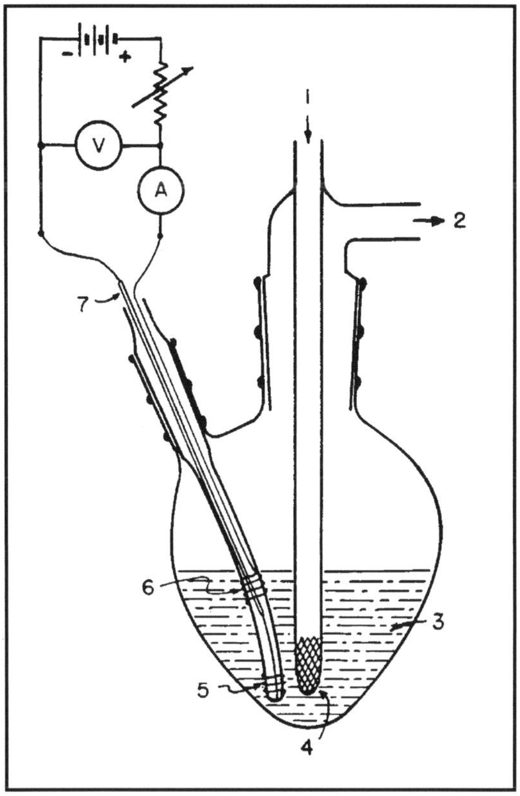

Figure 16.15 — Electrolytic generator for arsine or stibine. 1: inlet for purified airstream; 2: outlet for gas mixture; 3: electrolyte; 4: fritted tube end; 5: cathode; 6: anode; 7: insulating tube. (Source: Reference 5)

bromine by aerating saturated bromine water in contact with a small amount of liquid bromine.[5] In all of these procedures it is, of course, desirable to thermostat the bubbler to provide constant concentrations.

An interesting technique for preparing highly reactive or unstable mixtures is to utilize chemical conversion reactions. A stable mixture of a suitable compound is passed over a solid catalyst or reactant to produce the desired substance in the airstream. A table of reactions indicated some of these possibilities.[7] Others may be determined from the chemical literature. Multistep conversions also may be used.

Illustrative Calculations for Flow-Dilution Systems

The variables involved in flow-dilution systems are the source strength, the desired concentration, and the flow rates. The following examples illustrate some of the calculations.

Table 16.2 (continued) — Permeation Rates (ng/min cm) for Various Compounds

Material	*Temp (°C)*	*Wall Thickness (Inches)*	*G (Rate)*	*Life (Months)*
Ethylene oxide	30	.030	128	23
	30	.030TFE	560	5.3
Ethyleneimine	50	.030	46	61
Ethyl mercaptan	30	.030TFE	64	44
Formaldehyde	70	.030TFE	29	60
	100	.030TFE	320	6
Halothane	30	.030TFE	625	10
Hexane	70	.030	160	14
Hydrazine	70	.030TFE	140	24
Hydrogen cyanide	30	.030	80	54
	30	.030TFE	330	13
Hydrogen fluoride	30	.062	120	12
	45	.062	400	3.7
Hydrogen sulfide	30	.062	240	6
	35	.062	330	4.4
Isopropylamine	70	.030TFE	550	4.3
Isopropyl mercaptan	70	.030	74	37
	70	.030TFE	300	9.2
Methanol	70	.030	216	12
Methyl amine	30	.030	136	17
Methyl bromide	30	.030	225	26
Methyl ethyl ketone	70	.030	100	27
	30	.030TFE	34	80
Methyl ethyl sulfide	70	.030	130	21
Methyl hydrazine	70	.030TFE	198	14
Methyl iodide	30	.030	33	234
	30	.030TFE	200	39
Methyl isocyanate	30	.030TFE	1780	1.8
	30	.062	125	11.3
Methyl mercaptan	30	.030	65	46.7
	30	.030FTE	270	11.2
Nitrogen dioxide[A]	30	.062	1000	2
Perchloro methyl mercaptan	70	.030TFE	125	46
Phosgene	30	.062	400	5
	30	.030	1250	3.8
Propane	30	.030	100	20
	30	.062	37	53
Propanol	70	.030	17	160
Propylene oxide	30	.030TFE	186	15
Styrene	70	.030	72	43
Sulfur dioxide[A]	30	.062	220	9.5
	30	.030	710	6.7
	35	.062	365	5.7
Tetrachloroethene	70	.030	300	18
Tetrahydrothiophene	70	.030TFE	64	52
Thiophene	70	.030	143	25
Toluene	70	.030	120	24
	30	.030TFE	22	133
1,1,1 Trichloroethane	70	.030	113	40
1,1,2 Trichloroethane	70	.030TFE	274	18
Trichloroethene	70	.030	1060	4.7
Trichlorofluoro	30	.062TFE	480	4.4
methane (F11)	30	.030TFE	1700	2.7
Trimethyl amine	30	.030TFE	215	10
Trimethyl phosphite	70	.030TFE	93	38
Vinyl acetate	70	.030	700	4.5
Vinyl chloride	30	.062	120	11
	30	.030	400	7.8
m-xylene	70	.030	44	67
o-xylene	70	.030	40	76

Note: Data from Analytical Instrument Development, Inc. Material is FEP Teflon unless TFE is specified. Rates are for 0.25 inch o.d. tubes.
[A]Also supplied with vial to extend life.

Example 3. Air is passed over mercury in a heated saturation unit and then equilibrated in a thermostated bath at 20°C at which its vapor pressure is 0.00120 mm Hg. What will the mercury concentration be in ppm and mg/m³ in the airstream warmed to 25°C?

Answer. Applying Equation 16-5:

$$\text{ppm} = 10^6 \left(\frac{0.00120}{760} \right) = 1.58 \text{ ppm}$$

Applying Equation 16-6:

$$\text{mg/m}^3 = 1.58 \left(\frac{200.61}{24.45} \right) = 12.9 \text{ mg/m}^3$$

Example 4. A gas stream of 50 mL/min is passed over a sulfur dioxide FEP Teflon permeation tube of 0.25-inch od × 0.030-inch wall thickness × 4.0 cm long, maintained at 30°C. The stream is mixed with a sufficient flow of clean air to total 500 mL/min at 25°C. What is the final concentration of sulfur dioxide in ppm?

Answer. The value of G from Table 14.2 for these dimensions and 30°C is 710 ng/min cm. The molecular weight is 32.06 + 2 × 16.00 = 64.06. The value of $K = V_m/MW = 24.47/64.06 = 0.382$. Applying Equation 16-7:

$$C = \frac{G\,L\,K}{F} = \frac{710(4.0)(0.382)}{500} = 2.17 \text{ ppm}$$

Example 5. Estimate the concentration that would be produced if the permeation tube temperature in Example 4 were raised to 35°C. Assume that the activation energy, E, is 18.8 Kcal/g mol.

Answer. Applying Equation 16-9:

$$\log \left(\frac{G_2}{G_1} \right) = \log \left(\frac{C_2}{C_1} \right) =$$

$$\left(\frac{18{,}800}{2.303 \times 1.9885} \right) \left(\frac{1}{303.2} - \frac{1}{308.2} \right) = 0.2197$$

Thus, $C_2/C_1 = 1.66$ and $C_2 = 2.17 \times 1.66 = 3.60$ ppm

Caution: Tubes may explode if heated beyond their design limits.

Source Devices for Aerosols

Preparation of aerosol mixtures is much more complex and difficult than that of gas and vapor mixtures. A major consideration is the size distribution of the particles. Commonly, a lognormal distribution describes the values; this is characterized by a geometric mean and a geometric standard deviation. The usual aerosol source device supplies a range of sizes. However, certain special types supply uniform-sized particles. If the geometric standard deviation is less than 1.1, the particles are considered homogeneous, or monodisperse. There is also a great variety of particle shapes, including spherical, crystalline, irregular, plate-like, spiked, and rod-shaped or fibrous. If the material is a mixture of compounds, the composition may vary with size. Certain substances may be present on the surfaces, which also can be electrostatically charged. All of these properties are affected by the source devices and methods of treatment. In the generation of known concentrations of aerosols, the choices of the operating parameters are determined by the objectives of the study, which may be to duplicate and study a complex aerosol existing naturally or in industry, or to prepare a simple pure aerosol for theoretical examination. A good general treatment of this subject with 257 references is available.(45) Extensive discussions of 28 papers of an aerosol symposium were published.(14) Useful standards for sizing particles by microscopic measurements using latex spheres and pollen of ragweed and mulberry have been suggested.(46)

Another major problem is the proper design of an exposure chamber from which to use or sample the aerosol. Because of settling, impaction, and inertial forces, the spacial distribution of the aerosol or of its different size fractions may not be uniform. One recommended design(47) places the instruments to be calibrated on a turntable in the chamber, and allows them to sample nonisokinetically from a quiescent atmosphere. Alternatively, the aerosol may be produced in a wind tunnel and sampled by the instrument isokinetically. If the aerosol is constituted of different size fractions, the two methods will likely give different results.

Dry Dust Feeders

Methods of producing solid aerosols have been comprehensively described.[48] One of the most convenient and widely used methods is to redisperse a dry powder. Standard test dusts are available, such as road dust, fly ash, silicates, silica, mineral dust, and many pigment powders and chemicals. Because these may tend to agglomerate, the degree of packing of the powder must be controlled and reproducible. A simple method consists of shaking the powder on a screen into the airstream. Mechanical systems attempt to provide a constant feed rate by use of moving belts or troughs, or by rotating turntables, screws, or gears. Because of the erratic behavior of loosely packed dust, the popular Wright dust feed mechanism (Figure 16.16) achieves closer control by compressing the dust in a tubular cup into a uniform cake. A rotating scraper advanced by a screw slices off a thin layer of cake continuously. In all of these devices the dust is dispersed by an air jet, which also serves to break up some aggregates. The dusty cloud is passed into a relatively large chamber, which serves to smooth out any rapid fluctuations. Concentrations may fluctuate ±20% over a period of a half hour, because of variations in the packing of the dust or laminations in the cake. Settling chambers, baffles, or cyclones may be added to the system to remove coarse particles, and ion sources to remove electrostatic charges.

Another system utilizes a fluidized bed to disperse a dry powder[49] as illustrated in Figure 16.17. A chain conveyer feeds the dust through an air lock into a chamber containing 100- to 200-μm glass or brass beads. An upward airstream at 9–30 L/min suspends and agitates the beads and blows the dust into the system. Electrostatic charges are produced and are neutralized with an ion source. After 1–3 hours a steady state concentration ±5% is achieved.

Producing fibrous aerosols of desired lengths and diameters is especially difficult. Glass wool fibers have been oriented in a parallel direction in a glycol methacrylate histological embedding medium and sliced

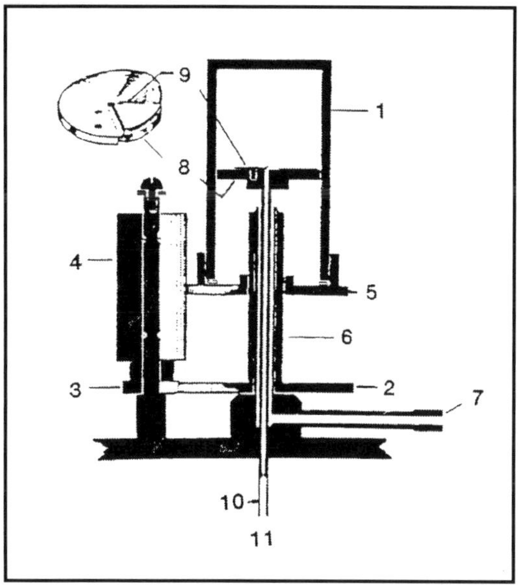

Figure 16.16 — Schematic diagram of Wright dust feeder 1: compressed dust cup; 2, 3, 4, 5: differential gear train that rotates and lowers cup on threaded spindle; 6, 7: compressed air inlet; 8: scraper head; 9: scraper blade; 10: dust outlet; 11: location for impaction plate.

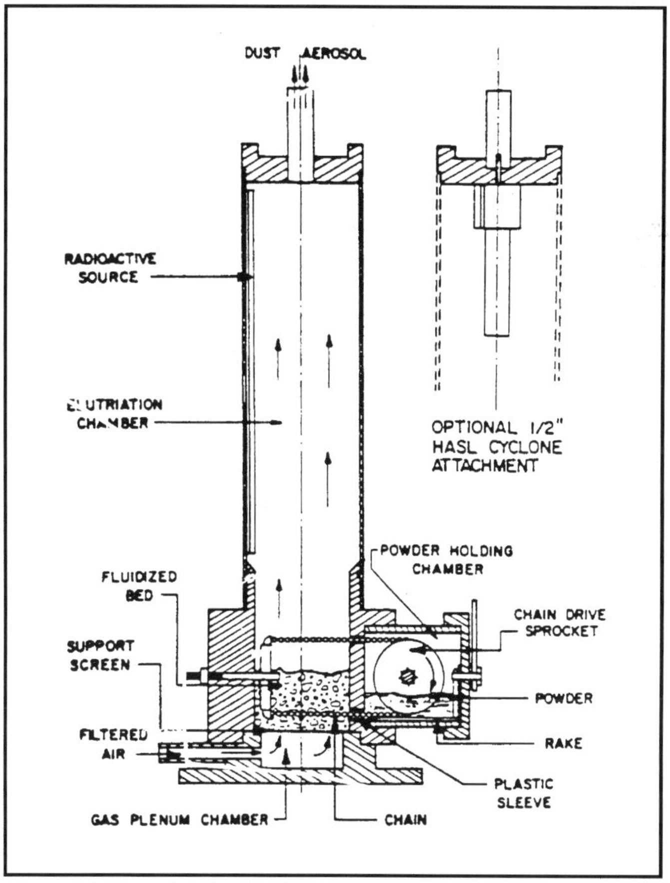

Figure 16.17 — Fluidized bed aerosol generator. (Source: Reference 49)

into desired lengths with a microtome.[50] The plastic medium is then ashed and the fibers separated from any debris by liquid elutriation. A later study[51] used frozen polyethylene glycol for sectioning on the microtome, subsequently dissolved in hot water. The fibers are suspended into an airstream from a fluidized bed.

Nebulizers

The compressed air nebulizer, Figure 16.18, is a convenient and useful device to produce aerosols from liquids. The liquid stream is drawn through a capillary tube and shattered into fine droplets by the air jet. The DeVilbiss nebulizer is simple, but holds only about 10 mL of liquid. Modifications can be added[45] such as utilizing a recirculating reservoir system for the liquid (Lauterbach), providing baffles to intercept and return coarse droplets (Collison, Dautrebande), droplet shattering baffles (Lovelace), and nozzle controls. The characteristics of these devices have been described in detail.[52]

Rather coarse sprays are obtained by pumping the liquid mechanically through tangential nozzles, as is done in fuel oil burners. The airflow merely carries off the droplets. Commercial aerosol cans use a mixture of liquid to be atomized and a liquified volatile propellant (such as dichlorodifluoromethane). The rapid evaporation of the propellant from the liquid emerging from the nozzle orifice shatters the stream into droplets having a broad size range. Electrostatic dispersion also has been utilized to break up a liquid stream by electrically charging the orifice. The droplets should be discharged by passage near an ion source soon afterward.

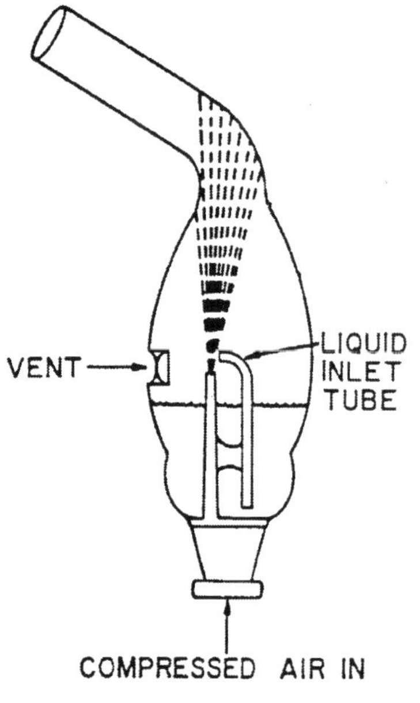

Figure 16.18 — DeVilbiss compressed air nebulizer (Source: Reference 52)

Somewhat different is the popular vibrating orifice generator, Figure 16.19, which uses an intense acoustic field to produce a monodisperse aerosol. In the version illustrated the pressurized liquid is ejected from the orifice as a fine stream, which is disrupted by the vibrations of the piezoelectric ceramic orifice plate into very uniform-sized droplets (coefficient of variation < 1%).

Spinning Disc Aerosol Generators

A very useful generator for monodisperse aerosols is based on feeding the liquid continuously onto the center of a rapidly spinning disc (60,000 rpm). When the droplet on the edge of the disc grows to a sufficient size, the centrifugal force exceeds that of surface tension and the droplet is thrown off. A commercial version,[22] illustrated in Figure 16.20, produces liquid droplets in the 1 to 10 micron size range. Smaller satellite drops are diverted down by an airstream into a compartment around the disc. The larger particles escape to the outer compartment and are passed around a sealed radioactive ion source to remove the electrostatic charges, then to the outlet.

These liquid sources can be readily applied to supply solid aerosols by dispersing a solution or colloidal suspension. The solvent evaporates from the droplets naturally or on warming, leaving a smaller particle of crystalline solute, or a clump of one or more colloidal particles according to their theoretical probabilities of occurrence in the volume of the droplet. The sizes of the particles are controlled by varying the concentrations. The nature of the materials and of the drying process often affects the nature of the particles, which may exhibit shells or crusts. Passing the particles through a high temperature zone may be employed to decompose them chemically (e.g., production of metal oxides from their salts[53]) or to fuse them into spherical particles.

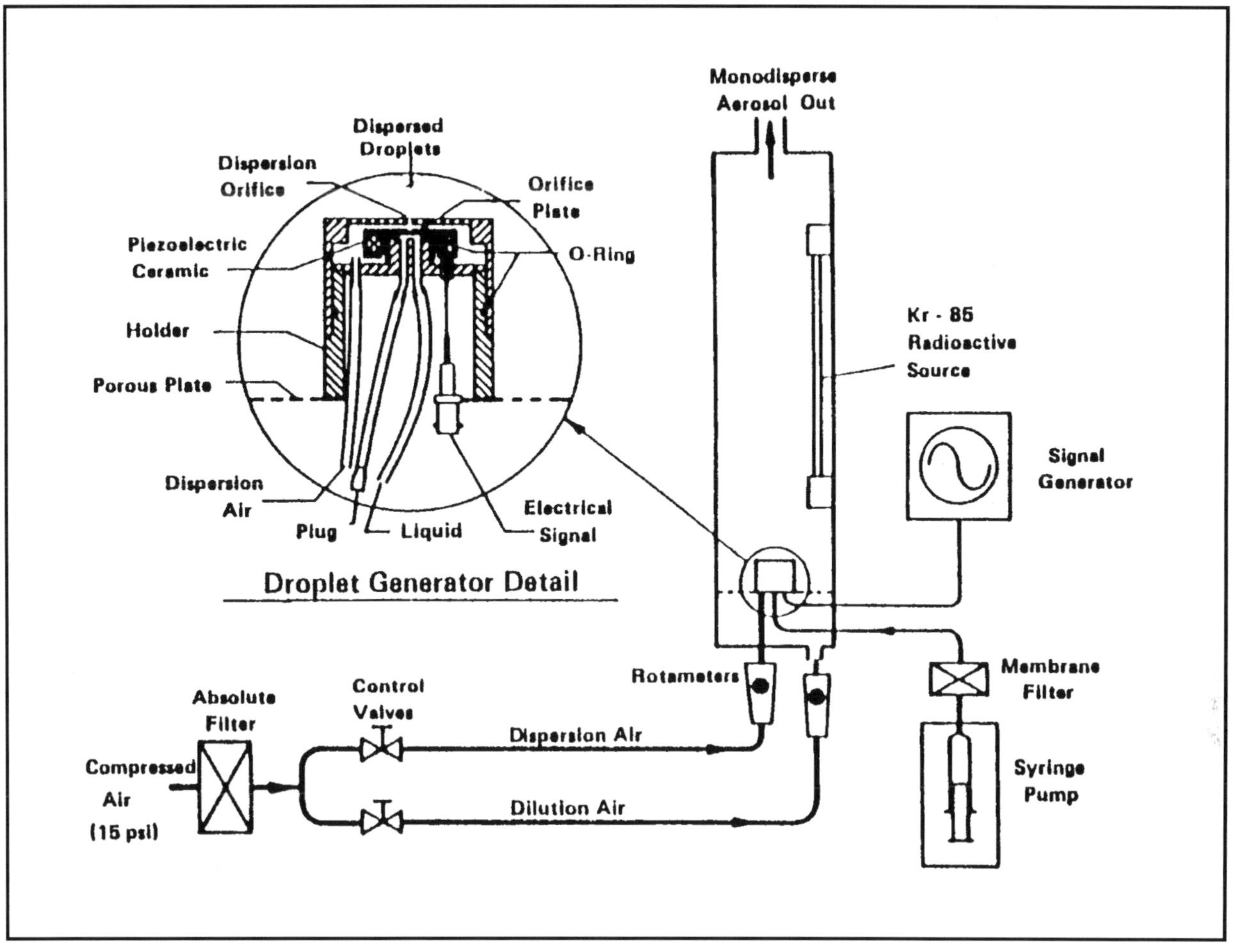

Figure 16.19 — Schematic of vibrating orifice aerosol generator. (Source: Reference 14)

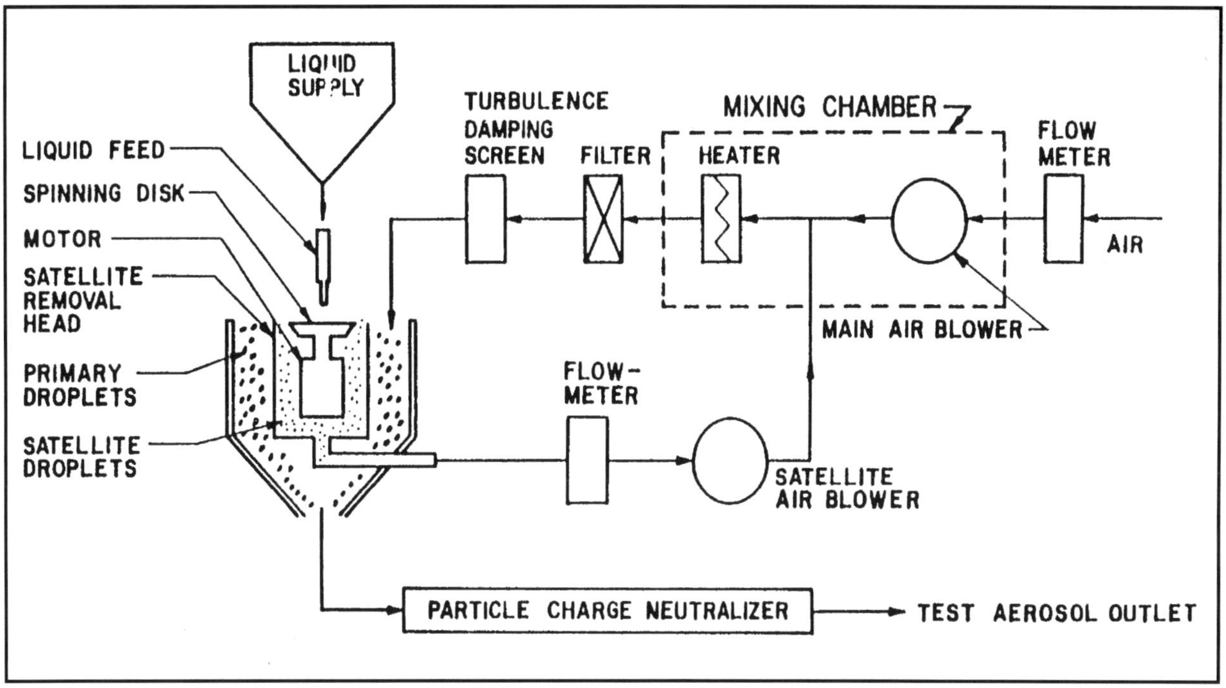

Figure 16.20 — Spinning disc aerosol generator. (courtesy of Environmental Research Corp., St. Paul, Minn.)

Vaporization and Condensation of Liquids

The principle of vaporization and condensation was utilized in the Sinclair-LaMer generator for materials such as oleic acid, stearic acid, lubricating oils, menthol, dibutyl phthalate, dioctyl phthalate, and tri-o-cresyl phosphate, as well as for sublimable solids. The system is illustrated in Figure 16.21.[8] Filtered air or nitrogen is bubbled through the hot liquid in the flask on the left (1). Another portion of the entering air is passed over a heated filament (2) coated with sodium chloride, to provide fine condensation nuclei. The vapor passes into the empty superheater flask (3), in which any droplets are evaporated, and then up the chimney (4) in which it is slowly cooled. The supersaturated vapor condenses on the sodium chloride particles to produce a monodisperse aerosol. Although the condensation nuclei vary in size, they have only a slight effect on the final aerosol droplet size, which is much larger. The aerosol is blended with clean air in a mixer (5). This system has been widely used as a convenient monodisperse source in the 0.02 to 30 micron size range.

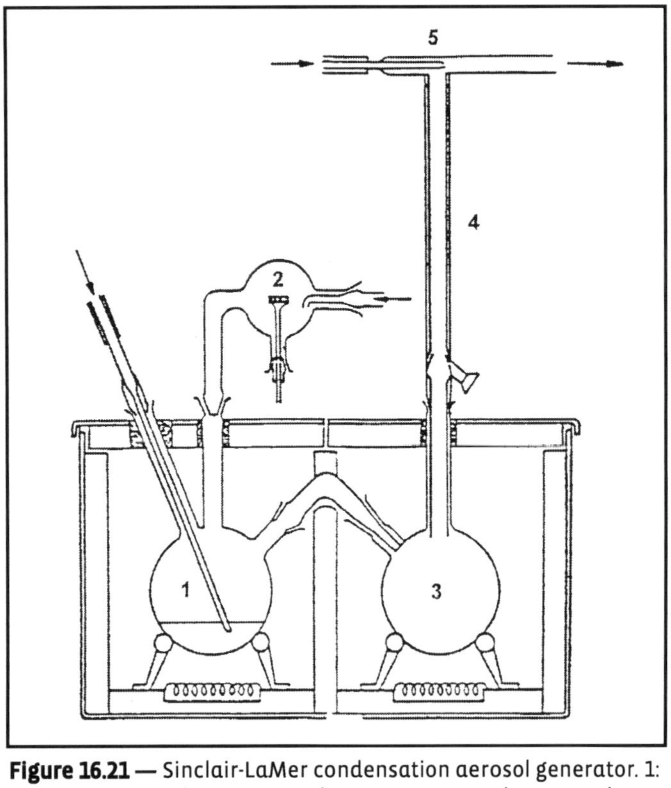

Figure 16.21 — Sinclair-LaMer condensation aerosol generator. 1: vaporizer; 2: condensation nuclei source; 3: superheater; 4: double-walled air cooler; 5: dilution mixer. (Source: Reference 8)

Miscellaneous Generation Systems

Many dusts can be produced by means duplicating their natural formation. Thus, hammer or impact mills, ball mills, scraping, brushing, and grinding of materials have been employed. Combustion (e.g., tobacco smoke), high voltage arcing, and gas welding or flame cutting torches can be used. Organic metallic compounds (e.g., lead tetraethyl) may be burned in a gas flame. Metal powders can be fed into a flame or burned spontaneously (thermit and magnesium). Molten metals may be sprayed from metallizing guns. Metal wires can be vaporized by electrical discharges from a bank of condensers. Gaseous reactions also may be employed to produce aerosols, such as reaction of sulfur trioxide with water vapor[54] or of ammonia and hydrogen chloride. Finally, photochemical reactions can be utilized. The natural process for producing oxidative smog has thus been duplicated by irradiating automobile exhaust.

Multipurpose Calibration Components and Systems

A variety of components and systems have been constructed and are commercially available for testing analytical methods and calibrating instruments.[22] Clean air sources for filling respiratory air tanks, as well as for instruments, include oil filters in the air system or use oil-free compressors. Heatless air dryer-scrubbers are available to remove water and contaminants. These utilize two absorption beds alternately. While one is used the other is purged with a portion of the clean air. For ultra pure requirements, a heated catalytic oxidizer can be provided to burn off organic impurities. An automated flow-temperature-humidity control system has been described.[55]

In the Standards Completion Program, the 516 methods were evaluated by two National Institute for Occupational Safety and Health contract laboratories. Each set up a multipurpose system[3] for simultaneously producing several test concentrations in the desired range. Figure 16.22 illustrates schematically the one used mostly for testing charcoal tube sampling methods. The test substance was generated at a high concentration and passed through a manifold. Three taps were provided for 0.5, 1, and 2 times the PEL concentrations. To the flow from each the necessary dilution air was added at the throat of a Venturi tube, and the mixed flow was passed to the corresponding sampling manifold having six taps. The flows through the charcoal tubes connected at these taps were controlled by calibrated critical orifices. Thus, the system provided 18 simultaneous samples at three desired concentrations.

The numerous commercial sources of air analyzing instruments[22] commonly provide means for their calibration. Concentrations at the high end of the range (span gas) and at the bottom of the range (zero gas) are used alternately to adjust the electronics of the instrument to provide the proper readings. Quality assurance procedures describe these requirements in detail.[4,10,11] An elaborate computer controlled system also has been described[56] capable of providing mixtures in various desired concentration patterns.

Summary

Preparation of accurately known low concentrations of air contaminants is essential for testing and validating analytical methods associated with control regulations, for calibrating monitoring instruments, and for conducting scientific studies of effects, needed to develop control standards. Batch methods prepare a fixed volume of mixture in an appropriate container, such as a sealed chamber, a glass carboy, a plastic bag, or a compressed gas cylinder. Careful choices and tests must be made to ensure that substantial quantities of the contaminants are not adsorbed or lost on surfaces. If a large volume is prepared there is also a potential danger of toxic exposure from accidental release or of explosion of combustible contaminants. Flow-dilution methods accurately meter and mix a flow of the contaminant and of clean diluent air. They have the advantages of compactness, ability to change concentrations rapidly in a properly designed system, and ability to provide a large quantity of mixture. Any losses of contaminant on the surfaces cease after equilibrium occurs, and a steady state is reached in the operation of the system.

Recommendations for the design of flow-dilution systems include use of inert materials such as glass and Teflon.

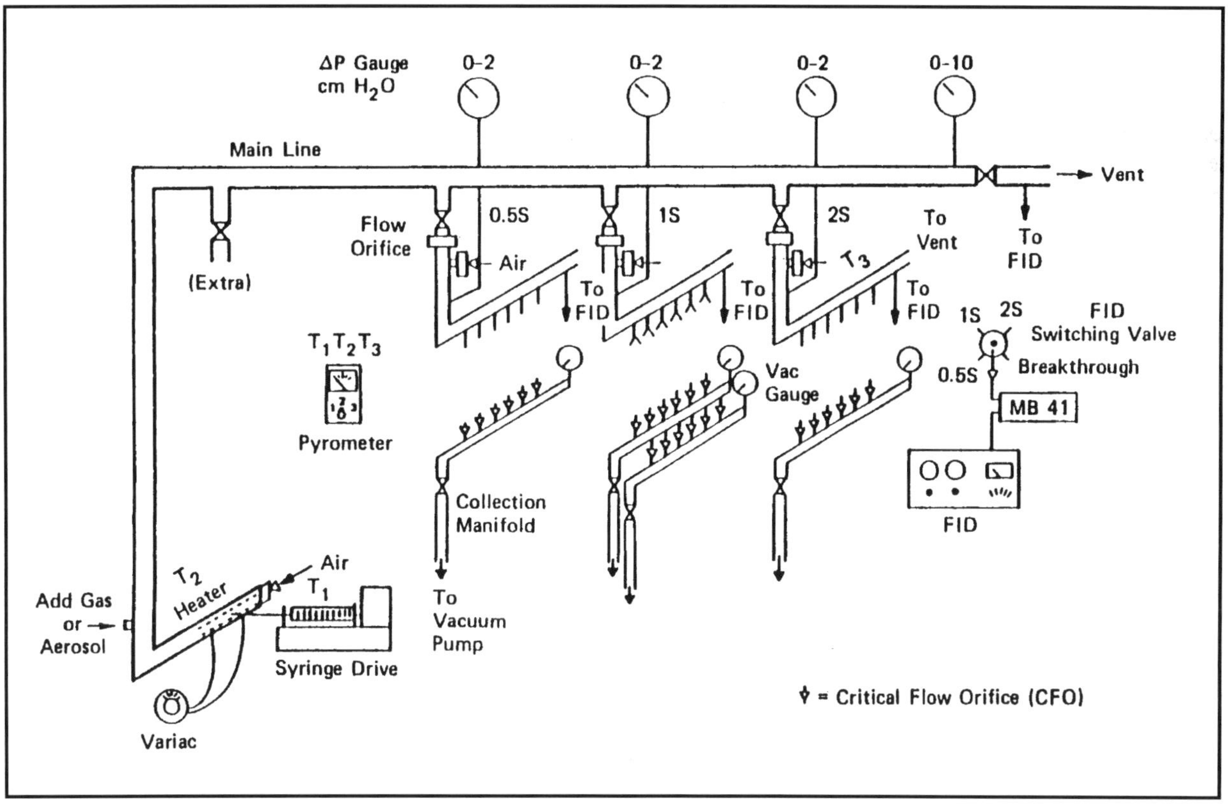

Figure 16.22 — Calibration system for generating multiple concentrations simultaneously. (Source: Reference 3)

Connections should preferably be with ball and ground glass joints. Plastic tubing may be used if not exposed to the contaminant in butt-to-butt glass tubing connections. A variety of sources of known flows of contaminants is described, such as devices relying on equilibrium vapor pressures, diffusion, motor-driven syringes, and permeation tubes. Preparation of known aerosol concentrations is a more difficult and complex operation. A number of systems is described.

Theoretical equations are given for calculating concentrations of contaminants in batch and flow dilution systems. Illustrative examples are presented. A few multipurpose test and calibration systems are described. This chapter is designed to give the reader state of the art knowledge of how to design and apply accurate systems for preparation of known concentrations of air contaminants.

References

1. **Hill, J.W. and R.H. Petrucci:** *General Chemistry.* Upper Saddle River, NJ: Prentice Hall, 1996.
2. **Taylor, D.G., R.E. Kupel, and J.M. Bryant:** *Documentation of NIOSH Validation Tests* (DHEW [NIOSH] pub. 77-185). Cincinnati, OH: U.S. Dept. of Health, Education, and Welfare, National Institute for Occupational Safety and Health, 1977.
3. **Gunderson, E.C. and C.C. Anderson:** *Development and Validation of Methods for Sampling and Analysis of Workplace Toxic Substances* (DHHS [NIOSH] pub. 80-133). Cincinnati, OH: U.S. Dept. of Health and Human Services, National Institute for Occupational Safety and Health, 1980.
4. **Environmental Monitoring Systems Laboratory:** *Quality Assurance Handbook for Air Pollution Measurement Systems,* vol. I, *Principles* (EPA 600/9-76-005); vol. II, *Ambient Air Specific Methods* (EPA 600/4-77-027a); vol. III, *Stationary Source Specific Methods* (EPA 600/4-77-027b). Washington, DC: U.S. Environmental Protection Agency, 1976–1977. (Superseded in 1990 by the EPA Electronic Bulletin Board System at (301) 589-0046; system questions answered at 202-382-7671.)
5. **Saltzman, B.E.:** Preparation and analysis of calibrated low concentrations of sixteen toxic gases. *Anal. Chem. 33*:1100–1112 (1961).
6. **Cotabish, H.N., P.W. McConnaughey, and H.C. Messer:** Making known concentrations for instrument calibration. *Am. Ind. Hyg. Assoc. J. 22*:392–402 (1961).
7. **Hersch, P.A.:** Controlled addition of experimental pollutants to air. *J. Air Pollut. Control Assoc. 19*:164–172 (1969).
8. **Fuchs, N.A. and A.G. Sutugin:** Generation and use of monodisperse aerosols. In *Aerosol Science,* C.N. Davies (ed.). New York: Academic Press, 1966.
9. **Silverman, L.:** Experimental test methods. In *Air Pollution Handbook,* P.L. Magill, F.R. Holden, C. Ackley, and F.G. Sawyer (eds.). New York: McGraw-Hill Book Co., 1956. pp. 12-1 to 12-41.
10. **American Society for Testing and Materials (ASTM):** *Calibration in Air Monitoring* (ASTM Spec. pub. 598). Philadelphia, PA: ASTM, 1976.
11. **American Society for Testing and Materials (ASTM):** *1987 Annual Book of ASTM Standards,* vol. 11.03. Philadelphia, PA: ASTM, 1987.
12. **Green, H.L.:** *Particulate Clouds: Dusts, Smoke and Mists.* 2nd ed., Chap. 2. Princeton, NJ: Van Nostrand, 1964.
13. **Nelson, G.O.:** *Gas Mixtures—Preparation and Control.* Chelsea, MI: Lewis Publishers, Inc., 1992.
14. **Willeke, K. (ed.):** *Generation of Aerosols and Facilities for Exposure Experiments.* Ann Arbor, MI: Ann Arbor Science Publishers, Inc., 1980.
15. **Woodfin, W.J.:** *Gas and Vapor Generation Systems for Laboratories* (DHHS [NIOSH] pub. 84-113). Cincinnati, OH: National Institute for Occupational Safety and Health, 1984.
16. **Chang, Y.S. and B.T. Chen:** Aerosol sampler calibration. In *Air Sampling Instruments,* 8th ed. Cincinnati, OH: American Conference of Governmental Industrial Hygienists, 1995.
17. **Moss, O.R.:** Calibration of gas and vapor samplers. In *Air Sampling Instruments,* 8th ed. Cincinnati, OH: American Conference of Govern-mental Industrial Hygienists, 1995.
18. **John, W.:** The characteristics of environmental and laboratory-generated aerosols. In *Aerosol Measurement,* K. Willeke and P. Baron (eds.). New York: Van Nostrand Reinhold, 1993.
19. **Baker, R.A. and R.C. Doerr:** Methods of sampling and storage of air containing vapors and gases. *Int. J. Air Water Pollut. 2*:142–158 (1959).
20. **Wilson, K.W. and H. Buchberg:** Evaluation of materials for controlled air reaction chambers. *Ind. Eng. Chem. 50*:1705–1708 (1958).
21. **Mokler, B.V. and R.K. White:** Quantitative standard for exposure chamber integrity. *Am. Ind. Hyg. Assoc. J. 44*:292–295 (1983).
22. **Cohen, B.S. and S.V. Hering (eds.):** *Air Sampling Instruments,* 8th ed. Cincinnati, OH: American Conference of Governmental Industrial Hygienists, 1995.

23. **Clemons, C.A. and A.P. Altshuller:** Plastic containers for sampling and storage of atmospheric hydrocarbons prior to gas chromatographic analysis. *J. Air Pollut. Control Assoc. 14*:407–408 (1964).
24. **Altshuller, A.P., A.F. Wartburg, I.R. Cohen and S.F. Sleva:** Storage of vapors and gases in plastic bags. *Int. J. Air Water Pollut. 6*: 75–81 (1962).
25. **Connor, W.D. and J.S. Nader:** Air sampling with plastic bags. *Am. Ind. Hyg. Assoc. J. 25*: 291–297 (1964).
26. **Schuette, F.J.:** Plastic bags for collection of gas samples. *Atmos. Environ. 1*:515–517 (1967).
27. **Smith, B.S. and J.O. Pierce:** The use of plastic bags for industrial air sampling. *Am. Ind. Hyg. Assoc. J. 31*:343–348 (1970).
28. **Samimi, B.S.:** Calibration of MIRAN gas analyzers: extent of vapor loss within a closed loop calibration system. *Am. Ind. Hyg. Assoc. J. 44*:40–45 (1983).
29. **Polasek, J.C. and J.A. Bullin:** Eval-uation of bag sequential sampling technique for ambient air analysis. *Environ. Sci. Tech. 12*:708–712 (1978).
30. **Posner, J.C. and W.J. Woodfin:** Sampling with gas bags I: Losses of analyte with time. *Appl. Ind. Hyg. 1*:163–168 (1986).
31. **Kelly, N.A.:** The contamination of fluorocarbon-film bags by hydrocarbons and nitrogen oxides. *J. Air Pollut. Control Assoc. 33*:120–125 (1983).
32. **Saltzman, B.E. and A.F. Wartburg:** Precision flow dilution system for standard low concentrations of nitrogen dioxide. *Anal. Chem 37*: 1261–1264 (1965).
33. **Laviolett, P.A. and P.C. Reist:** Improved pulsation damper for respirable dust mass sampling devices. *Am. Ind. Hyg. Assoc. J. 33*:279–282 (1972).
34. **Treaftis, H.N., T.F. Tomb, and H.F. Carden:** Effect of altitude on personal respirable dust sampler calibration. *Am. Ind. Hyg. Assoc. J. 37*:133–138 (1976).
35. **Altshuller, A.P. and A.F. Wartburg:** Interaction of ozone with plastic and metallic materials in a dynamic flow system. *Int. J. Air Water Pollut. 4*: 70–78 (1961).
36. **Ash, R.M. and J.R. Lynch:** The evaluation of gas detector tube systems: carbon tetrachloride. *Am. Ind. Hyg. Assoc. J. 32*:552–553 (1971).
37. **Scheide, E.P., E.E. Hughes, and J.K. Taylor:** A calibration system for producing known concentrations of mercury vapor in air. *Am. Ind. Hyg. Assoc. J. 40*:180–186 (1979).
38. **Miller, R.R., R.L. Letts, W.J. Potts, and M.J. McKenna:** Improved methodology for generating controlled test atmospheres. *Am. Ind. Hyg. Assoc. J. 41*:844–846 (1980).
39. **Decker, J.R., O.R. Moss, and B.L. Kay:** Controlled-delivery vapor generator for animal exposures. *Am. Ind. Hyg. Assoc. J. 43*:400–402 (1982).
40. **Altshuller, A.P. and I.R. Cohen:** Application of diffusion cells to the production of known concentrations of gaseous hydrocarbons. *Anal. Chem. 32*:802–810 (1960).
41. **Avera, C.B., Jr.:** Simple flow regulator for extremely low gas flows. *Rev. Sci. Instrum. 32*:985–986 (1961).
42. **O'Keeffe, A.E. and G.C. Ortman:** Primary standards for trace gas analysis. *Anal. Chem. 38*:760–763 (1966).
43. **Saltzman, B.E.:** Permeation tubes as primary gaseous standards. In *International Symposium on Identification and Measurement of Environmental Pollutants*, B. Westley (ed.). Ottawa, Ontario, Canada: National Research Council of Canada, 1971. pp. 64–68.
44. **Saltzman, B.E., W.R. Burg, and G. Ramaswami:** Performance of permeation tubes as standard gas sources. *Environ. Sci. Tech. 5*:1121–1128 (1971).
45. **Raabe, O.G.:** Generation and characterization of aerosols. In *Conference on Inhalation Carcinogenesis* (CONF-691001). Gatlinburg, TN: Oak Ridge National Laboratory, 1969.
46. **Fairchild, C.J. and L.D. Wheat:** Calibration and evaluation of a real-time cascade impactor. *Am. Ind. Hyg. Assoc. J. 45*:205–211 (1984).
47. **Marple, V.A. and K.L. Rubow:** Air aerosol chamber for instrument evaluation and calibration. *Am. Ind. Hyg. Assoc. J. 44*:361–367 (1983).
48. **Silverman, L. and C.E. Billings:** Methods of generating solid aerosols. *J. Air Pollut. Control Assoc. 6*:76–83 (1956).
49. **Marple, V.A., B.Y.H Liu, and K.L. Rubow:** A dust generator for laboratory use. *Am. Ind. Hyg. Assoc. J. 39*:26–32 (1978).
50. **Esmen, N.A., R.A. Kahn, D. LaPietra, and E.P. McGovern:** Generation of monodisperse fibrous glass aerosols. *Am. Ind. Hyg. Assoc. J. 41*:175–179 (1980).
51. **Carpenter, R.L., J.A. Pickrell, K.S. Sass, and B.V. Mokler:** Glass fiber aerosols: preparation, aerosol generation, and characterization. *Am. Ind. Hyg. Assoc. J. 44*:170–175 (1983).
52. **Mercer, T.T., M.I. Tillery, and H.Y. Chow:** Operating characteristics of some compressed air nebulizers. *Am. Ind. Hyg. Assoc. J. 29*:66–78 (1968).
53. **Crisp, S., W.A. Hardcastle, J.M. Nunan, and A.F. Smith:** An improved generator for the production of metal oxide fumes. *Am. Ind. Hyg. Assoc. J. 42*:590–595 (1981).
54. **Chang, D.P.Y. and B.K. Tarkington:** Experience with a high output sulfuric acid aerosol generator. *Am. Ind. Hyg. Assoc. J. 38*:493–497 (1977).

55. **Nelson, G.O. and R.D. Taylor:** An automated flow-temperature-humidity control system. *Am. Ind. Hyg. Assoc. J. 41*:769–771 (1980).

56. **Koizumi, A. and M. Ikeda:** A servomechanism for vapor concentration control in experimental exposure chambers. *Am. Ind. Hyg. Assoc. J. 42*:417–425 (1981).

Appendix A. Temperature and Pressure Effects

(Written by Salvatore R. DiNardi)

Introduction

Many disciplines have their own set of definitions for a standard condition. Table A16.1 summarizes the standard conditions that occupational hygienists deal with regularly. Using guidance from the design of industrial exhaust ventilation systems[1] gives a range of temperature and pressure changes that can be tolerated before corrections are applied to the volume of air sampled during an exposure assessment. The tolerable range is described in following paragraphs.

All occupational exposure limits (OELs) and environmental exposure standards and limits are expressed at 25°C and 1 atmosphere (760 mm Hg), the normal temperature and pressure (NTP). Any occupational or environmental exposure assessment data should be corrected to the NTP condition at which the limits and standards are derived so that meaningful comparisons between exposures and limits can be made.

This appendix describes how to apply temperature and pressure differences between NTP conditions and field conditions into a program to monitor exposure to air contaminants. The volume of air changes if the temperature and the pressure acting on the air volume differs from the standard temperature and pressure (NTP). To compare an individual's exposure with OELs (e.g., threshold limit values [TLVs®], permissible exposure limits, recommended exposure limits, workplace environmental exposure limits) established at NTP occupational hygienists must correct the volume of air sampled in the field to the NTP standard condition. Examples of substantial variations from NTP will be given later.

Boyle's, Charles', Gay-Lussac's, and Dalton's laws form the basis for understanding temperature and pressure effects on air sample volume.[2] It is assumed that air behaves as an ideal gas.[2] This assumption introduces a small error, less than 0.5% at concentrations less than 5000 ppm by volume.[3] The assumption that air behaves as an ideal gas, a statement that makes physical chemists cringe, enables occupational hygienists to calculate the concentration of air contaminants in the workplace and the ambient environment.

Combined Temperature and Pressure Effect on Volume

Recall the ideal gas equation:

$$PV = nRT \qquad \text{(A16.1)}$$

where:

- P = atmospheric pressure (mm Hg or atmospheres)
- V = volume that the ideal gas occupies (cubic meters or liters)
- n = number of moles of the ideal gas (recall n = mass/molecular weight or m/M)
- T = absolute temperature in Kelvin (K = °C + 273.15)
- R = universal gas constant; units selected based on the units selected for P and V (R = 0.082 L atmosphere/mole Kelvin)

If Equation A16.1 is written at two conditions, the standard condition (symbolized as a subscript "S"), and the field condition (symbolized as a subscript "F"), the equation becomes:

Table A16.1 — Standard Conditions for Various Disciplines

Discipline	*Symbol*	*Temperature Standard*	*Absolute Temperature*	*Pressure Standard*
Occupational hygiene	NTP	25°C	298.15 K	101 325 Pa, 1 atm
Air pollution	NTP	25°C	298.15 K	101 325 Pa, 1 atm
Industrial ventilation	IEVSTP[A]	70°F, 21.1°C	529.67°R	29.921 inches Hg
ASHRAE[B]	ASHRAE	15°C, 59.0°F	288.15 K	101 325 Pa, 1 atm
Chemistry/physics	STP	0°C	273.15 K	760 mm Hg, 1 atm

[A]Abbreviation suggested by author (dry air only, 28.96 g/mole)
[B]American Society of Heating, Refrigeration and Air-Conditioning Engineers (ASHRAE), *ASHRAE Handbook of Fundamentals* (Atlanta, Ga.: ASHRAE, 1993), p. 6.1.

$$P_S V_S = nRT_S \quad (A16.2)$$

And,

$$P_F V_F = nRT_F \quad (A16.3)$$

Combining Equations A16.2 and A16.3 yields the following equation:

$$\frac{P_S V_S}{T_S} = \frac{P_F V_F}{T_F} \quad (A16.4)$$

The volume of air sampled in the field (V_F) must be adjusted from the field condition (V_F) to the air volume at the standard condition (V_S) by applying the temperature and pressure adjustment factor. Solving Equation A16.4 for V_S yields the volume of air that exists at NTP when a volume of air sampled at field conditions is at NTP.

$$V_S = \frac{P_F V_F T_S}{T_F P_S} \quad (A16.5)$$

Example 1a. Determine the NTP volume of air collected for a dust sample at a molybdenum ore handling facility in Leadville, Colo. The sample pump runs at 1.9 L/min for 480 minutes. The elevation at the sampling location is 12,000 feet, the atmospheric pressure (which the U.S. Weather Bureau often refers to as the local station pressure because it is not corrected to sea level) is 499.8 mm Hg. The ambient temperature is –40°F.

The given or assumed data:

Q_F = volume flow rate at the calibration and field condition
t_F = time interval at the field condition
V_F = volume delivered at the field condition = $(Q_F)(t_F)$(1.9 L/min)(480 min) = 912 L
T_F = temperature at the field condition = –40 °F = –40 °C = 273.15 K + (–40 °C) = 233.15 K
P_F = barometric pressure at the field condition in Leadville, Colo. = 499.8 mm Hg

Solution 1a. VS can be calculated using Equation A16.5. If the changes to temperature and pressure are considered separately:

$$\frac{P_S}{P_F} = \frac{499.8 \text{ mmHg}}{760.0 \text{ mmHg}} = 0.66$$

This means that as the volume of air moves from Leadville, CO, at a local station pressure of 499.8 mm Hg, it will shrink to two-thirds of its original volume due to the increase in pressure as sea level is approached.

$$\frac{T_S}{T_F} = \frac{298.15 \text{ K}}{233.15 \text{ K}} = 1.28$$

As the volume of air moves from Leadville, Colo., at –40°F, it will increase to 1.28 times its original volume due to the increase in temperature to the standard condition. Combining these two changes due to temperature and pressure effects results in a volume (V_S) of 770.5 L from the sampled air volume of 912 L (using Equation A16.5).

$$V_S = \frac{P_F V_F T_S}{T_F P_S}$$

$$V_S = (912.0)(0.66)(1.28) = 770.5 \text{ L}$$

The percentage difference from NTP can be determined:

$$\%\text{difference} = \left(\frac{V_S - V_F}{V_F}\right) \times 100$$

$$\%\text{difference} = \left(\frac{770.5 - 912}{770.5}\right) \times 100 = -15.5\%$$

This result shows that the extreme pressure and temperature condition yield an air sample volume that is 15.5% smaller when corrected to normal pressure compared to pressure at an altitude of 12,000 feet, and when warmed to normal temperatures of 25°F from the initial temperature of –40°F. This volume change must be considered in subsequent calculations to assess workers' exposure.

Example 1b. Using the standard volume (V_S) calculated in the first part of this example determine the concentration of dust collected at the molybdenum ore handling facility. Laboratory analysis of the sample showed that 3.3 mg of dust was collected in the sample.

Solution 1b. Recall that concentration is the ration of the mass of the contaminant to the volume of air sampled. Therefore, the concentration can be determined using:

$$C = \frac{m}{V_S}$$

$$C = \frac{3.3 \text{ mg}}{0.770} = 4.3 \text{ mg/m}^3$$

If the air volume were not adjusted to standard conditions, the calculated concentration (using the air volume of 912 L) would have been 3.6 mg/m³. The difference between the concentration calculated using V_F and the concentration calculated using V_S is related directly to the 15.5% difference in the volume between field conditions and standard conditions.

Range of Temperatures Requiring a Volume Correction

Temperature correction is the adjustment of the volume (the volume flow rate multiplied by time) brought about by the difference between the field sampling temperature (T_F) and the desired standard temperature (T_S) of 25°C (298.15 K). The volume existing at the standard condition (V_S at NTP) either increases or decreases the ratio of the field and standard temperature (the temperature effect factor, T_S/T_F).

A temperature change ranging from 10°C (283.15 K or 50°F) to 40°C (313.15 K or 100°F), results in a change in volume of ±5% (Table A16.2). If an error of ±5% in volume can be tolerated in an exposure assessment, then a change in temperature between 15 and 40°C will not require a volume correction. The volume change should be evaluated to determine the effect of temperature difference on volume before the decision is made to ignore the effect of temperature on the volume sampled.

Range of Pressures Requiring a Volume Correction

Pressure correction is the adjustment of the volume (the volume flow rate multiplied by time) brought about by the difference between or field sampling pressure (P_F) and

Table A16.2 — The Temperature Range with a Minimum Effect on Volume

T_F[A]	T_S[B]	T_S/T_F	*Percentage Change from Normal Temperature*
(°C/K)	(°C/K)		(%)
10/283.15	25/298.15	1.05	+5
40/313.15	25/298.15	0.95	-5

[A]T_F is the temperature at the field condition.
[B]T_S is the temperature at normal conditions (NTP) (25°C or 298.15 K).

Table A16.3 — Effect of altitude on the atmospheric pressure

Altitude Above Sea Level *feet*	*meters*	*Absolute Barometer* *inches Hg*	*mm Hg*
-5000	-1524	35.7	914
-4500	-1372	35.1	898
-4000	-1219	34.5	882
-3500	-1067	33.9	867
-3000	-914	33.3	852
-2500	-762	32.7	837
-2000	-610	32.1	822
-1500	-457	31.6	807
-1000	-305	31.0	793
-500	-152	30.5	779
0 (sea level)	0	29.9	765
500	152	29.4	751
1000	305	28.9	738
1500	457	28.3	724
2000	610	27.8	711
2500	762	27.3	698
3000	914	26.8	686
3500	1067	26.3	673
4000	1219	25.8	661
4500	1372	25.4	649
5000	1524	24.9	637
6000	1829	24.0	613
7000	2134	23.1	590
8000	2438	22.2	568
9000	2743	21.4	547
10,000	3048	20.6	526
15,000	4572	16.9	432
20000	6096	13.8	352
25000	7620	11.1	284
30000	9144	8.89	227
35000	10,668	7.04	180
40000	12,192	5.52	141
45000	13,716	4.28	109
50000	15,240	3.27	83.6

the desired standard pressure (P_S) of one atmosphere (760 mm Hg). The volume existing at the standard condition (V_S) either increases or decreases by the ratio of the field pressure to the standard pressure (the pressure effect factor, P_F/P_S).

The effect of pressure (elevation) on volume should be determined before a decision is made to ignore the effect of pressure on the volume sampled. A pressure change ranging from 722 mm Hg (1500 feet in elevation) to 798 mm Hg (–1500 feet below sea level) results in a pressure effect on volume of ±5% (Table A16.3). So, a change in volume of ±5% will occur for atmospheric pressure between 722 and 798 mm Hg. Table A16.4 shows the relationship between altitude above sea level and the atmospheric pressure.

Example 2. Determine the normal standard (NTP) volume of air collected at 0.2 L/min for 20 minutes when an air sampling pump is operating at a sampling location that is at an elevation of 1000 feet above sea level. The pump was calibrated at the field location.

Given or assumed data:

Q_F = Volume flow rate at the calibration and field condition
t_F = Time interval at the field condition
V_F = Volume delivered at the field condition = $(Q_F)(t_F)$(0.20 L/min)(20 min) = 4.0 L
T_F = Temperature at the field condition=25°C=298.15 K
P_F = Barometric pressure at the field condition at 1000 feet =733.9 mm Hg

Solution 2. At constant temperature (isothermal condition) Equation A16.5 reduces to:

$$V_S = V_F \left(\frac{P_F}{P_S} \right)$$

So,

$$V_S = (4.0\ \text{L}) \left(\frac{733.8\ \text{mmHg}}{760.0\ \text{mm Hg}} \right) = 3.86\ \text{L}$$

In this example the volume flow rate measured is 0.20 L/min. The volume delivered is (0.2 L/min)(20 min) = 4.0 L. When corrected the field volume becomes the pressure-corrected standard volume (V_S) of 3.86 L. This volume (3.86 L) would exist if the air moving through the system were at the standard condition (one atmosphere).

The percentage difference from NTP can be determined:

$$\%\text{difference} = \left(\frac{3.86 - 4.0}{4.0} \right) \times 100 = -3.5\%$$

In this case the volume change between field and standard conditions is less than 5% and may be considered too small to correct, however this is not always the situation.

Example 3. Determine the NTP volume of air collected at 0.2 L/min for 20 minutes when an air sampling pump is operating at a sampling location that is at an elevation of 5000 feet above sea level. The pump was calibrated at the field location.

Given or assumed data:

Q_F = Volume flow rate at the calibration and field condition
t_F = Time interval at the field condition
V_F = Volume delivered at the field condition = $(Q_F)(t_F)$(0.20 L/min)(20 min) = 4.0 L
T_F = Temperature at the field condition = 25°C = 298.15 K
P_F = Barometric pressure at the field condition at 5000 feet = 638.2 mm Hg

Solution 3. At constant temperature (isothermal condition) Equation A16.5 reduces to:

$$V_S = V_F \left(\frac{P_F}{P_S} \right)$$

So,

$$V_S = (4.0\ \text{L}) \left(\frac{638.2\ \text{mmHg}}{760.0\ \text{mm Hg}} \right) = 3.36\ \text{L}$$

This large volume change is produced by the large difference in barometric pressure when an air sample volume is brought to sea level from an altitude of 5000 feet. This produces a 16% decrease in the volume. This volume change must be considered in subsequent calculations to assess worker exposure if a comparison of workers' exposure to an OEL expressed at NTP is desired. When corrected to the standard pressure conditions this results in a pressure corrected standard volume (V_S) of 3.36 L. This is the volume (3.36 L) that would exist if the air moving through the system were at the standard condition, rather than the actual conditions in the field.

Example 4. Determine the NTP concentration of a gaseous contaminant in parts per million (ppm). The 8-hour sample was collected in a field location at an elevation of 6000 feet above sea level where the air temperature was 10° C. The sampling pump used to collect the sample was calibrated at the field location at a flow rate of 0.25 L/min. Analysis of the sample determined that the sample contained 98 micrograms of the contaminant.

Given or assumed data:

Q_F = Volume flow rate at the calibration and field condition

t_F = Time interval at the field condition = 8-hr = 480 min

V_F = Volume delivered at the field condition = $(Q_F)(t_F)$(0.25 L/min) (480 min) = 120 L

T_F = Temperature at the field condition = 10°C = 283.15 K

P_F = Barometric pressure at the field condition at 5000 feet = 613 mm Hg

m = mass of contaminant in the sample = 98 µg

MW = molecular weight of the contaminant = 58 g/mole

Solution 4. V_S can be determined using Equation A16.5:

$$V_S = \frac{(613\text{ mmHg})(120\text{ L})(298.15\text{ K})}{(283.15\text{ K})(760\text{ mmHg})} = 101.9\text{ L}$$

This large volume change results from the difference in barometric pressure and temperature between the sample site and normal conditions. This standard volume is used in subsequent calculations to assess worker exposure so that the concentration can be compared to an OEL expressed at NTP. Recall that concentration can be expressed as the mass of contaminant per volume of air. So, for this example:

$$C = \frac{m}{V_S} = \frac{98\ \mu g}{101.9\text{ L}} = \frac{98\text{ mg}}{101.9\text{ m}^3} = 0.962\text{ mg/m}^3$$

Concentration expressed as mass per volume can be converted to a concentration in parts per million (for gas and vapor contaminants) using Equation 16.6a:

$$\text{ppm} = \frac{24.45 \times \left(\frac{\text{mg}}{\text{m}^3}\right)}{\text{MW}}$$

$$\text{ppm} = \frac{24.45 \times \left(0.962\ \frac{\text{mg}}{\text{m}^3}\right)}{\text{MW}}$$

This is the concentration that would be compared to any applicable occupational exposure limits to determine if the exposure to the worker is acceptable.

Temperature and Pressure Correction to Mass Concentration

In the ideal gas law, Equation 16-1, substitute for n, the number of moles (n = mass/molecular weight) of gas or vapor A, $n_A = m_A/MW_A$, and the ideal gas equation can be written as:

$$PV_A = \frac{m_A RT}{MW_A} \qquad \text{(A16.7)}$$

Solving this equation for V_A, the volume of gas or vapor A, the impurity that is in the air that is to be sampled, yields the ideal gas expanded value for V_A:

$$V_A = \frac{m_A RT}{M_A} \qquad \text{(A16.8)}$$

Recall that the definition of concentration in parts per million by volume, for concentrations less than 5000 ppm, yields:

$$C_{PPM} = \left(\frac{V_A}{V_F}\right) 10^6 \qquad (A16.9)$$

Substituting the ideal gas expanded value for VA into the above equation for CPPM yields:

$$C_{PPM} = \left(\frac{m_A RT}{MW_A P V_\Gamma}\right) 10^6 \qquad (A16.10)$$

where:

m_A = mass of contaminant gas or vapor A
V_F = volume of air in which the mass (m_A) of contaminant gas or vapor A is contained
MW_A = molecular weight of the gas or vapor A
R = universal gas constant (0.082 L atmosphere/mole K)
T = absolute temperature (Kelvin)
P = barometric pressure (atmospheres)

In Equation A16.10 the mass of contaminants (m_A) in a volume of air (V_B) is the mass concentration:

$$C_{M/V} = \left(\frac{m_A}{V_F}\right) \qquad (A16.11)$$

By substituting Equation A16.11 into Equation A16.10 the concentration in parts per million becomes:

$$C_{PPM} = \left(\frac{C_{M/V} RT}{MW_A P}\right) 10^6 \qquad (A16.12)$$

At NTP, Equation A16.12 becomes:

$$C_{PPM} = \left(\frac{C_{M/V} \times 0.082\ \text{Latm} \times 298.15\ \text{K}}{1\text{atm} \times MW_A \times P}\right) 10^6 \qquad (A16.13)$$

which reduces to:

$$C_{PPM} = \left(\frac{C_{M/V} \times 24.45\ \text{L}}{\text{mole} \times MW_A}\right) 10^6 \qquad (A16.14)$$

$C_{M/V}$ can be expanded as mass of impurity, or contaminant, per volume of air supplied, corrected to the standard condition, and the above equation written as:

$$C_{PPM} = \left(\frac{m \times 24.45\ \text{L}}{V_F \times \text{mole} \times MW_A}\right) 10^6 \qquad (A16.14)$$

The volume of air sampled in the field (V_F) must be adjusted to normal conditions (V_S) by applying the temperature and pressure correction as shown in Equation A16.4.

$$C_{PPM} = \left(\frac{m \times 24.45\ \text{L}}{V_S \times \text{mole} \times MW_A}\right) 10^6 \qquad (A16.15)$$

Then, substituting Equation A16.5 into Equation A16.14 yields:

$$C_{PPM} = \left(\frac{m \times 24.45\ \text{L}}{V_F\left(\frac{P_F T_S}{P_S T_F}\right) \times \text{mole} \times MW_A}\right) 10^6 \qquad (A16.16)$$

The units of volume may have to be reduced to a standard volume (e.g., cubic meters) from liters or cubic centimeters. The units of mass may have to be reduced to milligrams from whatever value the laboratory reported. Apply conversions to givmge the final concentration in milligrams per cubic meter, micrograms per cubic meter, and so on:

$$C_{PPM} = \left(\frac{m \times 24.45\ \text{L} \times P_S T_F}{V_F (P_F T_S) \times \text{mole} \times MW_A}\right) 10^6 \qquad (A16.17)$$

$$C_{PPM} = \left(\frac{m \times 24.45\ \text{L} \times 760\text{mmHg} \times (t + 273.15)\text{K}}{V_F \times P_F \times 298.15\text{K} \times \text{mole} \times MW_A}\right) \times 10^6 \qquad (A16.18)$$

The National Institute for Occupational Safety and Health[5] uses following the relationship to calculate the concentration in parts per million from mass per volume concentration (mg/m^3):

$$C_{PPM} = \frac{mg}{m^3} \times \frac{24.45}{MW} \times \frac{760}{P} \times \frac{(t+273)}{298} \quad (A16.19)$$

where:

P = barometric pressure (mm Hg) of air at the sampling location
t = temperature (°C) of the location where the air is sampled

The temperature correction factor (T_S/T_F) and the pressure correction factor (P_F/P_S) are applied to the air sample volume in cubic meters and not to the molar gas volume. However, if the molar gas volume is corrected to the same temperature and pressure condition that the air sample volume was corrected to the resulting concentration in parts per million will be identical. Because concentration in parts per million is independent of temperature and pressure (i.e., it is calculated on a volume-per-volume basis) and both volumes are expressed at the same condition, the concentrations are identical.

It is an individual choice to decide whether to write the conversion equation at 25°C and one atmosphere and to correct the temperature and pressure of air sample volume or to use the general equation and substitute the temperature and pressure into the general equation if and only if the concentration is expressed at the same temperature and pressure.

Example 5. An industrial hygienist collected an air sample of a gaseous contaminant at an industrial facility. Laboratory analysis of the sample revealed a concentration of 25 mg/m³. The temperature and atmospheric pressure at the field location where the sample was collected were 28°C and 745 mmHg, respectively. Determine the concentration of the air contaminant in parts per million at standard conditions.

Given or assumed data:

C = Concentration = 25 mg/m³
T_F = Temperature at the field condition = 28°C = 301.15°C
P_F = Barometric pressure at the field condition = 745 mmHg
MW = molecular weight of the contaminant = 58 g/mole

Solution 5. The conversion of concentration from a mass/volume relationship to a volume/volume relationship can be completed using Equation A16.9. This equation includes the conversion of temperature and pressure from field conditions to standard conditions.

$$C_{PPM} = \left(25\ \frac{mg}{m^3}\right) \times \frac{24.45}{58} \times \frac{760}{745} \times \frac{(28+273)}{298}$$

$$C_{PPM} = 10.9\ ppm$$

Conclusion

Apply the temperature and pressure correction [(P_F/P_S)(T_S/T_F)] to the field air sample volume and not the molar gas volume. Applying the temperature and pressure correction [(P_F/P_S)(T_S/T_F)] to the air sample volume returns it to the volume at NTP. The mass per volume concentration (mg/m³) can then be converted to parts per million.

Appendix References

1. **American Conference of Governmental Industrial Hygienists (ACGIH®):** *Industrial Ventilation, A Manual of Recommended Practice*, 24th edition. Cincinnati, OH: ACGIH®, 2001.
2. **DiNardi, S.R.:** *Calculation Methods for Industrial Hygiene*. New York: John Wiley & Sons, 1995.
3. **Nelson, G.O.:** *Control Test Atmospheres*. Ann Arbor, MI: Ann Arbor Science Press, 1971.
4. **American Conference of Governmental Industrial Hygienists (ACGIH®):** *Threshold Limit Values and Biological Indices 1993–1994*. Cincinnati, OH: ACGIH®, 1993.
5. **National Institute for Occupational Safety and Health (NIOSH):** *Manual of Analytical Methods, in NIOSH Pocket Guide to Chemical Hazards and Other Databases* (CD-ROM; DHHS [NIOSH] Publication no. 2000-130). Washington, D.C.: NIOSH, 2000.

Additional References

Caravanos, J.: *Quantitative Industrial Hygiene: A Formula Workbook*. Cincinnati, OH: ACGIH®, 1991.

Stewart, J.H.: *Industrial-Occupational Hygiene Calculations: A Professional Reference*, 2nd edition. Westborough, MA: Millennium Publishing, 2005.

Fleeger, A.K. and D.L. Lillquist: *Industrial Hygiene Reference and Study Guide*, 3rd edition. Fairfax, VA: AIHA®, 2011.

Burton, D.J.: *Useful Equations — Applied Computations for OH&S Professionals*, 3rd edition. Bountiful, UT: IVE, Inc., 2010.

Finucane, E.W.: *Definitions, Conversions, and Calculations for Occupational Safety and Health Professionals*, 3rd edition. Boca Raton, FL: CRC Press, 2006.

Outcome Competencies

After completing this chapter, the reader should be able to:

1. Define underlined terms used in this chapter.
2. Explain the principles of operation of selected direct-reading survey instruments.
3. Select direct-reading instruments based on fundamental scientific principles to satisfy occupational hygiene objectives.
4. Describe the need for calibration procedures for selected direct-reading instruments.
5. Discuss the basic chemical and physical phenomenon underlying the operation of sampling and analysis instruments.

Key Terms

Aerosol photometers • combustible gas indicators • computed tomography • condensation nucleus counters • detector tube • direct-reading instruments • electrochemical sensors • electron capture detectors • fibrous aerosol monitors • flame ionization detectors • Fourier transform infrared spectrometry • gas chromatograph • infrared gas analyzers • ionization potential • metallic oxide semiconductor (MOS) sensors • multiple particle monitors • optical particle counters • photoacoustic spectroscopy • photoionization detectors • piezoelectric mass sensors • quartz crystal microbalances • real-time monitors • thermal drift • thermal conductivity • Wheatstone bridge • tapered element oscillating microbalance

Prerequisite Knowledge

Basic Chemistry
Basic Physics

Prior to beginning this chapter, the user should review the following chapters:

Chapter Number	Chapter Topic
15	Principles and Instrumentation for Calibrating Air Sampling Equipment

Mention of particular instruments in this chapter does not imply endorsement by AIHA. Mention of such instruments is for example purposes only.

Key Topics

I. Introduction

II. Direct-Reading Gas and Vapor Monitors
   A. Electrochemical Sensors
   B. General Survey Monitors for Gases and Vapors
   C. Monitoring Multiple Gases and Vapors

III. Direct-Reading Aerosol Monitors
   A. Optical Techniques for Determining Aerosol Size and Count
   B. Optical Techniques for Determining Aerosol Mass
   C. Electrical Techniques for Determining Aerosol Size
   D. Electrical Techniques for Determining Aerosol Count
   E. Resonance Techniques for Determining Aerosol Mass
   F. Bata Absorption Techniques for Determining Aerosol Mass

IV. Future Directions

Direct-Reading Instruments for Determining Concentrations of Gases, Vapors and Aerosols

17

Lori Todd, PhD, CIH

Introduction

Direct-reading instruments are among the most important tools available to occupational hygienists for detecting and quantifying gases, vapors, and aerosols. These instruments permit real-time or near real-time measurements of contaminant concentrations in the field, thus eliminating the lag time encountered when samples are collected on media and analyzed by a laboratory. Using direct-reading instruments, air contaminants are sampled and analyzed within the instrument in a relatively short time (seconds to minutes). Results are usually indicated on an analog or digital display, a graph, or by a color change that is compared with a calibrated scale. Real-time monitors generally can be used to obtain short-term or continuous measurements. Some monitors have data-logging capabilities that allow digital storage of data. While a data logger does not enhance the accuracy of a measurement, it frees the occupational hygienist from manually recording data and allows for a variety of statistical analyses.

Direct-reading instruments range in size from small personal monitors to hand-held monitors to complex stationary installations with multi-point monitoring capability. Field monitoring instruments are usually lightweight, portable, rugged, weather and temperature insensitive, and are simple to operate and maintain. While very versatile, there is no magic black box that can be used to measure all contaminants in air; in addition, instruments used for gases and vapors cannot be used for aerosols, and vice versa.

Direct-reading instruments provide powerful on-the-spot information and are ideal for situations where the occupational hygienist wants immediate information that is temporally resolved into short time intervals. Personal direct-reading instruments, which can be placed on lapels or pockets, can be used for personal exposure monitoring and are available for a limited number of chemicals, particularly for gases that have high acute toxicity, such as carbon monoxide and phosgene.[1] Direct-reading monitors can profile information on fluctuations in contaminant concentrations that is lost when performing traditional integrated sampling. These measurements can estimate instantaneous exposures, short-term exposures, and time integrated exposures, to compare with ceiling limits, short-term exposure limits (STELs), and time-weighted averages (TWAs), respectively.

Direct-reading instruments can be used as educational and motivational tools in the workplace. Workers can obtain immediate feedback on exposure concentration and they can see the impact on exposure when work practices are modified. When direct-reading instruments are combined with the use of video cameras, workers and management can use the information for training, exposure documentation and, ultimately, to reduce exposures.[2,3]

Direct-reading instruments for gases and vapors are designed to (1) monitor a specific single gas or vapor, (2) monitor specific multiple gases and vapors, or (3) monitor multiple gases and vapors without differentiating among them. All instruments are designed to be used within a designated detection range and should be calibrated before field use. A variety of detection principles are used in direct-reading instruments for gases and vapors including infrared (IR), ultraviolet (UV), flame ionization, photo-ionization, colorimetric, and electrochemical reactions. Table 17.1 has a partial list of commonly used measurement techniques.

In conjunction with traditional integrated sampling methods, direct-reading instruments for gases and vapors can be used in developing personal sampling strategies and for obtaining a comprehensive exposure evaluation. Used to perform an initial survey of the workplace, direct-reading instruments can document the types of contaminants and the range of concentrations in the air. This information would allow a better choice of chemicals to sample, pump flow rates to use, and the representative subset of workers to monitor. When the sample probe of a

Table 17.1 — Commonly Used Direct-Reading Instruments for Gases and Vapors

Instrument	*Common Analytes*	*Principle of Operation*	*Range*
Combustible gas detectors	combustible gases and vapors (nonspecific)	hot wire—test gas is passed over a heated wire (sometimes in the presence of a catalyst). The test gas burns, changing the temperature of the filament, and the electrical resistance of the filament is measured.	Usually measured in percentage of the lower explosive limit. Some models measure down to 1 ppm.
Colorimetric detectors	various vapors including formaldehyde, hydrogen sulfide, sulfur dioxide, toluene diisocyanate (specific)	reaction of the test gas with a chemical reagent (either as a liquid or in some cases an impregnated paper or tape) and measurement of the color produced	Variable
Electrochemical sensors	carbon monoxide, nitric oxide, nitrogen dioxide, hydrogen sulfide, sulfur dioxide (specific)	chemical oxidation of test gas	1 to 3000 ppm
Infrared gas analyzers	organic and inorganic gases and vapors (specific)	measures infrared absorbance of test gas	sub-ppm to low percentage levels
Metal oxide sensors	hydrogen sulfide, nitro, amine, alcohol, and halogenated	metal oxide sensor is chemically reduced by the gas, increasing its electrical resistance hydrocarbons (specific)	1 to 50 ppm
Thermal conductivity sensors	carbon monoxide, carbon dioxide, nitrogen, oxygen, methane, ethane, propane, and butane	uses specific heat of combustion of a gas or vapor	percentage gas
Portable gas chromatographs	organic and inorganic gases and vapors (specific)	uses a packed column to separate complex mixtures of gases; detectors available include flame ionization, electron capture, thermal conductivity, flame photometric, and photoionization	0.1 to 10,000 ppm
Detectors for gas chromatographs			
Electron capture detector	halogenated hydrocarbons, nitrous oxide, and compounds containing cyano or nitro groups	uses a radioactive source such as 63Ni to supply energy to the detector that monitors the intensity of the electron beam arriving at a collection electrode. When an electron-capturing species passes through the cell the intensity of the electron beam decreases.	0.1 ppb to low ppm
Flame ionization detectors	organic compounds including aliphatic and aromatic hydrocarbons, ketones, alcohols, and halogenated hydrocarbons	creates organic ions by passing a hydrogen gas through flame. Measures conductivity of the flame.	0.1 to 100,000 ppm
Photoionization detectors	most organic compounds, particularly aromatic compounds	creates ions by exposing test gas to ultraviolet light. Measures conductivity of the gases in the light field.	0.2 to 2000 ppm

direct-reading instrument is placed in the breathing zone of a worker, peak exposures to chemicals can be evaluated.

Direct-reading instruments can be used for evaluating the effectiveness of local exhaust ventilation systems and other controls, detecting leaks, monitoring source emissions, emergency response, and monitoring hazardous waste sites. Carbon monoxide exposures and explosive and oxygen deficient atmospheres create life-threatening situations requiring immediate feedback of concentrations; they cannot wait for laboratory analyses. Some chemicals are difficult to collect on traditional media and for them, real-time instrumentation is the best solution. Direct-reading instruments used in stationary installations are used to provide early warning of high contaminant concentrations resulting from process leaks, spills, failure of ventilation systems, or other catastrophic releases.

The selection of the appropriate direct-reading instrument depends on the application for which it will be used. For monitoring employee exposures to gases and vapors, an instrument would probably be chosen that has high selectivity and can detect and quantify target chemicals in a specific concentration range. For hazardous waste sites or some emergency situations where there are unknown contaminants, a nonspecific general survey instrument, which can respond to a range of contaminants, would be needed. Other factors that impact instrument choice include price, portability, weight, size, battery operation and life, and requirements for personnel training.

While manufacturers have been simplifying operation, direct-reading instruments all require the user to understand the limitations and conditions that can affect performance and calibration, and also to understand maintenance requirements and interpret results. Measurements of gases and vapors can be adversely affected by interferences from other contaminants; therefore, the occupational hygienist needs to be aware of the sampling environment before selecting an instrument. Environmental conditions such as temperature extremes, humidity, elevation above sea level, barometric pressure, presence of particulates, and oxygen concentration can affect instrument performance and accuracy. In addition, electromagnetic fields in the environment can interfere with instrument performance and cause a wide variety of problems including intermittent operation, changes in pump flow rates, illogical displays, and total shut downs.(4)

Potential sources of error should be minimized through proper quality control practices. All instruments require calibration before use. Calibration of gas and vapor monitors includes comparison of instrument readings to known concentrations of gases. Ideally, a multi-point calibration should be performed using specific contaminants that will be measured in the field over the range of expected concentrations. In some cases it may be important to calibrate the instrument for interferences. Interferences can result in false-positive or false-negative results by interfering with collection, detection, or quantification of contaminants. For nonspecific instruments, calibration is usually performed using a relatively nontoxic gas, such as isobutylene. A few instruments are calibrated electronically and do not require the use of a calibrant gas.

For potentially explosive atmospheres, direct-reading instruments need to be intrinsically safe or explosion-proof. Intrinsically safe means that instruments cannot release thermal or electrical energy that could cause ignition of hazardous chemicals. Explosion-proof means that there is a chamber within the instrument that is designed to contain and withstand any explosion caused by contaminants entering the instrument. Minimum standards for inherent safety in hazardous environments has been defined by the National Fire Protection Association in its National Electrical Code.(5) Testing and certification of equipment is performed by the Underwriters Laboratory or Factory Mutual Research Corp., and other international testing agencies.

Direct-reading instruments for aerosols can be used for surveying the workplace to prioritize sources of exposure to dusts, for respirator fit-testing, for asbestos monitoring, and as an educational tool to evaluate work practices and identify dust generating sources. Aerosol monitoring has been combined with videotaping to evaluate the influence of different operations and activities on exposure.(3)

Measuring aerosols is complicated and, in many ways, more difficult than measurement of gases and vapors. Measurement is

Table 17.2 — Commonly Used Aerosol Monitors

Instrument	*Sample Flow*	*Size Range*	*Concentration Range*
Light-scattering photometers	passive to 100 L/min	0.1 to 20 µm	0.0001 µm/m³ to 200 g/m³
Light-scattering particle counters	0.12 L/min to 28 L/min	0.1 to 8000 m (up to 32,000 µm for drop size analyzers)	1 particle/L to 10^5 particles/cm³
Condensation nucleus counters	0.003 L/min to 4.2 L/min	1.6 nm to 20 nm	0.1 to 10^6 particles/cm³
Single Particle Aerosal Relaxation Time (SPART)	0.5 to 5 L/min	< 0.3 to 10 µm	
Beta attenuation aerosol mass monitors	15 L/min	< 10 µm	10 mg/m³ max
Piezoelectric crystal microbalance	0.24 to 1 L/min	0.05 to 35 µm	100 g/m³ to 100 mg/m³
Tapered Element Oscillating Microbalance (TEOM)	0.5 to 35 µm		5 µg/m³ to 2000 mg/m³
Fibrous aerosol monitor fibers/cm³	2 L/min	0.2 µm 2 to 200 µm	0.0001 to 30

affected by many factors such as particle size and shape, particle settling velocity, wind currents, and sampling flow rates. Accurate and defensible measurement of aerosols depends on careful calibration of direct-reading aerosol monitors. While some monitors can be calibrated using fundamental theories of operation, it is more common to establish an empirical relationship using a set of calibrated test aerosols. Calibration may involve testing the system with suspensions of known sizes of nebulized, monodisperse polystyrene latex spheres or aerosols generated using a vibrating-orifice generator.[6]

In general, direct-reading instruments for aerosols cannot differentiate between types of aerosols. The type of information provided by the instruments includes particle size distribution, particle count, and total and respirable mass concentration. However, there is no single instrument that can provide all of these measurements. Direct-reading instruments for aerosols primarily operate using four techniques: (1) optical, (2) electrical, (3) resonance oscillation, and (4) beta absorption. Table 17.2 is a partial list of commonly used measurement techniques for aerosols.

Different properties of aerosols (such as optical, physical and electrical) are measured by the direct-reading instruments. For example, if instruments measure particle size, the size may be derived from one of the many properties of aerosols such as its optical, aerodynamic, mechanical or electrical behavior. Thus, direct comparisons of measurements between instruments may be difficult.

This chapter describes the principles of operation, applications, limitations, and calibration procedures for some commonly used direct-reading instruments.

Direct-Reading Gas and Vapor Monitors

Electrochemical Sensors

A variety of instruments dedicated to monitoring specific single gas and vapor contaminants use electrochemical sensors. Electrochemical sensors are available for up to 50 different individual gases including oxygen, carbon monoxide, nitric oxide, nitrogen dioxide, hydrogen sulfide, hydrogen cyanide, and sulfur dioxide (see Table 17.3).[7–9] These sensors can be incorporated into a compact design and used as lightweight personal monitors that are small enough to fit into a shirt pocket. They have low power requirements and can operate continuously for up to four months without needing replacement batteries.

Carbon monoxide can be monitored using electrochemical cells (the most common detection method), solid-state sensors, and IR methods. Carbon monoxide is produced as a by-product of fuel combustion and is associated with motor vehicle exhaust; therefore, human exposures may be encountered in inadequately ventilated

Table 17.3 — Gases Detectable by Electrochemical Sensors

Ammonia	Formic acid	Hydrogen sulfide	Phosphine
Arsine	Freon	Nitric acid	Silane
Bromine	Germane	Nitric oxide	Silicon tetrafluoride
Carbon dioxide	Hydrazine	Nitrogen dioxide	Sulfur dioxide
Carbon monoxide	Hydrochloric acid	Nitrogen oxides	Tetrachloroethylene
Chlorine	Hydrogen	Nitrous oxide	Trichloroethylene
Ethylene oxide	Hydrogen chloride	Oxygen	Tungsten hexafluoride
Fluorine	Hydrogen cyanide	Ozone	
Formaldehyde	Hydrogen fluoride	Phosgene	

Sources: References 1 and 7

buildings with attached automobile garages. Garage workers and traffic police are particularly prone to such exposures. Carbon monoxide poisoning can produce symptoms ranging from headaches and dizziness to unconsciousness and death.

Hydrogen sulfide can be monitored using electrochemical cells and solid-state sensors. It is commonly measured using real-time instruments rather than integrated methods because of its high toxicity, the fact that it causes olfactory fatigue, and its prevalence in confined spaces. Hydrogen sulfide is the primary toxic contaminant that causes death in confined spaces.[10]

Oxygen can also be monitored using electrochemical cells; measurements are usually taken in conjunction with combustible gas measurements for confined space entry where the air can be oxygen deficient. The Occupational Safety and Health Administration defines oxygen deficient atmospheres as concentrations of 19.5% or lower; normal air contains 20.9% oxygen.[11,12] It is important to verify adequate oxygen levels to ensure that the combustible sensor is functioning properly. Oxygen deficient atmospheres can be hazardous to health; the hazard can be compounded if the gas displacing the oxygen in the air is toxic. A life-or-death safety hazard may also exist in this atmosphere if the chemical displacing the oxygen is flammable or explosive.

A typical electrochemical sensor (see Figure 17.1) uses a coarse particulate filter, an electrochemical cell with two electrodes, an electrolyte (liquid, gel, or part of a solid matrix), and a porous membrane (normally Teflon). The monitored gas diffuses into the cell, dissolves in the electrolyte, and reacts with a sensing electrode. Charged ions and electrons are produced from this reaction and diffuse across the electrolyte to a counting electrode. This results in a change in the electrochemical potential between the electrodes. The associated electronic circuitry measures, amplifies, and controls the resulting electronic signal and converts it into a meter reading. The electrolytic solutions and composition of electrodes in the sensors can be modified to achieve chemical specificity, sensitivity, and range of detection.

Measurements obtained using electrochemical sensors may be inaccurate due to interferences and contamination. Gases of similar molecular size and chemical reactivity can interfere with measurement by reacting with the electrode and can result in false positive results. This lack of specificity is important to realize when monitoring atmospheres with multiple unknown toxic chemicals. The sensors can be contaminated by acidic or alkaline gases that neutralize the electrolytic solution, which can result in decreased sensitivity. The membrane can become clogged with particulates, and with condensed aerosols, water vapor, and hot gases. A clogged membrane will limit the diffusion of gases into the sensor and will result in underestimation of concentrations.

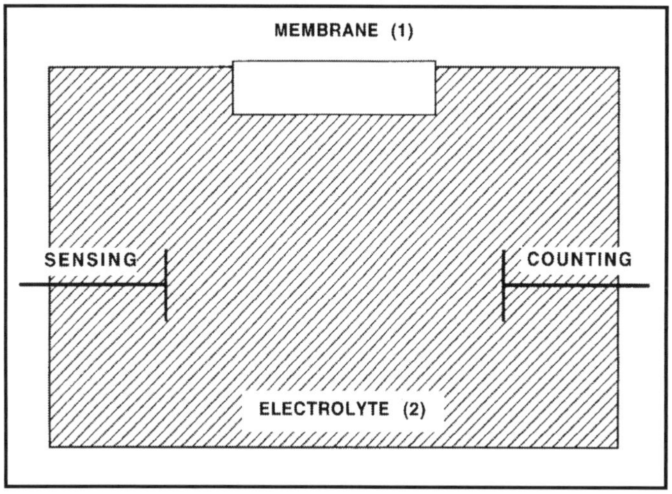

Figure 17.1 — A typical electrochemical sensor.

The electrochemical sensors themselves can be hazardous if they contain a corrosive liquid electrolyte; if the solution leaks, it can cause chemical burns on contact with the skin or eyes. The electrochemical cells used in oxygen monitors usually contain a sensing electrode of lead or zinc, a counting electrode of gold or platinum, and an alkaline electrolyte of potassium hydroxide and water. The chemical reaction in the cell is proportional to the concentration (partial pressure) of oxygen and is displayed as percentage by volume oxygen within a range of 0 to 25%. Electrochemical cells used to monitor oxygen deteriorate over time, whether they are used or not, because they are exposed to ambient air that contains oxygen. Therefore, replacement is required within a year. Usually, oxygen monitors have an alarm that is activated at 19.5% oxygen.

Oxygen meters must be calibrated with clean air containing 20.9% oxygen at the same altitude and temperature that they will be used. Meters calibrated above sea level (in Denver, for example) and used at a lower elevation (for example, Boston) will overestimate oxygen concentrations. Calibration of oxygen monitors is simple and involves placing the instrument in fresh ambient air and adjusting the potentiometer until it reads the specific oxygen percentage indicated by the manufacturer (20.8% or 20.9%). This should be performed immediately before field use. To check the ability to measure oxygen deficient atmospheres, manufacturers supply gases containing 10 to 15% oxygen.

The DrägerSensor® XS-2 (Draeger Safety Inc., Pittsburgh, Pa.) has sensors for carbon monoxide, hydrogen sulfide and oxygen. The carbon monoxide sensor can detect concentrations up to 2000 ppm in 20 seconds. The hydrogen sulfide filter measures up to 100 ppm in 30 seconds. The oxygen sensor measures up to 25% by volume oxygen in 20 seconds.

General Survey Monitors for Gases and Vapors

General survey instruments are capable of measuring a wide range of air contaminants but cannot distinguish among them. They are usually used as area samplers to measure concentrations that are immediately dangerous to life and health, and concentrations that are within occupational exposure limits, in the ppm range. Commonly used monitors include combustible gas indicators, photoionization and flame ionization detectors, and solid-state sensors.

Combustible Gas Instruments (CGI)

Combustible gas instruments (CGI) were the first direct-reading instruments to be developed and were used to detect methane in underground mines in Great Britain.[7] CGIs are currently used to measure gases in confined spaces and atmospheres containing combustible gases and vapors (methane and gasoline).[8] These instruments are capable of measuring the presence of flammable gases in percentage of lower explosive limit (LEL) and percentage of gas by volume. A few CGIs are equipped with sensors that allow reliable measurement of low ppm concentrations for a limited number of gases and vapors. The CGI is primarily a safety meter used to detect hazardous concentrations up to 100% of the LEL. When 100% of the LEL is reached, flammable or explosive concentrations are present. In terms of concentrations that relate to occupational exposure limits, a relatively low percentage LEL corresponds to a high concentration. For example, the LEL of methane is 5.3%. Therefore, an LEL of 10% is equivalent to 5300 ppm ($0.10 \times 5.3\% = 0.53\%$ or 5300 ppm). This level is much greater than any threshold limit value or permissible exposure limit. Thus, most CGIs cannot be used to determine compliance with occupational exposure limits.

Virtually all CGIs in use today are based on catalytic combustion. The air containing the contaminant passes over a heated catalytic filament, which is incorporated into a Wheatstone bridge (see Figure 17.2).

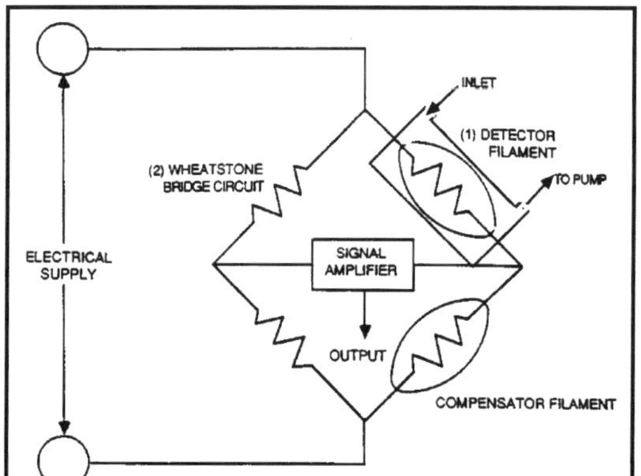

Figure 17.2 — A Wheatstone bridge.

A Wheatstone bridge is a circuit that measures the differential resistance in an electric current. The catalytic sensor has two filaments; one is coated with a catalyst (usually platinum) to facilitate oxidation or combustion of very low concentrations of a gas. The other filament, the compensating filament, operates at the same voltage as the catalyst, but does not cause oxidation and, therefore, does not increase in temperature.

When the meter is turned on, a current is applied to the Wheatstone bridge and the filaments are heated to a very high temperature. The gas is passed through a coarse metal filter, comes in contact with the heated filaments, and ignites on the filament coated with the catalyst. The burning gas causes the filament to heat; however, there is no temperature change in the compensating filament. The increase in temperature causes an increase in resistance and a decrease in current flow relative to the compensating filament. The heat of combustion changes the temperature in the sensor chamber in proportion to the amount of combustible gas present in the sample stream; this is translated into a meter reading. The greater the change in resistance, the greater the concentration. Catalytic sensors are usually sensitive to concentrations as low as 0.5 to 1% of the LEL.

Thermal conductivity (TC) is another method used for detecting explosive atmospheres that uses the specific heat of combustion of a gas or vapor as a measure of its concentration in air. TC is used in instruments where very high concentrations of flammable gases are expected-greater than 100% of the LEL-and measures percentage of gas as compared with percentage of the LEL. This method is not sensitive to low concentrations of gases. Typical applications include pipeline leaks, tank farms, and landfills. A TC filament is substituted into a Wheatstone bridge. The combustible gases in the sample cool this filament instead of heating it, which decreases the resistance across the Wheatstone bridge and produces a meter reading. The meter reading represents how cool the TC filament is relative to the hot compensating filament. When this equipment samples gases, they will cool the filament even if they are not flammable.

Semiconductor sensors are also used to detect combustible gases and vapors. Sensors consist of a semiconductor, such as silica, covered with a metallic oxide, such as zinc oxide or aluminum oxide. The oxide forms a porous surface that traps oxygen and provides a base level of conduction through the sensor. A conductor is any material that has many free electrons and allows electrons to move through it easily. A heated coil embedded in the semiconductor maintains a constant temperature, controls the number of free electrons, and prevents condensation of water vapor. The sensor is attached to a Wheatstone bridge. When the sensor is exposed to a contaminant, the gas reacts with the trapped oxygen in the sensor, which causes the release of electrons and a decrease in the resistance across the Wheatstone bridge. This results in a meter reading proportional to concentration.

All CGI readings are relative to the gas used to calibrate the equipment in the factory, which may be methane, pentane, propane, or hexane. When the CGI is exposed only to the calibrant, it will respond accurately. When a CGI is calibrated, the instrument response depends on the calibrant gas as well as the type of catalyst employed in the sensor. It is very important to understand the implications of using one calibrant gas over another and the way to interpret the meter readings, because CGIs are used to detect situations where an explosive atmosphere could be present.

Ideally, when the CGI is calibrated, the calibrant gas should have a heat of combustion that is similar to the chemical being monitored. To provide a wide margin of safety, if there are several potential explosive gases in the environment, the instrument should be calibrated for the least sensitive gas. Therefore, a gas should be selected that would require a very high concentration to get the lowest percentage LEL. Thus, all the other gases would overestimate the percentage LEL. For example, methane has a heat of combustion of 55.50 millijoules (mj)/kg and pentane has a heat of combustion of 48.64 mj/kg. Therefore, higher concentrations are required in air for methane to create a potentially explosive atmosphere. If a CGI is calibrated to methane and encounters pentane, it will be more sensitive to pentane and read high. Therefore, the occupational hygienist will be conservative in the interpretation of the measurements and will be provided with a margin of safety. In addition, most CGIs have alarms set for 20 to 25% of the LEL because of the inherent uncertainty when sampling unknown explosion hazards.

When sampling a gas in air that is not the calibrant, the gas may burn more readily on the filament, creating a hotter filament at a lower concentration. This would result in the recording of a higher than actual percentage LEL on the meter. These gases are called hot burning gases. Conversely, when sampling a gas that burns less readily on the filament than the calibrant, this creates a cooler filament at a higher concentration. This would result in the recording of a lower than actual percentage LEL on the meter. These gases are called cool burning gases.

Many manufacturers of CGIs provide instrument response curves to allow conversion of a meter reading to concentration when a specific gas other than the calibrant is being sampled. The response curves are created in the laboratory by using known concentrations of gases and recording the meter readings over the entire LEL range. In the field, if the identity of the vapor to be sampled is known, the response curve can be used to approximate the actual concentration (see Figure 17.3). For example, a 60% LEL reading for the hotter burning gas B would actually represent 40% of the LEL. A 60% LEL reading for the cooler burning gas C would actually represent 75%.

Conversion factors are also used to convert meter readings of specific chemicals into concentrations. The conversion factor is a single number provided by the manufacturer that is used to describe the entire

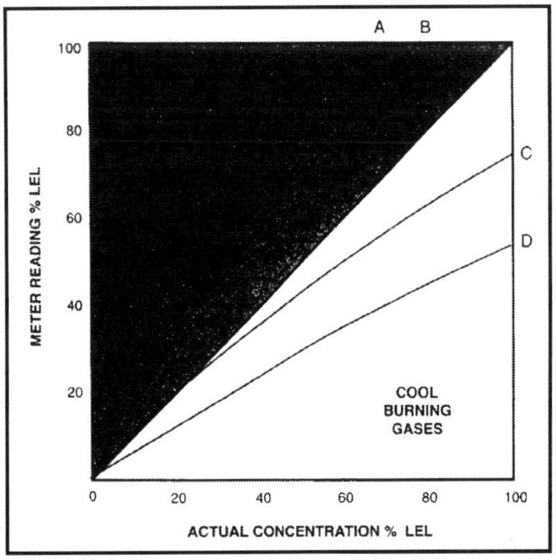

Figure 17.3 — Combustible gas instrument response curve for conversion of a meter reading to concentration.

response curve; therefore, it is only a conservative approximation. If a conversion factor is 0.9 and the readout is 50% LEL, the estimated concentration is 45% (0.9 ± 50%) of the LEL. When response curves or conversion factors are used, an accuracy of ±25% should be factored into the interpretation of the measurement. Manufacturer supplied conversion factors and response curves should only be used for the model and calibrant for which they were generated. Without response curves or conversion factors, the instrument cannot be used to estimate concentrations.

As with all direct-reading instruments, CGIs should be calibrated under the same conditions as those in the field. In the field, the calibration check involves using a single concentration of a gas in the middle of the response range. The response should be within acceptable limits as described by the manufacturer. After the check with the calibrant gas, the user can sample known concentrations of other gases and check the calibration using the response curves or conversion factors.

While CGIs appear relatively simple to use, they have limitations that could result in dire outcomes if not fully understood. Sensors need to be replaced periodically because every time the instrument is used the catalyst deteriorates. It is important for a user to know the response time of an instrument, as response time varies and improper readings may be obtained. CGIs that use a catalytic sensor require the sample air to be oxidized or burned on the filament. Therefore, the occupational hygienist must know the minimum oxygen requirement for oxidation. If the concentration of oxygen in ambient air is too low, the signal obtained will be too low. For confined spaces, in particular, CGIs should always be used in conjunction with oxygen meters. The oxygen concentration should be obtained first, since CGI performance depends on oxygen availability.

Oxygen deficiency may be created when there are concentrations of gases and vapors above the upper explosion limit. In this situation many CGIs will initially peg 100% LEL and then quickly return to zero (see Figure 17.4). Therefore, the meter reading must be observed as soon as measurements are started. For some cool gases, the reading may not peg at 60% rather than 100% before dropping.

When concentrations are above the upper explosion limit, the atmosphere is too rich to burn, and oxidation cannot occur. In this case the temperature of both filaments will decrease.

Although CGIs can measure a wide variety of flammable gases and vapors, they cannot measure all materials and can give false-positive or false-negative results. On the other hand, some CGIs have catalysts that enhance the oxidation of chlorinated hydrocarbons, which can result in overestimation of concentrations and meter readings that represent flammable atmospheres when there are none.[7]

High concentrations of some compounds can poison catalysts such as organic heavy metals, silicates, silicones, and silanes. They can coat the catalyst and result in a decreased response of the instrument to other chemicals. Corrosive gases can corrode the sensors, which will ultimately result in depressed readings.

TIF Instruments, Inc (Owatonna, MN) makes the TIF 8800 Combustible Gas Detector. It measures hydrocarbons, halogenated hydrocarbons, alcohol's ethers, ketones and other compounds with a minimum detection level of 5 ppm. Thermo Electron (Franklin, MA) makes the Innova ™ Portable Gas Meter that measures combustible gases in the 0–1000 ppm range. It measures hydrocarbons, oxygen, and a choice of one or two toxic chemicals.

Solid-State Sensors

Solid-state sensors are used to detect ppm and combustible concentrations of gases. These metallic oxide semiconductor (MOS) sensors can be used to detect a variety of compounds including nitro, amine, alcohol, and halogenated hydrocarbons, as well as a limited number of inorganic gases.

When mixtures are present in air, MOS sensors are best used as general survey instruments because they lack specificity and cannot distinguish between chemicals. The sensor will respond to a number of interfering gases and result in inaccurate meter readings. For example, sensors designed to monitor carbon monoxide may be sensitive to sulfur dioxide and hydrogen sulfide as well.

The advantages of MOS sensors include small size, low cost, and simplicity of operation. Disadvantages include lack of specificity,

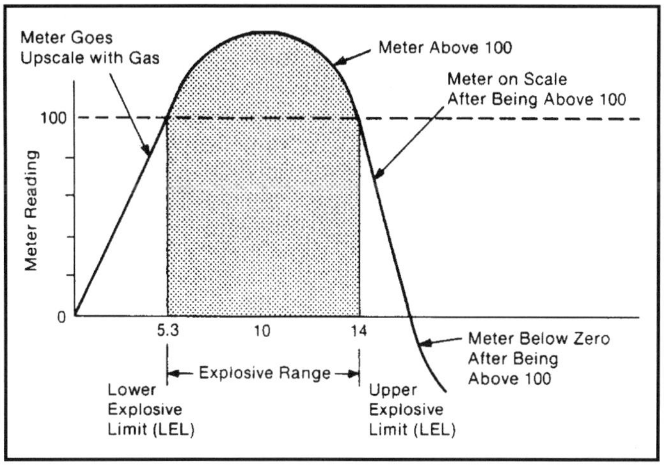

Figure 17.4 — Sensor response range from lower explosive limit to upper explosive limit.

low sensitivity, and low. The Millenium II series from Net-Safety (Calgary, Alberta) can be fitted with a solid-state sensor for H2S and NH3. These sensors can detect concentrations over their entire range in less than 20 seconds under a wide variety of environmental conditions, including hot dry conditions. The sensors can be separated from the unit by a distance of up to 600 meters. The sensors have been designed to increase sensitivity and stability.

Instruments with solid-state sensors are initially calibrated in the laboratory; field checks are performed for individual chemicals over several concentrations. Calibration of MOS sensors can be time consuming and more complicated than for other direct-reading instruments. Multiple concentrations must be tested several times over a range of concentrations because MOS sensors are not linear.

Photoionization Detectors (PIDs)

Portable photoionization detectors (PIDs) are general survey instruments used for detecting leaks, surveying plants to identify problem areas, evaluating source emissions, monitoring ventilation efficiency, evaluating work practices, and determining the need for personal protective equipment for hazardous waste site workers. These instruments are nonspecific and are often used to give qualitative information on the amount and class of chemicals present in air. Immediate qualitative results can be obtained for unknowns and mixtures of chemicals. A portable PID can be used around the perimeter of a leaking industrial operation or a hazardous waste site to determine airborne releases of total hydrocarbons into the community. PIDs can be used at hazardous waste sites to determine whether decontamination procedures are effective and for screening of air, water, soil, and drum bulk samples to determine priorities for further sampling.

Quantitative analysis by photoionization is based on the fact that most organic compounds and some inorganic compounds can be ionized when they are bombarded by high-energy UV light. These compounds absorb the energy of the light, which excites the molecule and results in a loss of an electron and the formation of a positively charged ion. The number of ions formed and the ion current produced is directly proportional to mass and concentration. Some compounds are ionized easily while others are not. The amount of energy required to displace an electron is called the ionization potential (IP). Each chemical compound has a unique IP; the higher the IP, the greater the amount of energy required to ionize the material. PIDs operate by collecting the ions on an electrode, amplifying the ion current formed (measured in electron volts), and translating the current into concentration. This process is represented by Equation 17-1.

$$RH + hv \rightarrow RH^{+} + e^{-} \quad (17\text{-}1)$$

where

RH = test gas
hv = photon with UV light energy greater than or equal to the IP of the test gas
RH^{+} = positively charged ion
e^{-} = electron

PIDs use a pump or fan to draw the air sample into a UV lamp that is either contained within the housing of the instrument or is located in a separate probe. Lamps of different energies are available; the energy of the lamp determines whether a particular chemical will be ionized. When the UV light energy is greater than the IP of the chemical, ionization will occur. In theory, if the UV light energy is less than the IP of the chemical, there will be no ionization. In practice, a lamp can detect chemicals with IPs that are higher than the rating on the lamp because the rating (in eV) refers to the major emission line of the lamp. However, sensitivity drops off rapidly and is not easily defined or quantified.

The lamps contain a low-pressure gas through which a high potential electrical current is passed. By varying the composition of the gas in the lamp, manufacturers can develop lamps with different energy levels. Hydrogen is used to emit 10.2 eV, nitrogen for 10.6 eV, and argon for 11.7 eV. There are only a few lamps available: 9.5 eV, 10.0 eV, 10.2 eV, 10.6 eV, 11.7 eV, and 11.8 eV. When the sample is ionized, the electrical signal is displayed on an analog or digital output. The output does not distinguish between chemicals; it just detects an increase in the ion current.

To use PIDs, the occupational hygienist must know the IP of the chemicals suspected of being present in the air and the IP (eV capacity) of the lamp in the PID. The instrument should not be used to detect compounds with IPs greater than the lamp's capacity. The IPs of most organic compounds are less than 12 eV (see Table 17.4). The IPs of the atmospheric gases nitrogen, oxygen, water, carbon monoxide, and carbon dioxide are greater than 12 eV, and the IP of methane is 12.98 eV. Thus, measurements of contaminants in ambient air will not be affected by these major components of air.

It is possible to use PIDs quantitatively if only one chemical is present in air or if a mixture of chemicals is present and each chemical has the same IP. PIDs are more sensitive to complex compounds than to simple ones. They can detect a range of organic chemicals and some inorganic chemicals, including aromatics, unsaturated chlorinated hydrocarbons, aldehydes, ketones, ethylene oxide, hydrogen sulfide, and glycol ether solvents. Sensitivity increases as carbon number increases and is affected by the functional group (alcohol, amine, halide), structure (straight, branched, cyclical), and type of bond (saturated, unsaturated). In addition to chemical structure, the lamp intensity will also affect the sensitivity of the instrument to a given contaminant. For example, an 11.7 eV lamp is one tenth as sensitive to benzene, which has an IP of 9.25 eV, as a 10.2 eV lamp. Manufacturers usually have charts that list the sensitivity of their lamps to various chemical compounds. The sensitivities are related to a meter response at a known concentration (usually 10 ppm) of the contaminant.

The choice of which UV lamp to use in the instrument depends on the contaminants present in the air as well as the required stability of the lamp. Using lamps with different energies can achieve some degree of selectivity. The 11.7 eV lamp is capable of ionizing the largest number of chemicals and detecting the most chemicals; thus, it has the least selectivity. However, it can be used to selectively detect chemicals with IPs greater than 10.6 eV, such as chlorinated hydrocarbons (methylene chloride, chloroform, and carbon tetrachloride). A 9.5 eV lamp will selectively detect aromatic hydrocarbons such as benzene, xylene, and toluene in atmospheres where there are alkanes and alcohols that have IPs of greater than 10 eV.

In terms of lamp stability, the 11.7 eV and 11.8 eV lamps have the shortest usable lives. The windows in these lamps are made of lithium fluoride, which can transmit high energy, short wavelength UV light; however, lithium fluoride is hygroscopic and is degraded by UV light. Therefore, the windows will absorb water and swell, and light transmission will decrease, even when the instrument is not in use. The more the instrument is used, the greater the damage by UV light. The combination of water vapor and UV damage results in a service life of 3–6 months. Lamps emitting 9.5 eV, 10.2 eV, and 10.6 eV are made of magnesium fluoride; the 10.0 eV lamp has windows made of calcium fluoride. These windows are much more stable than lithium fluoride, are not degraded by UV light, and are not hygroscopic.

All PID readings are relative to the factory calibrant gas; the manufacturer adjusts a span setting (potentiometer) so that the PID reads directly for a defined concentration of a known chemical. For chemicals other than the calibrant gas, the meter reading is not the actual concentration. Therefore, meter responses to chemicals other than the calibrant gases should be recorded as ppm-calibrant gas equivalents, not as ppm. PIDs cannot detect all contaminants present in air; therefore, when there is no meter reading it does not mean all contaminants are absent. The typical range of concentrations that can be detected is 0.2 to 2000 ppm for the calibration gas, and readings are usually linear to about 600 ppm. Measurements above 600 ppm are usually not linear and may underestimate actual concentrations. Benzene and isobutylene are most often used to calibrate PIDs.

Table 17.4 — Ionization Potentials of Selected Chemicals

Compound	*IP (eV)*
Acetaldehyde	10.21
Acetic acid	10.37
Acetone	9.69
Acrolein	10.10
Allyl alcohol	9.67
Allyl chloride	10.20
Ammonia	10.15
Aniline	7.70
Benzene	9.25
Benzyl chloride	10.16
1,3-Butadiene	9.07
n-Butyl amine	8.71
Carbon disulfide	10.13
Chlorobenzene	9.07
Crotonaldehyde	9.73
Cyclohexane	9.98
Cyclohexanone	9.14
Cyclohexene	8.95
Diborane	11.4
1,1-Dichloroethane	11.06
Dimethyl amine	8.24
Ethyl acetate	10.11
Ethyl amine	8.86
Ethyl benzene	8.76
Ethyl bromide	10.29
Ethyl butyl ketone	9.02
Ethyl chloride	10.98
Ethylene chlorohydrin	10.90
Heptane	10.07
Hydrogen cyanide	13.91
Hydrogen sulfide	10.46
Isoamyl acetate	9.90
Isoamyl alcohol	10.16
Isopropyl acetate	9.99
Isopropyl alcohol	10.16
Isopropyl amine	8.72
Isopropyl ether	9.20
Methanol	10.85
Methyl acetate	10.27
Methyl acrylate	10.72
Methyl ethyl ketone	9.53
Methyl mercaptan	9.44
Morpholine	8.88
Nitrobenzene	9.92
Octane	9.9
Pentane	10.35
2-Pentanone	9.39
Phosphine	9.96
Propane	11.07
n-Propyl acetate	10.04
n-Propyl alcohol	10.20
Propylene dichloride	10.87
Propylene oxide	10.22
Styrene	8.47
Toluene	8.82
Triethylamine	7.50
Vinyl chloride	10.00
Water	12.61
m-Xylene	8.56

Factory calibration is performed under optimal conditions; therefore, if the lamp ages or becomes contaminated, the instrument must be recalibrated. The only way to ensure the instrument is working properly is to use the span gas (factory calibrant gas) at multiple concentrations. Some models have microprocessor-controlled calibration procedures. If a single compound is known to be present in the air, it is possible to calibrate the instrument to that chemical to make the readings relevant. Another option is to take the manufacturer's response factor for that chemical and use it to adjust the concentration obtained with the PID. For example, if a chemical has a response factor of 0.5 when using a particular lamp, the user would multiply the meter reading (for example, 50) by 0.5 to get 25 ppm.

PIDs are adversely affected by humidity, particulates, and hot and corrosive atmospheres. Although water vapor has an IP of 12.59, it can cause lamp fogging and deflect, scatter, or absorb light.[13] When UV light is scattered, less light reaches contaminants for ionization, resulting in lower meter readings. It is particularly important to calibrate PIDs in the environment where the equipment will be used (outdoors versus an air-conditioned interior). Dust particles can cover a UV lamp and decrease the amount of UV light transmitted; therefore, most PIDs have an inlet filter to decrease the possibility of particulates entering the ionization chamber. However, if small particles pass through the filter, they can scatter the light and decrease ionization. If the particles are charged, they can act as ions and result in elevated readings or erratic measurements. Hot gases can condense on the lamp or within the instrument and decrease meter readings. Corrosive gases can permanently fog or etch the lamp window or deteriorate the electrodes.

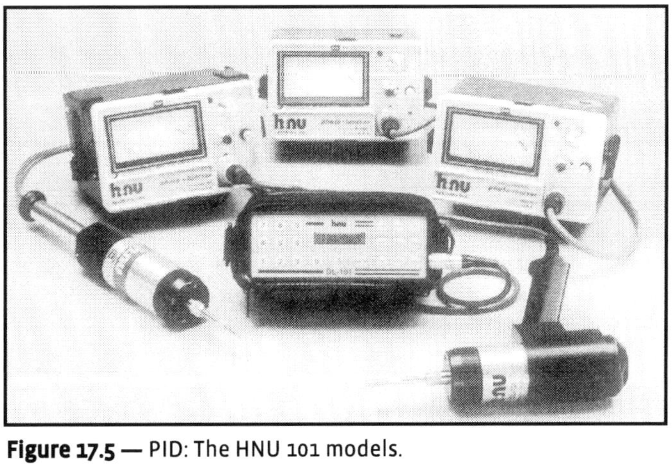
Figure 17.5 — PID: The HNU 101 models.

The instruments should be zeroed in the field before obtaining measurements. Clean air always contains some ionizable materials, and readings will always vary depending on what is in the air. However, readings will usually be approximately 0.2 units. If background readings are very high, non-contaminated factory air (zero or hydrocarbon free air) should be used. There are several manufacturers of PIDs including Perkin-Elmer, Inc., MSA, Thermo Environmental Instruments, RAE, and HNU.

PIDs from HNU Systems, Inc. (Newton, Mass.) are factory calibrated to benzene, have a separate probe that houses the UV lamp, and a box that contains the readout display and controls (see Figure 17.5). The HNU 101 models have three interchangeable lamps (11.7 eV, 10.2 eV, and 9.5 eV) and three ranges selected by the user (0–20, 0–200, and 0–2000 units). The instruments weigh from 7 to 13 pounds and have a lead-acid gel rechargeable battery that provides at least eight hours of continuous use. The UV probe and readout are factory calibrated together, and it is important that they remain together, or the instrument may not be accurately calibrated. HNU (Pembroke, MA) makes a detector with interchangeable heads including three PID lamps (9.5, 10.6 or 11.7 wavelengths). The instrument can measure from 1–3000 ppm with an optional 1–20,000 ppb range for one of the models. The response time is under a second.

For most of the units, a small fan inside the probe draws air in, and the response is read on an analog display. The HW-101 model is designed for hazardous waste site monitoring and has a moisture-resistant ion chamber that uses a positive displacement pump and inlet filter to draw the samples into the probe. The DL-101 model is microprocessor controlled and has data-logging ability.

The Photovac 2020 (Photovac, Waltham, MA) does not have a separate probe and meter. It has a single, lightweight unit with a pump, in-line filter, and digital LCD readout. The Photovac 2020 has an advanced microprocessor that can store and receive data for up to 12 hours of sampling (see Figure 17.6). Photovac units offer a range of lamps

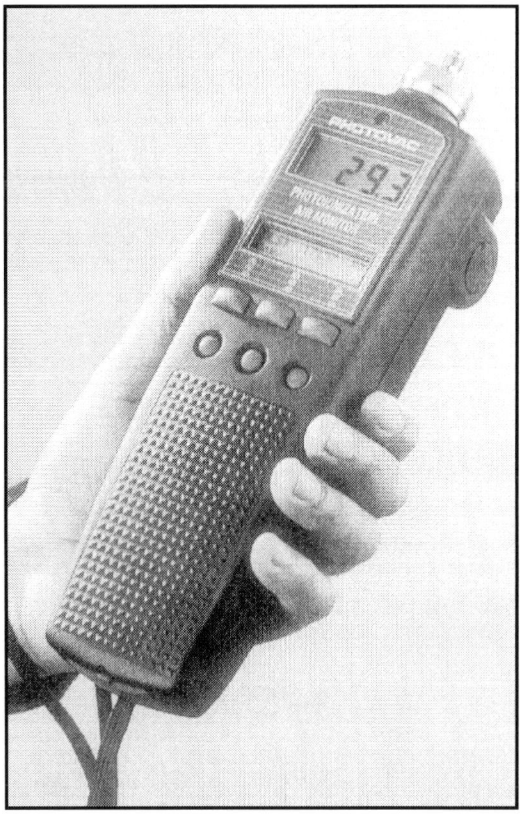

Figure 17.6 — PID: The Photovac 2020.

Table 17.5 — Relative Response of the OVA (FID Instrument) to Different Chemicals (if Calibrated to Methane)

Compound	*Relative Response (%)*
Acetaldehyde	25
Acetic acid	80
Acetone	60
Acetylene	225
Acrylonitrile	70
Benzene	150
n-Butane	63
1,3-Butadiene	28
Carbon tetrachloride	10
Chloroform	65
Cyclohexane	85
Diethylamine	75
Diethyl ether	18
Ethane	110
Ethanol	25
Ethyl acetate	65
Ethylene	85
Ethylene oxide	70
Hexane	75
Isopropyl alcohol	65
Methane (calibrant)	100
Methanol	12
Methyl ethyl ketone	80
Methylene chloride	90
Octane	80
Phenol	54
Tetrachloroethylene	70
Toluene	110
Trichloroethylene	70
Vinyl chloride	35
o-Xylene	116

including, 10.6 eV, and 11.7 eV. It can perform in a variety of environmental conditions and has a response time of less than 3 seconds.

Passive PID monitors are now available. These units do not use an active sampling pump and are typically much smaller and lighter than other units. RAE Systems (Sunnyvale, Calif.) offers a personal PID that can be mounted in the worker's breathing zone. A new instrument from RAE combines PID with LEL, O2, and toxic sensors (five-gas monitor).

Flame Ionization Detectors (FIDs)

Portable flame ionization detectors (FIDs) use a hydrogen flame as the means to produce ions, instead of the UV light used by PIDs. FIDs can be used in similar situations as PIDs, with the exception of landfill sites because of sensitivity to methane, and when inorganic chemicals are expected. In general, FIDs tend to be more difficult to operate than PIDs; however, FIDs are less sensitive to the effects of humidity. FIDs respond to a greater number of organic chemicals than PIDs and are linear over a greater range.

Using a hydrogen flame, the energy is sufficient to ionize materials with IPs of 15.4 eV or less. FIDs respond to virtually all compounds that have carbon-carbon or carbon-hydrogen bonds; therefore, they respond to nearly all organic vapors. The sensitivity of the FID to vapors depends on the energy required to break chemical bonds (the sensitivity of PIDs is related to the IP of the contaminant). Similar to PIDs, the response of the FID will vary depending on the particular chemical. The presence of functional groups will affect sensitivity because they alter the chemical environment of the carbon atom. For example, FIDs respond well to aromatic hydrocarbons, moderately to chlorinated hydrocarbons, poorly to short-chained alcohols, and not at all to formaldehyde (see Table 17.5). Although the detector response is proportional to the number of molecules, the relationship is not linear and is even skewed with organic compounds containing oxygen, nitrogen, sulfur, or chlorine.

The FID has a burner assembly in which hydrogen is mixed with the incoming sample gas stream, and this is fed to the jet where ignition occurs (see Equation 17.2). FIDs are essentially carbon counters; the organic chemicals present in the gas sample stream form carbon ions. The positively charged carbon ions formed are collected on a negatively charged electrode. The current generated is proportional to the number of ions and concentration.

$$RH + O_2 \rightarrow RH^+ + e^- \rightarrow CO_2 + H_2O \quad (17\text{-}2)$$

where

- RH = test gas
- O_2 = is necessary for combustion to occur
- RH^+ = positively charged ion
- e^- = is an electron.

The FID is insensitive to water, nitrogen, oxygen, and most inorganic compounds, and has a negligible response to carbon monoxide and carbon dioxide. This insensitivity to ambient gases makes the FID extremely useful in the analysis of atmospheric samples.

As with the PID, measurements using the FID are relative to the factory calibrant gas, methane. The meter responds accurately to methane but does not distinguish between methane and other gases. When an FID meter reads 75, it means either that there is 75 ppm of methane in the air or another chemical that is equivalent to 75 ppm of methane. Therefore, readings for all other chemicals should be recorded as ppm-methane equivalents. Methane is used because it is less expensive than most other hydrocarbon gases and is linear over a wide range of concentrations.

It is possible to perform qualitative analysis only when the atmosphere is complex and contains two or more organic compounds. The FID response will not represent the concentrations of specific organic compounds, but rather an estimate of the total concentration of volatile organic compounds. If only one organic contaminant is present, it may be possible to quantify the contaminant if the FID has been calibrated for that specific contaminant.

Before field operation, FIDs should be calibrated with a methane concentration within the concentration range expected in the field. A one-point calibration curve is usually sufficient because the instruments are linear up to 10,000 ppm. However, if concentration ranges larger than 1 to 10,000 ppm are expected, or for instruments with several measurement ranges, then a multipoint calibration should be performed. This large dynamic range (up to 107) permits field analysis over a wide range of concentrations without need for the sample to be diluted.

To zero FIDs in the field, a background reading is first obtained without the flame being lit. The user zeros the instrument on the most sensitive setting; a stable meter reading denotes proper operation of the collecting electrode in the combustion chamber. After the instrument has been stable for one minute, the flame can be ignited. To minimize contamination, it is important to use fuel that is ultra high purity; for hydrogen this corresponds to 99.999% hydrogen and less than 1% total hydrocarbon contamination. After ignition the meter reading will rise quickly then fall and should stabilize within 15 minutes. The background reading will depend on the location and is usually is 1–5 ppm as methane. This corresponds to approximately 1–1.5 ppm from methane in ambient air and 2–4 ppm from contaminants in the fuel. If clean, ambient air is not available, an activated charcoal filter can be attached to the sample inlet to remove all hydrocarbons except methane and ethane with molecular sizes too small to be trapped. When compared with a PID, the background reading for an FID will be higher because an FID responds to more contaminants.

FIDs usually have inlet particulate filters to prevent large particles from entering the combustion chamber. These filters should be changed frequently, or the particulates can adsorb contaminants and then slowly desorb and release them into the air. This will impact recovery of the instrument after sampling and background measurements. During combustion, fine particulates can be formed in the combustion chamber; over time, these charged particles can build up and attach themselves to the collecting electrode. This will result in erratic meter readings before the flame is ignited.

Some FIDs come equipped with a gas chromatography column so that they can be operated in a general survey mode (FID only) or a gas chromatograph (GC) mode. The GC mode is used for identification and quantification when there are a limited number of known contaminants in the air. The user must first calibrate the GC, as discussed in the section on portable GCs, to establish a calibration curve and peak retention times.

Thermo Environmental Instruments, Inc. (Franklin, Mass.) makes the TVA1000B which is an over-the-shoulder portable vapor analyzer that offers both PID and FID. It has an 8-hour battery life and can operate under a range of environmental conditions. The FID can measure from 0.5 ppm to ten thousand ppm or higher depending on compound.

Table 17.6 — Specific Infrared Absorption Bands for Hydorcarbons

Chemical Groups	*Absorption Band (μm)*
Alkanes (C-C)	3.35–3.65
Alkenes (C=C)	3.25–3.45
Alkynes (C_C)	3.05–3.25
Aromatic	3.25–3.35
Substituted aromatic	6.15–6.35
Alcohols (-OH)	2.80–3.10
Acids (C-OOH)	5.60–6.00
Aldehydes (COH)	5.60–5.90
Ketones (C=O)	5.60–5.90
Esters (COOR)	5.75–6.00
Chlorinated (C-Cl)	12.80–15.50

Source: Reference 7

Monitoring Multiple Gases and Vapors

IR Gas Analyzers

Direct-reading infrared gas analyzers are versatile, can quantify hundreds of chemicals, and are capable of being used for continuous monitoring, short-term sampling, and bag sampling. Advantages of portable IR analyzers are that they can measure a wide variety of compounds at concentrations in the low ppm to ppb range, are easy to use, can be set up quickly, and are relatively stable in the field. These systems have been used to detect leaks of ethylene oxide in hospital sterilization units, and nitrous oxide and other anesthetic gases in hospitals and dentists' offices.(14) IR analyzers are often used in indoor air investigations to measure the buildup of carbon dioxide; carbon dioxide used as a tracer gas can indicate whether the ventilation system is operating efficiently.

While portable IR monitors can be used for personal exposure monitoring, they are better suited to source monitoring because their size usually restricts their use to a fixed position. However, they can be used to supplement personal monitoring when air samples collected in Tedlar bags from the breathing zone of a worker or a source are analyzed with an IR monitor. IR analyzers also have been combined with videotaping to evaluate work practices and to train workers on the impact of work practices on exposure.

While it is possible to identify and quantify unknowns, most instruments are used to quantify known gases and vapors. Identification of unknowns requires a great deal of expertise in interpreting IR spectra. For some instruments, this identification can require a large IR spectral library of compounds.

Quantitative analysis by IR spectrometry is based on the principle that compounds selectively absorb energy in the IR region of the electromagnetic spectrum. The mid-IR region (2.5–20 microns) is the commonly used wavelength range for quantification. Each compound is comprised of atoms that bend, twist, rotate, and impart a vibrational energy unique to the compound. Many of the vibrational energy transitions observed in IR spectra are characteristic of certain functional groups (see Table 17.6). When a compound interacts with IR radiation, the pattern of energy absorption, called the absorption spectrum, represents vibrational patterns from the atoms and the functional groups. The characteristic absorption spectrum that is produced can be used to identify the chemical and is considered to be a fingerprint. Figure 17.7 shows an infrared spectrum for the chemical sulfur hexafluoride. The selective absorption of light at specific wavelengths allows the user to focus on defined areas of the absorption spectrum, especially where absorption is optimal and where there are no potential interferences from other chemicals.

While a compound can be identified from the spectral pattern of absorption, quantification of a compound from a spectrum is possible because the intensity of the IR absorption is proportional to the concentration of the chemical and the distance (path length) that the light travels through the chemical. The longer the path length that the IR light travels before it reaches the

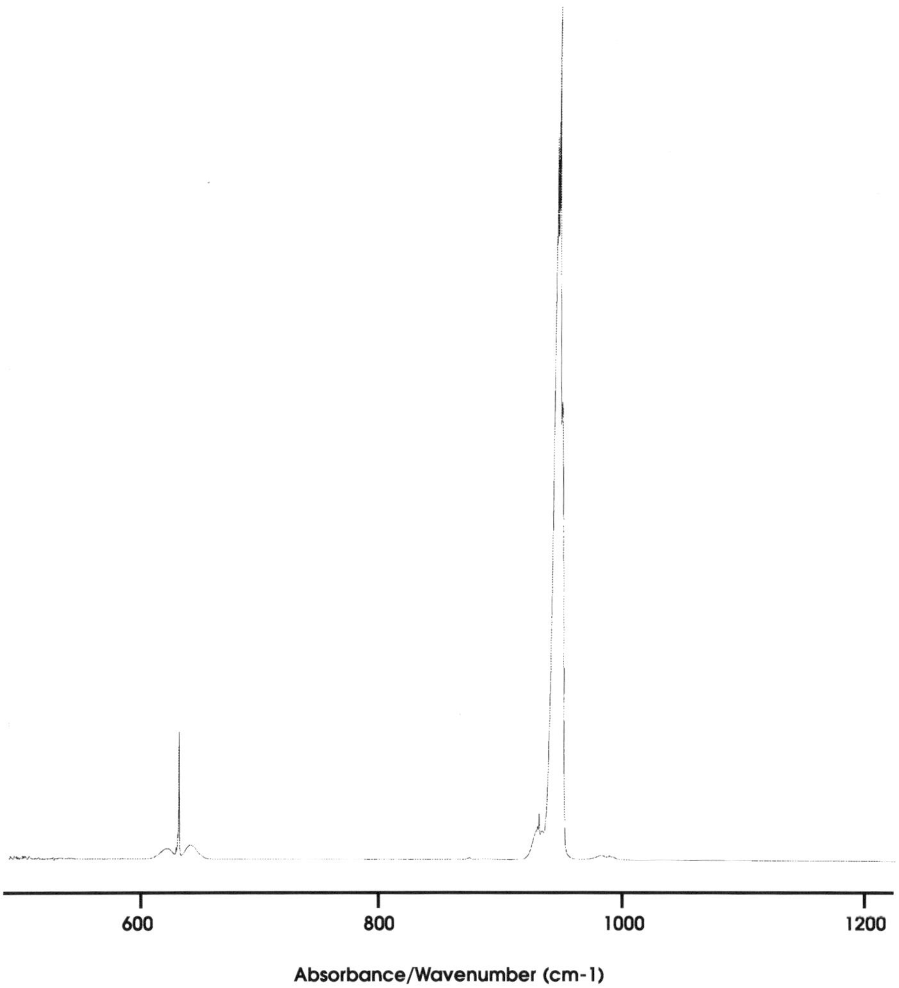

Figure 17.7 — An infrared spectrum for the chemical sulfur hexafluoride. Y axis is absorbance unit.

detector, the greater the sensitivity and the lower the limit of detection. This is described mathematically by the Bougher-Beer Lambert law as shown in Equation 17-3.

$$\frac{I}{I_0} = e^{-\mu CL} \tag{17-3}$$

where

- I = intensity of IR light with molecular absorption
- I_0 = intensity of IR light without molecular absorption
- μ = molecular absorption coefficient of the chemical
- C = concentration of the chemical
- L = path length of the IR radiation through the chemical

IR spectrometers fall into two categories: dispersive and nondispersive. Dispersive instruments use gratings or prisms to disperse the transmitted beam of IR radiation and are most often used in the laboratory. Nondispersive instruments do not use gratings or prisms; the IR beam usually passes through a band-pass filter that limits the frequency range of the light passing through the sample to the detector. The instrument detects species that absorb IR energy in the selected range. Commercially available portable IR gas analyzers are nondispersive, single beam instruments with a sample inlet, an IR radiation source (usually a Nichrome™ wire resistor), single or multiple filters to select the wavelength of radiation that passes through the sample, a closed sample cell with a fixed or variable path length, and a detector. Path lengths are achieved from 1 to 20 m using mirrors to reflect or fold the IR radiation within the sample cell. This variability in path length is used to compensate for the differences in absorption coefficients of chemicals that affect the detection limits. In the field, the instrument is first zeroed in contaminant-free air before the sample air is drawn into the gas cell by the pump. If contaminant-free air is not available, a charcoal canister, or zeroing charcoal cartridge, can be used to filter the air before it enters the instrument. This cartridge is similar to the cartridges used in respirators. The cartridge must be kept in a plastic bag to avoid contamination. If the zeroing cartridge is saturated with contaminants, and the concentration in air is lower than the concentration through the cartridge, the concentration of contaminant in the sample air may appear negative. IR analyzers are usually equipped with particulate filters to keep dust out of the sample cell, because dust will decrease sensitivity of the instrument by scattering IR light and settling on the mirrors and windows.

IR analyzers are relatively simple to operate and can be dedicated to a single compound or used to detect multiple compounds. For multiple compounds, identification and quantification using portable IR analyzers is usually performed by selecting a limited region in the IR where the compound absorbs strongly and ideally does not interfere with other compounds present in the air. If the compounds in mixtures have overlapping peaks, concentrations will appear falsely elevated. This problem may be overcome by taking a measurement at a secondary peak where the compounds do not overlap. Instruments are usually provided with a chart containing suggested path lengths and wavelengths for specific compounds at specific limits of detection. Therefore, the occupational hygienist must know the nature of both the target compounds and the environment being monitored. With this knowledge it may be possible to select wavelengths with minimal interferences. Fortunately, neither oxygen nor nitrogen interferes with IR measurements; however, water vapor is a major interferer. Measuring a compound in the region where water vapor absorbs infrared light can result in overestimation of concentrations.

IR analyzers need to be calibrated with chemicals when they are first purchased as well as before field use with a multipoint calibration curve. The pump flow meter also needs to be calibrated when the instrument is first purchased and at regular intervals. The initial calibration ensures that the sample cell and mirrors have not been damaged and the alignment has not changed during shipping. A multipoint calibration curve of absorbance versus concentration (ppm) is created by either flowing a known concentration of a gas through the cell or by generating concentrations by injecting small amounts (microliter) of a known concentration of a gas into the cell using a closed loop system. Small amounts are injected to minimize pressurization of the cell. Calibration curves should be prepared using the same instrument settings that will be used in the field.

Thermo Environmental Instruments, Inc. (Franklin, Mass.) manufactures the Miran SapphIRe line of IR analyzers. The analysis takes from 20–165 seconds depending on number of wavelengths measured. The air samples are drawn into a glass cell by a pump that can be used to measure over 100 different chemicals. The path length can be adjusted to allow for a range of sensitivities that, for some compounds, can measure sub ppm concentrations. The battery life of the instrument is approximately 4 hours.

Photoacoustic Analyzers

Quantification of air contaminants by photoacoustic spectroscopy (PAS) involves the use of sound and UV or IR radiation to quantify air contaminants. This type of spectroscopy uses the fact that molecules vibrate at a particular frequency called the resonance frequency. The number and types of atoms determine a chemical's unique resonance frequency. The resonance frequency of most molecules is about 1013 Hz or 1013 vibrations per second. When molecules are exposed to IR radiation of the same frequency as the resonance frequency, energy is transferred to the molecule, and the molecule gains energy and vibrates more vigorously. The excess energy is then quickly transferred to the surrounding medium, which is usually air or helium, in the form of heat. The transfer of energy causes an increase in the temperature of the medium and produces an increase in pressure; this increase in pressure waves, or sound waves, is detected by a microphone. The intensity of the sound emitted depends on the concentration of the contaminant and the intensity of the incident light.

Similar to analysis by infrared spectroscopy, when a contaminant is irradiated with IR light in the mid-IR region (2.5–15.4 microns), the pattern of energy absorption at specific wavelengths (the fingerprint) can be used to identify the chemical. The intensity of the absorption is proportional to the concentration of contaminants. The fundamental difference between IR spectroscopy and PAS is that in PAS the amount of light energy that is absorbed is measured directly by measuring the sound energy emitted. Interferences by carbon dioxide, water vapor, and other chemicals present in the air, which absorb at wavelengths similar to those used to measure the chemical, will compromise both the limit of detection and the accuracy of the measurement.

A typical photoacoustic analyzer consists of a radiation source that is emitted in pulses, an optical filter or filters to select wavelengths specific for the chemical, a photoacoustic cell filled with air or helium, a microphone, amplifier, recorder, and readout display. The use of optical filters limits the number of chemicals that can be evaluated at one time. Photoacoustic analyzers are usually set up to detect a single chemical or up to five known contaminants. The filters are selected to coincide with a strong absorption band in the IR for the specific gas. Detection limits are chemical-specific and are reported to be between 0.001 and 1 ppm.[15]

Both portable and fixed PAS systems are available. Portable systems are frequently used to evaluate indoor air problems by measuring the growth or decay of tracer gases in air. This measurement can be used to calculate air exchange rates and study airflows in a building. Typical tracers include carbon dioxide and sulfur hexafluoride. Tracers can also be used to evaluate the efficiency of local exhaust ventilation systems. Fixed systems can be set up to collect data from multiple points in a workplace and can be used with an alarm to signify elevated concentrations of specific highly toxic contaminants.

CAI (Orange, CA) makes a bench top or rack mounted photo acoustic analyzer that can run on batteries. It has a one-hour warm up time prior to operation and can measure five gases at a time down to the ppb range. The instrument can compensate for changes in temperature and pressure.

Portable GCs

Traditionally, GCs have been laboratory-based instruments; however, portable versions of the GC are increasingly being used as on-site monitoring devices for hazardous waste sites and for environmental and occupational hygiene monitoring. A portable GC can be transported to the field and used under battery power. The use of portable GCs has allowed on-site measurements of vapor and liquid samples; this eliminates the need to collect samples on separate media, ship them to a laboratory, store them over time, and desorb them with other chemicals. Portable GCs are particularly good for identification of specific chemicals in mixtures and unknown chemicals and are best for monitoring volatile compounds.

To date, portable GCs have not been used for compliance monitoring by the Occupational Safety and Health Administration, and generally have not replaced personal sampling methods using collection media. The use of portable GCs for occupational hygiene monitoring is likely to increase in the future; in fact, NIOSH has developed several analytical methods that rely on portable GCs.

In general, a GC consists of an injection system, a GC column, and a detector (see Figure 17.8). An ambient air or liquid sample is usually injected into the system through a septum using a gas-tight syringe, or air is pulled directly into a sampling loop using a vacuum pump. Heated injection ports are

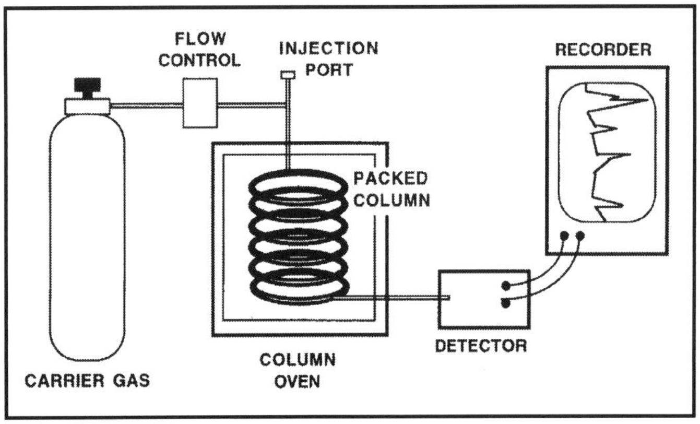

Figure 17.8 — Schematic for a typical gas chromatograph.

used to prevent condensation of chemicals with low volatility and high boiling points, or when ambient temperatures are low.

A carrier gas stream moves compounds from the injection port or sampling loop into the heart of the GC system, the gas chromatography column. The carrier gas can be high-purity air, hydrogen, helium, or nitrogen. The column is filled with packings and coatings that physically interact with the chemicals in the sample and enable separation of complex mixtures into individual compounds. Ideally, each compound will have a different affinity for the column material and will be slowed down to a different extent. The result is that individual compounds will be eluted from the column at different rates and, therefore, reach the detector at different retention times. The retention time of a contaminant depends on the type of column packing material, the length of the column, the flow rate of the carrier gas, and the temperature of the column.

There are two different types of columns: packed and capillary. The choice of the appropriate column is essential to adequate resolution of the contaminants. Selection of an improper column can result in inadequate peak separation, broad peaks, tailing, or shouldering. Packed columns consist of a fine, inert, solid material (the support phase) that has a large surface area for holding a thin film coating of a nonvolatile liquid (stationary phase). Some columns have no liquid phase, and the solid material also serves as a solid adsorbent phase. Capillary columns are hollow tubes; the specially treated glass or fused silica walls of the tube serve as the support phase. The liquid stationary phase is coated or bonded to the walls. Columns vary in length from 6 inches up to 30 feet and are usually coiled to allow their length to fit into a portable instrument.

The operating temperature of a column can affect the performance of a GC. Portable GCs with unheated columns are susceptible to changes in ambient temperatures, which can affect retention times and reproducibility of results. A rule of thumb is that column temperatures should be kept at least 5 degrees above ambient temperatures. Lack of temperature control will limit the resolution of compounds eluting from the column, the reproducibility of the results, the range of possible analyses that can be detected, and cause thermal drift. Thermal drift is the change in retention time of a compound over time. To minimize thermal drift, unheated columns should be used only for compounds with short retention times. Heated columns result in stable operating conditions and reproducible results within a large range of ambient temperatures. GCs that have columns enclosed in a temperature-controlled oven offer isothermal operation and enable regulation of temperature in 1°C increments.

Most field GCs use a technique called backflushing of a column to allow rapid clearing of residual chemicals with long retention times so that the components do not contaminate the column and interfere with subsequent analyses. Two columns are used when backflushing, a short precolumn and a longer analytical column. The precolumn is used to trap heavy, less volatile compounds. After the volatile compounds have cleared the precolumn, the carrier gas flow is reversed, and the remaining contaminants are flushed out away from the detector. Backflushing can significantly shorten the required analytical time.

Most field GCs come with a single detector; the most commonly used detectors are the FID, PID, and electron capture detectors (ECD). The detectors vary in sensitivity, selectivity, and linearity. Table 17.1 lists the characteristics of these detectors. The choice of detector depends on the chemicals for which monitoring is needed, the presence of other contaminants, and the required sensitivity. A strip chart recorder or microprocessor is usually attached to the GC; the separated components detected are represented as peaks. Concentration is then determined automatically using microprocessors that integrate the area under the peak or manually by directly measuring the peak height, calculating the area under the peak using the formula for triangles, counting the number of squares underneath the peak, or cutting out and weighing each peak. In the field, retention time and area of the peaks are then compared with peaks generated during calibration of the instrument. Field operation of GCs requires that they be calibrated with the chemical of interest under the same conditions as the chemical that will be measured in the field.

One limitation of using a portable GC is that it requires a high degree of skill to operate. The operator must calibrate the instrument and know the relative retention times and peak height characteristics of each contaminant of interest. Therefore, known concentrations of individual calibration gases or calibration gas mixtures must be used. Calibration gases can be obtained from specialty gas suppliers and should be introduced into the GC to obtain retention times, sensitivities, and peak heights. Calibration should be repeated when operating conditions are changed.

When evaluating field samples, the operator must be aware that a single peak may represent multiple contaminants that have the same retention time; organic chemicals do not all have unique retention times. Peaks may be detected that cannot be identified without using other analysis methods. The absence of a peak does not ensure that the contaminant is absent; therefore, one of the operating parameters (column, gas flow, temperature) should be changed to confirm the negative results.

If syringes are used to inject low concentration standards or samples, the occupational hygienist should use glass syringes with stainless steel plungers. The sealing ring of the plunger should be Teflon or another material that has little or no affinity for organic compounds. Syringes need to be checked regularly for leaks or blockages and need to be purged with clean air. To avoid cross-contamination, syringes used for injecting calibration gases should not be used for injecting sample gases.

The most important aspect of making accurate GC measurements is repeatability and reproducibility. Therefore, operators should have a thorough quality assurance and quality control program. Proper field operation requires the use of correct carrier and calibration gases and a detector. Some instruments use internal gas cylinders that must be charged before going to the field or external gas cylinders and regulators. Transporting gas cylinders to and from the field can pose logistical problems, particularly when flammable gases such a hydrogen are needed for the FID. Regulations regarding air or land transportation of hazardous compressed gases must be taken into consideration when planning a survey. To reduce contamination of the sample, tubing that is used to connect gas cylinders to GCs should be made of Teflon or stainless steel.

The Voyager (Photovac, Waltham, MA) can measure a wide range of organic compounds and can operate in a wide range of temperature and humidity conditions. The detection limits are typically in the 5–50 ppm range and can be operated for up to 8 hours on a battery depending on the column temperature needed. HNU (Pembroke, MA) makes a portable GC, Model 312. Detection limits range from 0.5–50 ppm depending on the chemical and can handle a wide range of environmental conditions. It has a battery life of 3–4 hours and can run off cigarette lighter adapter. The 312 has 3 ranges with computer-controlled autoranging. Set points can be programmed for each point and/or compound.

Fourier Transform IR (FTIR) Spectrometers

Direct-reading instruments based on Fourier transform infrared spectrometry are on the forefront of monitoring technology for occupational hygiene and environmental applications.[16] These instruments have the potential to monitor a wide range of compounds simultaneously at very low limits of detection (ppb). An FTIR spectrometer can monitor the same IR wavelength regions that a conventional filter-based IR spectrometer measures; however, it is much more efficient at collecting and analyzing the radiation, resulting in higher spectral resolution, greater specificity, higher signal-to-noise ratio, and lower limits of detection.[17] Spectral data obtained with the FTIR spectrometer can be used to identify unknown as well as known contaminants and can quantify chemicals in mixtures. Compounds are identified by their pattern of absorption, their "fingerprint."

At the heart of the FTIR spectrometer is the interferometer; most models use a Michelson interferometer to simultaneously detect the entire spectral region at once. Most other IR techniques scan the entire wavelength region one wavelength at a time. A simple schematic is provided in Figure 17.10. In its simplest form, the Michelson interferometer consists of a beam splitter and two mirrors, one of which is moveable. For the highest accuracy, the two mirrors should be perpendicular to one another. When a plane monochromatic wave is incident on the beam splitter of the Michelson interferometer, the amplitude of the light is evenly split into two paths toward the mirrors. The light is then reflected by the mirrors back to the beam splitter where they are recombined; interference results from the phase difference in the two IR beams. The phase difference depends on the wavelengths of light present in the beams. The detector records the intensity difference created between the stationary and moving mirrors as a function of the path difference between the two mirrors (the position of the moving mirror); this results in an interferogram (see Figure 17.10). When a Fourier transform is performed on the interferogram, a single beam spectrum is obtained, which is a plot of the intensity versus wave number (cm^{-1}) (see Figure 17.11).

When obtaining data, a clean air background spectrum is first obtained before taking the sample spectrum. A transmission spectrum is created by dividing the single beam of the sample spectrum by the background spectrum obtained in clean air. The clean air spectrum ideally removes spectral features due to chemical interferers and instrument characteristics. An absorbance spectrum is then obtained by taking the negative logarithm of the transmission spectrum. This absorbance spectrum is used for quantitative analysis by comparing it with a reference absorption spectrum for the chemicals of interest at known concentrations. Several techniques are used for quantification, including classical least squares and partial least squares.[18,19]

FTIR systems can be used in extractive or open-path modes. Extractive modes are more commonly used; open-path modes are currently being evaluated and developed. In the extractive mode the FTIR spectrometer is set up similar to IR spectrometers and uses a closed long-path gas cell. The sample is drawn into a cell using a pump, and the cell can use mirrors to create multiple reflections of IR light through the sample to create a long path length. The FTIR measurements represent the concentration of contaminants in the sampled air. Extractive FTIR spectrometers have been used for a variety of industrial and environmental applications

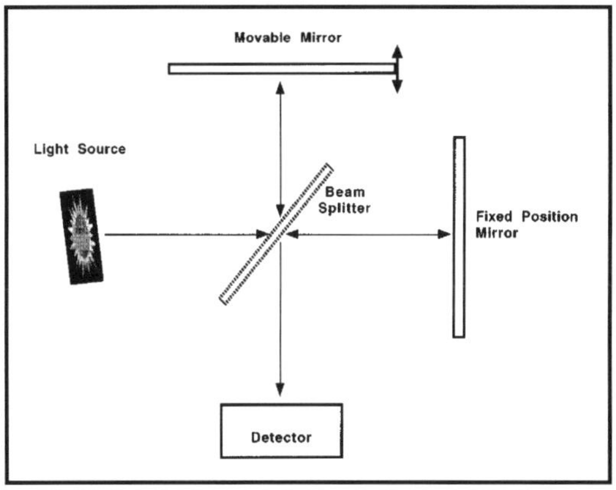

Figure 17.9 — A simple schematic of an FTIR interferometer.

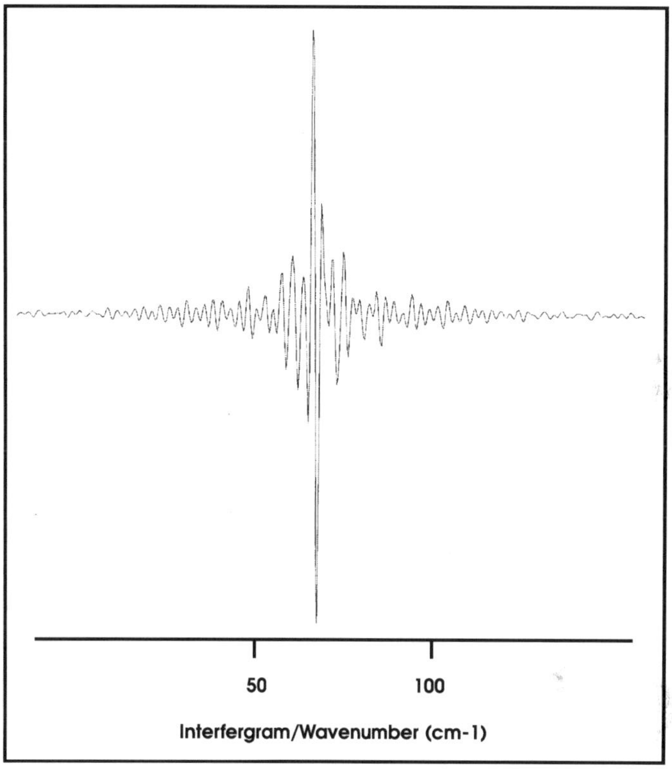

Figure 17.10 — A typical interferogram obtained with an FTIR spectrometer. Y axis is signal strength.

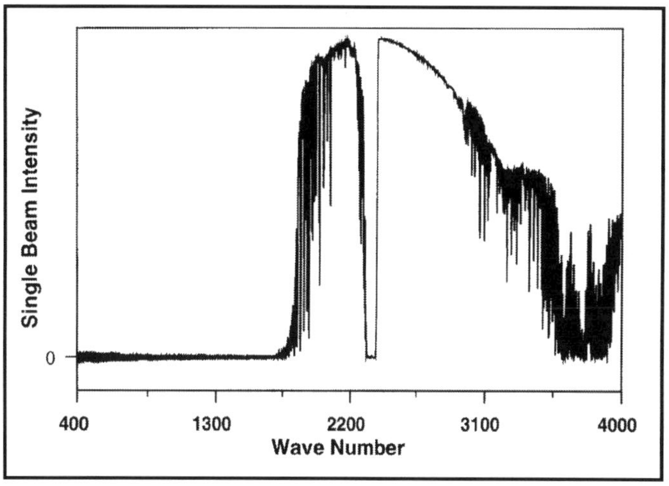

Figure 17.11 — A typical single beam spectrum obtained with an FTIR spectrometer.

including near real-time monitoring of chemicals in a semiconductor industry, auto exhaust emissions, stack gases, chemical processes, and air pollution.[20,21] Extractive systems are calibrated by generating a multipoint calibration curve for known concentrations of calibration gases before field use.

In the open-path (remote sensing) mode, the gas cell is replaced by the open atmosphere. In the bistatic configuration, the IR source is placed at opposite ends of the optical path (as far as 500 m apart) from the detector. In the monostatic configuration, the light source and detector are positioned at the same end of the path; the beam is sent out to a retroreflector placed at the physical end of the path, which reflects the light directly back to the detector. Telescopes can be used to send and receive the beam to and from the interferometer to the retroreflector (monostatic systems) or to receive the light at the detector (bistatic systems); see Figure 17.12.

When pollutants present in the optical path are measured, the concentration is integrated over the entire length of the optical path and is reported as the product of concentration and path length (ppm-meters). The concentration is then divided by the path length to obtain a path-averaged concentration (ppm).

Open-path FTIR spectrometers have only recently been used for environmental and occupational sampling. In the environmental arena, open-path FTIR spectrometers can provide real-time monitoring of industrial

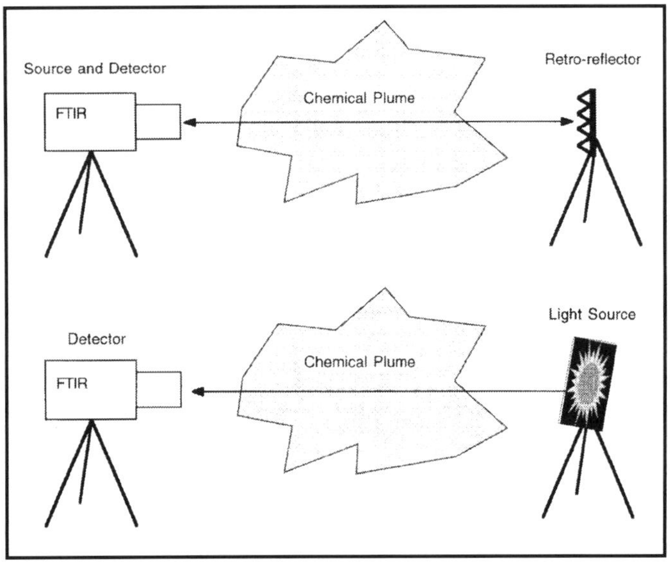

Figure 17.12 — Monostatic (top) and bistatic (bottom) open-path FTIR spectrometer systems.

fence-line and stack emissions and process leaks. In the occupational arena, open-path FTIR spectrometers have the potential to provide the temporal resolution and sensitivity required for measuring short-term exposures to acutely toxic chemicals, and the spatial coverage to detect leaks of toxic chemicals and obtain TWA concentrations of complex mixtures over large areas in a room.[22–25] This technology is attractive because these instruments can simultaneously measure a wide variety of compounds non-invasively, in real-time, and over large areas that would normally require the use of large numbers of point sampling devices. There is no contact of the instrument with the sample, and there are no sampling lines, bags, or canisters that can adsorb compounds and result in unpredictable contaminant losses.

Calibration of open-path FTIR spectrometers poses a challenging problem. Unlike the extractive FTIR, there is no gas cell that can be purged with clean air to obtain contaminant-free background data and filled with known concentrations of contaminants to determine accuracy. A custom designed calibration cell, placed in the open-path, is one of the methods being developed for field calibration and verification.

In the field, a second challenge facing users of remote sensing equipment is the acquisition of a clean background spectrum under the same experimental conditions as those taken for the sample spectrum.[26,27] The clean air spectrum ideally removes spectral features present due to chemical interferences and instrument characteristics. However, in most occupational and environmental applications, it is difficult to find air that is free of target analytes. Even if a clean air background can be obtained at the start of the day, instrument fluctuations and changing environmental conditions (e.g., partial pressure of water vapor) over the course of the day, may require obtaining additional backgrounds for greater accuracy. In the workplace, during a work shift, it may be impossible to obtain a new background spectrum once the chemical processes are underway. The impact on accuracy of using a background taken under different environmental conditions from the sample will depend primarily on the chemical being detected. For example, changes in the partial pressure of water vapor during a day can result in a significant quantification error for toluene because absorption peaks are located in regions where there is considerable water absorption.[25] Research is underway to develop quantification methods that do not require the acquisition of a clean background spectrum.

Although open-path FTIR spectrometers can provide good temporal resolution of concentrations, spatial resolution is limited because of the long optical path length over which the concentration of chemicals are averaged to provide a path-integrated output of the instrument. However, when a network of intersecting open-path FTIR spectrometers are used in a room, a technique called computed tomography can be applied to the measurements to create both spatially and temporally resolved concentration distribution maps (see Figure 17.13). These maps could be used for exposure assessment, source monitoring, leak detection, and ventilation evaluation. This technique is currently being evaluated and developed for the occupational hygiene application.[28-32]

Midac (Costa Mesa CA) makes a range of field ready open-path FTIRs. These FTIR's can be made in a bistatic or monostatic configuration with a resolution of 0.5 wave numbers with a cooled detector. Telescopes are available for long distances. The analysis software provided uses a Classical Least Squares method to quantify the concentrations. Midac FTIR's use both uncooled DTGS and cooled MCT detectors. OPTRA (Topsfield MA) makes a compact FTIR with an 8.0 wave number resolution with an uncooled pyroelectric detector and a plastic injection molded retroreflector array. The software uses an artificial neural network and partial least squares method to identify and quantify 105 different compounds common to industrial settings.

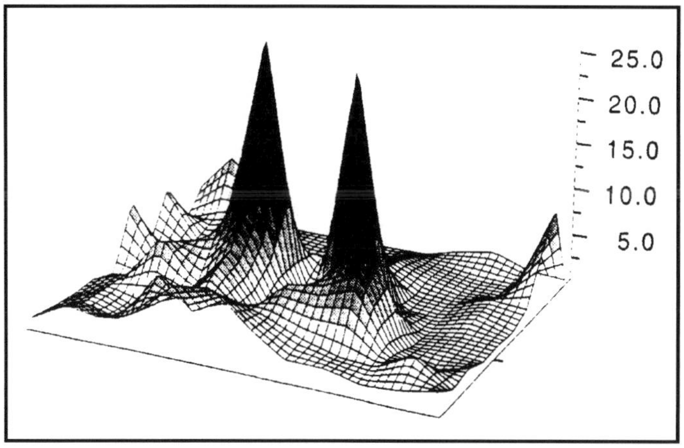

Figure 17.13 — An example of a concentration distribution map created with a computed tomography system. The height of the peaks (z axis) represents the concentration of a chemical in a room. The xy location is the location of the peaks in a room.

Detector Tubes

Detector tubes, or colorimetric indicator tubes, are the most widely used direct-reading devices due to their ease of use, minimum training requirements, fast on-site results, and wide range of chemical sensitivities. The first detector tube was developed in 1917 at Harvard University for measuring concentrations of carbon monoxide.[7] Since then detector tubes have been developed for the rapid detection, identification, and quantification of hundreds of chemicals.

A detector tube is a hermetically sealed glass tube containing an inert solid or granular material such as silica gel, alumina, pumice, or ground glass. The inert material is impregnated with one or more reagents that change color when they react with a chemical or group of chemicals. The reagents used in the tubes are selected for specific chemicals or classes of chemicals and may vary by manufacturer. When air is drawn through the tube, the length of the resulting color change (or stain), or the intensity of the color change, which occurs in 1 to 2 min, is compared with a reference to obtain the airborne concentration. There are three methods used to convert color change to concentration: (1) use the calibration scale marked directly on the detector tube, (2) use a separate conversion chart, or (3) use a separate comparison tube. The easiest tubes to use are those with a concentration scale marked directly on the tube (see Figure 17.14).

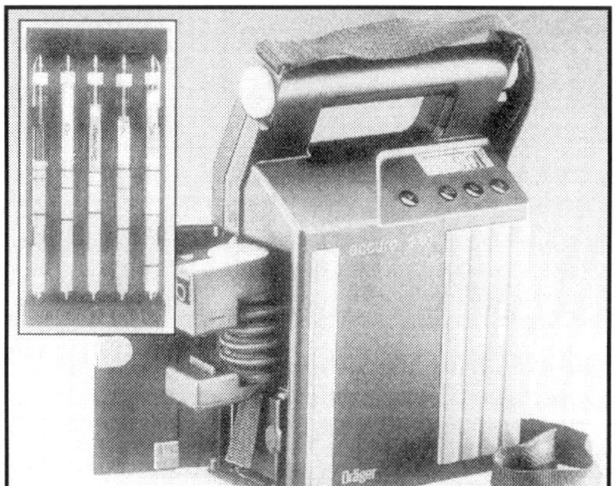

Figure 17.14 — Detector tubes, or colormetric indicator tubes, and pumps from National Draeger.

Most detector tubes contain a glass wool or cotton filter at each end to prevent particulates or aerosols from entering the tubes. Some tubes contain a prelayer that adsorbs interferences, such as water vapor or other chemicals. To use a detector tube, the ends of the tube are broken, and the tube is placed in a bellows, piston, or bulb-type pump. Both the tubes and the pumps are specially designed by each manufacturer; therefore, interchanging equipment from different manufacturers will result in significant measurement errors. When a pump stroke is performed, air is drawn through the tube at a flow rate and volume determined by the manufacturer. A specified number of strokes are used for a given chemical and detection range. Total pump stroke time can range from several seconds to several minutes. A new color detection system from National Draeger (Pittsburgh, PA) uses a battery-operated constant mass flow pump and chemical-specific chips that contain 10 capillary tubes. The color change in the capillary tube is read electronically; the concentration is displayed as a digital readout. A limited number of chemicals can be measured with this system at this time (see Figure 17.15).

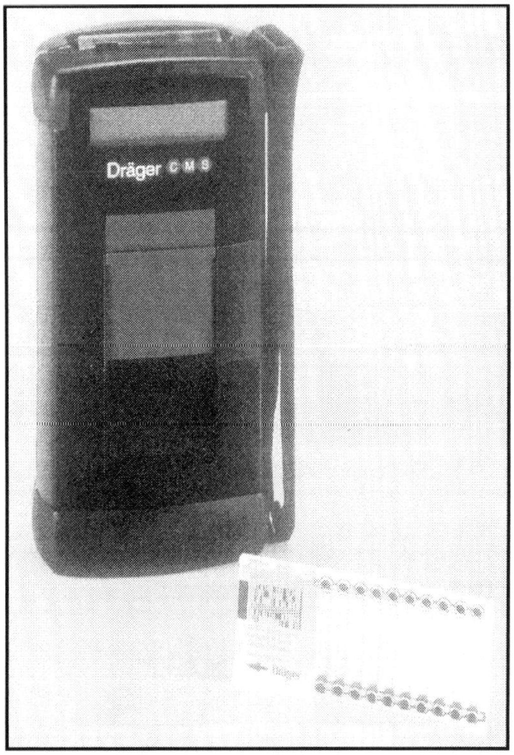

Figure 17.15 — A new generation of tubes and pumps from National Draeger.

Selection of a detector tube depends on the chemical or chemicals to be monitored and the concentration range. While tubes may be used to measure a single contaminant, most tubes react with more than one chemical, usually chemicals that are structurally similar. These interferers are documented by the manufacturer and should be understood by the occupational hygienist when evaluating the results. Usually, for a given chemical there are several tubes available to cover different measurement ranges For some chemicals there are multiple ranges available in a single tube. All manufacturers offer qualitative indicator tubes that simply record the presence or absence of a contaminant. These tubes, called poly tubes, are designed to detect a large number of organic or inorganic gases and vapors. Qualitative tubes should not be used to estimate airborne concentrations.

Detector tubes are most effective when used for determining the presence in the air of a chemical or class of chemicals. This information can then be used to choose a more accurate and complex sampling method, such as a real-time continuous monitor or personal sampler. In cases where detector tubes are the only sources of information, multiple readings should be taken successively in one location throughout the day to account for temporal variability and over several locations to account for spatial variability of concentrations and contaminant species in air. Detector tubes are not recommended for compliance monitoring of personal exposures unless there are no other alternatives. In this case, detector tubes may be placed in the breathing zone to evaluate ceiling concentrations or STEL concentrations. Detector tubes can be used for source monitoring to evaluate peak exposures; however, many tubes would need to be used to sample adequately for a long enough time period.

Detector tubes are used at hazardous waste sites for measurement of leaks and spills because they offer a wide range of specificities. Inaccessible regions can be sampled using detector tubes by attaching the detector tube to a flexible tube that is then attached to a pump. Several manufacturers have developed Hazmat kits using a variety of tubes to rapidly measure classes of contaminants. These kits have a decision matrix that enables end-users to choose the next appropriate tube or tubes depending on the reading of the previous tubes.

Detector tubes are limited by being sensitive to temperature, humidity, atmospheric pressure, light, time, and the presence of interfering chemicals. The reagents in the detector tubes are chemically reactive and can be degraded over time by temperature and light; therefore, shelf life is limited. Most tubes carry an expiration date of two to three years, which represents the maximum shelf life when stored under optimal conditions specified by the manufacturer. Chemicals in tubes exposed to sunlight, heat, and ultraviolet light can significantly degrade in a matter of hours.

Generally, detector tubes are recommended to use in the range of 0 to 40°C. However, most tubes are calibrated at 20–25°C, 760 mm Hg, and 50% relative humidity. Sampling under conditions that deviate from the calibration conditions may require corrections or conversions supplied by the manufacturer.

The primary limitation of detector tubes is their susceptibility to interferences, both positive and negative, from other chemicals. Negative interferences will result in no color change. Positive interferences can result in overestimation of concentrations, or false positives. Sometimes interferences can result in a different color change. Usually, the manufacturer documents the known interferences. Interferences can be used to the advantage of the occupational hygienist, and several different tubes can be used to screen a class of chemicals to determine what chemicals are in the air.

Some detector tubes have been designed to perform integrated sampling over long monitoring periods of up to eight hours and use low-flow peristaltic or diaphragm sampling pumps (normally at a flow rate of 10–20 cc/min). With these tubes the length of stain is usually calibrated in microliters. Using the sample volume, flow rate, and time, the measurement can be converted to a TWA concentration. Long-term tubes that rely on diffusion are also available with results indicated in ppm-hrs. Dividing by the exposure time will allow for TWA determinations. Long-term results must be corrected for temperature and pressure. Long-term tubes are subject to the same cross-sensitivities as the short-term tubes and may be more affected by environmental conditions because of the long sampling time.

Long-term tubes are effective for investigating sensitive employee concerns that require immediate attention. The tubes are usually selected for a concentration range that includes the PEL or American Conference of Governmental Industrial Hygienists' threshold limit value. The tube can be attached to the clothing of an individual and placed in the breathing zone. Long-term tubes can be used as a screening device and can detect significantly lower concentrations than their short-term counterparts. Lower limits of detection are obtained by sampling for longer periods of time.

Detector tubes and pumps were once certified by the National Institute for Occupational Safety and Health (NIOSH) to meet specific performance standards (described in the Code of Federal Regulations Title 42, Part 84), which include specifications for accuracy at four concentrations, standard deviations of the tube readings, and variation of the stain length. A program administered by the Safety Equipment Institute (SEI) now voluntarily certifies a number of tubes. The SEI publishes an annual list of tubes that have been validated by this program (SEI, McLean, Va.). The accuracy of detector tubes has been found to vary among tubes and manufacturers. To be considered acceptable, a detector tube usually must be accurate to within ±25%. Some tubes have not met these specifications and have been found to be accurate to within ±35%.

Detector tube pumps should be calibrated quarterly to ensure proper volume and flow rate measurement. Care must be taken to see that leak-proof valves and connections are maintained. Leak checks should be performed when the pump is first purchased and periodically when the pumps are idle for long periods of time. Leak checks involve inserting an unopened tube into the pump and compressing the bellows or pulling the piston back and locking it (depending on the type of pump). After 2 minutes if the bellows type pump has expanded noticeably, this indicates leakage. In the case of the piston type pump, if the piston on release does not return to a fully closed position, this indicates leakage.

Direct-Reading Aerosol Monitors

Optical Techniques for Determining Aerosol Size and Count

Optical Particle Counter

The most popular direct-reading aerosol monitors are light-scattering devices (also called aerosol photometers). They operate by illuminating an aerosol as it passes through a chamber (sensing volume) and by measuring the light scattered by all the particles at a given scattering angle relative to the incident beam. As the number of particles increases, the light reaching the detector increases. The detector can be a solid-state photodiode or a photomultiplier tube.

Scattering angle has a great influence on aerosol measurements. The smaller the scattering angle, the greater the detection of large particles. A scattering angle of 90 degrees provides the greatest sensitivity for small particles. Scatter depends on the size and shape of the particle, the refractive index of the particle, the wavelength of light, and the angle of scatter. For multiple particles, scatter depends on the particle size distribution, changes in the refractive indices with aerosol composition, dust density, and dust concentration.[33]

Light-scattering monitors are factory and field calibrated. Factory calibration is performed to ensure proper instrument response as compared with similar instruments. Field calibration is performed to improve the specificity of the monitor for particular aerosols and processes. Factory calibration is usually performed by measuring a calibrated aerosol such as Arizona road dust, oil mist, or cement dust. Field calibration involves testing the instrument with a monodisperse test aerosol of known size and refractive index or with a dust with a similar size distribution of the aerosol to be sampled. A side-by-side comparison using a gravimetric method is then performed.

Single-particle techniques based on light scattering cover a size range of 70 nm to more than 100 m and are capable of measuring concentrations of less than 1 particle/L (clean-room monitoring) to about 105 particles/cm^3 (aerosol research). Multiple-particle scattering techniques are applicable for concentration measurements of atmospheric aerosols ranging from a few micrograms per cubic meter to several hundred milligrams per cubic meter.

Single-particle, direct-reading instruments, or optical particle counters (OPCs), use monochromatic light such as a laser or light-emitting diode or a broad band light source such as a tungsten filament lamp to illuminate aerosols. In an OPC, aerosol is drawn into the instrument and light scattered by individual particles is measured by a photodetector. From the count rate and pulse height of the photoelectric pulses, the number concentration and size of particles can be determined.

Condensation Nucleus Counter

Condensation nucleus counters (CNCs) can measure very small particles (<1.0 µm) and have been used to study atmospheric aerosols for many years. They are currently used for testing high-efficiency particulate air filters in clean rooms and for quantitatively fit-testing respirators.[34] The CNC has a fast response time, is lightweight and portable, and can be used for real-time measurement. The CNC works by enlarging the particles to a size suitable to measure photometrically. The incoming air stream is first saturated with a vapor such as water or alcohol and is then cooled to induce a super-saturated solution. Vapors then condense on the particles and the particles grow in size. Using CNCs, individual particles can be counted or the intensity of the scattered light can be used to measure concentration (particles/cm^3).

Several types of CNCs have been developed that vary in the method by which the super-saturation is induced and in the method of particle detection. For example, an expansion-type CNC humidifies the aerosol with water vapor at room temperature and then cools by volume expansion or pressure release. The conductive cooling type CNC uses alcohol to saturate the aerosols and then uses conductive cooling for super-saturation; particles are measured by light scattering. The mixing-type CNC combines an aerosol stream at room temperature with a hot air stream of dibutyl-phthalate or dioctyl sebacate. The resultant mixed air is cooled down adiabatically and vapor condenses on particles at a steady-state continuous flow.

Optical Techniques for Determining Aerosol Mass

Multiple Particle Monitors

Multiple particle optical monitors are real-time dust monitors used to measure aerosol concentrations. They have been used in filter testing, atmospheric monitoring, and mine aerosol measurement. The light source used in a photometer can be monochromatic, such as a light-scattering diode or a laser, or a broad-wavelength light source, such as a tungsten filament lamp. The detector can be either a solid-state photodiode or a photomultiplier tube. When particles are drawn into the instrument, the intensity of light scattered into the detector can be used to estimate concentration. As the number of particles increases, the light reaching the detector increases.

The amount of light scattered by a particle into the detector (which determines its sensitivity and the relative response for different types of particles), depends on the size, shape, and refractive index of the particle. These instruments usually use a forward-scattering geometry, and the angle of scattering (theta) is defined relative to the light source. For most instruments, this angle is approximately 90 degrees; however, in some instruments the angle may be as small as 12 degrees.

The advantage of light-scattering methods is that they provide a linear response over a large concentration range. Concentration measurements are not affected by the sampling flow rate; however, sampling rate influences instrument response rate. These instruments actually measure particle count and not mass; therefore, to determine mass the optical properties, density of the dust, and size distribution of the dust must be constant and understood. For quantitative measurements these instruments must be calibrated with an aerosol similar in refractive index and particle size to the one being measured. The instrument must be operated in its linear range, where the number of particles detected is linearly correlated with the photometer signal. This range of linearity is limited at high concentrations by multiple scattering and at low concentrations by the stray-light background in the chamber.

An example of a portable, direct-reading respirable dust photometer designed to detect concentrations of dusts present in workplace air is the tyndallometer TM digital µP (H. Hund GmbH, Wetzlar, Germany). This instrument measures the IR light scattered by airborne dust particles at a mean scattering angle of 70 degrees. The photometer value obtained for dusts can be linearly converted into mass values of respirable dust.

A respirable aerosol monitor (GCA, Bedford, Mass.) allows real-time assessment of respirable dust by light scattering after aerodynamic separation of this fraction by a 10-mm cyclone. These instruments have been used extensively for mineral dust aerosol measurements.

A personal dust monitor, Haz-Dust II, from Environmental Devices (Haverhill, Mass.) can display inhalable, thoracic, and respirable dust levels and collect the specific size fraction by attaching a size-selective device to the sensor. This instrument uses near-forward light scattering of IR radiation to measure the concentration of airborne dust particles; IR light is positioned at a 90degree angle from a photodetector. The amount of light received by the photodetector is directly proportional to the aerosol concentration.

Electrical Techniques for Determining Aerosol Size

Several instruments combine optical detection techniques with manipulation of particle motion to measure the aerodynamic diameter of a particle. Aerodynamic diameter can then be used to describe the behavior of particles in gravitational settling, filtration, and respiratory deposition.

One instrument, the E-SPART (single particle aerosol relaxation time) (Hosakawa Micron International, Osaka, Japan) determines particle size by subjecting particles to either a superimposed acoustic and DC electric field or only an AC electrical field.[35,36] Aerosol samples are drawn into the instrument using a vacuum pump at a flow rate of 0.5 L/min. In the acoustic/electric mode, particles are subjected to sinusoidal force by an acoustic transducer at a specific frequency that induces an oscillatory velocity component in the horizontal direction. In addition, particles are subjected to a DC electric field that induces a migration velocity component, which depends on the polarity and the magnitude of the electric charge of the particle and the field strength. A differential laser Doppler velocimeter (LDV) measures the horizontal oscillatory component, and a microphone measures the acoustic field. The motion of the particle, detected by the LDV optics, lags behind the acoustic field by an amount that depends primarily on the particle aerodynamic diameter. Aerodynamic diameters are measured for both electrically charged and uncharged particles using the acoustic mode. Electrical charge is determined from the electrical migration velocity and the aerodynamic diameter. The manufacturer states that the range of aerodynamic diameters measurable with acceptable sensitivity and resolution is 0.2 to 10.0 µm.[37]

In the second mode, particles are only subjected to an AC electric field, and this mode is only applicable to electrically charged particles. A charged particle experiences an oscillatory motion in the electric field, and the oscillatory velocity component will lag behind the electric field by an amount that depends primarily on the particle aerodynamic diameter. The amplitude of the oscillations is directly proportional to the electric charge on the particles. Data generated includes number of particles counted, average charge on the particles, a plot of the size distribution of the particles, and aerodynamic diameter.

Although instrument response can be calculated theoretically, particle size calibration is usually performed using aerosolized monodisperse polystyrene latex spheres (that are less than 10 µm), or using particles greater than 10 µm generated using a vibrating-orifice aerosol generator. Calibration is performed under known conditions of temperature and humidity. Charge calibration is more difficult to perform because it is difficult to generate particles with both a known size and charge.[38] The electric field can be calculated from the distance between the electrodes and the applied voltage across the electrodes.

The Aerodynamic Particle Sizer (APS) (TSI, Inc., St. Paul, Minn.) is a relatively portable instrument that rapidly and precisely sizes most particles by measuring their velocity relative to the air velocity within an acceleration nozzle.[39] When particles are introduced into an accelerated velocity field, small particles follow the motion of the air, while large particles lag behind. This creates an increase in the relative velocity between the air and the particles. This velocity is compared with a calibration curve created using monodisperse spheres.

Aerosols are introduced into the instrument at a flow rate of 5 L/min. Air at the rate of 4 L/min is diverted through a filter and becomes clean sheath air. The remaining 1 L/min aerosol-laden air is fed into a focusing nozzle, recombined with the sheath air, and fed into an acceleration nozzle. At the exit of the acceleration nozzle each particle passes through two laser beams; light scattered from each particle causes two pulses, which are detected by a photomultiplier. The time lag between these pulses is used to calculate particle size.

Calibration of each APS instrument is unique due to variations in the nozzle sizes, laser spacing, and laser beam locations. Biases, which can be on the order of 25%, can be caused by particle density, particle shape factor, gas viscosity, and gas density.

Electrical Techniques for Determining Aerosol Count

Fibrous aerosol monitors (FAMs) (MIE, Inc.) are modified light-scattering monitors that are direct-reading devices designed to measure airborne concentrations of fibrous materials with a length-to-diameter aspect ration greater than three, such as asbestos and fiber glass. Results are reported as a fiber count rather than mass concentration. FAM instruments are extensively used for asbestos removal operations to provide real-time measurement of fiber concentrations to ensure the integrity of asbestos removal engineering control systems. At least two FAMs are used for asbestos monitoring: one inside and one outside the containment area. FAMs are usually equipped with alarms to warn of "containment barrier" failures. Conventional methods for measuring the concentration of airborne asbestos and other fibers involve time-integrated collection on filters and analysis with either a light microscope or an electron microscope.

FAMs operate by drawing air through a tube, using a diaphragm pump, where two pairs of electrodes create electric fields perpendicular to each other and to the axis of the tube. The two electric fields oscillate, which causes fibers to align and oscillate as they travel through the tube. A laser beam shines parallel to the direction of the airflow and illuminates the fibers. The fibers scatter the light in directions perpendicular to their long axes; a photomultiplier tube, positioned in the wall of the flow tube, detects the resulting pulses of scattered light. Fiber count is digitally displayed as fibers per cc and is determined from these pulses. Compact particles do not align in the oscillating field and do not produce pulses synchronous with the oscillating electric field.

One of the limitations of this method is that measurements assume that ideal cylindrical fibers are being detected. However, fibers may not have an ideal cylindrical or even ellipsoidal shape. For example, asbestos fibers may have a noncylindrical cross section, a curvature, or may exist as clumps of fibers. Fibers with curvatures or that have other attached particles may not align at 90 degrees to the detector axis as required for optimum detection geometry. FAMs cannot differentiate among fibers of different materials such as asbestos, fiberglass, cotton, or paper. Another limitation is that the laser beam has a Gaussian illumination of the detection volume; therefore, fibers in the center of the beam scatter more light than fibers at the edge of the beam. Large diameter fibers may settle and go undetected.[40]

Instrument response is calibrated by the manufacturer using a side-by-side comparison with NIOSH Method 7400, which uses a filter to collect amosite aerosol and phase contrast microscopy to count fibers. The manufacturer recommends that this type of calibration be repeated yearly. Field calibration is not possible for testing fiber count accuracy; however, FAMs can be tested for integrity of the electronics, laser alignment, and accurate flow rate.

Resonance Techniques for Determining Aerosol Mass

Piezoelectric Mass Sensors

Piezoelectric quartz crystal microbalances (QCMs) enable quick measurement of aerosol mass, particularly for respirable aerosols, and have been used in occupational hygiene and environmental monitoring for measuring welding and tobacco smoke.[41]

Piezoelectric mass sensors are based on the principle that when crystalline materials are mechanically stressed by compression or tension they produce a voltage proportional to the stress. When these crystals are subjected to an electric current, they oscillate, and the natural vibrational frequency depends on the thickness and density of the crystal. Piezoelectric quartz crystals used in QCMs are usually cut and polished on specific crystallographic planes to produce a single vibrational mode. Most clean quartz crystals vibrate at a natural frequency of 5 or 10 MHz.[42] The crystal is attached to electrodes and is part of an oscillator circuit. When particles are deposited on the crystal, the oscillation frequency decreases in direct proportion to the mass of particles. Concentration is determined from the sample flow rate, sampling time, and mass deposited. Piezoelectric aerosol sensors collect particles on a quartz crystal primarily by electrostatic precipitation or inertial impaction. Commercially available instruments may incorporate size-selective impactors upstream of the sensor to selectively measure respirable aerosols.[43,44] After deposition, most instruments have a mechanism for cleaning the crystal.

Sampling efficiency is affected by both the mass and size of particles. QCM monitors have low sensitivity when particles larger than 10 µm in diameter or large masses of particles are collected. In addition, large, elastic, or spherical particles may bounce or migrate off the crystal surface after deposition. This loss may be eliminated or decreased by applying a specialized sticky coating to the surface of the crystal. Excessive overloading of the instrument by aerosols can cause the vibration of the sensing crystal to cease altogether. Manufacturers usually provide procedures to prevent overloading and clean the crystal.

Piezoelectric mass sensors are complex and time consuming to operate. They are initially calibrated by the manufacturer, which sets the display to correspond to a measured aerosol concentration for known changes in the frequency of vibration of the quartz crystal. In the field, instruments should be calibrated by the occupational hygienist using a well-characterized aerosol such as polystyrene latex spheres or, if possible, against the expected challenge aerosol.

Tapered Element Oscillating Microbalance

Another instrument that determines aerosol mass using resonance oscillation is the tapered element oscillating microbalance

(TEOM®). In this instrument a specially tapered hollow tube constructed of a glass-like material is used instead of a quartz crystal. The narrow end of the tube supports the collection medium, usually a filter, and is made to oscillate at its natural frequency when driven by an amplifier. Aerosol-laden air is drawn into the instrument, travels first through the filter where the particles are deposited, and then through the hollow tube. As mass is collected on the filter, the natural frequency decreases and is recorded by the oscillation amplifier.

Sampling efficiency is not particularly affected by particle size; particles that are not collected by the filters do not represent a significant mass. Particle size can affect wall losses, which are common to all aerosol sampling devices. Collection of sufficient mass on the filter can conceivably result in particle bounce or migration and damping of oscillations; however, the filters would probably clog before particle loading became too great.[45]

Calibration is performed by adding a known mass to the tapered element and by measuring the change in the oscillating frequency. Rupprecht and Patashnik, (Vorheesville, N.Y.) manufactures a variety of TEOM devices for measuring diesel exhaust, emissions from underground mine fires, and chemicals in ambient air.[46]

Beta Absorption Techniques for Determining Aerosol Mass

Another instrument that measures aerosol mass uses the beta absorption method. This method is well suited to evaluate fume concentrations and chemicals in indoor air.[47] Beta absorption instruments function by measuring differential absorption of beta radiation before and after collection of particulates on a filter or an impactor. An aerosol is drawn into the instrument, sometimes through a cyclone, and collected on a surface that is positioned between a radioisotope source and an electron counter, which measures intensity. As the mass deposited increases, there is a near exponential decrease in the number of beta particles transmitted through the sample, as shown in Equation 17.4.

$$\frac{I}{I_0} = e^{-\mu x} \qquad (17.4)$$

where

I = transmitted flux of continuous beta particles
I_0 = incident flux of beta particles
μ = mass absorption coefficient for beta absorption (cm^2/g)
x = mass thickness of sample (g/cm^2)

Advantages of this technique include simplicity of instrument design, ease of automation, and a dynamic range of sensitivity that is matched to the mass range normally of interest in aerosol monitoring.

Radioisotope sources are selected using beta particle emissions with sufficient half-lives so that frequent source replacements are unnecessary, and sufficient source strengths are available to provide adequate precision. Most beta gauges use ^{14}C or ^{147}Pm isotopes, with half-lives of 5730 and 2.62 years, respectively.[48] Detectors must be sensitive to counting the beta particles at a sufficient rate to perform measurements in a short time interval. Systematic measurement errors may be due to fluctuations in atmospheric density, changes in relative humidity, and long- and short-term drift in the detector.[49]

Future Directions

As industrial processes advance and new technology is incorporated into the workplace, new challenges in direct reading instruments will be required. An example of this is nanotechnology. Nanoparticles are typically defined as any particle from 1–100 nanometers in diameter. The EPA has recently drafted a white paper nanotechnology.[50] NIOSH is investigating nanotechnology in the workplace.[51] NIOSH has identified 10 critical topics including research into new instruments to measure nanoparticles in the workplace. There are several concerns with nanoparticles. Due to their very small size they appear to be more biologically active than larger particles of the same composition. In addition, the manufacture and use of nanotechnology is increasing and it is estimated that over 2 million workers will be employed in these industries over the next 15 years. The types of current uses of this technology include: water filtration, dental bonding, and protective coatings on many materials. Additionally, while some particle counters typically used will detect the mass of the particles the issues with surface area and particle count of the nanoparticles may be inadequate to protect workers.[52]

References

1. **Ness, S.A.:** *Air Monitoring of Toxic Exposures: An Integrated Approach.* New York: Van Nostrand Reinhold, 1991.
2. **Gressel, M.G., W.A. Heitbrink, and P.A. Jensen:** Video exposure monitoring-a means of studying sources of occupational air contaminant exposure, part 1-video exposure monitoring techniques. *Appl. Occup. Environ. Hyg. 8*:334–3383. (1993).
3. **Gressel, M.G., W.A. Heitbrink, J.D. McGlothlin, and T.J. Fischbach:** Advantages of real-time data acquisition of exposure assessment. *Appl. Ind. Hyg. 3*:316–320 (1987).
4. **Feldman, R.F.:** Degraded instrument performance due to radio interference: criteria and standards. *Appl. Occup. Environ. Hyg. 8*:351–355 (1993).
5. **National Fire Protection Agency (NFPA):** National Electrical Code. Quincy, MA: NFPA, 1996.
6. **Berglund, R.N. and B.Y.H. Liu:** Generation of monodisperse aerosol standards. *Environ. Sci. Technol. 7*:147–153 (1973).
7. **Maslansky, C.J. and S.P. Maslansky:** *Air Monitoring Instrumentation: A Manual for Emergency, Investigatory, and Remedial Responders.* New York: Van Nostrand Reinhold, 1993.
8. **Snee, T.J.:** An instrument for measuring the concentration of combustible airborne material. *Ann. Occup. Hyg. 29*:81–90 (1985).
9. **Ashley, K.:** Developments in electrochemical sensors for occupational and environmental health applications. *J. Haz. Mat. 102*:1–12 (2003).
10. **Schivon, G., G. Zotti, R. Tonioloi, and G. Bontempelli:** Electrochemical detection of trace hydrogen sulfide in gaseous samples by porous silver electrodes supported on ion-exchange membranes (solid polymer electrolytes). *Anal. Chem. 67*:318–323 (1995).
11. "Hazardous Waste Operations and Emergency Response" Code of Federal Regulations, Title 29, Part 1910.120. 2009.
12. "Permit-required Confined Spaces" Code of Federal Regulations, Title 29, Part 1910.146. 2009.
13. **Barsky, J.B., S.S. Que Hee, and C.S. Clark:** An evaluation of the response of some portable, direct-reading 10.2eV and 11.8eV photoionization detectors, and a flame ionization gas chromatograph for organic vapors in high humidity atmosphere. *Am. Ind. Hyg. Assoc. J. 46*:9–14 (1985).
14. **Elias, J.D., D.N. Wylie, A. Yassi, and N. Tran:** Eliminating worker exposure to ethylene oxide from hospital sterilizers: an evaluation of cost and effectiveness of an isolation system. *Appl. Occup. Environ. Hyg. 8*:687–692 (1993).
15. **Ekberg, L.E.:** Volatile organic compounds in office buildings. *Atmos. Environ. 28*: 3571–3575 (1994).
16. **Simonde, M., H. Xiao, and S.P. Levine:** Optical remote sensing for air pollutants-review. *Am. Ind. Hyg. Assoc. J. 55*:953–965 (1994).
17. **Levine, S.P., Y. Li-Shi, C.R. Strong, and X. Hong Kui:** Advantages and disadvantages in the use of Fourier transform infrared (FTIR) and filter infrared (FIR) spectrometers for monitoring airborne gases and vapors of individual hygiene concern. *Appl. Ind. Hyg. 4*:180–187 (1994).
18. **Haaland, D.M.:** Improved sensitivity of infrared spectroscopy by the application of least squares methods. *Appl. Spectrosc. 34*:539–548 (1980).
19. **Haaland, D.M. and R.G. Easterling:** Application of a new least-squares method for the quantitative infrared analysis of multicomponent samples. *Appl. Spectros. 36*:665–672 (1985).
20. **Herget, F.W. and S.P. Levine:** Fourier transform infrared (FTIR) spectroscopy for monitoring semiconductor process gas emissions. *App. Ind. Hyg. 1*:110–112 (1986).
21. **Ying, L.-S., S.P. Levine, C.R. Strang, and W.F. Herget:** Fourier transform infrared (FTIR) spectroscopy for monitoring airborne gases and vapors of industrial hygiene concern. *Am. Ind. Hyg. Assoc. J. 50*:78–84 (1989).
22. **Xiao, H.K., S.P. Levine, W.F. Herger, J.B. D'arcy, et al.:** A transportable remote sensing, infrared air monitoring system. *Am. Ind. Hyg. Assoc. J. 52*:449–457 (1991).
23. **Spellicy, R.L., W.L. Crow, J.A. Draves, W.F. Buchholtz, et al.:** Spectroscopic remote sensing-addressing requirements of the Clean Air Act. *Spectroscopy 8*:24–34 (1991).
24. **Yost, M.G., H.K. Xiao, R.C. Spear, and S.P. Levine:** Comparative testing of an FTIR remote optical sensor with area samplers in a controlled ventilation chamber. *Am. Ind. Hyg. Assoc. J. 53*:611–616 (1992).
25. **Todd, L.A.:** Evaluation of an open-path Fourier transform infrared (OP-FTIR) spectrophotometer using an exposure chamber. *Appl. Occup. Environ. Hyg. 11*:1327–1334 (1996).
26. **Grant, W.B., R.H. Kagan, and W.A. McClenny:** Optical remote measurement of toxic gases. *J. Air Waste Manag. Assoc. 42*:18–30 (1992).
27. **Russwurm, G.M. and J.W. Childers:** *FT-IR Open-Path Monitoring Guidance Document,* 2nd edition. Research Triangle Park, NC: ManTech Environmental Technology, Inc., 1993.

28. **Todd, L.A.:** Computed Tomography in Industrial Hygiene. In *Patty's Industrial Hygiene*, 5th edition, Volume 1. Harris, R. (ed.). Hoboken, NJ: John Wiley & Sons, Inc., 2000. pp. 411–446.
29. **Todd, L. and D. Leith:** Remote sensing and computed tomography in industrial hygiene. *Am. Ind. Hyg. Assoc. J. 51*:224–233 (1990).
30. **Todd, L.A, S.K. Farhat, K.M. Mottus, and G.J. Mihlan:** Experimental Evaluation of an Environmental CAT Scanning System for Mapping Chemicals in Air in Real-time. *Appl. Occup. Env. Hyg. 16(1)*:45–55 (2001)
31. **Bhattacharyya, R. and L.A. Todd:** Spatial and temporal visualization of gases and vapours in air using computed tomography: numerical studies. *Ann. Occup. Hyg. 41*:105–122 (1997).
32. **Yost, M.G., A.J. Gagdil, A.C. Drescher, Y. Zhou, et al.:** Imaging indoor tracer gas concentrations with computed tomography: experimental results with a remote sensing FTIR system. *Am. Ind. Hyg. Assoc. J. 55*:395–402 (1994).
33. **Gebhart, J.:** Optical direct-reading techniques: light intensity system. In *Aerosol Measurement Principles, Techniques, and Applications*. Willeke, K. and P.A. Baron (eds.). New York: Van Nostrand Reinhold, 1993. pp. 313–344.
34. **Baron, P.A.:** Modern real-time aerosol samplers. *Appl. Ind. Hyg. 3*:97–103 (1988).
35. **Mazumeter, M.K., R.E. Ware, and W.G. Hood:** Simultaneous measurements of aerodynamic diameter and electrostatic charge on single-particle basis. In *Measurements of Suspended Particles* by Quasi-elastic Light Scattering. Dahneke, B. (ed.). New York: John Wiley & Sons, 1983.
36. **Renninger, R.G., M.K. Mazumder, and M.K. Testerman:** Particle sizing by electrical single particle aerodynamic relaxation time analyzer. *Rev. Sci. Instrum. 52*:242–246 (1981).
37. **Mazumder, M.K., R.E. Ware, J.D. Wilson, R.G. Renniger, et al.:** SPART Analyzer: its application to aerodynamic size distribution measurement. *J. Aerosol Sci. 10*:561–569 (1979).
38. **Mazumder, M.K., R.E. Ware, T. Yokoyama, B.J. Rubin, et al.:** Measurement of particle size and electrostatic charge distributions on toners using E-SPART analyzer. *IEEE Trans. Ind. Appl. 27*:611–619 (1991).
39. **Wilson, J.C. and B.Y.H. Liu:** Aerodynamic particle size measurement by laser-Doppler velocimetry. *J. Aerosol Sci. 11*:139–150 (1980).
40. **Baron, P.A., M.K. Mazumder, and Y.S. Cheng:** Direct-reading techniques using optical particle detection. In *Aerosol Measurement: Principles, Techniques, and Applications*. Willeke, K. and P.A. Baron (eds.). New York: Van Nostrand Reinhold, 1993. pp. 381–409.
41. **Swift, D.L. and M. Lippmann:** Electrostatic and thermal precipitators. In *Air Sampling Instruments for Evaluation of Atmospheric Contaminants*, 7th edition. Hering, S.V. (ed.). Cincinnati, OH: ACGIH®, 1989. pp. 387–403.
42. **Williams, K., C. Fairchild, and J. Jaklevic:** Dynamic mass measurement techniques. In *Aerosol Measurement: Principles, Techniques, and Applications*. Willeke, K. and P. Baron (eds.). New York: Van Nostrand Reinhold, 1993. pp. 296–312.
43. **Samimi, B.:** Laboratory evaluation of RDM-201 respirable dust monitor. *Am. Ind. Hyg. Assoc. J. 47*:354–359 (1985).
44. **Sem, G.J., K. Tsurubayashi and K. Homma:** Performance of the piezoelectric microbalance respirable aerosol sensor. *Am. Ind. Hyg. Assoc. J. 38*:580–588 (1977).
45. **Williams, K.L. and R.P. Vinson:** *Evaluation of the TEOM Dust Monitor.* (Bureau of Mines Information Circular 9119). Washington, DC: U.S. Department of the Interior, Bureau of Mines, 1986.
46. **Shore, P.R. and R.D. Cuthbertson:** *Application of a Tapered Element Oscillating Microbalance to Continuous Diesel Particulate Measurement* (Rep. 850,405). Warrendale, PA: Society of Automotive Engineers, 1985.
47. **Glinsmann P.W. and F.S. Fosenthal:** Evaluation of an aerosol photometer for monitoring welding fume levels in a shipyard. *Am. Ind. Hyg. Assoc. J. 46*:391–395 (1985).
48. **Klein F., C. Ranty, and L. Sowa:** New examinations of the validity of the principle of beta radiation absorption for determinations of ambient air dust concentrations. *J. Aerosol Sci. (U.K.) 15*:391–395 (1984).
49. **Courtney W.J., R.W. Shaw, and T.C. Dzubay:** Precision and accuracy of beta gauge for aerosol mass determinations. *Environ. Sci. Tech. 16*:236–239 (1982).
50. **U.S. Environmental Protection Agency (EPA):** EPA 100/B-07/001 U.S. Environmental Protection Agency. Nanotechnology White Paper. February 2007.
51. **National Institute for Occupational Safety and Health (NIOSH):** Nanotechnology at NIOSH. Available at www.cdc.gov/niosh/topics/nanotech/. [Accessed on October 9, 2009].
52. **Schulte P., C. Geraci, R. Zumwalde, M. Hoover, and E. Kuemple:** Occupational risk management of engineered nanoparticles. *J. Occup. Env. Hyg. 5*:239–249 (2008).

Outcome Competencies

After completing this chapter, the reader should be able to:

1. Define underlined terms used in this chapter.
2. Describe indoor air quality (IAQ) impacts on health.
3. Describe the building environment.
4. Discuss future trends in building design and energy conservation and their impact on IAQ.
5. Describe building HVAC systems.
6. Discuss ASHRAE ventilation standards.
7. Describe how HVAC systems impact air quality.
8. Anticipate and recognize IAQ problems.
9. Describe the planning and conduct of an IAQ survey.
10. List pollutant categories.
11. Describe two procedures for sampling indoor air contaminants.

Prerequisite Knowledge

College chemistry and biology

Prior to beginning this chapter, the reader should review the following chapters:

Chapter Number	Chapter Topic
4	Occupational Exposure Limits
5	Occupational Toxicology
6	Occupational Epidemiology
7	Principles of Evaluating Worker Exposure
9	Comprehensive Exposure Assessment
14	Sampling and Sizing Particles
22	Biohazards and Associated Issues
28	Occupational Health Psychology
32	Ergonomics
43	Hazard Communication
45	Risk Communication

Key Terms

β(1,3)d-glucans • air quality • allergen • building-related disease • endotoxin • hypersensitivity diseases • Legionella • multiple chemical sensitivity • mycotoxins • ozone • pollutants • psychosomatic • radon • radon progeny • sick building syndrome • toxicoses • volatile organic compounds

Key Topics

- I. Health Effects Related to IAQ
  - A. Overview
  - B. Building-Related Disease
  - C. Asthma and other Hypersensitivity Diseases
  - D. Infections
  - E. Toxicoses
  - F. Cancer
  - G. Sick Building Syndrome
  - H. Psychosomatic Symptoms
  - I. Multiple Chemical Sensitivity
- II. Buildings and Building Environments
  - A. Thermal Comfort
  - B. Relative Humidity
  - C. Odors and IAQ
  - D. Trends in Building Design, Materials and Furnishings
- III. Ventilation
  - A. Heating, Ventilating, and Air-Conditioning Systems
  - B. Ventilation Standards
  - C. Indoor/Outdoor Relationships
  - D. Filtration
  - E. Problems with Maintaining Standard Ventilation
  - F. Ventilation System Contamination
  - G. Insulation in Ventilation Systems
  - H. Assessing Ventilation Problems
- IV. Pollutant Categories
  - A. Standards and Guidelines for Indoor Air Contaminants
  - B. Chemical Agents
  - C. Biological Agents
- V. IAQ Problem Investigation, Remediation and Prevention
  - A. IAQ Investigation Strategies
  - B. Preventative Measures and Maintaining Good IAQ
- VI. IAQ Around the World
- VII. Concluding Remarks
  - A. State of the Art
  - B. Controversial Topics and Research Needs
  - C. Summary
- VIII. Acknowledgements

Indoor Air Quality

18

Ellen C. Gunderson, CIH, CSP and Catherine C. Bobenhausen, CIH, CSP, LEED AP

Introduction

Buildings, and especially homes, are often considered safe havens, sheltering people not only from harsh weather, but also from air pollution, and people spend nearly 90% of the time indoors. However, recent experience shows that the indoor environment is not always comfortable, problem-free, or even equal to the outside environment.[1,2] Over the past few decades, industrial hygiene practitioners have been spending a growing proportion of their time responding to health and comfort issues associated with buildings. Indoor air quality (IAQ) research and the collective experience with numerous and varying IAQ cases has led to the maturation of this relatively new field of practice.[3] The common approach of sampling for specific contaminants and comparing airborne concentrations to occupational exposure levels is not sufficient to diagnose and resolve IAQ problems. The traditional role of the industrial hygienist as a "detective in the workplace" bears great relevance to the practice of IAQ problem resolution. At the present time, it is generally recognized that good IAQ makes good business sense and that proactive measures to prevent IAQ problems are cost effective. This is illustrated by the current trend in green, sustainable and high performance building programs that include IAQ components.[4]

Practitioners should have a fundamental knowledge base — which includes knowing common sources of IAQ problems (Table 18.1), potential chemical and biological contaminants and their health effects, and also a keen understanding of buildings and ventilation systems. While developing a general knowledge of heating, ventilating and air conditioning (HVAC) systems and how they are maintained and operated, the IAQ investigator must also know the limits of their practice, and enlist the help of professionals, such as engineers and HVAC specialists, when needed. A professional, objective demeanor is essential when working with building owners, managers and occupants.

As HVAC equipment, systems and controls have grown more complex, organizations like the American Society of Heating, Refrigerating and Air-Conditioning Engineers (ASHRAE) and the U.S. Green Building Council (USGBC) have placed greater importance on the need to prevent IAQ problems from the outset, by ensuring that systems are designed to deliver sufficient outside air to building occupants, and that, once installed, the equipment is commissioned to ensure that it will operate as designed. More emphasis is placed on establishing building operating and maintenance procedures and on training building staff. Still, industrial hygiene practitioners, in the course of investigating IAQ complaints in new buildings as well as old buildings, encounter obvious deficiencies, such as chemical storage in mechanical rooms, fans running backwards, and HVAC systems running with little or no outside air.

The typical office environment — a fluorescent-lit, carpeted landscape flanked by rows of computer workstations under a ceiling of acoustical tile, inside a sealed office tower — if not outright inhospitable to people, is arguably not the most delightful place for people to be. Surveys have found that daylit spaces, openable windows, and individual control of temperature and light

Table 18.1 — Common IAQ Issues/Pollutants and Potential Sources

IAQ Issues and Pollutants	*Potential Sources*
Inadequate ventilation (insufficient outside air, nsufficient airflow, inadequate circulation)	Energy-saving and maintenance measures, improper system design or operation, occupant tampering with HVAC system, poor office layout, system unbalanced
Temperature and humidity extremes	Improper placement of thermostats, poor humidity control, inability of the building to compensate for climate extremes, tenant-added office equipment and processes
Combustion contaminants	Furnaces, boilers, generators, gas or kerosene space heaters, tobacco products, outdoor air, vehicle exhaust
Volatile organic compounds (VOCs)	Paints, stains, varnishes, solvents, pesticides, adhesives, wood preservatives, waxes, polishes, cleansers, lubricants, sealants, dyes, air fresheners, fuels, plastics, copy machines, printers, tobacco products, perfumes, dry cleaned clothing, carpets, furnishings
Formaldehyde	Particle board, pressed wood products, plywood, insulation, cabinetry, furniture, wallpaper, fabrics
Biological contaminants	Wet or damp materials, cooling towers, humidifiers, cooling coils or drain pans, damp duct insulation or filters, condensation, re-entrained sanitary exhausts, bird droppings, cockroaches or rodents, dustmites on upholstered furniture or carpeting, body odors
Soil gases (sewer gas, VOCs, methane)	Contaminated soil, sewer drain leak, dry drain traps, leaking underground storage tanks, landfill
Radon	Uranium-bearing soil under buildings, groundwater, construction materials
Ozone	Infiltration of outdoor air, some electrical air cleaners, office machines
Pesticides	Termiticides, insecticides, rodenticides, fungicides, disinfectants, herbicides
Particles and fibers	Printing, paper handling, smoking and other combustion, outdoor sources, deterioration of materials, construction/renovation, vacuuming, insulation, carpets, housekeeping
Environmental tobacco smoke (ETS)	Lighted cigarettes, cigars, pipes
Asbestos	Building materials in older buildings deteriorated or disturbed during renovation
Lead	Lead-based paint deterioration or improper removal, contaminated soil

levels, often contribute to a heightened sense of well-being indoors, and new building designers are taking note, with a rising trend towards high performance, "green," building design which incorporates such features. Attention to chemicals used in paints, sealants, floor finishes, and other potentially noxious products used during interior fit-out has led to alternative, lower-emitting products and technologies. The carpet and rug industry has embraced a labeling program which is based on meeting specific criteria to limit off-gassing.[5] Composite wood products such as medium density fiberboard and particleboard used in cabinetry, furniture, doors, and other wood-based products, are available without added urea-formaldehyde, commonly used in resin and adhesive. Each of these initiatives helps to reduce recognized sources of discomfort in the indoor environment. However, current understanding of the complex chemistry associated with emissions from building materials, cleaners, air fresheners, and consumer products remains incomplete.

IAQ testing can be requested by building owners, and architects, to achieve credit under the USGBC's Leadership in Energy and

Environmental Design (LEED) green building rating systems.[6] The purpose of such testing is to determine the acceptability of indoor air prior to occupying the building, by comparing air quality in newly-constructed spaces against criteria for certain contaminants.

It has been known for hundreds of years that infectious disease is more readily transmitted indoors, but the knowledge about the consequences of long-term exposure to trace levels of airborne chemicals indoors and their chemical interaction is still evolving.[7,8] Advances in analytical chemistry and sampling methodology are leading to greater knowledge about the chemical makeup of indoor air, and the health consequences are still being discovered. Research into IAQ-related health effects and building environments not only adds to the understanding of IAQ problems, but also helps define what is "normal" and what is not. And so, the basis for developing standards for specific contaminants indoors comes from the growing knowledge of what is "normal" or "acceptable" in buildings.

ASHRAE in its standard for ventilation for acceptable indoor air quality defines acceptable IAQ as "air in which there are no known contaminants at harmful concentrations as determined by cognizant authorities and with which a substantial majority (80% or more) of the people exposed do not express dissatisfaction."[9] The ASHRAE standard also cites various guidelines and standards including those for outside air quality, as relevant to indoor air. The "majority" or "80% rule" — while perhaps helpful as the basis of design — is less useful for the industrial hygiene practitioner in that it does not account for IAQ effects on absenteeism or reduced productivity or a medical diagnosis of disease for one person (let alone up to 20%), which cannot be ignored if it might be related to air quality in the work environment.[10] There are also special occupancies that demand stricter standards because of the occupants' susceptibilities, such as hospitals, health care facilities and schools. Such occupancies are addressed by specific guidelines set by ASHRAE and others, including the Joint Commission on Accreditation for Healthcare Organizations, for hospitals.

It should be noted that, in spite of increasing knowledge (noted by the many publications cited in this chapter), there are still many issues in the area of IAQ that are not fully resolved and will require further research. The future holds many new questions as well. How will lowering energy consumption in buildings (to save money and in some cases in response to global climate change concerns) affect IAQ? Does green building design really improve IAQ, or is there still an overly simplistic view of what is needed? In many investigations the actual causes of complaints remain elusive. Ongoing epidemiologic research into building-related complaints and laboratory-based studies on the relationships between exposure and disease for specific agents offer promise for the future.

Health Effects Related to IAQ

Overview

Air pollutants can irritate the mucus membranes of the eyes, nose, throat, and upper airway, and cause coughing, sneezing, and/or nasal irritation. Depending on their size and solubility, they may be inhaled and drawn in to the upper or lower respiratory tract, where they can impact the membrane. From there, they may be absorbed and affect other target organs. Some are stored inside the body — in the bone, fat, kidneys or liver, creating the potential for adverse health effects over time, even in the absence of acute effects at the time of exposure. In addition, some pollutants cause skin rashes and itching. The health impact of some indoor air contaminants may be more pronounced in residential settings because of specific sources such as secondhand smoke, also known as environmental tobacco smoke (ETS), and radon, both of which are known human carcinogens. Lead is another serious residential hazard, particularly problematic for young children, primarily from lead-based paint, which is found in dust which can be handled and eaten as well as inhaled from the air.

Building-Related Disease

Diseases related to building occupancy include allergic asthma, and allergic rhinitis; infectious diseases such as legionellosis, tuberculosis, influenza, measles; hypersensitivity diseases such as hypersensitivity pneumonitis (also called allergic alveolitis), and humidifier fever; and toxic effects resulting from exposure to specific chemicals (e.g., carbon monoxide, pesticides, or microbial toxins). Long term (years) exposure to indoor air pollutants, such as radon and ETS, may result in increased risk of lung cancer.

Asthma and Other Hypersensitivity Diseases

The hypersensitivity diseases important with respect to indoor air all result from specific immune system responses to environmental challenges.[11] There are two general categories: the IgE-mediated diseases (asthma, allergic rhinitis, or hay fever) and hypersensitivity pneumonitis, which is mediated by IgG and the cellular immune system. All hypersensitivity diseases require an initial series of sensitizing exposures during which the immune system becomes activated. Symptoms occur on subsequent exposures in response to stimulation of the previously activated immune response. Most cases of hypersensitivity disease are caused by proteins or glycoproteins, although some highly reactive chemicals can bind to larger molecules to cause hypersensitivity pneumonitis.

The prevalence of asthma has significantly increased over the past few decades, and researchers are concerned that the indoor environment may play a role in this increase. According to the American Academy of Allergy, Asthma and Immunology (AAAI), asthma's primary cause is inflammation of the airways in the lungs. This inflammation makes the airways smaller, which makes it more difficult for air to move in and out of the lungs. It is considered the most common serious chronic disease in children.[12] Table 18.2[13] defines the different types of asthma and lists indoor allergens and irritants that may exacerbate asthma symptoms or trigger asthma attacks. Some of the most common include ETS, dust mites, mold, cockroaches and other pests, cat and dog dander, and nitrogen dioxide from combustion sources. Exposures to formaldehyde and other VOCs (from fragrances and cleaning products), and ozone have also been associated with asthma symptoms in more recent studies. Damp conditions in buildings are also seen as a contributing factor.[14–16]

Numerous studies into the actual cause of asthma have shown that dust mite allergen is strongly associated with the development of asthma in susceptible children. Findings also suggest that ETS is associated with asthma development in preschool age children.[14]

Even though much of the asthma research has focused on residential environments and the effects on children, the practitioner should be aware that asthma trigger findings also apply to office environments and to sensitized individuals.

Infections

The most common of building-related diseases are contagious illnesses, which are readily transmitted through indoor air, especially in crowded environments.[17] These diseases include influenza, the common cold, and tuberculosis. The only infectious disease that is commonly spread from environmental reservoirs is Legionnaires' disease. A form of pneumonia, Legionnaire's disease is considered to be fairly common and serious in the U.S.[18] Pontiac fever is a non-pneumonia, flu-like disease which is also associated with Legionella bacteria. All of the environmental-source infections are opportunistic, requiring some deficit in the immunity of the host before infection can occur. By definition, all infections are caused by biological agents.

Toxicoses

Most of the common indoor air pollutants are toxins that exert their effects in a dose-response manner, for the most part without regard to host susceptibility. Many are inflammatory agents that act directly on the contacted cells. Some are absorbed and exert effects on organ systems distant from the site of exposure. Some cross the blood-brain barrier to cause central nervous system effects. Most toxicoses associated with indoor air are caused by exposures to chemicals derived from combustion such as carbon monoxide (CO), nitrogen dioxide (NO_2) or from activities or materials used in the environment (e.g., the VOCs). With the exception of endotoxin and the glucans, exposure to biological toxins in levels sufficient to cause disease is rare in non-industrial indoor environments.

Cancer

A number of indoor air pollutants have been classified as known human carcinogens. This includes ETS, formaldehyde, benzo(a)pyrene and other polycyclic aromatic hydrocarbons (PAHs), benzene, chlorinated

Table 18.2 — Types of Asthma[13]

Type of Asthma	*Definition*	*Triggers*	*Prevalence*
Allergic Asthma	• Characterized by airway obstruction associated with allergies and triggered by substances called allergens.	• Airborne pollens • Molds • Animal dander • House dust mites • Cockroach droppings	• Allergic asthma accounts for nearly 60% of all asthma cases.
Non-Allergic Asthma	• Caused by viral infections, certain medications or irritants found in the air, that aggravate the nose and airways.	• Airborne particles (e.g., coal, chalk dust) • Air pollutant (e.g., tobacco smoke, wood smoke) • Strong odors or sprays (e.g., perfumes, household cleaners, cooking fumes, paints or varnishes) • Viral infection (e.g., colds, viral pneumonia, sinusitis, nasal polyps) • Aspirin-sensitivity • Gastroesophageal reflux disease (GERD)	• About one-third of all asthma sufferers have non-allergic asthma.
Exercise-Induced Asthma (EIA)	• Triggered by vigorous physical activity. Symptoms of EIA occur to varying degrees in a majority of asthma sufferers and are likely to be triggered as a result of breathing cold, dry air while exercising.	• Breathing airborne pollens during exercise • Breathing air pollutants during exercise • Exercising with viral respiratory tract infections • Exercising in cold, dry air.	• Exercise can cause symptoms in up to 80% of people with asthma. • 35–40% of people with seasonal allergies also have EIA and symptoms worsen during the spring and fall.
Occupational Asthma	• This type of asthma is directly related to inhaling irritants and other potentially harmful substances found in the workplace.	• Fumes • Chemicals • Gases • Resins • Metals • Dusts and vapors • Insecticides	• As many as 15% of all asthma cases in the U.S. have work-related causes. • Occupational asthma is the most prevalent work-related lung disease in developed countries.
Nocturnal Asthma	• Also known as sleep-related asthma, this type of asthma occurs when a person is sleeping regardless of the time of day. However, symptoms worsen between midnight and 4 a.m.	• Temperature changes in the body • Allergen exposure in the bedroom • Gastroesophageal reflux disease (GERD) • Low circulation of adrenal gland hormones • Delayed reactions to allergens exposed to during the day	• Nocturnal asthma occurs in as many as 75% of asthma patients.

solvents such as tetrachloroethylene, and radon gas. Studies have shown that carcinogens, especially formaldehyde, are routinely found in homes, often at higher concentrations than concurrent outdoor levels, due to the presence of indoor sources. Primary sources are emissions from building materials and furnishings and consumer products.[15] The actual cancer risk is unclear for long term exposures to low level concentrations of many indoor pollutants such as formaldehyde. Conversely, significant lung cancer risks have been shown for long term indoor exposures to ETS and radon gas. ETS even produces a synergistic effect with radon exposure.

Sick Building Syndrome (SBS)

SBS is the term used to describe situations in which building occupants experience acute health and comfort effects that appear to be linked to time spent in a building, but no specific illness or cause can be identified.

SBS can include symptoms associated with acute discomfort, such as headache; eye, nose, or throat irritation; dry cough; dry or itchy skin; dizziness and nausea; difficulty in concentrating; fatigue; and sensitivity to odors. The cause of the symptoms is not known, and most of the complainants report relief soon after leaving the building. The symptoms are subjective, rarely associated with objective clinical findings, and are typically present in some occupants of all buildings at some time. To be considered an outbreak of SBS, the reported incidence should be at least 20%, there should be some commonality among the symptoms, and a clear temporal association between symptoms and building occupancy should be apparent.

Outbreaks of SBS have been attributed to exposure to VOCs, low relative humidity, endotoxin, some factor within dust, and unknown exposures resulting from underventilated air.

Psychosomatic Symptoms

In cases where there are no objective clinical findings, it can be difficult to separate environmentally-caused symptoms from those created by suggestion, or those that are the result of either on-the-job or other stress. Media focus can elevate concern. Fear can lead to psychosomatic symptoms that mimic illness. A good strategy in these cases is to map reported complaints in space and time. Features to examine are shifting incidence in time and/or space not associated with ventilation system parameters, an epidemic curve consistent with person-to-person rather than common-source transmission, and consistent lack of medical correlates of exposure. Involving medical professionals is valuable in situations where cancers are unrelated and yet building occupants suspect a "cluster." Exploring possible causes of widespread worker dissatisfaction is also of help in assessing questionable cases of SBS. On the other hand, poor air quality is a general stressor and can trigger complex psychological reactions including changes in mood, motivation, and problems with interpersonal relations.

Multiple Chemical Sensitivity (MCS)

Multiple chemical sensitivity (MCS) has been defined as a condition in which a person reports sensitivity or intolerance (as distinct from an allergic reaction) to a number of chemicals and other irritants at very low concentrations.[19] It is frequently associated with indoor environments, with symptoms similar to those of SBS. There are different views among medical professionals about the existence, causes, diagnosis, and treatment of this condition. Many recognized medical groups and societies, including the Centers for Disease Control and Prevention (CDC), the American Medical Association and the American Academy of Allergy, Asthma and Immunology, do not consider MCS a distinct physical disorder. The basis for this conclusion is the absence of clinical evidence to support a physical cause for the symptoms, and the absence of antibodies which would suggest a response to chemical exposure, as is the case with an immune response, or allergic reaction. In addition, many MCS patients appear to have other psychological disorders that may contribute to the symptoms.

There is consensus however, that complaints of MCS should not be dismissed as psychogenic, and a thorough workup is essential.[20] The IAQ investigator should take MCS issues seriously, respond quickly to complaints, implement appropriate corrective actions and work with medical professionals as needed. Given the prevalence of MCS and chemical sensitivity cases and the need to standardize the diagnosis, researchers and clinicians developed the following six consensus criteria for the diagnosis of MCS.[21]

1. The symptoms are reproducible with repeated (chemical) exposures.
2. The condition is chronic.
3. Low levels of exposure (lower than previously or commonly tolerated) result in manifestations of the syndrome.
4. The symptoms improve or resolve when the incitants are removed.
5. Responses occur to multiple chemically unrelated substances.
6. Symptoms involve multiple organ systems.

A number of resources are available that expand on the MCS debate, present case studies and diagnostic tests, and summarize research on opposing sides of the issue.[22–24]

Buildings and Building Environments

IAQ concerns have called industrial hygienists into a wide range of buildings — among them schools, apartment buildings, offices, hospitals, medical centers, hotels, retail establishments, government buildings, nursing homes, and the administrative offices of manufacturing facilities. The profession has played roles in all phases of new construction, as well as in maintenance, renovation and demolition of buildings.

The primary objective for involving an industrial hygienist is to prevent health effects and to ensure comfortable conditions for people in the building, whether they are children, immunocompromised patients, or the public at large. This review will describe many of the common problems in buildings today, actions needed to help solve IAQ problems, discuss some issues related to specific building types and occupancies, and speculate on future trends and challenges.

Thermal Comfort

The greatest source of dissatisfaction with IAQ in offices is with temperature, which is highly subjective and subject to individual preference. Indeed, ASHRAE defines thermal comfort as "that condition of mind which expresses satisfaction with the thermal environment."[25] Personal activity, clothing, fitness level, air temperature, air movement, and relative humidity (RH) can influence the perception of thermal comfort. Small swings in temperature (on the order of 1–2°F) can affect thermal comfort. Personal control over temperature settings in work areas is often a means of increasing satisfaction.

For sedentary workers, air temperature, air movement, and clothing are the most important factors, while RH has little effect on thermal comfort. In fact, it has been shown that sedentary people are unable to perceive changes in RH over a relatively wide range. Lowering RH in the presence of active workers has a cooling effect. In environments where both active and sedentary workers coexist, a slightly warm air temperature at low RH might provide comfort for most, although it is rarely possible to satisfy everyone. Increasing air movement decreases body temperature and people feel cooler. However, minimal air movement can lead to complaints of still, stale air and poor air exchange.

Aside from thermal comfort issues, elevated temperatures (as well as elevated RH) have been shown to heighten perceptions of poor IAQ and result in more complaints, as temperature and humidity increase.[26,27] Additionally, formaldehyde and other VOCs tend to be emitted at greater rates from building materials and furnishings at higher indoor temperature and humidity.

Relative Humidity (RH)

Extremes in RH have been associated with poor IAQ. Low RH has been blamed for some of the symptoms of SBS, for increased susceptibility to infectious disease, and for exacerbation of asthma. Eye irritation, throat irritation, and cough are often blamed on low RH, but it is becoming clear that most people are comfortable at RH levels that routinely occur even in cold winter climates (<25%), if adequate ventilation is provided to control odors and other air pollutants.

Some evidence indicates that host susceptibility to airborne infectious agents is not as affected by RH as was once thought. Usually, the increased incidence of colds and influenza in winter has been used as evidence for the role of RH in susceptibility to infections. The dry air is considered either to damage mucous membranes or to damage the infectious agents themselves. Damage to mucous membranes at other than extremely low RH (<5%) has not been documented.

Available moisture, expressed as water activity, or the amount of water available in a material, is more important than RH with respect to microbial growth, since microorganisms grow on surfaces and in materials, not in the air.[28] Growth of microorganisms on surfaces and the survival of the house dust mite, a source for potent asthma-inducing allergens, is facilitated by high RH (>60%). Even at lower RH, cool surfaces may lead to condensation that can support fungal and/or dust mite amplification. There is growing evidence that moisture problems and dampness in buildings lead to adverse respiratory health effects. Damp conditions are associated with asthma and may lead to its development and/or exacerbate the condition. Other conditions such as the presence of dust mites and fungal allergens that are common to damp buildings may be contributing factors in such cases.[14]

Odors and IAQ

Mechanical ventilation standards were first established on the basis of controlling human body odor. More recently, body odor has become of less concern because of improvements in both personal hygiene and in HVAC equipment. Perception of almost any odor in a supposedly clean environment will elicit a negative response in some people. Especially problematic are odors that are unexpected in the environment. For example, paint odors that might be acceptable at home would be perceived as disturbing in a work environment, especially where stress or unrelated illness has lowered the threshold for tolerance. Cigarette smoke is perceived as offensive in most places in the U.S., as the result of smoking bans for most building occupancies.

Inadequate ventilation can cause adverse effects in the absence of any perceptible odor. On the other hand, odor can be used as a very rough indication of the concentration of a pollutant in the environment[29], although minor differences in concentration are beyond olfactory discrimination. For many pollutants (e.g., acrolein, formaldehyde, formic acid, acetic acid, acetone) the odor threshold is either close to or above that for the irritant and/or health effects concentrations, and the perception of the odor is a clear indication of a problem. For other pollutants, the odor threshold is well below that for concentrations causing known health effects, and symptoms could be psychologically induced. For most normal, healthy adults, this is probably the case for odors associated with VOCs released from fungi and bacteria.

Trends in Building Design, Materials and Furnishings

An interest in designing more environmentally conscious buildings has gained prominence in the past 10 years. Using high performance, "green" or "sustainable" building practices has become common. This has also led to a greater awareness of occupant IAQ issues and ways in which to prevent them. The U.S. Green Building Council (USGBC) and its Leadership in Energy and Environmental Design (LEED®) rating systems incorporate IAQ performance standards. These include requiring that design engineers meet the current ASHRAE 62.1 ventilation standard and control or eliminate smoking in the new building, and assigning credits for such measures as outdoor air delivery monitoring, increased ventilation, IAQ management plans, use of low VOC emitting materials (adhesives, sealants, paints, coatings, carpet and composite wood), system controls for lighting and thermal comfort, and ensuring access to daylight and views. One component of a construction IAQ management plan includes a "before occupancy" air testing option that specifies maximum concentrations of certain airborne contaminants (Table 18.3).[6]

The EPA has developed construction guidelines with a primary focus on IAQ in schools. *IAQ Design Tools for Schools (DTfS)* provides guidance and resources to help design new schools as well as repair, renovate and maintain existing facilities.[30] The concept of designing "high performance schools" includes addressing IAQ, energy efficiency, daylighting, materials efficiency and safety in an economical manner. Some states have developed similar initiatives.[31,32]

ASHRAE has also developed guidelines, publications and certifications on design and operation of residential and commercial high performance buildings, geared toward building owners, facility managers, architects, contractors and engineers.[33]

Table 18.3 — LEED Pre-Occupancy Air Testing Limits[6]

Contaminant	*Maximum Concentration*
Formaldehyde	50 ppb
Particulates (PM_{10})	50 µg/m^3
Total Volatile Organic Compounds (TVOC)	500 µg/m^3
*4-Phenylcyclohexene (4-PCH)	6.5 µg/m^3
Carbon Monoxide (CO)	9 ppm and no greater than 2 ppm above outdoor levels

*This test is only required if carpets and fabrics with styrene butadiene rubber (SBR) latex backing material are installed as part of the base building systems.

Initiatives to combat global climate change will have a significant effect on how buildings are designed and operated. According to the USGBC, in the U.S., buildings account for 72% of electricity consumption, 39% of energy use, 38% of all carbon dioxide (CO_2) emissions, 40% of raw materials use, 30% of waste output (136 million tons annually), and 14% of potable water consumption. Climate change initiatives focus on reducing the carbon footprint of buildings, through modifications to their design, including producing net zero energy consumption. Besides using sustainable building practices as discussed above, existing buildings as well as new buildings may need to meet more stringent energy efficiency requirements. To accomplish this without adversely affecting IAQ will be challenging. A balanced approach may be needed.[34] ASHRAE's Advanced Energy Design Guide series of publications offer contractors and designers practical tools and recommendations for achieving 30% energy savings compared to code minimum. This is the first step in the process toward achieving a net-zero energy building, which ASHRAE defines as a building that, on an annual basis, draws from outside resources equal or less energy than it provides using on-site renewable energy sources.[35]

Natural ventilation systems have seen increased use in European commercial buildings, and interest in applying these systems in U.S. commercial buildings (low- to mid-rise) is growing. Hybrid (or mixed-mode) ventilation systems may offer energy savings, IAQ and climate control through the combination of natural ventilation systems with mechanical equipment.[36]

Ventilation

SBS apparently occurs most often in mechanically ventilated, air-conditioned buildings in which the amount or distribution of outdoor (fresh) air is inadequate. In buildings lacking sufficient outdoor air supply, bioeffluents, emissions from building materials and other sources can build up to levels where occupants notice odors and experience discomfort.

Heating, Ventilating, and Air-Conditioning (HVAC) Systems

HVAC systems in mechanically ventilated buildings control IAQ by providing outdoor air; filtering, mixing, and distributing both outdoor and indoor air to the occupied space; and providing some level of temperature and humidity control. In addition, ventilation systems may act as sources for specific pollutants including VOCs, fibers, dust and bioaerosols.

Major components of HVAC systems (Figure 18.1) include outdoor air intakes (for makeup air), intake fans, and filter banks;

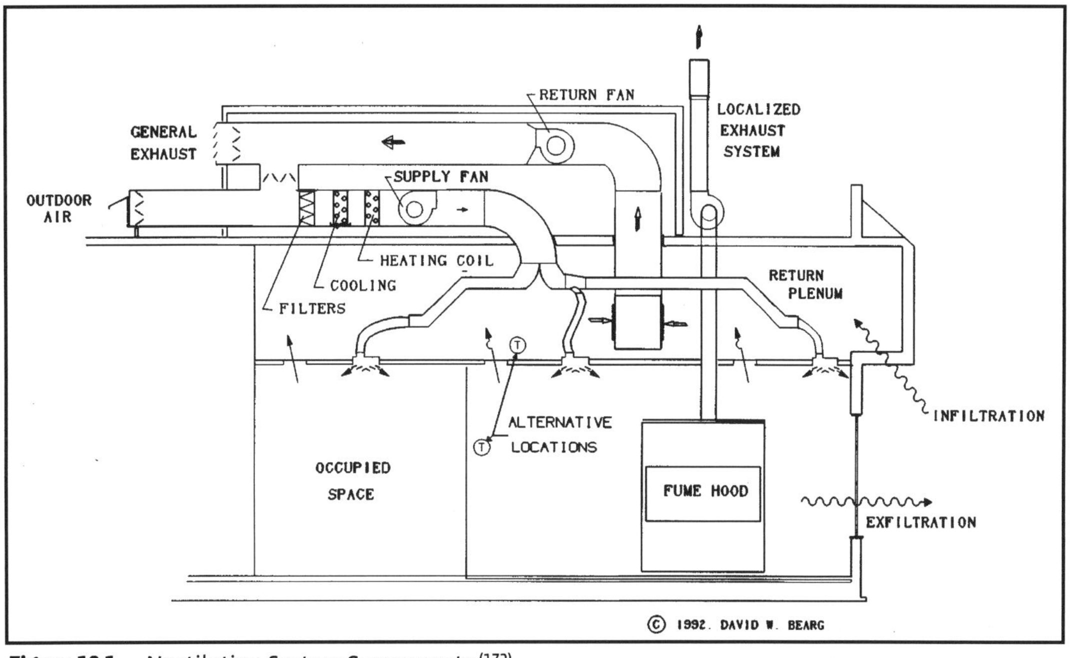

Figure 18.1 — Ventilation System Components.[172]

heat exchangers to provide heating or cooling; distribution fans and ductwork; diffusers to provide mixing in the occupied space; and a system for returning air to the central system. The design intent of such a system should be the delivery of air quality that is acceptable to a majority of building occupants. If this intent is to be achieved, the system must be installed, operated and maintained correctly.

Design factors that may adversely impact air quality include:

- insufficient provision for outdoor air;
- inefficient filtration;
- poorly designed or located fresh air intakes;
- inadequate cooling (and dehumidification);
- improperly designed drip pans;
- water spray humidification systems;
- use of porous insulation near water sources;
- limited access to HVAC components that require maintenance;
- use of materials that release VOCs or fibers; and
- ineffective distribution of air within the occupied space.

Neglect and poor maintenance may result in inoperable fans, closed dampers, clogged filters, slimy condensate pans, and dirty ductwork.

Many of the causes of poor IAQ that result from design, operation and maintenance of HVAC equipment are addressed in the current version of ASHRAE 62.1, Ventilation for Acceptable Indoor Air Quality.[9] For example, to meet ASHRAE 62.1, air handling and fan coil units are now designed for easy access to facilitate inspection and preventive maintenance. While this voluntary standard can be adopted by State and local codes, which would make it enforceable for new construction, most buildings have not implemented any of the improvements included in the current version of ASHRAE 62.1.

Ventilation Standards

Most ventilation systems are designed to provide the minimum amount of ventilation air (i.e., outside air) required by building code. State building codes vary by jurisdiction, often referencing the ASHRAE standard that was current at the time. Industrial hygienists should be aware that many older buildings where problems arise, have ventilation systems that were designed to meet outmoded ventilation requirements. In response to the first energy crisis of 1973, ASHRAE's outside air requirement for ventilation was set at 5 cubic feet per minute (cfm) per person to save money by cutting demand for heat and air conditioning. In the 1980s, complaints about poor IAQ led to arguments for increased use of outside air (15 cfm per person or more). However, many older buildings still retain the equipment designed to deliver minimum outside air. To make matters worse, renovations to interior layouts may have resulted in even lower amounts of outside air delivery to specific areas of the building.

The current ASHRAE 62.1[9] sets the standard of care for ventilation system design. Unlike earlier versions of the standard, it also incorporates guidance for construction, startup, operation, and maintenance of HVAC systems. It also addresses source management, humidity control, and air filtration. It specifies minimum maintenance activities and frequencies to achieve system cleanliness and avoid fouling and microbial growth. It also indicates that, in instances where microbial contamination and/or water intrusion or accumulation is observed, the situation, at a minimum, should be investigated and rectified.

ASHRAE 62.1 gives specific procedures for determining ventilation rates for different types of facilities, and IAQ procedures for achieving minimum contaminant concentrations. The standard calls for the calculation of outdoor air requirements based on both the occupant density and the square footage of the space. For example, for offices, the outdoor air requirement is 5 cfm per person, plus 0.06 cfm/ft^2. So a 1000 ft^2 office occupied by five people would require 85 cfm of outdoor air, or 17 cfm/person.[9] The standard recommends that if ventilation air does not meet EPA National Ambient Air Quality Standards, the ventilation system must be designed to clean or filter the incoming air. The standard discusses a common situation where some ventilation air bypasses occupants, moving from supply to exhaust without fully mixing in the occupied space, and dictates that ventilation effectiveness should approach 100 percent (i.e., all the outdoor air delivered to the space should actually reach the zone where the occupants are located). Supply air diffusers with good throw characteristics are essential in achieving well-mixed air without short-circuiting or "dumping" of ventilation air.

Guidance related to the heating and cooling and dehumidification of ventilation air is provided in the current ASHRAE Standard 55, Thermal Environmental Conditions for Human Occupancy. The standard recommends maintaining indoor temperatures between 68 to 75°F in winter, and between 73 to 79°F in summer, and keeping relative humidity below 60%. The standard states that there is no established lower humidity limit for thermal comfort; consequently it does not specify a minimum humidity level. Since the human body uses evaporative cooling to regulate temperature, people normally feel warmer in high RH than low. If the air temperature is 75°F and the relative humidity is 0%, the air temperature will feel like 69°F. But if the relative humidity is 100%, it feels more like 80°F. ASHRAE 55 does acknowledge that non-thermal comfort factors, including skin drying, mucous membrane irritation, dryness of the eyes, and static electricity generation, may place limits on what is acceptable in terms of very low humidity environments.[25]

Indoor/Outdoor Relationships

The primary source for some indoor air pollutants is the outdoor air. Fungal spores, some kinds of bacteria, combustion particles and gases, and ozone are all present in outdoor air. For most air pollutants, levels indoors should be lower than those outdoors (providing no indoor source exists). Outdoor air quality is, therefore, a necessary and useful control for determining whether a potential pollutant has an indoor or outdoor source.

Vapor intrusion from beneath buildings, from petroleum-contaminated groundwater or soil, and chemical trespass from such businesses as dry cleaners, nail salons and parking garages, are also potential sources of indoor air pollutants.

Filtration

Even typical inexpensive disposable filters used on home furnaces will remove a percentage of all particles from air. In general, removal rates depend on the size of the particle. While many gaseous pollutants are unobstructed by ventilation system and other barriers to entry, many will adsorb to indoor surfaces or react with indoor substances and thereby be removed from the air. Residence times (expressed by decay rates) for gaseous pollutants vary with the pollutant, lighting, reactive substrates available, temperature, and dilution rate.

In most large buildings, air-handling units bring in outside air, mix it with building air, and circulate the mixture through the building, either through a ducted system or through the ceiling plenum. The air mixture is usually passed through filters that are designed to protect the air-handling equipment from accumulations of dirt. Although filter media are available that remove most particles from air, most buildings use filters of minimal efficiency that do not prevent entry of smaller, inhalable particles (i.e., those less than one micron in diameter) that can pose potential health issues.

Innovations in filter technology and advances in testing methodologies have resulted in new devices such as extended surface pleated air filters which capture smaller size particles (i.e., those of greatest health consequence) without significantly impacting fan horsepower requirements. ASHRAE 52.2–2007, *Method of Testing General Ventilation Air-Cleaning Devices for Removal Efficiency by Particle Size*, establishes a performance standard that sets a Minimum Efficiency Reporting Value (MERV) for filtration media based on removal efficiency by particle size.[37] To maintain the filter efficiency, significant air leakage between or around the filters must be avoided.

Special measures are being taken in the construction of some new high-performance buildings to protect building occupants from fine particles.[6] For example, during construction, HVAC filters with a MERV rating of 8 are used to protect the HVAC equipment, and once the building is finished, new filters are installed with a MERV of at least 13. An example of a MERV 8 filter is a disposable extended surface pleated filter, 1 to 5 in. thick with cotton-polyester blend media in a cardboard frame. An example of a MERV 13 filter is a rigid style cartridge box filter 6 to 12 in. deep which uses lofted (air laid) or paper (wet laid) media. These types of filters are typically used in high performance commercial buildings, and they are designed to control particles in the range of 0.30 to 1.0 micron size.

Handling dust-loaded filters can release clouds of particles into the air, so it is incumbent on maintenance personnel to use appropriate work practices to safeguard IAQ. Mechanical rooms should not be used for storage of used filters, or other materials (cleaning supplies, pesticides, etc.) that may impact building air quality. If filters become wet, viable microorganisms (fungal spores and bacteria) can germinate, grow, and produce new spores that are introduced into the airstream either because fungi grow through the filter to the downstream side, or during filter change or other disturbance. Such growth also can lead to the release of microbial VOCs (MVOCs) and odors characteristic of microbial growth.

For optimum IAQ the most efficient filters should be used based on the system design. The filters should be maintained properly and changed at recommended intervals, or when the resistance to airflow measured across the filters meets manufacturers' replacement guidelines.

Problems with Maintaining Acceptable Ventilation

Air-handling systems can be designed to deliver a specified amount of outdoor air of acceptable quality and to provide effective distribution so that each occupant receives a full measure of ventilation air. As long as the system is designed appropriately, built as designed, operated according to design specifications, maintained in top condition, and not modified, providing adequate ventilation should theoretically be achievable over the life of the building. Unfortunately, it is rare that all of these conditions are met. Pressure imbalances within the building (caused, for example, by the piston-like action of elevators) may bring contaminated air from underground parking garages, restrooms, or loading docks into occupied spaces. Unplanned airflows through buildings can be the source of moisture, mold or inadvertent contamination of indoor air.[38] The quality of the outside air may deteriorate (e.g., heavy traffic may elevate CO levels, or nearby cooling towers may impact building air intakes). Budget cutting measures may reduce the degree of maintenance and operation of the system. Renovation of tenant spaces may have unforeseen consequences on the delivery of ventilation air to building occupants, and tenant-specific contaminants (e.g., nail or hair salons or drycleaners) may adversely affect other occupants' air quality.

On any given day, subtle effects on the quality of delivered air to building occupants may result from the way that air flows through the building. The amount and direction of airflow through the building will depend on how well the air handling equipment is operating, the quality of the construction, the temperature difference between outdoors and indoors, radiant heat load, the wind direction and speed, the position of doors and windows, the position of dampers, and the location of supply diffusers and return/exhaust grilles.

Ventilation System Contamination

Some of the more serious outbreaks of building-related disease (e.g., hypersensitivity pneumonitis) have involved microbial contamination of the ventilation system downstream of any filtration. Such microbial contamination is always associated with water in the system. Water sources can include cooling coil condensate that drips into and collects in poorly drained pans, humidification and water spray air-cleaning systems, and condensation on cold surfaces including those in ductwork. Air handlers and terminal units with cooling coils have historically been designed with flat drain pans. The majority of buildings still have these types of systems — the pans allow water and mineral scale to collect and stagnate, slowing or completely blocking their drains, thereby fostering microbial growth. This may cause slimy condensate to overflow into the base of the air handler or leak onto the floor of the mechanical room. Additionally, the microbial slime can be a source for degraded air that is then circulated throughout the building. While the necessity of draining condensate pans should be obvious, many systems have not been designed to drain adequately or at all. These types of pans need to be cleaned and periodically disinfected. The major manufacturers of HVAC equipment, supported by ASHRAE in the most recent versions of its ventilation standard, have made improvements to new HVAC equipment. For example, condensate drain pans in new equipment are sloped, often in two directions, to allow for positive drainage and eliminate ponded water. Drain pans are being constructed of non-corrosive materials like stainless steel, galvanized steel, or polymeric material, to resist deterioration and facilitate cleaning.

Humidifiers and water spray air cleaners are not designed to be maintained in a sterile condition, and the benefits of their use should be carefully weighed against the risk of contamination and subsequent disease-causing exposures. Water spray systems are especially risky because they not only become contaminated, but also actively aerosolize contaminated droplets. Filters and other surfaces downstream from these units can be constantly wet and support further microbial growth. Evaporative humidifiers are less likely to release particles (including intact microorganisms), although humidifier fever has been shown to result from contamination of evaporative units.

Condensation in ventilation system components occurs when cool surfaces are in contact with warm humid air. If ventilation system components are maintained at the same temperature as the airstream, even RH near saturation is unlikely to lead to microbial problems. The accumulation of dirt on ventilation system surfaces tends to slow drying after condensation has occurred, produces an increased surface area for microbial growth, and provides nutrient material for the organisms.

Insulation in Ventilation Systems

Porous, matte-faced fiber glass has often been used in HVAC equipment and ductwork for acoustical attenuation and thermal insulation. The uneven surface of the insulation can become dirty, and, if moisture is present (which is particularly likely downstream of the cooling coil, where the RH is nearly 100%), microbial growth can result. Cleaning microbial growth from insulation is difficult and not recommended. Generally the insulation must be removed and replaced. In addition to problems related to microbial growth, fiber glass may be subject to abrasion and physical degradation, potentially causing fibers to be released into the airstream.

ASHRAE has established specific requirements for the types of materials to be used in new equipment and ductwork, to reduce the potential for microbial growth and fiber release. HVAC equipment is now available with double-wall construction (fiber glass insulation sandwiched between two layers of metal). Closed-cell foam or foil-faced insulation, considered a "cleanable surface", is being used in sections of air handlers and ductwork that may become wet during system operation (e.g., outdoor air intakes and mixing boxes, cooling coil sections and humidifier sections). Even with these improvements, it is critical that the IAQ investigator inspect the air handler and duct system for signs of moisture and microbial growth.

Assessing Ventilation Problems

As part of an IAQ investigation, the investigator may choose to develop an IAQ profile for the building, including a basic understanding of the HVAC system. Such a profile is developed using these types of records:

- HVAC system design information including planned and actual ventilation air per occupant (typically expressed in cubic feet per minute);
- Updated schedules and procedures for facility operations and maintenance, and manufacturers' equipment manuals;
- Maintenance records for HVAC system components;
- Material Safety Data Sheets (MSDSs) for chemicals used in system operation and maintenance;
- "As built" drawings;
- Updated information on major space use changes and on significant increases or decreases in occupant density including current floorplans;
- Occupant surveys and temperature and relative temperature records;
- The most recent testing and balancing (TAB) report;
- Commissioning documents; and
- Documentation of HVAC control system set points and ranges.

This review of records is supplemented with a walkthrough inspection of occupied areas, mechanical rooms, and outdoor air intakes to identify IAQ problem indicators (as recorded on floor plans). IAQ problem indicators would include:

- Odors;
- Dirty or unsanitary conditions;

- Visible fungal growth;
- Evidence of moisture in inappropriate locations;
- Staining or discoloration of building materials;
- Smoke damage;
- Presence of hazardous substances;
- Potential for soil gas entry;
- Outdoor air intakes located near exhausts or loading docks;
- Poorly maintained filters;
- Uneven temperatures or temperature/RH extremes;
- Overcrowding;
- Personal air cleaners or fans;
- Inadequate ventilation;
- Inadequate exhaust air flow;
- Blocked vents; and
- Inadequately draining condensate drain pans.

During the site walkthrough, there should be an inspection for signs of water damage or microbial contamination. Building management should be immediately notified of observed deficiencies so that conditions can be properly rectified.

A good IAQ investigator must be cognizant of the many factors involved in delivery of adequate ventilation air to building occupants, and be adept at identifying the true nature of the problem in the building they are investigating.

Pollutant Categories

Standards and Guidelines for Indoor Air Contaminants

Although there are no enforceable standards in the U.S. that are appropriate for indoor air exposures, the IAQ investigator has a number of useful consensus standards and guidelines to reference. The workplace occupational exposure levels which have been established by OSHA, NIOSH and ACGIH® are normally considered too lenient for use in non-industrial settings, where chemicals are not routinely handled. Table 18.4[9,39–52] lists several agencies and organizations that have standards and guidelines that may be useful for IAQ purposes. It should be noted that available guidelines do not adequately take into account exposure to multiple contaminants at low levels, which is recognized as a common problem in interpreting IAQ data. Some of the more restrictive numerical standards and guidelines from the cited resources and others are summarized in Table 18.5 along with typical levels found indoors.

Also relevant are comparative IAQ data from "non-problem" buildings, such as the data obtained by EPA in their Building Assessment Survey and Evaluation (BASE) study, which involved collection of chemical and biological sampling data from approximately 100 non-problem commercial buildings across the U.S. The BASE data and publications of studies that have evaluated the BASE data are available on the EPA website (http://www.epa.gov/iaq/base/). New publications are posted as they become available.

Efforts have also been made to develop indoor environmental quality (IEQ) metrics which incorporate factors such as thermal comfort, lighting, and noise, with single or multiple contaminant concentrations. Some individual indoor contaminants have specific guidelines and recommendations such as those for radon and lead.[53,54] EPA researchers developed an Environmental Relative Moldiness Index (ERMI) scale for U.S. homes based on mold-specific analysis of dust samples collected in a national study.[55]

There are also no federal regulations pertaining to indoor microbiological contamination at this time, although some states have regulations applicable to fungal growth in the indoor environment. The interpretation of microbiological sampling results is more complex than assessing chemical data. Not only is there a natural background of bioaerosols outdoors and indoors, but both are highly variable geographically and seasonally, as well as on a daily and hourly basis.

Details on exposure guidelines and assessment of individual contaminants are given in the following subsections. It should not be concluded from this discussion that it is incumbent on the IAQ investigator to conduct extensive sampling in order to resolve IAQ issues. Sampling may not be needed at all in some cases. Whether sampling should be conducted will be based on an informed evaluation of occupant complaints and symptoms, as well as the air quality and physical conditions in the building. A thorough knowledge of the nature of possible chemical and biological contaminants, their sources, and standards and guidelines, as

Table 18.4 — IAQ Standards and Guidelines Resources

Government Agency Standards/Guidelines	*Resource*
Ambient air	U. S. Environmental Protection Agency (EPA): National Ambient Air Quality Standards (NAAQS)[39]
	California Air Resources Board: Ambient Air Quality Standards[40]
Indoor Air	Health Canada: Exposure Guidelines for Residential Indoor Air Quality[41], Formaldehyde[42], Moulds[43]
	National Research Council Canada: Indoor Air Quality Guidelines and Standards[44]
	California Office of Environmental Health Hazard Assessment (OEHHA): Chronic Reference Exposure Levels (CRELs), [45]
	Texas Department of Health: Texas Voluntary Indoor Air Quality Guidelines for Government Buildings[46]
Occupational	Occupational Safety and Health Agency (OSHA): Permissible Exposure Limits (PELs)[47]
	National Institute for Occupational Safety and Health (NIOSH): Recommended Exposure Levels (RELs)[48]
Consensus Standards	*Resource*
Indoor Air	American Society of Heating, Refrigeration and Air-Conditioning Engineers (ASHRAE): ANSI/ASHRAE Standard 62.1: Ventilation for Acceptable Indoor Air Quality[9]
Occupational	American Conference of Governmental Industrial Hygienists (ACGIH): Threshold Limit Values (TLVs®)[49]
	American Industrial Hygiene Association (AIHA): Workplace Environmental Exposure Levels (WEELs)[50]
Other Guidelines	*Resource*
Indoor Air	World Health Organization (WHO): WHO Guidelines for Indoor Air Quality: Selected Pollutants[51]
	American Society of Testing and Materials (ASTM): ASTM Standards on Indoor Air Quality[52]

discussed below, will further sharpen the skills of the investigator.

Chemical Agents

Indoor air contaminants of a chemical nature can come from a variety of sources including combustion, smoking, building materials and furnishings, cleaning agents, paints, adhesives, and natural sources such as radon from radium-containing soil. They include typical outdoor air pollutants and also chemicals that may be generated by indoor activities.

Carbon Dioxide (CO_2)

Although not a pollutant per se, CO_2 is frequently measured to assess the adequacy of ventilation, or as a means of controlling ventilation to auditoriums or other spaces with variable occupancy.

Nature and Sources. CO_2 is present in exhaled air, and humans are its main source indoors. Unvented or poorly vented combustion appliances and ETS may be additional sources.

Health Effects. At levels typically encountered indoors (ranging from 500 to several thousand parts per million), CO_2 is important not as a cause of health effects, but as a surrogate for other indoor pollutants, or an indicator of inadequate ventilation air. At CO_2 levels above 800 ppm, air quality complaints may increase. In general, these levels are an indication of a lack of fresh air or inadequate mixing of air in an occupied area.

Monitoring/Sampling. CO_2 is easily measured and has been used as an indicator of ventilation rates in IAQ investigations. Note that this method works only for spaces where there are enough people to serve as a source, and when they have been present long enough that CO_2 levels have reached equilibrium. Such measurements are often inappropriate because CO_2 and ventilation rates may not in fact have stabilized, producing erroneous results. Other methods, using tracer-gas techniques and actual air velocity measurements, are more accurate.

CO_2 testing can be accomplished by use of real time non-dispersive infrared (NDIR) analyzers with output logged over time, which permits evaluation of short or long term trends associated with occupancy

Table 18.5 — Selected Standards and Guidelines for Common Indoor Air Pollutants

Pollutant	*Standard (S) or Guideline (G)*	*Source*	*Remarks*	*Levels Commonly found Indoors**
Carbon Monoxide	9 ppm (S)	EPA	8 hr avg outdoor	ND to 4 ppm**
	15 ppm (G)	CPSC	1 hr avg indoor	
	9 ppm (G)	LEED	and not > 2 ppm above outdoor levels; indoor preoccupancy limit	
Formaldehyde				
	0.05 ppm (G)	LEED	Indoor preoccupancy limit	< 0.03 ppm
	0.04 ppm (G)	Health Canada	8 hr avg indoor residential	
	0.1 ppm	Health Canada	1 hr avg indoor residential	
	0.016 ppm (S)	FEMA	8 hr avg indoor trailer	
	0.014 ppm (G)	CA-r	School building materials emission limit (Ref 44)	
	0.002 ppm (G)	CA-r	No significant health risk with indefinite exposure	
Nitrogen Dioxide	0.053 ppm (S)	EPA	Annual avg outdoor	ND to 0.3 ppm**
	0.18 ppm (S)	CA	1 hr avg outdoor	
Ozone	0.075 ppm (S)	EPA	8 hr avg outdoor	ND to 0.03 ppm
	0.07 ppm (S)	CA	"	
	0.05 ppm (S)	CA-ac	Limit on output of air cleaners	
	0.05 ppm (S)	FDA	Limit on output of indoor medical devices	
Respirable Particulates (PM_{10})	150 μg/m³ (S)	EPA	24 hr avg outdoor	3 to 35 μg/m³
	50 μg/m³ (S)	CA	"	
	50 μg/m³ (G)	LEED	Indoor preoccupancy limit	
Fine Particulates ($PM_{2.5}$)	35 μg/m³ (S)	EPA	24 hr avg outdoor	1 to 25 μg/m³
	15 μg/m³ (S)	EPA	Annual avg	
	12 μg/m³ (S)	CA	"	
Lead	0.15 μg/ m³ (S)	EPA	3 mo rolling avg	—
Radon	4 pCi/L (G)	EPA	Annual avg indoor	0.7 to 1.3 pCi/L (homes)
Sulfur Dioxide	0.03 ppm (S)	EPA	Annual avg outdoor	**
	0.04 ppm (S)	CA	24 hr avg outdoor	
	0.25 ppm (S)	CA	1 hr avg outdoor	
Hydrogen Sulfide	0.03 ppm (S)	CA	1 hr avg outdoor	—

ND – none detected using standard sampling methods
EPA – EPA National Ambient Air Quality Standard
CPSC – U.S. Consumer Product Safety Commission
CA – California Ambient Air Quality Standard
CA-r – California Chronic Reference Exposure Level
CA-ac – California standard for non-industrial air cleaners
FEMA – Federal Emergency Management Administration
FDA – U.S. Food and Drug Administration
LEED – U.S. Green Building Council LEED certification IAQ preoccupancy limits for new construction
PM_{10} – particles with diameters of 10 μm or less
$PM_{2.5}$ – particles with diameters of 2.5 μm or less
pCi/L – pico-curies/liter
* outside levels may affect indoor levels
** depending on fuel sources used indoors; levels are normally less than outdoors, unless a significant indoor source exists

patterns and operation of the HVAC equipment. A multitude of instruments specifically marketed to the IAQ practitioner are available. Colorimetric detector tubes are also used. Detection limits are approximately one order of magnitude below the ambient outdoor level (300–400 ppm). Air samples may also be collected in Tedlar bags for subsequent analysis.

Standards and Levels Measured. The OSHA permissible exposure limit (PEL) for CO_2 is 5000 ppm, as is the ACGIH® Threshold Limit Value (TLV®). This limit has been set to protect against CO_2's ability to act as a simple asphyxiant at levels not normally encountered in non-industrial settings. ASHRAE notes that if levels of CO_2 can be maintained at less than 700 ppm above the outdoor air concentration, then comfort criteria with respect to human bioeffluents (odor) will likely be satisfied. Although 1000 ppm is calculated to represent a ventilation rate of approximately 15 cfm outdoor air per person in commercial buildings, where the ventilation rate is adequate to dilute human-source air pollutants, CO_2 levels are usually below 800 ppm. In some buildings, a permanent CO_2 monitoring system is integrated with the building automation system to adjust HVAC operation based on feedback on occupancy patterns/space ventilation performance. These systems are used specifically for conference rooms, auditoriums and other spaces with the capacity for high density occupancy.

Control. Control of CO_2 in the nonindustrial environment depends almost entirely on the use of increased ventilation with outside air. It should be noted that CO_2 concentration is measured and used in "demand controlled ventilation" as an energy saving mechanism based on adjusting the supply air to rooms with variable occupancy (e.g., auditoriums, meeting rooms, gymnasiums).

Carbon Monoxide (CO)

CO is a very dangerous gas that can cause serious illness and death.

Nature and Sources. CO is an odorless, tasteless, colorless gas that is produced by the incomplete combustion of any fuel containing carbon atoms. CO exposure usually occurs combined with other combustion products, many of which have distinctive odors. The most common sources for CO in nonindustrial environments include vehicular exhaust from indoor garages or inappropriately placed air intakes, smoking, and, in residential environments, unvented or improperly operated combustion appliances. Backdrafting and spillage are ways that combustion byproducts including CO can be life-threatening indoors. Depressurization of the building and the design and condition of chimneys/air shafts both play roles in backdrafting and spillage accidents.

Health Effects. CO is an asphyxiant that converts hemoglobin to carboxyhemoglobin (COHb), thus competitively decreasing the amount of oxygen transported to tissues and resulting in tissue hypoxia. Exposure results in fatigue, shortness of breath, headache, nausea, and at high levels, death. COHb levels above 4–5% can exacerbate symptoms of cardiovascular disease, and extreme altitudes may exacerbate the detrimental effects of CO on persons with this disease. Health effects of low-level CO exposure resulting in less than 3% bound hemoglobin are not well established, but probably include effects on the heart and brain. In the general nonsmoking population when CO exposure levels do not exceed 25 ppm, COHb levels are generally in the range of 0.3–0.7%, while for smokers 2–3% COHb is considered normal.

Monitoring/Sampling. Active and passive direct reading electrochemical CO monitors, sensitive to levels as low as 1 to 5 ppm, are commonly used. Output from real-time analyzers can often be logged to evaluate trends over time. Since low concentrations are of interest, selecting an instrument which is sensitive over a low concentration range is preferable to one that is not as sensitive. Colorimetric detector tubes are also available.

Standards. The current National Ambient Air Quality Standard for CO is 9 ppm maximum for 8-hour average exposure, or 35 ppm maximum for 1-hour average exposure. These levels are intended to provide a margin of safety for people with cardiovascular disease. Mean CO concentrations in nonindustrial indoor environments (excluding garages and other automobile service facilities) range from 1.2–4.2 ppm. The ACGIH® time-weighted average (TWA) TLV® for CO is 25 ppm.

Control. Control of CO depends on removing sources in the indoor environment and ensuring that the location of the outside air intake is suitable for supplying outdoor air that (at a minimum) meets the National Ambient Air Quality Standard of 9 ppm. Control of indoor sources includes controlling or eliminating smoking, proper ventilation of indoor garages, and placement of air intakes such that exhaust fumes from loading docks, garages, and adjacent traffic are not entrained in building air. Most of these approaches also apply to the residential environment. In addition, heating and cooking appliances that burn carbon-containing fuel (e.g., gas ovens, ranges, water heaters, gas fireplaces, space heaters) should be tested for CO output under all operating conditions. Gas space heaters and hot water heaters should be power vented, have sealed combustion, or be installed outside the conditioned space. Gas appliances should not be located where they can be affected by building pressurization or by other combustion appliances. These types of appliances must be properly maintained and vented. For example, their operation may be coupled with a fan-powered exterior exhaust. The use of CO detectors with alarms are becoming more prevalent in homes and also in mechanical rooms of buildings as early warnings of potentially hazardous CO levels. Demand-controlled ventilation is employed in parking garages using CO sensors to control fans. The state of Massachusetts passed regulations to control CO levels in indoor ice rinks with proper maintenance and use of ice resurfacing machines and ventilation.

Nitrogen and Sulfur Oxides (NO_2, SO_2)

Nature and Sources. NO_2 is associated with emissions from automobiles, diesel trucks, electrical power-generating stations, and industrial processes. Indoor sources include emissions from unvented appliances that use fossil fuels, including gas stoves and space heaters. These occur primarily in residences and are uncommon in the occupational or commercial environment. Cigarette smoke is also a source of NO_2. SO_2 is derived from combustion of sulfur-containing fossil fuels, which are not commonly used indoors. Most indoor exposure results from misuse of equipment, including inadequate venting of oil-burning combustion appliances. While SO_2 is an important pollutant in outdoor air, levels indoors rarely exceed 30% of those outdoors unless an unvented kerosene burner is used with an extremely low grade of fuel.

Health Effects. NO_2 is rarely associated with acute building-related disease except in cases where entrainment from outdoor air occurs or in conjunction with ETS exposure. Exposure to NO_2 at high concentrations (>200 ppm) is associated with acute pulmonary edema and death. Exposure to levels encountered in nonindustrial interiors can lead to a decrease in pulmonary function in asthmatics and may cause effects on lung defenses, biochemistry, function, and structure. Chronic exposure is considered a significant cause for concern, especially for children. In addition, NO_2 is likely to have additive or synergistic effects with other indoor pollutants.[56,57]

SO_2 is an irritant that causes bronchoconstriction in asthmatics, especially during exercise. Levels that cause these effects are in the range of 0.25–0.5 ppm.

Monitoring/Sampling. Passive monitors using a triethanolamine sorbent are available for NO_2, and colorimetric and chemiluminescent real-time detectors for both NO_2 and SO_2. Grab-sample detector tubes are available for measurement of SO_2. It should be emphasized that unless an apparent source for NO_2 or SO_2 is present, it is rarely helpful to monitor for these pollutants in most IAQ investigations.

Standards and Levels Measured. NO_2 is regulated in ambient air by the EPA at 0.053 ppm (annual average), and ACGIH® recommends a TWA-TLV® of 3 ppm. The EPA is required to issue a public alert at ambient NO_2 levels of 0.6 ppm, and 1.6 ppm is considered a public emergency. A concentration of 2.0 ppm NO_2 causes significant harm and widespread health effects in the general population. Average outdoor levels range from 0.001 ppm in rural areas to 0.03 ppm in urban air. Indoor levels are almost always below those outdoors unless a significant source is present. In homes with gas-fired stoves, ovens, or heaters, NO_2 levels as high as 0.55 ppm have been measured.

The National Air Quality Standards for SO_2 are 0.03 ppm (annual average) and 0.14

ppm (24-hour average). The TLV® for SO_2 is 2.0 ppm. Levels reported in houses range from 0.03–0.65 ppm depending on the type(s) of combustion sources present.

Control. Control of NO_2 and SO_2 depends primarily on removing sources.

Environmental Tobacco Smoke (ETS)

Nature and Sources. ETS, sometimes referred to as "secondhand smoke", has been one of the most frequent causes of complaints for building occupants. Burning tobacco releases a complex mixture of chemicals and particles into the air, a mixture that changes as it ages. In addition to CO and particles, nitrogen oxides, CO_2, hydrogen cyanide, and formaldehyde are produced along with a wide variety of other gases and VOCs. Although always diluted by room air, side-stream smoke contains the same kinds of toxic and carcinogenic substances as inhaled smoke.

Health Effects. Active cigarette smoking has been clearly established as a major and preventable cause of life threatening diseases including heart disease and lung cancer. In addition, exposure to ETS clearly increases risk of lung cancer. ETS is estimated to cause approximately 3,400 lung cancer deaths and from 22,700 to 69,600 heart disease deaths annually among adult nonsmokers in the U.S.[58]

Exposure of young children to ETS from maternal smoking increases rates of respiratory tract infections, chronic ear infections and middle-ear effusions, and leads to decrements in pulmonary function and predisposes susceptible children to the development of asthma. It has been reported that nonsmoking pregnant women exposed to ETS daily for several hours are at increased risk of producing low-birth-weight babies. The U.S. Environmental Protection Agency, the National Institutes of Health National Toxicology Program, and the International Agency for Research on Cancer have concluded that ETS is a known human carcinogen. NIOSH has concluded that ETS is an occupational carcinogen.

The U.S. Surgeon General has reported that there is sufficient evidence to infer a causal relationship between exposure to ETS and Sudden Infant Death Syndrome, and, among lifetime nonsmokers, lung cancer and increased risk of coronary heart disease morbidity and mortality. The U.S. Surgeon General has concluded there is no risk-free level of ETS exposure; even brief exposures can be harmful.[59]

ETS contains more than 50 cancer-causing chemicals. Nonsmokers who are exposed to ETS are inhaling many of the same cancer-causing substances and toxins as smokers. Exposure to ETS may also increase heart rate, blood pressure response, and oxygen consumption, especially in nonsmokers, and result in eye and throat irritation, headache, rhinitis, coughing, and bronchoconstriction in asthmatics.

Odor is associated with volatile components of ETS. Given the extremely emotional situations that can be generated where smokers and nonsmokers must coexist, it is logical to assume that a variety of psychological symptoms may be traced to ETS, especially in nonsmokers.

Monitoring/Sampling. Respirable particles are currently the most commonly used indicator to determine ETS impacts on IAQ.[60] In this case, samples are collected on filters and analyzed by high pressure liquid chromatography (HPLC). Nicotine, 3-ethenylpyridine and solanesol are other components of ETS that have also been analyzed in air to determine ETS contamination of indoor air. Alternatively, evaluation of indoor exposure to ETS can be done through biological monitoring. Nicotine and cotinine are unique to tobacco products and can be measured in saliva, blood, or urine.

Levels Measured. Concentrations of ETS components in air depend on frequency and amount of smoking, outdoor air ventilation rates, presence and efficiency of air cleaning devices, and patterns of air distribution and recirculation. ETS aerosols adsorb readily to surfaces and can release volatile constituents long after smokers have left a room. In the presence of ETS, CO levels ranging from 2 to 35 ppm, and particle concentrations ranging from 10–1000 $\mu g/m^3$ have been measured. The mean impact of smoking a pack of cigarettes in a fully air-conditioned building with recirculation is to increase particle levels by approximately 41 $\mu g/m^3$. Urinary nicotine measurements in nonsmokers exposed to ETS have ranged from <10 to >80 µg/hour of exposure.

Standards. Other than outright bans on smoking, there are no standards that delineate acceptable levels of ETS in indoor air. There are standards that cover some specific components not unique to ETS.

Control. The best control option for preventing exposure to ETS is to completely ban smoking. Many municipalities in the U.S. now ban smoking in public buildings and areas, and smoking in workplaces is increasingly prohibited. Short of a complete ban, smoking can be confined to areas that are separately ventilated so that recirculation does not spread ETS into the general environment. Properly designed ventilation systems can lessen the impact of ETS on building occupants, but such design carries a considerable energy penalty, since the exhausted air should be wholly discharged to the outside. Ventilation rates must be high, and in reality, it is impractical to provide ventilation rates that will reduce the odor in an average smoking environment to a level that will satisfy the majority of nonsmokers. Air cleaning for control of ETS exposures, such as filtration and electrostatic precipitation, has not been shown to be effective. Reducing ETS exposure in the home, particularly for children, is a major focus that will require education and voluntary efforts by the public.[61]

Particulate Matter

Nature and Sources. Airborne particulate matter includes a broad range of substances that are small enough to remain suspended in air. In many references, it is noted that particles designated "respirable" are less than 10 μm in diameter and they fall into two general categories: larger than 2–3 μm, and smaller than 2–3 μm. More recent designations (notably by standard setting agencies and organizations) use the term "inhalable" to describe particles equal to or less than 10 μm in diameter (PM_{10}), and "respirable" for particles equal to or less than 2.5 μm ($PM_{2.5}$). Ultrafine particles are generally described as particles less than 0.1 μm in diameter. In nonindustrial occupational environments, the principal sources of fine and ultrafine particles are cigarette smoke and possibly aerosols from spray air fresheners or cleaning materials. Larger particle aerosols include particles and fibers from carpets, building materials and furnishings, dirt carried in from outdoors, particulate generated from office activities, equipment and supplies (i.e., paper, toner, etc.) and most of the biological particle fraction of the air. Outdoor air could also be a significant source for fine particles in naturally ventilated buildings.

Health Effects. In the indoor environment, health effects related to particle exposures include those discussed for ETS, radon, and biological particles, and in general may cause eye, skin and respiratory system irritation. Respirable particles can be especially irritating for asthmatics. Lung-damaging particles that may be retained in the lung are 0.2 to 5 μm in size.[9] Exposure to fine particles in outdoor air at levels below the current National Ambient Air Quality Standard has been associated epidemiologically with acute respiratory distress. The health effects related to the ultrafines are actively under study. The relationship between indoor ultrafine particles generated in homes and childhood asthma is of concern.[62] It is well known that the ultrafine particles represent the greatest number of particles in a given air sample, although their total mass may be only a fraction of the total sample mass. Also, the ultrafines may penetrate more deeply into the lungs than larger particles.[63]

Monitoring/Sampling. Particulate matter can be sampled using gravimetric methods that require laboratory analysis or by continuous monitors based on optical methods. Aerosol size distribution can be determined using an inertial impactor to separately deposit size fractions.

Standards. The National Ambient Air Quality Standard for PM_{10} particles is 150 μg/m^3 (24-hour average); and for $PM_{2.5}$ particles, 35μg/m^3 (24-hour average) and 15 μg/m^3 (annual average). These levels are much lower than the 8-hr occupational exposure limits for inert or nuisance dusts. Both the OSHA PEL and the ACGIH® TLV® are 10 mg/m^3 for inhalable particles and 3 mg/m^3 for respirable particles.

Control. Control of fine-particle aerosols in the indoor environment is best achieved by banning smoking or restricting smoking to smoking lounges with dedicated exhaust ventilation. In addition to having good air filtration in well-maintained HVAC systems, regular cleaning and maintenance of the building environment is key to controlling indoor particulate levels.

Asbestos and Other Fibers

Asbestos and fiber glass (synthetic vitreous fibers) are two fibers that have caused serious concern in the nonindustrial environment. Although not as serious, other fibers, natural and synthetic, may cause IAQ problems. They can originate from carpet, building materials and furnishings, and clothing and activities of building occupants.

Asbestos

Nature and Sources. Asbestos is defined as a group of naturally occurring magnesium silicate minerals that are in fibrous form. The three species, chrysotile, amosite and crocidolite, have been used commonly between the 1920s and mid 1970s in a variety of building construction materials and commercial products for insulation, as a fire-retardant, and as a binder and strengthener in plastics, cement and insulation. The EPA has banned several asbestos products and manufacturers have also voluntarily limited uses of asbestos, but not all products are banned. Today, asbestos is most commonly found in older buildings and homes (pre-1978) — in pipe and furnace/boiler insulation materials, asbestos shingles, millboard, textured paints and coating materials, and vinyl floor tiles and sheeting. Elevated concentrations of airborne asbestos fibers can occur when asbestos-containing materials (ACM) are deteriorating, damaged, or disturbed by cutting, sanding or other renovation activities. Improper removal of ACM can release asbestos fibers into the air increasing asbestos levels and endangering building occupants.(64)

Health Effects. Studies show that the majority of people who have developed an asbestos-related disease were asbestos workers. Workers in factories and shipyards breathing high levels of airborne asbestos fibers were found to have an increased risk of:

- lung cancer;
- mesothelioma, a cancer of the lining of the chest and the abdominal cavity; and
- asbestosis, in which the lungs become scarred with fibrous tissue.

Some people developed disease from exposure to clothing and equipment brought home from job sites. The symptoms of these diseases do not usually appear until about 20 to 30 years after the first exposure to asbestos. The risks of non-occupational and ambient exposures are not well understood.(64) It is believed that any exposure to asbestos involves some health risk. No safe level of exposure has been established.(65)

Monitoring/Sampling. The most common methods for determination of airborne asbestos fiber concentrations include sampling on cellulose ester filters and analysis by phase contrast microscopy (PCM) in occupational settings; and analysis by transmission electron microscopy (TEM) in non-occupational settings. TEM can identify the smallest fibers and is specific for asbestos, whereas PCM counts total fibers of a specific aspect ratio which provides an index of total asbestos concentration. In a building where occupant exposure is a concern after an asbestos abatement project, "clearance" samples, usually collected and analyzed by TEM, must pass a standard before reopening the project area to the building.

Standards and Levels Measured. There are numerous regulations pertaining to asbestos at national, state and local levels. EPA and OSHA are primarily responsible for generating standards and regulations for asbestos control.(66,67) The OSHA 8-hr TWA PEL for all forms of asbestos is 0.1 f/cc for respirable fibers, and 1.0 f/cc for a 30-min short term exposure. The ACGIH® 8-hr TLV® is 0.1 f/cc of respirable fibers. These standards are based on the PCM method of analysis. The EPA has established a level of 0.01 f/cc as a standard for clearance of asbestos abatement projects, primarily using the TEM method. Levels measured by TEM in outdoor air across the U.S. ranged from below detection limits to 0.008 f/cc and mean concentration of 0.00039 f/cc, with levels being higher in urban areas and lower in suburban and rural areas. Average concentrations found in public buildings, schools and residences were 0.00059-0.00099 f/cc, 0.0002 f/cc, and 0.0001 f/cc, respectively. Insignificant differences were noted for buildings with or without ACM.(68)

Control. If asbestos in building materials is in good condition it should not present a health hazard or adversely affect IAQ. Proper surveys and the implementation of asbestos management plans are needed to maintain ACM in schools and public and commercial buildings. Persons in residences should be aware of potential asbestos problems before doing renovations.

After the WTC Disaster

On the morning of September 11, 2001 in lower Manhattan, the South and North towers of the World Trade Center (WTC) collapsed after being hit by two commercial airplanes. Massive dust clouds rose from Ground Zero, engulfing the southern tip of the island and traveling downwind to the south and east towards Brooklyn, enveloping the area for three days, and then ultimately settling, coating streets and buildings. Fires smoldered at the site through mid-December, adding combustion-related air contaminants to the mix.

In the years following this unprecedented tragedy, industrial hygienists and related professionals have worked on identifying what was in the dust, establishing thresholds for cleanliness inside buildings, and seeking to learn from it. In addition to a death toll of more than 2,600, many firefighters, emergency workers, residents and others continue to suffer persistent health-related consequences as a legacy of the event.

The collapse pulverized the buildings and their contents — estimated to include 6 million cubic feet of masonry, 5 million square feet of painted surfaces, 7 million square feet of flooring, 600,000 cubic feet of glazing, and 200 elevators, exposing hundreds of thousands of people. WTC dust was found to consist predominantly (95%) of coarse particles, and included pulverized cement, glass fibers, asbestos, lead, polycyclic aromatic hydrocarbons (PAHs), polychlorinated biphenyls (PCBs), and polychlorinated furans and dioxins.(174) The pH of the dust was highly alkaline (pH 9.0-11.0), producing bronchial hyperreactivity, persistent cough, and increased risk of asthma and other illnesses.(175–178)

The EPA had to establish air quality benchmarks for the area, and set screening levels for asbestos (70 or fewer structures per square millimeter based on AHERA), benzene (20 ppb based on the assumption of continuous exposure over a year), $PM_{2.5}$ (40 μg/m^3, 24 hour average exposure for sensitive groups), PM10 (150 μg/m^3, 24 hour average exposure for sensitive groups), PCBs (730 ng/m^3 based on the assumption of continuous exposure over a year) and dioxin (0.16 ng/m^3 based on the assumption of continuous exposure over a year).(179)

The Lower Manhattan Test and Clean Program, whose final report was completed in November 2008, used cleanup benchmarks for asbestos and man-made vitreous fibers in indoor air (0.0009 s/cc for asbestos and 0.01 f/cc for man-made vitreous fibers). For accessible surfaces, dust benchmarks included 5,000 s/cm^2 for asbestos, 5,000 f/cm^2 for man-made vitreous fibers, 40 μg/ft^2 for lead and 150 μg/m^2 for PAHs.(180) These benchmarks are sure to be valuable indicators for future use by industrial hygienists.

Fiber Glass

Nature and Sources. Fiber glass (or fibrous glass) generally includes particles composed of glassy, amorphous material with an aspect (length/width) ratio greater than 3. Fiber glass is used in textiles and fabrics; as reinforcement in plastics, rubber, and paper; and as thermal insulation material. The insulating properties of fiber glass vary inversely with the particle diameter, so that while most fiber glass fibers are in the range of 4–9 μm in diameter, those with the best insulating properties are 1 μm and less. Fiber glass is used for both thermal insulation and sound insulation in walls, ceilings, and in ventilation system ductwork and is ubiquitous in the work environment.

Health Effects. The health effects associated with fiber glass are under considerable debate. Although some studies have shown higher lung cancer risks for workers in industrial settings, measurements of airborne vitreous fiber levels in commercial buildings indicate insignificant risk to occupants.(69) Lung tumors have been induced in animals by implantation of very small-diameter glass fibers of a sort not common in buildings. Aside from possible chronic health effects, fiber glass has been reported to cause epidemics of rash and itching in office workers. Respiratory and eye irritation may be present.

Monitoring/Sampling. Air monitoring for fibers is done using filter cassettes with microscopic evaluation as for asbestos as discussed above. Real time fibrous aerosol monitors are also used. However, fiber glass is rarely detected in air in nonindustrial environments. Wipe samples have been a more effective means for documenting exposure.

Standards and Levels Measured. In epidemics of skin rash that have been traced to fiber glass, measures of total suspended particles (presumably including any fiber glass) have been below the pre-1996 occupational standards (TLV-TWA 10 mg/m^3) and even below detectable limits. The current TLV-TWA established by ACGIH® limits exposure to 1 fiber/cc for defined respirable fibers, and 5 mg/m^3 for the inhalable mass fraction. In most cases where air measurements have been attempted, fiber glass has been undetectable. Wipe samples of surfaces have confirmed the presence of fiber glass, and in most cases sources were discernible.

Control. Control of exposure to airborne fiber glass involves preventing its introduction into the air. This is accomplished by ensuring that fiber glass subject to abrasion is covered and maintained in good condition, and by using care in fiber glass installation and removal operations. Regular cleaning of the indoor environment is needed to minimize a buildup on surfaces of fibers of all types, natural and synthetic.

Lead

Nature and Sources. Before it was known how harmful lead could be, it was used in paint, gasoline, water pipes, and many other products. Old lead-based paint is the most significant source of lead exposure in the U.S. today. Most buildings built before 1960, and some built as recently as 1978, contain leaded paint. Harmful exposures to lead can be created when lead-based paint is improperly removed from surfaces by dry scraping, sanding or open-flame burning. High levels of airborne lead particles can also result from lead dust from outdoor sources, including contaminated soil tracked inside. Soil by roads and highways may be contaminated from years of exhaust from cars and trucks that used leaded gas.[(70)]

Health Effects. Lead affects practically all systems within the body. At high levels it can cause convulsions, coma and even death. Lower levels of lead can adversely affect the brain, central nervous system, blood cells, and kidneys. Young children are especially vulnerable to the damaging effects of lead since lead is more easily absorbed into growing bodies and internal organs, and children may have more contact with lead sources. There is no known safe level of lead in the body.[(70,71)]

Monitoring/Sampling. Airborne lead is commonly collected on filters and analyzed by inductively coupled plasma atomic emission spectrometry (ICP-AES), flame atomic absorption (FAA) or graphite furnace atomic absorption spectrometry (GFAAS) for increased sensitivity. Surface dust wipes and paint samples are analyzed using similar methods. Field screening techniques to estimate the lead content of paints and other environmental matrices include portable x-ray fluorescence (XRF) and chemical spot test kits. Portable XRF is the most commonly used method for screening for lead-based paint in residences and is the method recommended by HUD and EPA.

Standards and Levels Measured. The national lead ambient air quality standard established in 1978 of 1.5 µg/m^3 (total suspended particulates), as a quarterly average, was revised in 2009 to 0.15 µg/m^3 because of numerous health study findings. The averaging time was also changed to a "rolling" 3-month period. Nationwide, the average ambient lead concentration has dramatically decreased since the phase out of lead in gasoline. In 1980, the mean concentration of all 22 monitoring sites (maximum 3-month average at each site) in the U.S. was 1.39 µg/m^3, compared to 0.12 µg/m^3 in 2007.[(72)] The occupational standards for lead are much higher; the OSHA PEL and the ACGIH® TLV® for an 8-hr TWA is 0.05 mg/m^3. *The HUD Guidelines for the Evaluation and Control of Lead-Based Paint Hazards in Housing* addresses lead hazards posed by paint, dust, and soil in the residential environment.[(54)] The concentration of airborne lead indoors is influenced by the outdoor levels and any significant indoor sources, but typically, indoor levels are lower than outdoor levels.

Control. Key to control is knowing if and where lead is present in the indoor environment. If materials are in good condition they may just need to be maintained. If lead-based paint is present, control methods include frequent cleaning of surfaces using wet methods (damp mopping, wiping, etc.), vacuuming carpets with vacuum containing a HEPA filter, taking precautions to avoid creating lead dust during repairs, maintenance and renovations, and using proper procedures during lead abatement. In homes, special precautions should be taken to protect children from exposures.

Ozone (O_3)

Nature and Sources. Ozone is a colorless gas with a characteristic odor that is produced in ambient air during the photochemical oxidation of combustion products such as the nitrogen oxides and hydrocarbons. It can also result from the operation of electrical motors, photocopy machines, and electrostatic air cleaners in occupational environments. Many portable indoor air cleaning devices (types such as electrostatic precipitators, ionizing and photocatalytic oxidation devices) used in homes, businesses or by individuals can emit ozone. The State of California is requiring manufacturers to certify that air cleaners for non-industrial use do not emit more than 0.05 ppm ozone.(73) The U.S. Food and Drug Administration already regulates medical devices to emit no more than 0.05 ppm ozone.

Health Effects. Symptoms associated with exposure to ozone include cough, upper airway irritation, tickle in the throat, chest discomfort including substernal pain or soreness, difficulty or pain in taking a deep breath, shortness of breath, wheezing, headache, fatigue, nasal congestion, and eye irritation. Symptoms usually disappear within 2–4 hours of cessation of exposure. For sedentary people (e.g., office workers) ozone concentrations in excess of 0.1 ppm are likely to result in symptoms such as dryness of upper respiratory tract and throat and nose irritation, and 0.5 ppm will induce decrements in pulmonary function. Symptoms occur at lower ozone levels in exercising individuals.

Monitoring/Sampling. The characteristic odor of ozone is detectable well below the level at which symptoms are induced. Therefore, in the absence of this odor, IAQ issues are unlikely to be due to ozone exposure. Typical ozone monitors are based on ultraviolet absorption. Others include those based on chemiluminescence, electrochemistry or colorimetry. Colorimetric methods actually measure total oxidants, and ultraviolet absorption may be susceptible to interference by organics that absorb at the same wavelength.

Standards and Levels Measured. The National Ambient Air Quality Standard for ozone is 0.075 ppm (8 hour average). ACGIH® has set limits based on workloads averaged over 8 hours: 0.05 ppm for heavy work, 0.08 ppm for moderate work, 0.10 ppm for light work, and 0.20 ppm average for less than or equal to 2 hours of any type work. The OSHA PEL is 0.1 ppm averaged over 8 hours. Domestic and nonindustrial exposures are usually in the 0.02 to 0.03 ppm range. The odor of ozone can be detected by some people at levels as low as 0.001 ppm, and by most at 0.02 ppm.

Control. Control of ozone in nonindustrial occupational environments depends on adequate ventilation to dilute internal sources and proper maintenance of electrical equipment and other potential sources.

Formaldehyde (HCHO)

Nature and Sources. HCHO is a very volatile organic compound that, due to its continued use in a variety of manufacturing processes, is ubiquitous indoors. HCHO is used in pressed wood products, bonding/laminating agents, adhesives, paper and textile products. It is also used in cosmetics and toiletries as a preservative. In the 1970s, HCHO was recognized as a major contributor to indoor air problems in mobile homes, which led to HUD setting a target ambient level standard of 0.4 ppm in manufactured homes, achieved through product emission standards.

Health Effects. HCHO in excess of 1–3 ppm will cause mucous membrane irritation. Chronic, direct skin exposure may induce an immunologically mediated reaction, as can intravenous exposure (e.g., during dialysis). HCHO is a suspected carcinogen, and chronic exposure to levels above 1 ppm should be cause for concern.

Monitoring/Sampling. HCHO is generally measured by collection on 3,4-dinitrophenylhydrazine (DNPH)-coated silica gel cartridges, with analysis by HPLC. Passive indoor air samplers have been developed for long-term studies (over 5 to 7 days) with subsequent colorimetric analysis to measure levels typically found in residential or office environments. Direct reading instruments based on electrochemical techniques are available but usually not practical in IAQ investigations because of their higher limit of detection.

Standards and Levels Measured. The OSHA 8-hour workplace limit is 0.75 ppm, with a 2 ppm limit for a short term exposure. The ACGIH® ceiling exposure limit is 0.3 ppm. The ASHRAE standard for providing a comfortable indoor environment is 0.1 ppm. Similar guidelines for acceptable HCHO levels in indoor air range from 0.05–0.10 ppm. Data from CDC suggest 0.01–0.03 ppm as a common range found indoors. HUD standards for composite wood (emissions of 0.2 ppm from plywood and 0.3 ppm from particle board) in mobile homes were established to limit the overall airborne HCHO concentration to 0.4 ppm. FEMA established its own HCHO standard for trailers of 0.016 ppm based on an 8-hr sample of indoor air that must be met prior to occupancy.

Control. Control of HCHO depends on selecting building materials that are low in HCHO content, increasing ventilation particularly when formaldehyde-containing products are first installed, applying sealants to exposed edges and surfaces of countertops and cabinets, and controlling temperature and humidity. At high temperature and humidity HCHO emissions increase from these products.

Other VOCs

Nature and Sources. Potential indoor sources of VOCs include human bioeffluents, personal care products, cleaning chemicals, paints, lacquers, varnishes, pesticides, pressed wood products, building materials, furnishings and insulation. In homes, sources also include dry-cleaned clothes, cosmetics and air fresheners. Table 18.6 lists some commonly encountered VOCs and potential sources. Microorganisms also release volatiles ("microbial volatile organic compounds" or MVOCs) that are responsible for musty, moldy odors.

VOCs may also enter a building by "vapor intrusion", which is defined as the migration of volatile chemicals from contaminated soil or groundwater into overlying buildings. In extreme cases the vapors may accumulate in homes or occupied buildings to levels that may pose a safety or health hazard. In most cases however, the levels are low or not detectable. The EPA and various state agencies have developed guidance documents to help in vapor intrusion investigations.[74] Studies have suggested that certain types of VOCs (e.g. terpenes, d-limonene, ethylene-based glycol ethers) emitted from cleaning products, air fresheners and building materials, may react with ozone in the air to form secondary pollutants such as formaldehyde

Table 18.6 — Commonly Encountered VOCs and Potential Sources

Chemical	*Potential Sources*
Formaldehyde	Particle board, furnishings, fabrics
Acetone, isopropanol	Paint, coatings, finishes, paint remover, thinner, caulking
Aliphatic hydrocarbons (octane, decane, undecane, hexane, isodecane, petroleum mixtures)	Paint, adhesives, gasoline, combustion sources, carpet, linoleum, caulking
Aromatic hydrocarbons (toluene, xylenes, ethylbenzene, benzene, styrene)	Combustion sources, paint, adhesive, gasoline, linoleum, wall coating
Chlorinated solvents (dichloromethane, methylene chloride, trichloroethane, tetrachloroethylene, trichloroethylene)	Upholstery and carpet cleaner or protector, paint, paint remover, lacquers, solvents, dry-cleaned clothing
n-Butyl acetate	Acoustic ceiling tile, linoleum, caulking
Dichlorobenzene	Carpet, moth crystals, air fresheners
4-Phenylcyclohexene (4-PC)	Carpet, paint
Terpenes (limonene, α-pinene)	Deodorizers, cleaning agents, polishes, fabrics, fabric softener, cigarettes
2-Butoxyethanol, ethanol, isopropanol	Cleaners, disinfectants

In the Spotlight: Reducing Formaldehyde from Indoor Air

Formaldehyde in manufactured homes comes primarily from resins and adhesives in composite wood. Spurring federal action, and responding to growing concern, California set stringent, production-based emissions limits. Since 2009, manufacturers of hardwood, plywood, particleboard, medium density fiberboard, and furniture and other finished products made with composite wood have had to meet "Phase 1" formaldehyde emission standards as part of California's airborne toxics control measure (ATCM). More stringent "Phase 2" standards are being phased in through 2012. To meet Phase 2 standards, manufacturers use modified urea-formaldehyde resin systems, no-added formaldehyde (NAF) or ultra-low-emitting-formaldehyde (ULEF) resin systems.[182] An NAF resin may include resins made from soy, polyvinyl acetate, or methylenediisocyanate. A ULEF resin may include melamine-urea-formaldehyde resin, phenol formaldehyde resin and resorcinol formaldehyde resin. The California requirements include third-party testing and certification, labeling, chain-of-custody documentation, and recordkeeping.

On July 10, 2010, the federal Formaldehyde Standards for Composite Wood Products Act became law, under the Toxic Substances Control Act (TSCA). This act established formaldehyde emission limits identical to those of California. EPA must establish regulations for labeling and emissions standards by January 1, 2013, and they will take effect 180 days later.[183]

and ultrafine particles that may contribute to sensory irritation.[75–77]

Health Effects. Of the VOCs typically found indoors, only a few, such as formaldehyde and acrolein, are irritants at levels typically measured. A few of the VOCs commonly found in indoor environments are known carcinogens (e.g., benzene), although evidence for carcinogenicity is extrapolated from high-level exposures in industrial environments.[78] Others (e.g., carbon tetrachloride, chloroform) have produced cancer in laboratory animals, but no direct evidence exists for human effects.[79] Most VOCs are lipid soluble, readily cross the blood-brain barrier, and are easily absorbed through the lungs. Most are neurotoxic and, in levels in excess of occupationally acceptable limits, may cause central nervous system depression, vertigo, visual disorders, and occasionally tremors, fatigue, anorexia, and weakness. Potential genotoxic effects are still under investigation. Effects of low-level exposures to VOC mixtures over long periods of time are still being researched.

Monitoring/Sampling. Multisorbent tubes combining Tenax GC with synthetic charcoals and other sorbents are generally used to sample for a broad range of VOCs. Summa™ canisters and passive dosimeters may also be an option for VOC sampling. Analysis is typically by gas chromatography/mass spectrometry (GC/MS). Methods for measuring VOCs have been reviewed by Hodgson.[80]

Levels Measured. VOC levels in buildings are usually reported either as totals derived from summing all the individual peaks on a gas chromatogram or as individual species identified by separate peaks. For summed reports, the total VOC concentration is usually referenced to toluene or hexane. Typical total VOC concentrations range from 50 to 1000 μg/m³ over long periods, with levels reaching up to hundreds of mg/m³ over short term periods. There are often dozens, sometimes hundreds, of individual compounds present at concentrations of approximately 1 μg/m³ or more.[81,82] Table 18.7[83] summarizes VOCs most frequently found in the EPA BASE study of 56 normal public and private office buildings. Twelve VOCs with the highest median concentrations are presented. Overall, indoor VOC concentrations ranged from below the limit of detection to 450 μg/m³. All detectable VOCs had median indoor/outdoor concentration ratios greater than one, suggesting that all detectable VOCs had indoor sources. Five of the VOCs (d-limonene, 2-butoxyethanol, n-undecane, n-dodecane, and hexanal) had median indoor/outdoor concentration ratios near or greater than 10.[83]

Standards. There are no standards for total VOCs. Many individual VOCs have TLVs and regulatory occupational exposure limits. (Refer to Chapter 4, Appendix A for methods of determining compliance with PELs or TLVs for mixtures of VOCs.) However, the measured indoor concentrations of individual compounds are nearly always lower than levels of known concern. Results from the EPA BASE study where "non-problem" public and private office buildings were studied, indicated the average concentration of total VOCs in 41 buildings was only 2.1 mg/m³.[82,84]

Control. Three approaches are of use in reducing indoor VOC exposure: source prevention or removal, dilution ventilation, and air cleaning. Controlling sources of VOCs involves selecting low emission materials where available, treating high emission sources before installation, and proper storage of organic chemicals. Based on extensive chamber testing studies of VOC emissions from building materials and furnishings over the past several years, many manufacturers and organizations have developed standards and labeling practices that have helped to reduce VOCs emissions from those products. Office furnishings, carpet, fabrics, wall coverings and paints are examples of materials that may be designated

Table 18.7 — VOCs Commonly Found in Normal Indoor Air of Office Buildings[83]

VOC	*Concentration Range (μg/m³)*	*VOC*	*Concentration Range (μg/m³)*
Acetone	7.1–220	d-Limonene	0.3–140
Toluene	1.6–360	Benzene	0.6–17
m- & p-Xylenes	0.8–96	1,1,1-Trichloroethane	0.6–450
n-Undecane	0.6–58	Hexanal	0.8–12
n-Dodecane	0.5–72	2-Butoxyethanol	0.7–78
Nonanal	1.2–7.9	n-Hexane	0.6–21

"low VOC" or "green" labeled if manufacturers subscribe to such programs. California's Section 01350, Special Environmental Requirements Specification references its *Standard Practice for the Testing of Volatile Organic Emissions from Various Sources Using Small-Scale Environmental Chambers* defines testing protocols and sets VOC emission limits based on the following chemicals of concern as listed by Cal-EPA[85]:

1. Chemicals with established Chronic Reference Exposure Levels (CRELs). A CREL is an airborne concentration level that would pose no significant health risk to individuals indefinitely exposed to that level. CRELs are based solely on health considerations and are developed from the best available data in the scientific literature.
2. Chemicals listed as: (a) probable or known carcinogens, or (b) reproductive toxicants.
3. The ten most abundant compounds emitted from the test material.

The Collaborative for High Performance Schools[31] has assessed building products certified to meet the Section 01350 low-emitting materials criteria, and is developing a High Performance Products Database as a source for materials with low emissions, recycled content, rapidly renewable materials, organic, certified wood, life cycle and multiple attributes.

Dilution ventilation is often successful in ameliorating some of the symptoms of VOC-suspected SBS, providing strongly emitting VOC sources are not present, and providing the ventilation system itself does not constitute a source. Increasing ventilation rates in the presence of strongly emitting sources may increase emission rates by enhancing vaporization. The use of activated charcoal and catalytic oxidation to scrub VOCs from the air is used in submarines, but is not known to be effective in situations where levels are already low.

Endocrine Disruptor Compounds (EDCs)

Nature and Sources. Endocrine disrupters, are substances that alter the normal function(s) of the endocrine systems of animals and humans. The air and dust inside buildings may contain a wide variety of chemicals, some of which have been identified as endocrine disrupting substances. The focus in recent years has been on two groups of chemicals[15]:

- *Polybrominated diphenyl ethers (PBDEs).* PBDEs are flame retardants added to plastics and textiles to meet fire safety regulations. They are commonly used in polyurethane foam products and electronics, and are included in mattresses, seat cushions, upholstered furniture, carpet padding, office machines, computers, circuit boards, appliance casings, televisions, upholstery fabrics, office furniture, rigid insulation, and building materials.
- *Phthalates.* Phthalates are plasticizers used to create flexible plastic products such as vinyl upholstery, vinyl sheet flooring, shower curtains, and garden hoses.

Both types of these chemicals are reported to be ubiquitous in indoor environments, especially in homes, where they are emitted from host materials.

Health Effects. Since EDCs are considered persistent in the environment and bioaccumulate in humans, there is much concern about adverse effects on growth, development and reproduction. It is felt that children are most susceptible. More research is needed on the health effects of exposure to PBDEs and phthalates.

Monitoring/Sampling. Air and dust samples of the PBDEs have been collected with passive PUF (polyurethane foam) samplers and active sampling with filters with analysis by high resolution GC/MS. Air and dust samples of the phthalates have been collected by various methods including OVS-Tenax sorbent tubes and filters with analysis by GC/FID or GC/MS or HPLC.

Levels Measured. Rudel, et. al., conducted extensive sampling for EDCs in indoor air and dust in 120 homes. The most abundant compounds in air included phthalates (plasticizers, emulsifiers), o-phenylphenol (disinfectant), 4-nonylphenol (detergent metabolite), and 4-tert-butylphenol (adhesive) with typical concentrations in the range of 50–1500 ng/m^3. The penta- and tetrabrominated diphenyl ethers (flame retardants) were frequently detected in dust, and 2,3-dibromo-1-propanol, the carcinogenic intermediate of a flame retardant banned in 1977, was detected in air and dust. Many pesticides were detected in air and dust, the most abundant being permethrins and the synergist piperonyl butoxide. Frequently finding previously banned pesticides suggested limited indoor degradation. Finding compounds of relatively low volatility in air indicated that air contaminants do not have to be volatile; they can be adsorbed on dust particles and suspended in the air.[86]

Standards. There are few guidelines or standards on these chemicals. Some risk based guidelines have been developed in EPA studies.[87] Penta- and octa- forms of PBDEs have been taken off the market since 2005, but deca-PBDE is still in use. Some bans on materials containing some forms of PBDEs have been put in place in several states.

Control. Reported preventative measures to minimize exposures include increased ventilation, routine cleaning, use of HEPA vacuums, use of low VOC emitting materials and less plastic and synthetic materials.

Radon

Nature and Sources. Radon is a noble gas that emits alpha particles with a half-life of 3.8 days. It is a decay product of radium 226, which is a decay product of the uranium 238 series. Radon progeny, two of which emit alpha particles, have half-lives of less than 30 min. See the decay scheme in Figure 18.2. Radon equilibrates rapidly with its decay products so that without a replenishing source, significant concentrations cannot be maintained. Prior to about 1983, radon was considered a problem only in such high risk areas as contaminated areas near inactive uranium mines. On the other hand, uranium 238, and hence radium 226, is a constituent of nearly all soils and rocks, although there is considerable geographic variation in concentration. The EPA publishes guidelines and recommendations for testing and remediation of radon problems[88,89], as well as detailed maps showing areas with the potential for radon emissions.[90] Groundwater in contact with radium-bearing granite can be a source of radon exposure, as can building materials made of such granite, or when contaminated with uranium or radium mill tailings. Elevated radon levels are most likely in below-grade spaces, especially in granitic areas. Residential exposure is almost always higher than that in multi-story buildings, and the highest residential levels are in basements, where levels have been measured that carry the same risk of lung cancer as that ascribed to heavy smoking. Nevertheless, commercial buildings supplied with contaminated groundwater or built of radium-containing building materials can also present some risk of radon exposure. More information about Radon is in Chapter 26, Ionizing Radiation.

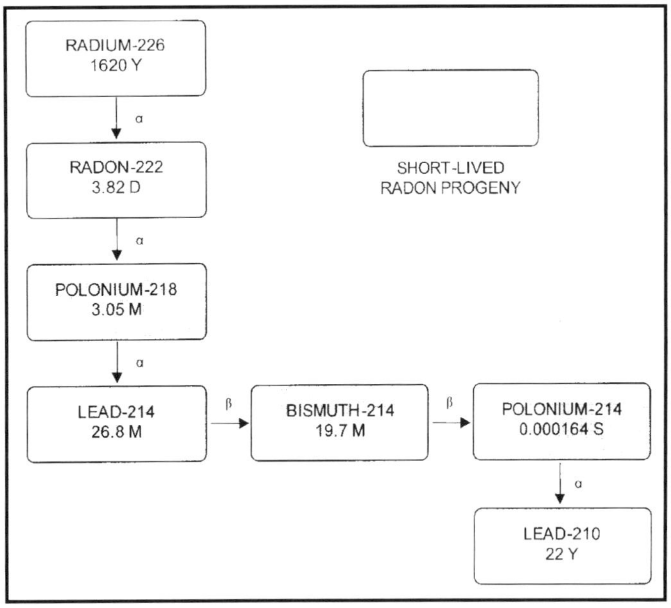

Figure 18.2 — Decay pathway from radium-226 to lead-210 by year, day, minute, and second (adapted from Ref. 169).

Health Effects. The major risks from exposure to radon decay products include lung cancer, some nasal cancers, and stomach cancer from ingestion of radon-containing water. It is estimated that 5,000 to 20,000 deaths per year are due to exposure to radon.[53,91] It has been reported that radon is the second leading cause of lung cancer in the U.S. and 12% or more of lung cancer deaths are linked to radon.[92] Lung cancer risk is increased in smokers. Radon decay products are present in the environment attached to particles as well as in a free state. Unattached radon decay products are small enough to reach the unciliated bronchiolar or alveolar regions of the lung where, due to long residence times, they cause damage by killing epithelial cells or transforming them into cancer precursors. Particles with attached radon progeny can lodge in the tracheobronchial tree emitting alpha particles that cause similar damage at this site.[93,94] Radon is not an irritant or acutely toxic and is therefore not of concern in acute epidemics of SBS or building-related disease.

Monitoring/Sampling. EPA has published guidelines for the use of continuous monitors (scintillation cell), 3- to 5-day integrating charcoal canisters, alpha-track detectors, and grab-sample scintillation cells that provide reasonable accuracy and precision. Passive radon samplers containing activated charcoal are readily available for monitoring most indoor environments, but must be exposed an extended time, to achieve sufficient detection. Active charcoal samplers provide sufficient detection in a much shorter time period.

Levels Measured. According to the EPA, the average indoor radon level in the U.S. is 1.3 pCi/L. As discussed above this varies geographically and seasonally. The average outdoor ambient radon level is 0.4 pCi/L.[88,95]

Standards. EPA guidelines suggest that radon levels be maintained below 4 pCi/L.

Control. Ventilation is the most economical method for removing radon. This practice, combined with the use of radium-free building materials and sealing of below-grade access points to prevent entry of radon from surrounding soil and rock, is effective in minimizing radon exposure in most interiors. If the water supply is contaminated, either changing the supply or removing radon by aeration or absorption with activated charcoal is effective.[53] In buildings where contaminated materials were used for construction, it may be helpful to seal surfaces with epoxy paint. The EPA provides guidance documents for radon reduction in existing and new construction.[89,96]

Biological Agents

Biological agents are living organisms or by-products from living organisms. They are ubiquitous in nature, and all persons are exposed to a wide variety of biological materials daily, indoors as well as outdoors. The term *biological agent* can be defined as a substance of biological origin that is capable of producing a host effect, for example, an infection or a hypersensitivity, irritant, inflammatory, or other response.[28] Some people will not experience health reactions to a given biological agent, while others may experience one or more of the following reactions:

- Infection
- Allergy effects
- Toxic effects

Specific biological agents are grouped here by these types of reactions for the purpose of discussion. Microbial VOCs do not fall into any of these categories and are discussed at the end of this section.

Agents of Infection

Infectious diseases caused by bacteria and viruses, examples being flu, measles, chicken pox, and tuberculosis, may be readily spread indoors. Most infectious diseases pass from person to person through physical contact. Crowded conditions with poor air circulation can promote this spread. Under certain conditions, some bacteria and viruses thrive in buildings and circulate through HVAC systems. For example, *Legionella Pneumophila*, the bacterium causing Legionnaire's disease (a serious and sometimes fatal infection) and Pontiac Fever (a flu-like illness) is known to thrive in and be disseminated by large HVAC systems or their cooling tower water. Although some illnesses have been linked to biological agents in the indoor environment, many also have causes not related exclusively to the indoor environment.

Nature and Sources. Viruses, bacteria, fungi, and (rarely) protozoa can grow in other organisms to cause disease. Many of the most common infectious diseases are airborne. This means that the agent becomes airborne in sufficient numbers to result in disease, survives transport through the air, and can cause infection readily via inhalation.

Sources for viral agents are nearly always infected people, and the airborne diseases are usually spread by coughing, sneezing, talking, or by aerosol generating processes. Sources for airborne bacterial infectious agents are also usually infected people or animals, although a few bacterial pathogens are spread primarily from environmental reservoirs (e.g., Legionella). The common environmental reservoirs for infectious bacteria are all associated with liquid water and include cooling towers, humidifiers, hot water systems, and recirculating water wash systems. The fungi and protozoa that cause infectious disease are always released from environmental reservoirs. The fungi require gaseous oxygen for growth and are usually found in damp environments or on the edges of liquid water reservoirs, whereas the protozoa are found only in water.

Table 18.8 — Disease Types, Agents of Infection, and Reservoirs

Type of Disease	*Agent*	*Disease*	*Reservoir(s)*
Contagious disease	Influenza viruses	influenza	infected people
	measles virus	measles	infected people
	Mycobacterium tuberculosis	tuberculosis	infected people
Virulent environmental infections	*Histoplasma capsulatum*	histoplasmosis	wet soil enriched with bird droppings
	Coccidioides immitis	coccidioidomycosis	dry soil (deserts)
	Legionella pneumophila	Pontiac fever	hot water systems, cooling towers, etc.
Opportunistic environmental infections	*Legionella pneumophila*	Legionnaires' disease	hot water systems, cooling towers, etc.
	Mycobacterium avium	atypical tuberculosis	natural water reservoirs
	Cryptococcus neoformans	cryptococcosis	dry bird droppings
	Aspergillus fumigatus	aspergillosis	self-heating plant-based organic matter

Health Effects. The infectious diseases can be classified into three groups: contagious diseases, virulent environmental-source infections, and opportunistic infections. The contagious diseases are caused by viruses and bacteria and are always transmitted from one person to another. Both the virulent and opportunistic environmental-source infections result from exposure to aerosols produced from environmental reservoirs. Examples of diseases within each of these categories are presented in Table 18.8.

Contagious and virulent diseases can infect all exposed people who are not specifically immunized (either artificially or by having had the infection). Theoretically, a single organism can penetrate to the appropriate site in the respiratory system and initiate the disease process, although exposure to many organisms (i.e., an infectious dose) is necessary before this event can occur.[97] By definition, opportunistic infections require that the host's natural immunity be impaired to some degree. Infection with Cryptococcus and Legionella require relatively little immune dysfunction (heavy smoking may be sufficient). Infection with *Mycobacterium avium* or *Aspergillus fumigatus* requires major damage to the immune system, and these agents are hazardous principally for patients with immunosuppresive diseases such as AIDS, some kinds of cancer, or those being treated with immunosuppressants (e.g., to prevent transplant rejection).[98]

Monitoring/Sampling. Air sampling for infectious viruses is difficult and seldom conducted as part of IAQ investigations. Confirmed infection in people may be sufficient evidence that a specific virus was present. Researchers have collected air samples for the detection of specific infectious agents with high-volume air samplers with filters, liquid impingers, cyclones and impactors. Samples have been analyzed by cell or tissue culture or by the detection of specific nucleotide sequences using polymerase chain reaction (PCR) technology. Bacterial sampling methods are similar, but include direct-agar impaction. Laboratory culture or PCR are the primary methods of analysis.

The opportunistic environmental agents, such as *Legionella pneumophila* and *Aspergillus fumigatus*, can be sampled using culturable techniques with subsequent identification of the organisms using either traditional morphological and physiological criteria, or using immunological or genetic tracers. Monitoring is usually not appropriate unless there is some reason to suspect the presence of a particular organism, or unless an especially sensitive population is likely to be exposed.

Levels Measured. For the opportunistic infections host risk factors are far more important than level of exposure. Thus, a relatively normal person will not become infected in the presence of millions of *Aspergillus fumigatus* spores, whereas for a severely immunocompromised person, a single spore is theoretically sufficient.

Standards. Several groups have proposed standards for levels of *Legionella pneumophila*, which can be found quite frequently in cooling tower water. One guideline suggests that recovery of culturable *Legionella* in concentrations exceeding 1000 CFU/mL of cooling tower water should prompt immediate remediation.[99] Lower levels are more difficult to interpret in the absence of reported cases. Miller and Kenepp[100] suggest that a dominance of *Legionella* (i.e., >50%) in a water sample should prompt concern. There are strict government mandates in the U.K.[101] and Australia[102] for cleaning cooling towers and testing for *Legionella*. Similar legislation may occur in the U.S in the future. Currently there are no uniform guidelines, rules or regulations regarding *Legionella* in the United States. The proposed ASHRAE Standard 188, Prevention of Legionellosis Associated with Building Water Systems, is under review. This standard is based on *ASHRAE Guideline 12–2000, Minimizing the Risk of Legionellosis Associated with Building Water Systems*.

Control. Control of contagious disease involves breaking the "chain of infection", as detailed in Chapter 22. Generally, exposure to aerosols from environmental sources (where the reservoir is known) can be prevented using isolation or, as a last resort, respiratory protection. For man-made reservoirs, biocides can be used to kill or at least limit the numbers of residual organisms following thorough cleaning of the reservoir. This approach is well established for *Legionella*. Additional preventive measures for *Legionella* include proper siting of cooling towers and other water mist sources so that emitted aerosols are not entrained into building air intakes, and ensuring that the systems are properly maintained. This is especially important in facilities such as hospitals that have susceptible occupants.[18,103,104] To protect patients from acquiring infections during hospital stays ("nosocomial" infections), it is important to incorporate safeguards into the actual design of new health care facilities, including special measures related to ventilation. Increasingly, industrial hygienists are invited to participate in the early planning stages. Several references are available to aid the practitioner.[103,105,106]

Allergens

Allergic reactions, one of the most common health problems related to IAQ, can range from being mildly uncomfortable to life-threatening, such as in anaphylatic shock or triggering of a severe asthma attack.

Nature and Sources. Allergens are proteins with the ability to trigger immune responses and cause allergic reactions, and they can be found in the indoor environment adhered to very small particles, either in the air or in settled dust (e.g., in carpets and on surfaces). Exposure to allergens indoors occurs mainly through inhalation of airborne particles.[107] A few very highly reactive chemicals can bind to serum proteins following exposure and stimulate antibody production. The major sources for allergens in indoor air are arthropods (cockroaches, dust mites), mammals (cats, dogs, rodents), birds, fungi, and actinomycetes. Some common airborne allergens and their biological sources are given in Table 18.9. Accumulated pollen grains provide a source for some of the most common indoor allergens. Natural rubber latex is a potent, at times debilitating occupational allergen that may be abundant in some hospital or cleanroom environments. Arthropod allergens are borne on fecal material or body parts, while the mammalian and avian allergens are borne on skin scales, particles of dried urine, saliva, or serum. The fungal allergens are often enzymes that are contained in fungal spores or produced as the spores germinate.[108] All of these organisms can occupy indoor environments and shed allergen-containing particles directly into the air or into dust that is subsequently aerosolized. Fungal spores are also abundant in outdoor air, as are pollen grains. To date, fungal allergens have not been extensively found in indoor environments.[109] Latex allergens are carried on latex gloves and other products, and become airborne on the powder used to facilitate the products' use.

Reservoirs for allergens in the indoor environment include dust (arthropods, fungi, vertebrate dander), water reservoirs from which aerosols are released (e.g., humidifiers), and surfaces supporting growth of organisms that readily release spores or other kinds of aerosols (e.g., dry-spored fungi).

Health Effects. The hypersensitivity diseases are caused by specific responses of

Table 18.9 — Some Common Airborne Allergens[28]

Agent	*Antigenic Product*	*Common Sources*
Pollen	Soluble antigens	Outdoor air, settled dust
Bacteria	Organisms, soluble antigens	Outdoor air, settled dust, indoor growth, humidifiers
Amebae	Soluble antigens	Humidifiers, wash waters
Fungi	Organisms, spores, fragments, soluble antigens	Outdoor air, settled dust, indoor growth, humidifiers
Arthropods		
Dust mites	Fecal pellets, dried body fragments	Settled dust
Cockroaches	Fecal particles, saliva, dried body fragments	Settled dust
Birds	Dried eggs, droppings, serum	Settled dust
Mammals		
Cats	Skin dander, saliva	Settled dust
Dogs	Skin dander, saliva, urine	Settled dust
Rodents	Urine	Settled dust, bedding

the immune system and require a two-step exposure process: initial exposures that stimulate the immune system, and a second set of exposures that result in mediator release and symptoms. Levels of allergens that induce each of these steps may differ.[11]

Airborne allergens cause diseases such as hypersensitivity pneumonitis, allergic rhinitis, and allergic asthma. Symptoms of hypersensitivity pneumonitis include fever, chills, shortness of breath, malaise, and cough. The disease mimics influenza initially, then pneumonia, but symptoms resolve with cessation of exposure. Long-term exposure can result in permanent lung damage.

Symptoms of allergic rhinitis include runny or itchy nose and eyes and sinus congestion, while those of allergic asthma are wheezing and chest tightness resulting from bronchiolar constriction. It is often difficult to separate these hypersensitivity conditions from vasomotor rhinitis and bronchoconstriction related to chemical or cold air exposures.[110] Allergic rhinitis and allergic asthma are controlled by a particular genotype borne by about 20–40% of the U.S. population. Approximately 6% of the U.S. population is sensitive to the nearly ubiquitous house dust mite, 2% to various animal danders, and less than 1% to various microbial allergens.[111]

Monitoring/Sampling. Samples for measurement of allergens can be collected either as bulk dust or directly from air. Dust sampling is preferentially used for the arthropod and mammalian allergens, while microorganisms are usually assessed using air sampling. Dust is considered to represent cumulative exposure over time, while air sampling represents only levels at the time of sampling. This distinction is particularly important for the allergens (including dust mite) that are borne on relatively large particles that remain in the air for only short periods after disturbance of reservoirs. The relevance of dust as a surrogate for airborne exposure remains to be clearly documented. At least for the fungi, there is a poor correlation between dust samples and simultaneously collected air samples.

Analysis of samples collected for allergen measurement is best performed using specific immunoassays. Such assays are available for major allergens derived from dust mites, cockroaches, cats, and dogs, and some fungi.

For the bacteria, culture followed by traditional methods is typically done, but other approaches are used.[28] Many bacteria may not be culturable, and culturability is not a prerequisite for allergenicity. For the fungi, culture is also a commonly used analytical method and the only method that ensures that all viable species of fungi collected can be identified. While PCR methods for microbials have been licensed, they currently detect fewer than 100 specific agents. Culturing is essential if patient treatment is to include immunotherapy. For total fungi, spore counts overcome the culturability problem, and some fungi can be identified from spore characteristics alone.

A combination of culture and microscopy can provide reasonably accurate quantitation of fungal aerosols.

Several analytical chemistry-based methods have been proposed for assessing total fungal load in indoor environments. Measurement of β(1-3)d-glucans or of ergosterol (the principal fungal sterol) have been used.[112] Both correlate well with culturable fungal counts, but provide no information on the kinds of fungi present.

Levels Measured. Levels of the arthropod and mammalian allergens in residences range from essentially undetectable to in excess of 10,000 µg/g of dust. Levels below 2 µg/g are considered low, between 2 and 10 µg/g moderate, and in excess of 10 µg/g sufficiently high that most sensitized people will experience symptoms. Results from the EPA BASE study show that cat allergen was found in almost all buildings sampled, and dust mite allergens were detected in approximately half of the samples. Although common, the concentrations found rarely exceeded accepted threshold levels associated with sensitization or symptom provocation.[113]

Levels of allergen-bearing bacteria (i.e., actinomycetes) in buildings are usually very low (<1/m³ of air), so that recovery of any of these organisms should stimulate a search for potential sources. Fungal levels in indoor environments are strongly related to the kind of ventilation, levels outdoors, seasonal variation, reservoirs indoors, and disturbance of the reservoirs.[28] Table 18.10 lists the most common fungi and bacteria found indoors in normal buildings, although sampling results may typically report numerous additional genera for any given sample. The taxa of fungi isolated from indoor and outdoor air should be similar and the concentration of airborne fungi should be lower indoors than outdoors. Outdoor airborne fungal concentrations (total culturable or countable fungi) are reported to exceed 1000 CFU/m³ routinely, and concentrations near 10,000 CFU/m³ are not uncommon in summer months. With these factors in mind, guidelines of acceptable ranges for non-industrial indoor environments are difficult to give without numerous qualifications. In specialized environments where immunosuppressed persons are present, levels of any saprophytic fungus below 100 CFU/m³ were reported as not of concern. The dominance in indoor air of specific fungi that are not common in outdoor air may signal problems at lower levels.[28] It is commonly recommended that visual identification or odor perception, confirmed by source sampling, is very reliable evidence of fungal growth and the potential for exposure.

Table 18.10 — Common Indoor Fungi and Bacteria

Fungi	Bacteria
Alternaria	Staphylococcus
Aspergillus	Micrococcus
Cladosporium	Flavobacterium
Penicillium	

Standards. There are no published standards for allergens in air or in reservoirs. Many governmental agencies and groups have proposed guideline upper limit levels that range from 50 to 2,000 total CFU/m³ for fungi in non-contaminated environments. However, these guidelines are not based on health effects, nor are they consistent with finding that average levels in normal non-air-conditioned homes during the growing season often exceed 2,000 CFU/m³.[114,115] A literature review reported an average fungal concentration of 1252 CFU/m³ (range 17 to 9100 CFU/m³) in 820 non-complaint residential structures. This review also noted that fungal concentrations found in residential buildings were consistently higher than those in commercial buildings.[116] The comparative approaches discussed above are generally preferred.

Comparisons of total bacteria levels indoors versus outdoors may not be as useful as for fungi, since natural bacteria reservoirs exist in both places. Comparisons of the specific types of bacteria present, excluding those of known human origin, can help determine building-related sources.[117] EPA BASE study results for airborne culturable bacteria suggest that 175 CFU/m³ may serve as an upper bounds guideline for

Table 18.11 — Proposed Risk Thresholds for Allergens in Dust Samples[113,119,120]

	Low	*Moderate*	*High*
Cat	< 1 µg/g	1–8 µg/g	> 8 µg/g
Fel d1	77.7%	21.5%	0.8%
Dust mite	< 2 µg/g	2–10 µg/g	> 10 µg/g
Der f1, Der p1	98%, 99.2%	1.2%, 0.4%	0.8%, 0.4%
Cockroach		2 U*/g	

* U – unit of allergen

office environments.[118] In the EPA BASE study, settled dust samples were collected for allergen analysis from 93 normal (non-complaint) office buildings. Table 18.11 shows the percentage of BASE samples by allergen concentration ranges proposed as relative risk thresholds for sensitization to cat and dust mite allergen.[113] A risk threshold for cockroach is listed based on published studies.[119,120]

Control. Cockroach allergen exposure is best achieved by eradicating cockroaches and by sealing the indoor environment to prevent their reinfestation. Dust mites can be controlled by keeping humidity within reservoirs consistently below 60%, by limiting the use of carpeting and upholstered furniture in humid environments, by encasing mattresses and other soft furnishings in plastic, and by washing bedding in hot water. Mammalian and avian allergens are best controlled by keeping animals and birds out of the indoor environment. Regular cleaning of indoor environments also aids in control of these allergens. Exposure to allergen-bearing bacteria (actinomycetes) usually results from aerosolization of spores from heated reservoirs. Keeping water out of ventilation systems, limiting the use of water spray humidification, and venting clothes dryers outdoors all will prevent their amplification. In commercial buildings, fungi grow primarily on material that is water-soaked or on which condensation is consistently present. Eliminating these water sources will essentially prevent fungal amplification. Water-damaged carpets, furnishings and building materials should be thoroughly cleaned and dried within 48 hours of any significant water intrusion event, or discarded, to prevent fungal growth. Moisture control is necessary through proper ventilation of areas where water is present and diligent maintenance of building HVAC systems.

Biological Toxins

The health effects of biological toxins in non-industrial environments and homes are not well understood and more research is needed. Many different kinds of organisms produce potent toxins. Notable among these are endotoxins (produced by some kinds of bacteria), β(1-3)d-glucans (part of the cell wall of most fungi), and the mycotoxins (secondary metabolites produced by many fungi).

Endotoxin

Nature and Sources. Endotoxin is a lipopolysaccharide that forms the outer cell wall of gram-negative bacteria. The lipid portion of the molecule is responsible for its toxicity.[121] Endotoxin is invariably present in ambient air and is a consistent component of house dust.

Health Effects. Endotoxin was first recognized as an air quality problem in the cotton processing industry, where it plays a role in diseases such as byssinosis. Exposure to endotoxin can result in acute bronchoconstriction, shortness of breath, cough, fever, and nausea, depending on the level and duration of exposure.[122,123] Disease-causing exposures (>50 ng/m^3) usually occur in association with recirculating water systems that produce aerosols and in agricultural and industrial environments where organic material is handled.[124] Some evidence suggests that endotoxin may also play a role in SBS; however, a dose-response relationship is not well documented in the non-industrial workplace.[125,126] Endotoxin also acts as a stimulant to the immune system and may play a role in sensitization to some allergens. There is also some evidence of lowered lung cancer rates in people routinely exposed to high levels of endotoxin.[127,128]

Monitoring, Levels. Endotoxin can be measured using the Limulus amoebocyte bioassay, or by using GC/MS methods. The Limulus method, which is most commonly used, is quite sensitive and measures biologically active endotoxin rather than actual amounts of lipopolysaccharide. GC/MS methods document total lipopolysaccharide and provide information on component structures, but are less sensitive than the Limulus method. Both bulk and air samples can be evaluated using these assays. Air samples are usually collected on filter media. Milton[121] proposed a standard method for sampling and analysis of airborne endotoxin that takes into account the variables associated with its ubiquity in the environment and its ability to adhere firmly to many sample collection media.

Levels of endotoxin in ambient air are usually <1 ng/m^3. Levels as high as 7 µg/m^3 have been measured in cotton mills, industrial settings where recirculating wash water is used, and in agricultural environments. In residential dust, median levels of 1.1 ng/mg have been reported.[121] Reported residential air levels have ranged from undetectable to 18 ng/m^3.[129]

Standards, Control. There is currently no standard for endotoxin in any environment. Control measures specific to endotoxin usually involve removal of source water or, where this is impossible, use of unrecirculated potable water. In some environments (e.g., machining shops where water-based lubricants/coolants are used) local exhaust ventilation or respiratory protection may be the only alternatives.

β(1-3)d-glucans

Nature and Sources. β(1-3)d-glucans form the major portion of most fungal cell walls and may be chemically bound to chitin (and hence insoluble), or may form a soluble matrix in which the chitin fibrils are embedded. Most fungi that are common in indoor environments contain β(1-3)d-glucans. Exceptions are the common black bread molds (Rhizopus sp.) and the mirror yeasts (Sporobolomyces).

Health Effects. β(1-3)d-glucans act as immunostimulants in a similar manner to endotoxin and may be involved in the development of hypersensitivity pneumonitis.[130,131] Their antitumor activities are well-recognized.[60] Soluble glucans appear to have an effect on the lung similar to that of endotoxin.[132]

Monitoring, Levels. The β(1-3)d-glucans act similarly to endotoxin in some Limulus assays. However, enzyme-linked immunosorbent assays have been developed that are sensitive and accurate.[133]

Control. Control measures separate from those discussed for the fungi have not been proposed.

Mycotoxins

Nature and Sources. Mycotoxins are secondary products of fungal metabolism. The chemical structures of mycotoxins are quite diverse, ranging from that of moniliformin ($C_4H_2O_3$) to complex polypeptides with molecular weights over 2,000. Although only a few have been studied, most fungi probably produce these secondary metabolites, the kinds and amounts depending on the fungal strain and the food source being metabolized. Mycotoxins probably play an ecological role in colony formation, and their production may depend on the presence of competing organisms. Mycotoxins can be present in either viable or nonviable fungi, in spores or mycelia; this is important for investigators to realize if they plan to draw conclusions based on viable fungi only.[134]

Exposure to mycotoxins occurs when moldy food is eaten, when contaminated materials are handled so that skin contact occurs, or when spores, mycelial fragments, or materials supporting growth are disturbed and become airborne.

Health Effects. The mycotoxins of primary concern with respect to IAQ are the potent cytotoxins that cause cell disruption and interfere with essential cellular processes. Some are carcinogenic (e.g., the aflatoxins produced by *Aspergillus flavus* and *A. parasiticus*). Others cause damage to the immune system or specific organs. The macrocyclic trichothecene toxins (produced by *Stachybotrys atra, Mycrothecium verrucaria*, and other fungi) fall into this latter class.

Toxicological data on mycotoxins is nearly all derived from ingestion exposures. For some trichothecene toxins, doses well below 1 mg/kg body weight are lethal for experimental animals by ingestion. Medical opinion does not support the proposition that human health has been adversely affected by inhaled mycotoxins in the home, school, or office environment.[135,136]

Monitoring/Sampling. Mycotoxins in indoor environments are assessed using either air or reservoir sampling with cultural or microscopic analysis for known toxigenic fungi. Rarely, analysis for specific mycotoxins is performed. Mycotoxins probably become airborne on particle sizes ranging from approximately 2–10 µm in diameter. Methods for collecting air samples depend on the kind of analysis to be performed. For cultural analysis, culture plate impactors are generally used. It should be noted that this kind of analysis detects only viable (culturable) propagules and may lead to serious underestimates in the potential for mycotoxin exposure under field conditions.

Microslide impactors can be used to sample for fungi such as *Stachybotrys chartarum* with spores that are readily identifiable microscopically. These have the advantage of reasonable sensitivity with no reliance on viability. Both culturable and slide impactors are generally used as short-term grab samplers and provide only a limited picture of the potential for exposure over time.

For most of the mycotoxins, methods for chemical analysis require more sample volume than is generally available from most air samples (except the most contaminated of environments). Immunoaffinity methods are available for aflatoxin, while analysis of the trichothecenes depends on either GC/MS or HPLC methods.

Standards and Levels Measured. Risk assessment is usually based on the presence of potentially toxigenic culturable fungi. No standards exist for mycotoxins in indoor air.

Control. Approaches for the control of exposure to mycotoxins rely on control of source fungi.

Microbial VOCs

VOCs are produced by all microorganisms, and to the extent such VOCs result exclusively from microbial growth, are termed MVOCs. A very wide range of different MVOCs are produced, ranging from ethanol and butanol to 8 and 9 carbon alcohols, aldehydes and ketones. These compounds cause odors readily associated with mold and decay. The role of MVOCs in human health is unknown and merits investigation. It is probable that microbial contamination in indoor environments with inadequate ventilation will at the very least exacerbate irritant symptoms and contribute discomforting odors.

Sampling. MVOCs can be monitored in the same way as other VOCs with the provision that the methods used must be sensitive, and samples must usually be collected near sources. Samples have been collected using adsorbents and canisters with analysis using GC/MS methods.

Levels Measured. Data from a limited number of MVOC studies show that levels of MVOCs found indoors are typically lower than VOC levels. Table 18.12[137–139] compares MVOC levels found in "non-complaint buildings" to those found outdoors and in "complaint buildings". MVOC levels in non-complaint buildings were essentially representative of outdoor air. In complaint buildings, where odor and eye, nose, and throat irritation complaints were common, MVOC levels were approximately 7 times higher than typical outdoor levels.[137–139]

Standards. There are no standards for MVOCs.

IAQ Problem Investigation, Remediation and Prevention

IAQ Investigation Strategies

Steps to resolving an IAQ problem may range from a simple common sense approach to a very complex action plan involving a team of professionals from various disciplines over an extended time period. The following discussion is general in nature, and more specific information should be obtained from references cited to develop effective investigation strategies. Most IAQ investigations are the result of occupant health or comfort concerns, and the approach presented focuses on this. Other investigations may include addressing specific problems in buildings, such as odors, microbial growth, or suspected building-related disease. Investigations as part of a building maintenance program may also be conducted to ensure, improve, or certify good IAQ.

Table 18.12 — MVOCs From Comparative Field Studies

Location	MVOC	Concentration Avg. and/or Range Found (µg/m^3)
Non-Complaint Buildings		
23 Homes[139]	1-Octen-3-ol	4.1
	2-Pentylfuran	3.7
132 Homes[138]	1-Octen-3-ol	1.8
	Pentan-2-ol	0.2
	3-Methyl-1-butanol	0.7
30 Buildings[137]	Total	2.2 – 8.8
Complaint Buildings		
30 Buildings[137]	Total	10.1 – 85.7 (avg. 29.2)
Outdoors		
27 Samples[137]	Total	1.1 – 9.5 (avg. 4.5)

Table 18.13 — Resources for IAQ Practitioners

Building Owners Guides	
Building Air Quality: A Guide for Building Owners and Facility Managers[140]	EPA and NIOSH — http://www.epa.gov/iaq
Building Air Quality — Action Plan[141]	EPA and NIOSH — http://www.epa.gov/iaq
Indoor Air Quality Tools for Schools Action Kit[142]	EPA — http://www.epa.gov/iaq
Investigation and Diagnosis	
Indoor Air Quality Building Education and Assessment Model (I-Beam) Software[143]	EPA — http://www.epa.gov/iaq
OSHA Technical Manual Sec. III, Chapter 2, Indoor Air Quality[144]	OSHA — http://www.osha-slc.gov/SLTC/indoorairquality/index.html
The IAQ Investigator's Guide[145]	AIHA — http://www.aiha.org/market
Ventilation and HVAC Systems	
ASHRAE Standard 62.1 Ventilation for Acceptable Indoor Air Quality[9]	ASHRAE http://www.ashrae.org
62.1 User's Manual[146]	ANSI/ASHRAE http://www.ashrae.org
The IAQ and HVAC Workbook, 5th ed.[147]	Burton, DJ http://www.aiha.org/market
IAQ Guidelines for Occupied Buildings Under Construction, 2nd ed.[148]	Sheet Metal and Air Conditioning Contractors National Association http://www.smacna.org
Biological Contaminants and Remediation	
Bioaerosols: Assessment and Control[28]	ACGIH — http://www.acgih.org
Field Guide for Determination of Biological Contaminants in Environmental Samples[134]	AIHA — http://www.aiha.org/market
Mold Remediation in Schools and Commercial Buildings[149]	EPA — http://www.epa.gov/iaq/molds
Guidelines on Assessment and Remediation of Fungi in Indoor Environments[150]	New York City Department of Health — http://www.nyc.gov/html/doh/downloads/pdf/epi/epi-mold-guidelines.pdf
Recognition, Evaluation, and Control of Indoor Mold[151]	AIHA — http://www.aiha.org/market
Standard and Reference Guide for Mold Remediation (S520)[152]	Institute of Inspection, Cleaning and Restoration Certification (IICRC) — http://www.iicrc.org
High Performance/Sustainable/Green Building and Energy Practices	
International Performance Measurement & Verification Protocol — Volume II Concepts and Practices for Improved Indoor Environmental Quality[153]	US Department of Energy (DOE) — http://www.ipmvp.org
CHPS Best Practices Manual[31]	Collaborative for High Performance Schools — http://www.chps.net/manual/index.htm
Leadership for Energy and Environmental Design (LEED)[6]	U.S. Green Building Council (USGBC) — http://www.usgbc.org
Advanced Energy Design Guide series[35]	ASHRAE — http://www.ashrae.org/publications/page/1604
Green Guide for Health Care[154]	Center for Maximum Potential Building Systems — www.gghc.org

A number of publications and resources are essential for the IAQ practitioner. No single resource fully addresses all the complexities of IAQ issues that one may encounter. Many are available on the internet at governmental agency websites. Table 18.13 lists several useful resources categorized by specific IAQ subject matter.

Initial Screening. When initially responding to complaints by building occupants, it is important to respond quickly, conduct interviews of affected individuals, and inspect the areas of concern. The goal is to characterize the complaints and identify any obvious causes of the problem. Typical questions to ask may include:

- What is the problem (e.g., odor, irritation)?
- When and where have you noticed it?
- What do you think is the cause?
- Do you have any symptoms (what are they, when do they occur, where)?
- How long do symptoms persist after leaving the building?
- Are there any recent changes in the area (chemicals, equipment, processes, building renovations)?
- Do you have allergies, wear contact lenses?
- Have you seen a doctor for these complaints?

Although rare, if potentially serious health problems are reported, the person should be referred to a medical professional for diagnosis and treatment. Likewise, if a serious environmental condition is found, people should be advised to leave the area, and the cause of the problem addressed immediately. Sometimes the concerns are not related to the building, so it is critical to gather sufficient information about the issues and the building environment. Questionnaires should be used with caution to avoid biased responses.

A walk-through inspection should be conducted in the area of concern and adjacent areas, and HVAC system that supplies air to the area. A number of resources give thorough checklists and guidance in inspecting these areas.[140,143] In general, the following should be considered:

- Are there odors in or near the area?
- Is there evidence of water intrusion, including dampness and staining?
- Is the area clean (dusty surfaces, housekeeping, proper food storage)?
- Are occupants near office equipment that may generate contaminants?
- Are temperature, humidity, and carbon dioxide levels in the normal range?
- During the HVAC inspection, determine if the system is operating properly, if filters are maintained, if fresh air is adequate, and if there are potential sources at air intakes. Are drip pans draining and is there microbial growth?

Many times complaints may be resolved by HVAC adjustments or improved cleaning of the area. It has been reported that most common IAQ complaints are related to temperature and air movement: The air is either too hot or too cold, or the air is too drafty or too still. Other common complaints are related to odors or dust. If deficiencies are found that may be related to the complaint, corrective actions can be made before considering more extensive evaluation. Sources of odors should be identified when possible. Based on observations, the need for any sampling can be determined. The whole environment should be considered in the initial screening since the complaints may not be building related, but only perceived as such. Other factors to consider are lighting, potential ergonomic problems, noise and vibration.

In an investigation where water intrusion or microbial growth is found, it is important to address such issues as quickly as possible. Water damaged materials should be dried completely within 24 to 48 hours or discarded to prevent potential microbial growth. Visual confirmation of microbial growth is usually enough evidence to proceed with a remediation plan. Specific guidance documents should be consulted for planning and removal of microbial growth and cleaning or disposing of contaminated materials.[149–152] Depending on the size of the contamination, specific recommendations are given for removal procedures, personal protective equipment and containment of the area.

The investigator should work closely with the building owner or building maintenance personnel to agree on corrective actions, both short term and long term. This should be communicated to area occupants so that they know what is being done and when. Involving the occupants early on, and enlisting their help if possible, can benefit

Table 18.14 — Typical Equipment and Monitors for Testing IAQ Parameters

IAQ Parameters	*Equipment and Monitors*
Ventilation	Temperature/relative humidity monitor Air velocity meter Smoke tubes/bottles Balometer Micromanometer Carbon dioxide monitor Moisture meter
Chemical Contaminants	Carbon monoxide monitor Electronic gas sensors Photoionization detector for VOCs (with ppb sensitivity) Sampling pumps, sorbent tubes, filters, impingers Passive monitors, detectors Gas sample bags, evacuated canisters Colorimetric detector tubes (CO, CO_2, NO_X, others with appropriate sensitivity)
Biological Contaminants	Moisture meter Sampling pumps, filters, treated filters, glass slide and media samplers Particle size selective samplers (impactors, cyclones) Surface wipe samplers, swabs
Particulates	Sampling pumps, filters, particle size selective samplers (impactors, cyclones) Surface wipe samplers, swabs Particle size selective samplers and monitors measuring concentration or particle count

the investigation. Timely follow up after corrective actions have been completed will determine if actions resolved the problem.

Detailed Assessment. When the initial screening is inconclusive or corrective actions fail to fix the problem, more extensive investigation may be needed. This may involve more thorough evaluation of the HVAC system and its maintenance, further checking for contaminant sources and sampling for suspect pollutants. Commonly used equipment and monitors for testing IAQ parameters are summarized in Table 18.14.

Assistance from other professionals may be needed to further characterize the problem, such as a mechanical engineer for evaluating the HVAC system, or a medical professional for health evaluations.

Sampling should only be conducted when it is clear how the data is to be used, and always with a well organized plan. This is especially important in IAQ investigations where microbial growth is concerned. Extensive baseline samples, control area samples, and indoor/outdoor comparison samples are needed when conducting air sampling. Sampling for extended periods of time using datalogging capabilities of monitors is sometimes needed to fully characterize some environments. Source sampling requires the same degree of planning. Guidelines for interpreting chemical and microbial data are not always consistent, so multiple resources should be consulted before drawing conclusions. Understanding what is "normal", or typically found in similar environments, is very important. Just as in the initial screening, communications to area occupants and timely follow up are very important, especially if corrective actions do not quickly resolve the issues.

IAQ Investigations in Certain Environments. The investigative approach discussed above is most applicable to a standard office building with mechanical HVAC systems. However, the investigator should be aware of special IAQ concerns in additional types of facilities and environments they may encounter. While the approach and methodologies presented earlier may still apply, the investigator may be challenged further with select populations, unusual living and work spaces, or conditions that require the development of more creative investigation and solution strategies. Table 18.15 presents a number of special environments with unique IAQ issues.

Table 18.15 — IAQ Considerations for Certain Environments

Environment	*Considerations*	*Resources*
Hospitals, health care facilities	Sensitive patients/residents; immunocompromised patients may not resist infection; potential for BRI (aspergillosis, Legionellosis, tuberculosis); hazardous chemicals, sensitizers, anesthetic gases, latex allergen, other allergens may be present in labs, sterilizers, pharmacies	IAQ in Healthcare Orgs Guideline — JCAHO[155] Infection Control — CDC[156] Infection Control in Design, Construction — Hansen[157], Health Canada[106] Legionella — CDC[103], OSHA[18], ASHRAE[104]
Schools	Low budgets; preventative maintenance low priority; overcrowding; natural ventilation and humidity issues; children sensitive to contaminants, allergens, asthma triggers	"Tools for Schools" IAQ guides — EPA[142] IAQ in Schools — WA state[32] Ventilation — ASHRAE 62.1[9] Design for IAQ — CHPS[31], EPA[30]
Recreational facilities	Humidity from swimming pools, locker rooms, saunas, human respiration; CO and NO_2 from ice rink care vehicles; food service areas	Ventilation — ASHRAE 62.1[9] Ice Rinks — MA state[158], PA state[159]
Transportation	Combustion products from various vehicles; security issues affecting building maintenance, construction activities; ventilation, disease transmission in aircraft	Ventilation — ASHRAE 62.1[9] Aircraft — ASHRAE 161[160], Hocking[161]
Residential buildings	Combustion sources for cooking and heating; ETS; allergens from pets, poor housekeeping; moisture sources; chemicals for cleaning, air fresheners, pesticides, crafts, hobbies	IAQ in Homes — EPA[162], CPSC[163] Ventilation — ASHRAE 62.2[164] and 24[165]
Basic living environments	Emissions from unvented cooking and heating stoves; solid fuels or biomass; possible overexposure to particulates, CO, VOCs, PAHs	IAQ Guidelines — WHO[51] Ventilation — ASHRAE 62.1[9]
Correctional and custodial care facilities	Security concerns; communication issues; sanitary conditions; moisture control; tuberculosis transmission control	Tuberculosis Control in Correctional Facilities — CDC[166] Ventilation — ASHRAE 62.1[9]
Libraries and museums	Ventilation and humidity control different for collections and occupants; chemicals in preservation, restoration, research areas	Ventilation — ASHRAE 62.1[9]

Preventative Measures and Maintaining Good IAQ

One of the best ways to prevent IAQ problems is to design buildings with IAQ in mind from the beginning. The same applies to building renovations. Given the opportunity, the very successful industrial hygienist is one who prevents IAQ problems from happening, and working closely with architects and construction professionals can foster such success. In the last several years the concepts of "healthy buildings", "green buildings", "sustainable buildings" and "high performance buildings" have evolved and become common practice. Guidelines and certifications that accompany these specific designations are not consistent nor is the IAQ component in such programs. Achieving good IAQ should be a major component in designing a "healthy" or any new building. Good IAQ should not be sacrificed for poorly planned energy reduction initiatives. Some of the factors in healthy building design and renovation will be discussed below, but more information should be obtained from selected resources.[167,168] Good ventilation system design is critical, as well as proper layout of the interior space. The exterior layout is also very important, including locating supply air intakes for HVAC systems away from potential contaminant sources, and the proper location of cooling towers. Using building materials and furnishings that do not emit excessive VOC's, and choosing low odor, non-toxic adhesives, sealants and paints will help ensure such necessary materials have minimal impact on building occupants. There is a perception that high performance or green buildings come with a cost premium. Initial construction cost may be higher than a conventional building, but in the longer term they can show a cost benefit because of occupant productivity. A number of studies suggest substantial economic benefits if better IAQ is provided in new and existing buildings because of occupants' improved health and productivity. Higher ventilation rates, reduced occupant density and reduced space sharing have resulted in statistically significant reductions in respiratory illnesses, such as influenza and common colds. Improved indoor temperature control, better lighting quality and increased daylighting have all been linked to productivity gains.[169]

Scheduling building renovations and repairs, such as roofing, painting and carpeting, during non-working hours also prevents IAQ problems. Occupants should be notified of projects that may impact their area, so that they are aware of the cause of any residual odors, and may relocate if necessary.

Proper maintenance of buildings cannot be overemphasized. This includes maintaining and inspecting HVAC systems on a regular basis, utilizing routine and thorough cleaning and housekeeping services, and addressing moisture problems and water leaks quickly. The use of chemicals, cleaning products and pesticides in buildings should be limited, and only those that have the least impact on occupants should be selected. To this end, facility managers and personnel need to be trained so that they can prevent IAQ problems, and also respond to IAQ issues when they occur.

Since occupants themselves can contribute to or be the source of an IAQ problem, they should be informed of what they can do to help maintain good IAQ. This includes not bringing in or using chemicals, pesticides or consumer products that may impact the work environment. They should also know to clean up small water spills promptly, store food properly, maintain good housekeeping, and not to block air vents or grills. They should know whom to contact to report temperature or ventilation problems, evidence of water leaks, or building cleaning and maintenance issues.

IAQ Around the World

Buildings in modern urban environments throughout the world, especially office buildings, tend to have similar construction and also similar IAQ problems. Variations depend on factors such as outdoor contaminant concentrations, sources of pollutants indoors and ventilation. Natural ventilation of buildings is used exclusively in some areas of the world, while mechanical ventilation is common in other areas.

Dramatic differences in IAQ problems are seen when comparing developed countries with less developed countries. The most significant IAQ issue for developing countries is exposure to pollutants released during combustion of solid fuels, including biomass (wood, animal waste and crop residues), charcoal and coal, used for cooking and heating in household settings. The WHO estimates over half of the world's population uses solid fuels in simple open or poorly ventilated stoves resulting in incomplete combustion and very high exposures. Children and women are predominantly affected. Studies have shown that the levels of emitted respirable particles and gases (including CO, NO_2, VOCs and polycyclic aromatic hydrocarbons) can be 10–20 times higher than common international air quality guidelines. If coal is used additional pollutants may be emitted, including oxides of sulfur and toxic substances such as arsenic and fluorine. The health effects associated with exposure to solid fuels (mainly biomass) from studies in developing countries indicate an increased incidence of chronic bronchitis in women, acute respiratory infections in children and, where coal is used, lung cancer. In addition, evidence is now emerging of links with a number of other conditions, including perinatal mortality, low birth weight, asthma, pneumonia, tuberculosis, chronic obstructive pulmonary disease, cataracts, and cancer of the upper airways.[51,170]

Recognizing that limited data is currently available to recommend numerical IAQ guidelines for developing countries, WHO has proposed a phased approach for developing guidelines to address the need for urgent action pragmatically. Measures include improving cooking/heating arrangements so that smoke is vented to the outside, switching to cleaner fuels, and improving stove design.[51]

According to the World Health Organization, tuberculosis kills more adults than any other infectious disease in the world. Since this airborne infection is believed to be transmitted between persons almost exclusively indoors, TB may qualify as the most deadly of all indoor air hazards.[170] TB is usually prevalent in poorer countries or poor communities where there are crowded living conditions, poor health care, malnutrition, and other diseases associated with TB. Although declining in the U.S., Canada and Western Europe with effective testing, treatment and control since the 1940s, a resurgence of TB cases has occurred in recent years. Persons in these countries, who were born in high prevalence countries, appear to contribute to a significant portion of the cases. TB control remains a substantial public health challenge in a number of settings, such as health care facilities (with immunocompromised and susceptible patients) and correctional institutions (with crowded and diverse populations).[51]

Concluding Remarks

State of the Art

Indoor air pollution and related health questions have been the subject of continuing research since the late 1970s. As the scope of knowledge advances, the astute investigator must stay current, and be equipped with the latest information before embarking on any investigation. Sources of reputable information include the proceedings of the most recent scientific meetings focusing on IAQ, training courses sponsored by professional organizations, and publications and resources from regulatory agencies and professional organizations that address IAQ issues.

Controversial Topics and Research Needs

Despite progress in the field of IAQ, uncertainties remain in some areas, generating controversy. Some of these issues include symptom complexes that remain unclear (MCS), the role of mycotoxins and MVOCs in building-related complaints, and the role of routine monitoring and control measures in the absence of clearly defined problems (especially with respect to *Legionella*). Reference to the most recent literature on these topics is essential before initiating investigations, interpreting data, or recommending remedial measures.

Interdisciplinary research is needed to help resolve questions that linger. Asthma causalities related to IAQ need to be clarified. For microbiological agents the dose-response characteristics and human susceptibility factors need to be more clearly understood. The role of EDCs in IAQ and chronic disease needs more study. The chemistry of mixtures of air contaminants indoors is not the same as it is outdoors, and studies on these mixtures and chemical interactions may draw attention to potentially harmful atmospheres. More sophisticated IAQ exposure models need to be developed and validated to predict performance of building and ventilation designs.

Summary

Air quality varies widely both outdoors and in. Indoor air is a complex mixture of outdoor air (with its entrained contaminants) and particulates, aerosols and gases released indoors. Indoor contaminants can include fine particulate from lead-based paint, infectious bioaerosols released by people or environmental reservoirs, combustion-related fumes from cooking/heating fuel or candle-burning, aerosol spray, allergens from dust mites, cockroaches, pets, and microbial toxins from bacteria and fungi. Gases include carbon dioxide (primarily from exhaled breath), carbon monoxide, nitrogen oxides, sulfur oxides (from combustion), ozone (from electrical equipment), formaldehyde (from building materials), other VOCs (released from building materials, furnishings, occupant activities, and microbial growth) and radon.

Health effects can range from discomfort to infections, allergic diseases (asthma, allergic rhinitis, hypersensitivity pneumonitis), toxicoses (cancer, asphyxiation, skin rash, mucous membrane irritation), and psychosomatic issues. Successful IAQ investigations often involve collaboration among specialists. Before sampling or monitoring, the investigator functions first as a detective, to establish the facts of the case. Problem resolution often involves improvements to the HVAC system, which may include testing, balancing, and commissioning. More diligent building maintenance and cleaning may be required. Lessons learned in problem buildings have led to improvements in design practices for new buildings. Acceptable levels of air contaminants in non-industrial settings have developed from a variety of sources, including data from "non-problem" buildings, standards established for outdoor air, and research studies. Even with these benchmarks, the investigator is called upon to contribute their skills in determining sources and proposing practical solutions to IAQ issues they encounter.

Acknowledgements

The authors would like to acknowledge the contributions of the original authors of the first edition of this chapter, Dr. Harriet A. Burge and Dr. Marion E. Hoyer.

References

1. **Samet, J.M., J.D. Spengler:** Indoor Environments and Health: Moving into the 21st Century. *Am. J. Public Health 93(9):*1489–1493 (2003).
2. **American Society of Heating, Refrigerating and Air-Conditioning Engineers (ASHRAE):** Indoor Air Quality Position Document. Atlanta, GA: ASHRAE, 2005.
3. **Mendell, M.J., et al.:** Causes and prevention of symptom complaints in office buildings: Distilling the experience of indoor environmental quality investigators. *Facilities (26)11/12:*436–444 (2006).
4. **Epstien, B., J. Panko and E. Horner:** State of the Science: Resolving Indoor Environmental Quality Concerns — Where Have We Been? Where Are We Now? Where are We Going? Presented at American Industrial Hygiene Conference and Expo, June, 2008. (Abstract).
5. **The Carpet and Rug Institute (CRI):** Green label testing protocol and product requirements. Retrieved from http://www.carpet-rug.org/commercial-customers/green-building-and-the-environment/green-label-plus/carpet-and-adhesive.cfm
6. **U.S. Green Building Council (USGBC):** LEED® for New Construction & Major Renovations. Washington, DC: USGBC, 2011. Retrieved from http://www.usgbc.org.
7. **Spengler, J.D., T. Platts-Mills, C. Mitchell, M. Hodgson, and E. Storey:** What is the scientific evidence for health problems associated with the indoor environment? 2005 Surgeon General's Workshop on Health Indoor Environment. Bethesda, MD: National Institutes of Health, 2005.
8. **Weschler, C.J. and J.C. Little:** Chemical and physical factors that influence pollutant dynamics in indoor atmospheric environments. *Atmospheric Env. 41:*3109–3110 (2007).
9. **American Society of Heating, Refrigerating and Air-Conditioning Engineers (ASHRAE):** Standard 62.1–2010: Ventilation for Acceptable Indoor Air Quality. Atlanta, GA: ASHRAE, 2010.
10. **Milton, D.K., P.M. Glencross, M.D. Walters, S. Kumar, and W. Fisk:** IEQ and the impact on employee sick leave. *ASHRAE J. 44(7):*97–98 (2002).
11. **Cookingham, C.E. and W.R. Solomon:** Bioaerosol-induced hypersensitivity diseases. In *Bioaerosols.* Burge, H. (ed.). Boca Raton, FL: CRC/Lewis Publishers, 1995.
12. **Center for Managing Chronic Disease:** Asthma Health Outcomes Project. University of Michigan, Dec. 2007. Retrieved from http:// asthma.umich.edu/media/ahop_autogen/AHOP_2-21-08.pdf
13. **American Academy of Allergy, Asthma and Immunology (AAAI):** Types of Asthma. AAAI website. Retrieved from http://www.aaai.org/patients/allergic_asthma/types.stm
14. **National Academy of Sciences (NAS):** *Clearing the Air: Asthma and Indoor Air Exposures.* Washington, D.C.: National Academy Press, 2000.
15. **California Air Resources Board (ARB):** Indoor Air Pollution in California, Report AB1173. Sacramento, CA: ARB, July 2005. Retrieved from http://www.arb.ca.gov/research/indoor/ab1173/finalreport.htm
16. **U.S. Environmental Protection Agency (EPA):** Indoor Environmental Asthma Triggers. EPA website, Retrieved from http://www.epa.gov/asthma/triggers.html
17. **Burge, H.A.:** Airborne Contagious Disease. In *Bioaerosols.* Burge, H.A. (ed.). Boca Raton, FL: CRC/Lewis Publishers, 1995.
18. **Occupational Safety and Health Administration (OSHA):** OSHA Technical Manual, Section III, Chapter 7, Legionnaires' Disease. Retrieved from http://www.osha.gov/dts/osta/otm/otm_iii/otm_iii_7.html. Washington DC: OSHA, 1999.
19. **U.S. Environmental Protection Agency (EPA):** Indoor Air Quality Glossary of Terms. EPA website. Retrieved from http://www.epa.gov/iaq/glossary.html

20. **U.S. Environmental Protection Agency (EPA):** Indoor Air Pollution: An Introduction for Health Professionals, EPA 402-R-94-007. Washington, DC: 1994. Retrieved from http://www.epa.gov/iaq/pubs/hpguide.html
21. **Bartha, L., et al.:** Multiple Chemical Sensitivity: A 1999 Consensus. *Arch. Environ. Health 54(3)*:147–49 (1999).
22. **Ashford, N. and C. Miller:** *Chemical Exposures: Low Levels and High Stakes*, 2nd edition. New York: John Wiley & Sons, 1998.
23. **Standenmayer, H:** *Environmental Illness: Myth and Reality.* Boca Raton, FL: CRC/Lewis Publishers, 1998.
24. **The Interagency Workgroup on Multiple Chemical Sensitivity:** A Report on Multiple Chemical Sensitivity (Predecisional Draft). Atlanta, GA: Agency for Toxic Substances and Disease Registry, 1998. Retrieved from http://www.health.gov/environment/mcs/toc.htm
25. **American Society of Heating, Refrigerating, and Air-Conditioning Engineers (ASHRAE):** ANSI/ASHRAE Standard 55–2010, Thermal Environmental Conditions for Human Occupancy. Atlanta, GA: ASHRAE, 2010.
26. **Fang, L., G. Clausen, and P.O. Fanger:** Impact of Temperature and Humidity on Acceptability of Indoor Air Quality During Immediate and Longer Whole-Body Exposures. Proceedings of Healthy Buildings/IAQ'97, Vol. 2:231–236, Washington, DC (1997).
27. **Molhave, L., Z. Sui, A.H. Jorgensen, O.F. Pedersen, S.K. Kjaergaard:** Sensory and Physiological Effects on Humans of Combined Exposures to Air Temperatures and Volatile Organic Compounds. *Indoor Air 3(3)*:155–169 (1993).
28. **American Conference of Governmental Industrial Hygienists (ACGIH®):** *Bioaerosols: Assessment and Control.* Cincinnati, OH: ACGIH®, 1999.
29. **American Industrial Hygiene Association (AIHA®):** *Odor Thresholds for Chemicals with Established Occupational Health Standards.* Fairfax, VA: AIHA®, 1989.
30. **U.S. Environmental Protection Agency (EPA):** IAQ Design Tools for Schools. Washington, DC: EPA, 2010. Retrieved from http://www.epa.gov/iaq/schooldesign/
31. **Collaborative for High Performance Schools (CHPS):** *CHPS Best Practices Manual.* San Francisco, CA: CHPS, 2006. Retrieved from http://www.chps.net/dev/Drupal/node/288
32. **Washington State Department of Health:** *School Indoor Air Quality Best Management Practices Manual.* Olympia, WA: 2003. Retrieved from http://www.doh.wa.gov/ehp/ts/IAQ/schooliaqbmp.pdf
33. **American Society of Heating, Refrigerating, and Air-Conditioning Engineers (ASHRAE):** *High Performance Building Design.* Atlanta, GA: 2009. Retrieved from http://www.ashrae.org/certification/page/1683
34. **Levin, H.:** Systematic Evaluation and Assessment of Building Environmental Performance (SEABEP). Presented at Buildings and Environment, 2nd International Conference, June 1997.
35. **American Society of Heating, Refrigerating and Air-Conditioning Engineers (ASHRAE):** *Advanced Energy Design Guides.* Atlanta, GA: ASHRAE, 2010. Retrieved from http://www.ashrae.org/publications/page/1604
36. **Emmerich, S.J.:** Simulated Performance of Natural and Hybrid Ventilation Systems in an Office Building. HVAC & R Research. Oct, 2006.
37. **American Society of Heating, Refrigerating and Air-Conditioning Engineers (ASHRAE):** *Standard 52.2–2007: Method of Testing General Ventilation Air-Cleaning Devices for Removal Efficiency by Particle Size.* Atlanta, GA: ASHRAE, 2007.
38. **Brennan, T., J.B. Cummings and J. Lstiburek:** Unplanned Airflows and Moisture Problems. *ASHRAE Journal. 44(11)*: 44–52 (2002).
39. **U.S. Environmental Protection Agency (EPA):** National Ambient Air Quality Standards (NAAQS), 40 CFR part 50. Washington, DC: EPA, 2011. Retrieved from http://www.epa.gov/air/criteria.html.
40. **California Air Resources Board:** Ambient Air Quality Standards (California Code of Regulations, Title 17, Section 70200). Sacramento, CA: ARB, 2010.
41. **Health Canada:** Exposure Guidelines for Residential Indoor Air Quality. Ottawa, Ontario: Health Canada, 1989.
42. **Health Canada:** Residential Indoor Air Quality Guideline, Formaldehyde. Ottawa, Ontario: Health Canada, 2006. Retrieved from http://www.hc-sc.gc.ca/ewh-semt/pubs/air/formaldehyde-eng.php
43. **Health Canada:** Residential Indoor Air Quality Guidelines, Moulds. Ottawa, Ontario: Health Canada, 2007. Retrieved from http://www.hc-sc.gc.ca/ewh-semt/pubs/air/mould-moisissure-eng.php
44. **National Research Council Canada:** *Indoor Air Quality Guidelines and Standards*, RR-204. Ottawa, Ontario: National Research Council Canada, 2005. Retrieved from http://irc.nrc-cnrc.gc.ca/pubs/rr/rr204/rr204.pdf
45. **State of California, Office of Environmental Health Hazard Assessment (OEHHA):** Chronic Reference Exposure Levels (CRELs). Sacramento, CA: OEHHA, 2008. Retrieved from http://www.oehha.org/air/chronic_rels/AllChrels.html

46. **Texas Department of Health (TDH):** Texas Voluntary Indoor Air Quality Guidelines for Government Buildings (Pub. No. 2-10). Austin, TX: TDH, 2003. Retrieved from http://www.dshs.tx.us/iaq/SchoolsGuide.shtm
47. **Occupational Safety & Health Administration (OSHA):** Limits for Air Contaminants (Standard 1910.1000 Table Z-1). Washington, D.C.: OSHA, 2006.
48. **National Institute for Occupational Safety and Health (NIOSH):** *NIOSH Pocket Guide to Chemical Hazards* (NIOSH Pub. No. 2010-68). Cincinnati, OH: NIOSH, 2010.
49. **American Conference of Governmental Industrial Hygienists (ACGIH®):** *2011 TLVs® and BEIs®*. Cincinnati, OH: ACGIH®, 2011.
50. **American Industrial Hygiene Association (AIHA®):** *2010 Workplace Environmental Exposure (WEEL™) Values.* Fairfax, VA: AIHA®, 2010. Retrieved from http://www.aiha.org/1documents/Committees/weel-levels.pdf
51. **World Health Organization (WHO):** Guidelines for Indoor Air Quality: Selected Pollutants. Copenhagen, Denmark: WHO, 2010. Retrieved from http://www.euro.who.int/_data/assets/pdf_file/0009/129169/e94535.pdf.
52. **American Society for Testing and Materials (ASTM):** ASTM Standards on Indoor Air Quality (various). West Conshohocken, PA: ASTM, 2007.
53. **U.S. Environmental Protection Agency (EPA):** Technical Support Document for the 1992 Citizen's Guide to Radon (EPA/400-R-92-011). Washington, D.C.: EPA, 1992.
54. **U.S. Department of Housing and Urban Development (HUD):** HUD Technical Guidelines for the Evaluation and Control of Lead-Base Paint Hazards in Housing. Washington, DC: HUD, 1995. Retrieved from http://www.hud.gov/offices/lead/lbp/hudguidelines/index.cfm
55. **Vesper, S.J., et al.:** Development of an Environmental Relative Moldiness Index for U.S. Homes. *J. Occup. Env. Med. 49(8)*:829–833 (2007).
56. **Lee, S.D.:** Nitrogen Oxides and Their Effects on Health. Ann Arbor, MI: Ann Arbor Science Publishers, 1980.
57. **Ahmed, T., I. Danta, R.L. Dougherty, R. Shreck, et al.:** Effect of NO2 (0.1 ppm) on specific bronchial reactivity to ragweed antigen in subjects with allergic asthma. *Am. Rev. Respir. Dis. 127*:160 (1983). [Abstract]
58. **California Air Resources Board (ARB):** Proposed Identification of Environmental Tobacco Smoke as a Toxic Air Contaminant. Final report, September 29, 2005, approved by Scientific Review Panel on June 24, 2005. Sacramento, CA: ARB, 2005. Retrieved from http://www.arb.ca.gov/toxics/ets/ets.htm
59. **Centers for Disease Control and Prevention (CDC):** *The Health Consequences of Involuntary Exposure to Tobacco Smoke: A Report of the Surgeon General.* Atlanta, GA: CDC, 2006.
60. **American Society of Testing and Materials (ASTM):** Standard D 5955-02 (2007), *Standard Test Methods for Estimating Contribution of Environmental Tobacco Smoke to Respirable Suspended Particles Based on UVPM and FPM.* West Conshohocken, PA: ASTM, 2007.
61. **Samet, J.M. and S.S. Wang:** Environmental Tobacco Smoke. In *Indoor Air Quality Handbook.* Spengler, J.D., J.M. Samet and J.F. McCarthy (eds.). New York: McGraw-Hill, 2001. pp. 30.1–30.30.
62. **Weichenthal, S., A. Dufresne and C. Infante-Rivard:** Indoor ultrafine particles and childhood asthma: Exploring a potential public health concern. *Indoor Air 17(2)*:81–91 (2007).
63. **Fogarty, R. and P.A. Nelson:** Tracking Ultrafine Particles in Building Investigations. In *Indoor Air Quality Handbook.* Spengler, J.D., J.M. Samet and J.F. McCarthy (eds.). New York: McGraw-Hill, 2001. pp. 50.1–50.18.
64. **U.S. Environmental Protection Agency (EPA):** *An Introduction to Indoor Air Quality, Asbestos.* Washington, DC: EPA, 2008. Retrieved from http://www.epa.gov/iaq/asbestos.html
65. **National Institute for Occupational Safety and Health (NIOSH):** Asbestos Bibliography (Revised), DHHS(NIOSH) Pub. No. 97-162. Cincinnati, OH: NIOSH, 1997. Retrieved from http://www.cdc.gov/niosh/pdfs/97-162.pdf
66. **U.S. Environmental Protection Agency (EPA):** Laws and Regulations, Asbestos. Washington, D.C.: EPA website, 2010. Retrieved from http://www.epa.gov/asbestos//pubs/asbreg.html
67. **Occupational Safety and Health Administration (OSHA):** Asbestos, OSHA Standards. Washington, D.C.: OSHA website, 2008. Retrieved from http://www.osha.gov/SLTC/asbestos/standards.html
68. **World Health Organization (WHO):** Environmental Health Criteria 203, Chrysotile Asbestos. Geneva, Switzerland: WHO, 1998.
69. **Vallarino, J.:** Fibers. In *Indoor Air Quality Handbook.* Spengler, J.D., J.M. Samet and J.F. McCarthy (eds.). New York: McGraw-Hill, 2001. pp. 37.1–37.22.
70. **U.S. Environmental Protection Agency (EPA):** Indoor Air Quality in Homes/Residences, Lead-Based Paint. Washington, D.C.: EPA website, 2011. Retrieved from www.epa.gov/iaq/homes/hip-lead.html

71. **U.S. Environmental Protection Agency (EPA):** Lead in Air, Regulatory Actions. Washington, D.C.: EPA website, 2008. Retrieved from http://epa.gov/air/lead/actions.html
72. **U.S. Environmental Protection Agency (EPA):** Air Trends, Lead. Washington, D.C.: EPA website, 2010. Retrieved from http://www.epa.gov/air/airtrends/lead.html
73. **State of California Air Resources Board (ARB):** Final Regulation Order for Limiting Ozone Emissions from Indoor Air Cleaning Devices. Sacramento, CA: ARB, 2008. Retrieved from http://www.arb.ca.gov/regact/2007/iacd07/finalreg07.pdf
74. **U.S. Environmental Protection Agency (EPA):** Draft guidance for evaluating the vapor intrusion to indoor air pathway from groundwater and soils (Subsurface vapor intrusion guidance). Washington, D.C.: EPA, 2002. Retrieved from http://epa.gov/osw/hazard/correctiveaction/eis/vapor/complete.pdf
75. **Nazaroff, W.W., B.K. Coleman, H. Destaillats, A.T. Hodgson, et al.:** Indoor air chemistry: Cleaning agents, ozone and toxic air contaminants, ARB Contract No. 01-336. Berkeley, CA: University of California, 2006. Retrieved from http://www.arb.ca.gov/research/apr/past/indoor.htm
76. **Singer, B.C., H. Destaillats, A.T. Hodgson and W.W. Nazaroff:** Cleaning products and air fresheners: emissions and resulting concentrations of glycol ethers and terpenoids. *Indoor Air 16*:179–91 (2006).
77. **Wolkoff, P, C.K. Wilkins, P.A. Clausen, and G.D. Nielsen:** Organic compounds in office environments- sensory irritation, odor, measurements and the role of reactive chemistry. *Indoor Air 16*:7–19 (2006)
78. **Rinsky, R.A., A.B. Smith, R. Hornung, T.G. Filloon, et al.:** Benzene and leukemia: an epidemiologic risk assessment. *N. Engl. J. Med. 316*:1044–50 (1987).
79. **Rodricks, J.V.:** Assessing carcinogenic risks associated with indoor air pollutants. In *Indoor Air and Human Health*, 2nd edition. Gammage, R.B. and B.A. Berven (eds.). Boca Raton, FL: CRC/Lewis Publishers, 1996.
80. **Hodgson, A.T.:** A review and a limited comparison of methods for measuring total volatile organic compounds in indoor air. *Indoor Air 5(4)*:247–257 (1995).
81. **Brown, S., M.R. Sim, M.J. Abramson, and C.N. Gray:** Concentrations of volatile organic compounds in indoor air-a review. *Indoor Air 4*:123–134 (1994).
82. **Tucker, W.G.:** Volatile Organic Compounds. In *Indoor Air Quality Handbook*. Spengler, J.D., J.M. Samet and J.F. McCarthy (eds.). New York: McGraw-Hill, 2001. pp. 31.1-31.20.
83. **Girman, J.R., G.E. Hadwen, L.E. Burton, S.E. Womble, and J.F. McCarthy:** Individual volatile organic compound prevalence and concentrations in 56 buildings of the building assessment survey and evaluation (BASE) study. Proceedings of Indoor Air 1999. pp. 460–465.
84. **U.S. Environmental Protection Agency (EPA):** Building Assessment, Survey and Evaluation Study (BASE). Information available at http://www.epa.gov/iaq/base. Washington, DC: EPA, 2011.
85. **California Dept. of Health Services (DHS):** Standard Method for the Testing and Evaluation of Volatile Organic Chemical Emissions from Various Indoor Sources Using Environmental Chambers. Sacramento, CA: DHS, 2010.
86. **Rudel, R.A., D.E. Camann, J.D. Spengler, L.R. Korn and J.G. Brody:** Phthalates, alkylphenols, pesticides, polybrominated diphenyl ethers, and other endocrine-disrupting compounds in indoor air and dust. *Environ. Sci. Technol. 37(20)*: 4543–53 (2003).
87. **U.S. Environmental Protection Agency (EPA):** Endocrine Disruptor Screening Program (EDSP). EPA website, 2011. Retrieved from http://www.epa.gov/endo/
88. **U.S. Environmental Protection Agency (EPA):** A Citizen's Guide to Radon (EPA 402-K-09-001). Washington, D.C.: EPA, 2009. Retrieved from http://www.epa.gov/pdfs/citizensguide.pdf
89. **U.S. Environmental Protection Agency (EPA):** EPA Model Standards and Techniques for Control of Radon in New Residential Buildings. Washington, DC: EPA, March 1994. Retrieved from http://www.epa.gov/radon/pubs/newconst.html
90. **U.S. Environmental Protection Agency (EPA):** EPA Map of Radon Zones. EPA website, 2011. Retrieved from http://www.epa.gov/radon/zonemap.html.
91. **Nero, A.:** Indoor Concentrations of Radon 222 and its Daughters: Sources, Range and Environmental Influences. In *Indoor Air and Human Health*, 2nd edition. Gammage, R.B. and B.A. Berven (eds.). Boca Raton, FL: CRC/Lewis Publishers, 1996. pp. 43–67.
92. **National Academy of Sciences (NAS):** *Health Effects of Exposure to Radon*. Washington, D.C.: National Academy Press, 1999.
93. **Samet, J.M.:** Radon and Lung Cancer Revisited. In *Indoor Air and Human Health*, 2nd edition. Gammage, R.B. and B.A. Berven (eds.). Boca Raton, FL: CRC/Lewis Publishers, 1996. pp. 325-340.
94. **Ellet, W. and N. Nelson:** Epidemiology and Risk assessment: Testing Models for Radon-Induced Lung Cancer. In *Indoor Air and Human Health*, 2nd edition. Gammage, R.B. and B.A. Berven (eds.). Boca Raton, FL: CRC/Lewis Publishers, 1996. pp. 79-129.

95. **National Academy of Sciences (NAS):** *Biological Effects of Ionizing Radon* (BEIR) VI Report. Washington, D.C.: NAS, 1998.
96. **U.S. Environmental Protection Agency (EPA):** Consumers Guide to Radon Reduction (402-10/005). Washington, D.C.: EPA, 2010. Retrieved from http://www.epa.gov/radon/pubs/consguid.html
97. **Riley, R.L.:** Indoor airborne infection. *Environ. Int. 8*:317–320 (1982).
98. **Rhame, F.S., A.J. Streifel, K.H. Kersey, and P.B. McGlave:** Extrinsic risk factors for pneumonia in the patient at high risk of infection. *Am. J. Med. 76*:42–52 (1984).
99. **Morris, G.K., and J.C. Feeley:** Legionella: impact on indoor air quality and the HVAC industry. In *Proceedings of the American Society of Heating, Refrigerating and Air-Conditioning Engineers' (ASHRAE) Annual Meeting*. Atlanta, GA: ASHRAE, p. 77 (1990). [Abstract]
100. **Miller, R.D., and K.A. Kenepp:** Legionella in Cooling Towers: Use of Legionella-Total Bacteria Ratios. In *Aerobiology*. Muilenberg, M. and H. Burge (eds.). Boca Raton, FL: CRC/Lewis Publishing, 1996. pp. 99–107.
101. **Health and Safety Executive (HSE) (UK):** The Control of Legionella Bacteria in Water Systems. Approved code of practice and guidance. London, UK: HSE, 2000.
102. **Australian/New Zealand Standard:** Air handling and water systems of buildings, microbial control. AS3666, Parts 1,2,3. Sydney, AU: Standards Australia, 2002.
103. **Centers of Disease Control and Prevention (CDC):** *Guidelines for Environmental Infection Control in Healthcare Facilities*. Atlanta, GA: CDC, 2003. Retrieved from http://www.cdc.gov/mmWR/preview/mmwrhtml/rr5210a1.htm.
104. **American Society of Heating, Refrigerating and Air-Conditioning Engineers (ASHRAE):** ASHRAE Guideline 12–2000, *Minimizing the Risk of Legionellosis Associated with Building Water Systems*. Atlanta, GA: ASHRAE, 2000.
105. **Bartley, J.M.:** *APIC State-of-the-Art Report: The Role of Infection Control During Construction of Health Care Facilities*. Retrieved from http://www.apic.org/pdf/srconst.pdf. Washington, D.C.: Association for Professionals in Infection Control and Epidemiology, Inc., 2000.
106. **Health Canada:** *Construction-Related Nosocomial Infections in Patients in Health Care Facilities — Decreasing the Risk of Aspergillus, Legionella and Other Infections*. Retrieved from http://hc-sc.gc.ca/hpb/lcdc. Ottawa, Canada: Canadian Medical Association, 2001.
107. **U.S. Dept. of Housing and Urban Development (HUD):** *Healthy Homes Issues: Asthma, Healthy Homes Initiative (HHI) Background Information*, Version 3. Washington, D.C.: HUD, 2006. Retrieved from http://portal.hud.gov/hudportal/documents/huddoc?id=DOC_12480.pdf
108. **Sporik, R.B., L.K. Arruda, J. Woodfolk, M.D. Chapman, et al.:** Environmental exposure to Aspergillus fumigatus allergen (Asp f I). *Clin. Exper. Allergy 23(4)*:326–31 (1993).
109. **Ryan, T.J., L.W. Whitehead, T.H. Connor, and K.D. Burau:** Survey of the Asp f 1 Allergen in Office Environments. *Appl. Occup. Environ. Hyg. 16*:679–84 (2001).
110. **Pope, A.M., R. Patterson, and H. Burge (eds.):** *Indoor Allergens*. Washington, D.C.: National Academy of Sciences Press, 1993.
111. **Gergen, P., P. Turkeltaub, and M. Kovar:** The prevalence of allergic skin test reactivity to eight common aeroallergens in the U.S. population: Results from the second National Health and Nutrition Examination Survey. *J. Allergy Clin. Immunol. 80*:669–79 (1987).
112. **Axelsson, B., A. Saraf, and L. Larsson:** Determination of ergosterol in organic dust by gas chromatography-mass spectrometry. *J. Chromatogr. B 666*:77–84 (1995).
113. **Macher, J.M., F.C. Tsai, L.E. Burton, and K-S Liu:** Concentrations of Cat and Dust Mite Allergens in 93 U.S. office buildings. Proceedings from Indoor Air 2002. Monterey, CA, 2002.
114. **Rao, C.Y., H.A. Burge, and J.C. Chang:** Review of quantitative standards and guidelines for fungi in indoor air. *J. Air Waste Manag. Assoc. 46*:899–908 (1996).
115. **Burge, H.A.:** An update on pollen and fungal spore aerobiology. *J. Allergy Clin. Immunol. 110*:544–52 (2002).
116. **Gots, R.E., N.J. Layton, and S.W. Pirages:** Indoor health: Background levels of fungi. *Am. Ind. Hyg. Assoc. J. 64*:427–38 (2003).
117. **American Industrial Hygiene Association (AIHA®):** The Facts about Mold. Fairfax, VA: AIHA®, 2009. Retrieved from http://www.aiha.org/news-pubs/newsroom/Pages/ConsumerBrochures.aspx
118. **F.C. Tsai and J.M. Macher:** Concentrations of airborne culturable bacteria in 100 large US office buildings in the BASE study. *Indoor Air. 15(Suppl 9)*:71–81 (2005).
119. **Rauh, V.A., G.L. Chew, and R.S. Garfinkel:** Deteriorated Housing Contributes to High Cockroach Allergen Levels in Inner-City Households. *Environ. Health Perspect. 110(2)*:323–27 (2002).
120. **Gelber, L.E., L.H. Seltzer, et al.:** Sensitization and exposure to indoor allergens as risk factors to asthma among patients presenting to hospital. *Am. Rev. Respir. Dis. 147*:573–78 (1993).

121. **Milton, D.M.:** Endotoxin. In *Bioaerosols.* Burge, H.A. (ed.). Boca Raton, FL: CRC/Lewis Publishing, 1995.
122. **Sandstrom, T., L. Bjermer, and R. Rylander:** Lipopolysaccharide (LPS) inhalation in healthy subjects increases neutrophils, lymphocytes, and fibronectin levels in bronchoalveolar lavage fluid. *Eur. Respir. J. 5(8)*:992–96 (1992).
123. **Milton, D.K., D. Kriebel, D. Wypij, M. Walters, et al.:** Acute and chronic airflow obstruction and endotoxin exposure. *Am. J. Respir. Crit. Care Med. 149*:A399 (1994). [Abstract]
124. **Milton, D.K., J. Amsel, C.E. Reed, P.L. Enright, et al.:** Cross-sectional follow-up of a flu-like respiratory illness among fiber glass manufacturing employees: endotoxin exposure associated with two distinct sequelae. *Am. J. Ind. Med. 28*:469–88 (1995).
125. **Teeuw, K.B., C.M. Vandenbroucke-Grauls, and J. Verhoef:** Airborne gram-negative bacteria and endotoxin in sick building syndrome. A study in Dutch governmental office buildings. *Arch. Intern. Med. 154*:2339–45 (1994).
126. **Reynold, S.J., D.W. Black, S.S. Borin, et al.:** Indoor environmental quality in six commercial office buildings in the midwest United States. *Appl. Occ. Env. Health J. 16*:1065–77 (2001).
127. **Hodgson, J.T. and R.D. Jones:** Mortality of workers in the British cotton industry in 1968–1984. *Scand. J. Work Environ. Health 16*:113–20 (1990).
128. **Rose, C.S., L.S. Newman, J.W. Martyny, D. Weiner, et al.:** Outbreak of hypersensitivity pneumonitis in an indoor swimming pool: clinical, pathophysiologic, radiographic, pathologic, lavage and environmental findings. *Am. Rev. Respir. Dis. 141*:A315 (1994). [Abstract]
129. **Rylander, R., S. Sorensen, H. Goto, K. Yuasa, et al.:** The importance of endotoxin and glucan for symptoms in sick building. In *Present and Future of Indoor Air Quality.* Proceedings of the Brussels Conference. Bieva, C.J., Y. Courtois, and M. Govaerts (eds.). New York: Excerpta Medica, 1989.
130. **Fogelmark, B., H. Goto, K. Yuasa, B. Marchat, et al.:** Acute pulmonary toxicity of inhaled beta 1,3-glucan and endotoxin. *Agents Actions 35(1-2)*:50–56 (1992).
131. **Fogelmark, B., M. Sjostrand, and R. Rylander:** Pulmonary inflammation induced by repeated inhalations of beta(1,3)-D-glucan and endotoxin. *Int. J. Exp. Pathol. 75*:85–90 (1994)
132. **Kiho, T., M. Sakushima, S.R. Wang, K. Nagai, et al.:** Polysaccharides in fungi. XXVI. Two branched (1-3)-d-glucans from hot water extract of Yu Er. *Chem. Pharm. Bull. 39(3)*:798–800 (1991).
133. **Douwes, J., G. Doekes, D. Heederik, B. Brunekreef, et al.:** Measurement of environmental ß(1,3)-glucans by enzyme immunoassay. *Am. J. Respir. Crit. Care Med. 151*:A142 (1995).
134. **American Industrial Hygiene Association (AIHA®):** *Field Guide for the Determination of Biological Contaminants in Environmental Samples*, 2nd edition. Hung, L.L., J.D. Miller, and H.K. Dillon (eds.). Fairfax, VA: AIHA®, 2005.
135. **American College of Occupational and Environmental Medicine (ACOEM):** Adverse Human Health Effects Associated with Molds in the Indoor Environment (Evidence Based Statement). Arlington Heights, IL: ACOEM, 2011.
136. **Centers for Disease Control and Prevention (CDC):** State of the Science on Molds and Human Health (Statement for the Record). Retrieved from http://www.cdc.gov/nceh/airpollution/images/moldsci.pdf. Atlanta, GA: CDC, 2002.
137. **Strom, G., J. West, B. Wessen, and U. Palmgren:** Health implications of fungi in indoor environments: Quantitative analysis of microbial volatiles in damp Swedish houses. *Air Qua. Mon. 2*:291–305 (1994).
138. **Elke, K., J. Begerow, et al.:** Determination of selected microbial volatile organic compounds by diffusion sampling and dual-column capillary GC-FID—a new feasible approach for the detection of an exposure to indoor mould fungi. *J. Environ. Mon. 1*:445–52 (1999).
139. **Ryan, T.J. and C. Taylor:** Dominant MVOCs in 23 US Homes. Presented at American Industrial Hygiene Conference & Exposition, Chicago, IL. May, 2006.
140. **U.S. Environmental Protection Agency (EPA)/NIOSH:** *Building Air Quality: A Guide for Building Owners and Facility Managers* (EPA Pub. No./400/1-91/033, DHHS (NIOSH) Pub. No.91-114. Washington, D.C.: EPA, 1991.Retrieved from http://www.epa.gov/iaq/largebldgs/baqtoc.html.
141. **U.S. Environmental Protection Agency (EPA)/NIOSH:** *Building Air Quality Action Plan* (EPA Pub. No. 402-K-98-001). Washington, D.C.: EPA, 1998. Retrieved from http://www.epa.gov/iaq/largebldgs/pdf_files/baqactionplan.pdf
142. **U.S. Environmental Protection Agency (EPA):** Indoor Air Quality Tools for Schools (IAQ TfS) Action Kit. Washington, D.C.: EPA, 2008 Retrieved from http://www.epa.gov/iaq/schools/actionkit.html
143. **U.S Environmental Protection Agency (EPA):** Indoor Air Quality Building Education and Assessment Model (I-BEAM) Software. Washington, D.C.: EPA, 2008. Retrieved from http://www.epa.gov/iaq/largebldgs/i-beam/index.html

144. **U.S. Occupational Safety and Health Administration (OSHA):** OSHA Technical Manual, Section III, Chapter 2, Indoor Air Quality. Washington, DC: OSHA, 1999. Retrieved from http://www.osha-slc.gov/SLTC/indoorairquality/index.html.
145. **American Industrial Hygiene Association (AIHA®):** *The IAQ Investigator's Guide*, 2nd edition. Gunderson, E.C. (ed.) Fairfax, VA: AIHA®, 2006.
146. **American Society of Heating, Refrigerating and Air-Conditioning Engineers (ASHRAE):** 62.1 Users Manual. Atlanta, GA: ASHRAE, 2007
147. **Burton, D.J.:** *IAQ and HVAC Workbook*, 5th edition. Bountiful, UT: IVE, Inc., 2005.
148. **Sheet Metal and Air Conditioning Contractors National Association, Inc. (SMACNA):** *IAQ Guidelines for Occupied Buildings Under Construction*, 2nd. Chantilly, VA: SMACNA, 2007.
149. **U.S. Environmental Protection Agency (EPA):** *Mold Remediation in Schools and Commercial Buildings*. Washington, D.C.: EPA, 2001. Retrieved from http://www.epa.gov/mold/mold_remediation.html
150. **New York City Department of Health:** Guidelines on Assessment and Remediation of Fungi in Indoor Environments. New York: New York Dept. of Health, 2008. Retrieved from http:// home2.nyc.gov/html/doh/html/epi/moldrpt1.shtml
151. **Prezant, B., D.M. Weekes, and J.D. Miller (eds.):** *Recognition, Evaluation, and Control of Indoor Mold*. Fairfax, VA: AIHA®, 2008.
152. **Institute of Inspection, Cleaning and Restoration Certification (IICRC):** *Standard and Reference Guide for Mold Remediation* (S520). Vancouver, WA: IICRC, 2008.
153. **U.S. Department of Energy (DOE):** International Performance Measurement and Verification Protocol – Volume II Concepts and Practices for Improved Indoor Environmental Quality. Retrieved from http://www.evo-world.org/index.php?option=com_form&form_id=12.
154. **Center for Maximum Potential Building Systems (CMPBS):** *Green Guide for Health Care: Best Practices for Creating High Performance Healing Environments*. Version 2.2, January 2007. Updated Operations Section, 2008 Revision, December 2008. Retrieved from http://www.gghc.org
155. **Joint Commission on Accreditation of Healthcare Organizations (JCAHO):** A Guide to Managing IAQ in Healthcare Organizations. Oakbrook Terrace, IL: JCAHO, 1997.
156. **Centers for Disease Control and Prevention (CDC):** Guidelines for Environmental Infection Control in Health-care Facilities. Atlanta, GA: CDC, 2003. Retrieved from http://www.cdc.gov/mmwr/preview/mmwrhtml/rr5210a1.htm
157. **Hansen, W., ed.:** *Infection Control During Construction Manual,* 2nd edition. Marblehead, MA: HC Pro, Inc., 2004.
158. **Massachusetts Dept. of Public Health:** *Requirements to Maintain Air Quality in Indoor Skating Rinks* (105CMR675.000). Boston, MA: MA Dept. of Public Health, 1997.
159. **Pennsylvania Dept. of Health:** *Guidelines on Ice Skating Rink Resurfacing Machine and Indoor Air Quality Issues.* PA: PA Dept. of Health, 2003. Retrieved from http://www.dsf.health.state.pa.us/health/cwp/view.asp?A=171&Q=234573
160. **American Society of Heating, Refrigerating and Air-Conditioning Engineers (ASHRAE):** 161-2007, *Air Quality within Commercial Aircraft.* Atlanta, GA: ASHRAE, 2007.
161. **Hocking, M.B.:** *Air Quality in Airplane Cabins and Similar Enclosed Spaces.* Germany: Springer Science & Business, 2005.
162. **U.S. Environmental Protection Agency (EPA):** IAQ in Homes/Residences (website). Washington, D.C.: EPA, 2011. Retrieved from http://www.epa.gov/iaq/homes/index.html
163. **Consumer Product Safety Commission (CPSC):** Indoor Air Quality Publications (website). Bethesda, MD: CPSC, 2011. Retrieved from http://www.cpsc.gov/cpscpub/pubs/iaq.html
164. **American Society of Heating, Refrigerating and Air-Conditioning Engineers (ASHRAE):** 62.2-2010, *Ventilation and Acceptable Indoor Air Quality in Low-Rise Residential Buildings.* Atlanta, GA: ASHRAE, 2010.
165. **American Society of Heating, Refrigerating and Air-Conditioning Engineers (ASHRAE):** Guideline 24-2008, *Ventilation and Indoor Air Quality in Low-Rise Residential Buildings.* Atlanta, GA: ASHRAE, 2008.
166. **Centers for Disease Control and Prevention (CDC):** *Prevention and Control of Tuberculosis in Correctional and Detention Facilities: Recommendations from CDC,* Report 55(RR09). Atlanta, GA: CDC, 2006. Retrieved from http://www.cdc.gov/mmwr/PDF/rr/rr5509.pdf.
167. **Spengler, J.D., Q. Chen and K.M. Dilwali:** Indoor Air Quality Factors in Designing a Healthy Building. In *Indoor Air Quality Handbook.* Spengler, J.D., J.M. Samet and J.F. McCarthy (eds.). New York: McGraw-Hill, 2001. pp 5.1–5.29.
168. **Levin, H.:** Indoor Air Quality by Design. In *Indoor Air Quality Handbook.* Spengler, J.D., J.M. Samet and J.F. McCarthy (eds.). New York: McGraw-Hill, 2001. pp 60.3–60.21.

169. **Fisk, W.J.:** How IEQ Affects Health, Productivity. *ASHRAE J. 44(5)*:56–60 (2002).
170. **Fullerton, D.G., N. Bruce, and S.B. Gordon:** Review: Indoor air pollution from biomass fuel smoke is a major health concern in the developing world. *Trans. Royal Society of Trop. Med. and Hyg. (102)*:843–51 (2008).
171. **Nardell, E.A.:** Tuberculosis. In *Indoor Air Quality Handbook*, J.D. Spengler, J.M. Samet and J.F. McCarthy, eds. New York: McGraw-Hill, 2001. p 47.1.
172. **Bearg, D.W.:** *Indoor Air Quality and HVAC Systems*. Boca Raton, FL: CRC/Lewis Publishers, 1993.
173. **Samet, J.M.:** Radon. In *Indoor Air Quality Handbook*. Spengler, J.D., J.M. Samet and J.F. McCarthy (eds.). New York: McGraw-Hill, 2001. pp 40.2.
174. **Centers for Disease Control and Prevention (CDC), NIOSH Science Blog:** *Respiratory Health Consequences Resulting from the Collapse of the World Trade Center.* Contribution by Dr. David Prezant of the World Trade Center Medical Monitoring and Treatment Program and the Albert Einstein College of Medicine, September 8, 2008. Retrieved from http://www.cdc.gov/niosh/blog/nsb090808_wtc.html
175. **Lioy, P.J., C.P. Weisel, J.R. Millette, et al.:** Characterization of the dust/smoke aerosol that settled east of the World Trade Center (WTC) in lower Manhattan after the collapse of the WTC September 11, 2001. *Environ Health Perspect. 110(7)*:703–14 (2002).
176. **Prezant, D.J., S. Levin, K. Kelly, and T.K. Aldrich:** Overview: Health Consequences of the World Trade Center Disaster. *Mt. Sinai Med. J. 75*:89–100 (2008).
177. **Brackbill, R., L. Thorpe, L. DiGrande, M. Perrin, J. Sapp, D. Wu., et al.:** Surveillance for World Trade Center Health Effects Among Survivors of Collapsed and Damaged Buildings. *MMWR 7 55(2)*:1–18 (2006).
178. **Landrigan, P.J., P.J. Lioy, et.al., and NIEHS World Trade Center Working Group:** Health and Environmental Consequences of the World Trade Center Disaster. *Environ. Health Perspect. 112(6)*:731–39 (2004).
179. **U.S. Environmental Protection Agency (EPA):** *EPA Response to September 11: Benchmarks, Standards and Guidelines Established to Protect Public Health.* Last updated July 24, 2007. Retrieved from http://www.epa.gov/wtc/benchmarks.htm
180. **U.S. Environmental Protection Agency (EPA) Region 2:** Lower Manhattan Test and Clean Program. November 2008. Retrieved from http://www.epa.gov/wtc/testandclean/Lower%20Manhattan%20Test%20ə%20Clean%20Program%20Final%20Report.pdf
181. **Centers for Disease Control and Prevention (CDC):** Fact Sheet: Final Report on Formaldehyde Levels in FEMA-Supplied Travel Trailers, Park Models, and Mobile Homes. Atlanta, GA: CDC, 2008. Retrieved from http://www.cdc.gov/nceh/ehhe/trailerstudy/residents.htm#final
182. **California Air Resources Board (ARB):** 93120-93120.12, title 17, California Code of Regulations, § 93120. Airborne Toxic Control Measure to Reduce Formaldehyde Emissions from Composite Wood Products. Sacramento, CA: ARB, 2008. Retrieved from http://www.arb.ca.gov/toxics/compwood/compwood.htm.
183. Toxic Substances Control Act (15 U.D.C. 2601 et seq.) Title VI — Formaldehyde Standards for Composite Wood Products, July 10, 2010. Retrieved from http://www.gpo.gov/fdsys/pkg/PLAW-111publ199/pdf.

Outcome Competencies

After completing this chapter, the reader should be able to:

1. Define underlined terms used in this chapter.
2. Anticipate when biological monitoring is appropriate.
3. Assess the limiting factors to biological monitoring.
4. Provide justification for the concept of biological monitoring.
5. Provide justification for recommendations based on biological monitoring.

Key Terms

absorbed dose • adducts • antibodies • antigens • biochemical epidemiology • biologically effective dose • biological exposure indices (BEIs) • biological monitoring • biomarker • blood • breast milk • chemical • conjugates • determinant • ear wax • elimination • end-exhaled breath (alveolar exhaled breath) • endogenous • enzyme • excretion • feces • flatus • fluids • hair • half-times (pseudo first order) • health surveillance • immune response • macromolecules • markers • medical monitoring • medical surveillance • menses • metabolites • midstream urine • mixed exhaled breath • nail • plasma (blood) • saliva • sebum • semen • serum (blood) • sputum • sweat • uptake • urine

Prerequisite Knowledge

TLV®–TWAs and PELs and the documentation that forms their basis

Undergraduate biology; human metabolism and physiology; toxicology; undergraduate chemistry; epidemiology; biostatistics; undergraduate kinetics as a part of physical chemistry; undergraduate arithmetic using logarithms, exponentials, differentials, and integration.

Basic biology; physiology; chemistry; biostatistics; algebra; and epidemiology.

Key Topics

I. What is Biological Monitoring?

II. Hygienists and Biological Monitoring

III. When to Use Biological Monitoring
   - A. Federally Mandated Biological Monitoring: The Lead Standard
   - B. Federally Mandated Biological Monitoring: The Cadmium Standard
   - C. Biological Monitoring Recommendations
   - D. Compounds Without Recommendations
   - E. Routes of Exposure Other Than Inhalation
   - F. Presence of Personal Protective Equipment
   - G. Unanticipated Exposures
   - H. Adjunct to Current Environmental Sampling Activities

IV. Factors for Biological Monitoring Data Interpretation Using the BEIs
   - A. Vapor Inhalation Predominates as the Route of Exposure
   - B. When Vapor Inhalation is Not the Major Route of Exposure

V. Biological Monitoring Sampling/Quality Assurance and Quality Control
   - A. Breath Sampling
   - B. Urine Sampling
   - C. Other Noninvasive Biological Monitoring Media

Appendix I. Illustrated Examples for Xylene Relative to Workload, the BEI® and Inhalation Conditions

Biological Monitoring

19

By Shane S. Que Hee, PhD

What is Biological Monitoring?

Biological monitoring is the measurement in human body media of chemical markers resulting from exposure to chemical, physical, and biological agents.[1] These markers can be: (1) the original exposing chemical; (2) metabolites of a single exposing chemical; (3) conjugates caused by interaction of a single exposing chemical or its metabolites with non-macromolecular components of endogenous biochemical cycles; (4) adducts formed by reaction of a single exposing chemical or its metabolites with endogenous macromolecules (proteins, nucleic acids, lipids, and sugars), antigens, and antibodies; or (5) an endogenous enzyme or biochemical affected by chemical, physical, or biological agents. Biological monitoring markers are a subset of biomarkers, a general term that describes chemical, biochemical, physical, and physiological markers in, of, or from, living organisms, tissues, organs, or cells. Biomonitoring is the measurement of biomarkers or living things. Thus, while microbial air sampling is part of biomonitoring, it is not biological monitoring.

The biological media can be: exhaled breath, flatus; urine, blood, blood serum, blood plasma, sebum, ear wax, semen, the menses, breast milk, sweat, hair, nail, teeth, tears, feces, saliva, fat, skin, sputum, and internal organs. The media used most in the workplace are urine, blood, and exhaled breath because of known relationships between the marker and the environmental concentration of the exposing chemical. Marker concentrations in the rest of the above media are difficult to interpret except in a qualitative manner. Another consideration is that monitoring should be as noninvasive of the worker as is possible, this favoring urine and breath sampling over blood sampling.

The markers may be of dose and/or effect. The markers of effect are subdivided into those of adverse effect (medical monitoring), potentially adverse effect or predictive of effect (health surveillance), and markers of susceptibility (including genetic markers and markers of genetic deficiency). Overseeing markers of dose and effect of workers in a workplace or ambient setting is part of a medical surveillance program according to NIOSH and OSHA, although the American College of Occupational and Environmental Medicine considers only markers of effect to be categorized as medical surveillance. Correlating markers within epidemiological studies is termed "biochemical epidemiology" or "molecular epidemiology."

Both marker types may have to be identified and quantified in samples, so that laboratories which can analyze for the marker in the biological medium must be known and available as well as sampling methods. Whereas reference ranges for healthy people may exist for markers of effect, the critical concentration of a marker of dose is mostly keyed, for example in the United States, Australia, and the European Community, to a air standard reference level like an action level or a permissable exposure limit (PEL), or a recommended occupational air exposure limit such as a threshold limit value-time weighted average (TLV®-TWA), workplace environmental exposure level (WEEL™), or similar limit. The use of such reference air levels to anchor markers of dose produces equivalent biological monitoring results when inhalation is the only major (>70%) route of exposure, and when only the exposing chemical is involved.

The concentrations found in biological monitoring reflect absorption into the body from all routes of exposure: namely, inhalation, oral ingestion, eye, ear, and skin exposure. Different chemicals and their markers take different times to appear in the same body medium as characterized by different half-times. The same chemical and its markers also take different half-times to appear in different body media. The same chemical and its markers usually have different half-times to appear in the same body media after exposure through different exposure routes. The excretion and clearance characteristics are responsible for different recommended sampling times for markers in biological media.

Hygienists and Biological Monitoring

The legal authority of industrial/environmental hygienists (hygienists) does not include invasive sampling of the human body, unless they are also certified in plebotomy. Sampling that is invasive of the body is the province of medical personnel like licensed physicians, nurses, and dentists since they already have the legal authority to inject medications. Certified plebotomists can also draw blood, and hygienists must obtain this additional certification to draw blood samples in the U.S. Thus actual medical monitoring and monitoring for markers of susceptibility and effect are usually outside the practicing scope of hygienists. Hygienists must, however, be able to explain the relevance of medical surveillance including blood and urine sampling during worker training or counseling, and how the marker data relate to environmental sampling results. The advent of a home self-fingerstick blood sampling test for AIDS in 1996 was a precedent that may eventually allow workers to sample blood analogously, and then to give samples to the hygienist or send directly to the analytical laboratory. A hygienist must be able to refer workers to a physician not only for taking blood samples, but also for medical emergency, disabling injuries, workers' compensation situations, and to follow-up on signs of chronic health problems. Therefore, the field use of biological monitoring for hygienists who are not also certified phlebotomists is limited at present to methods that involve collection of biological media by means that are noninvasive of the human body. The major body media that can be sampled non-invasively from the body are: ear wax, exhaled breath, flatus, feces, hair, nails, saliva, sebum, semen, sputum, sweat, tears, and urine. Of these media, only urine and exhaled breath have gained general acceptance. External contamination with an exposing chemical is problematic with hair, nails, saliva, sebum, and sweat. To assess what is inside or outside of hair or nails is difficult because there is no generally accepted washing technique. Ear wax, feces, flatus, sebum, semen, sputum, sweat, and tears are awkward or inconvenient to sample, and not enough data are available to interpret what the concentrations signify relative to exposure. Feces, sebum, semen, and ear wax are also complex media requiring skilled expensive analyses. Tears, flatus, feces, and sweat are difficult to procure on demand. Saliva sampling in industrial settings is comparatively unexplored although it is being increasingly used in medicine.

The training of hygienists in air sampling and analysis makes breath analysis feasible (Chapter 11, Sampling of Gases and Vapors; Chapter 12, Analysis of Gases and Vapors; Chapter 15, Principles and Instrumentation for Calibrating Air Sampling Equipment, and Chapter 17, Direct-Reading Instrumental Methods for Gases, Vapors, and Aerosols).

Analytical methods and laboratories able to do the analyses of the collected sample must be available. Lists of laboratories are provided in such references as: (1) the Annual Buyer's Guide for *Industrial Hygiene News* under Medical Testing Laboratory; (2) the annual Directory for *Occupational Hazards* under Laboratory Testing Services for Environmental Management and under Medical Screening and Recordkeeping Services for Occupational Health; (3) the annual Purchasing Sourcebook of *Occupational Health and Safety* under the Services Section: Air Monitoring and Analyses-Exterior; Biological Monitoring; Consultants-Environmental Health Laboratories Analysis; Environmental Health — Laboratory Analysis Service; Health Monitoring; Laboratory Analysis Service —

General; and Screening Services; and (4) the annual Lab Guide edition of *Analytical Chemistry* under the heading Services, Elemental Analysis, Inorganic; Elemental Analyses, Organic; and Forensic Analyses.

Information about state-certified analytical laboratories is available from the list of state OSHA Regional Offices and State Safety and Health Agencies in the Resource Finder Section of the annual Directory of *Occupational Hazards*. The ACGIH® BEI® Committee and the American Industrial Hygiene Association (AIHA®) Biological Monitoring Committee www.aiha.org are two other informational resources. Since laboratories change, hygienists are urged to be up to date.

An alternative to analytical laboratory analysis is to employ methods that measure markers directly in excreted body fluids like urine and breath in the workplace. This aspect of biological monitoring is hardly developed, although dipstick technologies now being used for urinalysis and blood analyses in medicine are analogous to detector tube methods of contaminant air analysis. Thus for example, dipstick technology is available for urines for specific gravity, nitrite, pH, protein, glucose, ketone, acetoacetic acid, bilirubin, urobilogen, and hemoglobin. Intense research efforts are ongoing to produce direct reading colorimetric methods for human biomarkers to produce in-vitro diagnostic medical devices (iVDs) for personalized medicine. If detector tubes are used for breath samples, the higher breath water vapor and carbon dioxide concentrations than in workplace air must also be considered. Since a breath BEI® is much lower in concentration than its corresponding TLV®-TWA, the current short-term detector tube technology is often not sensitive enough for breath analysis except in cases of gross overexposure near IDLH concentrations. Some of the long-term detector tube types may be suitable for exhaled breath detection as long as a before shift breath sample is used as a comparison and the appropriate high humidity and high carbon dioxide blanks are also done. The advantage of using detector tubes is that hygienists are trained to use them, and they can be used directly in the field or with Tedlar bag breath samples.

Another alternative to sampling of excreted body fluids is to employ direct reading instruments and devices to measure excretion on external parts of the human body or to sample these parts by wiping or rinsing.[2] Differentiating between external exposure and excretion is a major difficulty for breath and skin sampling, and before shift evaluation is also essential. Noninvasive detection of substances on the skin is also not very developed at present[2], but colorimetric wipes are commercially available for a small number of specific compounds. The use of ionizing radiation methods like X-ray fluorescence for bone lead[1,3] may be potentially harmful, and can only be used under medical supervision.

When to Use Biological Monitoring

The major uses of biological monitoring occur when:

- Biological monitoring is mandated (for example, blood lead keyed to a critical air concentration) or recommended (for example, BEI or BEEL documentation exists or individual states or countries require it);
- Routes of exposure other than inhalation are important (contribute greater than 30%);
- Personal protective equipment (PPE) such as respirators, gloves, and protective garments are worn;
- Unanticipated exposures occur in the workplace or outside it, especially when air monitoring is not performed; and
- A confirmatory technique to air sampling is required

There are just three mandated biological monitoring U.S. federal criteria. One since 1993 is by the Centers for Disease Control and Prevention (CDC) defining people with Acquired Immune Deficiency Syndrome or AIDS (<200 CD_4^+ (T-helper lymphocyte) cells/mm3 blood plus human immunodeficiency virus (HIV) infection). Detailed discussion of this is beyond the present scope of this chapter since it properly is medical monitoring. However, the criterion is relevant to measurement of HIV in first responders tending worker injuries and to cleanup personnel of medical waste and human biological fluids to fulfill the requirements of the OSHA bloodborne pathogens standard (29 CFR 1910.130). HIV testing is to occur at least 6 weeks, 12 weeks, and 6 months after exposure to a HIV-infected person along with CD_4^+ counting, and Western Blot and HIV antigen tests if the Enzyme Linked Immunosorbent Assay (ELISA) test for HIV antibodies is positive. A saliva rapid test is now also available. In common with many drug testing systems, a positive rapid screening test result has to be subsequently confirmed.

The other two U.S. federal criteria concern worker medical removal under OSHA from exposure to two metals: lead and cadmium. In either case, methods for sampling, preservation, storage, and transport must be proper. All biological samples must be analyzed in a laboratory that is proficient in the analysis of each marker.

Federally Mandated Biological Monitoring: The Lead Standard

The current OSHA biological monitoring standard for blood lead is a maximum concentration of 50 µg Pb/100g blood for administrative removal from the workplace of a worker exposed at or above the air action level of 30 µg/m³.[5] Lead is defined in the standard in terms of lead equivalent for elemental lead, all inorganic lead compounds, and organic lead soaps. Medical removal occurs at (1) a blood lead level of 60 µg/100 g or greater is obtained and confirmed by a second follow-within two weeks after the employer receives the results of the first blood sampling test; (2) the arithmetic mean of the last three blood sampling tests or the arithmetic mean of all tests conducted over the previous six months (whichever is longer) is calculated to be at or above 50 µg/100 g (excepting if the most recent blood test is at or below 40 µg/100g). Medical removal is to continue until two consecutive blood lead levels are 40 µg/100 g or less. The OSHA PEL is 50 µg/m³. Blood sampling analysis is mandated every six months for workers above the air action level for more than 30 days per year; at least every two months for blood lead concentrations >40 µg/100g together with at least one annual medical examination; and at least monthly for medically removed workers but at least two weeks after the initial blood test, together with a medical examination. The blood lead testing must be done by an analytical laboratory currently licensed by the CDC, that produces results within 95 % confidence and/or within an accuracy of ±15 % or ± 6 µg/100g, whichever is greater. Employees must be notified by the employer in writing within 5 working days after receipt of biological monitoring results concerning what the blood lead level is when it exceeds 40 µg/100g, and that the lead standard requires temporary medical removal with worker benefits of up to 18 months for each removal.

Medical examination requirements are the responsibility of the licensed physician but are worth quoting in detail because hygienists may have to assist in some of the aspects, and the topic must be covered during worker training by hygienists. The lead standard medical surveillance was the model for subsequent medical surveillance of other chemicals.

Medical examinations require a detailed work history and medical history with particular attention to past occupational and nonoccupational lead exposures, personal habits (smoking, alcohol consumption, hygiene), and past gastrointestinal, renal, cardiovascular, and neurological symptoms. Pulmonary status must be evaluated if negative pressure respirators are to be used. A physical examination must pay particular attention to teeth, gums, hematologic, gastrointestinal, renal, cardiovascular, and neurologic systems. Blood pressure must be measured. A blood sample must be taken and analyzed for blood lead, hemoglobin (the major pigment of red blood cells), hematocrit (the % volume of blood cells to total blood volume), red cell indices, peripheral smear morphology, zinc protoporphyrin, blood urea nitrogen, serum creatinine, routine urinalysis with routine microscopic examination, and "any laboratory or other test deemed necessary by sound medical practice". If a physician is of the opinion that a state of lead intoxication exists from the physical examination alone (for example, observation of blue "lead line" at the tooth/gum interface, acute encephalopathy, lead colic, peripheral neuropathy, impotence, and abnormal menstrual cycles), the worker known to be exposed at or above the air action level can be removed immediately. An employee can also request pregnancy testing or laboratory evaluation of male fertility, and also counseling on the effects of past/current exposure to lead. If the employer selects the first physician, the employee has the right of a second opinion within 15 days of receipt of the written findings of that first physician, but must signify intent to do this in writing to the employer. A third physician may be designated by the involved physicians in the event of irreconcilable disagreement. Hygienists make physician recommendations effective, as they are the key on-site personnel.

The key participation of hygienists in the lead standard comes with worker training, workplace signs, air sampling, and record-keeping. For the lead standard, the content of specific parts of the standard must be given to all employees potentially exposed to ANY level of airborne lead. Initial training must be started within the first 180 days of employment but before the time of initial job assignment, and refresher training offered at least annually thereafter for all potentially or actually exposed above the air action level, or for whom the possibility of skin or eye irritation exists. This training involves imparting the content of the lead standard and its appendices; explanations of the specific natures of the unit processes which could cause lead exposures at and above the air lead action level; the purpose, proper selection, fitting, use, limitations, and maintenance of respirators; the purposes and description of the lead medical surveillance program, the lead medical removal criteria, adverse health effects of lead with particular attention to adverse male and female reproductive effects; the engineering controls and work practices associated with the worker's job; the contents of any compliance plan including air monitoring; and instructions to the employee that any chelating agent like EDTA should not be routinely used to remove lead from the body unless this is under the direction of a physician.

Relative to air sampling, air monitoring must occur at least every six months for workers over the action level but under the PEL, whether they wear respirators or not. If the PEL is exceeded, air monitoring must be repeated every three months. Air monitoring may be discontinued if two samplings at least two weeks apart are below the action level. Any production, process, control, or personnel change triggers air monitoring. Workers may request respirators even if the PEL is not exceeded. Other PPE, change rooms, showers, the requirements for filtered air lunchrooms and housekeeping and engineering controls are beyond the scope of this discussion. Observing hygienists must have had at least the same medical surveillance and PPE program as the employees they are monitoring.

There are four sets of records to be kept:

(1) The air sampling record must contain dates, number, duration, locations and results for each of the samples taken, including a description of the sampling procedure used to determine representative employee exposure where applicable; a description of the sampling and analytical chemistry methods used and evidence of their accuracy; the type of respirator worn; name, social security number, and job classification of the monitored employee, and of all other employees whose exposure the measurement is intended to represent; and the environmental variables that could affect the measurement of employee exposure;

(2) The medical surveillance record similarly must include: name, social security number, and description of employee job duties; a copy of the physician's written opinions; results of any air sampling for that employee and representative exposure levels supplied to the physician; and any employee medical complaints about lead exposure. Both records must be maintained by the employer for at least 40 years (30 years in later OSHA recommendations for different chemicals) or for the duration of employment plus 20 years, whichever is longer;

(3) The employer must keep or ensure that the licensed physician must similarly maintain: a copy of the medical examination results including medical and work histories; a description of any laboratory procedures, and a copy of the standards/guidelines used to interpret the test results or references to that information; and a copy of the results of biological monitoring; and

(4) The employer must also maintain an accurate record for each employee medically removed. The record must include: employee name and social security number; the dates of medical removal and the corresponding date of return; a brief explanation of how each removal was or

is being accomplished; and a statement with respect to each removal indicating whether or not the reason for the removal was an elevated blood lead. This record must be maintained for at least during the worker's employment.

When the air PEL is exceeded in each work area, a specific sign must be posted in addition to signs required by other ordinances, regulations or statutes:

WARNING
LEAD WORK AREA
POISON
NO SMOKING OR EATING

The above information has been provided as a complete package since air monitoring, biological monitoring, hygienic considerations, record-keeping, and preventative measures all must be done simultaneously by the hygienist.

Federally Mandated Biological Monitoring: The Cadmium Standard

The cadmium standard (29 CFR 1910.1027 for general industry and 29 CFR 1926.1127 for construction) includes biological monitoring provisions (29 CFR 1910.1027 Appendix F). The standard first came into effect in 1994, and amendments that included lower biological monitoring thresholds went into effect on January 1, 1999. Decision-making logic re biological monitoring thresholds is available in a free computer Experts Systems software package, OSHA GOCAD 2.0, (available at http://www.osha.gov) under cadmium biological monitoring advisor. This software prepares and saves: a letter to the employee; a memorandum for the employer; notes for the physician's records; and a serial log. The first version, GOCAD 1.0, is obsolete.

The acute symptoms of cadmium overexposure are metal fume fever (flu-like symptoms of weakness, fever, headache, chills, sweating, and muscular pain 1–10 h after exposure with maximum severity between 1–3 days); tightness of the chest and throat; coughing; and fluid accumulation in the lungs. Subacute effects include loss of smell; anemia; and discoloration of the teeth. Cadmium is a carcinogen (lung and prostate), but the major target organ for chronic toxicity is the kidney (excess protein in urine ["proteinuria"] is a marker of adverse effect) and then the bone ("itai-itai" disease).

The current OSHA thresholds are provided in 29 CFR 1910.1027 Appendix A. The 8 h-TWA Permissible Exposure Limit (PEL) for cadmium is 5 µg Cd/m^3 air for a total dust sample. The upper limits for normal levels of cadmium in the body are 3 µg Cd/g creatinine (CdU) in a post-shift spot urine sample, and 5 µg Cd/L of whole blood (CdB) in a post-shift sample. If kidney damage is present a post-shift spot urine will show a marker of 300 µg β_2-microglobulin/g creatinine.

Mandatory medical removal occurs above 750 µg β_2-microglobulin/g creatinine if either CdB exceeds 5 µg Cd/L of whole blood or CdU exceeds 3 µg Cd/g creatinine. The presence of Cd must be demonstrated since β(2)-M increase also is also caused by myeloma and influenza. Workers with acidic urines (pH<6) are more susceptible to kidney damage, and physicians/sam-ple collectors must measure fresh urine pH. An immediately dangerous air concentration over an 8-h exposure period is agreed to be 1 mg/m^3 to cause enhanced mortality (55 Fed Regist 4052).

The biological monitoring results are classified as Category A, B, or C in Table 19.1. Category A (CdU ≤3 µg Cd/g creatinine; β(2)-M ≤300 µg β_2-microglobulin/g creatinine; CdB ≤5 µg Cd/L of whole blood) requires a biennial medical examination and annual biological monitoring. Category B (any of CdU >3 to <7 µg Cd/g creatinine; β(2)-M >300 to <750 µg β_2-microglobulin/g creatinine; CdB >5 and <10 µg Cd/L of whole blood) requires semiannual biological monitoring; a medical examination within 90 days of the sampling; an additional annual medical examination; a series of environmental measures to be assessed within 2 weeks of the sampling (Table 19.1); and the physician is provided with the discretion to remove the worker from the workplace. Category C (any of CdU >7 µg Cd/g creatinine; β(2)-M >750 µg β_2-microglobulin/g creatinine; CdB > 10 µg Cd/L of whole blood) triggers quarterly biological monitoring; a medical examination within 90 days of the sampling; additional semiannual medical examinations; and the same set of environmental assessments to be completed within 2 weeks of the sampling as for Category B with the additional provisions for periodic assessment of exposures, and worker mandatory workplace removal for β(2)-M >750 µg β_2-microglobulin/ g creatinine with Cd U >3 µg Cd/g creatinine or CdB >5 µg Cd/L. A consistent increase of the marker concentrations above the critical lower thresholds is more serious than marker concentrations that revert to below reference range upper thresholds. The chance of developing kidney disease is greatly enhanced above the upper thresholds of Category C; however, cases are also known where kidney disease has not developed under such conditions. The time needed to gauge these changes for each marker will differ because of different worker inter-individual susceptibility that is a complex interaction of genetic, environmental, aging, gender, medicinal, dietary, and personal lifestyle factors.

Table 19.1 — Employer Actions for the OSHA Cadmium Standard

Required Actions	Monitoring A[1]	Result B[1]	Category C[1]
Biological monitoring			
Annual	+		
Semi-annual		+	
Quarterly			+
Medical Examination			
Biennial	+		
Annual		+	
Semiannual			+
Within 90 days of sampling		+	+
Assess within 2 weeks			
Excess Cd exposure (air, surface)		+	+
Work practices		+	+
Personal hygiene		+	+
Respirator usage		+	+
Smoking history		+	+
Correct within 30 days		+	+
Periodically assess exposures			+
Discretionary medical removal		+	+
Mandatory medical removal			+[2]

(1) Category A: Requirements of paragraph (1)(3) (i)(B) and (1)(4)(v)(A) of the Cd standard. Category B or C: Requirements of paragraph (1)(4)(v)(B)-(C)

(2) B2-M >750 µg β_2-microglobulin/g creatinine if either CdB exceeds 5 µg Cd/L of whole blood or CdU exceeds 3 µg Cd/g creatinine.

+, specified

Sample collection and analysis of the biological monitoring media involve either atomic absorption, inductively coupled plasma (ICP) atomic emission spectroscopy, neutron activation, isotope dilution mass spectrometry (MS), and ICP-MS, after digestion. Though OSHA does not recommend any official biological monitoring methods, NIOSH Method 8005 for metals in blood or tissue, and NIOSH Method 8310 for metals in urine are available. Employers and hygienists must ensure that analytical laboratories know the analytical quality assurance/quality control requirements for biological monitoring of the OSHA cadmium standard at 29 CFR 1910.1027 Appendix F. These can be summarized as:

Cd B >2 µg/L: <20% coefficient of variation CV (100 x standard deviation/arithmetic mean for the same sample)
: ±1 µg/L accuracy to the consensus mean or within 15% of the consensus mean

CdU >2 µg/g creatinine: <20% CV precision
: accuracy within 15% of the consensus mean

β(2)-M ^{3}100 µg/g creatinine: ≤5% CV
: accuracy within 15% of the consensus mean

The consensus mean is the mean for all participating laboratories in the quality assurance/quality assurance interlaboratory evaluation. All laboratories must have documentation for at least two years of analyses for each marker in their interlaboratory collaboration programs.

Relative to urine samples, workers are recommended to empty their bladders, drink a large glass of water, and then provide one spot urine sample within one hour. Sterile 250 mL polypropylene or polyethylene urine collection cups should be used and accessories are small sealable plastic bags, preprinted labels, 15-mL polyethylene or polypropylene screw cap tubes, and powderless metal-free laboratory gloves to be used during voiding. The sealed collection cup should be kept in a plastic bag until collection time. Workers must wash their hands with soap and water before receiving the sealed collection cup. The collection cup should not be opened until just before voiding, and the cup must be sealed immediately after filling. The inside of the container and cap must not be touched by or come into contact with the body, clothing, or other surfaces. The cup is swirled gently to re-suspend any solids, and the 15-mL screw cap tube is filled with 10–12 mL urine by decanting. The screw-cap tube sample to be analyzed for Cd and creatinine does not need to be refrigerated for storage or transport, though the CDCP recommends adding 0.1 mL concentrated nitric acid as preservative, and then freezing. The pH of the rest of the contents of the cup should be adjusted to 8.0 with a metal-free plastic eye dropper using 0.1 M sodium hydroxide solution (use another eye dropper or a plastic rod to test the pH indicator paper after swirling the solution after each addition of base). The cup should then be sealed, labeled, and frozen/stored at -20°C for storage/transport until testing is to be done for β(2)-M and creatinine.

Biological Monitoring Recommendations

OSHA Recommendations

Although OSHA has only promulgated two standards that mandate biological monitoring as the basis for worker medical removal, the OSHA Medical Records Rule[6] defines "employee exposure record" to include all biological monitoring as "exposure records" by specific OSHA standards. OSHA includes as "exposure records" all "tests as are needed according to a physician's professional judgment"[6,7,23], a common part of all OSHA standards with medical surveillance. Sometimes special biological monitoring tests are mentioned directly in the guidelines.

OSHA distinguishes between medical screening and medical surveillance.[23]

- Medical screening, according to OSHA, is "a method for detecting disease or body dysfunction before an individual would normally seek medical care. Screening tests are usually administered to individuals without current symptoms, but who may be at high risk for certain adverse health outcomes." This is very close to the above stated definition for medical surveillance used in its predictive guise for supposedly healthy people. OSHA further states: "The fundamental purpose of medical screening is early diagnosis and treatment of the individual and thus has a clinical focus." This purpose reinforces the primacy of the physician in the testing.
- Medical surveillance, according to OSHA, is "the analysis of health information to look for problems that may be occurring in the workplace that require targeted prevention, and thus serves as a feedback loop to the employer." OSHA elaborates further: "Surveillance may be based on a single case or sentinel event, but more typically uses screening results from the group of employees being evaluated to look for abnormal trends in health status. Surveillance can also be conducted on a single employee over time. Review of group results helps to identify potential problem areas and the effectiveness of existing worksite preventive strategies." This definition of medical surveillance therefore involves both single cases, single sentinel events, or prospective epidemiology-type studies at one point in time or through time. OSHA adds: "The fundamental purpose of medical surveillance is to detect and eliminate the underlying causes (i.e. hazards/exposures) of any discovered trends and thus has a prevention focus." This purpose broadens the scope of medical surveillance to the whole program that prevents, identifies, controls, and manages health effects in the workplace, even though prevention is stated to be the supposed focus. This broadened scope for medical surveillance is identical to that of NIOSH. Thus, personal air sampling, ventilation, hygiene, training, safety, and administrative rotation of workers to lower exposures are included in addition to specific clinical and health issues related to chemical, physical, and biological exposures. This purpose of medical surveillance allows hygienists and safety engineers to be the primary decision-makers relative to preventative measures in the workplace.

OSHA provides the major medical screening and medical surveillance endpoints together in its guidance. Table 19.2 summarizes these markers for the 14 specific chemical hazards that are relevant to biological monitoring. The tabulated endpoints are for medical screening except for the ones required for fitness to wear respirators ("Pulmonary function testing" and "Evaluation of ability to wear a respirator"), and "Additional tests if deemed necessary". The category "Other required tests" often also contains specific medical monitoring markers for the exposure chemical. The category "Additional tests if deemed necessary" allows the full range of health surveillance markers to be used "if deemed necessary" by a physician.

Table 19.2 — Major Nonconstruction Industry Medical Screening and Surveillance Endpoints Recommended by OSHA for Chemical Hazards that Cause Systemic Effects[(6)]

Endpoint	*Chemical*[A,B]													
	1	*2*	*3*	*4*	*5*	*6*	*7*	*8*	*9*	*10*	*11*	*12*	*13*	*14*
Preplacement exam	+a	+a	+a,k,l	+a,k,l	+a,k,l	+	+a	+	+a	+a,l	+	+a,k,l	+a,l	+a
Periodic exam	+a,b	+a	+b,l	+b,l	+b,l	+b	+a	+a	+b	+a,l	+a,l	+a,b,l	+a,l	+a
Emergency/exposure exam/tests	+	+	+b,l,m	+b,l,r	+b,l	+a,z	-	+F	+a	+l	+a,l	+a,l	+a,l	+
Termination exam	+	+h	-	+s	+a	-	+h	-	+a	-	-	-	+h	-
Exam emphasis	c	I	n	t	w	A	C	G	I	K	L	P	R	T
Work and medical history	+d	+b,j	+o	+b,d	+d	+d	+a	+d	+d	+d	+d,M	+d	+d	+d,U
Chest X-ray	+	+	-	-	+	-	+	-	-	-	-	-	-	-
Pulmonary function tests	-	-	+p	-	+	-	+	-	-	+	-	-	-	-
Other required tests	e	-	q	u	x	-	D	H	J	-	N	Q	S	V
Evaluate ability to wear respirators	+	+	+	+	+	+	+	+	+	+	+	+	+	+
Additional necessary tests	+	+	+	+	+	+	+	+	+	+	+	+	+	+
Written medical opinion	+f	+f	+f	+g,v	+f	+B	+f	+f	+f	+f	+f	+f	+g,v	+f
Counseling	+g	+g	+g	+g,v	+g,y	-	+g,E	+g	+g	+g	+g,O	+g	+g,v	-
Medical removal plan	-	-	+	-	+	-	-	-	-	+	+	+	+	+

[A]+, required;-, not required

[B]**a:** Standard specifies specific factors such as personal air exposures and/or years of exposure, biological indices, employee age, amount of time/year, and periodic exams may be required at varying time intervals depending on exposure circumstances. **b:** Annual. **c:** Lung, gastrointestinal tract, thyroid, skin, neurological (peripheral and central). **d:** Standard requires focus on specific body systems; symptoms; personal habits; family history; environmental history; and occupational history. **e:** Fecal occult blood. **f:** Physician to employer; employer to employee. **g:** By physician. **h:** If no exam within 6 months of termination. **i:** Skin, nose. **j:** Smoking history included. **k:** No examination is required if previous exam occurred within a specific time frame and provisions of the standard were met. **l:** Additional medical review by specialist physician(s) may be necessary for workers with abnormalities. **m:** Includes urinary phenol. **n:** Blood cell forming system, cardiopulmonary (if respirators used at least 30 days/year initial year, and then every 3 years). **o:** Required for initial and periodic exams, and the preplacement exam requires a special history. **p:** Initially and every 3 years if respirators worn 30 days/year and with special requirements. **q:** Complete blood count and differential, specific blood tests repeated as required. **r:** Within 48 hours of exposure. **s:** If 12 months and beyond from last exam. **t:** Liver, spleen, lymph nodes, skin. **u:** Complete blood count with differential count and platelet both annually and 48 hours after exposure in an emergency situation and then repeated monthly for 3 more months. **v:** Other licensed health care professional. **w:** Lung, cardiovascular system, kidney and urine, and for males over 40 prostate palpation. **x:** Annually—cadmium in urine, ß-2-microglobulin in urine, cadmium in blood, complete blood count, blood urea nitrogen, serum creatinine, urinalysis. **y:** Specific requirements. **z:** Special medical surveillance occurs within 24 hours. **A:** Determination for increased risk for example, target organs, reduced immune system competence, reproductive/developmental system competence, and known interacting factors such as smoking. **B:** Physician to employer. **C:** Skin. **D:** Weight, urine cytology, urinalysis for sugar, albumin, hemoglobin. **E:** Employer must inform employee of possible health consequences if employee refuses any required medical exam. **F:** Male reproductive repeated every 3 months. **G:** Male reproductive and genitourinary system. **H:** Sperm count, follicle stimulating hormone, luteinizing hormone, total estrogen for females and males. **I:** Nose/lung, skin, neurological, blood, reproductive, eyes. **J:** Complete blood count with differential, hematocrit, hemoglobin, red cell count; if requested by the employee, pregnancy testing and male fertility testing "as deemed appropriate by the physician." **K:** Skin irritation or sensitization; lung/nose; eyes; shortness of breath. **L:** Teeth, gums, blood cell forming system, gastrointestinal, kidney, cardiovascular, and neurological. **M:** Includes reproductive history, past lead exposure (work and nonwork), and history of specific body systems. **N:** Blood hemoglobin, hematocrit, zinc protoporphyrin, urea nitrogen, serum creatinine, lead, peripheral blood cell smear morphology, red cell indices; urinalysis with microscopic examination; also, if requested by the employee, pregnancy testing or male fertility testing. **O:** Includes advising the employee of any medical condition, occupational or nonoccupational, requiring further medical examination or treatment. **P:** Skin and liver. **Q:** Liver function tests and urinalysis. **R:** Lungs, cardiovascular (including blood pressure and pulse), liver, nervous, skin; extent and depth depends on employee's health status, work, and medical history. **S:** Pre- and postshift tests are included in the standard. **T:** Enlargement of kidneys, spleen, and liver or their dysfunction; abnormalities in skin, connective tissue, and lungs. **U:** Includes alcohol intake, history of hepatitis, exposure to compounds that cause liver damage, blood transfusions, hospitalizations, and work history. **V:** Blood tests for total bilirubin, alkaline phosphatase, serum glutamic-oxalotransaminase (aspartate aminotransaminase), glutamic-pyruvic transaminase (alanine aminotransferase), and -glutamyl transferase (-glutamyl transpeptidase).

For example, the 1987 benzene OSHA guidelines[8] (PEL 1 ppm with STEL of 5 ppm and action level of 0.5 ppm) refer to emergency situations (for example, benzene air concentrations that approach the IDLH of 500 ppm or that cause adverse symptoms) after which a spot urine sample is to be analyzed within 72 hr for urinary phenol normalized to a urine specific gravity of 1.024. The critical urinary phenol level is 75 mg/L. At or above this concentration, complete blood counts at monthly intervals for three months following the emergency exposure are mandated triggering further actions if discrepancies in complete blood counts occur (hemoglobin levels or hematocrits are outside the 95% confidence level of reference ranges; the platelet count is at 20% or more below the worker's most recent values or falls below the 95% confidence limit of the lower limit of the reference range; the leukocyte (white blood cell) count is <4,000/mm^3 or there is an abnormal differential leukocyte count relative to reference ranges). Any further persistent (repeatable within two weeks) decrease in any of these variables is cause to refer the worker to an internist or hematologist, an act which triggers medical removal of the worker from the areas of benzene exposure with up to 6 months of benefits. It might be noted that benzene biological monitoring with phenol is only to gauge the likelihood of adverse benzene effect for benzene air concentrations above 10 ppm 8-hour TWA, and thus is definitely medical surveillance. ACGIH® has recommended urinary S-phenylmercapturic acid and trans, trans-muconic acid as markers for intrinsically safe air exposures at or below its 8-h TLV®-TWA of 0.5 ppm.[10] See the section on ACGIH® Recommendations for more detail on the latter.

It might be noted in Table 19.2 that the suspect carcinogens and their 29 CFR parts are: 2-acetylaminofluorene (1910.1015); 4-aminodiphenyl (1910.1011); benzidine (1910.1010); bis-chloromethyl ether (1910.1008); 3,3'-dichlorobenzidine (and its salts) (1910.1007); 4-dimethylaminoazobenzene (1910.1015); ethyleneimine (1910.1012); methyl chloromethyl ether (1910.1008); alpha-naphthylamine (1910.1004); beta-naphthylamine (1910.1009); 4-nitrobiphenyl (1910.1003); N-nitrosodimethylamine (1910.1019); and beta-propiolactone (1910.1013).

OSHA also provides medical screening and medical surveillance guidance (Table III) for general chemical exposure related to the following situations:

- Asbestos in General Industry (29 CFR 1910.1001(l)) and in Construction and Shipyards (29 CFR 1926.1191(m)/1915.1001)
- Hazardous wastes in HAZWOPER (29 CFR 1910.120(f)/1926.65)
- Hazardous chemicals in laboratories (29 CFR 1910.1450(g))
- Respiratory protection (29 CFR 1910.134(e)/1926.103).

Tables 19.2 and Tables 19.3 together summarize OSHA guidance on medical screening and medical surveillance related to chemical exposure. It should be noted that medical screening and surveillance guidelines also exist for bloodborne pathogens, compressed air environments, cotton dust, noise, and ionizing radiation (as contained in 10 CFR 835 for the Department of Energy and as memorialized between OSHA and the Nuclear Regulatory Commission OSHA Directive CPL 2.86 of 1989). Any known toxicologic interactions with the toxic effects of chemicals (e.g. leukemia from benzene exposure and ionizing radiation absorption) bring these other medical screening and medical surveillance endpoints into effect also. Directives also exist for microwave popcorn processing plants (National Emphasis Program), and genetic testing (OSHA Medical Surveillance Regulations).

According to 29 CFR 1904.39, the employer must orally report to OSHA (nearest office or 800-321-6742) within 8 hours a fatality or hospitalization by three or more employees as a result of a work-related incident. This includes heart attacks, and any fatality or multiple hospitalization within 30 days of the incident. Employers must record in the OSHA 300 log new work-related injuries and illnesses that meet one or more of the general recording criteria or meet the recording criteria for specific types of conditions. An injury or illness is an abnormal condition or disorder. Injuries include cases such as, but not limited to, a cut, fracture, sprain, or amputation. Illnesses include both acute and chronic illnesses, such as, but not limited to, a skin disease, respiratory disorder, or poisoning. Regardless of where signs or symptoms surface, a case is recordable in the

OSHA 300 log only if a work event or exposure is a discernable cause of the injury or illness or of a significant aggravation to a pre-existing health condition. Recordable work-related injuries and illnesses are those that result in one or more of the following: death; days away from work; restricted work; transfer to another job; medical treatment beyond first aid; loss of consciousness; or diagnosis of a significant injury or illness. Work is considered restricted when, as a result of a work-related injury or illness, (a) the employer keeps the employee from performing one or more of the routine functions of his or her job (job functions that the employee regularly performs at least once per week), or from working the full workday that he or she would otherwise have been scheduled to work, or (b) a physician or other licensed health care professional recommends that the employee not perform one or more of the routine functions of his or her job, or not work the full workday that he or she would otherwise have been scheduled to work. Medical treatment means any treatment not contained in the list of first aid treatments. Medical treatment does not include visits to a healthcare professional for observation and counseling or diagnostic procedures. First aid means only those treatments specifically listed in 29 CFR 1904.7. Examples of first aid include: the use of non-prescription medications at non- prescription strength, the application of hot or cold therapy, eye patches or finger guards, and others.

OSHA in its Hazard Communication Final Rule[9] defines industrial hygienists to be "health professionals" along with licensed physicians, toxicologists and epidemiologists (but not nurses) and therefore are able to ask manufacturers for the identity of chemicals that are trade secrets for non-emergency health and safety reasons, including biological monitoring purposes. Any health professional must be given trade secret data immediately by manufacturers in an emergency situation.[9] The corresponding state agencies may mandate biological monitoring tests when OSHA or the U.S. EPA do not. Hygienists should always check the regulations of the state of which they are resident.

Because of its broad nature, OSHA's General Duty Clause can also be used to ensure all workplaces are safe. OSHA has, under this Clause, cited employers for failing to protect workers from dermal exposure that led to health effects, even though air concentrations were below the PEL and respiratory PPE were properly used. Since biological monitoring could have led to the detection of the exposure but not air sampling, biological monitoring could be required to test the effectiveness of any control measures.

Table 19.3 — OSHA Medical Screening and Medical Surveillance Endpoints for Generalized Chemical Exposures and to Asbestos[6]

Endpoint	*Chemical Exposure*[A,B]				
	1	*1A*	*2*	*3*	*4*
Preplacement exam	+a,b	+a,b	+a	-q	+s,t
Periodic exam	+c	+c,l	+c,l	-q	+t,u
Emergency/exposure exam/tests	-	-	+a	+a	-
Termination exam	+d	-	+n	-	-
Exam emphasis	e	m	o	-q	+a,t
Work/medical history	+f	+f	+p	-q	+a
Chest X-ray	+g	+g	-,o	-q	-v
Pulmonary function tests	+h	+h	-,o	-q	-v
Other required tests	-	-	-,o	-q	-v
Evaluate ability to wear respirators	+	+	+	+q	+
Additional necessary tests	+	+	+	+	+
Written medical opinion	+i	+i	+i	+r	+w
Employee counseling	+j,k	+j,k	+j	+j	+x
Medical removal plan	-	-	-	-	-

[A]+, required; -, not required

[B]**a:** Standard specifies specific factors such as personal air exposures and/or years of exposure, biological indices, employee age, amount of time/year, and periodic exams may be required at varying time intervals depending on exposure circumstances. **b:** No examination is required if previous exam occurred within a specific time frame and provisions of the standard were met. **c:** Annual. **d:** Within 30 days of termination. **e:** Respiratory, cardiovascular, gastrointestinal. **f:** Standard form required. **g:** Specialized requirements. **h:** B reader, board eligible/certified radiologist or physician with expertise in pneumoconioses required for X-ray interpretation and classification. **h:** Forced vital capacity (FVC) and forced expired volume in one second (FEV1) measurements. **i:** Physician to employer; employer to employee. **j:** By physician. **k:** Includes informing employee of increased risk of lung cancer from combined effect of smoking and asbestos exposure. **l:** Can be more frequent if determined to be necessary by physician. **m:** Pulmonary and gastrointestinal. **n:** If no exam within 6 months of termination/reassignment: **o:** Determined by physician. **p:** Emphasis is on symptoms related to handling and exposure to hazardous substances and health hazards, fitness for duty, and ability to wear PPE. **q:** When required by specific standards in Table 13.2 or others. **r:** Physician to employer. **s:** Evaluation questionnaire or exam required, or follow-up exam when deemed necessary by physician or other licensed health professional. **t:** Specific protocol required. **u:** Specific protocol required. **v:** As determined by physician or other licensed health care professional. **w:** By physician or other licensed health care professional to employer and to employee. **x:** By physician or other licensed health care professional

ACGIH® BEIs®

The American Conference of Governmental Industrial Hygienists (ACGIH®) has issued 75 Biological Exposure Indices (BEIs®) for 47 compounds or groups of compounds, with 2 Notices of Intended Changes in 2008[10] (Table

IV). Each annual update of the TLV®-TWAs and BEIs® should be consulted as well as their most recent Documentations since they all change. For example, methyl isobutyl ketone has a 2008 notice for intended change to its TWA (50 to 30 ppm) that will eventually impact its BEI®.

Up to 2008, BEIs for single chemicals have been set mostly on the air TLV®-TWA for each chemical and therefore on workplace inhalation exposure only, over 8 hr/day for 5 d/week for the toxic effect on which the TLV®-TWA is based. This effect is discussed in the Documentation of the latter[11] and cited in the TLVs® and BEIs® booklet for that calendar year. BEIs® have not yet been issued based on a cancer criterion, though cancer classifications are now established for TLV®-TWAs. BEIs® that use non-specific markers of effect include: red blood cell cholinesterase activity for acetylcholineesterase inhibiting pesticides (organophosphate and organocarbamate pesticides); carboxyhemoglobin in blood for carbon monoxide (dichloromethane is the major positive interference); and methemoglobin in blood for methemoglobin inducers like nitrobenzene. A TLV®-TWA is not designed to protect the health of all workers. The hygienist must use professional judgment to assess if TLV®-TWAs and BEIs® are truly protective for each worker under consideration.

Each BEI® documentation is organized into the following sections for the exposing compound: Recommended BEI®; Properties; Absorption; Elimination; Metabolic Pathways and Biochemical Interactions; Possible Nonoccupational Exposure; TLV®-TWA; and Summary. Then for each index the subheadings are generally (but not always): Analytical Method; Sampling and Storage; Biological Levels without Occupational Exposure; Kinetics; Factors Affecting Interpretation of Measurements; Justification; Current Database Available; Recommendations; Reference Values Recommended by Other Organizations; and Other Indicators of Exposure. There may be more than one BEI® for each exposing compound.

Since adverse effects on internal organs after xenobiotic absorption are dependent on the biologically effective dose exposing them, the absorbed dose is more correlated to the adverse health effects caused by an internal target organ than the external exposure dose. For irritative compounds, the exposure dose is related to the irritative effect directly. Many irritants have ceiling air values rather than TLV®-TWAs, some amines, aldehydes and ketones being the exceptions. Thus the Documentation of the TLV® must be consulted to see if the critical health effect keyed to the TLV®-TWA is based on internal target organs or not. The workload or physical activity at which the TLV®-TWA was set is then its reference workload condition. Usually the Documentation of the TLV® for a compound is not explicit about the type of workload, but moderate workload (100 watt) is generally assumed. The compound's BEI® Documentation is essential for the hygienist to assess whether biological monitoring is feasible or necessary, and to be able to interpret the results. The other piece of necessary documentation is an appropriate NIOSH[17] or other sampling and chemical analysis method.

AIHA® Biological Environmental Exposure Levels (BEELs)

The American Industrial Hygiene Association® in 2006, funded its Biological Environmental Exposure Level (BEEL) Project Team within the Biological Monitoring Committee to formulate Guidelines and their documentations for chemicals that did not have ACGIH® TLV®-TWAs and that especially were absorbed through the skin. BEELs for chemicals that also have AIHA® Workplace Environmental Exposure Levels (WEELs™) based on systemic effects would have the same relationship as BEIs® do to their corresponding TLV®-TWAs. It is envisaged to propose the following BEEL types: Analytical, one-tenth of the Hygienic BEEL to define the lower quantifiable concentration for analytical methods for the marker in its biological medium; Action, one-half of the Hygienic BEEL to protect sensitive people and to start control measures; Hygienic BEEL (analogous to a BEI® set on its specific TLV®-TWA); and Removal from Exposure BEEL, the marker concentration at which the worker must be removed from the exposure. This is a modified Control Banding approach that spans at least 2 orders of magnitude.

The first proposed BEEL is for p,p'-methylene dianiline (MDA) whereby the Hygienic BEEL is 41 µg total MDA/g creatinine for spot end-of-shift urine samples, and the corresponding Removal From Exposure BEEL of

Table 19.4 — Biological Exposure Indices (BEIs) Recommended by the ACGIH® in 2010[10]

Exposing Chemical	*Marker/Medium*	*Sampling Time*	*BEI*	*Other Notations*
Acetone	Acetone/U	ES	50 mg/L	Ns
Acetylcholinesterase Inhibiting Pesticides	Cholinesterase activity/RBC	D	70% of individuals baseline	Ns
Aniline	Aniline*/U	ES	—	Nq
	Aniline released from hemoglobin in blood	ES	—	Nq
	p-Aminophenol*/U	ES	50 mg/L	B, Ns, Sq
Arsenic (As), Elemental and Soluble Inorganic Compounds	Inorganic arsenic plus methylated metabolites/U	EWK	35 μg As/L	B
Benzene	S-Phenylmercapturic acid/U	ES	2.5 ug/g creatinine	B
	t,t-Muconic acid/U	ES	500 μg/g creatinine	B
1,3-Butadiene	1,2-Dihydroxy-4-(N-acetylcysteinyl) butane/U	ES	2.5 mg/L	B, Sq
	Mixture N-1 and N-2-(hydroxybutenyl)valine hemoglobin (Hb) adducts/B	NC	2.5 pmol/g Hb	Sq
2-Butoxyethanol	Butoxyacetic acid/U	ES	200 mg/g creatinine	—
Cadmium and Inorganic Compounds	Cadmium/U	NC	5 μg/g creatinine	B
	Cadmium/B	NC	5 μg/L	B
Carbon Disulfide	2-Thiothiazolidine-4- carboxylic acid/U	ES	0.5 mg/g creatinine	B, Ns
Carbon Monoxide	Carboxyhemoglobin/B	ES	3.5% of hemoglobin	B, Ns
	Carbon Monoxide/EEA	ES	20 ppm	B, Ns
Chlorobenzene	4-Chlorocatechol*/U	ES-EWK	100 mg/g creatinine	Ns
	Total p-chlorophenol*/U	ES-EWK	20 mg/g creatinine	Ns
Chromium (VI), Water-soluble fume	Total Chromium/U	ES-EWK	25 μg/L	—
	Total Chromium/U	IDS	10 μg/L	—
Cobalt (Co)	Cobalt/U	ES-EWK	15 μg/L	B
	Cobalt/B	ES-EWK	1 μg/L	B, Sq
Cyclohexanol	1,2-Cyclohexanediol*/U	ES-EWK	—	Nq, Ns
	Cyclohexanol*/U	ES	—	Nq, Ns
Cyclohexanone	1,2-Cyclohexanediol*/U	ES-EWK	80 mg/L	Ns, Sq
	Cyclohexanol*/U	ES	8 mg/L	Ns, Sq
Dichloromethane	Dichloromethane/U	ES	0.3 mg/L	Sq
N,N-Dimethylacetamide	N-Methylacetamide/U	ES-EWK	30 mg/g creatinine	—
N,N-Dimethylformamide	N-Methylformamide/U	ES	15 mg/L	—
	N-Acetyl-S-(N-methylcarbamoyl) cysteine/U	PLS-EWK	40 mg/L	Sq
2-Ethoxyethanol and 2-Ethoxyethanolacetate	2-Ethoxyacetic acid/U	ES-EWK	100 mg/g creatinine	—
Ethyl Benzene	Sum of mandelic and phenylglyoxylic acids/U	ES-EWK	0.7 g/g creatinine	Ns, Sq
	Ethyl benzene/EEA	NC	—	Sq
Fluorides	Fluorides/U	PS	3 mg/g creatinine	B, Ns
		ES	10 mg/g creatinine	B, Ns

(continued on next page.)

Table 19.4 — Biological Exposure Indices (BEIs) Recommended by ACGIH® in 2010 (continued)[10]

Exposing Chemical	*Marker/Medium*	*Sampling Time*	*BEI*	*Other Notations*
Furfural	Furoic acid/U	ES	200 mg/L	Ns
n-Hexane	2,5-Hexanedione°/U	ES-EWK	0.4 mg/L	—
Lead	Lead#/B	NC	30 µg/100 ml	—
Mercury	Total inorganic mercury/U Total inorganic mercury/B	PS ES-EWK	35 µg/g creatinine 15 µg/L	B B
Methanol	Methanol/U	ES	15 mg/L	B, Ns
Methemoglobin Inducers	Methemoglobin/B	DS or ES	1.5% of hemoglobin	B, Ns, Sq
2-Methoxyethanol and 2-Methoxyacetic acetate	2-Methoxyethyl acid/U	ES-EWK	1 mg/g creatinine	
Methyl n-Butyl Ketone	2,5-Hexanedione°/U	ES-EWK	0.4 mg/L	—
Methyl Chloroform	Methyl chloroform/EEA Trichloroacetic acid/U Total trichloroethanol/U Total trichloroethanol/B	PLS-EWK EWK ES-EWK ES-EWK	40 ppm 10 mg/L 30 mg/L 1 mg/L	— Ns, Sq Ns, Sq Ns
4,4-Methylene bis(2-chloroaniline) (MBOCA)	Total MBOCA/U	ES	—	Nq
Methyl Ethyl Ketone (MEK)	MEK/U	ES	2 mg/L	—
Methyl Isobutyl Ketone	Methyl Isobutyl Ketone/U	ES	1 mg/L	—
N-Methyl-2-Pyrrolidone	5-Hydroxy-N-methyl-2-pyrrolidone/U	ES	100 mg/L	—
Nitrobenzene	Total p-nitrophenol/U Methemoglobin/B	ES-EWK ES	5 mg/g creatinine 1.5% of hemoglobin	Ns B, Ns, Sq
Parathion	Total p-nitrophenol/U Cholinesterase activity/RBC	ES D	0.5 mg/g creatinine 70% of individual's baseline	Ns B, Ns, Sq
Pentachlorophenol (PCP)	Total PCP/U Free PCP/Plasma	PLS-EWK ES	2 mg/g creatinine 5 mg/L	B B
Phenol	Phenol*/U	ES	250 mg/g creatinine	B, Ns
Polycyclic Aromatic Hydrocarbons (PAHs)	1-Hydroxypyrene*/U	ES-EWK	—	Ns
2-Propanol	Acetone/U	ES-EWK	40 mg/L	B, Ns
Styrene	Mandelic plus phenylglyoxylic acids/U Styrene/venous B	ES ES	400 mg/g creatinine 0.2 mg/L	Ns Sq
Tetrachloroethylene	Tetrachloroethylene/EEA Tetrachloroethylene/B	PS PS	3 ppm 0.5 mg/L	— —
Tetrahydrofuran	Tetrahydrofuran/U	ES	2 mg/L	—
Toluene	Toluene/B Toluene/U o-Cresol*/U	PLS-EWK ES ES	0.02 mg/L 0.03 mg/L 0.3 mg/g creatinine	— — B
Trichloroethylene	Trichloroacetic acid/U Trichloroethanol/B Trichloroethylene/B Trichloroethylene/EEA	ES-EWK ES-EWK ES-EWK ES-EWK	15 mg/L 0.5 mg/L — —	Ns Ns Sq Sq
Uranium	Uranium/U	ES	200 µg/L	—

Table 19.4 — Biological Exposure Indices (BEIs) Recommended by ACGIH® in 2010 (continued)[10]

Exposing Chemical	*Marker/Medium*	*Sampling Time*	*BEI*	*Other Notations*
Xylenes	Methylhippuric acids/U	ES	1.5 g/g creatinine	—

Marker/Medium Column: B - Blood; RBC - Red Blood Cells; EEA -End Exhaled Air; MEA - Mixed Exhaled Air; U - Urine, * - with Hydrolysis, ° - without Hydrolysis, # - see reference 10 for additional information for women of childbearing potential

Sampling Time Column: D - Discretionary after a minimum of two weeks of exposure; DS - During the Shift within the last two hours of exposure; ES - End of Shift; EWK - End of Workweek; ES-EWK - End of Shift at the End of the Workweek; IDS - Increase During the Shift; NC - Not Critical if prior exposure has occurred for more than two weeks

Other Notations Column: B - Background, there is an endogenous background in unexposed individuals; Nq - No number is set due to insufficient data; Ns - Nonspecific, other exposing chemicals give the same marker; Sq - Semiquantitative, there is an ambiguous dose response

410 µg total MDA/g creatinine. The corresponding respective Glove BEELS were 0.9 mg and 9 mg; the respective Skin Exposure BEELs were 0.45 µg/cm² and 4.5 µg/cm²; and the respective Oral Exposure BEELs were 13 mg/kg body weight and 130 mg/kg. The BEEL Guide (Documentation) is similar in organization to that for a WEEL Guide but with only the most sensitive toxicology endpoints provided, plus more emphasis on biological monitoring, analytical methods, and skin sampling methods.

The other chemicals under investigation are: Methamphetamine; n-Octanol; Dimethyl Sulfoxide; Capsaicin; D-Limonene; Polypropylene glycol; 1-Butoxy-2-propanol; Ecstasy; and Gamma-Hydroxybutyrate.

Other Recommendations

Non-U.S. biological monitoring guidelines for the workplace usually are similar to BEIs®. These include: German BATs (Biological Tolerance Values)[14]; and draft recommendations of the Scientific Committee for Occupational Exposure Limits to Chemical Agents under European Council Directive 98/24. The biological monitoring guidelines of many non-European countries are often based on the BEIs®.

NIOSH has no formal biological monitoring recommendations for workers but has developed a "skin exposure" notation system that flags chemicals for which biological monitoring may be useful that will be part of its Pocket Guide. NIOSH has published an online compendium of literature medical tests that include biological monitoring for specific OSHA-regulated chemicals at http://www.cdc.gov/niosh/nmed/medstart.html.

Another approach is not to use health risk assessment but to define a goal that is achievable in a defined percentage of a country's workplaces. In the United Kingdom, the Health Safety Executive uses the 90% percentile of the available validated data from representative workplaces with good industrial hygiene practices. This is termed the Hygienic Benchmark Guideline value. For example, the latter value for MDA is 88 µg/g creatinine.[24]

Compounds without Recommendations

For those compounds without recommendations, other literature sources must be consulted for any guiding critical biological equivalent values. The most useful references are the latest editions of books by Lauwerys and Hoet[12], Baselt [13], La Dou et al.[15], the textbook by Que Hee[1], and the AIHA® *Biological Monitoring — A Practical Field Manual.*[26] Other than these, the primary journal literature can be searched through computer and hand searches of Chemical Abstracts, Biological Abstracts, Medline, Index Medicus, the Hazardous Substances Data Bank (HSDB), the *Toxicological Profiles* of individual chemicals published by the Agency for Toxic Substances and Disease Registry (ATSDR), the criteria documents of EPA and NIOSH, National Toxicology Program material, and other U.S. government agency websites. Biological monitoring publications of the World Health Organization, and of the European Union can also be consulted. Biological monitoring markers and their appropriate analytical methods would be useful additional information by manufacturers in their material safety data sheets (MSDSs).

Routes of Exposure Other than Inhalation

The hygienist must observe whether a worker handles or spills specific solvents and which parts of the skin are exposed, and for how long. Any gloves and garments that are worn when spills occur must be known to be protective against chemical degradation and permeation through consulting standard references.[4]

Hot dusty environments where many chemicals are also used may pose an ingestion hazard through the licking of lips, and inhalation of particulates larger than respirable size that are then cleared through the ciliary locomotor into the stomach from the upper airways, and from the nose and throat. Workers should shower after work and don clean clothes. Improper storage/cleaning of respirators may cause contaminated dusts to accumulate and lead to both inhalation and ingestion exposures. Food in any workplace unit process area where toxic chemicals are in use should be forbidden. Workplace smoking may enhance both inhalation and oral exposure of workplace contaminants and their pyrolysis products.

A major signal to consider biological monitoring occurs when workers feel ill when air sampling results are below mandated or recommended concentrations. The worker may be hypersensitive, or other major routes of exposure may exist. The worker should be sent to a physician to check the former condition, and the work practices of the worker observed relative to nearness to exposure sources for the latter in addition to determining the extent of use and functioning of personal protective equipment (PPE). MSDSs must be initially consulted to identify the specific compounds involved in the exposures and which are likely to pose inhalation, dermal absorption, and oral ingestion potential. The unit processes in the specific workplace must also be known and understood. Toxic interaction information should be obtained.

Those compounds that have a "skin" notation with their TLV® are those for which skin absorption and/or toxicity data by liquid, solid, or vapor exposures have been published and adjudged important by the TLV® Committee. ACGIH® has a general policy[10] of defining as "skin" a chemical whose animal dermal acute LD_{50} is less than or equal to 1 g/kg body weight; where "dermal application studies have shown absorption that could cause systemic effects following exposure"; or when "potential significant contribution to the overall exposure can occur by the cutaneous route including mucous membranes and the eyes". The OSHA "skin" designation is assigned only in cases where dermal exposure has been shown to cause systemic poisoning or where skin exposure leads to an absorbed dose greater than that permitted to be absorbed by inhalation at the PEL. NIOSH in its current Pocket Guide[25] merely states the notation reflects "potential for skin absorption". NIOSH is currently revising its skin notation. Although these "skin" notations are not equivalent, ACGIH®, NIOSH, and OSHA emphasize that the dermal route should be considered in control measures for such designated chemicals. The air TLV®, PEL, or REL are based only on inhalation exposure and do not account for skin or oral exposure over a 8-hr exposure/16-h no exposure day, for 5 day/week followed by 2 days of no exposure regimen for a healthy worker for a working lifetime. ACGIH® cautions: "The Skin notation also alerts the industrial hygienist that overexposure may occur during dermal contact with liquid and aerosols, even when airborne exposures are at or below the TLV®."[10]

The absence of a "skin" notation does not mean that the chemical is not absorbed through the skin or is not toxic. Most nonpolar organic and organometallic liquids that are not miscible with water have water solubilities in the > ppm range, and will potentially pass through the skin, as will compounds in solution with such liquids. How relevant potential skin absorption is has to be assessed visually and directly by hygienists on a case-by-case basis. Such evaluations may also require skin patches, skin sampling, or tracer studies[2], as well as biological monitoring.

Presence of Personal Protective Equipment

The presence of PPE creates a barrier to the hazardous agent so that the agent is prevented from body access. The final test for effectiveness of PPE is that markers for the exposing compound are NOT detected in biological media above critical concentrations that correspond to critical air concentrations for air exposure, whether or not expensive engineering controls, PPE, hygienic, and administrative measures may have been instituted in the workplace or environment. If marker levels do not decrease after controls are instituted, then either the controls are ineffective, a non-workplace source of the marker is present, or there may be worker connivance. The hygienist needs then to sleuth out the cause.

Quantitative fit testing is essential to maximize protection of negative pressure respirators in addition to appropriate cartridge selection, worker training, and qualitative fit testing. Positive pressure respirators must maintain a protective flow of air across the nose and mouth to prevent entry of exposing chemicals. Gloves and garments must not be degraded or permeated by the exposing chemicals. All PPE must be maintained appropriately.

Unanticipated Exposures

One of the advantages of biological monitoring is that its integrative nature allows warning of unexpected exposures. Thus while postshift or end-of-shift sampling are generally recommended in the BEIs, preshift sampling will allow assessment of carryover from previous work exposures or from non-workplace exposures. Carryover is not likely for compounds of half-times less than 6 hours. However the excretion of chemicals is usually at least biphasic, consisting of a fast exponential period and then a slower exponential period. Buildup can be addressed by administrative rotation, improving respirator or engineering control protection, and worker hygienic controls. Nonoccupational exposures, not being under the control of the worker's employer, are difficult to handle, but the responsibility is the worker's, once informed.

Another common workplace situation is when PPE are doffed but the worker unknowingly is still near an emission source of vapor, or puts a bare hand on spilt solvent, for example, on the PPE itself. Biological monitoring may indicate whether a potentially hazardous amount of chemical has been absorbed that is equivalent to a hazardous inhalation exposure as embodied in a TLV®.

Adjunct to Current Environmental Sampling Activities

Health effects are related to the absorbed dose from all routes and all environments rather than that just contributed by the workplace, unless the dose contributed by the latter dominates. Control plots showing the variation of marker and exposure concentrations with time are invaluable to assess whether individual worker exposure trends are stable and under control, and if more attention needs to be given to control of non-inhalation routes of exposure. This might have ramifications on worker and management training, management support, the written biological monitoring program and its role in the occupational and environmental health program, and when to start and end the biological monitoring program for a specific worker. Clear objectives and decision points are necessary in any biological monitoring program.

Factors for Biological Monitoring Data Interpretation Using the BEIs®

In this section we will focus attention on compounds with BEIs® as representative of most guidelines based on a personal breathing zone 8-h air sampling concentration.

Any marker concentration sampled under BEI end-of-shift conditions that exceeds 0.7 its BEI® concentration reflects a threshold above which almost all healthy workers irrespective of exposure routes might experience systemic health effects upon which the corresponding TLV®-TWA is based. The appropriate baseline sample (preshift for end-of-shift sampling; pre-shift on first work day after the weekend for end-of-week sampling) should always be subtracted to obtain the workplace contribution if it is known that it is caused by holdover from the previous work exposures. If this difference still exceeds 0.7 the BEI®, the workplace is then definitely the source of overexposure. If the baseline sample shows a contribution from recent non-occupational exposure, the elimination will be in its fast phase and should not be subtracted from the end-of-shift value.

For effective control, the most important routes of exposure must then be prioritized through a time-and-motion study relative to job proximity to known sources of the suspected chemical.

If volatile solvents (vapor pressure >3.0 x 10^{-3} mm Hg), gases, or hot processes are present, then inhalation of vapor may be a major exposure route. If hot processes are involved or the environment is dusty, inhalation of particulates may also be major. If there is little respirable dust (<3 mg/m^3 of particulates containing no asbestos and <1 % crystalline silica ["PNOC", particles not otherwise classified, below aerodynamic diameters of 10 µm]), or little "total dust" or "inhalable dust" (<10 mg/m^3 for PNOC of aerodynamic diameters <100 µm), particulate inhalation exposure should be minor. Aerosols in the thoracic size range (<25 µm aerodynamic diameter) deposit in the lung with the fraction between 10–25 µm depositing in the upper lung (bronchioles upwards to the bronchi) where the ciliary locomotor process can sweep particles up to the trachea and larynx, and then into the stomach by the saliva flow, thus facilitating absorption through ingestion. Particles between 25 to 100 µm aerodynamic diameter are more likely to deposit in the nasal conchae and pharynx from where some ingestion is also expected. If particulate chemicals are soluble in saliva and if there is nasal drip, ingestion of part of them will occur. Whole particles will also be ingested during swallowing and mouth air breathing. Hot and dusty environments may cause dusty faces and lips, and licking of lips and contamination of food and tobacco products may cause oral exposures. Dermal exposures become important when solvents are handled in the absence of PPE, and when PPE are not protective. This route of exposure is especially important for moderately volatile and nonvolatile chemicals of high octanol/water coefficients (K_{ow}) of 10 to 10,000 that contact the skin with water solubilities above ppm values (See Reference 1 Chapter 3, and the BEI® Documentation BEI®-4 to BEI®-11). Hygienic considerations are the key controls for oral and skin exposure in the absence of engineering controls and PPE. They are key for full compliance with the lead standard also (see Lead Standard section).

Vapor Inhalation Predominates as the Route of Exposure

The major parameter to account for when inhalation exposure is dominant (>70% of the total absorbed dose) is physical activity or workload. If a worker is exposed to within 30% of the TLV®-TWA concentration in a TWA breathing zone personal air sample, a concentration above 0.70 of the BEI of the marker should result if inhalation dominates after correction for any baseline concentration.

Table 19.5 gives some physiological data that depend on workload.[15] The alveolar ventilation rate is the volume of air per minute inspired into the alveoli, and increases linearly up to 150 watt work. If the same vapor concentration of a substance is being inspired at these different work rates relative to moderate workload using the data of Table V over the same exposure period, heavy work potentially exposes (38/27) = 1.41 times, light workload (16/27) = 0.59 times, and at rest (5/27) = 0.185 times the inhaled mass at moderate workload, the usual physical activity assumed in setting TLV-TWAs. These values represent extremes since expiration rate generally increases correspondingly but never matches inspiration rate except during hyperventilation.

The difference obtained between mass potentially breathed in minus that breathed out when divided by the mass potentially breathed in is termed the uptake for that time period at a specific physical activity, and is usually expressed in units of percent.

Table 19.5 — Some Physiological Parameters Influenced by Physical Activity[10]

Workload (watt)[1]	*Oxygen Demand (L/min)*	*Alveolar Ventilation (L air./min)*	*Heart pump rate (L/min)*	*Blood Flow (L/min)*			*Signs*
				Muscles	*Liver*	*Brain*	
At rest; sedentary (0)	0.3	5.0	6.0	1.0	1.5	0.6	Slow regular breaths
Light work (50)	0.8	16.0	9.0	3.6	1.3	0.7	Ribcage visibly rises and falls
Moderate work (100)	1.3	27.0	13.0	7.9	1.2	0.7	Noisy breath; light sweating
Heavy work (150)	1.8	38.0	19.0	13.0	1.1	0.7	Heavy breathing and sweating

[1]The watts cited are the midpoints with +/- 25 watt range. More complicated schemes with different watts relative to resting also exist (see Chapter 25, "Thermal Standards and Measurement Techniques")

Uptake is usually determined in bicycle ergometer, treadmill, or step-testing studies where watts of work expended can be measured directly along with biological markers and physiological parameters. The literature values of parameters in Table V for these different regimens vary.

The uptakes of chemically inert solvent vapors such as aliphatic (for example, hexane), alicyclic (for example, cyclohexane), and aromatic (for example, benzene) hydrocarbons and their chlorinated analogs have been found[16] to obey similar correlational relationships but not hydrogen-bonding solvents like alcohols (for example, n-butanol). The relationship for chemically inert solvent vapors that is obeyed for % uptake over 2-hr of exposure (workbreak to workbreak conditions) at a defined concentration near a TLV®-TWA in a bicycle ergometer study was[16]:

$$\%\ \text{Uptake} = \frac{-86 \times AAC_{20\text{–}30}}{\text{inspired air concentration}} + 79.3 \quad (1)$$

where AAC_{20-30} is the alveolar air concentration determined 20 to 30 minutes after the 2-hour exposure has ended at a given physical activity.

Correlational equations such as Equation (1) must be applied with caution since they are valid only for the chemicals and exposure scenarios investigated. In addition a boundary conditions analysis is recommended to illustrate the utility of such equations. Thus in Equation (1), the % uptake is zero at (AAC_{20-30}/inspired air concentration)=0.992, and 100% at -0.241, the latter being completely unrealistic. When AAC_{20-30} is zero, the % uptake is 79%. Thus the real maximum uptake is 79% for the compounds and exposure conditions investigated. An equation is not necessarily meaningful for all parameter values.

Appendix 1 contains examples of the calculations for xylene[15] relative to its BEI® at different workloads and exposure conditions. Appendix 1 gives some idea of the strengths and weaknesses of the urinary BEI of metabolite markers relative to exposure conditions at its reference physical activity. Hygienists must ascertain whether the BEI is protective or not for a given exposure scenario rather than rely solely on the urinary concentrations determined by analytical chemistry laboratories. The same may be said for air sampling results.

Workers do not work at one physical activity, nor do they inhale the same concentration of a single chemical as occurs in studies with volunteers. Females always have greater uptakes than males for challenges to the same concentration of nonpolar compound vapors at the same physical activity.[1] The xylenes BEI® documentation[15] also states that ethylbenzene causes up to 20% inhibition of the metabolism of m-xylene, the major xylene isomer in technical xylene. The Xylenes BEI® is valid only for exposure to technical grade xylene containing ethylbenzene and not for exposure to pure xylene isomers. The metabolism of m-xylene is also inhibited up to 50% by alcohol consumption or the ingestion of aspirin. The hygienist must identify whether such latter additional factors are important for each worker through questionnaires or directly. The Documentations must therefore be consulted to define such questions when a BEI® is exceeded. Methylhippuric acids are also relatively specific urinary markers since xylenes, or methyl alkyl benzenes where the alkyl is a normal (unbranched) aliphatic hydrocarbon chain containing an odd number of carbon atoms (beta-oxidation cuts off 2-carbon units from the sidechain) are the only solvent type precursors that will produce methylhippuric acids on metabolism. Such long chain alkyls have a much lower vapor pressure than the corresponding methyl analogs, but this factor may be outweighed in petroleum fractions having high concentrations of long-chain derivatives relative to their methyl analogs.

Urinary markers are often much less specific than methyl hippuric acids as a marker for xylene. Hippuric acid, a urinary marker for toluene[15], is also produced by workplace exposure to benzaldehyde (or to almond-flavored foods), benzyl alcohol, benzoic acid, benzyl halides, and monosubstituted aromatic hydrocarbons with a side chain containing a normal aliphatic side chain of an odd number of carbon atoms (through β-oxidation), and to sodium benzoate preservative in foods. Another positive interference is that hippuric acid is produced endogenously as an end product of nitrogen metabolism, with much interindividual variation. For such cases, baseline sampling is essential to discern the workplace contribution. If the exposed worker cannot be distinguished from nonexposed workers, then a new marker must be selected. This was the case when the toluene TLV®-TWA was lowered progressively over the years so that now end-of-shift urinary o-cresol at 0.5 mg/L is better than 1.6 g hippuric acid/g creatinine for urine even though hippuric acid is the major metabolite. The urine markers for toluene are still favored over the toluene blood BEI® of 0.050 mg/L because they are non-invasive.

It is important to realize that a sedentary worker exposed to an atmosphere at TLV®-TWA conditions that were set on an internal target organ effect is at much lower health risk than a worker exposed at higher physical activities because the absorbed dose is lower relative to the absorbed dose at which the TLV®-TWA was set. The sedentary worker who has the same urinary concentration of a marker as a worker of high physical activity still has the same potential adverse health effects. This shows that air exposure monitoring alone is not sufficient to adjudge health risk except when reference conditions are met, and the basis of the TLV®-TWA thoroughly understood. Every hygienist therefore needs to consult the current Documentations of both TLV®-TWAs and BEIs®.

When the personal breathing zone sample cannot (<70% of TLV®-TWA) apparently account for the concentration of the marker in the biological fluid after baseline correction, inhalation during physical activity above that operating in setting the TLV® could still account for the biological monitoring results. For example, if the breathing zone personal air sample is 0.5 the TLV®-TWA, and a worker exposed to xylenes is adjudged to be doing hard work, the ratio of absorbed mass at an air concentration 0.5 the TLV®-TWA relative to moderate physical activity at the TLV®-TWA is (ratio of air concentrations) × (ratio of absorbed masses for heavy to moderate workload at the TLV®-TWA) = 0.5 × 1.24 = 0.62 that absorbed at moderate workload at the TLV®-TWA, that is, for xylenes from Appendix 1, 2,244 × 0.62 = 1,391 mg equivalent is absorbed. If it is known that the exposure was acute (for example, a time and motion study indicated only one short visit to an area where xylene was being used), the critical acute exposure time would be

$$-\ln\left[\frac{(1391-263)}{1391}\right] = 0.811 \times \frac{3.6}{0.693}$$

= 1.1 hr before sampling

This should agree with the time actually observed in the workplace, if the assumption is valid and assuming no urination between the exposure and urine sampling. Similarly, if the air concentration instead was 0.1 the TLV®-TWA at heavy workload, the critical acute exposure time now becomes:

$$-\ln\left[\frac{[(0.1 \times 2244 \times 1.24) - 263]}{(0.1 \times 2244 \times 1.24)}\right] = 0.54 \times \frac{3.6}{0.693}$$

=15 hr before sampling

This is an impossible answer in terms of workplace exposures on the same day unless longer shifts are being worked or there are non-occupational sources of the exposing chemical or there are non-acute workplace exposures. A direct reading instrument investigation to detect organic vapors may then allow direct confirmation of the correct exposure scenario. The critical acute exposure times lengthen with lengthening of marker half-time, so that each marker of an exposing compound is a distinct case, having its own uptake, and half-time as major controlling factors.

Half-times are only reliable in the above calculations over a period of zero to double the half-time. Most chemicals are eliminated in three distinct phases, fast (α), moderate time (β), and slow (δ), each with its pseudo first order rate constant, half-time, and boundary times. End-of-shift sampling is only reliable for fast excretion periods, and end-of-week sampling is best for long half times but not when bioaccumulation occurs.

When Vapor Inhalation is not the Major Route of Exposure

Once heavy workload has been examined and discounted as an inhalation exposure factor, other modes of exposure should then be investigated.

If the environment is dusty, the respirable fraction of dusts may contain adsorbed organics. These may be liberated on particle deposition but they may also be phagocytosized along with the particle by pulmonary alveolar macrophages and then be eventually transported by the lymph to lymph nodes where they are liberated with lysates spilling into the venous system for further systemic distribution. A personal breathing zone filter sample for respirable dust can be analyzed for the exposing compound. If this shows negligible exposing compound or there is little respirable dust, a "total dust" air sample should also be taken, and analyzed similarly to the respirable dust for exposing compound. A similar thoracic dust air sample might also be taken. If worker faces are dusty, the oral exposure route may be important from inhaling large particles and subsequent deposition in the nose, mouth, and upper airways to allow the ciliary locomotor process to waft particles into the stomach aided by mucus flow. If this analysis does not account for the biological monitoring data, skin exposure routes should then be further investigated.

While a full treatment of dermal exposure is presented elsewhere in this book, it is pertinent to summarize the most important points relevant to the present discussion:

1. Dermatitis and skin absorption may not be related. Often dermatitis is caused by a buildup of acidic or basic or skin cuticle damaging agents on the skin surface because they are not efficiently absorbed. Dermatitis can also be caused by high applied exposing concentrations. Similarly, a high skin coverage for an agent does not mean that high skin absorption efficiency has occurred or will occur. However, detectable skin coverage does mean that the agent is bioaccessible, that is, the skin has been exposed. Whether the agent has been absorbed and/or excreted or not is not evident from skin sampling coverage data alone.
2. Absorption of a chemical that contacts the skin varies with skin surface area exposed; distance of blood vessels from the surface; temperature; state of desiccation of the skin; whether the skin is abraded or not; and the thickness of the epidermis, dermis, and hypodermis layers. Thus, for the same apparent application area and agent coverage, the skin of the scrotum will allow more efficient absorption than the skin on the palm of the hand because the actual skin exposure contact area is larger because of the crinkled surface, and the blood vessels are very close to the skin surface.
3. Whether absorption through the epidermis occurs is dependent on how bioavailable the agent is, and this is a balance between the water solubility s and the lipophilicity as expressed through the octanol/water partition coefficient K_{ow}.

The best current mathematical model is called the Revised Robinson Method[27] as embodied in Equation (2) to calculate skin permeation flux Fl for a pure liquid specific chemical:

$$Fl = sKp \qquad (2)$$

where, Fl is in units of mg $cm^{-2}\ h^{-1}$

Kp is a characteristic constant that consists of a stratum corneum component Kp_{sc} (same as the revised Potts and Guy constant) reflecting compound transfer through a lipid layer, a stratum corneum protein transfer component Kp_{ol}, and a epidermal-dermal layer water transfer component K_{aq}.

$$Kp = \left[\frac{1}{\dfrac{1}{Kp_{sc} + Kp_{ol}} + \dfrac{1}{K_{aq}}}\right] \qquad (3)$$

$$\log Kp_{sc} = b1 + b2 \times \log K_{ow} + b3 \times M^{0.5} \qquad (4)$$

$$Kp_{ol} = \frac{b4}{(M^{0.5})} \qquad (5)$$

$$K_{aq} = \frac{b5}{(M^{0.5})} \qquad (6)$$

In Equations 2 through 6, M is the molecular weight, s is water solubility in mg/L, K_{ow} is the ratio of the molar solubility of the agent in n-octanol to that in water at body temperature, and b1, b2, b3, b4, b5 are chemical-specific constants.

From Equation (2), when Kp_{ol} and K_{aq} approach zero, Kp —> Kp_{sc},the revised Potts and Guy constant.that treats the stratum corneum lipid layer as the sole resistance. It might be noted that each constant has a dependence on $M^{0.5}$.

A skin permeation calculation program that includes both the Potts and Guy and Modified Robinson models, as well as the Frasch model is available at the NIOSH website.

4. Gases and vapors can also be skin absorbed, but usually at a much lower fluxes than neat liquids or solids dissolved in solvents that can permeate skin. The absorption rates become higher when IDLH vapor and gas concentrations are approached. Whole body flux rates are rarely applicable to real situations. The bioavailability of the agents is also important, short chain ketone and amine vapors being more efficiently absorbed than water vapor. Pure solids generally are not absorbed unless they are basic, acidic, deliquescent, or react with the epidermis.

Biological Monitoring Sampling/Quality Assurance and Quality Control

The practicing hygienist is advised at present to initiate biological monitoring only for those compounds that have guidelines like BEIs® (that is, a numerical value that can be backed with a Documentation) so that the importance of other sources of the markers, baseline values, genetic factors, antagonisms, synergisms, half-times, and the basic metabolic pathways are available. The hygienist needs to be able to prepare an initial questionnaire for the worker in the event of biological monitoring results that exceed the guideline, cannot be explained by vapor inhalation, and for biological monitoring interpretation purposes.

The hygienist must think through the objectives of the biological monitoring first, and it is useful to prepare a document similar to a Human Consent Form that sets out these objectives along with what samples are to be taken for what purpose and what will be done with the data. Such material should also be part of a worker training program. A generalized such form may be initially required by the employer as a condition of worker employment to the effect that the worker gives permission for taking non-invasively sampled biological media like urine and breath to be analyzed for purposes of ascertaining the worker's health risk relative to health standard recommendations, and that the data will be confidential but open to the worker who also has the right of a medical opinion, and counseling. The ethics aspect of the worker-hygienist interaction is important, and is explored elsewhere.[26]

A licensed physician, certified nurse, or certified phlebotomist must be utilized for blood sampling. The blood BEIs® are for methemoglobin (aniline, methemoglobin inducers, nitrobenzene), red cell acetylcholinesterase (acetylcholinesterase inhibiting pesticides; parathion), 1,3-butadiene (hemoglobin adduct); cadmium; carboxyhemoglobin (carbon monoxide), cobalt, lead, mercury, total trichloroethanol (methyl chloroform), free pentachlorophenol (plasma), styrene, tetrachloroethylene, toluene, and trichloroethylene (free trichloroethanol and trichloroethylene). The hygienist must be certified as a nurse or phlebotomist to draw blood samples. The lead and cadmium OSHA standards are the models for decision logic once blood concentrations are known.

An alternative is to leave all biological monitoring and environmental sampling to physicians and personnel certified for blood sampling. This is more common in Europe and Japan. The problem with that is that U.S. physicians and these personnel are generally not trained to do air or breath sampling or are not familiar with biological equivalent values. While hygienists are trained to do air sampling, they are usually not for breath sampling. However it is far easier for them to learn breath sampling since this is related to air sampling for which they are trained than it is for physicians. The hygienist's familiarity with NIOSH[17] and OSHA[18] methods and with the actual environment of the workplace are major advantages.

No matter the sampling method chosen or who does it, the analytical chemistry laboratory must be consulted for sampling, storage, and transport procedures, if it provides the relevant sampling containers, appropriate preservatives, or any transport containers, and the timeline for sampling and analysis. Time taken before actual sampling to optimize such factors will result in less expensive analyses caused by invalid sampling and analyses.

The appropriate negative control sample (usually baseline before exposure) must also be provided to aid in chromatographic resolution problems and peak assignments, and to be able to interpret the results relative to workplace exposures. The appropriate blanks should also be sent. Some examples include: an empty container; a container filled with isotonic (0.9%) saline or standard reference urine of the same volume as the urine sample; a gas bag filled with pure air; a blood vacutaner tube of the same color top and filled with the same volume of isotonic saline or standard reference blood as the actual blood sample; an unused blank vacutaner tube of the same colored top; and field blanks of all of these.

The hygienist is urged to also send appropriate spiked samples ("positive controls") to ensure laboratory quality control/assurance at the user level. The chemical form and concentration of the spike must be that found in the biological medium. For example, urinary total trichloroethanol as a marker for methyl chloroform is actually present as free trichloroethanol and its -glucuronide, the latter dominating. The positive blank preferred here is both compounds spiked in two separate tubes in a standard urine (or nonexposed worker's baseline urine) at the BEI® equivalent with the unspiked urine itself also analyzed. Alternatively, a urine of high known marker content could be aliquoted into specific volumes that are then frozen, one being then included as a blind sample in a batch of samples. Standard reference materials from the National Institute for Standards and Technology (NIST) or from specimen banks with materials characterized through interlaboratory collaboration are also encouraged to prove confidence in the whole biological monitoring sampling and analysis process.

If the BEI® is exceeded, in addition to the types of calculations referred to in Appendix 1, the sampling should be repeated at least three times to confirm the results before action on a medical front or on control measures is initiated. Sometimes if the exposures of a group of workers is adjudged to be equivalent, group analyses may be useful to indicate a common problem. However, interindividual variability may be a confounding factor.

Breath Sampling

The physiological basis of breath sampling can be consulted in the BEI® Documentation[15] BEI®-12 to BEI®-14, in Reference 1 Section 6.3, and pages 44–63 of reference 19, with pages 364–387 of reference 20 providing some specific breath sampling methods.

The easiest method is with a clean, nonleaking Tedlar bag. "Clean" means filled and then evacuated three times with pure air from a compressed air cylinder or other certified air source and applying a hot-air hair dryer during each evacuation (or being held in an incubator oven at 50°C for 5 minutes). A "nonleaking" bag is one that is air-filled which does not make bubbles when lightly pressed down upon in a tub of water and no water also enters the bag.

The bag is connected to the sidearm of a clean (soaked overnight in 10% nitric acid with copious water rinsing before drying) Pyrex vacuum flask by a clean (by blowing hot about (50°C) pure air through it for at least 30 min after rinsing with a solvent known to solubilize the marker) FEP Teflon tube (0.25" inner diameter) by leakproof butt-to-butt joints (using Tygon collars). The flask is rubber-stoppered with the inside of the stopper coated with Teflon tape. The stopper should also contain a clean (10% nitric acid washed) glass tube that almost reaches the flask bottom. The top of the glass tube above the stopper is similarly connected butt-to-butt to similar clean Teflon tubing connected to a Teflon 0.5" to 0.25" adapter. Alternatively, the latter Teflon tubing can be worked through the stopper to be near the flask bottom. The setup must be leak-proof (use soap bubble fluid to detect leaks during sampling), and the transfer tubing must be as short as possible. The function of the flask is to collect any drool, spittle, or saliva that will inevitably occur. Sampling occurs by pursing the mouth lips and blowing through the 0.5" part of the adapter tube, and the bag manipulated to distribute the sample to the distal end of the bag. If the tubing still has too much resistance, the inner diameter should be increased, and the length shortened as much as possible. The trap minimizes the amount of condensed water vapor in the gas bag, especially important if normalization to breath carbon dioxide concentrations is required or intended. The use of desiccants is not recommended since the intended analyte is often also adsorbed or absorbed resulting in loss.

Mixed exhaled breath is sampled after normal air inspiration by the worker holding the nose by the fingers (or by noseclip) and then breathing out normally at the usual expiration rate but through the mouth into the 0.5" adapter and its attachments, and repeating this operation until the desired bag volume is obtained (full is best but more than half-full may suffice depending on the compound). End-exhaled breath is obtained by breathing out normally into the air and then pursing the lips to blow the forced expiration component into the adapter and its attachments.

The use of evacuated Pyrex or stainless steel bottles and canisters is discouraged unless they can be evacuated to a known pressure and are equipped with an air-tight on/off valve. If these latter containers are not evacuated the volume of breath sampled is uncertain because of dilution with air already in the container even if a wet test meter is also connected to record the volume.

Another alternative is replace the Tedlar bag with a solid sorbent tube connected to a wet-test meter by Tygon tubing. The solid sorbent must be one that can allow water vapor to pass through like Tenax GC, the Poropak series, the Chromosorb 101 through 106 series, or the XAD resins. A charcoal tube will be inadequate. However, wet test meters are heavy and expensive and are not accurate on nonlevel surfaces. The solid sorbent can then be analyzed by standard NIOSH, OSHA or EPA methods, as described later for taking solid sorbent samples from Tedlar gas bag samples.

The hygienist has several options for Tedlar gas bag analysis. If direct reading instruments or devices are available, they can be calibrated using clean Tedlar gas bags in a matrix of mixed or end-exhaled breath generated by the hygienist using the above apparatus. The marker is then added by a gas-tight syringe using the calculated injected volume for the known volume of breath matrix. If detector tubes are used, any relevant interferences should be noted in their handbooks, and the appropriate number of strokes utilized to achieve a reading at the BEI® concentration. The latter may not be attainable since short-term detector tubes are designed for the higher concentrations about the TLV®-TWA in general, and long-term detector tubes developed for sampling at hazardous waste sites may be better. The prior evaluation of a breath control (baseline) relative to a known Tedlar Bag sample at the BEI concentration is recommended before any breath is evaluated with this method. The same applies for measurement with a gas/vapor infrared (IR) spectrophotometer of variable wavelength/pathlength where the interfering IR absorption of water vapor and carbon dioxide of the control must be subtracted. The high instrument flow rate is also a major disadvantage.

The hygienist must do prior calculations to define the correct volume gas bag, and to assess feasibility. For example, the mixed exhaled BEI® for benzene in breath in 1996 was 0.08 ppm and the end-exhaled BEI was 0.12 ppm. If 0.10 ppm is chosen as the first concentration (to simplify calculations), this is equivalent to 0.32 mg benzene/m^3 air at 25 oC and 760 mm Hg. A 10-L gas bag must contain 320 (µg) × 10 (L)/1000 (L) = 3.2 µg benzene. The liquid density of benzene is 0.879 g/mL or 879,000 µg/1000 µL benzene liquid. Therefore 3.2 µg benzene is a liquid benzene volume of 3.6 nL. This is an impossible volume for a 10-µL syringe. Multiple dilutions of 10-L gas bags are required. Thus 1 µL of liquid benzene of mass 879 µg is injected into a gas bag with 10 L mixed exhaled air. The gas bag is placed in an oven at 50°C or exposed to a hot air dryer for a few minutes to mix the vapors thoroughly. This creates a benzene concentration of 87.9 µg/L or 27.5 ppm at 25°C and 760 mm Hg, and should be checked with a calibrated direct reading instrument for stability and accuracy. A 3.2 µg benzene mass is then contained in 3.2 (µg) 1000 (mL)/87.9 (µg) = 36.4 mL of this 27.5 ppm concentration which can now be injected into a gas bag filled with 9,963.6 mL of mixed exhaled air by a gas-tight syringe, and again mixed. Four other concentrations bracketing the 0.10 ppm concentration can then be prepared.

The best calibrated direct reading instruments to use for benzene and other aromatics are photoionization detectors (PID) with lamp energies 10.2 eV or 10.6 eV. Aliphatics are best detected by PID detectors with 11.6 eV lamps. These still may not be sensitive enough if ppb (v/v) concentrations of aliphatics are to be measured. If portable capillary column gas chromatography (GC) with PID detection (for example with a 10.6 eV arc) is available with a gas sampling valve, then this can be easily calibrated by these gas bags and the background resolution of breath peaks optimized before the worker breath sample is to be analyzed along with a bag sample of the worker breath when not exposed to benzene. If there is no gas sampling valve, Tedlar gas bag samples have to be injected using a gas-tight syringe of appropriate volume. The quantitation is then by interpolation on the external or internal standards curve generated through these gas bags. This is the basis of NIOSH method 3700[17] which uses a portable GC/PID of method working range of 0.1–500 ppm, and which is designed for Tedlar bag air samples. The advantage is that answers can be obtained on-site and almost immediately, and injection of samples into the air carrier gas of the column dilutes the effects of humidity and excess carbon dioxide.

If the hygienist does not have the resources to do this type of quantitation, then sampling a known volume of the breath sample for benzene from the Tedlar Gas Bag through a large (200 mg/100 mg) charcoal tube (to minimize breakthrough caused by high humidity) may suffice for hydrophobic organic markers using a calibrated personal sampling pump. How much volume is necessary? Firstly the NIOSH[17] or OSHA[18] method should be consulted for the marker. For benzene, NIOSH Method 1501 states that the flow rate should be <0.20 L/min for an air volume of 2 (10 min sample) to 30 L for the TLV®-TWA of 10 ppm or 32 mg/m^3. The meaningful lower limit for this method therefore is a sampled benzene mass of 32,000 (μg) × 2 (L)/1000 (L) = 64 μg benzene. If this is desorbed in 1 mL of carbon disulfide and 5 μL injected, the absolute lower limit on-column is 64,000 (ng) × 5 (μL)/1000 (μL) = 320 ng using flame ionization detection (FID). A 10-L gas bag of 0.1 ppm benzene contains 3.2 μg so that the standard NIOSH carbon disulfide desorption technique is impractical unless the analytical laboratory can be 64/3.2 = 20 times more sensitive or the gas bag should be 20 times larger (that is, 200 L), a rather impractical size, or some combination of larger bags and enhanced laboratory sensitivity. The hygienist must ask the certified analytical laboratory whether this specific degree of enhanced sensitivity is possible before going ahead with this method. If so, nearly the entire bag can be sampled by the pump through the charcoal tube, as long as the volume sampled is accurately known. Such analyses by the standard NIOSH method using carbon disulfide for desorption and GC/FID frees up hygienist time at the expense of when the results are procured. Such tubes may be broken during transport and storage as discussed elsewhere.

The hygienist should also send an accompanying worker control breath sample of the same volume obtained without analyte exposure so as to facilitate background resolution from analyte peaks, and to confirm no nonworkplace exposure to analyte. Other blanks include bags, vacuum containers, or solid sorbent tubes that contain or have sampled an equivalent volume of pure air, as well as unused solid sorbent tubes, and field blanks. Positive controls consisting of sampled known air concentrations at the BEI concentration from gas bags should also be sent for analysis. Hygienists should remember that all analyses are relative to the appropriate negative control, the latter being as essential as the breath sample suspected of containing the marker. Potential utilization of all NIOSH, OSHA, and EPA air sampling and analysis methods is a very big advantage for breath sampling.

If standard charcoal tube sampling is not possible due to sensitivity problems, a known volume of the 10-L gas bag contents has to be sampled onto an appropriate solid sorbent which then has to be analyzed by thermal desorption so that all the sample is placed on-column, using the appropriate GC columns and detectors. For the case of benzene above, the absolute lower limit on-column for the standard GC/FID NIOSH method is 320 ng, well below the contents of the 10-L gas bag containing 0.10 ppm benzene. Therefore a laboratory specializing in thermal desorption, for example one that is also EPA-accredited to do purge-and-trap or headspace analyses for the exposing compound in ground and surface waters, should be consulted for the solid sorbent of choice. For benzene, this is the solid sorbent used in the purge-and-trap technique of EPA Methods 502.2, 503.1, 524.1, 524.2, 602, 624, 5030, and 8020 [60/80 mesh 2,6-diphenylene oxide polymer commonly called Tenax GC, Tenax TA, or equivalent (XAD-2, etc)]. The hygienist should ensure that the solid sorbent tube has the same geometry as that used for the particular laboratory's thermal desorption technique after purge and trapping or headspace analysis. Commonly, GC-mass spectrometry (GC-MS), GC-FID, and GC-PID are used for quantitation purposes for benzene depending on the desired sensitivity. These are more expensive analyses than standard industrial hygiene analyses. Some investigators have sampled breath directly onto such tubes. The

Tedlar bag method has the advantage of allowing a precision analysis, and being familiar to hygienists.

The above sampling techniques should suffice for other organic solvent breath samples depending on sensitivity, for example, ethyl benzene, n-hexane, methyl chloroform, perchloroethylene, and trichloroethylene (Table 19.4). The aromatics can be sampled and analyzed sensitively by the same analytical techniques as benzene. For chlorinated aliphatic analyses, GC-electron capture detection (ECD) has better sensitivity than FID or PID. Some BEI® breath tests (ethylbenzene and trichloroethylene) are qualitative or screening tests. Carbon monoxide, methyl chloroform, and tetrachloroethylene have numerical BEIs®.

Carbon monoxide in end-exhaled air cannot be analyzed by the above techniques but can be by a calibrated portable electrochemical cell involving oxidation to carbon dioxide at a Teflon-bonded diffusion electrode similar to the carbon monoxide Ecolysers familiar to most hygienists and using NIOSH method S340[17] which is designed for Tedlar gas bag samples over the carbon monoxide range from 1-120 ppm.

Urine Sampling

The hygienist must provide a wide-mouth clean container with volume markings (polyethylene for metals, cleaned by overnight soaking in 10% nitric acid with subsequent distilled water rinsing and dried; an acid-washed pyrex vessel for organics, fitted with a Teflon-lined screw-capped lid) of the appropriate volume (250 mL should suffice for spot samples if the bladder is emptied before the shift; otherwise the volume should be 500 mL) fitted with screw cap lids (they spill less than other lid types), and containing any indicated preservative [BEI® Documentation recommendations are: copper sulfate for pentachlorophenol; thymol for urinary phenol; hydrochloric acid for mandelic acid (styrene); hydrochloric acid or quinoxalinol or zinc chloride for phenylglyoxylic acid (styrene); thymol or hydrochloric acid for hippuric acid (toluene) and methylhippuric acid (xylenes)]. The addition of acidic agents like thymol, hydrochloric acid, copper sulfate, and quinoxalinol can cause conjugate hydrolysis. The worker should be asked to shower and then provide a midstream urine sample before putting on clothes if possible, though this is usually impractical in most cases. The hygienist should note the sampling time following that recommended by the BEI® Documentation (Table 19.4), the urine volume (a container should never be filled entirely), and measure the urine specific gravity with a hydrometer (urinometer) or dipstick. Urine samples should be stored and transported (with adequate insulation) frozen in dry ice with no preservatives unless recommended otherwise, and stored in laboratories at -20°C. Such precautions ensure that conjugates are not hydrolysed, that microorganism growth is prevented, and volatile constituents are not lost. Labels and screw caps should be duct-taped. Urine samples taken similarly before the workshift (baseline sample) should also be analyzed at the beginning of a biological monitoring program or whenever a change in process or control occur in the workplace. Such a sample reflects nonworkplace factors if taken after a nonworking weekend on the first day of the workweek. A baseline should also be taken when the BEI® is exceeded to ensure that the exposure source is not external to the workplace, or if there is holdover from the previous exposure. Urine baseline samples also empty the bladder before the shift and allow later spot samples to be more representative of shift exposures. The appropriate baseline sample for an end-of-week BEI® is the before shift spot sample after a weekend. Creatinine concentrations must also be requested if recommended. The latter accounts for worker fluid intake and urine dilution, but the marker must also be excreted through kidney glomerular filtration rather than through the distal or proximal tubules. The usual blank samples (empty container; container with preservative; container with preservative with standard reference control urine or isotonic saline) and positive controls (container with preservative with a standard reference urine containing spiked marker at the BEI® concentration; container with preservative with the same standard reference urine as used for spiking; or a urine of known marker concentration from an exposed person stored appropriately) should also be sent for analysis.

To collect urine samples for measurement of excretion rates at the end of shift, the worker should empty the bladder completely about 3–4 hours before the end of the shift (the time should be noted) before providing the next void for analysis (the time and urine volume should also be noted and specific gravity measured). The volume divided by the elapsed time should then be provided along with the sample but not the specific gravity since the latter is user quality assurance.

The correction for specific gravity should be performed as follows:

corrected specific gravity =

$$24 \times \frac{\text{observed value}}{\text{last two digits of observed value}} \quad (7)$$

The BEI® Documentation[15] defines concentrated urine to be any of the following: specific gravity >1.03; creatinine >3 g/L. Dilute urine is defined as: specific gravity <1.01; creatinine <0.5 g/L.

Such urines cannot be used and resampling must be done. Hygienists should always request specific gravity and creatinine determinations by the laboratory that analyzes the urine samples. If the samples have not precipitated, the specific gravity measured by the laboratory should be close to that measured by the hygienist when the urine is fresh. If the specific gravity is measured by the hygienist, this will allow resampling if the sample is too dilute or concentrated without needless expenses involved with transporting and analyzing invalid samples, and of course, not wasting further time while invalid results are awaited. Reference 1 Section 6.2 should be read to supplement the BEI® Documentation[11] account of Urine Sampling at BEI®-16 to BEI®-19.

Sampling methods that involve 24-hour urines involve larger containers that can be kept in a home refrigerator freezer. Such samples may be necessary with pesticides or other compounds of longer half-times than 6 hours depending on the compound and the guideline. Often analytical laboratories provide them as part of the analysis costs.

The compounds for which urinary BEI® markers are recommended include: acetone; aniline; arsenic; benzene; 1,3-butadiene; 2-butoxyethanol; cadmium; carbon disulfide; chlorobenzene; chromium VI; cobalt; cyclohexanol; dichloromethane; NN-dimethylacetamide; N,N-dimethylformamide; 2-ethoxyethanol/2-ethoxyethyl acetate; ethyl benzene; fluorides; furfural; n-hexane; mercury; methanol; 2-methoxyethanol/2-methoxyethyl acetate; methyl-n-butyl ketone; methyl chloroform; 4,4'-methylene bis(2-chloroaniline); methyl ethyl ketone; methyl isobutyl ketone; N-methyl-2-pyrrolidone; nitrobenzene; parathion; pentachlorophenol; phenol; polycyclic aromatic hydrocarbons; 2-propanol; styrene; tetrachloroethylene; tetrahydrofuran; toluene; trichloroethylene; vanadium pentoxide; and xylenes. In fact the only compounds without an urinary BEI are: acetylcholinesterase inhibiting pesticides; carbon monoxide; lead; and methemoglobin inducers.

There are many analytical methods for urine metals, including NIOSH Method 8310 which uses inductively coupled plasma atomic emission spectroscopy (ICP-AES) for multielemental analyses[17] and Method 8003[17] for lead by atomic absorption spectroscopy (AAS). For fluorides, there is Method 8308. For organic BEI® markers that have NIOSH methods for urine, Method 8300 is for hippuric acid; Method 8301 is for hippuric and methylhippuric acids; Method 8302 is for 4,4'-methylenebis (2-chloroaniline) or MBOCA; Method 8303 is for pentachlorophenol; and Method 8305 for phenol and o-cresol. Non-BEI® marker urinary NIOSH methods[17] include ones for benzidine (Method 8304 and 8306), with the other methods being for markers in blood (delta-aminolevulinic acid dehydratase for lead; 2-butanone, ethanol and toluene; elements; lead; and pentachlorophenol) and serum (polychlorinated biphenyls). In addition to references 3 and 13, specific methods for biological monitoring are also in references 19 through 22. The NIOSH methods are preferred, and their sampling directions should be followed closely by hygienists. EPA methods usually use 24-h hour urines for monitoring pesticides.

Other Noninvasive Biological Monitoring Media

Hygienists are advised not to sample these if possible. If it is necessary to do so, hygienists should read the relevant sections of Reference 1, Chapter 6, for the sampling and analysis methods, and references therein. Of these alternative media, saliva samples are probably the most promising although hair samples are sometimes used to confirm retrospective exposures for forensic purposes.

The case studies in the AIHA's publication, *Biological Monitoring — A Practical Field Manual*[26] should be read to assess the use of alternative and traditional sampling methods.

APPENDIX I. Illustrated Examples for Xylene Relative to Workload, The BEI®, and Inhalation Conditions

Using Equation (1), about 63 % uptake of 200-ppm of inspired xylene occurs at rest (0 watt) for 2-hours or at light exercise (up to 50 watt) for 90 minutes compared with 50 % at 150 watt. An uptake of about 57% might be expected at 100 watt (moderate work) from the alveolar ventilations of Table 19.2. Uptake decreases while the absolute absorbed dose increases with increasing physical activity. Thus working at moderate physical activity at the xylene 2008 TLV®-TWA of 100 ppm (434 mg/m³) has an absorbed dose of [434 (mg/m³) × 0.027 (m³/min) × 120 (min)) × 0.57 (uptake)] = 802 mg every two hours. This has to be corrected for the content of ethylbenzene in the technical xylene, usually about 10-50 (mean 30) % since ethylbenzene does not produce a methylhippuric acid in urine. Thus the xylene isomer content absorbed every two hours is about (802 × 0.70 = 561) mg. Assuming no change in alveolar ventilation after each 20-30 min break nor in uptake, an eight hour workday consisting of four two hour work periods will cause about 561 × 4= 2,244 mg of xylene isomers to be absorbed. The BEI® Documentation for xylenes[15] states that pulmonary retention for volunteers is 60–65% of the inhaled amount using mixed exhaled air, independent of exposure concentration or pulmonary ventilation.

The BEI® Documentation for xylenes[15] further states that about 93–95 (mean 94) % of the absorbed xylenes are metabolized to methyl benzoic acids with 3–6 (mean 4.5) % exhaled (half-times of 1 hr and 20 hr), and <1–2 (mean <1.5) % metabolized to xylenols after 6 hr of inhalation of volunteers at 100 ppm m-xylene. The BEI® marker is total methylhippuric acids with pseudo first-order half-times of 3.6 hr and 30.1 hr. Baselt[13] states, however, that the first half-time is about 1.5 hr. The urinary BEI is 1.5 g total methylhippuric acids/g creatinine for a spot urine sample at the end-of-the-shift.

The molecular weight of methylhippuric acid is 193 compared with 106 for xylene. Thus 1.5 g of methylhippuric acid is equivalent to 1,500 (mg)/193 = 7.77 mmoles of methylhippuric acids which is the same as the number of moles of methyl benzoic acids if all of the latter are conjugated by glycine. The original absorbed xylene equivalent can now be calculated by correcting for xylenol production and xylene exhalation (7.77/0.94 = 8.27 mmoles). This is a mass of 8.27 × 106 = 876 mg xylene equivalent. Thus the urine BEI® concentration is equivalent to 876 mg absorbed xylene/g creatinine. The volume and creatinine content of the spot urine can be factored in if known. Spot urines are about 300-800 mL in volume (the same as the capacity of the bladder), most being towards the lower volume end, especially if earlier urination has occurred. The daily urine volume is 0.6–2.5 L/day with mean 1.2 L/day.[15] Since the creatinine excretion rate is 1.0–1.6 (mean 1.2) g/day, the mean creatinine urinary concentration is 1.0 g/L.[15] The mean specific gravity of urine is taken to be 1.024 and the volume of urine should be corrected to this specific gravity if the latter for the spot sample is different. A 300 mL urine sample corrected to specific gravity 1.024 is therefore expected to contain about 0.3 g creatinine and 0.3 × 876 = 263 mg xylene equivalents at the BEI® at 1 g creatinine/L urine. Since 2,244 mg of xylene is absorbed over 8 hr, only a fraction of the absorbed xylene equivalents (263/2,244 = 0.117) needs to be excreted in the 300 mL spot sample to meet the BEI condition.

Assuming a pseudo first-order process:

$$C_t = C_O \times e^{-kt} = C_O \times e^{\frac{-0.693t}{t_{0.5}}} \qquad \text{(A1)}$$

where c_t and c_0 are the equivalent moles/urine volume of untransformed xylene at times t and at the initial exposure time t_0 respectively; and $t_{0.5}$ is the pseudo first-order xylene equivalent half-time relative to the marker, here for methylhippuric acids.

An acute TLV®-TWA critical exposure (c_0 = 2,244 mg) time t corresponding to c_t / c_0 = 1 - 0.117 = 0.883 must occur in -ln 0.883 × 3.6 (hr)/0.693 = 0.65 hr before sampling. All acute TLV®-TWA exposure times before then cause higher transformed xylene equivalents than the BEI® concentration, and the BEI® is protective. The other extreme case is acute exposure at the TLV®-TWA at the beginning of the first shift. The absorbed xylene that remains in 8-hr is: ct = 2,244 (mg) exp (-0.693 × 8 (hr)/3.6 (hr)) = 481 mg so that 2244-481 = 1,763 mg of xylene equivalents is lost. Thus 1,763 × 0.94 (efficiency of metabolism to the BEI® marker) = 1,657 mg xylene equivalents might be found in the spot sample assuming no other urination. This is 1,657/263 = 6.3 times the BEI critical xylene equivalent mass in a 300 mL spot urine sample assuming no other urination.

TWA exposures are generally not acute single dose. If the work day is 8a-12 noon, and 1p-5p and if 0.25 of the total xylene mass is exposed at the midpoint of the first 2-hr exposure period (561 mg xylene absorbed) with sampling at 5p with no urination in between t = 8 hr:

$$C_t = 561 \times e^{\frac{-0.693 \times 8}{3.6}} = 120 \text{ mg} \qquad (A2)$$

That is, (561-120) = 441 mg of xylene was transformed and 441 × 0.94 = 415 mg of this xylene forms methylhippuric acids. If this same procedure is done for the second 2 hr exposure, then for the two 2-hr exposures after the one-hr lunch (exposure periods with t = 6, 3 and 1 hr respectively), the corresponding respective transformed xylene masses are: 361, 231, and 92 mg. This type of xylene exposure will cause approximately (415 + 361 + 231 + 92 = 1,099 mg absorbed xylene equivalents to have been excreted as methylhippuric acids, assuming no other urination during work. Thus the BEI® is protective for this exposure scenario since the calculated xylene equivalent mass in 300 mL of xylene was 263 mg at the BEI®, assuming 1 g creatinine/L urine. Even if urination occurred during lunch time, as long as no urination occurred between the last two work shifts the minimum excreted at the sampling time is 231 + 92 = 323 mg xylene equivalents, still >263 mg xylene equivalents at the BEI® for this 300 mL spot sample.. If urination occurred between the last two shifts (3p), then at t = 6, 4 and 1 hr, the xylene equivalents untransformed from the first three time periods would be: 177 + 260 + 463 = 900 × 0.94 = 846 mg of xylene still available for transformation to methylhippuric acids in the last two hours or 846- 846 exp -(0.693 × 2/3.6) = 270 mg plus the 92 mg from the last exposure of the last shift, making a total of 362 mg xylene equivalents in the final spot urine sample, still above the critical BEI® xylene equivalent mass. Thus to interpret the urine concentrations at a designated sampling time, a history of urinations must be known as well as duration and intensity of exposures. If the hygienist has direct reading instrument data, for example from detector tubes or organic vapor analysers or can infer exposure times by time-and-motion studies near exposure sources where personal air monitoring data over these times are also known, these exposure conditions can be similarly evaluated to assess if the BEI® is protective using the computational principles above.

The excretion rate of a marker is calculated[15] using the mean urine output of 0.05 L/hr and the urinary concentration corrected to a specific gravity of 1.024. Thus:

$$\text{Excretion Rate (mg/hr)} = 0.05C \qquad (A3)$$

where C is the concentration adjusted to specific gravity 1.024 in mg marker/L corrected urine volume or for creatinine excretion in mg marker/g creatinine assuming a mean concentration of 1 g creatinine/L urine. If the BEI® concentration is 1,500 mg/g creatinine, the excretion rate is (1,500 × 0.05/60 = 1.3 mg/min).

Apart from the case of having high exposure air concentrations near the TLV®-TWA within 0.65 hr of sampling, the BEI® is protective for all the above exposure scenarios.

A problem arises when physical activities less than the reference one occur. The worst case is for workers exposed to the TLV®-TWA at rest. It was shown above that 0.185 the mass is potentially absorbed relative to at moderate physical activity at an uptake 63/57 = 1.11 times that at moderate workload. Thus instead of 2,244 mg xylene being absorbed, only (0.185 x 1.11 × 2,244 = 461 mg) is absorbed for an exposure at the TLV®-TWA at rest, or 461/2,244 = 0.21 times the absorbed mass at moderate physical activity at the TLV®-TWA . Thus a 300 mL spot urine sample containing the BEI xylene equivalent mass of 263 mg at a creatinine concentration of 1 g/L is still protective if the TLV®-TWA is absorbed acutely [-ln (461-263)/461 × 3.6/0.693 = 4.4 hr before urine sampling if the worker is sedentary. Using the above four acute distributed exposure period scenario but with (461/4 = 115) mg xylene per exposure, the expected excreted xylene equivalent mass on urine sampling is now (85 + 74 + 47 + 19 = 225 mg, about 86 % of the BEI® xylene equivalent mass in a 300 mL spot urine sample. This also justifies an action level below the BEI® of about 30%. Note that the effect of previous urinations during lunch time and the last break before end-of-shift sampling is more important at low physical activities relative to BEI® considerations compared with at higher physical activities. Working at physical activities greater than the reference one at which the TLV®-TWA was set will result in higher urine concentrations on exposure to the TLV®-TWA. Thus the BEI® is still protective.

The above computational example for at rest workers will aid the hygienist in defining whether a sample that exceeds the BEI® is caused solely through enhanced physical activity through substituting the appropriate data related to high physical activity for those used for at rest physical activity. Thus, the absorbed equivalent mass of xylene at heavy work is (2,244 × 1.41 × 50/57 = 2,775 mg xylene equivalents at the TLV®-TWA, or (277,500/2,244 = 1.24) times that at moderate workload at the TLV®-TWA.

If the hygienist has some idea of the temporal frame of the exposures either through data logging capability of direct reading instruments or through time-and-motion studies relative to the known exposure sources then such data can be used instead.

REFERENCES

1. **Que Hee, S.S. (ed.):** *Biological Monitoring: An Introduction.* New York: Van Nostrand Reinhold, 1993.
2. **Ness, S.A.:** *Surface and Dermal Monitoring for Toxic Exposures.* New York: Van Nostrand Reinhold, 1994.
3. **Ellis, K.J.:** In-vivo monitoring techniques. In *Methods for Biological Monitoring: A Manual for Assessing Human Exposure to Hazardous Substances.* Kneip, T.J. and J.V. Crable (eds.). Washington D.C.: American Public Health Association, 1988. pp. 65–80.
4. **Forsberg, K. and Keith, L.H.:** *Chemical Protective Clothing: Permeation and Degradation Compendium.* Boca Raton, FL: Lewis Publishers, 1995. Also: **Forsberg, K., and Keith, L.H.,** *Instant Gloves + CPC Database Version 2.0,* Instant Reference Sources, Inc., Blacksburg, VA, 1999. Also: **Forsberg, K., and Keith, L.H.** *Chemical Protective Clothing Performance Index Book,* Second Edition, John Wiley; & Sons, New York, 1999.
5. **U.S. Dept. Labor, Occupational Safety and Health Administration:** Lead Standard. Title 29, Code of Federal Regulations, Part 1910.1025, Washington D.C.: U.S.D.L., 1989.
6. **U.S. Dept. Labor, Occupational Safety and Health Administration:** *Access to Employee Exposure and Medical Records; Proposed Modifications; Request for Comments and Notice of Public Hearing.* 29 CFR Part 1910. Fed. Regist. 47: 30420-30438, 1982.
7. **U.S. Department of Labor, Occupational Safety and Health Administration:** *Identification, Classification and Regulation of Potential Occupational Carcinogens 29 CFR Part 1990.* Fed. Regist., 45: 5001–296, 1980.
8. **U.S. Department of Labor, Occupational Safety and Health Administration:** *Benzene, Occupational Safety and Health, Chemicals, Cancer, Health, Risk Assessment 29 CFR Part 1910.* Fed. Regist., 52: 34562-34578, 1987.
9. **U.S. Department of Labor, Occupational Safety and Health Administration:** *Hazard Communication; Final Rule 29 CFR Part 1910. Fed. Regist., 48*:53280–348, 1983.
10. **American Conference of Governmental Industrial Hygienists (ACGIH®):** *2010 TLVs® and BEIs®.* Cincinnati, OH: ACGIH®, 2010.
11. **American Conference of Governmental Industrial Hygienists (ACGIH®):** *Documentation of the Threshold Limit Values and Biological Exposure Indices,* 7th edition. Cincinnati, OH: ACGIH®, 2001. www.acgih.org.
12. **Lauwerys, R.R. and Hoet, P.:** *Industrial Chemical Exposure: Guidelines for Biological Monitoring,* 3rd edition. Boca Raton, FL: Lewis Publishers, 2001.
13. **Baselt, R.C.:** *Biological Monitoring Methods for Industrial Chemicals,* 3rd Ed. Toxicology Institute, Foster City, CA, 1997.
14. **Commission for the Investigation of Health Hazards of Chemical Compounds in the Work Area:** *Maximum Concentrations at the Workplace and Biological Tolerance Values for Working Materials.* New York: VCH Publishers, 1991.
15. **La Dou, J., et al.:** *Occupational & Environmental Medicine.* 2nd edition. Norwalk, CT: Appleton and Lange, 1997.
16. **Astrand, I., J. Engstrom, and P. Ovrum:** Exposure to xylene and ethyl benzene. I: Uptake, distribution and elimination in man. *Scand. J. Work Environ. Health* 4:185–194 (1978).

17. **Schlecht, P.C. and O'Connor, P.F. (eds.):** *NIOSH Manual of Analytical Methods*, 4th edition. Cincinnati, OH: U.S. DHHS, 1994. Supplements 1996, 1998, and 2003. www.cdc.gov/niosh
18. **Carl Elskamp, C. and Hendricks, W. (eds.):** *OSHA Analytical Methods Manual*, 3rd edition. Salt Lake City, UT: U.S. Dept. of Labor, 2001. www.osha.gov
19. **Kneip, T.J. and J.V. Crable (eds.):** *Methods for Biological Monitoring: A Manual for Assessing Human Exposure to Hazardous Substances.* Washington D.C.: American Public Health Association, 1988.
20. **Sheldon, L., et al.:** *Biological Monitoring Techniques for Human Exposure to Industrial Chemicals: Analysis of Human Fat, Skin, Nails, Hair, Blood, Urine, and Breath.* Park Ridge, NJ: Noyes Publications, 1986.
21. **Carson, B.L., H.V. Ellis, III, and J.L. McCann:** *Toxicology and Biological Monitoring of Metals in Humans: Including Feasibility and Need.* Chelsea, MI.: Lewis Publishers, 1986.
22. **U.S. Environmental Protection Agency (EPA):** *Manual of Analytical Methods for the Analysis of Pesticides in Humans and Environmental Samples, EPA-600/8-80-038.* Research Triangle Park, N.C.: U.S. EPA, 1980.
23. **Occupational Safety and Health Administration (OSHA):** Screening and Surveillance: A Guide to OSHA Standards, OSHA 3162, US Dept Labor, Washington DC, 2000.
24. **Cocker, J.; Nutley, B. P.; and Wilson, H. K.:** A biological monitoring assessment of exposure to methylene dianiline in manufactures and users. *Occup. Environ. Med. 51*:519–522 (1994).
25. **National Institute for Occupational Safety and Health (NIOSH):** *NIOSH Pocket Guide to Chemical Hazards.* DHHS (NIOSH) Public. No. 2005-149, 2005.
26. **Que Hee, S.S. (ed.):** *Biological Monitoring: A Practical Field Manual.* Fairfax, VA: AIHA®, Fairfax, VA, 2004.
27. **Wilschut, A., W.F. ten Berge, P.J. Robinson, and T.E. McKone:** Estimating skin permeation. The validation of five mathematical skin permeation models. *Chemosphere 30*:1275–1296 (1995).

GLOSSARY

Absorbed dose: the mass or moles of exposing compound that actually enters into the bloodstream through any external routes of exposure; the absolute bioavailability

Adduct: the product of a reaction between an endogenous macromolecule and an exposing chemical or its metabolite

Antibody: the protein that a living organism is stimulated to make from the B lymphocytes when a foreign antigen is present

Antigen: a large macromolecule that triggers an immune response

Biochemical epidemiology: the correlation of chemical markers measured in bodily media with epidemiologic variates

Biologically effective dose: the absolute mass or moles of exposing compound that actually exposes a target organ internally after absorption

Biological monitoring: the measurement of chemical markers in body media that are indicative of external exposure to chemical and physical agents

Biomarker: the determinant to be measured in a biological system

Blood: the red fluid contained in arteries and veins

Breast milk: the white viscous fluid extruded from female breasts

Chemical: a single molecule or a mixture of molecules

Conjugate: the product of reaction of an exposing single chemical or a single metabolite with the endogenous biochemical pathways of the body

Determinant: the substrate or indicator to be measured in a biological system

Ear wax: the waxy discharge in the outer ear canal

Elimination: internal clearance of a marker from an internal organ

End-exhaled breath (alveolar exhaled breath): the exhaled breath forced from the lungs after natural exhalation

Endogenous: intrinsic; found naturally in the living system under study

Enzyme: an agent that catalyzes a biological reaction that is not itself consumed in the reaction

Excretion: appearance of a marker outside of the body

Feces: solid/liquid waste excreted from the anus

Flatus: sudden excretion of internal gas/vapor like a "burp", "cough", "sneeze" from the mouth, or a "fart" from the anus

Fluids: a state of matter that flows under pressure, that is, gas and liquid states

Hair: the flexible shaft of distinct coloring that protrudes from the skin surface.

Half-time (pseudo first order): $t_{0.5} = 0.693/k$ where k is the pseudo first-order process rate constant in units of time^{-1}

Health surveillance: the measurement of chemical markers in body media that are indicative of adverse and nonadverse health effects

Immune response: chemical/cellular response of the body to an antigen

Macromolecules: high molecular weight biochemicals such as proteins, phospholipids, glycosides, nucleic acids, and their mixed analogs like glycolipids, lipoproteins, and chromatin (nuclear protein/DNA complex)

Marker: the determinant to be measured in human body media

Medical monitoring: the measurement of chemical markers in body media known to be indicative of adverse health effects

Medical surveillance: the measurement of chemical markers in body media that may be indicative of external exposure to chemical and physical agents and/or of potentially adverse effects

Menses: the discharge from the vagina during the female period

Metabolite: the stable reduction/oxidation (redox) product of catabolism of an exposing chemical

Midstream urine: a urine sample taken with the first couple of mL discarded to eliminate potential microorganisms or semen

Mixed exhaled breath: the breath that is naturally exhaled without forcing

Nail: the horny covering at the upper tip of fingers and toes

Plasma (blood): the liquid that does not contain the cellular components of blood on sitting or mild centrifugation of a blood sample

Saliva: watery fluid in the mouth

Sebum: the waxy excretion on the skin surface

Semen: the viscous creamy fluid obtained from the penis on ejaculation

Serum (blood): the liquid that does not contain the cellular components of blood on coagulation

Sputum: watery fluid with solids excreted from the throat and upper lungs on expectoration

Sweat: the watery fluid excreted on the skin surface during high physical activity or in hot, humid environments

Uptake: [mass potentially breathed in - mass breathed out]/mass potentially breathed in after a specific time period

Urine: the watery non-viscous excretion voided by the penis in males and by the urethra in females

Outcome Competencies

After completing this chapter, the reader should be able to:

1. Define the underlined terms.
2. Define the various types of skin and surface sampling techniques available.
3. Understand the benefits and limitations of existing sampling techniques.
4. Outline the elements of a tiered approach to skin assessments in the workplace.
5. Describe available means for control of occupational skin exposures.

Key Terms

behavior • biomonitoring • contact dermatitis • dermis • diffusion coefficient • flux • flux rate • hapten complex • *in situ* techniques • interception techniques • Langerhans cells • partition coefficient • percutaneous absorption • permeability constant • personal protective equipment • pharmacokinetic modeling • primary irritants • removal techniques • skin • skin absorption • stratum corneum • skin designation • skin exposure assessment methodology • skin notation • skin sensitization • viable epidermis

Prerequisite Knowledge

Anatomy, physiology, immunology, differential calculus (basic knowledge), occupational sampling techniques, and industrial hygiene hierarchy of controls.

Key Topics

I. Introduction
   A. Concepts of skin exposure assessment methodology
   B. Guidance for understanding skin exposures
II. Skin Anatomy and Function
   A. Concepts of skin anatomy (stratum corneum, epidermis, dermis)
III. Adverse Reactions of the Skin to Industrial Agents
   A. Causes of occupational skin disorders and diseases
   B. Allergic reactions of the skin
IV. Measures of Skin Surface Contamination
   A. Limitations of current techniques
   B. Removal, interception, and *in situ* techniques
V. Skin Absorption
   A. Skin absorption and percutaneous absorption
   B. Fick's Law of diffusion
VI. Tiered Approach to Skin Exposure Assessment in the Workplace
   A. Qualitative information gathering
   B. Indices and estimates of exposure
VII. Management and Control of Occupational Skin Diseases
   A. Hierarchy of controls
   B. Behavioral aspects of skin exposure

Disclaimer: The findings and conclusions in this report are those of the authors and may not represent those of the National Institute for Occupational Safety and Health.

The Skin and the Work Environment

20

By Aleksandr B. Stefaniak, PhD, CIH, Gregory A. Day, PhD, M. Abbas Virji, ScD, CIH, Laura A. Geer, PhD, MHS, and Dhimiter Bello, ScD, MSC

Introduction

Human skin is a highly specialized and evolved organ that provides the primary barrier between the ambient environment and the internal human anatomy. Occupational exposure of the skin to chemicals, physical agents, or biological materials may result in numerous localized or systemic adverse health outcomes. Occupational skin diseases are widespread and potentially affect millions of workers in a wide array of industries. Affected workers may suffer from lost income earning potential, economic impact from incurred health care costs, and reduced quality of life. Unlike inhalation assessment, skin exposure assessment methodology is not nearly as well developed and is complicated by factors such as:

- The frequently variable and sporadic nature of skin exposure (airborne deposition, contact with contaminated surfaces, splashes, etc.);
- Uncertainties regarding skin absorption;
- Lack of relationship between sampling substrates and properties of human skin (e.g., retention characteristics of sampling substrates may differ from skin);
- Recovery of analyte from sampled skin or surfaces;
- Lack of biologically relevant sampling conventions (in contrast to inhalable, thoracic, and respirable aerosol fractions for the respiratory tract); and
- Lack of occupational exposure limits with which to compare sampling results.

Guidance is largely lacking from U.S. government agencies regarding selection of available methods for measuring and evaluating occupational skin exposures. In 2008, the Occupational Safety and Health Administration (OSHA) updated the OSHA Technical Manual (OTM), thereby providing some guidance for compliance officers on the available means for assessing and evaluating the extent of skin exposure.[1] The OTM advises that skin notations or skin designations for chemicals listed as threshold limit values (TLVs®) by the American Conference of Governmental Industrial Hygienists® (ACGIH®) or as permissible exposure limits (PELs) by OSHA are useful, but that many chemicals posing potential skin hazards are not designated as such. Importantly, skin notations or skin designations denote only the potential significant contribution to overall exposures by the cutaneous route[2], whereas TLVs® and PELs represent finite limits on airborne concentrations of chemical substances. The National Institute for Occupational Safety and Health (NIOSH) currently provides skin notations for 142 chemicals.[3] In 2008, NIOSH drafted the Current Intelligence Bulletin (CIB) #61: "A Strategy for Assigning the New NIOSH Skin Notations."[4] This document provides a strategic framework designed to provide scientifically valid skin notations and communicates that information to health professionals; however, the draft CIB did not include specific guidance on methods for measuring and evaluating skin exposures. In 2007, the U.S. Environmental Protection Agency (EPA) published a summary of approaches for assessing skin exposures in a wide range of circumstances, including during industrial production of chemicals, and exposures associated with consumer products, contaminated water, soil and sediment.[5] The report included descriptions of many different approaches (mostly modeling), but did not emphasize assessment of occupational skin exposures nor provide guidance regarding selection of an appropriate approach.

The need for assessment of occupational skin exposures may be clearly recognizable in some situations, (e.g., use of a lipophilic organic solvent or a persistent pesticide). In other situations, the need may be less clear, (e.g., skin exposure to contaminated residual dusts may remain long after the airborne release of an agent). Thus, the choice of whether to sample for skin exposure may be difficult, yet doing so is a necessary first step toward the design of a credible skin exposure assessment strategy. Considerations when deciding whether to assess skin or surface contamination and its extent include the following types of questions: What is known about the agent? Does it carry a skin notation? Is skin the primary target organ? Is skin exposure a pathway to another organ? What are the chemical properties (pH, lipophilicity, molecular weight, reactivity) and physical characteristics of the agent (form, vapor pressure)? Are the chemical and physical properties of the agent known to pose risk to the skin? Do work factors potentially affect exposures? Work-related factors include the nature of tasks involving the agent in the work environment and potential opportunities for skin contact (splashes, aerosolization, contact with vapors, contact with surfaces, and transfer from clothes or tools).

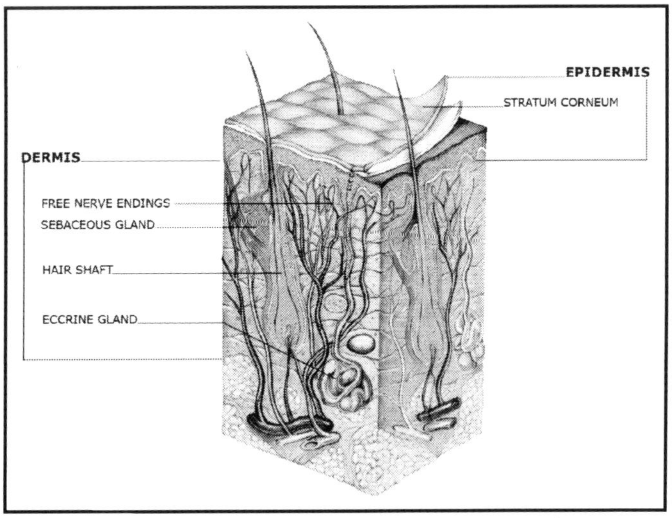

Figure 20.1 — The anatomy of human skin. (Courtesy of A.M. Stirnkorb, NIOSH).

The goals of this chapter are to provide occupational health and safety professionals with a state-of-the-art understanding of the anatomy and functions of the skin, to describe available methods for measuring and evaluating occupational skin exposures, to present a tiered strategy to skin exposure assessment in the workplace, and to describe options for management and control of skin exposures. Finally, real-world case studies are presented to illustrate the application of some concepts covered in this chapter.

Skin Anatomy and Function

Human skin is the largest organ in the human body and comprises three layers of stratified tissue (from outermost to innermost): stratum corneum (SC) which is the outer layer of the epidermis, the underlying viable epidermis, and the dermis. Figure 20.1 is an illustration of human skin that depicts the stratified layers of the skin. Functions of human skin include protecting against penetration of environmental and pathogenic micro-organisms and chemicals, facilitating the gripping of objects, providing self-maintenance and self-repair, providing mechanical protection from external pressures, and preventing water loss. In conjunction with other organs, skin functions include sensory (pain, temperature), temperature control (regulation of heat gain and loss), and immune defense.[6,7] Each anatomical skin layer has unique physiological functions and may act in conjunction with other skin layers or organs to provide functionality.

Stratum Corneum

The SC is 8- to 20-µm thick on most surfaces of the body (e.g., abdomen, back, forehead, volar forearm), but may be as thick as 400 µm (palms) and varies with age and gender. The SC is the outer nonviable layer of the epidermis and consists of several layers (commonly 15–20) of corneocytes, dead keratinocyte cells without nuclei and metabolic activity, joined tightly together by a tough intercellular matrix.[8–10] This structure is commonly referred to as the brick and mortar model, where corneocytes represent the bricks and intercellular matrix (keratin and lipids) the mortar. Each day, one new cellular layer appears on the inner face of the SC and one layer sloughs off the outer surface. The SC functions to maintain a water barrier across the skin, regulate skin surface pH, and provide elasticity. The water barrier function is dependent on the hydrophobic coating imparted by the intercellular lipids.[11] The skin pH gradient is maintained by sweat (water soluble electrolytes, amino acids, nitrogenous substances, etc.) and sebum (saturated and unsaturated lipid mixture) that is secreted onto the skin surface. Among healthy adults, skin surface pH is maintained by degradation of lipids and chemicals[12] and is generally acidic, with a median pH value of 5.3.[13] The SC contains about 5–20% water, much less than in the physiologically active skin layers (up to 70%).

Epidermis

The viable epidermis is the physiologically active skin layer directly beneath the SC and is made up of approximately 10 layers of keratinocyte cells, randomly stacked upon each other. This skin layer is 50- to 100-μm thick on most sites of the body. The viable epidermis continuously generates new basal cells on the inner face and keritanizes cells at the outer face to renew the SC.[14] The functions of the epidermis include protection against UV light, skin color, neurosensation, mechanical protection, water movement for barrier repair, and immune defense via Langherhans cells and T-lymphocytes.[11,14] Epidermal immune functions can either be innate (non-specific) or acquired (adapted) to specifically target foreign substances.

Dermis

Below the viable epidermis is the dermis, the thickest skin layer that amounts to about 7% of total bodyweight. The dermis provides elasticity, flexibility, strength and stability and comprises two types of connective tissue, the papillary/subpapillary dermis and the reticular dermis. The papillary/subpapillary dermis vasculature provides nutrition to the overlying epidermis and partly controls percutaneous absorption of chemicals to the blood. The papillary dermis, in conjunction with the epidermis, contributes to acquired immune responses of the skin by facilitating the migration of immune cells toward the lymph nodes.[15] The reticular dermis has vasculature; however, its function is mainly mechanical as it contains pilosebaceous units (sebum glands) and the coiled portion of sweat glands that function to secrete a precursor sweat solution.[15]

Adverse Reactions of the Skin to Industrial Agents

The potential exists in nearly all workplaces for adverse impact on the skin; however, skin hazards in the workplace are often overlooked due to the lack of health guidelines and under-developed methods of assessment.

The U.S. Bureau of Labor Statistics reported that skin diseases or disorders represented 18% of all nonfatal occupational illnesses in 2006.[16] Of the 41,400 cases of skin diseases and disorders, 13,200 occurred in the goods-producing industry (most cases in the manufacturing and construction sectors), while the remaining 28,100 occurred in the service-producing industry. Interestingly, more than one-third of all cases within the service-producing industry occurred in the education and health services sector. Of all occupational skin diseases, contact dermatitis, which may be either irritant (ICD) or allergic (ACD), is the most common, representing 90–95% of diseases.[17,18] ACD represents nearly half of all dermatoses; in the United States the cost of ACD in terms of lost productivity and treatment is estimated to be $1 billion per year.[19]

Adverse reactions of the skin to industrial agents may be acute such as cuts, scrapes, and mild burns or chronic such as development of ICD and ACD. The economic and psychological impacts of acute adverse effects to the skin often resolve quickly; however, for chronic skin diseases such as ICD and ACD, the effect is often long-lasting. Persons with ICD have a significant detrimental effect on quality of life, including decreased work productivity or loss of job and increased heath care costs.[20–22] For persons with ACD, only lifelong avoidance of the offending agent can prevent elicitation of disease.[19,23,24] People with ACD are forced to change jobs to avoid exposure, which may impact income-earning potential. Additionally, the psychological impact of ACD is great, with those with facial ACD reporting most impact on quality of life.[19]

Occupational Skin Disorders and Diseases

In the work environment, skin contact with agents may result in a wide range of adverse outcomes depending, in part, upon the specific agent and exposure conditions. Causes of occupational skin disorders and diseases include chemical, mechanical, physical, and biological agents. Reactions involving chemical and biological agents may also involve immunological factors.

Chemical

A diverse range of chemicals may cause adverse reactions to the skin; however, a thorough examination of all chemicals and mechanisms by which human skin may be damaged is beyond the scope of this chapter. Some chemicals cause damage by direct toxic damage to the skin while others act via immune-mediated mechanisms. Chemicals that cause direct toxic effects, also known as primary irritants, generally do not rely on the immune system to produce irritation, rather these chemicals act by damaging cells in the living layers of the epidermis. Mechanisms by which skin structure may be altered (Figure 20.2) include swelling of corneocytes due to excessive hydration; delipidisation of the lipid bilayer, fluidization of skin lipids, or denaturation of keratin in corneocytes due to organic solvents; and disordering of the SC lipid bilayer structure, reduced cohesion of the SC, or alteration of skin enzymatic activity at alkaline pH due to soaps and detergents. Most often, irritant effects to the skin are expressed locally at the site of contact, such as with exposure to cement and wood dusts; phosphates during the manufacture of fertilizer; and chlorothalinol during manufacture of pesticides.[25] However, evidence is emerging that a defective barrier can be a risk factor in development of allergic diseases such as asthma.[26]

Mechanical

Mechanically induced occupational skin diseases are often caused by trauma to the skin. Mechanical causes, which are a subset of physical factors, include friction, pressure, crushes, tears, contact with sharp objects (e.g., needles, blades), or any other impact that disrupts skin barrier function (Figure 20.3). While mechanical trauma such as a cut or abrasion may heal completely over time, any disruption of the skin barrier temporarily provides an unimpeded route of exposure that could result in more serious conditions such as immunologically mediated skin diseases or lead to systemic toxic effects. Additionally, some fibrous irritant materials such as glass fibers, in combination with friction, may cause mechanical dermatitis, (e.g., hyperkeratosis or acute dermatitis).[25]

Physical

Physically induced skin diseases may occur as the result of occupational exposure to temperature extremes and/or exposure to some forms of ionizing radiation (alpha and beta particulate) and non-ionizing radiation (lasers, ultraviolet light, etc.). Elevated temperatures often enhance perspiration (hence skin permeability), leading to greater absorption of exogenous agents. Cold temperatures may result in deadening of skin tissue (Figure 20.4), whereas overexposure to hot temperatures may cause skin burns. Ionizing radiation may cause burns to the skin and exposure to ultraviolet light may result in mild erythema (sunburn) or skin

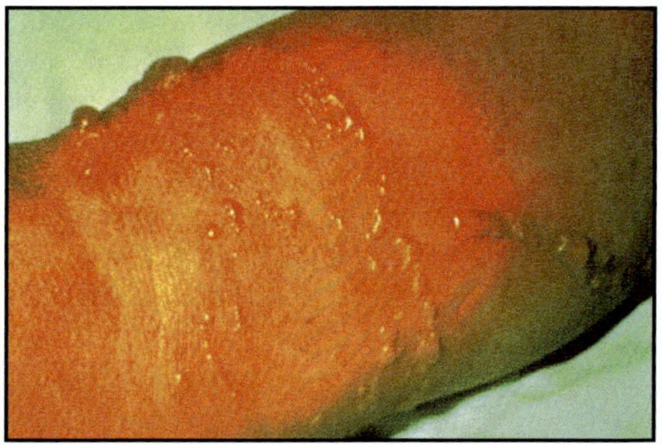

Figure 20.2 — Acute contact dermatitis from exposure to ethylene oxide.

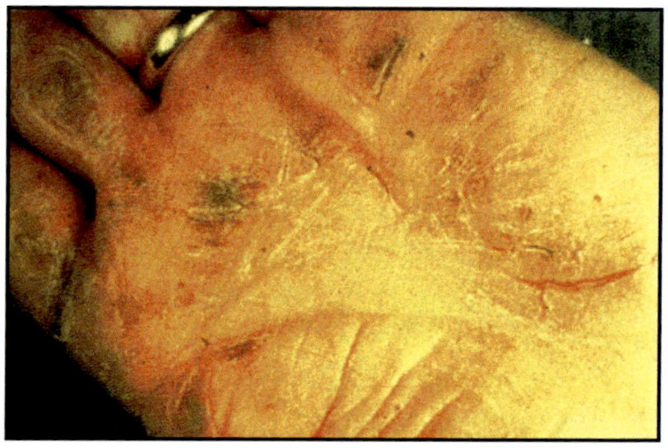

Figure 20.3 — Calluses and fissures caused by repetitive hand motion.

cancer. For example, Rosenthal, et al.[27] developed an exposure model for watermen on the Chesapeake Bay that was predictive of conditions known to be caused by excessive sun exposure to ultraviolet light, including skin elastosis and squamous cell carcinoma. In some cases, skin contact with a photosensitizing compound (called a chromophore) followed by exposure to ultraviolet light may result in photosensitization and manifest as either photoallergy (a specific immune reaction to a chromophore) or phototoxicity (an inflammatory reaction that depends on the chromophore concentration and ultraviolet light dose to the skin). Examples of photoallergens include carprofen and chlorpromazine, which may be encountered during the manufacture of some pharmaceuticals.[25] Occupational exposure to lasers is primarily an eye hazard, with skin being less vulnerable; however, from a probability standpoint, the likelihood of skin exposure is higher due to the large surface area of skin relative to the eye. Exposure to a laser may result in damage via photochemical or thermal mechanisms. Photochemical reactions include injury to the epidermis which manifest as erythema, whereas thermal mechanisms may result in a burn.[28]

Biological

Biological agents may cause a range of skin diseases and often occur among workers who handle, live, or work near livestock (Figure 20.5). Anthrax or wool-sorter's disease is an acute bacterial disease caused by skin (or ingestion and inhalation) exposure to *Bacillus anthracis* from herbivores such as cattle and sheep. Anthrax may be "weaponized" and has been used as a biowarfare agent to intentionally expose letter carriers in the U.S.[29] Additionally, , exposure to animal fluids such as urine and agricultural dusts such as mites, flax allergens, and molds may cause ACD. Contact urticaria can be either allergic or non-allergic, depending on the substance contacting the skin Compounds such as danders (e.g., goat) cause allergic contact urticaria, a localized swelling and redness that occurs on the skin immediately after direct contact with an offending compound.[25]

Immunological

Over 3,000 airborne chemicals have been shown to cause skin sensitization including plants and resins; plastics, rubbers, and glues; metals, industrial and pharmaceutical chemicals; and pesticides and feed additives.[25] In the occupational environment, cobalt, chromium (Figure 20.6) and nickel are among the most frequent and commonly encountered contact allergens.[30] Allergic reactions involve the acquired immune system and require three inputs: antigen, antigen-presenting cells, and T-lymphocytes. Development of an allergic skin reaction is a two-phase process, first a chemical must induce sensitization (i.e., priming of the immune system), and then repeat exposure to the same (or similar) chemical is needed to elicit a response. Most chemicals are too small to act as antigens, rather they must have appropriate lipophilicity to undergo percutaneous absorption into the epidermis then bind to macromolecules such as proteins to form a hapten complex. Note that compromised skin provides more direct access for chemical penetration to the epidermis. Within the epidermis, Langerhans cells (LC) capture, degrade, and present the hapten complex.[31] Once a hapten complex is internalized, the LC migrates from the

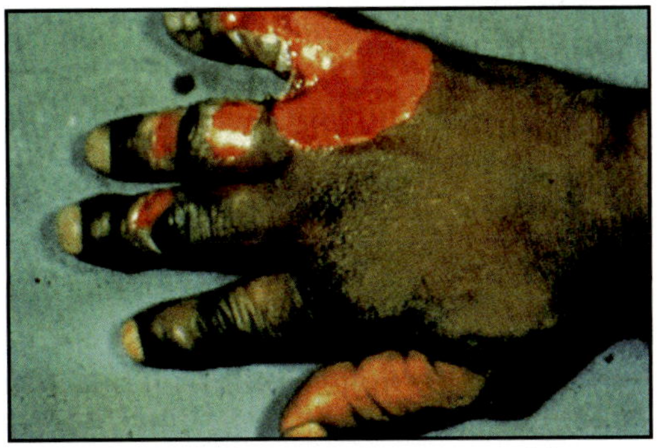

Figure 20.4 — Frostbite can be severe, with destruction of the skin and deeper tissues.

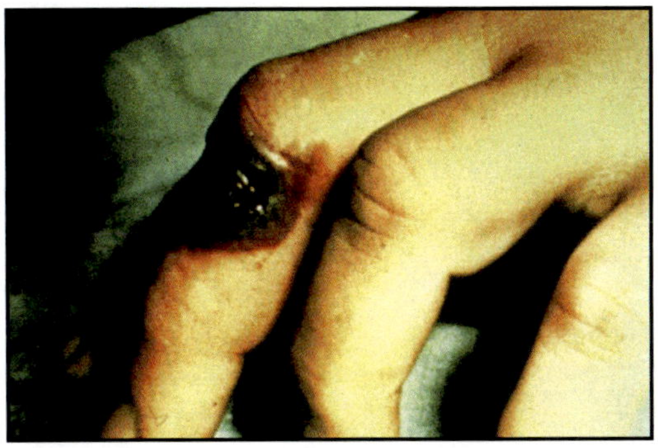

Figure 20.5 — Skin trauma caused by exposure to the biological agent anthrax.

epidermis to the draining lymph nodes via the afferent lymph vessels. Within the lymph nodes, LCs present the hapten to naïve CD4+ T-lymphocytes. Upon recognition of the hapten, these naïve T-lymphocytes differentiate to form memory CD4+ helper T-lymphocytes (i.e., a person becomes sensitized). Upon repeat contact with the same chemical, the CD4+ memory T-lymphocytes are recruited to the site of skin contact and interact with LCs in the epidermis to initiate inflammation responsible for ACD.[24,31,32] Note that an optimum concentration is generally required to stimulate LCs; too high a concentration will result in cytotoxity whereas too low a concentration may not be sufficient to elicit a response. Emerging evidence suggests that the skin is an important route of exposure resulting in systemic sensitization that contributes to further development of lung diseases upon inhalation exposure (e.g., isocyanate exposure and asthma).[26]

Measures of Skin and Surface Contamination

Chemicals may contact the skin in liquid or solid forms, resulting from aerosol or vapor deposition, sprays, direct immersion, spills and splashes, and/or transfer from contact with contaminated tools, equipment and other surfaces. Regardless of pathway, current approaches to measuring and evaluating skin exposures include removing contaminants from skin (or from work surfaces as surrogates of skin exposure) and interception of contaminants on substrates placed on top of the skin. Following collection, samples are analyzed using appropriate analytical techniques to quantify masses of contaminants for exposure estimation. The practicing industrial hygienist must be aware that the current sample collection and analysis paradigm underlying these techniques often does not account for:

1. The forms (chemical species, e.g. hexavalent chromium) of contaminants that can permeate through the skin (chemical analytical techniques provide estimates of total contaminant masses that may not provide biologically meaningful measures of the bioaccessible contaminants on skin or work surfaces); and
2. The adhesion characteristics of human skin (existing sampling substrates do not mimic furrows, microtopography, or adhesion and retention properties, which can result in under- or over-estimation of contaminants).

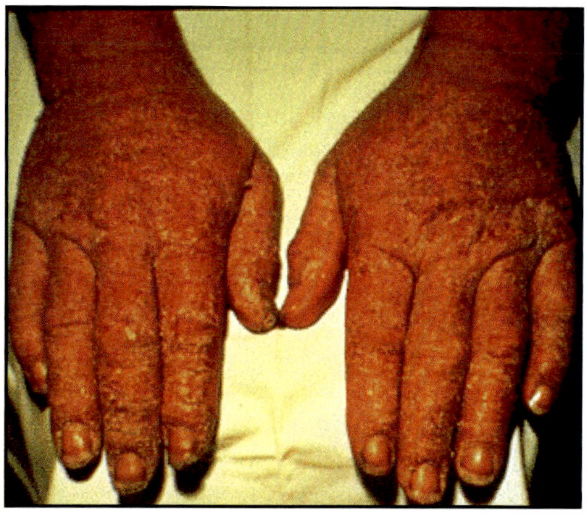

Figure 20.6 — Allergic contact dermatitis caused by skin exposure to compounds of chromium.

These shortcomings are important because only bioaccessible forms (lipophillic, etc.) of agents will undergo percutaneous absorption from the outside environment through the intact SC into the living epidermis layer of the skin. (If the SC barrier function is compromised, agents will readily access the epidermis and living tissue of the skin.) As such, current removal and interception sampling techniques provide only crude estimates of the skin or surface contamination. In other words, these current measures of exposure may not provide biologically relevant estimates of skin exposure.

Sampling to Estimate Contamination of Skin

Sampling to estimate contamination of skin currently includes three different techniques: <u>removal, interception, and *in situ*</u>. Additional details of techniques for measuring contamination of skin can be obtained from Ness[33] and from the European Committee for Standardization.[34]

Removal Techniques

Removal techniques include wiping, washing or rinsing, and tape stripping of the skin. The major assumption underlying all removal techniques is that the majority of the contaminant mass residing on skin is captured by the collection substrate. Removal efficiency of a contaminant is influenced by:

1. Pressure applied during sampling (i.e., wiping),
2. Accuracy in measuring the area from which to sample, and
3. Type of sampling substrate (e.g., pre-moistened wipes versus cotton swabs).

Skin sampling using removal techniques only collects the contaminant present on the skin surface at a given point in time and does not account for:

1. The fraction that may have volatilized or brushed off,
2. Material washed off by sweating or hygienic practices, or
3. The fraction of dissolved contaminant that may have permeated the skin prior to sample collection.

Skin Wiping

Sampling by wiping the skin is the most common removal technique. The general approach is to use a substrate, such as a pre-moistened commercial wipe material, to remove some fraction of available contamination from the skin. Ideally, demarcation of surface area allows calculation of the mass concentration of the contaminant removed from the skin. Que Hee et al.[35] observed experimentally that serial wipe sampling insufficiently removes all lead-containing dust from the hands of study subjects. Lidén et al.[36] reported that up to five serial wipes were needed to completely recover a soluble nickel salt intentionally applied to the skin. Thus, removal by wiping may underestimate the mass of contaminant on skin and results may be highly variable.

Liquid Washing or Rinsing

Estimating contamination of the hands can involve sampling by washing or rinsing of the skin. These techniques can be advantageous in certain sampling situations, particularly when estimating exposure to water-soluble chemicals such as pesticides or salts. One technique involves placing the hands into a liquid-filled container and washing contaminants from the skin by rubbing the hands together. Another technique involves holding the hands over a container while liquid is poured onto the hands, thus removing contaminants through liquid-skin contact. Wash and rinse liquids typically include water, sometimes combined with surfactants, and/or mild organic solvents. Connected to a tap-water supply, Marquart et al.[37] used a special apparatus to control the consistency of water pressure and volume when removing pesticides from the hands. Fenske et al.[38] reported that one washing removed six times more organic chemicals from skin than did wipe sampling. Note that using solvents, such as alcohols, may defat the skin, thereby compromising barrier properties and enhancing subsequent uptake of chemicals.

Tape Stripping

Tape stripping is a sampling method for removing contaminants not only from the skin surface, but also from within the SC. The technique is carried out by repeatedly placing an adhesive tape (three or more times) onto the surface of the skin and peeling it from the same area (e.g., hands, forearms, neck, and/or face). The surface area of the tape defines the area of the sample. Commercially available products used for tape stripping include Fixomull® (Smith and Nephew, Auckland, NZ), Blenderm™ (3M Corporation, St. Paul, MN, USA), D-Squame® and Sebutape® (CuDerm Corporation, Dallas, TX, USA). Each tape strip removes approximately one cell layer and sequential stripping allows estimation of permeation of the chemical deeper into the SC. The sampling procedure can vary, primarily depending on the properties of the contaminant of interest and the sampling objectives. Additional information regarding sampling by tape stripping can be obtained from Surakka et al.[39] and Kezic.[40]

Interception Techniques

Interception techniques (sometimes referred to as surrogate techniques and/or dosimeters) involve the use of gauzes, charcoal cloths, pads, patches or other types of substrates placed directly onto the surface of the skin and/or on the outside/underside of clothing. If appropriate, the clothing itself may be used as the sampling substrate (e.g., cotton gloves to evaluate exposures of the hands). The major assumption underlying all interception techniques is that the collection substrate captures and retains chemicals in a manner similar to that of the skin. Interception of skin contamination is influenced by:

1. Variability in deposition rates of contaminants onto the body
2. Type of clothing
3. The anatomical region of the body and actual duration of skin contact with chemicals
4. Retention and permeation of a chemical over time

Gauze patches or pads are often used to estimate skin contamination to pesticides because they are small, portable, inexpensive, and tend to absorb and retain materials like spray mists; however, the adsorption and retention properties of this substrate do not mimic human skin. Levels of contaminants on cotton gloves have been used as indices of skin exposure to cobalt[(41)] and beryllium.[(42)] Brouwer et al.[(43)] investigated the transfer of particles from contaminated surfaces to uncontaminated hands and to cotton gloves through a set of controlled laboratory experiments. Their results indicated that the mass of particles transferred from contaminated surfaces to cotton gloves was approximately 70-fold higher than was transferred to uncovered hands.

In Situ *Techniques*

Sampling to estimate contamination of the skin can also be accomplished using *in situ* techniques. These techniques generally involve measuring a fluorescent tracer on the skin surface or on clothing.[(44)] A qualitative approach is to add a fluorescing compound to the source of the hazardous substance and then visualize the dispersion of contaminants within the work environment using a light probe (e.g., ultraviolet). Ideally, the fluorescing compound has similar characteristics as the contaminant of interest regarding skin retention and permeation. The main advantage of this approach is that detection of the fluorescing compound is useful for identifying pathways from the source to contamination of surfaces (see below) and skin. Fluorescent tracers can also be used for quantitative evaluation of skin exposures. For example, Brouwer et al.[(45)] added a whitening agent (fluorescent tracer) to a colorless lacquer and measured deposition of the agent during spray painting on clothing and uncovered parts of skin. The authors then correlated deposited mass of the tracer with surface area exposed multiplied by duration of exposure (an alternative exposure metric). This approach involves the use of specially calibrated equipment, including a video camera, along with software for calculating surface area and intensity of illumination (i.e., mass). Another *in situ* approach involves reflectance of contaminants through the use of attenuated total reflectance Fourier transform infrared spectroscopy.[(46)] There is also additional information regarding quantitative *in situ* techniques.[(44,47–51)]

Sampling to Estimate Contamination of Surfaces

Techniques for evaluating surface contamination include wipe sampling, vacuuming, and direct-reading instruments. Additional details of these and other techniques can be obtained from Ness.[(33)] Clearly, levels of surface contamination are not direct measures of skin contamination. Rather, contaminated surfaces represent sources and, therefore, possible pathways of skin exposure resulting from either direct or indirect skin contact.

The most common approach to surface sampling is to use either a wet or a dry substrate while wiping and applying pressure. Detailed wipe sampling methods have been published by government agencies including NIOSH[(52)] and OSHA.[(53)] Despite this guidance, a high degree of variability is inevitable because the amount of pressure applied to surfaces while wiping may vary within and between surveyors (i.e., light, medium, and firm pressure); not all surveyors may use templates for delineating surface area; many surfaces do not allow the use of a template (i.e., irregular shapes); and the composition of surfaces may have very different properties (i.e., smooth, rough, porous). Such factors create inherent variability in not only the masses of contaminants removed from surfaces but also the estimated surface area sampled. This variability affects the accuracy of estimates of contamination; therefore, a prudent approach during a sampling campaign is to limit the number of surveyors collecting surface wipe samples.

Additional techniques include vacuuming and direct reading instruments. Vacuuming methods vary by several factors including the types of surfaces, flow rates (low- versus high-volume), collection times, and sampling substrates. Direct-reading techniques include chemical-specific colorimetric wipe indicators (e.g., for lead) and ionization detectors (e.g., for volatile chemicals). An in situ technique involves the use of fluorescent tracers (described above). Another technique for estimating surface contamination, also considered bulk sampling, is the use of a settling plate such as an uncovered Petri dish containing a filter substrate for collecting settled dust. The types of surfaces appropriate for settling plates are generally unobstructed surfaces including rafters, tops of bookshelves, and tops of room dividers.

Measures of Skin Exposure

Existing removal and interception sampling techniques provide crude estimates of biologically relevant skin exposure. While more accurate estimates of skin exposure to chemicals and other agents are desirable, such estimates are challenging due to a number factors including limitations of existing methods (types of substrates, collection techniques, and analytical issues) and variability associated with exposure patterns. Regarding the latter limitation, the level of skin contact with the contaminant may be variable and sporadic throughout the course of a work shift; skin loading may be cumulative throughout a work shift and/or accumulate for part of a shift followed by loss of contaminant due to brush off or wash off (sweating, hygienic cleansing, etc.). As described in the previous section, numerous sampling substrates exist and the choice of which to use is dependent upon the specific circumstances of the agent and workplace. Regardless of substrate chosen, the material does not mimic the furrows, microtopography, or adhesion and retention properties of human skin, which can result in under- or over-collection of contaminant. Available sampling techniques provide an estimate of contaminant mass on skin at a given point in time and do not account for the portion of contaminant that permeated into skin prior to sample collection (i.e., under-estimate exposure). Some techniques provide estimates of total skin loading, which is not necessarily a measure of biologically relevant loading. A portion of deposited contaminant mass may not become bioaccessible because it may not contact skin surface film liquids and dissolve; however, this mass could be captured during sample collection (i.e., over-estimating exposure). In addition to the relevant level of contaminant on skin and duration of exposure, consideration should be given to the area of exposed skin.[54] However, measures of exposed area are complicated by the irregular shape of appendages such as fingers. Finally, the total amount of contaminant on skin or a surface at the time of sample collection is never known, which prohibits determination of sample removal efficiency. Once collected, quantification of contaminant mass may be complicated by low recovery from a sample substrate by an analytical method. In addition, most analytical chemistry techniques provide estimates of total contaminant mass on a sample without regard to the biologically relevant (i.e., bioaccessible) form. Knowledge of the bioaccessible form of a contaminant and its permeability constant are necessary to estimate total mass uptake through the skin. Additionally, skin integrity may also affect mass uptake through the skin. An ideal quantitative measurement of skin exposure would accurately account for most, or all, of these factors; however, such an approach is currently lacking and novel methodologies are needed to quantify exposures in the workplace.

Skin Absorption

Skin absorption is the transfer of a compound from the outside environment into the living tissue. Absorption occurs via diffusion, the process whereby molecules spread from areas of high concentration to areas of low concentration, by three possible mechanisms: intercellular lipid pathway, trans-cellular permeation, and through hair follicles. Absorption is influenced by a number of factors, including duration and frequency of exposure, skin surface area and concentration, skin integrity, anatomical site and the characteristics of the chemical. As such, the rate of uptake of a chemical may vary within and between people.

The SC is the transport-rate limiting strata of the skin, thus knowledge of the movement (flux) of a chemical through the SC as a function of time (flux rate) is important for understanding the potential toxicity of a contaminant on skin. As the living tissue begins at the uppermost layer of the stratum granulosum, skin absorption is the transit of an agent through the SC. Percutaneous absorption applies to the passage beyond the epidermis for entry into the bloodstream. Between the SC and the blood vessels, the resistance to diffusion is about 10,000 times lower than through the SC.[55]

Various techniques exist for estimating penetration of contaminants through skin, including *in vitro* studies, *in vivo* animal studies (when inter-species differences are understood), or even human exposure studies. Among these approaches, *in vitro* techniques using various thicknesses (full thickness, SC only, etc.) of animal (porcine, etc.) or human skin are most often used to estimate permeation rates through the use of flow-through diffusion cells. Although many different designs have been used for diffusion cell studies, important considerations include the receptor volume, construction material, maintenance of physiological temperature, ease of assembly of skin, and mixing of receptor contents.[56] Regardless of cell type, the basic experimental approach is to apply a contaminant in a vehicle (donor fluid) such as artificial sweat to the outer surface of the skin section on the donor side of the cell. After a known period of time, the mass of contaminant that has entered the receptor fluid on the opposite side of the skin layer is measured and used to calculate a permeation rate.

Penetration of a dissolved chemical through the skin is related to its concentration in a particular solvent. According to Fick's law of diffusion, the rate of absorption of a chemical (assuming a single vehicle) is proportional to the applied concentration:

$$J \propto Cv \tag{20.1}$$

where

J = rate of absorption per unit area (also called flux)
C_v = Concentration of the penetrating chemical in a vehicle (g/m^3)

Absorption of a contaminant across the SC and into the living tissue can be divided into three phases. First, the contaminant leaves the vehicle and dissolves in the liquid film that coats the SC (lipids from the SC intercellular spaces, cellular debris, sebum, and sweat). This transfer is limited by the partition coefficient, K_m, which is defined as the ratio, at equilibrium, of the concentration of contaminant in the SC (C_{SC}) to the concentration of contaminant in the vehicle, C_v. Note that K_m takes into account the fact that the exclusive "motor" for net movement of contaminant molecules is the difference in concentration on each side of the SC. In the second phase, the contaminant enters the SC intercellular spaces and is distributed along a decreasing concentration gradient towards the deeper skin layers. The flow rate or mobility of a contaminant in the SC is determined by its diffusion coefficient, D_m. The filling of the SC by the flow of solute is limited by its maximum storage capacity and is theoretically independent from the contaminant vehicle, though in practice with *in vitro* cells this is not always true. A useful parameter that accounts for both the partitioning of contaminant on the skin surface and its movement through the SC is the permeability constant, k_p, which is the capacity of a solute to be absorbed from a given vehicle.

$$k_p = \frac{K_m \cdot K_d}{d} \tag{20.2}$$

where

k_p = permeability constant (cm/hr)
d = thickness of the skin layer in the *in vitro* cell (cm)

The utility of the permeability constant, k_p, is that it facilitates the relative comparison of permeation among different contaminants, even when data were collected using different vehicles or experimental conditions. By analogy, k_p can be thought of as the often cited measure miles per gallon, which is used to compare the relative fuel economy of various makes and models of vehicles. Caution is needed when using *in vitro* estimates of k_p as the values depend, in part, on experimental conditions (e.g., concentration-dependent changes in the SC itself caused by the contaminant). Values for permeability constants range from about a low of 10^{-6} cm/hr for water to a high of 10^{-2} cm/hr for very lipophilic chemicals. It follows that Eq. 20.1 can now be expressed as:

$$J = k_p \cdot C_v \qquad (20.3)$$

which is equivalent to:

$$J = -\frac{K_m \cdot C_v \cdot K_d}{d} \qquad (20.4)$$

where J is the flux having units of $\mu g \cdot cm^{-2} \cdot hr^{-1}$

Note that the negative sign in Eq. 20.4 indicates that the flux of contaminant is from a region of high concentration (SC surface) toward a region of lower concentration (epidermis).

After passing through the SC, compounds diffuse through the epidermis, the dermis, and finally enter the blood capillaries. Thus, the final absorption phase consists of the contaminant penetrating into the living tissue and begins before the second phase has ended. After a settling phase, absorption into the living tissue reaches a maximum flux which remains stable as long as the contaminant remains in sufficient quantity on the SC surface. During this phase of steady state flux, the amount of contaminant entering and leaving the SC are equal (as long as the contaminant concentration in the application remains unchanged); however, the amount stored inside the SC is continuously renewed at a constant maximal level. The amount absorbed during this phase is given by Fick's first law of diffusion:

$$Q = k_p \cdot A \cdot C_v \cdot t \qquad (20.5)$$

where

Q = quantity absorbed (g)
A = application area (cm^2)
t = time (hr)

Biomonitoring

Biological monitoring or biomonitoring is the measurement of a potentially toxic substance, its metabolite or a consequent biochemical effect in a biological specimen such as tissues, excreta or secreta (e.g., hair, blood and urine). Biomonitoring integrates all exposure routes including inhalation, skin and ingestion, for assessment of an actual rather than a potential dose and reflects individual variability in anatomy (body size) and physiology (such as metabolism and excretion). The comparison of skin exposure with biomonitoring is most informative when parameters of human metabolism and pharmacokinetics are characterized and available.[57–59] When biomonitoring is performed concomitant with personal air sampling, and a known correlation with air and biomonitoring exists, the excess excretion can be attributed to skin exposure, and thus an external skin exposure estimate can be approximated. Once this relationship is established for a specific compound, skin exposure can be modeled from biological monitoring and inhalation exposure values. Another more involved but advantageous alternative to assessing the relative contributions of each exposure route in the total internal dose is physiologically based pharmacokinetic modeling (PBPK). Interested readers may find more information on this approach in Kim and Nylander-French.[60]

Biomonitoring is an advantageous method because it confirms that uptake has occurred and provides a better measure of the magnitude of dose. As individual uptake, metabolism and excretion can be modulated by work conditions, these factors may not be accurately accounted for by simple skin exposure studies.[61] Additionally, personal hygiene can influence the association between exposure and absorption. Finally, biomonitoring can account for uncertainties associated with skin monitoring methods.

While biomonitoring has many advantages, there are also limitations to this method. Biomonitoring may not be desirable when the biological measures are highly variable or when the measurement methods are imprecise relative to other external exposure assessment techniques. Boogaard[62] points out that assuming 100% percutaneous absorption (worst-case) to obtain estimates for human health risk assessment is unreasonable in most cases and may lead to bias.

Tiered Approach to Skin Exposure Assessments in the Workplace

Assessment of potential skin contamination in the workplace requires a tiered approach to provide maximum protection for workers. As illustrated in Figure 20.7, this approach begins with simple qualitative observations and, if necessary, progresses to more complex semi-quantitative indices of exposure, and ultimately to complex quantitative exposure measures. The approach outlined in this section is written from the perspective of chemical hazards to the skin; however, the basic approach also applies to workplace assessments of mechanical, physical, biological, and immunological agents.

Qualitative Observation

The first step in the assessment approach is to qualitatively determine whether there is potential for contact with an agent that is toxic to the skin. This step involves review of the agent(s) encountered by workers and their work practices. Various resources can be utilized to understand the properties of agents used by workers, including Material Safety Data Sheets, industrial toxicology textbooks, professional association and governmental publications, case reports, and internet resources. Key questions that could provide important pieces of information include:

- Does the agent have a skin notation?
- Is skin the primary target organ?
- Is skin exposure a pathway to another organ?
- What is the primary form of the agent (powder, liquid, vapor, etc)?
- What are the chemical properties of the agent (pH, lipophilicity, molecular weight, reactivity)?
- What are the physical characteristics of the agent (form, vapor pressure)?
- Are the chemical and physical properties of the agent known to pose risk to the skin?

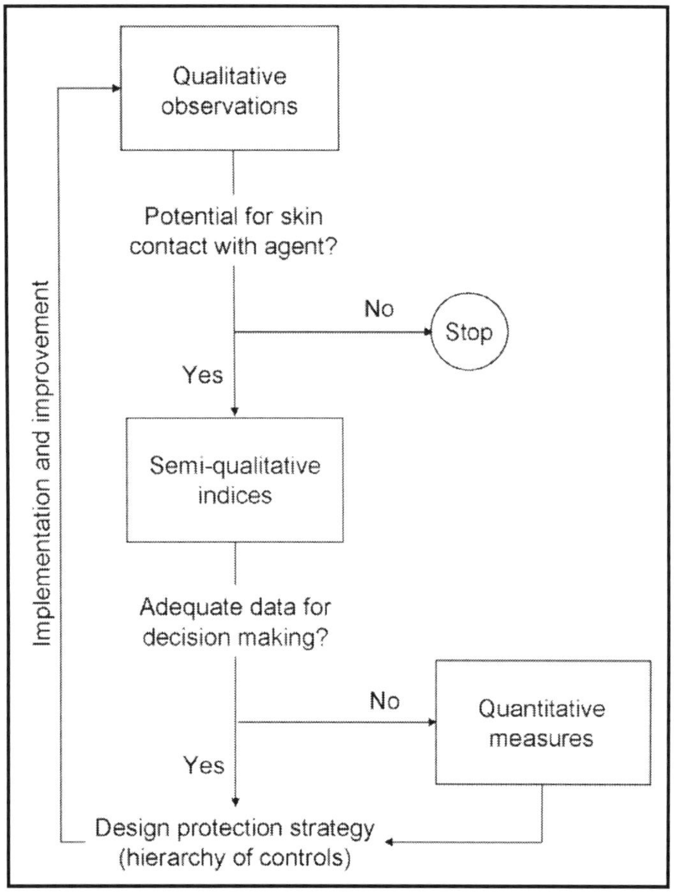

Figure 20.7 — A tiered approach to skin exposure assessment in the workplace.

Evaluation of work practices can vary in complexity and detail and may involve review of processes and job functions, discussions with workers on how tasks are performed, visual observation of work practices, and/or video recording and review of work practices. Important information on work practices may include:

- the nature of tasks involving the agent (pouring, mixing, etc);
- duration and frequency of tasks performed;
- amount/volume of agent encountered by a worker;
- frequency with which a worker may encounter the agent during a task;
- design of the process (e.g., enclosed, etc);
- design of the workspace and frequency of housekeeping;
- opportunities for skin contact (splashes, aerosolization, etc); and
- worker experience and training.

Upon review of the agent(s) and associated work practices, a preliminary decision can be made regarding whether the potential exists for skin contact in the workplace. If the results of the qualitative review indicate that there is not potential for skin contact with a hazardous agent, then no further action may be necessary; however, periodic re-evaluation is needed when the process, job or tasks are modified or when a new chemical is introduced.

Semi-Quantitative Indices of Exposure

If the observational data suggest that opportunities exist for skin contact with a hazardous substance, then it may be necessary to conduct semi-quantitative assessment of skin contamination to develop an understanding of exposure potential. Various models exist for semi-quantitative assessment of skin exposures, including RISKOFDERM[(63)] and DREAM.[(64)] Schneider et al.[(65)] developed a conceptual model of skin exposure that describes the transport of contaminants from the source to the surface of the skin. The model consists of six compartments and eight transport processes of the mass of contaminant. The six compartments include: 1) source of contaminant; 2) air; 3) surface contaminant layer; 4) outer clothing contaminant layer; 5) inner clothing contaminant layer; and 6) skin contaminant layer. The eight processes that describe the transport of mass from its source to the surface of the skin through the various compartments include: emission, deposition, re-suspension or evaporation, transfer, removal, re-distribution, decontamination and penetration or permeation. The parameters that need to be estimated in each compartment are defined.

van Wendel de Joode et al.[(64)] developed a structured dermal exposure assessment method (DREAM) based on the conceptual model of Schneider et al.[(65)] The DREAM model is a task-based model that requires the assessment of tasks and potential exposures for the jobs being evaluated. The assessment is performed for all the relevant body segments (nine in total from head to feet) and for all the tasks associated with a job. Total skin exposure of a worker to a contaminant is estimated by summing the exposure score from all the body segments and all the tasks for a job.

Factors are categorized into three general groups in the DREAM model. The first set of factors is associated with evaluating the mechanism of skin exposure, and includes emission (E), transfer (T) and deposition (D). For each of these mechanisms, scores are assigned for intensity (amount of substance on the surface); probability (frequency of occurrence); source weights (relative weights of each mechanism); and intrinsic emission (physical and chemical properties). Potential for skin exposure is obtained by summing the scores for the three mechanisms. A second set of factors is associated with the evaluation of the intrinsic emission mentioned above. Scores are assigned to these factors which include physical state, percent active ingredient, evaporation rate, viscosity, formulation, dustiness and stickiness. A third set of factors is associated with evaluating the protective effect of clothing. Scores are assigned to these factors which include clothing material, protection factor, replacement frequency, connection with other pieces of clothing, proportion of time, double clothing layer, replacement of inner clothing, and use of barrier cream. The score for clothing protection factor is multiplied by the potential skin exposure to obtain an estimate of actual skin exposure.

In the DREAM model, scores are assigned to the factors subjectively as described by Cherrie et al.[(66)], which range from 0–10 on a logarithmic scale. The model generates estimates of skin deposition in arbitrary scale, and does not assess uptake through the skin. van Wendel de Joode et al.[(67)] assessed the accuracy of the DREAM model by comparing the estimates derived from the DREAM model with measured levels; results indicated high variability using either approach. Geer at al.[(68)] utilized DREAM to examine skin exposure in nineteen U.S. manufacturing facilities and found results within the range of similar studies carried out in Europe.[(67,69)] Despite the high variability, DREAM is a promising instrument comparing tasks across a broad range of facilities and for prioritizing tasks for quantitative sampling.

Several other models exist for the assessment of skin exposure, for example models to assess deposition and uptake of solvents for spray painters.[(70,71)] The European research project RISKOFDERM has developed a generic model for dermal risk assessment by considering specific work situations, determinants of exposure, use of personal protective equipment (PPE), and activity time and area of body exposed.[(63,72–74)] Although the model provides quantitative estimates of skin exposure, its purpose is to identify gross exposure situations. A validation study indicated that the model is useful for distinguishing skin exposures among operations, but does not address differences within operations.[75]

If semi-quantitative assessment demonstrates skin contact with a hazardous agent, then a skin protection program that utilizes the industrial hygiene hierarchy of controls (see below) is necessary. Once implemented, a skin protection program should be reviewed to evaluate effectiveness and should be re-evaluated any time that the process is modified or a new chemical introduced. If assessment results are inconclusive or not sufficient to make a decision, then quantitative sampling approaches may be necessary.

Quantitative Exposure Estimates

In situations where semi-quantitative assessment cannot distinguish exposure estimates among exposure scenarios, quantitative measures are needed to allow identification and prioritization of tasks that require control measures. The goal of quantitative assessment is thus to collect sufficient data to permit a decision to be made regarding the level of controls necessary to protect workers' skin. Samples may be collected using removal, interception, and/or in situ techniques, any of which will provide quantitative estimates of exposure. Each of these sampling techniques has unique advantages and disadvantages and the choice will involve consideration for the goal of the skin assessment and the quality of data provided by a given technique. While guidance on the design of a skin sampling strategy is outside the scope of this chapter, the following factors are important to take into consideration. Quantitative measurements of the skin have been shown to vary between body segments (spatial), from day to day (temporal) and from worker to worker (personal).[61] Variability between tasks has also been noted as an important component of the total variability in skin exposure. The importance of the variance components may vary, in part, on the choice of the sampling method; hence, a sampling strategy should take into consideration the variability associated with the sampling method. Additionally, causes of exposure variability should also be taken into consideration; most causes arise from specific circumstances that are local to work settings, such as tasks and other determinants of exposure (i.e., contextual information regarding tasks). Therefore, in addition to the number of workers, the number of locations (body segments) and the number of repeated measurements, the sampling strategy should include consideration of these exposure determinants. The reader is referred to the European Committee for Standardization[76] for additional information on this topic.

Management and Control of Occupational Skin Exposures

Nearly one in five nonfatal occupational illnesses reported in the U.S. was a skin disease or disorder in 2006.[16] While some skin disorders may be relatively minor, many skin diseases such as ICD and ACD are chronic. Because the incidence of skin disorders and diseases is high, these reactions may provide sentinel outcomes that prompt the need for surveillance or indicate non-compliance with established occupational exposure prevention strategies. It must be emphasized that a skin protection strategy is just one component of a well-integrated comprehensive exposure prevention strategy that also accounts for inhalation exposures, housekeeping, maintenance activities and controls.

Hierarchy of Controls

The industrial hygiene hierarchy of controls applies to skin exposure prevention: elimination and substitution › engineering controls › administrative controls › PPE. Elimination or substitution of a hazard is the most effective primary prevention strategy and is especially pertinent for agents that cause immunological disease such as ACD because the effect is life-long. An example of elimination of a skin sensitizer is removal of water-soluble chromate content of cement through the addition of ferrous sulphate.[77] Another example involves the substitution of powdered natural rubber latex (NRL) gloves for non-powdered NRL gloves in the mid to late 1990s, which resulted in a decreased number of sensitized workers and asthma cases.[78–80] Next in preference is the use of engineering controls, which offer the advantage of being reliable because they require minimal operator interaction. Examples of engineering controls include enclosure of a process, use of local exhaust ventilation at an emission source, splash guards on a tank, and process automation or changes to avoid splashes or immersion. Administrative controls are considered a third-tier approach to skin exposure prevention because they do not prevent exposure from occurring in the first place and put some of the burden for skin protection on workers. For example, rotating workers among several processes, one of which includes wet work, may reduce the time each person is potentially exposed, but could increase the number of persons who may come in contact with the skin hazard of concern. The last, and least preferable, type of control for skin exposure prevention is PPE because it places nearly all the burden for skin protection on workers. Additionally, use of PPE is not as reliable as engineering controls. For example, organic chemicals may permeate through protective gloves without knowledge of the worker and splashes may absorb into clothing and provide a reservoir for a contaminant to contact the skin. Use of protective barriers such as clothing and some types of gloves may occlude the skin which will facilitate the permeation of chemicals[81], including potent allergens such as cobalt[82], chromium[83], and nickel.[84] Information on the permeation of chemicals through the gloves and breakthrough time from laboratory tests are published by most manufacturers; however, the published breakthrough times do not take into consideration workplace usage conditions including chemical mixtures and should be used with caution.[85,86] In general, while the use of gloves and PPE is common in many workplaces, the selection of PPE is not always appropriate and the PPE program is often poorly managed.[85] Thus use of gloves or other PPE should be part of a managed PPE program with appropriate management components.

Psychosocial/Behavioral Aspects of Skin Exposure

The dermal exposure route is a pathway driven by behavioral components, and thus examining behavior as an exposure determinant has specific utility in skin exposure assessment. In contrast with inhalation exposure, behavior is an important determinant of skin exposure due to heterogeneity in exposure, as well as the heightened importance of hygiene. Behavioral characteristics have been thought to account for most of the between-worker variability in skin exposure[87], and have been identified as a dominant factor in predicting skin exposure.[88,89] Lumens et al.[90] and Ulenbelt et al.[91] have examined the impact of hygienic behavior on external and internal lead and chromium levels. Accounting for hygienic behavior by determining factors such as whether the worker "washes hands before using the toilet," and by counting "the number of times gloves are taken on and off," nearly doubled the amount of internal dose variability explained by external measures of exposure.

Worker skin protection strategies rely more heavily on worker motivation and self-protective behavior, and less on industrial hygiene measures such as product substitutions and engineering controls. Because the burden of protection is placed heavily upon the worker, behavior becomes a significant determinant of skin exposure. Psychosocial factors that inform behavior include knowledge, attitudes, and perceptions. Geer et al.[92] designed a survey to assess worker knowledge, attitudes and perceptions (KAP) to examine predictors of worker precautionary behavior. The workers' belief in their own ability to control skin exposure using PPE, or PPE self-efficacy, was associated with increased odds of worker self-protective behavior.[68] Vaughan[93] found similar results in immigrant farm workers chronically exposed to pesticides, where self-protective behavior was more likely when workers: 1) felt informed about risks; 2) believed that precautionary methods were effective; and 3) had a greater perception about their own ability to control exposure. Thus increasing worker PPE self-efficacy, and perhaps additional behavioral factors, can increase worker precautionary behavior and greatly enhance worker protection.

Including consideration of relevant behavioral factors in skin exposure assessment may provide a means for better understanding exposure. Such evaluations will provide the basis for effective exposure reduction strategies such as worker education and training, and well-informed PPE selection and availability.

Case Studies

Skin Exposure to the Pesticide Chlorpyrifos

This case study reports on evaluating a range of occupational pesticide exposures through the use of multiple assessment approaches, including skin and inhalation sampling and biological monitoring, and is based on the publication by Geer et al.(94) For this study, a meta-analysis was performed on data accessed and compiled from the USEPA Pesticide Registrant Database under authority of the Federal Insecticide, Fungicide, and Rodenticide Act (FIFRA). Under FIFRA, USEPA has the authority to regulate the use of pesticides to prevent unreasonable adverse human health effects associated with pesticide exposure. Accordingly, the USEPA requires pesticide registrants to perform studies evaluating the potential for pesticide handler exposure. The current study provides such an assessment across a range of studies and job classes. Exposure was assessed using external sampling and biological monitoring, allowing the opportunity to not only evaluate the relative routes of exposure but also to examine the predictive association between the two methods of assessment.

The pesticide Chlorpyrifos (CAS # 2921-88-2), a type of organophosphate pesticide, was selected for this case study because of its prevalent use and toxicity, including neurophysiological effects(95-97) and quality and completeness of data among the registrant studies. In general, the process begins with the pesticide being mixed with water, followed by loading into equipment, and applying by spraying or automation. These activities can continue for several hours during a work shift. Water-based liquid may penetrate common clothing or protective clothing (e.g., pesticide can get under clothing during mixing, application, and post-application scouting). During mixing and loading, there is a high risk for skin exposure to the hands through direct contact with concentrated solutions or splashing. Application can generate a fine aerosol that may deposit on surfaces of the body, on workplace surfaces for cross-contamination, or can be inhaled. During scouting, a worker enters the field after application to check for efficacy, and may come into contact with sprayed surfaces thus contaminating their own skin.

Of approximately 100 registrant studies on file with the USEPA, five were selected for analysis based on inclusion criteria, such as exposure assessment in accordance with USEPA Guidelines[98], and inclusion of biological monitoring. Each worker was monitored once over a period of time representing a standard work shift or duration of application. Eighty workers across four job classes were included: mixer/loaders (M/L, n = 24), mixer/loader/applicators (M/L/A, n = 37), applicators (A, n = 9) and re-entry scouts (RS, n = 10).

Due to the varied nature of pesticide application leading to skin exposure over many regions of the body, a combination of methods was chosen: whole-body dosimetry (WBD) and hand wash sampling. The WBD substrate consisted of underclothing (a short-sleeved T-shirt and briefs). Additionally, all workers wore cotton coveralls. A ball cap was worn as a sampling substrate to estimate exposure to the neck and head. After collection, the coveralls and underclothing were cut into pieces representing potential exposure to body regions such as the arms, legs, front and back torso. Chlorpyrifos was extracted from the clothing and quantified. The amount of chlorpyrifos measured on the underclothing relative to the amount on the coveralls was used to estimate individual site-specific penetration factors (PFs) (i.e., the percentage of chlorpyrifos passing through the coveralls to the skin, for estimation of a skin exposure value). Hand wash samples were collected over the monitoring period during times when workers would typically wash their hands (i.e., before meals, before smoking, after using the bathroom, and at the end of the monitoring period) to assess surface deposition on the hands. Hand wash samples were also collected between tasks to note differences in task contribution. Inhalation exposure was evaluated by personal monitoring capturing both gas and particle phase Chlorpyrifos in workers' breathing zones. Biological monitoring of the primary chlorpyrifos urinary metabolite 3,5,6-trichloro-2-pyridinol (3,5,6-TCP) was performed to measure the absorbed dose of chlorpyrifos. Urine samples were collected one day prior to exposure (background), the day of exposure, and four days following exposure in twelve-hour composites.

Externally derived measures of worker exposure were compared with internal dose levels of the urinary biomarker in concurrently collected samples. The attribution of skin exposure to total exposure was determined. Overall, skin exposure was the predominant route of the combined inhalation and skin exposure in 44% of workers. Among the four job classes investigated, Applicators were consistently ranked as the most highly exposed based on median values of both total externally derived exposure levels and urinary derived dose estimates. Higher exposures among pesticide Applicators have been attributed to frequent spills on the body and improper use and poor condition of PPE. Applicators also had the highest median inhalation values, consistent with exposures due to aerosolization required for application. Skin exposure by itself tended to be highest among Mixer/Loaders where there is risk for hand exposure to concentrated solutions. The high skin exposure in this group was driven by extreme values among a small number of workers, implicating work practices as an exposure determinant.

The relationship between externally derived values and biological monitoring levels was examined in a simple linear regression. Total external estimates of dose (including inhalation and skin) was positively associated with, and accounted for 29% of the variability in the 3,5,6-TCP derived estimate of dose. The final multiple linear regression model including the variables skin dose, inhalation dose and application type (i.e., handwand, groundboom, aerial, or corn planter) explained 46% of the variability in the 3,5,6-TCP derived estimate of dose. The skin dose estimate was marginally significant ($P = 0.06$), while the inhalation dose estimate was not ($P = 0.57$).

The use of WBD to measure skin exposure alters (reduces) the amount of chlorpyrifos absorbed, thereby affecting urinary TCP levels. It is significant to note that despite the added protection afforded by the WBD, 75 of 80 workers had measurable levels of urinary 3,5,6-TCP associated with chlorpyrifos application. Additionally, although each of the registrant studies used a common set of methodological guidelines designed to minimize measurement differences across studies[98], each study was conducted independently and it is possible that there were subtle methodological differences in sampling and/or analysis that resulted in an unknown bias.

This case study highlights the need for skin exposure reduction strategies with a focus on jobs with the highest likelihood for exposure. Attempts at lowering worker exposure potential have included a focus on packaging (e.g., drip-less containers), integrated handling systems and other mechanical transfer systems, as well as enclosure of work processes. Overall, the USEPA Pesticide Registrant Database provided useful information for evaluating pesticide worker exposure and worker exposure assessment methods. These data help demonstrate the significance of the skin as a route of exposure in pesticide workers, and identify the need for methods and research to close the gap between external and internal exposure measures.

Skin Exposure to Isocyanates in the Auto Refinishing Industry

Isocyanates are important industrial chemicals used worldwide to produce a variety of polyurethane products (coatings, foams, adhesives, sealants, etc.). Isocyanates can cause irritation of the eyes, respiratory tract and skin, ACD, and hypersensitivity pneumonitis.[99,100] However, the primary health concern of isocyanate exposures is asthma. Isocyanates remain a leading cause of occupational asthma worldwide.[100–102] Historically, respiratory exposures have been reduced through improved hygiene controls and the use of less volatile isocyanates. Yet isocyanate asthma continues to occur, not uncommonly in settings with minimal inhalation exposure but opportunity for skin exposure.

Isocyanates are used in the auto body repair and refinishing industry for protective coatings in a two-component painting system. The isocyanate and the polyol are mixed in certain amounts in appropriate solvents and the mixture is sprayed onto the part to be coated. Spray painting typically takes place inside a spray booth, although smaller paint jobs may be completed on the shop floor. This industry is dominated by small family-owned businesses with limited financial and human (environmental health and safety) resources. Each auto body shop is a diverse and variable environment. The workflow in an auto body shop is irregular and highly variable between shops and from day-to-day.[103]

The Study of Painters and Repairers of Autobodies by Yale (SPRAY) study was designed as a cross-sectional epidemiologic study of isocyanate asthma in auto body shops, and its initial focus was on respiratory isocyanate exposures.[103–105] In response to field observations of abundant opportunities for isocyanate skin exposures in the auto body shops, the lack of skin exposure data and controls, and increased concerns about possible implications of skin exposure to isocyanates in sensitization and asthma[106], the SPRAY study was expanded to explore qualitative and quantitative skin exposure assessment methodologies and possible relationships with isocyanate asthma.

A task-based exposure assessment strategy was developed for this study, providing a cost-effective way of assessing exposures and identifying opportunities for exposure intervention. Detailed diary information was collected about daily task activities, their frequency, and duration, for each of the workers involved in the study every day during a one-week period. Information was also collected on possible determinants of exposure, such as shop size, business activity, materials and equipment used, engineering controls, work and hygiene practices, and PPE in use. Task-based inhalation and skin exposures to isocyanates were assessed.[103,105,107,108] Personal exposures of each worker for each day over the whole study week were estimated based on an algorithm that combined task frequency and exposure levels corrected for the use of PPE.[105,109,110] For each of the study participants, several health endpoints (respiratory, physiological, and immunological) were determined, including: a respiratory symptoms questionnaire, spirometry (FEV1, FVC, and PERF; forced expiratory volume in 1 sec, forced vital capacity, and peak expiratory flow rate, respectively) and methacholine challenge, and antibody testing (HDI-specific IgE and IgG).[104,111]

Extensive surface contamination and exposure of unprotected skin and under PPE was documented using both a colorimetric semi-quantitative technique[107] and a quantitative wipe method.[108] The highest skin exposures were found to be associated with painting and painting-related tasks, including during spray painting, paint mixing, and cleaning of painting equipment. Surprisingly, skin exposure to isocyanates was also documented during wet and dry sanding of recent paints. Frequent surface contamination (up to 80% of all samples) was documented along the trail of paint handling and use, from the mixing benches and cups to the spray guns and painted surfaces.[107,108] Face, neck, hands, and forearms were the body segments more frequently contaminated with isocyanates (30–40% of all samples). Skin exposure was found under gloves (the most common type being latex), coveralls (Tyvek®) and respirators (commonly half-facepiece).[107,112] The highest glove breakthrough rates were found during cleaning of the spray gun (80%) and spray painting tasks (~20–25%). The highest personal airborne isocyanate exposure levels, with a considerable margin from all other tasks, were measured during spray painting, followed by paint mixing.[103,105] The most important determinants of airborne isocyanate exposures included: task (especially spraying isocyanates), paint volume (size of painting job), spray booth type, and shop characteristics (such as shop size and annual income).[105] These same factors and surface contamination were also the most important determinants of isocyanate skin exposure.[107] The colorimetric indicators were found to be very useful and specific, although of limited sensitivity, for detection of potential surface and skin exposure to isocyanates and for guiding exposure interventions and controls. Both aerosol deposition during spray painting and contact with contaminated surfaces were important pathways resulting in skin contamination.

Using exposure algorithms that combined task-based exposure data, task frequency, and other exposure modifiers and determinants (type and efficiency of PPE, uncovered skin areas and likelihood for contamination, etc.), personal inhalation exposures and skin exposure indices were calculated for each worker.[109,110] Moderate correlation (rs =0.38; p<0.0001) was found between the inhalation and skin exposure estimates, justifying the use of both metrics in regression models of exposure and health outcomes.[110,111] In spite of some generally weak positive trend between inhalation and skin exposure estimates, there were clearly workers with little or no respiratory isocyanate exposures and significant skin exposures. Tasks such as wet sanding and mixing for example would result in substantial skin exposure but little respiratory exposures. Skin exposure was found to be an independent significant risk factor for isocyanate sensitization (development of isocyanate-specific IgG antibodies), in addition to inhalation exposures.[111] Pronk et al.[113] reported that isocyanate-specific IgG was prevalent in up to 50% of the painters and associated better with exposure than asthma (isocyanate-specific IgE antibodies, a more specific measure of asthma, were present in <4% of the spray painters). This is the first epidemiological evidence linking skin exposure to isocyanates with possible sensitization (IgG antibodies), further emphasizing the need for accurate assessments and control of skin exposures.

Acknowledgements

The authors thank Drs. L. Tapp, G.S. Dotson, and R.F. LeBouf at NIOSH for critical review of this chapter. The authors also thank N. Edwards and A.M. Stirnkorb at NIOSH for development of the figures.

References

1. **Occupational Safety and Health Administration (OSHA):** OSHA Technical Manual. Section II: Sampling, Measurement Methods and Instruments. Chapter 2: Occupational Skin Exposure. [Directive Number: 08-05 (TED 01), Updated Effective 06/24/2008]. Available online at http://www.osha.gov/dts/osta/otm/otm_ii/otm_ii_2.html.
2. **American Conference of Governmental Industrial Hygienists® (ACGIH®):** Threshold Limit Values® for Chemical Substances and Physical Agents and Biological Exposure Indices®. Cincinnati, OH: ACGIH®, 2008.
3. **National Institute for Occupational Safety and Health (NIOSH):** NIOSH Pocket Guide to Chemical Hazards. Department of Health and Human Services, Centers for Disease Control, NIOSH. DHHS (NIOSH) Publication No. 2005-149. Cincinnati, OH: National Institute for Occupational Safety and Health, 2005. Available online at http://www.cdc.gov/niosh/npg/default.html.
4. **Federal Register:** Review of NIOSH Draft Current Intelligence Bulletin, "A Strategy for Assigning the New NIOSH Skin Notations for Chemicals," 73(185): 54828-54829; September 23, 2008. Available online at http://www.cdc.gov/niosh/review/public/153/pdfs/DRAFT-CIB-Skin-Notation-Strategy.pdf
5. **U.S. Environmental Protection Agency (EPA):** Dermal exposure assessment: A summary of EPA approaches. National Center for Environmental Assessment, Washington, DC; EPA/600/R-07/040F. 2007. Available from NTIS, Springfield, VA, and online at http://www.epa.gov/ncea.
6. **Agache, P.:** The Human Skin: An overview. In *Measuring the Skin.* Agache, P. and P. Humbert (eds.). Berlin: Springer-Verlag, 2004. pp. 3–5.
7. **Agache, P. and D. Varchon:** Skin Mechanical Function. In *Measuring the Skin.* Agache, P. and P. Humbert (eds.). Berlin: Springer-Verlag, 2004. pp. 429–445.
8. **Pirot, F., Y.N. Kalia, A.L. Stinchcomb, G. Keating, A. Bunge, and R.H. Guy:** Characterization of the permeability barrier of human skin *in vitro. Proc. Natl. Acad. Sci. USA 94*:1562–1567 (1997).
9. **Rogiers, V.:** EEMCO guidance for the assessment of transepidermal water loss in cosmetic sciences. *Skin Pharm. Appl. Skin Physiol. 14*:117–128 (2001).
10. **Agache, P.:** Presentation of the skin surface ecosystem. In *Measuring the Skin.* Agache, P. and P. Humbert (eds.). Berlin: Springer-Verlag, 2004. pp. 21–31.
11. **Pirot, F. and F. Falson:** Skin barrier function. In *Measuring the Skin.* Agache, P. and P. Humbert (eds.). Berlin: Springer-Verlag, 2004. pp. 513–524.
12. **Parra, J.L. and M. Paye:** EEMCO guidance for the in vivo assessment of skin surface pH. *Skin Pharmacol Appl Skin Physiol. 16*:188–202 (2003).
13. **Stefaniak, A.B. and C.J. Harvey:** Dissolution of materials in artificial skin surface film liquids. Toxicol. *In Vitro 20*:1265–1283 (2006).
14. **Gentilhomme, E. and Y. Neveux:** Epidermal Physiology. In *Measuring the Skin.* Agache, P. and P. Humbert (eds.). Berlin: Springer-Verlag, 2004. pp. 165–172.
15. **Agache, P.:** Dermis connective tissue histophysiology. In *Measuring the Skin.* Agache, P. and P. Humbert (eds.). Berlin: Springer-Verlag, 2004. pp. 199–203.
16. **U.S. Bureau of Labor Statistics (USBLS):** Workplace Injuries and Illnesses in 2006. Washington, DC: U.S. Department of Labor, 2007. USDL 07-1562. Available online at http://www.bls.gov/news.release/pdf/osh.pdf.
17. **Lushniak, B.D.:** Occupational contact dermatitis. *Dermatol. Ther. 17*:272–277 (2004).
18. **Ingber, A and S. Merims:** The validity of the Mathias criteria for establishing occupational causation and aggravation of contact dermatitis. *Contact Derm. 51*:9–12 (2004).

19. **Forte, G., F. Petrucci, and B. Bocca:** Metal allergens of growing significance: Epidemiology, immunotoxicology, strategies for testing and prevention. *Inflamm. Allergy- Drug Targets 7*:145–162 (2008).
20. **Cvetkovski, R.S., et al.:** Relation between diagnoses on severity, sick leave and loss of job among patients with occupational hand eczema. *Br. J. Dermatol. 152*:93–98 (2005).
21. **Cvetkovski, R.S., R. Zachariae, H. Jensen, J. Olsen, J.D. Johansen, and T. Agner:** Prognosis of occupational hand eczema: A follow up study. *Arch. Dermatol. 142*:305–311 (2006).
22. **Fowler, J.F., et al.:** Impact of chronic hand dermatitis on quality of life, work productivity, activity impairment, and medical costs. *J. Am. Acad. Dermatol. 54*:448–457 (2006).
23. **Shelnutt, S.R., P. Goad, and D.V. Belsito:** Dermatological toxicity of hexavalent chromium. *Crit. Rev. Toxicol. 37*:375–387 (2007).
24. **Karlberg, A.-T., M.A. Bergström, A. Börje, K. Luthman, and J.L.G. Nilsson:** Allergic contact dermatitis- formation, structural requirements, and reactivity of skin sensitizers. *Chem. Res. Toxicol. 21*:53–69 (2008).
25. **Santos, R. and A. Goossens:** An update on airborne contact dermatitis: 2001–2006. *Contact Derm. 57*:353–360 (2007).
26. **Redlich, C.A. and C.A. Herrick:** Lung/skin connections in occupational lung disease. *Curr. Opin. Allergy Clin. Immunol. 8*:115–119 (2008).
27. **Rosenthal, F.S., S.K. West, B. Munoz, E.A. Emmett, P.T. Strickland, and H.R. Taylor:** Ocular and facial skin exposure to ultraviolet radiation in sunlight: a personal exposure model with application to a worker population. *Health Phys. 61(1)*:77–86 (1991).
28. **Sliney, D.H.:** Laser safety. *Lasers Surge Med. 16*:215–225 (1995).
29. **Zajkowska, J. and T. Hermanowska-Szpakowicz:** Anthrax as biological warfare weapon. *Med. Pr. 53(2)*:167–172 (2002).
30. **Walberg, J.E.:** Other Metals. In *Handbook of Occupational Dermatology*. Kanerva, L., P. Elsner, J.E. Wahlberg, and H.I. Maibach (eds.). Berlin: Springer-Verlag, 2000. p. 551.
31. **Aubin, F.:** Skin immune system. In *Measuring the Skin*. Agache, P. and P. Humbert (eds.). Berlin: Springer-Verlag, 2004. pp. 583–590.
32. **Arts, J.H.E., C. Mommers, and C. de Heer:** Dose-response relationships and threshold levels in skin and respiratory allergy. *Crit. Rev. Toxicol. 36*:219–251 (2006).
33. **Ness, S.A.:** Dermal Sampling Techniques. In *Surface and Dermal Monitoring for Toxic Exposures*. New York: Van Nostrand Reinhold, 1994. pp. 265–362.
34. **European Committee for Standardization (CEN):** Workplace Exposure. Measurement of Dermal Exposure. Principles and Methods. Brussels, Belgium: CEN, 2006. CEN/TS 15279.
35. **Que Hee, S.S., B. Peace, C.S. Clark, J.R. Boyle, R.L. Bornschein, and P.B. Hammond:** Evolution of efficient methods to sample lead sources, such as house dust and hand dust, in the homes of children. *Environ. Res. 38*:77–95 (1985).
36. **Lidén, C., L. Skare, B. Lind, G. Nise, and M. Vahter:** Assessment of skin exposure to nickel, chromium and cobalt by acid wipe sampling and ICP-MS. *Contact Derm. 54*:233–238 (2006).
37. **Marquart, H., D.H. Brouwer, and J.J. van Hemmen:** Removing pesticides from the hands with a simple washing procedure using soap and water. *J. Occup. Environ. Med. 44*:1075–1082 (2002).
38. **Fenske, R.A., N.J. Simcox, J.E. Camp, and C.J. Hines:** Comparison of three methods for assessment of hand exposure. *Appl. Occup. Environ. Hyg. 37*:618–623 (1999).
39. **Surakka, J., S. Johnsson, G. Rosén, T. Lindh, and T. Fischer:** A method for measuring dermal exposure to multifunctional acrylates. *J. Environ. Monit. 1*:533–540 (1999).
40. **Kezic, S.:** Methods for measuring in-vivo percutaneous absorption in humans. *Hum. Exp. Toxicol. 27*:289–95 (2008).
41. **Linnainmaa, M. and M. Kiilunen:** Urinary cobalt as a measure of exposure in the wet sharpening of hard metal and stellite blades. *Int. Arch. Occup. Environ. Health 69*:193–200 (1997).
42. **Day, G.A., et al.:** Exposure pathway assessment at a copper-beryllium alloy facility. *Ann. Occup. Hyg. 51*:67–80 (2007).
43. **Brouwer, D.H., R. Kroese, and J.J. van Hemmen:** Transfer of contaminants from surface to hands: experimental assessment of linearity of the exposure process, adherence to the skin, and area exposed during fixed pressure and repeated contact with surfaces contaminated with a powder. *Appl. Occup. Environ. Hyg. 14*:231–239 (1999).
44. **Cherrie, J.W., D.H. Brouwer, M. Roff, R. Vermeulen, and H. Kromhout:** Use of qualitative and quantitative fluorescence techniques to assess dermal exposure. *Ann. Occup. Hyg. 44*:519–522 (2000).
45. **Brouwer, D.H., C.M. Lansink, J.W. Cherrie, and J.J. van Hemmen:** Assessment of dermal exposure during airless spray painting using a quantitative visualization technique. *Ann. Occup. Hyg. 44(7)*:543–549 (2000).

46. **Doran, E.M., M.G. Yost, and R.A. Fenske:** Measuring dermal exposure to pesticide residues with attenuated total reflectance Fourier transform infrared (ATR-FTIR) spectroscopy. *Bull. Environ. Contam. Toxicol. 64(5)*:666–672 (2000).
47. **Fenske, R.A., S.M. Wong, J.T. Leffingwell, and R.C. Spear:** A video imaging technique for assessing dermal exposure. II. Fluorescent tracer testing. *Am. Ind. Hyg. Assoc. J. 47*:771–775 (1986).
48. **Archibald, B.A., K.R. Solomon, and G.R. Stephenson:** A new procedure for calibrating the video imaging technique for assessing dermal exposure to pesticides. *Arch. Environ. Cont. Toxicol. 26*:398–402 (1994).
49. **Roff, M.W.:** A novel lighting system for the measurement of dermal exposure using a fluorescent dye and an image processor. *Ann. Occup. Hyg. 38*:903–919 (1994).
50. **Bierman, E.P.B., D.H. Brouwer, and J.J. van Hemmen:** Implementation and evaluation of the fluorescent tracer technique in greenhouse exposure studies. *Ann. Occup. Hyg. 42*:467–475 (1998).
51. **Carden, A., M.G. Yost, and R.A. Fenske:** Noninvasive method for the assessment of dermal uptake of pesticides using attenuated total reflectance infrared spectroscopy. *Appl. Spectrosc. 59*:293–299 (2005).
52. **National Institute for Occupational Safety and Health (NIOSH):** Elements on Wipes: Method 9102. NIOSH Manual of Analytical Methods (NMAM), 4th edition, 3rd suppl., U.S. Department of Health and Human Services, Public Health Service, CDC, NIOSH. 2003. Available online at http://www.cdc.gov/niosh/nmam/new.html.
53. **Occupational Safety and Health Administration (OSHA):** Evaluation Guidelines for Surface Sampling Methods. T-006-01-0104-M. OSHA Salt Lake Technical Center, Salt Lake City UT. Page last updated 10/11/2007. Available online at http://www.osha.gov/dts/sltc/methods/surfacesampling/surfacesampling.html.
54. **Cherrie, J.W. and A. Robertson:** Biologically relevant assessment of dermal exposure. *Ann. Occup. Hyg. 39*:387–92 (1995).
55. **Agache, P.:** Skin absorption in man in vivo. In *Measuring the Skin.* Agache, P. and P. Humbert (eds.). Berlin: Springer-Verlag, 2004. pp. 525–548.
56. **Bronaugh, R.L.:** A flow-through diffusion cell. In *In Vitro Percutaneous Absorption: Principles, Fundamentals, and Applications.* Bronaugh, R.L. and H.I. Maibach (eds.). New York: CRC Press, 199. pp. 18–20.
57. **Chester, G.:** Evaluation of agricultural worker exposure to, and absorption of, pesticides. *Ann. Occup. Hyg. 37(5)*:509–523 (1993).
58. **Woollen, B.H.:** Biological monitoring for pesticide absorption. *Ann. Occup. Hyg. 37(5)*:525–540 (1993).
59. **Krieger, R.I.:** Pesticide exposure assessment. *Toxicol. Lett. 82-83*:65–72 (1995).
60. **Kim, D. and L.A. Nylander-French:** Physiologically based toxicokinetic models and their application in human exposure and internal dose assessment. *EXS 99*:37–55 (2009).
61. **Kromhout, H. and R. Vermeulen:** Temporal, personal and spatial variability in dermal exposure. *Ann. Occup. Hyg. 45(4)*:257–273 (2001).
62. **Boogaard, P.J.:** Biomonitoring as a tool in the human health risk characterization of dermal exposure. *Hum. Exp. Toxicol. 27(4)*:297–305 (2008).
63. **Oppl, R., F. Kalberlah, P.G. Evans, and J.J. van Hemmen:** A toolkit for dermal risk assessment and management: an overview. *Ann. Occup. Hyg. 47(8)*:629–640 (2003).
64. **van Wendel de Joode, B., D.H. Brouwer, R. Vermeulen, J.J. van Hemmen, D. Heederik, and H. Kromhout:** DREAM: a method for semi-quantitative dermal exposure assessment. *Ann. Occup. Hyg. 47(1)*:71–87 (2003).
65. **Schneider, T., R. Vermeulen, D.H. Brouwer, J.W. Cherrie, H. Kromhout, and C.L. Fogh:** Conceptual model for assessment of dermal exposure. *Occup. Environ. Med. 56*:765–773 (1999).
66. **Cherrie, J.W., T. Schneider, S. Spankie, and M. Quinn:** A new method for structured, subjective assessments of past concentrations. *Occup. Hyg. 3*:73–83 (1996).
67. **van Wendel de Joode, B., R. Vermeulen, J.J. van Hemmen, W. Fransman, and H. Kromhout:** Accuracy of a semiquantitative method for Dermal Exposure Assessment (DREAM). *Occup. Environ. Med. 62(9)*:623–632 (2005).
68. **Geer, L.A., et al.:** Survey assessment of worker dermal exposure and underlying behavioral determinants. *J. Occup. Environ. Hyg. 4(11)*:809–820 (2007).
69. **Tielemans, E., et al.:** Exposure profiles of pesticides among greenhouse workers: implications for epidemiological studies. *J. Expo. Sci. Environ. Epidemiol. 17(6)*:501–509 (2007).
70. **Brouwer, D.H., S. Semple, J. Marquart, and J.W. Cherrie:** A dermal model for spray painters. Part I: subjective exposure modeling of spray paint deposition. *Ann. Occup. Hyg. 45(1)*:15–23 (2001).
71. **Semple, S., D.H. Brouwer, F. Dick, and J.W. Cherrie:** A dermal model for spray painters. Part II: estimating the deposition and uptake of solvents. *Ann. Occup. Hyg. 45(1)*:25–33 (2001).

72. **Warren, N., H.A. Goede, S.C.H.A. Tijssen, R. Oppl, H.J. Schipper, and J.J. van Hemmen:** Deriving default dermal exposure values for use in a risk assessment toolkit for small and medium-sized enterprises. *Ann. Occup. Hyg. 47*:619–627 (2003).
73. **Marquart, J., D.H. Brouwer, H.J. Gijsbers, I.H.M. Links, N. Warren, and J.J. van Hemmen:** Determinants of dermal exposure relevant for exposure modelling in regulatory risk assessment. *Ann. Occup. Hyg. 47(8)*:599–607 (2003).
74. **Goede, H.A., et al.:** Classification of dermal exposure modifiers and assignment of values for a risk assessment toolkit. *Ann. Occup Hyg. 47(8)*:609–618 (2003).
75. **Kromhout, H., W. Fransman, R. Vermeulen, M. Roff, and J.J. van Hemmen:** Variability of task-based dermal exposure measurements from a variety of workplaces. *Ann. Occup. Hyg. 48(3)*:187–196 (2004).
76. **European Committee for Standardization (CEN):** Workplace Exposure. Strategy for the Evaluation of Dermal Exposure. Brussels, Belgium: CEN, 2006. CEN/TR 15278.
77. **Avnstorp, C.:** Risk factors for cement eczema. *Contact Derm. 25*:81–88 (1991).
78. **Charous, B.L., et al.:** Natural rubber latex allergy after 12 years: recommendations and perspectives. *J. Allergy Clin. Immunol. 109(1)*:31–34 (2002).
79. **Charous, B.L., S.M. Tarlo, M.A. Charous, and K. Kelly:** Natural rubber latex allergy in the occupational setting. *Methods 27(1)*:15–21 (2002).
80. **Zeiss, C.R., et al.:** Latex hypersensitivity in Department of Veterans Affairs health care workers: glove use, symptoms, and sensitization. *Ann. Allergy Asthma Immunol. 91*:539–545 (2003).
81. **Ramsing, D.W. and T. Agner:** Effect of glove occlusion on human skin (II): Long-term experimental exposure. *Contact Derm. 34*:258–262 (1996).
82. **Allenby, C.F. and D.A. Basketter:** Minimum eliciting patch test concentrations of cobalt. *Contact Derm. 20*:185–190 (1989).
83. **Gammelgaard, B., A. Fullerton, C. Avnstorp, and T. Menné:** Permeation of chromium salts through human skin *in vitro*. *Contact Derm. 27*:302–310 (1992).
84. **Fullerton, A., J.R. Andersen, A. Hoelgaard, and T. Menné:** Permeation of nickel salts through human skin *in vitro*. *Contact Derm. 15*:173–177 (1986).
85. **Evans ,P.G., J.J. McAlinden, and P. Griffin:** Personal protective equipment and dermal exposure. *Appl. Occup. Environ. Hyg. 16(2)*:334–37 (2001).
86. **Cherrie, J.W., S. Semple, and D. Brouwer:** Gloves and dermal exposure to chemicals: proposals for evaluating workplace effectiveness. *Ann. Occup. Hyg. 48(7)*:607–615 (2004).
87. **Vermeulen, R., P. Stewart, and H. Kromhout:** Dermal exposure assessment in occupational epidemiologic research. *Scand. J. Work Environ. Health 28(6)*:371–385 (2002).
88. **Rutz, R. and R.I. Krieger:** Exposure to pesticide mixer/loaders and applicators in California. *Rev. Environ. Contam. Toxicol. 129*:121–139 (1992).
89. **Wakefield, J.:** Human exposure assessment: find out what's getting in. *Environ. Health Perspect. 108(12)*:A559–565 (2000).
90. **Lumens, M.E.G.L., P. Ulenbelt, R.F.M. Herber, and T.F. Meyman:** The impact of hygienic behavior and working methods on the uptake of lead and chromium. *Appl. Occup. Environ. Hyg. 9(1)*:53–56 (1994).
91. **Ulenbelt, P., M.E.G.L. Lumens, H.M.A. Geron, R.F.M. Herber, S. Broersen, and R.L. Sielhuis:** Work hygiene behavior as modifier of the lead air-lead blood relation. *Int. Arch. Occup. Environ. Health 62*:203–207 (1990).
92. **Geer, L.A., B.A. Curbow, D.H. Anna, P.S. Lees, and T.J. Buckley:** Development of a questionnaire to assess worker knowledge, attitudes and perceptions underlying dermal exposure. *Scand. J. Work Environ. Health 32(3)*:209–218 (2006).
93. **Vaughan, E.:** Chronic exposure to an environmental hazard: Risk perceptions and self protective behavior. *Health Psychol. 12*:74–85 (1993).
94. **Geer, L.A., et al.:** Comparative analysis of passive dosimetry and biomonitoring for assessing Chlorpyrifos exposure in pesticide workers. *Ann. Occup. Hyg. 48(8)*:683–695 (2004).
95. **U.S. Environmental Protection Agency (EPA):** Full record for Chlorpyrifos. Integrated Risk Information System. 1988. Available online at http://www.epa.gov/iris/subst/0026.htm.
96. **Albers, J.W., et al.:** Analysis of Chlorpyrifos exposure and human health: expert panel report. *J. Toxicol. Environ. Health B. Crit. Rev. 2(4)*:301–324 (1999).
97. **U.S. Environmental Protection Agency (EPA):** Revised Human Health Risk Assessment for Chlorpyrifos and Agreement with Registrants. 2000. Available online at http://www.epa.gov/pesticides/op/chlorpyrifos.htm.
98. **U.S. Environmental Protection Agency (EPA):** Harmonized OPPTS Test Guidelines Series 875- Occupational and Residential Exposure Test Guidelines, Group B Post Application Exposure Monitoring Test Guidelines. Office of Prevention, Pesticides, and Toxic Substances. 1998.
99. **Goossens, A., T. Detienne, and M. Bruze:** Occupational allergic contact dermatitis caused by isocyanates. *Contact Derm. 47(5)*:304–308 (2002).

100. **Redlich, C.A., D. Bello, and A.V. Wisnewski:** Isocyanate Exposures and Health Effects. In *Environmental and Occupational Medicine.* Rom, W.N. (ed.). Philadelphia, PA: Lippincott-Raven, 2007. pp. 502–516.
101. **Di Stefano, F., S. Siriruttanapruk, J. McCoach, M. Di Gioacchino, and P.S. Burge:** Occupational asthma in a highly industrialized region of UK: report from a local surveillance scheme. *Allerg. Immunol. (Paris) 36(2)*:56–62 (2004).
102. **Wisnewski, A.V., C.A. Redlich, C.E. Mapp, and D.I. Bernstein:** Polyisocyanates and their Prepolymers. In *Asthma in the Workplace.* Bernstein, L.I., M. Chan-Yeung, J.-L. Malo, and D.I. Bernstein (eds.). London: Taylor & Francis, 2006. pp. 481–504.
103. **Redlich, C.A., et al.:** Subclinical immunologic and physiologic responses in hexamethylene diisocyanate-exposed auto body shop workers. *Am. J. Ind. Med. 39(6)*:587–597 (2001).
104. **Sparer, J., et al.:** Isocyanate exposures in autobody shop work: the SPRAY study. *J. Occup. Environ. Hyg. 1(9)*:570–581 (2004).
105. **Woskie, S.R., et al.:** Determinants of isocyanate exposures in auto body repair and refinishing shops. *Ann. Occup. Hyg. 48(5)*:393–403 (2004).
106. **Bello, D., et al.:** Skin exposure to isocyanates: reasons for concern. *Environ. Health Perspect. 115(3)*:328–335 (2007).
107. **Liu, Y., et al.:** Skin exposure to aliphatic polyisocyanates in the auto body repair and refinishing industry: a qualitative assessment. *Ann. Occup. Hyg. 51(5)*:429–439 (2007).
108. **Bello, D., et al.:** Skin exposure to aliphatic polyisocyanates in the auto body repair and refinishing industry: II. A quantitative assessment. *Ann. Occup. Hyg. 52(2)*:117–124 (2008).
109. **Woskie, S.R., et al.:** Comparison of task-based exposure metrics for an epidemiologic study of isocyanate inhalation exposures among autobody shop workers. *J. Occup. Environ. Hyg. 5(9)*:588–598 (2008).
110. **Liu, Y., et al.:** Skin exposure to aliphatic polyisocyanates in the auto body repair and refinishing industry: III. A personal exposure algorithm. *Ann. Occup. Hyg. 53(1)*:33–40 (2009).
111. **Stowe, M.H., et al.:** Cross-sectional SPRAY study of auto body workers expose to isocyanates: Effects of skin and respiratory exposures. Poster presented at the Intl. Conf. of Occupational and Environmental Exposure of Skin to Chemicals, Golden, CO, June 13–17, 2007.
112. **Liu, Y., et al.:** Qualitative assessment of isocyanate skin exposure in auto body shops: a pilot study. *Am. J. Ind. Med. 37(3)*:265–274 (2000).
113. **Pronk, A., et al.:** Respiratory symptoms, sensitization, and exposure response relationships in spray painters exposed to isocyanates. *Am. J. Respir. Crit. Care Med. 176(11)*:1090–97 (2007).

Outcome Competencies

After completing this chapter, the reader should be able to:

1. Define underlined terms used in this chapter.
2. Understand the anatomical and physiological characteristics of skin and describe the contribution of these characteristics to skin penetration.
3. Discuss the importance of the skin route of exposure.
4. Recognize conditions for skin exposure to occur.
5. Assess the variables associated with percutaneous absorption in an occupational setting.
6. Discuss the significance of industrial dermatoses.

Key Terms

acne • appendages • contact dermatitis • delayed hypersensitivity • dermatitis • desmosome • differential diagnosis • first-pass metabolism • hydration • intermediate filament • keratinocyte activation • occupational skin disease • perfusion • photosensitization • sensitization • skin care products • skin lesions • skin notation • skin penetration • stratum corneum • urticarial reactions • vehicle • wound healing

Prerequisite Knowledge

Anatomy (basic terminology; cell structure); physical chemistry (molecule structure, hydrophilicity and lipophilicity, ionization); biochemistry (membrane structure and function, xenobiotic metabolism, phase I and II enzymes, basics of gene regulation)

Key Topics

I. The Scenario of Occupational Skin Exposure

II. Macroscopic, microscopic, and molecular properties of skin
   A. Hypodermis
   B. Dermis
   C. Epidermis
   D. Cutaneous metabolism
   E. Stratum corneum
   F. Skin appendages

III. Biological differences and variations in skin properties
   A. Age
   B. Gender
   C. Race
   D. Biological conditions

IV. Environmental factors and skin penetration
   A. Physical Factors
   B. Chemical agents
   C. Disease
   D. Wound healing

V. Clinical evaluation of the skin
   A. Contact dermatitis
   B. Irritant reactions
   C. Allergic contact reactions
   D. Photosensitization
   E. Other reactions

The Development of Occupational Skin Disease

21

By Lutz W. Weber, PhD, DABT

The Scenario of Occupational Skin Exposure

One of the earliest works dealing clearly with matters of occupational medicine as well as health and safety is Georgius Agricola's (1494–1555) De Re Metallica(1), first published in 1556. Among many other matters this tome elaborates on descriptions of occupational ailments, protective clothing, workplace hazards, and safety. Agricola emphasized that "there is no compensation which should be thought great enough to equalize the extreme dangers to safety and life."[1] Even 450 years later, this perception stands up to any review.

In 1775, Percival Pott, a London physician, made his famous "Chirurgical observations relative to the cancer of scrotum in chimney sweeps", a first correlation of occupational exposure and skin-related disease. Industrial revolution brought large-scale chemical manufacturing, and in 1899, Herxheimer[2], while observing that many workers in the organochlorine industry suffered from a persistent skin disease, coined the term "chloracne." The true cause of this disease are polychlorinated aromatic hydrocarbons, in particular 2,3,7,8-tetrachlorodibenzo-p-dioxin (TCDD), first recognized by Schulz[3] on the occasion of an industrial accident in the 1950s. Schulz also noticed that the effects of this chemical, even when deposited on skin only, were systemic, asserting that skin penetration had occurred. Because of the diversity of toxicities it has proven challenging to develop best means of estimating dermal exposure across a broad panels of chemicals.

In 1997, a single incident riveted the attention of safety and health professionals on the seriousness of dermal absorption of toxicants. A distinguished professor of chemistry (a 48-year old woman) died following brief exposure in her laboratory to one or a few drops of dimethyl mercury that had leaked across a latex glove.(4) This incident emphasized in a striking fashion the importance of appropriate dermal protection, given the silent latency between exposure and symptoms for this and other compounds. Certainly, strategies for effective intervention must precede the accident investigation stage. These historical examples aim at giving the reader an idea of the importance of skin exposures in the occupational setting. Dermal issues figure prominently among major occupational or public health learning lessons. Skin disease and/or exposure are not arcane subjects, but rather represent issues of global proportions.

Despite the availability of personal protective equipment (PPE) it would be naïve to assume that it affords complete protection from workplace exposure. Materials of PPE construction fail after a certain time known as breakthrough time.[5,6] But not only the substance per se affects PPE breakthrough time, the vehicle and "inert" compounding agents can cause PPE materials to fail.[7] Furthermore, significant differences may exist between materials of identical specifications, but originating from different batches[8] or manufacturers.[9,10] Finally, the mechanical stress that goes along with the use of PPE, in particular, gloves, contributes to protection failure.[11] Thus, the choice of appropriate PPE has to be made on a case-by-case basis, considering the substance of interest and all pertinent workplace conditions.[12–14] For comprehensive treatments on PPE see.[15,16]

In this chapter the terms "epidermal" and "dermal" will be used to specifically refer to the skin layers of epidermis and dermis. When the combination of both layers and the stratum corneum, with or without hypodermis, is being referred to, the terms "skin," "cutaneous," or "percutaneous" will be used.

Skin absorption is the major route of occupational exposure[17] to a plethora of compounds such as industrial cleaners and solvents, chemical intermediates, lipid-soluble pesticides, and the historically important polychlorinated biphenyls (PCBs).[18] The American Conference of Governmental Industrial Hygienists (ACGIH®) therefore recognizes the importance of dermal exposure by designating some compounds with a "skin notation" attached to the Threshold Limit Value (TLV®).[19]

Occupational skin disease (OSD) ranks second among occupational diseases; repeated trauma disorders rank first. For reasons unknown, younger workers and women are at a higher than average risk of OSD. Data from the Bureau of Labor Statistics indicate that in the U.S. the overall incidence of OSD has declined from 8.2 cases in 1993 to 3.7 in 2007 per 10,000 full-time workers, corresponding to 62,900 and 35,300 total cases, respectively. The average absence from work due to reported OSD was about 7 days. About one-third of the cases had no time lost from work, another third resulted in 1 to 5 days lost. But more worrisome is the fact that close to 6%—one in fifteen— of the cases caused 1 month or more lost from work. In 2001, the highest incidence for OSD was observed in agricultural and forestry occupations, with 17.5 cases per 10,000 full-time workers, followed by manufacturing with 9.3 per 10,000; mining, surprisingly, showed an incidence of OSD of only 0.2 per 10,000. Very high (or maybe better recorded) rates of OSD occur among those working in industries where oil and grease exposures are common, in those where animals or their products are handled, in those classified as bakeries, and among hairdressers; incidences in excess of 100 per 10,000 full-time workers have been recorded. The resulting cost is high, both for the worker in terms of disability and for industry in terms of days lost and combined medical and compensation dollars spent (estimates go as high as $1 billion per year). Despite the recorded decline, there is still plenty of incentive to reduce the incidence of occupational skin disease even further. These figures for officially reported OSD may underestimate the true incidence, yet overestimate the days lost from work. It would be most helpful to know exactly why the rates of OSD have decreased over recent years in order to implement improved occupational safety measures.

Skin contact may be the toxicologically most significant route of exposure for comparatively small molecules (molecular weight of 500 or less[20]) exhibiting low volatility. As a general rule, when low volatility compounds elicit pronounced health effects, the possibility of dermal absorption must be factored into any risk estimate. Another factor that may enhance the dermal absorption of a chemical agent is a relatively high lipophilicity; compounds more soluble in oil than in water (partition coefficient >50) tend to penetrate the skin more readily. However, many more factors affect cutaneous penetration, and probably no other occupational health area requires the integration of such diverse exposure assessment and clinical skills to address what must be described as a multidimensional dermal absorption and disease problem.[21–23]

Skin absorption in an industrial setting can occur on direct dermal contact with solids, liquids, solutions, or on exposure to associated vapors. Although vapor absorption through the skin is important for high toxicity compounds, it represents a complex topic.[24] It is important to remember that the effective surface area for vapors almost invariably exceeds the estimated area for liquid exposure because of the difficulty of providing whole body protection and because personal protective equipment is typically provided for limited body surfaces, e.g., hands, arms, front of the trunk, and face.

The process of skin absorption is indeed critical, but the key question is whether there are any effects, either local (e.g., cutaneous irritation) or systemic (i.e., in target organs distant from the site of exposure). It is most important to keep in mind that skin absorption is likely to cause systemic exposure. When industrial chemicals are absorbed, one must evaluate first whether dermatitis occurs, and second, whether sufficient quantities have been absorbed to create a significant internal dose. The presence of dermatitis can often be readily determined by visual examination of the skin, but determining whether absorption will create a significant enough internal dose to be of concern is quite challenging. The fact that a chemical is transferred into the bloodstream does not necessarily make it toxic, and the fact that only small amounts are transported via blood does not necessarily render a chemical harmless.

Macroscopic, Microscopic, and Molecular Properties of Skin

In anatomical terms, the skin is very appropriately called the integument, or protective cover of the body. "The skin, the largest organ in the body, is covered by the epidermis — a multilayered, stratified, cornified epithelium that is highly specialized to protect the body from a diverse range of external insults that include mechanical trauma, microbial invasion, chemical damage and entry of allergens."[25] With a total weight of close to 4 kg and a surface area of almost 2 m^2 (19,400 cm^2; 3010 sq. inch; 20.9 sq. ft.), skin is indeed the largest organ in the body[26] (some surface values that are important in occupational assessment are compiled in Table 21.1).

The understanding of what "skin" means has evolved dramatically over the past four or five decades. From that of a vascularized matrix (dermis) covered by a dividing cell layer (epidermis) covered by a lipid membrane (stratum corneum), to a structured, fibril-enforced, extracellular matrix with marked metabolic capability covered by 3 layers of differentiating, fibril-linked cells that produce a cover layer described as "brick and mortar" structure, to an organ with multiple, highly specialized cell types, protected by a host of immunocompetent cells and an outer layer that, with the help of molecular biology methods, has been shown to be anything but just "a membrane." Thus, skin is a highly complex organ with important metabolic and immunological functions that can extend, on the molecular level, to specific responses to mechanical and chemical trauma mediated by epithelium-specific proteins, the keratins.

The skin consists of four layers: stratum corneum (SC) (aka the horny layer), epidermis or cuticle, dermis or corium (epidermis and dermis together are also called cutis), and hypodermis or subcutis (Figure 21.1). In humans all skin layers vary in thickness from one body region to another, in part as a reflection of exposure to mechanical stress, in part as the result of anatomical features. The thickness of the SC varies over a wide range, from as little as 5 µm at the eyelids or the scrotum to possibly more than 1000 µm in the palms and soles (Table 21.2). For most

Table 21.1 — Surface Areas of the Human Body with Thickness of the Stratum Corneum

	Surface, man (170 cm, 70 kg) m^2	Surface, woman (160 cm, 58 kg) m^2	Thickness of the stratum corneum µm
Total	1.94 (20.9 ft^2, 3010 inches^2)	1.69 (18.2 ft^2, 2620 inches^2)	20[A]
Trunk	0.57	0.54	15/10.5[B]
Arms	0.23	0.21	16
Hands	0.084	0.075	50/400[C]
Head	0.12	0.11	13[D]
Legs	0.51	0.49	15
Feet	0.11	0.098	50/600[E]
Scrotum	—	—	5

Note: Compiled from reference 24, where confidence intervals can be found.
[A]Average
[B]Abdomen/back
[C]Back/palm
[D]Forehead
[E]Back/sole

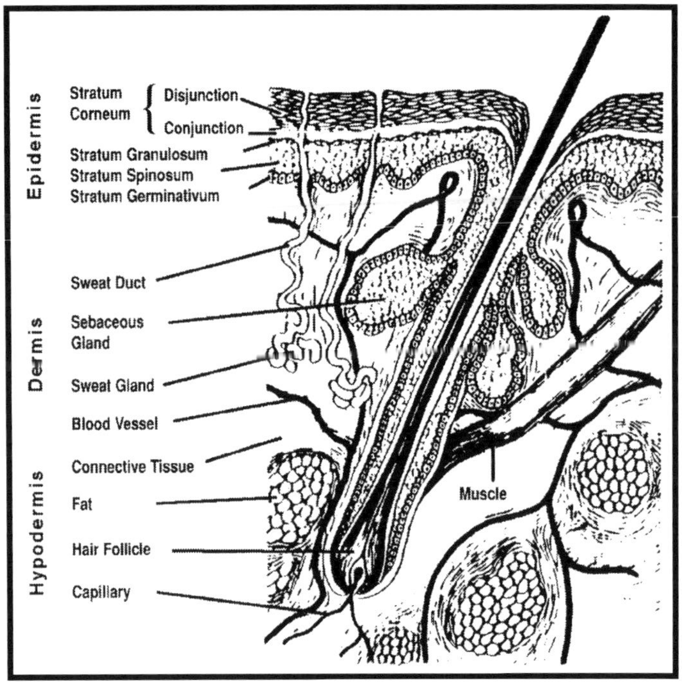

Figure 21.1 — Anatomy of the integument.

of the body surface (abdomen, back, thighs), however, SC thickness is rather uniform, namely, 10 to 20 µm. This layer is subject to constant renewal; the process is described later in connection with epidermis. The interface between epidermis and dermis is not a simple plane but more like a hill and valley structure in which the hills are known as papillae. epidermis varies also. To some extent the epidermis smoothes the numerous papillae that form the surface of dermis (Figure 21.1) and its thickness also changes somewhat with body area. In humans the epidermis is on average 160 µm thick. The border between dermis and subcutis is even less clearly defined, not the least on behalf of sweat glands and sebaceous glands and their respective ducts, all of which reach across the border of these two layers. The average thickness of dermis is given as 1250 µm but ranges from 300 to 3000 µm, often paralleling the thickness of the SC. Subcutaneous fat displays the most variation in thickness, not only between body regions, but also between individuals. It is about five times as thick in women as it is in men (Table 21.2)[(26)]. For the sake of following the course of physiological evolvement of skin, and in a reflection of the increasing complexity of the skin layers, the subsequent paragraphs will describe these layers from the deeper toward the superficial ones.

The epidermis and SC can be visualized as cells migrating outward: the cells proliferate; undergo terminal differentiation by producing keratin filaments to interconnect; increase keratin content and form lamellar bodies while losing water; extrude lipid into the intercellular space via exocytosis of lamellar bodies; die; compact; and are finally shed from the surface of the skin. One cycle of renewal, on average, lasts 28 days. The process advances at elevated speed in many skin diseases (e.g., psoriasis), allowing immature cells to become part of the SC, which impairs its barrier function severely. This has very practical implications in terms of removing psoriatic patients from the workplace in certain industries because of their much increased susceptibility towards many chemicals.

Hypodermis

Adipocytes are the major cellular component of the hypodermis, embedded in a strong extracellular matrix. This adipose layer not only provides thermal insulation to the organism, but also affords protection to mechanically stressed areas of the body, such as the palms and soles, and supplies lipids as a source of metabolic energy.

Table 21.2 — Layers of the Human Skin

	Thickness^A (µm)	Weight^B (g)	Blood Flow (L/min)
Stratum corneum (dead cells)	5<20>1000	—	N/A
Epidermis (living cells)	160^C	310; 270	N/A
Dermis (connective tissue, blood)	300<1250>3000	2400; 2100	0.2
Hypodermis (subcutaneous fat)	1375; 6600^B	2700; 111,500	0.15

Note: All weights in this table are calculated as thickness times surface area (from Table 21.2).
^A Values are given as minimum < average > maximum
^B Dual values refer to men; women
^C Average value; changes slightly with thickness of stratum corneum

The functional portions of sweat glands and of sebaceous glands can be found here as well as in the overlying dermis. The hypodermis is not known to contain any mentionable enzyme activities for metabolism of foreign substances (xenobiotics).

The subcutaneous fat melds together with the reticular layer of the dermis. Together with the rest of the adipose tissue it can represent a formidable reservoir for lipophilic material; otherwise, it has no known importance for skin penetration. Note that blood perfusion of adipose tissue, given its larger volume, is much less than that of dermis, making it a rather deep compartment in pharmacokinetic terms.

Dermis

In contrast to the epidermis, the dermis is richly vascularized. It is by far the thickest and thus largest portion of the skin, amounting to about 2.4 kg in men and 2.1 kg in women (Table 21.2). It has two layers, the stratum papillare or papillary layer on top, and the stratum reticulare or reticular layer below. The stratum papillare is the skin layer that is perfused; it also contains lymphatic vessels, sweat and sebaceous ducts, and tactile nerves. This layer is mainly made up of interlacing bundles of fine fibrils, whereas the reticular layer consists of fibroelastic connective tissue, mostly collagen. Dermal cells are typically fibroblasts and histiocytes that contain phase I and II enzymes similar to epidermis. Assuming that most material that penetrates the skin this far will be collected by blood and lymphatic vessels, the first-pass enzymes of the dermis may come into play only once the first-pass capacity of epidermis and the primary collecting capacity of the vessels have been overwhelmed.

In terms of toxicology this means that any effects of a substance that has penetrated the stratum corneum and reaches the epidermis will be local, while those effects can become systemic when a substance enters the bloodstream in the dermis. The dermis contains immunocompetent cells, the dendrocytes, that also partake in inflammatory reactions, and mast cells that are intricately involved in allergic reactions of the skin. There are also cells with macrophagic function in the skin: the dendrocytes, macrophages, and monocytes. Dermis also contains hair follicles, sebaceous glands, sweat glands, lymph ducts, and striated muscle (for piloerection). Hair follicles and sebaceous and sweat glands breach the barrier provided by the SC and thus constitute an important portal of entry for xenobiotics.

Epidermis

The epidermis is the uppermost layer of living cells in the integument (Figures 21.1 and 21.2) but lacks vascularity (blood vessels), thus it receives its nutrients through a diffusion from the dermis. It consists primarily of keratinocytes but there are also the Langerhans cells, a type of dendritic, immunocompetent cells that mostly serve the immune defense of the skin. Langerhans cells can

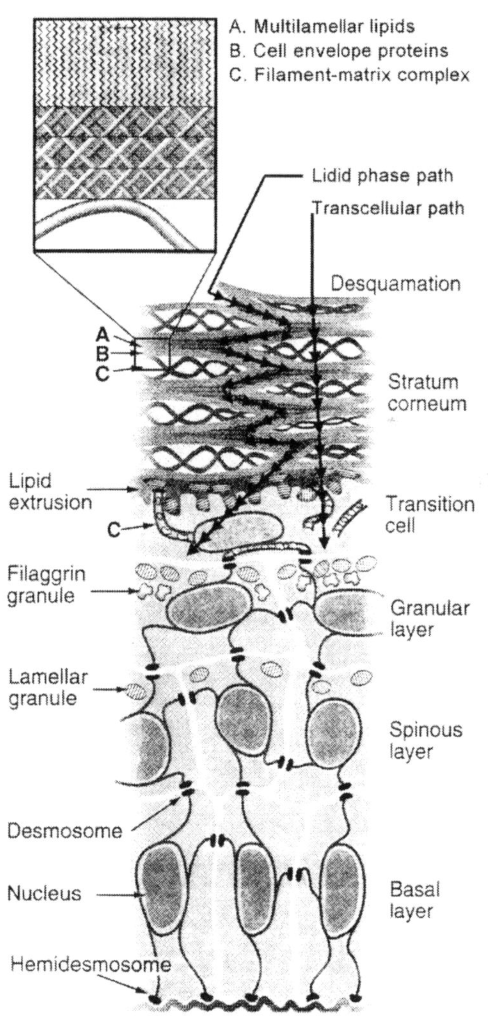

Figure 21.2 — The layers of the stratum corneum and routes of skin penetration. (Reprinted from Reference 27 with permission by the American Association for the Advancement of Science).

incorporate xenobiotic-protein conjugates and carry them into lymph nodes, where they trigger clonal expansion of antigen-specific T-cells. This process constitutes a (regional) systemic response to percutaneous absorption of a chemical. Melanocytes that contain the pigment of the skin are also located in the epidermis. There is evidence that certain substances can bind strongly to melanin, but it is as yet unclear whether this furthers or inhibits skin penetration or triggers any biologic responses. Finally, the epidermis contains Merkel cells, the sensory mechanoceptors of the skin.

The top cell layer of the epidermis is formed by the stratum granulosum or granular layer. This layer is topped by a zone of dying cells (in their state of terminal differentiation) that form the transition to the SC (Figure 21.2). The middle layer of the epidermis, the stratum spinosum or spiny layer, followed by the stratum germinativum or basal layer, that is, the layer where the cell division occurs that gives rise to the constant renewal of epidermis and SC.

The predominant proteins in epidermal cells are keratins. They are crucial components of all epithelia; their complexity of expression, to some extent, reflects the complexity of the epithelium, such as simple (one-layered) vs. stratified (multi-layered) epithelia. Absence of or mutation within any of the keratins results in damage to the epidermal barrier and a lack of mechanical strength, indicating that each keratin serves a highly cell-specific function. Expression of keratins within one cell type may change in the course of differentiation and will change during crucial events, such as injury followed by wound healing. The pattern of keratin gene expression in epidermal keratinocytes changes with each layer as they differentiate from the basal to spiny to granular layer cells.

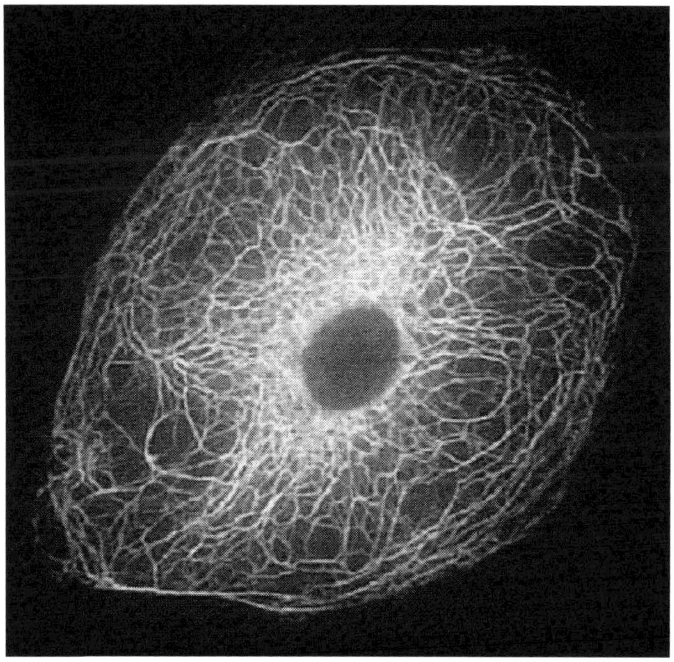

Figure 21.3 — The network of intermediate filaments inside a keratinocyte. (Fluorescence micrograph reprinted from Reference 25 with permission by the Ulster Medical Society).

There are several specific subcellular structures in keratinocytes: keratin or intermediary filaments, desmosomes, hemidesmosomes, keratohyalin or filaggrin granules, and lamellar bodies. Desmosomes provide dual anchor points for intermediary filaments to establish mechanical links between adjacent keratinocytes, and hemidesmosomes attach the filaments to the basement membrane between epidermal keratinocytes and the dermis (Figure 21.2). Thus, intermediary filaments and desmosomes form a three-dimensional network that imparts mechanical stability to the epidermis (Figure 21.3). The filaggrin granules and lamellar bodies (responsible for the term "granular layer") are part of the terminal differentiation process of keratinocytes where, along with the loss of water, the specific "brick and mortar" structure of the SC evolves. The granular layer contains filaggrin granules and lamellar bodies, the spiny layer contains lamellar bodies, intermediary filaments, and desmosomes. Next to the dermis the basal layer also contains intermediate filaments and desmosomes where they contact other spiny or basal layer cells; however, where the intermediary filaments of basal layer keratinocytes connect with the interface to the hypodermis, the link is established by hemidesmosomes (Figure 21.3).

Keratins are classified in two families, type I (acidic) and type II (neutral to basic), depending on their molecular weights (between 44 and 66 kDa) and physicochemical properties. Keratins are rich in simple amino acids, such as glycine and alanine, allowing hydrogen bonds to form easily between different protein chains to create strong fibrils. Currently at least 54 human keratins are known (28 type I and 26 type II overall, of which 13 type I and 15 type II occur in skin), displaying cell type- and differentiation-specific expression patterns that generally apply to one pair of type I and II keratins (however, a given cell may express multiple keratin pairs). Specific pairs of type I and II keratins spontaneously assemble in a strict 1:1 molecular ratio into heteropolymers that form fibrils called intermediate filaments that originate at the cell nucleus (the polymerization process may be aided by ionic milieu, pH, and specific kinases and phosphatases). The filaments are approximately 10 nm in diameter and extend through much of the cytoplasm, forming a network that is very tight around the nucleus but becomes more loose the closer it gets to the cell membrane (Figure 21.3). Keratin filaments are both flexible and elastic that harden (form stiff gels) when subjected to deformation stress but relax rapidly when the stress ceases.

Thus, keratins should not be viewed as a rigid protein scaffolds that only infer mechanical stability to the skin but also as linking molecules that regulate intra- and intercellular interactions to ascertain homeostatic cell behavior or that control developmental and adaptive processes. Gene expression levels and patterns of keratins affect cell size, proliferation, cell cycle regulation, apoptosis, cell migration, melanosome transport, stress response, and wound healing. However, a more detailed discussion of such processes is beyond the scope of this chapter. It may be added here that considerations of cytoskeleton, cellular architecture, shape, function, and differentiation as influenced by keratins apply not only to epidermal cells, but generally to all epithelia. A terminally differentiated epithelial cell's specific pattern of keratin expression is so constant that it can be used for typing of cells of epithelial origin (specifically, cancers). This surprisingly broad spectrum of keratin functions provides clues to the broad spectrum of physiological or toxic responses of the skin, such as blistering, callus formation, response to repetitive or mechanical trauma, irritation or allergy responses, and neoplastic growth, all of which may occur in an occupational setting.[27–30]

Cutaneous Metabolism

Contrary to popular belief, the epidermis and the dermis are capable of metabolizing foreign chemicals that have penetrated the stratum corneum ahead of a more systemic distribution and/or metabolism in the liver. Both epidermis and dermis express mRNAs for multiple Phase I and II xenobiotic-metabolizing enzymes, although there are differences in the specific expression patterns among the two skin layers. Although few experiments have been conducted to prove that specific mRNA expressions are accompanied by corresponding protein synthesis and enzyme activity, numerous studies have proven the ability of both epidermis and dermis to metabolize chemicals as well as to respond to enzyme inducers. Epidermal keratinocytes express mRNA and/or protein for CYP1A1, 1B1, 2B6, 2E1, 3A5, flavin monooxygenase-3, N-acetyltransferase-1, and several sulfotransferases. CYP3A4 mRNA is detectable only after exposure to enzyme inducers. Dermal fibroblasts express CYP1A1, 1B1, 2A6, 2C9, 2C18, 2C19, 2D6, 2E1, flavin monooxygenase-1, glutathione transferases M1 and P1, and N-acetyltransferase-1. The only xenobiotic-metabolizing enzyme that has consistently been shown not to be expressed in any skin cell type is CYP1A2.

It appears that the biotransformation capacity of epidermis exceeds that of the dermis; given the total weight of epidermis, about 0.3 kg, its first pass metabolism capacity can be substantial. Melanocytes also express many of the cytochrome isozymes that can be detected in keratinocytes or fibroblasts but, because of their comparatively low numbers, they likely play a lesser role in the xenobiotic-metabolizing capacity of the skin. In a comparison of the percutaneous absorption of chemical through viable (metabolically active) and non-viable (previously frozen) skin it was demonstrated that dermal metabolism can increase or decrease percutaneous absorption, depending on the chemical under investigation.[31] Thus, because enzymatic metabolism generally decreases the lipophilicity of a chemical, dermal first-pass metabolism is likely to affect a chemical's ability to permeate through skin.

It may be assumed that covalent binding of metabolically activated chemicals to proteins in the skin, or haptenation, plays an important role in the development of cutaneous allergic or hypersensitivity reactions; these reactions are mostly mediated by dendritic cells in the skin. Given the total mass of the skin its metabolic capacity is thought to equal or even exceed that of the liver, at least with respect to certain enzyme systems. This statement is of major importance when it comes to evaluating both local and systemic toxic effects due to chemical exposure of the skin. The situation may be different when high level exposure to an easily penetrating substance occurs in a limited area of skin that overwhelms the local first pass metabolism capacity: in such a case significant systemic exposure can occur that bypasses the first-pass metabolism accomplished by the liver following gastrointestinal exposure.[32–35]

Stratum Corneum

The SC was once thought to be a uniform layer with the essential characteristics of a lipid membrane, but this view has changed dramatically. SC consists of two layers, the stratum disjunctum and the stratum conjunctum (Figure 21.1). The stratum disjunctum is made up of loosely attached aggregates of dry, dead cell bodies. Due to the considerable amount of empty space between the aggregates, stratum disjunctum forms a remarkable sink for liquids or solutions. The stratum conjunctum constitutes the major barrier to skin penetration although it is not a membrane in the classical sense. It consists of densely packed dead cells, called corneocytes. To characterize their arrangement, such terms as "brick and mortar" structure[36] or "domain mosaic" structure[37] have been used (Figure 21.2).

The current view holds that corneocytes (brick) mostly consist of keratinous protein and lipids with little water. The intercellular spaces, or mortar, on the other hand, consist of lipid bilayers interspersed with water layers of fluctuating thickness, with varying physicochemical characteristics (Figure 21.2). Thus, the lipophilic or hydrophilic nature of either realm, brick or mortar, is not constant. If either of the components is absent, functionally deficient, or exists in excess, the function of the SC will be compromised.

A better understanding of the barrier function of the SC will arise from a closer look at its components, their development, and their interactions. SC has about 16–20 cell layers and is approximately 20 µm thick. The cells originate from the granular layer in the epidermis but change in size and appearance during their passage through the SC in a process called desquamation. This is a continuous process that may be seen as beginning with cell division in the basal layer of keratinocytes in the epidermis followed by differentiation and migration of the cells as described above, but desquamation as such comprises the fate of corneocytes, i.e., the death of granular keratinocytes, their compaction, and eventually the shedding of corneocyte aggregates from the surface of the skin. The cells become more and more flattened as they approach the surface of the skin, lose much of their moisture content, and, now called corneocytes, extrude lipid material into the extracellular space with the help of the lamellar bodies. These subcellular organelles, together with the filaggrin granules, give the name to the granular layer. Lamellar bodies take up various lipids synthesized in the granulocytes and modify them by means of endogenous enzymes into the final lipids as they are found in the extracellular space of the SC. The lamellar bodies leave the granulocytes via exocytosis, i.e., their outer membrane merges with the inner surface of the cell membrane, forming an opening in the cell membrane, and the lipid contents is released out of the cell. This unique structure of the SC, flattened, nonviable corneocytes enveloped in a multilayered lipid matrix, provides the original idea for the favored description of the SC as "brick and mortar" structure.[38] The structure of lipid bilayers in the SC can be disturbed by a variety of substances[39] that affect barrier function.

The extracellular lipids of the skin consist to approximately 50% of ceramides, 25% cholesterol, and 15% free fatty acids, the remainder made up by a multitude of other lipids, such as cholesteryl sulfate, but hardly any phospholipids. Maintenance of specific ratios of these lipids, within certain limits, is key to SC homeostasis. Lipid precursors are synthesized in the keratinocytes and transported into the extracellular space in lamellar bodies where they are further metabolized to their final forms as they exist in the lamellar membranes. Lamellar bodies appear first in keratinocytes at their transition from the spiny to the granular layer; contrary to the extracellular lipids these organelles contain significant amounts of phospholipids. Any defect in the synthesis of these lipids is likely to adversely affect the proper function of the lamellar lipid barrier.

In terms of dermal absorption a penetrating chemical appears to face two principal routes: through the mortar, or through the brick (Figure 21.2). However, chemicals use both routes to an extent that is determined by two basic variables: their own lipophilicity and the water content (hydration) of the SC, which can range from 10 to 70% of its mass. In this context it should be clear that skin penetration is also bi-directional: the body can evaporate water through the epidermis and SC, known as transepidermal water loss (TEWL). This is an important factor in the maintenance of SC moisture contents.[40]

Skin Appendages

The role of skin appendages in skin penetration is still a matter of controversy. Sweat glands and ducts, sebaceous glands and ducts, and hair follicles with shafts have little or no SC for protection. It has been shown that percutaneous absorption in normal rats is much stronger than in hairless rats, suggesting that appendages contribute significantly to skin absorption.[41] Huge regional and interindividual variations in the densities of appendages in humans make it hard to assess their true contribution to skin penetration, but they should not be overlooked in cases where their density is conspicuously high. Despite some indication that the total surface of hair follicles may entail racial or ethnic differences[42], the evident interindividual variations imply that such considerations should not bias any occupational evaluation.

To summarize, skin as an organ differs significantly from the other "outside" surfaces of the body, lung and intestinal tract, with respect to its metabolic capability (types and capacities of metabolic enzymes), reservoir function, and above all its main barrier against the environment, the stratum corneum. The structural and functional differences between the outermost skin layers and the fluid-covered epithelia of the lungs and intestinal tract are so fundamental that any attempt at using data and parameters for the lung or gastrointestinal tract to describe the movement of xenobiotics through the skin is likely to result in faulty estimates.

Biological Differences and Variations in Skin Properties

Age

Age has been said to reduce percutaneous absorption[43], most likely due to decreased water content of the epidermis and SC, but there is some indication that with very high age percutaneous absorption can increase substantially, probably through loss of protein components from the SC. Disruption of the skin barrier in humans >75 years of age is repaired more slowly than in younger people because of slow release of lamellar bodies. The reason is thought to be an age-related decrease in cholesterol synthesis. Because these changes may appear only at a very advanced age they are highly unlikely to play a role in an occupational setting. Systematic investigations of any correlation between age and percutaneous absorption have not been conducted.[44]

Gender

Variability of dermal absorption with the site of exposure has been mentioned; see Table 21.1 for data on the thickness of the SC with body region. Regarding gender, female rats display higher levels of percutaneous absorption than males.[24] The reason is thought to be a difference in thickness of SC and epidermis. Some studies suggest that gender differences also exist in humans, but comprehensive studies have not been performed. The thicker adipose tissue layer in female hypodermis may play a role in this finding.

Race

There are studies that suggest race- or ethnicity-related differences in the anatomy or physiology of human skin, e.g..[45,46] However, these studies are experimental investigations with a limited number of subjects or samples. At this point in time the general agreement appears to be that race or ethnicity play a minor role, if at all, in the properties of skin with respect to workplace exposures or occupational skin disease.[47,48]

Biological Conditions

The most likely biological condition to affect skin penetration is blood perfusion.

Strenuous work, mechanical stress, ambient temperature, inflammation, and vasoactive substances such as ethyl alcohol or organic nitro-compounds all can increase cardiac output and/or peripheral blood flow, affecting the rate of dermal absorption by increased skin temperature and accelerated removal of penetrating chemicals.

First-pass metabolism may increase dermal or systemic exposure when the resulting product is more water-soluble than the parent compound, allowing the metabolite to diffuse more easily through the epidermis and reach the blood vessels of the dermis. Lifestyle or environmental conditions, such as ethanol consumption, hunger, or diabetes, are known to increase cytochrome P450 activities (specifically, CYP2E1) and thus may exert some influence on percutaneous absorption. Covalent binding to skin constituents may inhibit or prevent percutaneous absorption.

The water content of the SC, as mentioned before, varies with ambient humidity or temperature, thickness and character of clothing, and possibly age. There are marked regional differences in TEWL, capacitance of the SC (a measure of its hydration), and the pH of the skin surface (approx. pH 5.5–5.9 in adults). Several of these factors are subject to circadian rhythms, such as transepidermal water loss (a basic measure for stratum corneum permeability), sebum secretion, pH (an important factor in the permeation of amphophilic substances), and capacitance (a measure of stratum corneum hydration). The rhythms may vary with skin location on the body and there may be two or three cycles every day. Transepidermal water loss and sebum excretion, which may be linked to each other, peak around midday and have their low points late in the day, around the onset of dark. The biological mechanisms that control these rhythms are not known.

Removal of contamination from the skin may be helpful if some caveats are observed. The first instinct, to shower with warm water, particularly with the ample use of soap, should be rejected: a thorough wash-in effect has been shown with substances such as lindane. OSHA and other protocols always specify use of a safety shower or eyewash fountain. Rubbing with dry paper or cloth results in increased local blood flow and, possibly, damage to the SC. Trying to wash contaminants away with solvents is even worse. The best is washing with plenty of cool water (prompting vasoconstriction) without soap. Corrosive materials form an exception because they dissociate when dissolved in water (alkali, anhydrous acids, phenol, etc.), thus exacerbating the damage. Such substances should be blotted or wiped off thoroughly before flushing the skin with copious amounts of cold water.[44,49]

To sum up, there are no reliable demographic correlates for age, gender, race, or genomic characteristics that can change the extent of skin protective programs, e.g., industrial hygiene control efforts. This generalization stands in contrast to medical investigations of both dermatitic (contact irritant, urticaric, or allergic) and non-dermatitic (psoriasis, infection, acne, vitiligo, or scleroderma) outbreaks in a workplace. In such circumstance there may well be clustering of cases according to one or more of these demographic variables. However, the significance of such findings should be determined for individual workers and should not rely upon broader generalizations. The references provided in this section are intended to be useful in the event of outbreak investigations but should never be used to modify the design or execution of skin protection programs that are intended to protect every worker regardless of age, gender, race, or genomic characteristics.

Environmental Factors and Skin Penetration

Physical Factors

The surface temperature of skin is normally around 32°C, but ambient temperature as well as thick or occlusive clothing can affect skin temperature significantly. Rule of thumb: a 10°C increase in skin surface temperature doubles the rate of percutaneous absorption.

Mechanical stress (vibration, tight clothing, repetitive movements, heavy loads) and ultraviolet radiation damage or destroy the SC locally, vastly increasing skin penetration. Several agents successfully used in transdermal drug delivery may also occur in a workplace setting: ultrasound, low-intensity currents (that may result in iontophoresis), or high-voltage pulsed currents (that may cause electroporation) increase skin penetration.[50,51] Another portal for enhanced skin absorption can arise when workers have used topical treatments that weaken the barrier function of the SC, such as urea in ointments or specific compounding agents in skin patches. This is not likely but should be noted in formal hazard communication series and adapted to workers using skin care products or wearing pharmaceutical patches.

The concentration of the penetrating chemical plays a role; both very high and very low concentrations reduce the rate of dermal absorption. Many industrial solvents are so volatile at the surface temperature of skin that they evaporate before substantial absorption occurs. On the other hand, liquids vaporized at high ambient temperature may condense on a relatively cooler skin.

Chemical Agents

Hydration of the SC, from immersion in water or extensive showering or bathing, from high ambient humidity, or from perspiration under tight or water-impermeable clothing, is thought to loosen the "mortar" structure (Figure 21.2) and increase dermal absorption. In addition, most skin care products or cosmetics contain effective moisturizers such as urea, glycerol, or surfactants (e.g., lauryl sulfate). Use of barrier creams or frequent washing with hand cleansers has been reported to increase rather than decrease the incidence of contact dermatitis. Heat and moisture combined are probably the most important external factors influencing skin penetration. A new generation of topical skin protectants as opposed to 'barrier creams' is currently being synthesized and evaluated as a result of interest in protecting against chemical warfare agents. At the time of this writing these should be regarded as investigational agents as opposed to those known to be effective and safe for industrial applications.[52]

The vehicle of skin penetration exerts much influence, depending on whether the penetrating chemical is a neat substance (liquid or solid), whether it is dissolved in water or organic material, or whether it is absorbed to particulate matter (e.g., dust). The pH value of the skin plays a role in the dermal absorption of chemicals that can ionize. Ionization of a chemical, or a molecular weight >500[20], may prevent skin absorption completely. Perspiration can dissolve chemicals and facilitate dermal absorption; if the resulting agent is a strong acid or base, that is, corrosive, it will destroy the SC. Other corrosives that destroy the SC include cement, alkylating agents such as ethylene oxide, and metal hydrides.

Many skin care products contain fatty acids that act as penetration enhancers by softening the lipid bilayers in the SC. The very common insect repellent DEET (N,N dieethyl-m toluamide) and many other organic solvents act similarly. However, aggressive solvents such as those used in paint stripper remove the lipids and destroy the SC, likely compromising its barrier function severely. They also further the invasion of microorganisms and the development of severe irritation.

Metalworking fluids (MWF) represent a special case. These water/oil emulsions are used in metal machining to cool and lubricate surfaces. With modern high-revving equipment there is considerable formation of mists, and MWF cause occupational health concern due to combined irritant and allergenic properties.[53,54]

Disease

Psoriasis is a disease that affects the SC, and thus skin penetration, significantly. Psoriasis involves increased keratinocyte proliferation and major changes in the pattern of keratin expression. The results is a much increased TEWL, up to 20 times higher than in healthy skin. Structural changes to the SC and a lack of intercellular lipid result in a scaly appearance and diminish the barrier function of psoriatic skin markedly. During psoriatic flares (also called pustular flares) it is not unusual for skin to bleed, crack and flake, limiting even common activities such as doing laundry or home care. It is critical that individuals not be exposed to chemicals during these periods.

Atopic dermatitis is characterized by reduced lipid content of the SC, above all ceramide, which affects barrier function in a negative way and allows for TEWL to be up to 10 times higher than in healthy skin.

As a side note with some significance for the occupational arena, there are a number of genetic diseases that affect the function of the SC. These diseases, classified as ichtyoses, modify the balance between epidermal proliferation and desquamation and affect the barrier function of the skin thoroughly. They cover a wide spectrum of phenotypes, from life-threatening (harlequin ichthyosis) to near unremarkable (ichthyosis vulgaris) but they all affect the structure of the epidermis and stratum corneum and thus the integrity of the cutaneous barrier.[27,30,55] All these disorders have in common an abnormality of the SC barrier associated with changes in the architecture of the lamellar membranes in the extracellular space of the SC resulting in visible scaliness of the skin that is a consequence of phase separation between lipid and non-lipid in the SC. This appearance is mostly the result of a hyperplastic response (more layers of corneocytes) of the epidermis attempting to compensate for the missing component(s). Secondary to the defective SC and the resulting signaling cascade that triggers compensatory reactions may be an inflammatory response that is commonly observed in ichthyotic skin. There are two main causes for ichtyoses: lipid synthesis or storage diseases, and keratin synthesis diseases. As a general rule these diseases affect the process of stratum corneum desquamation and result in some form of epidermal hyperplasia or hyperkeratosis because a lack or excess of one component in the epidermis or SC triggers compensatory reactions designed to reinstate homeostasis. These homeostatic mechanism aim at maintaining a uniform phase of the lamellar and non-lamellar portions of the stratum corneum; any disturbance is likely to cause phase separation with the resulting phenotype of ichthyosis, i.e., a scaly or flaky skin surface.

Currently, 11 mutation-based ichthyoses are known. Ichthyosis vulgaris, the result of a mutation in the filaggrin gene, is said to account for approximately 95% of all ichthyosis cases and occurs in every 250–1,000 people but may be more common among certain population segments (as high as 3.6% in the Chinese population). X-linked recessive ichthyosis has an incidence of about 1 in 2,000–6,000. The individual mutations are per se rare but, taken together, occur at an incidence that may become a confounding factor in the assessment of occupational skin disease.[56]

Any defect in the synthesis of these lipids is likely to adversely affect the proper function of the lamellar lipid barrier. For example, when linoleic acid in ceramides is replaced by oleic acid, the barrier function of the SC is compromised. By the same token, chemicals that affect the lipid composition of the SC, such as organic solvents or detergents, compromise its barrier function. However, the lipid synthesizing system of the keratinocytes and lamellar bodies is not static: it will adapt enzyme activities, when possible, to conditions of a compromised lipid barrier. This event triggers a rapid release (in a matter of minutes) of lamellar bodies into the extracellular space. Thus, the integrity of the SC can be reestablished rapidly unless the external insult persists. Keratinocyte express several types of lipid-sensitive receptors, such as peroxisome proliferator-activated receptors (PPAR) and liver X receptors (LXR), that not only regulate lipid synthesis, but also the synthesis of protein constituents of the cytoskeleton.[40]

The epidermal lipid synthesis system may also respond to extracellular delivery of lipid material, such as mineral oil, or components of skin care or medical products. This opens avenues to both damaging or improving the epidermal barrier function. Non-physiological lipids, such as Vaseline, will improve the barrier by passively filling empty space in the SC without affecting the synthetic apparatus of lamellar bodies or keratinocytes. However, this may construct an artificial permeability barrier and thus impede the repair of a damaged barrier. Extraneous application of lipids that are precursors to physiological lipids of the SC barrier may directly aid, or inhibit (if provided in non-physiological mixture ratios), the synthetic apparatus because they are actively taken up by the granulosa cells. However, not all pathologic conditions of a compromised SC barrier can be treated with topical lipid mixtures. UV or X-ray exposure, for example, blocks the uptake of lipid into lamellar bodies and thus cannot be treated with topical medication. As mentioned earlier, the epidermis is slightly acidic, and two of the key enzymes in epidermal lipid synthesis operate optimally in this limited pH range, 5.5–5.9. Thus, extended exposure to mild acid or alkali also may disrupt proper lipid synthesis.[40]

Wound Healing

Of major importance for the barrier function of skin is the role that keratins play in wound healing. These proteins serve this function in connection with a variety of other regulatory molecules, cytokines, and possibly vitamins.

Wound healing following topical injury is an important issue in maintaining the integrity of the skin. During their transition through the epidermis, keratinocytes undergo a preprogrammed course of differentiation. However, this process can be redirected temporarily by certain chemicals or by injury. The resulting "activation" allows an injured skin surface to heal or to adapt to changed environmental conditions. It appears that disruption of the SC allows water to leave the top layer of the epidermis, the granulose layer, carrying out calcium ions that exist at relatively high concentrations in the extracellular space. The keratinocyte activation can be suppressed by creating an artificial barrier on the skin. The injury-induced decrease in Ca^{2+} triggers the release of lamellar bodies from the granular cells. Other ions, such as potassium, may also be involved in this signaling process. Interleukins-1α or -6, or tumor necrosis factor-α, may serve as secondary signal transducers. In addition to lamellar body release, activation of keratinocytes induces a boost to cellular lipid synthesis (above all cholesterol and fatty acid syntheses), for which the granular cells are very well equipped.

The activated state, the differentiating state, and the basal (= proliferating) state are all characterized by the synthesis of specific keratin protein markers. The endogenous chemokines that trigger keratinocyte activation are typical mediators of pro- and anti-inflammatory, immune, allergic, proliferative, and acute phase processes as well as apoptosis, namely, interleukin-1 (produced by the immunocompetent cells of the skin and keratinocytes), tumor necrosis factor α (produced by macrophages, mast cells, and fibroblasts), transforming growth factors α and β (produced by macrophages and keratinocytes), and interferon-γ (produced by dendritic cells). The cell types in the skin where these chemokines are produced highlight an intricate autocrine and paracrine regulation network within or between cell types during the process of keratinocyte activation. Any of these cytokines binds to a specific receptor and triggers a signaling cascade that involves a multitude of gene regulatory factors and the production of one or several other cytokines.

The role of interleukin-1 in alerting surrounding cells (paracrine signaling) has been studied in order to better understand keratinocyte and dermal fibroblast activation. For both cell types activation means that the cells begin to proliferate and migrate, and their pattern of gene expression and protein production change in a manner specific for the changed conditions. The release of interleukin-1, as stated above, starts keratinocyte activation, but other chemokines are required to maintain the activated state, or terminate it and induce reversion to the basal state. An important position in the maintenance of keratinocyte activation comes to tumor necrosis factor α, which commands its own signaling cascade. Both interleukin-1 and tumor necrosis γ represent pro-inflammatory signals. Keratinocyte proliferation, another crucial part of maintaining keratinocytes in their active state, is regulated by transforming growth factor β, another chemokine at the beginning of a complex signaling cascade. Interferon-γ initiates an important step in wound healing, the keratinocyte-mediated contraction of newly formed basement membrane. Finally, transforming growth factor β causes keratinocytes to return to their basal state. It would go beyond the scope of this chapter to describe these highly complex processes in more detail; suffice it to say that there a many possibilities for exogenous chemicals or microorganisms to either trigger, or interfere with these processes.[40,57]

Clinical Evaluation of the Skin

This section attempts to provide only basic guidance to occupational hygienists who may share medical reports relating to skin disease and injury; far more thorough treatises can be obtained from, for example.[59–65] A thorough physical examination of the skin extends from head to toe, including nails and mucous membranes. Occupational exposure assessments must parallel such thoroughness. Occupational hygienists should be aware that physicians commonly find occupationally unrelated but significant skin lesions such as basal cell carcinomas or even melanomas of which the patient is totally unaware. The general assessment of the entire skin allows the examiner to determine a pattern of skin problems before focusing on individual lesions.

Occupational dermatitis is a multifactorial disease; frequently there are preexisting or exacerbating conditions that need to be taken into account[58] and some of them have been detailed in the preceding sections. Differential diagnosis is crucial and may require a biopsy and specialized histopathologic testing. Physicians assess where the patient's skin condition first appeared; what it looks like and what symptoms were initially associated with it; how the skin disease may have changed; and what is being done to treat the condition. Aging, trauma, nutrition, hygiene, and pigmentation leave critical signs, whereas color changes can also be related to underlying systemic conditions (e.g., jaundice: hepatobiliary conditions; cyanosis: cardiopulmonary diseases; diffuse hyperpigmentation: Addison's disease; paleness: anemia). Given that one's sense of well-being, appearance in fact, depends upon having healthy skin, it is not surprising that there are behavioral components to all but the most trivial of skin conditions. Because there are hundreds of dermatoses, a logical process of elimination is required to narrow the possibilities, first to specific groups of diseases and eventually to the exact few.

Occupational hygienists should be aware that repeated visits to dermatological specialists may be required. The careful review of exposures includes occupational chemicals (neat or as mixtures), materials (e.g., glass fibers), and exposure to mechanical forces or sunlight. Systemic medications, both prescription and over-the-counter; use of health care products or dietary supplements; nutrient hypersensitivities; preexisting disease such as tuberculosis; smoking and lifestyles (e.g., outdoors person); race; and pH of the skin must all be included in the differential diagnosis. Nutritional status plays a role as imbalance of vitamins A (deficiency predisposes for dermatosis, excess causes hyperkeratosis), B group (niacin deficiency and pellagra), and C (suppresses allergic reactions) are known to affect skin disease. The relationship of the onset time of a skin condition such as a rash to the use of drugs or chemicals is critical.

The history of atopic (allergic) diseases or skin cancer and a careful family history of skin problems may help to alert the physician to genetic (or familial) aspects of the dermatoses. When successive generations of family members work in the same plants, threading through the differential area between familial and occupational origins is tedious. Reports of a similar disease or disorder in other exposed workers often help to denote occupational origins of disease. A distinction is made between clinical impression and confirmatory laboratory testing and referral. This has proven difficult to understand for quantitative scientists, because some elements of skin disease seem to be remote in terms of occupational origin. Two terms are encountered frequently in connection with dermal disorders that per se do not represent disease pictures: (1) pruritus, the medical term for itching, is the irritation of sensory nerve terminals in the skin that is associated with many forms of skin disorder, and (2) eczema describes a manifestation mostly seen with contact dermatitis or mechanical trauma, involving erythema (redness), pruritus, and lesions with serous discharge followed by encrustation.

Contact Dermatitis

Contact dermatitis is generally confined to the areas actually touched by a chemical. It is by far the most common of occupational skin diseases, accounting for one-half to two-thirds of all cases. Clinical signs in affected human subjects may include one or more of erythema (reddening), edema (swelling), vesiculation (blisters), scaling, and thickening (see Figure 21.4), and may be accompanied by an itch or a burning sensation. When contact dermatitis is suspected, work and hobby history are the keys to identifying pertinent exposures to allergens or irritants. Outdoor workers in particular may experience sun, cold, and heat that can provoke skin reactions: season of the year should always be noted as well as other unusual patterns of occurrence (see Figure 21.4). Contact dermatitis is a term that comprises two different entities: direct irritant responses and cell-mediated allergic contact dermatitis. There is some controversy over the prevalence of irritant versus allergic contact dermatitis, with most recent figures suggesting that irritant dermatitis may be the more frequent type.

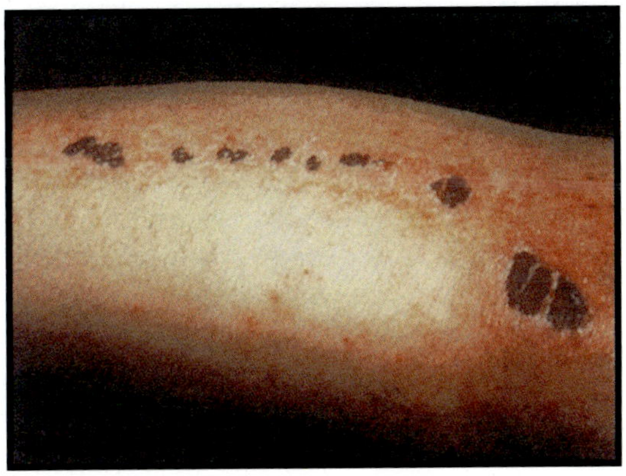

Figure 21.4 — Contact dermatitis. (All rights reserved. Reprinted with permission from the American Academy of Dermatology.)

Irritant Reactions

Skin irritants do not rely on an immunologic mechanism to produce a local response. Severity depends on (1) the potency of the irritant, (2) the circumstances of the contact, and (3) the skin site affected. Irritant response and dermal absorption are somehow related: factors enhancing one parameter likely enhance the other, this occurring through largely unknown mechanisms. Because irritation depends on damage to the lower, living layers of the epidermis, those factors that enhance penetration generally increase the severity of the irritant response. The distribution of dermatitis may be modified in that sites with a stronger barrier function (e.g., palms and soles) may show little or no dermatitis while other areas are more markedly affected (see Figure 21.5). Irritant contact dermatitis can be an acute effect, most commonly caused by detergents, soaps, or wet work, accounting for almost one-fourth of cases. Exposure to oils, greases, and MWF is to blame for a similar number of cases. Substances that dehydrate or remove lipids from the skin (aggressive solvents, paint stripper), or exert an oxidizing, reducing, or alkylating action also rank high among causes of irritation and chemical burns. Corrosive materials such as acids (hydrofluoric acid in particular), alkali, or phenol cause severe irritation and destruction of the SC. Repeated exposure to weaker agents can act in a cumulative fashion and result, over time, in the same outcome as a strong irritant. In the early stages of exposure the onset of disease can usually be prevented by simple washing with plenty of water and soap.

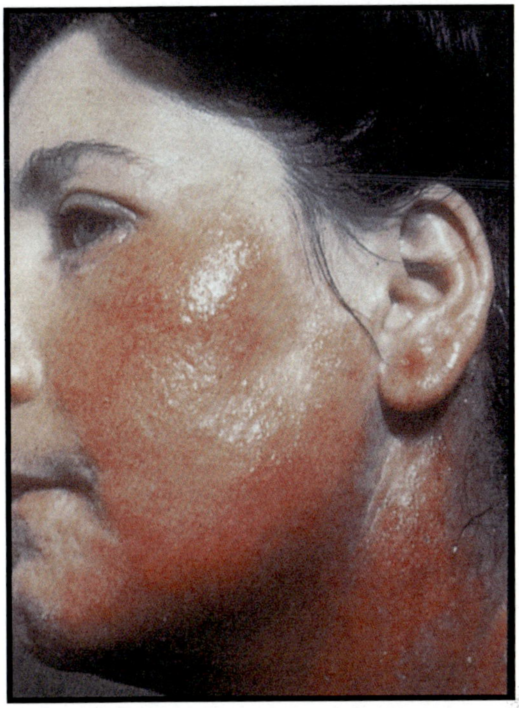

Figure 21.5 — Irritant reactions. (All rights reserved. Reprinted with permission from the American Academy of Dermatology.)

Allergic Contact Reactions

Allergic contact dermatitis (or delayed hypersensitivity, see Figure 21.6) occurs as a result of allergy to one or more specific substances (antigens) through type IV cell-mediated immunity. In sensitized persons such reactions can be provoked by minute amounts of the allergen. There are two main phases in cell-mediated immunity, the sensitization phase (in which the person becomes allergic to the antigen) and the elicitation phase. Sensitization usually takes at least 10 days. When sensitization has been achieved and the individual is then reexposed, a reaction is obvious after a characteristic delay of 12–48 hours; hence the term "delayed." Although there is some connection between skin and respiratory sensitization, it does not follow exact rules, and the dermal mode is much more common. This issue remains a dilemma for occupational standard-setters who must deal with both respiratory and dermal routes of exposure.

In a vicious circle, rubber components and additives leaching from protective gear are among the most frequent causes of occupational allergic dermatitis. Nickel and its salts, chromium and its salts, cobalt salts, organomercurials, and formaldehyde follow

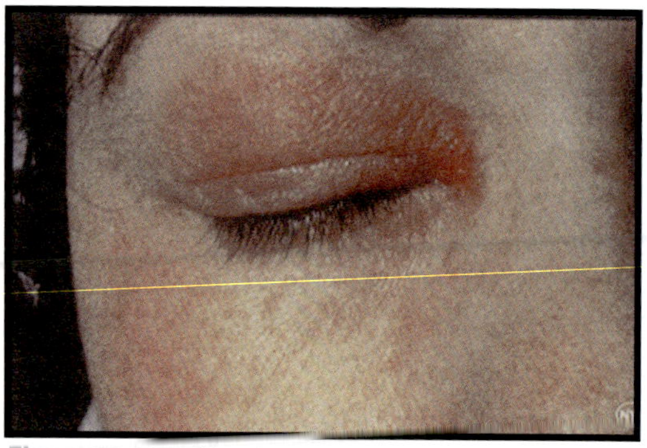

Figure 21.6 — Allergic contact reactions. (All rights reserved. Reprinted with permission from the American Academy of Dermatology.)

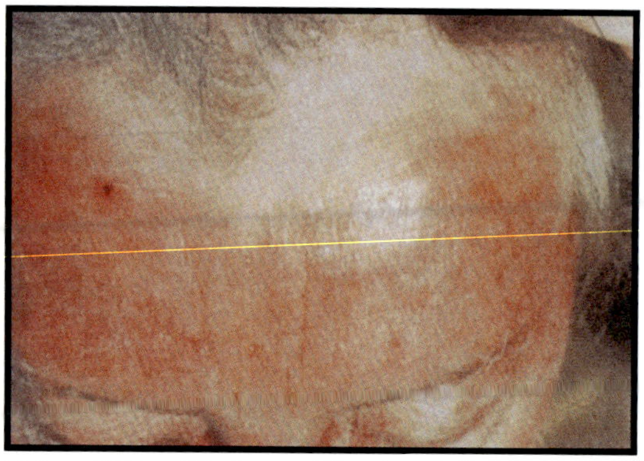

Figure 21.7 — Photosensitization. (All rights reserved. Reprinted with permission from the American Academy of Dermatology.)

close behind. Many aromatic compounds, above all substituted phenylamines, are causative agents, as are many monomeric ingredients of plastic polymers. Food stuffs, preservatives, and fragrances also rank high among agents causing skin allergies. Gardeners, grain mill workers, and people handling fruit or vegetables are prone to develop fungal or microbial allergies.

Photosensitization

Photosensitization is considered to be an adverse reaction to ultraviolet and/or visible radiation (see Figure 21.7). It may be produced by sunlight alone or by a number of substances, each having its own action spectrum. Although precise rules do not apply, the action spectrum usually approximates the chemical's absorption spectrum. There are several subgroups of photosensitivity, based on mechanistic considerations.

Phototoxicity does not involve the immune system, whereas photoallergy, like allergic dermatitis, is a type IV cell-mediated immune response. For photodynamic agents oxygen is required in addition to activation by light energy to elicit a toxic response. Other agents, typified by 8-methoxypsoralen, bind directly to cell constituents when activated by light. This emphasizes that phototoxic reactions can develop into skin cancer. Photosensitizers are typically chemicals that absorb short wavelength light well (action spectrum strongest in the UV-A range, 315–400 nm). These include polycyclic aromatic hydrocarbons, phenanthrene, and substituted phenylamines or salicylic acid derivatives. Because a large number of drugs induce photosensitivity, a careful differential diagnosis is most helpful.

A special case of photosensitization is represented by porphyrias (mostly porphyria cutanea tarda, or PCT). They are elicited by substances that interfere with porphyrin metabolism; because porphyrins are excellent UV absorbers, their deposition in skin causes the disease. PCT has been observed with accidental exposure to the insecticide, hexachlorobenzene.

Other Reactions

Urticaria ('Hives')

Urticarial reactions, that is, wheals and flares due to chemical contact, may be produced as direct reactions or as the result of an immediate hypersensitivity (see Figure 21.8). A number of substances directly trigger the release of vasoactive agents such as histamine. They include the biogenic polymers released by some plant species such as stinging nettles (Latin: urtica) and animals, for example, caterpillars and jellyfish. Other substances produce urticaria as a result of allergic sensitization with the production of immunoglobulin E. Such reactions usually occur within 30 to 60 min of contact with the offending agent (Figure 21.8). Urticarial reactions may go far beyond the dermal reaction and proceed to life-threatening conditions such as asthma and even anaphylaxis.

Bacterial and Fungal Infections

A wide variety of microorganisms can infect skin, causing widespread destruction of the barrier. This is clearly beyond the scope of this chapter.[59] However, it should be emphasized that dermal infections are very common with occupations related to agriculture or food and animal handling.

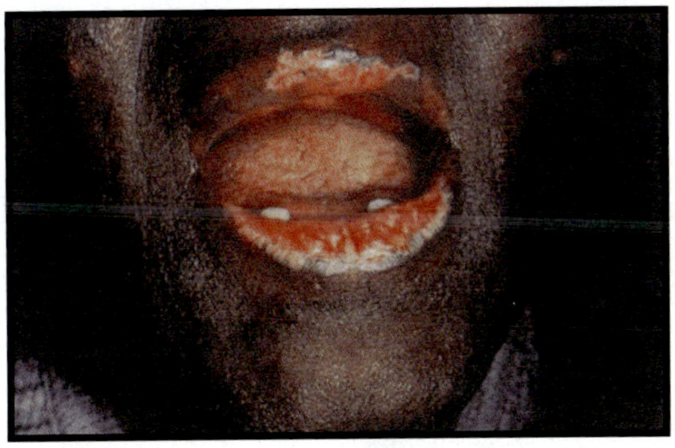

Figure 21.8 — Urticarial reactions. (All rights reserved. Reprinted with permission from the American Academy of Dermatology.)

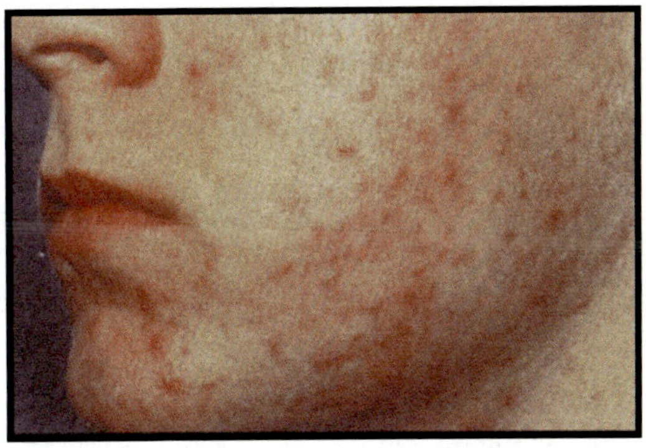

Figure 21.9 — Acne vulgaris. (All rights reserved. Reprinted with permission from the American Academy of Dermatology.)

They may be among the most underestimated occupational skin diseases, most likely because of poor recording. For example, cat scratch disease is a bacterial infection found in persons who occupationally handle cats. Because it develops only in immune-compromised individuals, it is rather a rare condition. It is also evident that preexisting conditions such as eczema increase the likelihood of bacterial or fungal infection of the skin.

Acne

The typical lesions of acne, namely comedones (blackheads) and inflammatory folliculitis, can be produced by coal-tar pitch, creosote, greases, and oils, particularly when acne vulgaris, the usual form of juvenile acne, is present.[66] Chloracne, on the other hand, is often associated with organochlorine compounds such as dioxins, PCBs, and various other chlorinated aromatic compounds.[67] It is important not only because of its refractory nature as a skin condition, but also because it may signal systemic exposure (See Figure 21.9).

Foreign Body Dermatitis and Granuloma

Foreign bodies such as fibrous glass, glass dust, silica, talc, beryllia, or zirconia can penetrate the skin and cause itching, papules, and urticarial reactions. In the case of fibrous glass, severity of the disease is related to both the diameter and length of the fibers; in the manufacture of composite materials this is frequently complicated by concurrent use of epoxy or resin monomers. With beryllia or zirconia as the causative agents, the cutaneous reaction may also involve an immunologic component.

Pigmentation

Hypopigmentation, depigmentation, or leukoderma are typically caused by substituted phenols and catechols. The chemical similarity of such agents to the amino acid tyrosine suggests that they interfere with the synthesis of melanin. Additives from rubber gloves have been known to cause leukoderma. Hyperpigmentation is a common result of heavy metals exposure, above all to arsenic, bismuth, mercury, or silver. Certain phenolic compounds may be oxidized in the skin by first pass metabolism enzymes or by light to form pigments. The process of photosensitization per se gives rise to hyperpigmentation from excessive melanin synthesis.

Alopecia

A number of chemicals either destroy the hair or the follicle, resulting in partial or complete hair loss. The best known causative agent is thallium. Alopecia universalis, the widespread loss of hair, needs to be differentiated from alopecia areata, or local hair loss, an asymptomatic, non-scarring form of hair loss. Alopecia areata is commonly localized to the scalp but may spread across the body. Several diseases have been associated with the development of alopecia areata, such as thyroiditis, atopy, vitiligo, or pernicious anemia (vitamin B12 deficiency).[68]

References

1. **Agricola, G.:** *De Re Metallica.* Translated from the first Latin edition of 1556 by Herbert C. Hoover and Lou H. Hoover. New York: Dover Publications, 1950.

2. **Herxheimer, K.:** Über Chlorakne [On chloracne]. *Münchner Med. Woschr. 46*:278 (1899).
3. **Schulz, K.H.:** Klinische und experimentelle Untersuchungen zur Ätiologe der Chlorakne [Clinical and experimental studies on the etiology of chloracne]. *Arch. Klin. Exp. Dermatol. 206*:589–596 (1957).
4. **Editorial:** An avoidable tragedy. *Occup. Hazards 59*:32 (1997).
5. **Harville, J., and S.S. Que Hee:** Permeation of 2,4-D isooctyl ester formulation through neoprene, nitrile and Tyvek protection materials. *Am. Ind. Hyg. Assoc. J. 50*:438–440 (1989).
6. **Silkowski, J.B., S.W. Horstman, and M.S. Morgan:** Permeation through five commercially available glove materials by two pentachlorophenol preparations. *Am. Ind. Hyg. Assoc. J. 45*:501–504 (1984).
7. **Mickelsen, R.L., M.M. Roder, and S.P. Berardinelli:** Permeation of chemical protective clothing by three binary solvent mixtures. *Am. Ind. Hyg. Assoc. J. 47*:236–240 (1986).
8. **Perkins, J.L., and B. Pool:** Batch lot variability in permeation through nitrile gloves. *Am. Ind. Hyg. Assoc. J. 58*:474–479 (1997).
9. **Mickelsen, R.L., and R.C. Hall:** A breakthrough time comparison of nitrile and neoprene glove materials produced by different glove manufacturers. *Am. Ind. Hyg. Assoc. J. 48*:941–947 (1987).
10. **Sansone, E.B., and Y.B. Tewari:** Differences in the extent of solvent penetration through natural rubber and nitrile gloves from various manufacturers. *Am. Ind. Hyg. Assoc. J. 41*:527–528 (1980).
11. **Rego, A., and L. Roley:** In-use barrier integrity of gloves: latex and nitrile superior to vinyl. *Am. J. Infect. Control 27*:405–410 (1999).
12. **Barker, R.L., and G.C Coletta, editors:** *Performance of Protective Clothing, ASTM STP 900*, pp. 207–213. American Society for Testing Materials, Philadelphia, 1986.
13. **Schwope, A., P. Costas, J. Jackson, and D. Weitzman:** Guidelines for the selection of chemical protective clothing. *American Conference of Governmental Industrial Hygienists*, Cincinnati, 1985.
14. **Stull, J.O., and D.F. White:** A review of overall integrity and material performance tests for the selection of chemical protective clothing. *Am. Ind. Hyg. Assoc. J. 53*:455–462 (1992).
15. **Anna, D.H. (ed.):** *Chemical Protective Clothing*, 2nd edition. Fairfax, VA: AIHA, 2003.
16. **Bromwich, D.:** *Chemical Protective Clothing: An Update.* Australian Institute of Occupational Hygienists Continuing Education Session (2005), 62 pp. Available online at http://dbohs.com/PDF/2005%20Bromwich%20CPC%20Workshop.pdf
17. **Wester, R.C. and H.I. Maibach:** Understanding percutaneous absorption for occupational health and safety. *Int. J. Occup. Environ. Health 6*:86-92 (2000).
18. **James, R.C., H. Busch, C.H. Tamburro, S.M. Roberts, J.D. Schell, and R.D. Harbison:** Polychlorinated biphenyl exposure and human disease. *J. Occup. Med. 35*:136–148 (1993).
19. **American Conference of Governmental Industrial Hygienists (ACGIH®):** 1996 *Threshold Limit Values® for Chemical Substances and Physical Agents.* Cincinnati, OH: ACGIH®, 1996.
20. **Bos, J.D. and M.M. Meinardi:** The 500 Dalton rule for the skin penetration of chemical compounds and drugs. *Exp. Dermatol. 9*:165–169 (2000).
21. **Hadgraft, J. and W.J. Pugh:** The selection and design of topical and transdermal agents: a review. *J. Investig. Dermatol. Symp. Proc. 3*:131–135 (1998).
22. **Roberts, M.S.:** Targeted drug delivery to the skin and deeper tissues: Role of physiology, solute structure and disease. *Clin. Exp. Pharmacol. Physiol. 24*:874–879 (1997).
23. **Franklin, C.A., D.A. Somers, and I. Chu:** Use of percutaneous absorption data in risk assessment. *J. Am. Cell. Toxicol. 8*:815-827 (1989).
24. **U.S. Environmental Protection Agency (EPA):** Dermal Exposure Assessment: Principles and Applications (preliminary rep. EPA/600/8- 91/011B). Washington, D.C.: EPA, 1992.
25. **McLean, W.H.I., and A.D. Irvine:** Disorders of keratinisation: from rare to common genetic diseases of skin and other epithelial tissues. *Ulster Med. J. 76*:72–82 (2007).
26. **Marks, J.G., and J. Miller (eds.):** *Lookingbill and Marks' Principles of Dermatology*, 4th edition. Philadelphia, PA: WB Saunders/Elsevier, Inc (2006).
27. **Roop, D.:** Defects in the barrier. *Science 267*:474–475 (1995).
28. **Koch, P.J. and D.R. Roop:** The role of keratins in epidermal development and homeostasis—going beyond the obvious. *J. Invest. Dermatol. 123*:x–xi (2004).
29. **Moll, R., M. Divo, and L. Langbein:** The human keratins: biology and pathology. Histochem. *Cell. Biol. 129*:705–733 (2008).
30. **Magin, T.M. , P. Vijayaraja, and R.E. Leube:** Structural and regulatory functions of keratins. *Exp. Cell Res. 313*:2021–2032 (2007).
31. **Kao, J., F.K. Patterson, and J. Hall:** Skin penetration and metabolism of topically applied chemicals in six mammalian species, including man: An in vitro study with benzo(a)pyrene and testosterone. *Toxicol. Appl. Pharmacol. 81*:502–516 (1985).

32. **Baron, J.M., T. Wiederholt, R. Heise, H.F. Merk, and D.R. Bickers:** Expression and function of cytochrome p450-dependent enzymes in human skin cells. *Curr. Med. Chem. 15*:2258–2264 (2008).
33. **Bashir, S.J., and H.I. Maibach:** Cutaneous metabolism of xenobiotics. In *Topical Absorption of Dermatological Products (Basic and Clinical Dermatology).* Bronaugh, R.L. and H.I. Maibach (eds.) Basel, Switzerland: Marcel Dekker, 2002. pp. 77–92.
34. **Bronaugh, R.L., M.E.K. Kraeling, J.J. Yourick, and H.L. Hood:** Cutaneous metabolism during in vitro percutaneous absorption. In: *Topical Absorption of Dermatological Products (Basic and Clinical Dermatology).* Bronaugh, R.L. and H.I. Maibach (eds.) Basel, Switzerland: Marcel Dekker, 2002. pp. 1–8.
35. **Svensson, C.K.:** Biotransformation of drugs in human skin. *Drug Metab. Dispos. 37*:247–253 (2009).
36. **Elias, P.M, K.R. Feingold, G.K. Menon, S. Grayson, M.L. Williams, and G. Grubauer:** The stratum corneum two-compartment model and its functional implications. In *Skin Pharmacokinetics,* Vol. I. Shroot, B. and H. Schaefer (eds.) Basel, Switzerland: S. Karger, 1987. pp. 1–9.
37. **Forslind, B., S. Engstrom, J. Engblom, and L. Norlen:** A novel approach to the understanding of human skin barrier function. *J. Dermatol. Sci. 14*:115–125 (1997).
38. **Herkenne, C., I. Alberti, A. Maik, Y.N. Kalia, F.-X. Mathy, V. Préat, and R.H. Guy:** In vivo methods for the assessment of topical drug bioavailability. *Pharm Res 25*:87–103 (2008).
39. **Marjukka Suhonen, T., J.A. Bouwstra, and A. Urtti:** Chemical enhancement of percutaneous absorption in relation to stratum corneum structural alterations. *J. Control. Release 59*:149–161 (1999).
40. **Feingold, K.R.:** The role of epidermal lipids in cutaneous permeability barrier homeostasis. *J. Lipid Res. 48*:2531-2546 (2007).
41. **Illel, B., H. Schaefer, J. Wepierre, and O. Doucet:** Follicles play an important role in percutaneous absorption. *J. Pharm. Sci. 80*:424–427 (1991).
42. **Mangelsdorf, S., N. Otberg, H.I. Maibach, R. Sinkgraven, W. Sterry, and J. Lademann:** Ethnic variation in vellus hair follicle size and distribution. *Skin Pharmacol. Physiol. 19*:159–167 (2006).
43. **Roskos, K.V., H.I. Maibach, and R.H. Guy:** The effect of aging on percutaneous absorption in man. *J. Pharmacokin. Biopharm. 17*:617–630 (1989).
44. **Buck, P.:** Skin barrier function: effect of age, race, and inflammatory disease. *Aromatherapy 14*:70–76 (2004).
45. **Rijken, F., P.L.B. Bruijnzeel, H. van Weelden, and R.C.M. Kiekens:** Responses of black and white skin to solar-simulating radiation: differences in DNA photodamage, infiltrating neutrophils, proteolytic enzymes induced, keratinocyte activation, and IL-10 expression. *J. Invest. Dermatol. 122*:1448–1455(2004).
46. **Weigland, D.A., C. Haygood, and J.R. Gaylor:** Cell layers and density of Negro and Caucasian stratum corneum. *J. Invest. Dermatol. 62*:563–568 (1974).
47. **Wesley, N.O., and H.I. Maibach:** Racial (ethnic) differences in skin properties: the objective data. *Am. J. Clin. Dermatol. 4*:843–860 (2003).
48. **Wester, R.C., and H.I. Maibach:** Percutaneous absorption of drugs. *Clin. Pharmacokin. 23*:253–266 (1992).
49. **Le Fur, I., A. Reinberg, S. Lopez, F. Morizot, M. Mechkouri, and E. Tschachler:** Analysis of circadian and ultradian rhythms of skin surface properties of face and forearm of healthy women. *J. Invest. Dermatol. 117*:718–724 (2001).
50. **Kanikkannan, N., K. Kandimalla, S.S. Lamba, and M. Singh:** Structure activity relationship of chemical penetration enhancers in transdermal drug delivery. *Curr. Med. Chem. 7*:593–608 (2000).
51. **Riviere, J.E. and M.C. Heit:** Electrically assisted transdermal drug delivery. *Pharm. Res. 14*:687–697 (1997).
52. **Eisenkraft, A., A. Krivoy, A. Vidan, E. Robenshtok, A. Hourvitz, T. Dushnitsky, and G. Markel:** Phase I study of a topical skin protectant against chemical warfare agents. *Mil. Med. 174*:1–47 (2009).
53. **Wigger-Alberti, W., U. Hinnen, and P. Elsner:** Predictive testing of metalworking fluids: A comparison of 2 cumulative human irritation models and correlation with epidemiological data. *Contact Derm. 36*:14–20 (1997).
54. **Sprince, N.L., J.A. Palmer, W. Popendorf, P.S. Thorne, M.I. Selim, C. Zwerling, and E.R. Miller:** Dermatitis among automobile production machine operators exposed to metal-working fluids. *Am. J. Ind. Med. 30*:421-429 (1996).
55. **Elias, P.M., M.L. Williams, W.M. Holleran, Y.J. Jiang, and M. Schmuth:** Pathogenesis of permeability barrier abnormalities in the ichthyoses: Inherited disorders of lipid metabolism. *J. Lipid Res. 49*:697–714 (2008).
56. **Oji, V., and H. Traupe:** Ichthyoses: Differential diagnosis and molecular genetics. *Eur. J. Dermatol. 16*:349–359 (2006).
57. **Freedberg, I.M., M. Tomic-Canic, M. Komine, and M. Blumenberg:** Keratins and the keratinocyte activation cycle. *J. Invest. Dermatol. 116*:633–640 (2001).

58. **Bos, P.M., D.H. Brouwer, H. Stevenson, P.J. Boogard, W.L. de Kort, and J.J. van Hemmen:** Proposal for the assessment of quantitative dermal exposure limits in occupational environments: Part 1. Development of a concept to derive a quantitative dermal occupational exposure limit. *Occup. Environ. Med. 55*:795–804 (1998).
59. **Adams, R.M.:** *Occupational Skin Diseases,* 3rd edition. Philadelphia, PA: Saunders, 1999.
60. **Allen, A.C.:** *The Skin: A Clinicopathological Treatise,* 2nd edition. New York: Grune and Stratton, 1967.
61. **Hogan, D.J.:** *Skin Lesions and Environmental Exposures (ATSDR Case Studies in Environmental Medicine).* Atlanta, GA.: Agency for Toxic Substances and Disease Registry, 1993.
62. **Luttrell, W.H., W.W. Jederberg, and K.R. Still (eds.):** *Toxicology Principles for the Industrial Hygienist.* Fairfax, VA: AIHA Press, 2008.
63. **Marzulli, E.N., and H.I. Maibach (eds.):** *Dermatotoxicology.* Washington, D.C.: Taylor & Francis, 1996.
64. **Percival, L., S.B. Tucker, S.H. Lamm, M.M. Key, B. Wilds, and K.S. Grumski:** A case study of dermatitis, based on a collaborative approach between occupational physicians and industrial hygiene. *Am. Ind. Hyg. Assoc. J. 56*:184–189 (1995).
65. **Rice, R.H., and T.M. Mauro:** Toxic responses of the skin. In *Casarett & Doull's Toxicology, The Basic Science of Poisons,* 7th edition. Klaassen, C.D. (ed.). New York: McGraw-Hill, 2007. pp. 741–760.
66. **Ancona, A.A.:** Occupational acne. *Occup. Med. 1*:229–243 (1986).
67. **Coenraads, P.J., A. Brouwer, K. Olie, and N. Tang:** Chloracne: Some recent issues. *Dermatol. Clin. 22*:569–576 (1994).
68. **Weitzner, J.M.:** Alopecia areata. *Am. Fam. Physician 41*:1197–1201 (1990).

Outcome Competencies

After completing this chapter, the reader should be able to:

1. Define underlined terms used in this chapter.
2. Describe characteristics of biohazards, and distinguish them from hazardous chemical or physical agents.
3. Identify risk factors of biohazardous and related agents.
4. Describe pathways of infection and their importance in control.
5. Understand risks associated with the Biosafety Levels as well as Animal Biosafety Levels.
6. Apply control strategies to biohazards and recognize their limitations, with an emphasis on biological safety cabinetry.
7. Describe general biohazardous waste issues and management practices.
8. Understand categories of sanitizers, decontaminants and sterilants.
9. Recognize federal regulatory requirements and guidelines for biohazards work.
10. Identify biological agents that are important in industrial processes.
11. Generate essential elements of a biohazards management program.
12. Draw process flow diagrams for biotechnology manufacturing.
13. Understand the issues and controls in place for biocrime and bioterrorism.
14. Be aware with emergency preparedness considerations involving biohazards and pandemic flu concerns.
15. Describe community concerns about gene therapies and genetically modified vectors, foods, or products.

Prerequisite Knowledge

None

Key Terms

bacteria • biohazard • biohazardous waste • bioterrorism • laminar flow biological safety cabinet • biological agent • biosafety • biosafety level • biotechnology • bloodborne pathogen • colonization • decontaminant • disinfectant • enzyme • etiologic agent • fungi • genetic engineering • genetically modified • infection • infectious agent • infectivity • microbe • mold • opportunistic pathogen • pandemic flu • pathogenicity • pathway of infection • personal protective equipment • primary barrier • prion • recombinant DNA • risk assessment • risk communication • secondary barrier • sterilant • transgenic • vector • virulence • virus • zoonotic infection

Key Topics

- I. Overview
  - A. Epidemics and Emerging Diseases
  - B. Categories of Agents
- II. Recognition and Evaluation of Biological Hazards
  - A. Nomenclature
  - B. Agent, Host, and Environment
  - C. Pathway of Infection
- III. Controls of Biohazards
  - A. Regulatory Environment
  - B. Approaches to Biological Safety
  - C. Biological Safety Cabinets
  - D. Biosafety Levels
  - E. Animal Use Biohazards
  - F. Transfer and Shipping Procedures for Biohazardous Agents
  - G. Decontamination, Disinfection, and Sterilization
  - H. Biotechnology and Industrial Biohazards
  - I. Enzymes in the Detergent Industry
  - J. Treatment and Disposal of Infectious Waste
- IV. Management Issues
  - A. Typical Program Elements
  - B. Emergency Planning and Risk Communication
- V. Summary

Biohazards and Associated Issues

22

Timothy J. Ryan, PhD, CIH, CSP

Overview

Epidemics and Emerging Diseases

The proven association of biologically active hazardous agents (i.e., biohazards) with human and animal diseases has existed for approximately 130 years. Yet for a variety of causes and reasons, including empirical research, genetic mutation, new technology, and novel laboratory techniques, new agents are still being discovered by scientists, and controlled by industrial hygienists. The interaction of a complex variety of factors is involved in each outcome associated with a specific biohazard. Recognizing and evaluating these factors is thus an imprecise, applied process that requires education, vigilance, experience, political savvy, and even luck, to effectively manage. Consider the form this process took in the following case.

In May 1993, an outbreak of an unexplained illness occurred in the southwestern United States, in the area of Arizona, New Mexico, Colorado and Utah known as "The Four Corners." The signal case of the imminent epidemic was a young, physically fit Navajo man suffering from shortness of breath. In reviewing the details of his death, investigators discovered the man's fiancée had died a few days earlier with similar respiratory symptoms. An investigation combing the entire Four Corners region was initiated which located an additional five cases, all of whom had died after acute respiratory failure. A series of laboratory tests failed to identify any known causes of the symptoms, such as bubonic plague, and after the first few patients died it became clear that a disease of unknown etiology was affecting people in the area, and that no one knew how it was transmitted. Widespread concern among the public ensued when the news media began extensively reporting on the outbreak.

During the next few weeks, as additional cases of the disease were reported in the region, physicians and other scientific experts came to believe some type of virus was potentially responsible for the mystery illness. Virologists at the Centers for Disease Control and Prevention (CDC) were able to link the pulmonary syndrome with a previously unknown type of hantavirus. Researchers knew that all other known hantaviruses were transmitted by rodents, and so began a program to trap as many different species of rodents living in the area as possible. In an action that might at first glance appear irresponsible to most industrial hygienists, especially given the high mortality associated with the presumed viral agent, public health practitioners decided not to wear protective clothing or masks during the trapping process. "We didn't want to go in wearing respirators, scaring ... everybody," one environmental disease specialist commented.[1] However, when the thousands of trapped specimens were dissected to prepare samples for analysis in CDC laboratories, industrial hygiene (IH) protocols mandating protective clothing and respirators were closely followed. The decision to offset the need for employee protection with minimizing public concern proved to be a lucky one in that no cases of what came to be called hantavirus pulmonary syndrome (HPS) were reported in health care workers who were exposed to either patients or specimens infected with related types of hantaviruses.

Among rodents trapped, the deer mouse (*Peromyscus maniculatus*) was found to be the main host to a previously unknown type of hantavirus. About 30% of the deer mice tested showed evidence of infection with hantavirus. Since the deer mouse often lives near people in rural and semi-rural areas—in barns and outbuildings, woodpiles, and even inside homes—researchers suspected that the deer mouse might be transmitting the virus to humans. By November, 1993, the specific hantavirus that caused the Four Corners outbreak was isolated. Using special laboratory containment equipment and other biological safety precautions, CDC used tissue from a deer mouse and grew the virus in the laboratory. The new virus was called Sin Nombre virus (SNV) and the symptoms it caused were associated with HPS. To put the rapid isolation of SNV in perspective, it took several decades for the first hantavirus discovered, the Hantaan virus, to be isolated. As part of the effort to locate the source of the virus, researchers located and examined stored samples of lung tissue from people who had died of unexplained lung disease. By this method, the earliest known case of HPS that has been confirmed was that of a 38-year-old Utah man in 1959. Interestingly, while HPS was not known to the established medical community, there is evidence that it was recognized in Navajo medical traditions, which associated its occurrence with mice.[2]

A compelling question to those interested in controlling biohazards and their diseases is why the HPS outbreak occurred at all. The answer is that environmental, agent, and host factors combined to allow case numbers to rise. During the outbreak period, there were many more mice than usual in the Four Corners area. In early 1993, heavy snows and rainfall helped drought-stricken plants and animals to revive and grow in larger-than-usual numbers. The area's deer mice had plenty to eat, and as a result they reproduced so rapidly that there were ten times more mice in May, 1993, than in the previous year. With so many mice, it was much more likely that mice and humans would come into contact with one another, and thus more likely that the hantavirus carried by the mice would be transmitted to humans.

This description of an emerging, heretofore unknown infectious disease (HPS) typifies the manner in which new hazardous microbes come to light as recognition and control issues for the IH profession. Other modern examples might include the spread of the West Nile virus, community acquired Methicillin resistant *S. aureus* (MRSA), Severe Acute Respiratory Syndrome (SARS) control, and pandemic avian influenza. The lack of understanding of hazards control of such newly discovered agents is typically high, and their potential for occupational exposure not always appreciated. Unlike biosafety professionals, laypersons have little scientific knowledge with respect to biological hazards. Their perceptions of what constitutes a biohazard are more influenced by media or entertainment sources, (e.g., the fact-based movie "The Hot Zone, about an Ebola virus hemorrhagic fever outbreak, or the Michael Crichton novels "The Andromeda Strain" and "Prey"). Spurred on by national or international accounts of would-be terrorists using microscopic agents to kill or injure the public, the formerly arcane term "biohazard" quickly found its way into such disparate discussions as Olympic events, New Year's celebrations at Times Square, the Congress of the United States, international airports, and even small town public water supplies.[3] Despite this newfound public interest, however, the proven hazards of microscopic life have taken some time to become recognized.

Antoni van Leeuwenhoek, a 17th century inventor of the water lens microscope, is credited with the first description ("little animals") of what we commonly refer to today as microbes. But it was not until the 19th century that Louis Pasteur, studying microbes and fermentation, suspected such microbes might also be responsible for illnesses. Eventually, in the 1880s, the German scientist Robert Koch identified the bacteria that cause anthrax, cholera, and tuberculosis.[4] Koch developed what are presently referred to as Koch's Postulates for linking a hazardous biological agent with the disease it is suspected of causing. His four step process entails: (1) tentatively identifying the causative agent, (2) finding that microbe in every case of the disease, (3) isolating the microbe under laboratory conditions, and (4) inoculating the agent to cause the disease in otherwise healthy study subjects. Koch's process is classic and still used in research and clinical microbiology laboratories, but the average person's understanding of what constitutes a biohazard is considerably less rigorous.

On occasion, the popular media, entertainment industry, and even professional training videos will erroneously label articles causing physical injury (e.g., broken glass) or chemical damage (e.g., chlorine gas) as biohazards. In professional nomenclature only an agent that is capable of interacting with living cells or tissues and as a result of that interaction propagating itself—or its effects—should be thought of as a biohazard. Broken glass from a clean syringe is not a biohazardous agent, yet that same glass, if contaminated with human blood, does constitute a biohazard. Note that the biohazardous agent need not be free-living under this definition, thus accounting for biohazardous viruses such as the human immunodeficiency virus (HIV; Figure 22.1), or Mad Cow Disease, attributed to a group of biohazards called prions (described later).

Categories of Agents

The industrial hygienist can potentially find biohazards anywhere on earth, and certainly anywhere human life is possible. As a practical concern, some industries such as health care, biotechnology, pharmaceuticals, and agriculture have more biohazards issues than others. But biohazards must also be addressed in less obvious locations or jobs, such as public trash containers or toilets, and among public service providers like police, fire, and sanitation workers.[5] While some causes of infectious diseases are so ubiquitous as to defy control (e.g., the common cold or flu viruses), to the extent controllable biohazards impact employees or the public at large, their management may be charged to the professional industrial hygienist.

Until the last several decades, the primary difference between biohazards and most other workplace hazards was that biohazards were naturally occurring agents whereas many occupational hazards were of human origin. Granted, numerous examples exist of toxic, naturally occurring chemicals and radiation in food, water and air. However, the vast majority of workplace stressors have some anthropogenic source. This is clearly the case with such classical industrial hygiene concerns as ergonomic issues related to assembly tools, hazardous or dangerous atmospheres in chemical refineries, noise and vibration stressors from machinery, and so forth. Until the advent of recombinant DNA (rDNA) technology in the early 1980s, biohazards were largely considered as naturally occurring hazardous microbes. Because of their biological diversity and vast numbers the classically trained industrial hygienist may find his or her foray into the study of biohazards complicated and quite challenging. Although biological agents are inherently different from chemical toxins, carcinogens, or physical agents, the IH paradigm of anticipation, recognition, evaluation, and control can still be applied.

Just as the controls of hazards related to ionizing radiation trace their roots to the basic science of physics, in an analogous manner the industrial hygienist must look to basic microbiology for the prescriptions and principles established for dealing with biohazards. Owing to the continued relevance of Koch's Postulates to the recognition of potentially hazardous microbes (vis a vis the prion diseases), the microbiology laboratory figures prominently in both presentation of biohazards and in the identification of their controls. One of the most significant organizations involved with microbiological safety is the CDC, which has published a very complete classification scheme for biohazards in its highly regarded and greatly expanded "Biosafety in Microbiological and Biomedical Laboratories", or BMBL.[6]

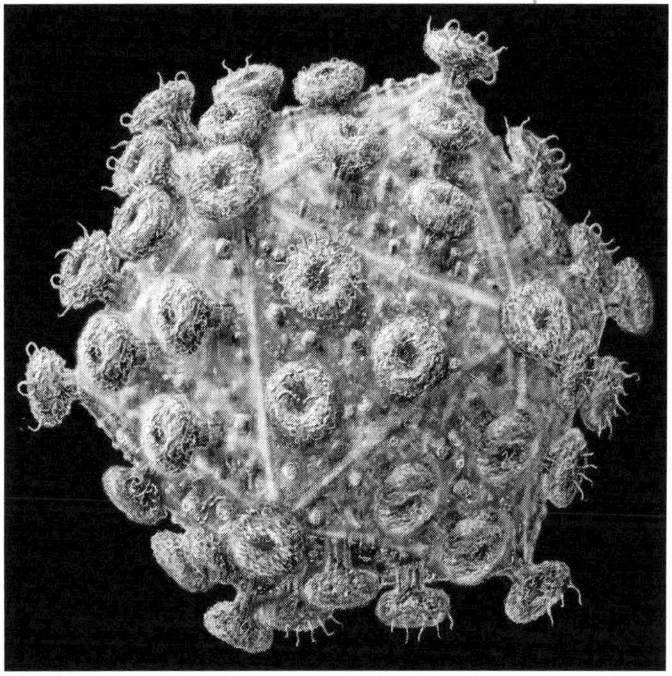

Figure 22.1 — Computer illustration of a fully-developed human immunodeficiency virus, causal agent of AIDS.

The CDC's BMBL currently lists eight categories of biohazardous agents. These are bacteria, fungi, parasites, rickettsia, viruses, arboviruses and related zoonotic viruses (with 597 specific entries, making it the largest single grouping), toxin agents, and prion diseases.[6] Specifically named biohazardous items encountered in field conditions—biohazardous wastes and "sharps", for example—are usually considered fomites, or objects that are contaminated with a biohazard from one of the eight categories. The basic biochemical or microbiological definition used to define these categories is increasingly subject to change as subtle nuances of the genetic code become better understood. Therefore, a discussion of the most current scientific naming conventions is better left to a current textbook of microbiology. For the purposes of this chapter, working definitions of biohazardous agents as listed in Table 22.1 will be employed. It is important to keep in mind that Table 22.1 lists only categories of agents as presently defined and excludes the very limited number of toxin agents. Until relatively recently, for example, prions were not specifically identified as such and were referred to as "unconventional filterable agents."[7] Another limitation of any purportedly complete listing of biohazardous agents is that associated or ancillary work done with biohazards may require additional precautions. Examples of such work includes that done with rDNA, primate or other cellular tissue cultures, and toxins of biological origin.

The diversity within each class of biohazardous agents requires an empirical approach to risk assessment rather than an analogous approach taken with hazardous materials like chemicals, radiation, or physical agents. Knowing that a chemical is an organic solvent gives the experienced industrial hygienist some idea of the health and safety hazards to expect from it. Yet knowing a biohazard is a virus tells little about the seriousness of exposure and infection from that virus. Infection may be asymptomatic or prove fatal. Furthermore, air sampling or the use of real-time, direct reading instruments for biological agents is not typical for assessing potential exposures. More often clinical specimens from workers or patients are collected to identify potential exposure to given etiologic agents. These results are then compared with bulk or wipe samples grown under laboratory conditions conducive for specific organisms. Finally, in terms of control for biohazards, administrative actions such as frequent hand washing and avoidance of foods in work areas can be just as important as engineering practices. The use of personal protective equipment (PPE) is considered a procedural fundamental since exposure to biohazards by inhalation, direct contact, and breaks in skin are important routes of transmission, and PPE provides crucial primary barrier protection from such direct exposures even when typical engineering controls are in place.

Although there are specially trained biological safety professionals, the number of such persons is only about 1,750 worldwide.[8] As a result, industrial or occupational hygienists may be called on to respond to complaints and to investigate exposure or other issues pertaining to biological agents. The purpose of this chapter is to assist such professionals in responding to such matters, whether they be in areas of hospital safety, industry, agriculture, research, education, public services, schools, communities, or defense.

Recognition and Evaluation of Biological Hazards

Nomenclature

Any risk assessment involving biohazardous materials must be firmly rooted in a clear understanding of biohazards nomenclature. A number of key biohazards definitions are provided in Table 22.2. As seen from the table "infection" does not always mean overt, symptomatic disease. Infections can be asymptomatic, resulting in the well known carrier-state epitomized by the infamous "Typhoid Mary" of 1906. In latent, or subclinical, infections the organism has interacted with the host in such a way that no signs or symptoms are displayed, yet an immune response is mounted (i.e., rise in antibody titer to the organism or its product). Other examples where subclinical infections are known to occur include exposures to *Mycobacterium tuberculosis* (TB) and Cytomegalovirus (CMV). Colonization is a state in which infection and establishment of an organism within a host has occurred

Table 22.1 — Categories of Biohazard Agents[6,7]

Agent Category	*Defining Characteristics*	*Occupationally Important Examples*
Bacteria	Bacteria are the oldest and most abundant life forms on Earth, and are found almost everywhere: in the soil and water, in plants and animals. Bacteria are one cell microbes lacking chlorophyll, and grow by simple division. Unlike the eucaryotes--animal and plant cells--bacterial cells are prcaryotes which lack a nucleus. They exist in three main morphologies: spherical (cocci), rod-shaped (bacilli), and spiral (spirilla). If conditions turn unfavorable, some bacteria can remain dormant in highly chemically resistant spores. Relatively few of the thousands of species of bacteria cause an infectious disease in humans.	Escherichia coli pathogenic strains such as E. coli 0157:H7, dubbed the "flesh eating" bacteria. Found in foods contaminated with fecal matter, destroys human cells and can cause fatal bleeding of the colon, bowel, and kidneys. TB, or tuberculosis, a lung disease caused by Mycobaterium tuberculosis. Historically a very significant U.S disease and now a re-emergent disease, placing healthcare workers at indigent or low-income clinics at particular risk. Spread from its human reservoir by droplet nuclei from coughing or sneezing.
Fungi	Fungi include mushrooms, molds, and yeasts, which are distinguishable from plants in that they do not make their own food. Occupationally important fungi get their nutrition by breaking down the remains of dead plants or necrosing tissue in at-risk patients.	Aspergillus species are commonly found degrading organic matter in nature. A. fumigatus and A. flavus are opportunistic human pathogens, causing Aspergillosis in immunocompromised (AIDS, transplant) patients. Histoplasmosis, a systemic mycosis caused by Histoplasma capsulatum infection, typically as the result of the disturbance of bird or bat droppings.
Parasites	Single or multicellular organisms living on or in a host from which they derive sustenance without providing benefit. In biohazard parlance, parasites are assumed to be detrimental if not wholly pathogenic.	Toxoplaxmosis caused by the coccidian protozoan of cats, Toxoplasma gondii. This agent may be spread via contaminated domestic cat feces to pregnant women, leading to fetal infection and death. Trichinellosis, caused by an intestinal roundworm, Trichinella spiralis. Spread by consumption of poorly cooked foods, especially pork.
Prions	PROteinaceous INfectious particles that lack nucleic acids; composed largely of an abnormal isoform of a normal cellular protein.	Creutzfeldt-Jakob disease, a fatal degenerative brain disease. Bovine spongiform encephalopathy, or "mad cow disease", known to affect only cows at this time.
Rickettsia	Eubacteria, very small gram negative intracellular parasites first described in 1909 by Harold Taylor Ricketts; non-motile, non-sporeforming, and nonencapsulated. Live in the cells of ticks and mites.	Clinically similar diseases transmitted by hard ticks, such as Rocky Mountain Spotted Fever caused by Rickettsia rickettsii and Queensland Tick Typhus caused by R. australis.

Table 22.1 — Categories of Biohazard Agents[6,7] (continued)

Agent Category	*Defining Characteristics*	*Occupationally Important Examples*
Viruses Other than Arboviruses	Ultramicroscopic pathogenic infectious agents characterized by multiplying in connection with living cells. Found in all living things including bacteria and fungi. They can appear as spirals, 20-sided figures, or more complex forms. Viruses are mostly genetic material—DNA or RNA—and may occur in a single or double strand. They are not presently considered cells, as they cannot carry out life functions independently.	Common colds Warts Influenza Viral Hepatitis A, B, C, D, and E Herpesviruses Poliovirus Rabies virus Human immunodeficiency virus, or HIV, targets then inhabits immune cells— T lymphocytes specifically. To cause full blown AIDS, HIV changes its genetic material from RNA to DNA. In doing so, HIV often genetically mutates such that an already weakened immune system has a more difficult task identifying and resisting the virus.
Arboviruses	Viruses transmitted by or borne by insects.	West Nile Fever, caused by the West Nile virus spread by mosquitoes preying on birds. Ebola virus, as caused 70% fatal outbreaks in equatorial Africa in 1995.

Table 22.2 — Selected Biohazards Nomenclature[7]

Colonization — Detectable presence of microbes

Communicable Disease — an Infectious Disease; due to a specific agent or its toxic products.

Etiologic Agent — A biohazardous material capable of causing infection and subsequent disease.

Fomite — Inanimate objects contaminated with infectious agents which serve to facilitate the spread of the agent to new hosts.

Herd Immunity — Immunity shared by all or most members of a group or community, which reduces invasive capacity of infectious diseases.

Inapparent Infection — Presence of infectious agents in a host that are detectable by laboratory means only; synonymous with asymptomatic, subclinical and occult infection.

Infection — Entry and growth of infectious agents in the host.

Infectious Disease — An infection that is clinically manifested in the host.

Infectious Dose — The empirically derived number of infectious agents required to cause infection in a normal, susceptible host.

Infectiousness, or Infectivity — Qualitative term used to describe the apparent ease by which an infectious agent is spread to a host.

Microbes — Microscopic agents, such as viruses, bacteria, parasites, and rickettsia.

Microflora — The unique microbial makeup characterizing a host or region of a host, or an artificial or natural environmental niche.

Pathogenicity — The ability of an infectious agent to produce infection and disease. See Virulence.

Sharps — Fomites such as used hypodermic needles, scalpel blades or broken glass likely to be, or potentially contaminated with infectious agents transmitted via the injection route.

Virulence — Qualitative term describing the case-fatality rates of an infectious agent, used to attribute the degree of pathogenicity of the agent. Relative infectiousness. See Pathogenicity.

Zoonosis — Diseases transmissible from animals to man under normal host-environment conditions.

without resulting in subclinical or clinical disease. Human examples of colonization include *Staphylococcus salivarius* and *Bacteriodaceae* spp., which colonize the mouth; *S. epidermidis* and *S. aureus*, which colonize the skin; and the presence of *Escherichia coli* and *Peptococcus* spp. in the large intestine.[9] Actual disease is characterized by a number of overt symptoms and analytical test results exhibited by the infected patient or in his or her personal samples. Such clinical infections are recognized by the display of symptoms and the presence of an immune response historically associated with the infectious agent.

Agent, Host, and Environment

With respect to evaluating biohazardous material risks, the three factors the industrial hygienist must understand and consider are the nature of the infectious agent or its products, the nature of the host (i.e., human physiology, including host immune responses), and environmental conditions. These three elements must be considered both in terms of their interrelationships and with respect to any external forces affecting them. Figure 22.2 depicts the interactive nature of the main components of risk assessment for biological hazards.[10]

The interactions among a biological agent, the environment, and a host can result in a continuum of effects across the population or workforce, from no infection to subclinical effects to disease and its concomitant host damage. For infection and illness to occur in a new host, Lee and Johnson[10] list six necessary and sufficient conditions that are related to the agent (A), environment (E), or host (H):

(1) The agent must be pathogenic (A);
(2) There must be a reservoir of sufficient number for the organism to live and reproduce (E);
(3) The agent must be able to escape from the reservoir (A, E);
(4) The organism must be transferable, or able to move or be moved through the environment by various means (A, E, H);
(5) There must be a portal of entry to the new host (e.g., broken skin, mucous membrane, inhalation, blood transfer) (H); and
(6) The new host must be susceptible to the agent (H).

If even one of the six elements is not fulfilled, then infection or disease cannot be spread beyond the reservoir. Just as time, distance and shielding are guiding principles for radiation exposure minimization, so is the control of biohazards based on eliminating one or more of these stepping-stones in the "pathway of infection".

Pathway of Infection

In practice every biosafety control strategy is intended to break one or more of the links in a pathway of infection, thus preventing the spread of disease. The acronym of RETER is sometimes employed in risk communication presentations of this concept, corresponding to Reservoir of the agent, means of Exit from the reservoir, method of Transmission, Entry to a susceptible host, and Re-infection.[11]

As an example application of the RETER model, consider the spread of rabies virus from mammals to humans. Rabies virus is clearly a pathogenic agent, responsible for 35,000 to 40,000 fatalities each year worldwide.[7] The virus sustains itself mostly in a reservoir of infected terrestrial mammals, including dogs, foxes, coyotes, skunks, and raccoons, although another reservoir for human exposure is bats, which are frequently infected and come in contact with humans during a variety of mostly outdoor activities. The agent exits the reservoir in virus-laden saliva of the rabid animal when it is transmitted in a bite, or is (very rarely) transmitted by aerosols. The host becomes

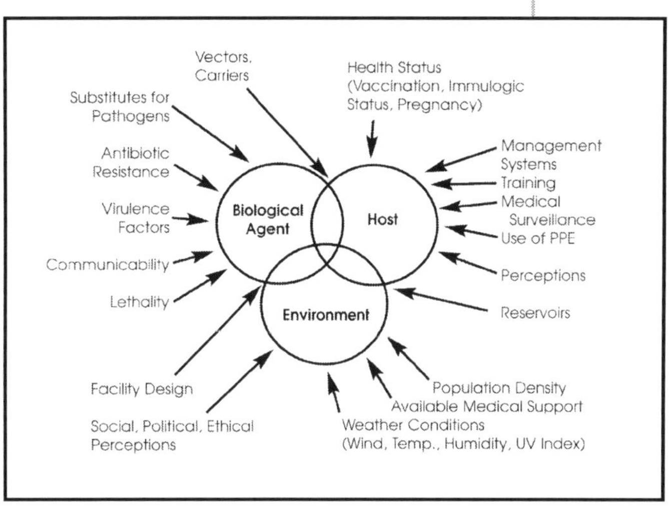

Figure 22.2 — Risk assessment involving biological agents: factors to consider.

infected upon virus entry from the animal's bite or inhalation of the viral particles, at which point re-infection can occur. Should any of these steps be blocked, rabies control is established. Specifically, if the reservoir is eliminated through such actions as immunizations of domestic dogs, or the removal of bat habitats, the pathway of infection is blocked. If there is no release from the reservoir or transmission through bites to the hosts, then there can be no disease.

The RETER concept is just as applicable in an occupational setting presenting biological hazards. In such environments the industrial hygienist may recommend procedures involving PPE when working in areas where rabies virus is prevalent. To control laboratory infections, administrative procedures that call for minimum container standing times post-agitation might be adopted to minimize the release of aerosols upon opening. The use of containment equipment such as laminar flow biological safety cabinets might be required to prevent virus release and transmission via the airborne route. Administrative procedures, such as the prohibition of sharps in proximity to combative patients, reduce the potential for transmission by the percutaneous route.

Insofar as agent factors are concerned, certainly the most significant issue is the pathogenicity (see Table 22.2) of the biological agent. Agents historically associated with high virulence, as demonstrated by elevated case-fatality rates, are readily recognized as high-risk biohazards. Similarly those for which there is significant morbidity but no preventive vaccine or known treatment must be given high priority. Several references provide lists[12–14] that place known biohazardous agents in categories according to their pathogenicity, virulence, and so forth. The least hazardous agents are not known to cause disease in healthy adults. Medium risk agents are associated with human disease, but are unlikely to be fatal, are mostly spread via direct contact, and there usually are curative medical treatments. Higher risk agents are indigenous or exotic agents with potential for difficult-to-control airborne transmission, and may produce diseases with serious or lethal consequences. The most hazardous exotic agents pose high risk of life-threatening disease, and there may be no known vaccine or treatment.[15]

Some of the most historically remarkable stories of disease prevention have come about through public health measures aimed at the destruction of habitats harboring disease-causing agents. Such was the case with the elimination of rats infested with rat fleas (acting as the reservoir and mode of transmission, respectively) during the infamous Bubonic Plague in Europe in 1348 AD.[16] With a case-fatality rate of upwards of 60%[7] this infectious disease caused by the bacillus *Yersinia pestis* is typically controlled by reducing the opportunity for humans to be bitten by infected fleas. Once hygiene measures were implemented to both decrease the rat population as well as minimize contact between rats and human hosts (and therefore fleas), control was achieved.

The now classical epidemiology employed by John Snow in his identification and correction of the great cholera epidemic in 1854 London[17] demonstrated conclusively the ability to control an infectious agent by controlling its exit from its reservoir. Cholera is caused by the bacterium *Vibrio cholerae*, with transmission to humans by water or food. The natural reservoir of the organism is not conclusively known but is believed to be humans or the aquatic environment.[18] In the London outbreak, Snow was able to effect control by eliminating the close proximity of human waste disposal to SoHo water wells, thereby preventing the exit of the infectious agent. To this day, many of the elements of modern plumbing codes are in place owing to the simple concept of waste and potable water separation first suggested by John Snow more than 150 years ago. Whether the agent is spread by airborne particles, direct contact with an infected host, or via intermediates termed vectors, eliminating the means of transmission of an infectious agent is perhaps one of the most critical approaches of direct biohazards control.

To further illustrate just how important interrupting the means of transmission can be, the industrial hygienist need only look to infamous control failures for examples. Such was the case with SARS, the viral respiratory illness first seen in China in 2002. Within months of the first reports of its existence, it had spread to North and South America, Europe, and Asia, leading to an epidemic by 2003.[19] Ultimately, over 8,000 persons worldwide would become infected, with close to 800 fatalities.[20] Transmission of SARS results primarily from direct patient contact or contact with large respiratory droplets in the close vicinity of an infected person, and so SARS was a major concern among healthcare workers. In April, 2003, a Toronto primary care physician (reportedly wearing no respiratory protection) contracted SARS after seeing a patient. In the course of treatment for the physician, as many as 11 healthcare workers who had treated him contracted SARS, presumably as a result of respirator selection failures and a lack of fit testing among those personnel wearing respirators.[21] As a result of this failure to control the transmission of the SARS virus (reentry in this instance), recommendations for the use of N95 respirators were strengthened. In addition, NIOSH conducted risk assessments that lead to safeguards directed at transmission control not only for healthcare workers, but for aircraft flight crews, cargo handlers, and cleaning personnel, and those transporting SARS patients.[19]

Routes of entry for biohazardous agents are many, but the most typical include direct contact with mucous membranes or breaks in the skin, by inhalation or ingestion, or by percutaneous injection. Intact skin provides an effective barrier to infection for almost all biohazards via direct contact (Leptospira, which can penetrate intact skin, is a notable exception). The protective nature of skin resides in its characteristic dry, slightly acidic nature (pH 5), and its capacity to support normal flora, which create a hostile and competitive environment for invading microbes. Use of gloves to prevent contact with bloodborne pathogens or respiratory protection against TB via inhalation are examples of barriers to eliminate the portal of entry.

The last two required conditions for infection are that a host receive an infectious dose through a portal of entry, and that the new host be susceptible to the agent. Theoretically, a single pathogenic microbe should be capable of causing infection. However, owing to host defense mechanisms—especially the immune response—and virulence factors related to the agent, an infectious dose may be as large as a million or more organisms. Such is the case for enteric pathogens like cholera. Conversely, the infectious dose may require very few organisms (e.g., 1–10), as in the case of respiratory organisms such as *Mycobacterium tuberculosis*. This wide variation in numbers required for infection is one of several reasons why biosafety professionals have relied on empirical experience and an understanding of the qualitative factors of disease spread in making meaningful risk assessments regarding biohazards work safeguards.

Many other host factors also play key roles in determining the outcome of an insult with a biohazardous agent. Mucous and other fluids (tears, urine, semen, vaginal secretions, saliva) bathe membranes associated with the urogenital tract, nasal passages, throat and respiratory tract, and eyes, and act to trap incoming invaders and mechanically carry them away from potential sites of adherence. Mucous also functions as a medium for the maintenance of indigenous beneficial microbes (i.e., the host's microflora) that prohibit colonization by entering pathogenic organisms. Without entry, interactions precipitating the infectious or toxic process cannot occur.

Finally, if the biological agent actually enters the host in sufficient numbers constituting an infectious dose, and if the host is susceptible, infection can occur if the agent can overcome biological competition. On ingestion, for example, the biological agent or microorganism is exposed to bile salts, peptidases, trypsin and numerous other enzymes, pancreatic and gastric acids, and a variety of indigenous and colonized intestinal microflora. Their role in defense against invading microorganisms is to compete for receptors on cells and for nutrients[22], or produce proteins that are bactericidal to invading pathogens.[23] Pathogens entering via the respiratory tract encounter cilia on the tracheal rings. The cilia forming the mucocilliary escalator beat toward the mouth, carrying particles up and out of potential target tissues such as the lungs. The very old, the very young, and persons with existing immune system deficiencies most often make up the population of susceptible hosts. Immunocompromised individuals in particular—transplant patients in hospitals, neonates, or persons with AIDS-related complex or AIDS—are susceptible to infections from organisms that most healthy adults can ward off. Termed opportunistic infections, these occurrences result from common molds and bacteria routinely present in the environment. Dust generated in construction projects in hospitals often contains *Aspergillus fumigatus* spores. Exposure to Aspergillus spores is not a problem for hospital staff, but can result in fatal infections for such immunocompromised individuals. Specialized industrial hygienists, infection control practitioners, and hospital engineering staff are all required in such scenarios to evaluate dust containment for the project, protection of ventilation systems, and maintaining the health status of such patients.

Control of Biohazards

There is no standard method for assessing biological risk, although the specific agent involved is obviously the first factor considered.[6] Quantitative models have been proposed, and certain models currently drive research in this area of concern, as in the case of aerosol transmission of TB.[24–27] Quantitative modeling for biological risk assessment is useful research, but applying a theoretical model to a specific situation may be of only limited utility. In applied, real world situations exposure models are likely to involve relatively small numbers of workers, making valid statistical analysis difficult. Furthermore, qualitative aspects of risk, such as effectiveness of training, human motivation for risk avoidance, and social or political influences are not quantifiable. Accordingly the approach put forth here is to evaluate and understand the characteristics of the agent, provide for physical containment whenever possible or mandated, and employ responsible management systems to ensure administrative safeguards and legal compliance.

Regulatory Environment

Required safeguards applicable to most biohazards operations (e.g., hospitals, research or clinical laboratories, production bioreactors) consist of a patchwork of guidelines, standards of practice, laws, and regulations resulting from a number of federal agencies, departments within agencies, state and sometimes local jurisdictions. Those working in the comprehensive practice of the IH profession sometimes only poorly understand the regulatory milieu pertaining to biohazards. On the other hand, the laws and guidelines for the safe handling, use, and disposal of etiologic agents are generally well understood by the certified biological safety professional (CBSP). That said, changes to the BMBL[28], in conjunction with passage of the US PATRIOT Act of 2001[29] and the Public Health Security and Bioterrorism Preparedness and Response Act of 2002[30], have produced complex, intertwined regulations that test the exactitude of even the most meticulous practitioner. Relatively recent regulations now criminalize the possession, shipment, or receipt of certain biological materials by restricted persons.[31] Thus it is now the domain of the safety professional to not only safeguard the employee or community from the biohazardous agent, but to ensure biosecurity measures are in place to safeguard and control access to high hazard agents.

The nature and scope of these changes is perhaps captured best in the Forward section of the latest edition of the BMBL[6], which states in part:

> "The events of September 11, 2001 and the anthrax attacks in October of that year re-shaped and changed, forever, the way we manage and conduct work in biological and clinical laboratories and draw into focus the need for inclusion of additional information in the BMBL. In an attempt to better serve the needs of our community in this new era, information on the following topics has been added in the 5th edition: Occupational medicine and immunization, Decontamination and sterilization, Laboratory biosecurity and risk assessment, Biosafety Level 3 (Ag) laboratories, Agent summary statements for some agricultural pathogens, {and} Biological toxins."[6]

Requirements for the safe handling and use of biohazardous agents vary by employer classification. In some workplaces (e.g., public or private colleges and universities receiving federal National Institutes of Health (NIH) funding), documents labeled as guidelines may be so important to continued funding of work as to require compliance. This is in fact the case with respect to NIH grant recipients, who must comply with the

National Institutes of Health Guidelines for Research (NIHG) involving rDNA.[32] In addition, the NIHG have sometimes been considered standards of practice in commercial biotechnology companies.[33] While the BMBL purports to make recommendations that are only advisory, the text goes on to state that the BMBL intent "...was and is to establish a voluntary code of practice."[25] Because BMBL recommendations are so widely accepted as a code of practice, any employer would be remiss in failing to adopt, or at least formally consider, the advisory recommendations they contain. In the event of a biohazards incident at a facility, management and possibly individuals could be held liable under U.S. or state statues.

In other biohazards use environments, regulatory controls are more prescriptive. In 1991, the Occupational Safety and Health Administration (OSHA) promulgated the first standard in its history aimed at healthcare workers exposed or potentially exposed to infectious agents.[34] The bloodborne pathogens standard (BBP) came on the heels of the CDC's then-new "universal precautions" recommendation[35] for handling all fluids from all patients as potentially infective for the then-unidentified causative agent of AIDS. At first interpreted relatively conservatively, the BBP has impacted a great many work and public places in the years since its passage. As a result, biohazards management programs can now be found not only in doctor and dentist offices, but in police and fire departments, in school nurse offices, and in organizations as diverse as intercollegiate sports (e.g., bloody noses or scrapes among athletes) to sanitation at large national airports (e.g., used insulin syringes). Until the advent of universal precautions and BBP, hospitals and most accredited clinical, teaching, treatment, and nursing employers had voluntarily submitted to community standards of practice concerning biohazardous agents, infection control, and waste disposal. Compliance with BBP practices is still highly visible at many healthcare organizations receiving outside funding, since under the terms of contracts for federal patient revenues, these organizations must comply with and submit to inspections by the Joint Commission for the Accreditation of Healthcare Organizations (JCAHO).[36]

Laws targeting high risk biohazards restrict the shipping, possession, and receipt of such agents.[29,30] The limitations of such efforts are readily apparent due to the fact that many biohazardous agents may be easily isolated from the natural environment. To create a pure culture of certain biohazardous agents, a reasonably careful and moderately informed person need only isolate the agent from ambient air or soil. Historically, CDC has had the responsibility for providing guidance to researchers and legislators concerning controls of biohazardous materials. The ominous sounding Antiterrorism and Effective Death Penalty Act of 1996[37] required the Secretary of Health and Human Services (HHS) to promulgate new regulations, expanding the CDC's role by placing additional controls on etiologic agents that could be used for terrorist purposes.[38] This was done in the aftermath of the bombings of the Alfred P. Murrah federal building in Oklahoma City and the first attack on the World Trade Center.

Since the second attack on the World Trade Center, and in the wake of the anthrax letter attacks of 2001, added safeguards have been implemented. The Public Health Security and Bioterrorism Preparedness and Response Act of 2002, Subtitle A of Public Law 107–188[30] requires HHS to establish and regulate a list of biological agents and toxins that have the potential to pose a severe threat to public health and safety. The Agricultural Bioterrorism Protection Act of 2002 requires the United States Department of Agriculture (USDA) to establish and regulate a list of biological agents that have the potential to pose a severe threat to animal health and safety, plant health and safety, or to the safety of animal or plant products. Agents so defined by HHS or USDA have been termed "select agents." CDC and USDA share responsibility for some agents because they potentially threaten both humans and animals (overlap agents). The laws require HHS and USDA to review and republish the lists of select agents and toxins on at least a biennial basis (see Table 22.3). Those who would possess or otherwise manage listed agents must register with The National Select Agent Registry Program. Covered facilities include government agencies, universities, research institutions, and commercial entities.[39] Under the current rules, CDC safeguards against the threats to public health and safety presented by biological agents, toxins, and delivery systems,

Table 22.3 — HHS Select Agents and Toxins and USDA Overlap Agents*

HHS SELECT AGENTS AND TOXINS

Abrin
Botulinum neurotoxins
Botulinum neurotoxin producing species of *Clostridium*
Cercopithecine herpesvirus 1 (Herpes B virus)
Clostridium perfringens epsilon toxin
Coccidioides posadasii/Coccidioides immitis
Conotoxins
Coxiella burnetii
Crimean-Congo haemorrhagic fever virus
Diacetoxyscirpenol
Eastern Equine Encephalitis virus
Ebola virus
Francisella tularensis
Lassa fever virus
Marburg virus
Monkeypox virus
Reconstructed replication competent forms of the 1918 pandemic influenza virus containing any portion of the coding regions of all eight gene segments (Reconstructed 1918 Influenza virus)
Ricin
Rickettsia prowazekii
Rickettsia rickettsii
Saxitoxin
Shiga-like ribosome inactivating proteins
South American Haemorrhagic Fever viruses
  Flexal
  Guanarito
  Junin
  Machupo
  Sabia
Staphylococcal enterotoxins
T-2 toxin
Tetrodotoxin
Tick-borne encephalitis complex (flavi) viruses
  Central European Tick-borne encephalitis
  Far Eastern Tick-borne encephalitis
  Kyasanur Forest disease
  Omsk Hemorrhagic Fever
  Russian Spring and Summer encephalitis
Variola major virus (Smallpox virus)
Variola minor virus (Alastrim)
Yersinia pestis

OVERLAP SELECT AGENTS AND TOXINS

Bacillus anthracis
Brucella abortus
Brucella melitensis
Brucella suis
Burkholderia mallei (formerly Pseudomonas *mallei*)
Burkholderia pseudomallei (formerly Pseudomonas *pseudomallei*)
Hendra virus
Nipah virus
Rift Valley fever virus
Venezuelan Equine Encephalitis virus

*This is a partial listing only which specifically excludes USDA-only listings

and provides facility management with guidance concerning restrictions for improper possession of such substances.

Possession of the majority of biohazardous agents is otherwise (and historically) regulated only indirectly, through individual apprehension and detention authorities granted to the Surgeon General and Secretary of HHS[40] for the purposes of preventing the spread of communicable diseases. Heretofore these powers were interpreted as necessary for the control of unintentional disease transmission, such as by carriers. With the new emphasis on sinister intent and the potential for use of biohazards in weapons of mass destruction, it is the stated goal of CDC to work with the Federal Bureau of Investigation (FBI) to craft criminal sanctions designed to capture and punish those who possess biohazardous agents for nefarious purposes.[41] Under the Homeland Security Act of 2002[42], the mandate for more cooperative, coordinated, and efficient information sharing with respect to possible terrorist use of biohazardous agents was created. Under this law, requirements related to biohazardous agents have been enacted on many fronts, including requirements for certain agricultural inspections, conduct of public health activities, coordination with HHS under the Public Health Services Act, as well as Smallpox vaccine development.

Insofar as packaging and shipping of biohazards is necessary, the federal government, most nations, and professional shipping associations have declared biological agents and materials suspected of containing them to be hazardous materials. Thus, the U.S. Department of Transportation (DOT)[43] mandates procedures for the legal shipping of biohazards and clinical specimens. Likewise, the U.S. Postal Service (USPS)[44] has enacted shipping mandates. The International Air Transport Association (IATA), representing both commercial and cargo airborne carriers of biohazards shipments, publishes requirements for shippers wishing to use member-carriers to transport biohazardous materials. Termed the "Dangerous Goods Regulations", these requirements are essentially obligatory inasmuch as most biohazards shipments are perishable and therefore require aircraft transport by IATA members. In addition, many USPS shipments are contracted to IATA-regulated carriers, effectively bringing virtually all biohazards shipments under some form of legally binding requirements for their shipment.[45–49]

The U.S. has historically regulated the import or other procurement of domestic plant and animal pathogens on the basis of economic crop or livestock protection, and not on the basis of threats to the populace. The USDA and Animal and Plant Health Inspection Service (APHIS) presently requires permits from all who would bring nonindigenous pathogenic biohazards into the U.S.[50,51] Export of plant or animal etiologic agents, as well as those affecting humans, is regulated by the U.S. Department of Commerce.[52] With respect to importation of human biohazardous agents, regulations of the CDC[53] apply, which require the approval of that agency in the form of a permitting-process before such materials may be legally transported into the country.

Prior to about 1988, disposal of biological waste was not of great public concern and so was loosely regulated, if at all. There was neither epidemiologic evidence that most hospital waste was any more infective than residential waste, nor evidence that hospital waste had caused disease in the community as the result of improper disposal.[54] Because infectious persons are dispersed within any community, control of biohazardous waste per se attracted little attention. With heightened fear of contracting AIDS, coincident with several highly publicized incidents of medical waste washing up on U.S. beaches in the early and mid-1980s, the public took greater interest in the fate of biomedical wastes. Outside of federal facilities operating under general exemptions from state laws, legal disposal of biohazardous waste is currently regulated by the individual states. The majority of such entities have generally defined biohazards as a category of hazardous waste. As such they are typically controlled by the state's environmental protection agency, department of natural resources, or department of public health. Biological wastes are discussed extensively later in this chapter.

Approaches to Biological Safety

The primary goal of any biosafety program is providing effective containment of hazardous viable agents in order to prevent the spread of infection. There are a number of well respected guides published and periodically updated on how to accomplish this goal. For example, the previously mentioned BMBL provides well-defined model laboratory, clinical, and animal-based biosafety programs. As noted, certification of compliance with these rules is required by government, academic, and industrial grantees, as well as contractors receiving funding from NIH. In patient care organizations, the infection control standards from the Accreditation Manual for Hospitals, published by JCAHO[36], will likely be the source of expected practices, in addition to any specific procedures mandated by OSHA for facilities under its jurisdiction.[55] For groups working with rDNA or on projects leading up to the environmental release of genetically engineered (recombinant) organisms, the NIHG[32] must be followed. Industrial biotechnology users not otherwise included in these categories have slightly more leeway in their approach, relying on guidance from AIHA's® *Biosafety Reference Manual*[56], the BMBL[6], or the WHO *Laboratory Biosafety Manual*.[57] Any reader with responsibilities in the settings mentioned should refer directly to these references for details of the recommendations, and how they apply to the particular operations of such workplaces.

Regardless of the specific program manual adopted by the industrial hygienist's organization, the paradigm for control of biohazardous material is containment. Both the NIHG and BMBL describe containment in terms of primary and secondary barriers. Primary barriers describe controls to protect the worker and immediate work area from potential exposure. Primary barriers include biological safety cabinets (BSC), sealed centrifuge rotors, glove boxes (termed isolators in some facilities), sharps containers, high efficiency particulate air (HEPA) filtered animal enclosures, etc. PPE such as gloves, eye protection, and respirators are important personal barriers. Primary containment is also provided by good microbiological technique. Secondary barriers refer to protections aimed at the external environment, such as non-laboratory work areas and the outside community. It is less clearly defined, and can refer to both additional appliances or devices, or to facility or other engineering controls installed to prevent migration of an uncontained biohazard. Thus, secondary containment is achieved by a combination of facility design (e.g., differential pressurization

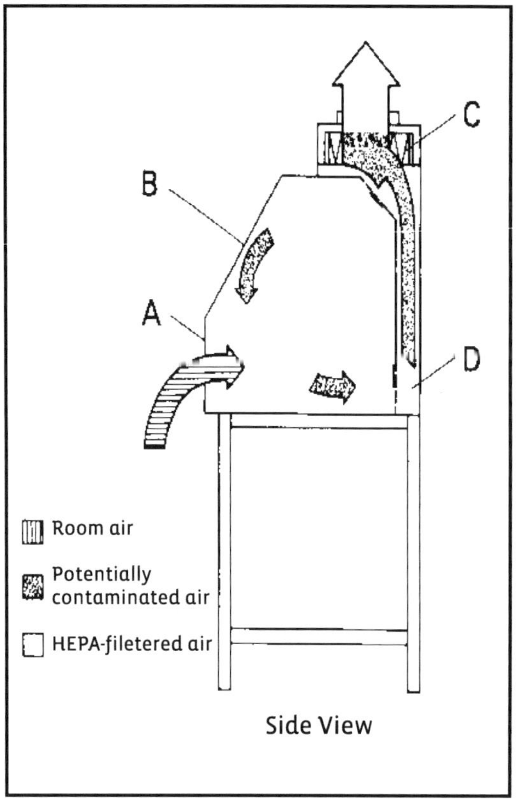

Figure 22.3 — Class I BSCL (A) front opening; (B) sash; (C) exhaust HEPA filter; (D) exhaust plenum. (Source: Reference 6)

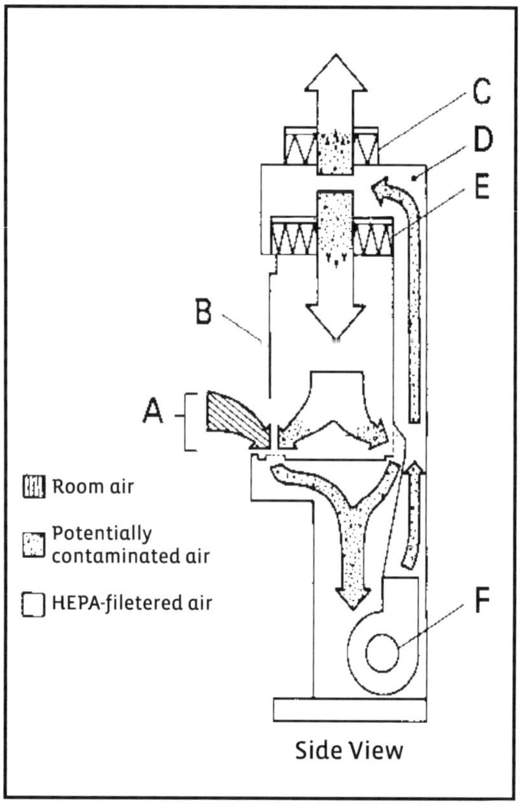

Figure 22.4 — Class II, type A, BSC: (A) front opening; (B) sash; (C) exhaust HEPA filter; (D) rear plenum; (E) supply HEPA filter; (F) blower. (Source: Reference 6).

of work areas, HEPA-filtered exhaust ventilation, anterooms and airlocks, sterilization of effluent liquids, etc.) in conjunction with work practices and procedures. As a side note it should be pointed out that when rDNA concerns were in their infancy, another level of containment referred to as "biological" was often described. In it, the intended host of the recombinant molecule was intentionally selected to be highly susceptible to ambient environmental conditions. In the event the host was inadvertently released, it would be short-lived outside the laboratory and its threat minimized. While no longer formally recognized, biological containment is still a functional option in some instances and should be considered whenever feasible.

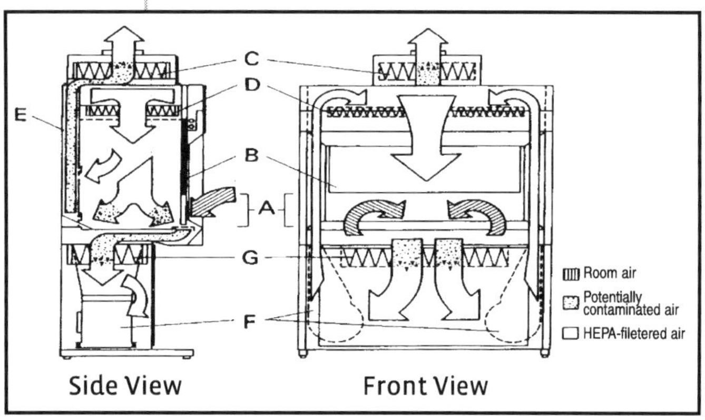

Figure 22.5 — Class II, type B1 BSC (classic design); (A) front opening; (B) sash; (C) exhaust HEPA filter; (C) supply HEPA filter; (E) negative pressure exhaust plenum; (F) blower; (G) additional HEPA filter for supply air. Note: The cabinet needs to be connected to the building exhaust system. (Source: Reference 6).

Biological Safety Cabinets

One of the most visible and effective engineering controls for those working with biohazards, whether in a research and development (R&D) laboratory, animal care facility, or clinical environment, is the BSC (Figures 22.3–22.8).[58] Intended to protect both the cabinet user and those in the secondary environment from airborne biohazards exposures, the BSC has become a staple in these areas. It is among the most effective and most commonly used engineering safeguards in laboratories manipulating known or suspected etiological agents.[59] There are six varieties of BSCs commercially available, consisting of three major classes (I–III) with 4 subtypes in class II (Table 19.4). The designations and types of BSCs can be confusing at first glance, but upon careful study of cabinet schematics the naming conventions are both logical and understandable.

For example, the level of overall protection from a cabinet class increases with increasing class number. Additionally, of the six varieties, all but class I cabinets (Figure 22.3) protect both the user and internal contents from cross contamination. All biosafety cabinets of class II are designed to create laminar airflows within the cabinet and so are more accurately described as laminar flow biological safety cabinets (LFBSC): Neither class I nor class III cabinets (Figure 22.8) utilize laminar airflow. Class 1 biosafety cabinets are negative-pressure, ventilated cabinets operated with an open front and a minimum face velocity at the work opening of at least 75 linear feet per minute (lfpm). The air entering the cabinet is not filtered but is exhausted through a HEPA filter either into the laboratory or to the outside. Because the air in most BSCs is recirculated within the cabinet and could therefore allow for the buildup of explosive vapors, only the 100 percent exhausted class II, type B2 cabinet (Figure 22.6) is suitable for use with flammable materials (and then only in "small" amounts). Incidental use of toxics and radionuclides is also allowed in class II, type B1 and class II, type A2 BSCs but only in "minute" amounts, and only when externally exhausted in the case of the latter (Table 22.4). Where volatile or radioactive materials use is permitted in either of these two BSC types, such items should be restricted to the back area of the BSC since air drawn from this point is exhausted, but air drawn by the front grill may be recirculated within the cabinet. It should be appreciated that BSCs are functionally very different from laboratory fume hoods and should not to be employed as local exhaust systems or integrated into variable air volume ventilation schemes or systems.

BSCs/LFBSCs are normally constructed to a design, materials, and performance standard issued by the National Sanitation Foundation (i.e., NSF 49).[60] NSF 49 also sets criteria for the testing, certification and

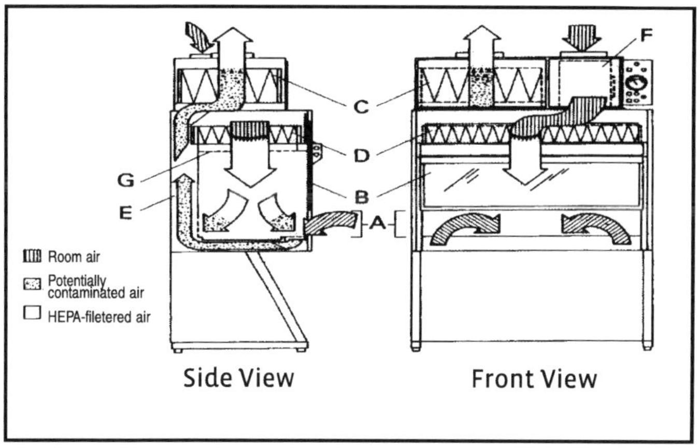

Figure 22.6 — Class II, type B2 BSC. (A) front opening; (B) sash; (C) exhaust HEPA filter; (D) supply HEPA filter; (E) negative pressure exhaust plenum; (F) filter screen. Note: the carbon filter in the building exhaust system is not shown. The cabinet exhaust needs to be connected to the building exhaust system. (Source: Reference 6).

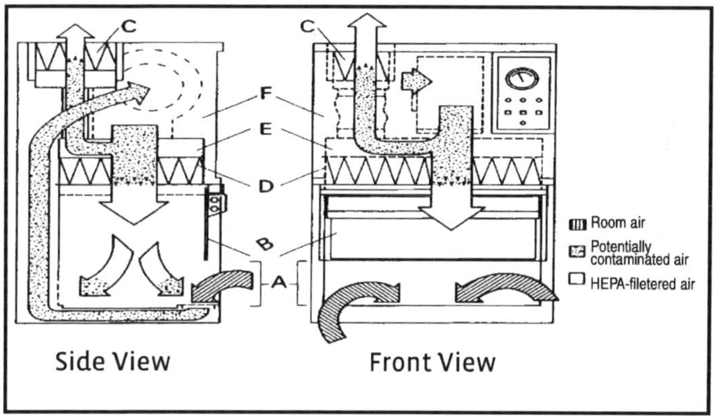

Figure 22.7 — Tabletop model of a Class II, type B3 BSC. (A) Front opening; (B) sash; (C) exhaust HEPA filter; (D) supply HEPA filter; (E) positive pressure plenum; (F) negative pressure plenum. Note: The cabinet exhaust needs to be connected to the building exhaust system. (Source: Reference 6).

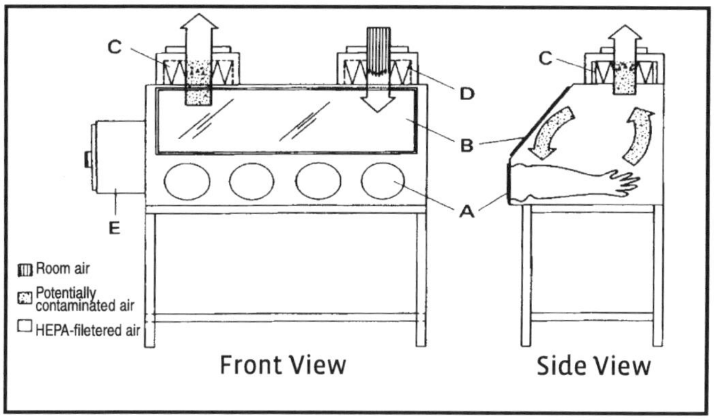

Figure 22.8 — Class III BSC. (A) Glove ports with O-ring for attaching arm-length gloves to cabinet; (B) sash; (C) exhaust HEPA filter; (D) supply HEPA filter; (E) double-ended autoclave or pass-through box. Note: A chemical dunk tank may be installed that would be located beneath the work surface of the BSC with access from above. The cabinet needs to be connected to an independent building exhaust system. (Source: Reference 6).

Table 22.4 — Comparison of Biosafety Cabinet Characteristics

BSC Class	*Face Velocity*	*Airflow Pattern*	*Applications Nonvolatile Toxic Chemicals and Radionuclides*	*Volatile Toxic Chemicals and Radionuclides*
I	75	In at front through HEPA to the outside or into the room through HEPA (Figure 2)	Yes	When exhausted outdoors [1,2]
II, A1	75	70% recirculated to the cabinet work area through HEPA; 30% balance can be exhausted through HEPA back into the room or to outside through a canopy unit (Figure 3)	Yes (minute amounts)	No
II, B1	100	30% recirculated, 70% exhausted. Exhaust cabinet air must pass through a dedicated duct to the outside through a HEPA filter (Figures 5A, 5B)	Yes	Yes (minute amounts) [1,2]
II, B2	100	No recirculation; total exhaust to the outside through a HEPA filter (Figure 6)	Yes	Yes (small amounts) [1,2]
II, A2	100	Similar to II, A1, but has 100 lfpm intake air velocity and plenums are under negative pressure to room; exhaust air can be ducted to outside through a canopy unit (Figure 7)	Yes	When exhausted outdoors (Formerly "B3") (minute amounts) [1,2]
III	N/A	Supply air is HEPA filtered. Exhaust air passes through two HEPA filters in series and is exhausted to the outside via a hard connection (Figure 8)	Yes	Yes (small amounts) [1,2]

1. Installation may require a special duct to the outside, an in-line charcoal filter, and a spark proof (explosion proof) motor and other electrical components in the cabinet. Discharge of a Class I or Class II, Type A2 cabinet into a room should not occur if volatile chemicals are used.
2. In no instance should the chemical concentration approach the lower explosion limits of the compounds.

decontamination of BSCs. CDC-NIH recommends that BSCs be certified in place, any time the unit is moved, and annually thereafter.[58] Perfor-mance certification is an involved procedure requiring mechanical expertise and moderately expensive, calibrated equipment. In some use settings, adjustments and testing of BSCs should not be attempted until the device is either decontaminated or internally sterilized. This is especially true for units used in clinical environments or used for the control of moderate to high-risk agents transmitted by the airborne route. Many HEPA filter compartments of BSCs are constructed so that old or leaking filters may be "bagged out" and new filters installed via the reverse process (i.e., bagged in). Although this concept is simple, experience has taught that equipment idiosyncrasies and model-by-model variations can result in filter change-out problems that can be both frustrating and potentially hazardous when such bags are breached. Since certification firms charge relatively modest rates for

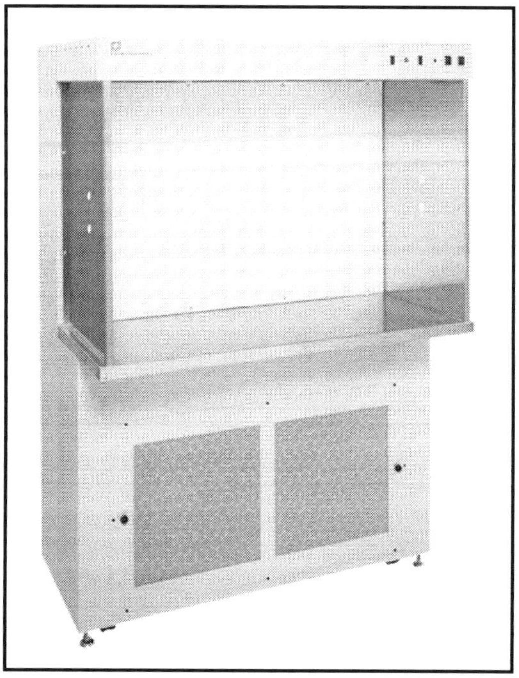

Figure 22.9 — Horizontal laminar flow clean bench.

their services, especially when contracted on an annual basis as opposed to a per-unit basis, BSC repairs and certifications are often left to firms specializing in such tasks.

Infrequently in applications such as sterile processing, pharmacy preparation, and electronics clean rooms, devices resembling BSCs may be encountered. Known as clean benches or sterile preparation hoods (see Figure 22.9), these units consist of a positively pressurized air plenum serving either a vertically or horizontally mounted HEPA filter. Because filtered air from the unit blows over the process toward the operator, clean benches are designed entirely for the purpose of product protection. They are not BSCs and their use should never be allowed where a BSC is in order.

Biosafety Levels

Equipment and approaches available for biohazards containment have been carefully considered, relative to the hazardousness of biohazard-specific operations, to create a widely accepted model for biohazards control referred to as Biosafety Levels (BSLs).[6] There are four biosafety levels (BSL-1 through BSL-4) describing combinations of laboratory practices and techniques, equipment, and facility design features that are recommended for operations involving hazardous etiologic agents. The BSLs, characteristics of agents used, practices, safety equipment, and facility requirements are summarized in Table 22.5. It must be appreciated that the reliance on BSLs for biohazards control is only ancillary to strict adherence to good standard microbiological practices and techniques. For this reason, it should be obvious that persons working with biohazards or potentially infected materials must be educated about the rationale for, and proficient in the performance of, these manipulations. It should also be noted that each of the BSLs include the same elements of good microbiological technique, and are additive to each other. That is, BSL-1 requires that the standard practices of Table 19.6 be utilized. BSL-2 requires all of these same standard practices, plus additional requirements such as the posting of the lab entrance with the biohazard symbol (Figure 19.10), as well as the use of special equipment and facilities. In similar fashion, BSL-3 and BSL-4 contain the requirements of the preceding BSL, plus additional facility, equipment and procedural safeguards. While the details of each BSL are beyond the scope of this chapter, they are summarized as follows.

Table 22.5 — Summary of Recommended Biosafety Levels for Infectious Agents

(1) Access to the laboratory is limited or restricted at the discretion of the laboratory director when experiments or work with cultures and specimens are in progress.
(2) Persons wash their hands after they handle viable materials, after removing gloves, and before leaving the laboratory.
(3) Eating, drinking, smoking, handling contact lenses, applying cosmetics, and storing food for human use are not permitted in the work areas. Persons who wear contact lenses in laboratories should also wear goggles or a face shield. Food is stored outside the work area in cabinets or refrigerators designated and used for this purpose only.
(4) Mouth pipetting is prohibited; mechanical pipetting devices are used.
(5) Policies for the safe handling of sharps are instituted.
(6) All procedures are performed carefully to minimize the creation of splashes or aerosols.
(7) Work surfaces are decontaminated at least once a day and after any spill of viable material.
(8) All cultures, stocks, and other regulated wastes are decontaminated before disposal by an approved decontamination method such as autoclaving. Materials to be decontaminated outside of the immediate laboratory are to be placed in a durable, leak-proof container and closed for transport from the laboratory. Materials to be decontaminated outside of the immediate laboratory are packaged in accordance with applicable local, state, and federal regulations be fore removal from the facility.
(9) A biohazard sign may be posted at the entrance to the laboratory whenever infectious agents are present. The sign may include the name of the agent(s) in use and the name and phone number of the investigator.
(10) An insect and rodent control program is in effect.

Source: Reference 6

Table 22.6 — Standard Microbiological Practices

Cleaning — Removal, by scrubbing or washing with soap and hot water, of infectious agents or organic matter in which such agents my survive or multiply

Contamination — The presence of a biohazardous agent on the body or inanimate objects including water and food

Decontamination — The process of disinfecting or sterilizing inanimate objects

Disinfection — Decrease in the number of pathogenic organisms to an acceptable level.

High-level — kills all biohazards with the exception of high numbers of spores. Accomplished by cleaning followed by application of disinfectants for at least 20-minute contact times.

Intermediate-level — does not kill spores. Accomplished by disinfectants or pasteurization.

Pasteurization — Heat treatment of fluids at specified temperatures for specified durations to kill human pathogens (e.g., milk: 167°F for a period of 30 minutes).

Sterilization — kills all forms of life. Accomplished by heat, gases (ethylene oxide or formaldehyde), irradiation, or chemicals.

Sanitized — Process of decreasing the overall count of microbes present on inanimate objects through chemical means exclusively.

Source: Reference 7

Biosafety Level 1 (BSL-1) represents a basic level of containment that is most reliant on standard microbiological practices as taught in most institutions of higher education. Special primary or secondary containment is not required, and the only essential facility requirement is provision of a sink with the express purpose of hand washing. BSL-1 applies to work with agents that are low risk and not known to cause disease in healthy adult humans. Work can be safely performed on open bench tops, windows may open if provided with screens, and the lab and furniture are easy to clean. Examples of work categories designated as BSL-1 include undergraduate and teaching laboratories, workplaces manipulating *B. licheniformis*, and *E. coli* K12 work. Known agents that are not classified at higher BSLs can be worked with under BSL-1 conditions so long as no evidence exists that the agent's virulence, pathogenicity, antibiotic resistance pattern, vaccine or treatment availability would suggest a higher BSL.

Biosafety Level 2 (BSL-2) practices apply to a broad spectrum of moderate-risk agents that are normally present in the community and which are associated with human disease. Primary hazards to BSL-2 personnel relate to accidental ingestion or contact exposures: BSL-2 agents are not known to be transmissible by the aerosol route although precautions against direct droplet exposures must be taken. If manipulations cause splashes or aerosols, primary containment by means of a LFBSC should be provided. Other facility characteristics at this level include the availability of an autoclave for disposing of infectious or contaminated articles, security features to restrict access, and a foot or knee operated hand washing sink. Agents in BSL-2 include bacteria such as *Salmonella typhi* and *Legionella pneumophila*, fungal agents including *Cryptococcus neoformans*, and the parasitic agents *Cryptosporidium* and *Toxoplasma* spp. Numerous contact-spread viruses are placed at BSL-2, including such recognized agents as hepatitis A, B, C, D, and E, Epstein Barr virus, influenza viruses, and HIV. Some manipulations with rickettsial and prion agents also have been placed in the BSL-2 category, but other procedures with these same agents are placed at BSL-3. The reader is therefore cautioned to stay current with the scientific literature for changes in recommendations based on evolving scientific evidence.

While it may at first seem surprising to see HIV allocated to BSL-2, since infection with the virus can potentially be fatal, defining characteristics of the agent's pathway of infection are its lack of aerosol transmission and extremely low incidence of laboratory-acquired infections. Nevertheless, a hybrid BSL termed Biosafety Level "2-plus" (BSL-2+) has evolved among biosafety professionals in certain settings to allay fears about HIV infection as well as more completely address risks of that agent. The exact control elements of BSL-2+ can vary by the individual in charge, but generally BSL-2+ refers to facilities appropriate for BSL-2, work practices and containment equipment developed for BSL-3, and the use of additional PPE (especially in the patient care setting). This combination provides better primary containment at the lab bench yet eliminates the need for a costly yet scientifically unjustifiable BSL-3 facility for secondary containment.

Biosafety Level 3 (BSL-3) agents are aerosol transmissible. They can be indigenous or exotic, and are associated with serious or lethal human disease for which preventive or therapeutic interventions may be available. Public health characteristics of these agents are that they pose high individual risk upon direct exposure, but low community risk upon release. Because of the qualitative nature of these risk descriptions, it is common to find some manipulations of a given biohazardous agent to be recommended at BSL-2, and other, aerosol-producing work at BSL-3. Examples of BSL-3 agents include *Mycobacterium tuberculosis, Histoplasma capsulatum,* West Nile virus, and human prion diseases. Activities involving industrial-scale quantities of HIV, or concentrated preparations thereof, are always to be done in BSL-3 facilities using practices and equipment of that level. Signature equipment of a BSL-3 facility includes a currently certified LFBSC, autoclave, self-closing laboratory doors, a sealed laboratory building envelope under negative air pressurization, and a ducted exhaust exclusively for laboratory air. Exhausted air must be dispersed away from other air intakes or occupied areas, or it must be HEPA filtered.

Work with exotic agents that pose a high risk of life-threatening disease, and for which preventive or therapeutic interventions are not usually available, must be conducted at BSL-4. These agents may be aerosol spread or possess an unknown risk of transmission. The most infamous agent in this class is the Ebola virus, with a case-fatality rate of almost 90%. BSL-4 laboratories are found in only a few places in the U.S., are preferably located on islands, and are usually related to government or military applications. In addition to the application of all BSL-3 requirements, BSL-4 laboratories require a medical surveillance program for all employees including the creation and maintenance of a baseline serum sample program. Building design characteristics and equipment unique to BSL-4 include airlocks, pass-through autoclaves for entry and exit of materials, class III BSCs (see Figure 22.8), dedicated non-recirculating ventilation systems, and HEPA filtered air to and from the operations rooms. BSL-4 laboratories can best be imagined as room-within-a-room containment, augmented by the use of glove boxes and sealed one-piece supplied-air suits as PPE. Operations involving this level of work are highly specialized, and they are used for only the most hazardous work. As such, they are not an appropriate training ground for either the scientist or biosafety professional, and should be under the close supervision of competent scientists who are trained and experienced in working with the agents involved. Neither occupational hygiene comprehensive practitioners nor biosafety professionals should be called on to manage a BSL-4 containment facility unless they have had extensive education, training, and work experience inside such a facility.

Animal Use Biohazards

Methods for the surveillance and control of the most important animal pathogens and diseases, as well as standards for laboratory diagnostics and vaccine production and control, have been published.[61] However, most routine hazards faced by individuals working with animals or their products in laboratories, veterinary clinics, and breeding facilities are not associated with infectious disease but with more pedestrian hazards. Handlers and caretakers run increased risks of back injury as a result of working with heavy equipment, unloading supplies, and moving large animals, and of animal inflicted injury such as bites, kicks, or scratches. In addition to the usual physical hazards like slips, trips, cuts and falls, animal facilities pose risks of electrocution, sensorineural hearing loss, allergy development, and exposure to strong cleaning agents. Yet it is infections from animals passed to man that have been of most academic interest and scientific study. A review of occupational zoonoses has been prepared by Fox and Lipman.[62]

Zoonotic infection has been and will continue to be one source of emerging and reemerging disease in humans. In a 25 year review of laboratory-acquired zoonotic infections at the National Animal Disease Center, 128 personnel infections were reportedly due to laboratory exposures to infected animals.[63] Among the more significant reasons for such infections is that workers fail to recognize the risk of acquiring zoonotic diseases from apparently healthy animals. With the documented aerosol transmission of Ebola strains by the airborne route from monkey to man[64], and human infections with *Herpesvirus simiae* (B virus)[65], this hazard has become more widely recognized. In addition, animals can only realistically be screened for those specific etiologic agents suspected to be present in that species for which diagnostic reagents are available. Since it is not always possible to know which animals present infectious hazards, protection against zoonotic infections should be universally applied. Key among these are approaches quite familiar to the industrial hygienist, such as substitution, engineering and administrative controls, and personal protective equipment. These controls should also be supported with rigorous training programs, medical surveillance efforts, and environmental monitoring.

Substitution

Wherever possible, buying and procurement practices should be in place to facilitate the use of pathogen free (or particular pathogen free) lab animals. While costly, this can be done in many instances. In some instances, though, procurement of known pathogen-free subjects is not feasible. Such is the case for the use of nonhuman primates, which are frequently caught in the wild. The quarantine of new animals before moving them into a clean colony is common practice to protect the colony from disease as well as to protect workers from some infections. However, quarantine is not a perfect practice. For example, primates often react negatively to repeated tests for TB throughout the quarantine period only to react positively later. Furthermore, effective quarantine depends on staff commitment to either treating or removing infected animals from the facility once they are identified.

Engineering and Administrative Controls

All organizations using animals should follow accepted standards of lab animal care. Recommendations for animal biosafety levels (ABSL) are available[57,66,67], as are regulations for animal care and welfare.[50,68] Adherence to these standards is important to keeping both animals and humans safe. Key practices include:

- Follow guidelines and standards with respect to containment, quarantine, separation of species and sexes, and breeding cages.
- Doors and cages should be clearly marked to indicate hazards that may be present and mitigation techniques.
- Facility design should have separate clean and dirty corridors and rooms to prevent spreading infections within the colony.
- Rooms should be designed for ease of cleaning with coved walls, smooth yet slip-resistant floors, pest control via tightly closing doors, screened windows, and well-maintained surfaces without holes in floors or walls.
- Floor drains should either be sealed or have their P-traps filled with water or an appropriate disinfectant.
- Exhaust air from animal facilities at any level should not be recirculated throughout the building due to the potential for dissemination of zoonotic agents, allergens, and undesirable odors. HEPA-filtered exhaust is required for Animal Biosafety Levels 3 and 4.[6]
- Animal cage rooms should be able to contain animals that have escaped from their enclosures or handlers, and prevent entry of unwanted pests and potential vectors.

PPE

Workers should have ready access to latex or vinyl gloves and filtering facepiece respirators at a minimum. They should be instructed to always wash their hands thoroughly after working with animals, materials containing animal proteins, or dirty equipment. It is recommended to provide workers with a change room, shower, and set of work clothing, in addition to a lab coat for use in animal areas. Such actions will prevent the contamination of street clothing with dander, dusts, hair, and pathogens. Respirators may be provided, in accordance with principles of good industrial hygiene practice and in compliance with OSHA standards for respiratory protection.

Training

Training for animal facility workers should include recognition of the potential for bites and scratches. Employees should be warned of the potential for developing allergies and contact dermatitis and their symptoms, as well as the risk of zoonotic illnesses. Training should include use and limitations of PPE, laboratory techniques to minimize formation of aerosols, and animal handling techniques to reduce the risk of bites and scratches. It should be emphasized that safe work practices and use of specialized equipment or PPE are to be followed at all times, even when working with apparently healthy animals in the absence of perceived risk. During this training, or as part of the medical surveillance activities, female employees of childbearing age should be cautioned about any specific zoonoses associated with the animals housed (e.g., toxoplasma and cats). Hearing conservation program compliance may be required for employees using mechanized animal cage washing equipment.

Medical Surveillance

Allergies and contact dermatitis can develop after prolonged work or within a relatively short period on the job. Usual causes are animals, latex-containing PPE, and animal waste. Immunocompromised or atopic individuals, whether or not they work directly with animals, should not be overlooked as an at-risk population since a number of zoonotic agents act as opportunistic pathogens. In the event complaints are made about odors, unusual illnesses, or allergies by individuals who do not normally work in the colony or near animals, qualitative IH surveys should be undertaken. If and where indicated, air, wipe, or bulk sampling for animal hair or dander may be collected and processed.[69] Complaints of illnesses made by animal handlers might best be investigated by a team comprised of veterinarians, epidemiologists, health care professionals, biosafety experts, and industrial hygienists. Workers in animal facilities should be vaccinated against moderate to severe disease-causing pathogens in instances where vaccines are available. If scientifically appropriate, or required by organizational policies, a serum bank for all animal care workers should be established and maintained. Where implemented employee samples should be collected as soon after hire as possible, and at periodic intervals thereafter.

Transfer and Shipping Procedures for Biohazardous Agents

The main objectives of the hazardous materials shipping standards and regulations are to anticipate and prevent accidents involving hazardous materials in transport, and mitigate the potential harm to individuals or the environment when accidents do occur.

These objectives can be accomplished by identifying the biohazardous agents and determining the correct shipping category; using proper packing and packaging materials and procedures; providing warning labels on the packages and documentation in the form of shipping papers; and by thorough training of persons involved in shipping biological materials. Continuing education for shippers is paramount in that regulations concerning the transportation of etiologic agents, biological toxins, and diagnostic specimens will only be tightened given the potentially catastrophic security threats to society posed in the past decade.

For example, in February of 1998, two men were arrested in Las Vegas, Nevada, after claiming to possess enough anthrax spores to "wipe out the city." One of those arrested had a previous conviction for illegally obtaining bubonic plague bacteria through the mail, and had laid out plans to attack New York City subways.[3] Though they were later discovered to have mislead authorities with their claims, the incident served to bring to light an essentially unregulated system by which persons or organizations could obtain certifiably pathogenic etiologic agents. Ultimately administrative control over suppliers of biohazardous materials was implemented by laws[28–30,35], and the regulations written to fulfill them.[31,38] Many regulations are aimed at ensuring that the change in possession (i.e., transfer) of biological materials is within the best interest of the public and the nation. Under such rules facilities or personnel wishing to legitimately receive biohazardous agents of human disease are required to register with the CDC, justify their need, and generate approved documentation for each transfer.

Specific actions by those who offer biohazardous materials for shipment include safe packaging, mandatory labeling, manifests or other shipping paper descriptions, and package handler training.[43] These regulations apply to all biohazardous shipments by common carrier via land, air, sea or rail. All etiologic agents should be packed and labeled to ensure the safety of the recipient as well as the carrier. Packages that are improperly packed may arrive damaged. If there are delays in transport due to paperwork discrepancies, the material may be unusable, as in the case of frozen material that has thawed. It is not the purpose of this chapter to detail all shipping regulations (the reader can consult applicable sources cited for further information), but some standard practices will be reviewed.

To ship biological materials that belong to BSL-2 through BSL-4, live vaccines, diagnostic samples, genetically modified pathogens, or biological toxins, packaging procedures for either biohazardous agents or clinical specimens must be followed. In the case of BSL-3 and BSL-4 agents, these requirements should be considered minimum standards. Both biohazardous agents and clinical samples must be contained in a group of three concentric containers. The first, primary receptacle makes intimate contact with the biohazardous material and is contained in spill-absorbent material within a watertight secondary container.

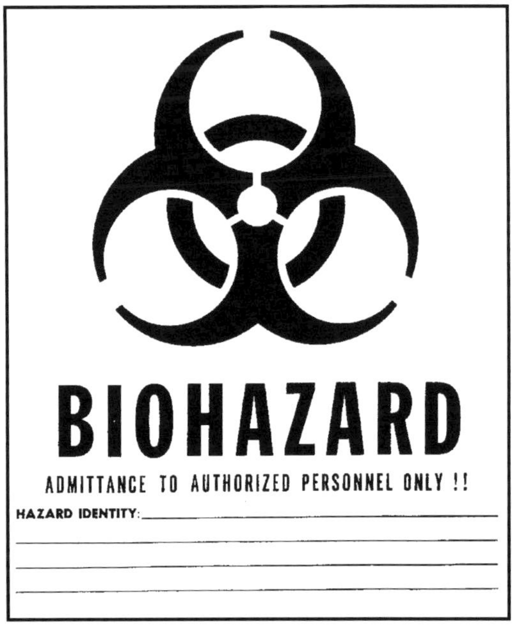

Figure 22.10 — Biohazard Symbol.

The secondary container is held by outer packaging meeting rigorous performance testing as mandated by DOT, USPS, IATA, or the US Public Health Service (PHS). For biological agents, the biohazards symbol (Figure 22.10) is required on the primary container and an "infectious substance" shipping label is required on the outer packaging. For clinical specimens, triple containerization is also required but the outer packaging is subject to less rigorous performance requirements and must bear the "clinical specimen" shipping label. So long as the specimens have only a low probability of containing an actual etiological agent, they may be shipped as described.

Incoming packages bearing the "infectious substance" or "clinical specimen" DOT shipping label should be carefully inspected upon receipt for signs of loss of containment.

Packages that are wet, leaking fluid or powder, or otherwise damaged to the extent that the contents of that or another package have been contaminated pose an ethical quandary for the receiving organization. Some may choose not to accept any damaged package, requiring the carrier to follow its standard procedures for handling returns or disposition of such items. In other cases, such as the anticipated arrival of an infectious substance or toxin, the receiving organization may need to control the potential biohazard immediately. Security safeguards for the receipt and supervised control of such packages are now also required.[28]

Written procedures should be in place for the following:

- **Routine Receipt.** Delays in transporting perishable contents must be avoided, and those expecting deliveries should be sensitive to possible security breaches in the event of significantly overdue packages. Give particular attention to items arriving on Fridays or before holidays or operational shutdowns. If delivery receipts or signed manifest copies are required, the procedure must detail how copies are handled to remain in compliance with applicable tracking laws.
- **Containment Precautions.** Any nonessential handling of a damaged package should be given careful consideration; it should most likely not be handled except by properly trained and

authorized personnel who have donned proper PPE. Inspection of adjacent packages and areas for signs of contamination should be performed. Non-essential personnel should leave the area until it has been adequately decontaminated, if necessary. The package should be secondarily contained (i.e., "over packed") for safe transport to a biosafety cabinet, where it may be decontaminated and opened.

- **Decontamination Procedures.** Once the immediate hazard posed by the package is abated, steps for cleaning and decontamination of the shipping/receiving area and any materials handling equipment should be followed. Responsibilities for area personnel, as well as the duties for internal specialists should be clearly spelled out. When and how to request assistance outside the organization should be stipulated.
- **Reporting.** Immediate notice of the problem to the organizational safety office and/or recipient should be given, fully documenting the problem. It may be advantageous to photograph the site and package, as well as its contents, should questions of liability arise in the future. Formal reports of the incident to the consignor, shipping company, and recipient company may be prudent.
- **First Aid.** Decontamination and follow-up medical evaluation of potentially exposed workers should be accomplished if appropriate.

Decontamination, Disinfection, and Sterilization(56,70–73)

As mentioned in the discussion of biosafety levels, good microbiological technique is expected from those manipulating biohazards in laboratory settings. Several such practices (see Table 22.6) indicate the use of decontaminating agents or procedures. Many other situations requiring inactivation of biohazardous materials are routinely encountered outside of the research setting. For example, spills or leaking packages labeled as biohazardous may need to have such hazards neutralized. Institutional care rooms which housed infectious patients need meticulous decontamination once the occupant has died or been discharged. Increasingly, concerns about the colonization of indoor spaces by bacteria or fungi may lead to a search for effective decontamination agents. "Decontamination" is a generic term, however, used in many industrial hygiene endeavors including radioisotope remediation, asbestos abatements, and HazMat operations. In the biohazards profession, decontamination is applied to both sterilization or disinfection. In the context of rendering materials noninfectious, it is necessary to precisely define a number of terms that are often, and incorrectly, used synonymously. Professionally accepted decontamination terms are listed in Table 22.6.

The size of an article, its heat sensitivity, corrosion resistance, propensity to absorb gases or liquids, unit cost, and end use all dictate the most suitable means of decontamination. Decontamination may be accomplished by physical means (heat, steam, and radiation) or by chemicals. Since sterilants and disinfectants are toxic to all viable cells, regardless of intended targets, it is important for users to be familiar with the hazards of the agents they select and to take the necessary precautions to prevent and monitor exposure.(74–77) Most chemical agents including ethylene oxide, formaldehyde, glutaraldehyde, and strong acids and bases require special handling techniques or PPE. Ionizing radiation devices, such as X- and gamma irradiators, may only be used within the context of federal or state licenses. Finally, environmental monitoring, performance testing, and medical surveillance may be required depending on the chemical. Several guidebooks are available for those interested in the many details of decontamination techniques.(56,70–73) The essentials of the most widely employed methods are reviewed here.(10)

Physical Agents

Steam. Used at 250°F (121°C) under pressure (15–18 psi, depending on altitude) in an autoclave, steam is the most widely used and convenient method of sterilization. Effective steam sterilization requires control of duration of exposure, configuration and size of the load, permeability and dimensions of the containers, and other variables to ensure sterility has been achieved. Indicators of effective sporocidal treatment (e.g., *Bacillus stearothermophilis* ampoules planted inside the treated equipment, or autoclave indicator tape wrapped outside of biohazardous waste loads) are frequently used on each load to validate the sterilization. Biological indicators may be used on a per-load, daily, weekly, or monthly basis to validate that the autoclave is functioning properly. Chemical indicators and autoclave tape do not give absolute assurance since they change appearance once the temperature set point has been achieved, but provide no indication that the proper holding time at that temperature was maintained.

Wet Heat. High temperatures cause denaturation of enzymes and kill organisms. Boiling (212°F for >30 minutes) and pasteurization (161°F for 15 seconds, or 143°F for 30 minutes) will kill vegetative cells but not bacterial spores.

Dry Heat. In clinical labs, open flames and Bacti-Cinerators(tm) (an electric device that dry-heats at 1600°F) are used to heat-sterilize inoculation loops. Hot air ovens (160–180°C for 2 hours) are used for anhydrous materials such as greases or powders. Incinerators are often employed to destroy infectious wastes.

Ionizing Radiation. Ionizing radiation is most often used for the sterilization of new, prepackaged medical devices, including operating room supplies such as syringes and catheters. It has also found applications in bulk package sterilization in the delivery and food industries.

Ultraviolet (UV) Radiation. In the past ultraviolet radiation has been used as a practical way to inactivate viruses, mycoplasma, bacteria, and fungi. It can be effective against airborne microorganisms and within biological safety cabinets to maintain low levels of contamination on exposed surfaces. Other common applications include air locks, animal holding areas, and laboratory rooms during periods of nonoccupancy. Its usefulness is limited by its low penetrating power; shadows and dust on the lamps can also reduce the effectiveness. UV radiation of 270 nm is necessary for greatest effectiveness, but many UV sources have been found to remain in service long after a diminution of output at that wavelength, thus giving users a false sense of effectiveness. UV radiation is among the least effective, least perfected methods of sanitization, and is not practical as a disinfectant of liquids.

Filtration. Membrane filters are used to remove bacteria, yeast, and molds from biologic and pharmaceutical solutions. Common pore sizes are 0.22 µm, 0.45 µm, and 0.8 µm.

Chemical Decontaminants

Chemical disinfectants inactivate microorganisms by chemical reaction. The effectiveness of the disinfectant against an infectious agent varies with the nature of the chemical, the concentration, contact duration, temperature, humidity, pH, and the presence of organic matter. Most disinfectant protocols require prewashing with soap and water to remove gross organic material.

Sodium hypochlorite (household bleach) is commonly used as a general disinfectant against a variety of bacteria, viruses, and fungi, including *Staphylococcus aureus, Mycobacterium tuberculosis*, and *Salmonella typhi.* Bleach treatments consistently find applications in indoor air quality remediation as a structural and ventilation system decontaminant although their usefulness in such applications is dubious and long-term efficacy unproven. A 1:100 dilution of household bleach to water creates a solution of greater than 500 ppm free available chlorine, which is effective against vegetative bacteria and most viruses. Efficacy is a time dependant function, based on biological load and free chlorine concentration. A 1:10 dilution (5000 ppm free available chlorine) is preferred by some for general applications. A major deficiency of bleach as a disinfectant is that precise concentrations of approximately 2500 ppm are needed for it to be effective against bacterial spores. Also, these solutions are corrosive and unstable over time. Fresh solutions need to be made daily.

Two aldehydes are currently of considerable importance as disinfectants: glutaraldehyde and formaldehyde. Glutaraldehyde is used in a 2% solution made alkaline before use. It is a highly reactive molecule and works well against bacteria and their spores, mycelial and spore forms of fungi, and various types of viruses. It is considered to be an effective antimycobacterial agent. Dried spores are considerably more resistant to disinfection. Organic matter is considered to have no effect on the antimicrobial activity of the aldehyde, which explains its wide use as a cold sterilant for medical equipment such as cystoscopes and anesthetic equipment which might otherwise be damaged by steam sterilization methods. Glutaraldehyde is used in the veterinary field for the disinfection of utensils and premises. It is an irritant and has potential mutagenic and carcinogenic effects.

Formaldehyde in solution (e.g., 8% formalin in 70% alcohol) is effective against vegetative bacteria, spores, and viruses. Its sporocidal activity is slower than glutaraldehyde, and it is less effective in the presence of proteinacious matter. Inhalation of formaldehyde vapor presents potential carcinogenic risk to humans. Paraformaldehyde flakes are vaporized by heating within sealed biological safety cabinets in a standard decontamination procedure. Vaporized paraformaldehyde may also be used to decontaminate entire rooms, but this procedure is highly hazardous because the gas is both extremely toxic and explosive at necessary concentrations. It requires rendering the room airtight during the procedure and neutralizing the gas prior to release. Personnel conducting this type of procedure must be highly trained, and conduct the work wearing self-contained breathing apparatuses. This technique is the primary option for decontaminating and decommissioning BSL-4 facilities. Gaseous formaldehyde treatment is increasingly finding applications in indoor air quality issues as an air duct or ventilation system decontaminant but like bleach treatments, its long-term value is suspect.

Ozone has a history of effective use as a gaseous fumigant and water purification reactant, but it is increasingly misrepresented to the lay public for its anti-microbial action in indoor settings. Presently there remains considerable controversy over the wisdom of introducing it into air ductwork because little research has been conducted to demonstrate its effectiveness and because it is a lung irritant. While some data suggest that low levels of ozone may reduce airborne concentrations and inhibit the growth of some biological organisms while ozone is present, effective use concentrations are 5–10 times higher than ambient standards of 0.05–0.10 ppm. Even at high concentrations, ozone may have no effect on biological contaminants embedded in porous material such as duct lining or ceiling tiles, and no biocides are currently registered by EPA for use on fiberglass duct board or in fiberglass lined ducts.(78,79) For these reasons ozone has not found widespread use by the professional community where disinfection, sterilization, or decontamination is required.

Iodophors (iodine-carrier) possess a wide spectrum of antimicrobial and antiviral activity. They are used for antiseptic and disinfectant purposes at different concentrations. Although not generally sporocidal, Povidone-iodine has been shown to be sporocidal and is important in preventing wound infections. Betadine in alcohol solution is widely used in the U.S. for disinfection of the hands and operation sites. Iodophors are usually carried in surfactant liquid; they are relatively harmless to man and have a built-in effectiveness indicator: a brown color. Iodophors are inactivated by organic matter, so preliminary surface cleaning may be needed in addition to iodophor disinfection.

Alcohols have rapid bactericidal activity, including acid-fast bacilli, but are not sporocidal and have poor activity against many viruses. Ethanol requires the presence of water for its effectiveness, but concentrations below 30% have little action. The most effective concentration is about 60–70%. Isopropanol and n-propyl alcohol are more effective bactericides than ethanol. However, they are not sporocidal. Seventy-percent (70%) alcohol is used for surface decontamination in biological safety cabinets. Solutions of iodine or chlorhexidine in 70% alcohol may be employed for the preoperative disinfection of the skin. All of these alcohols are flammable liquids and may be incompatible with some plastics and rubber.

Quaternary ammonium compounds, as their name implies, are substituted ammonium compounds. They are acceptable as general use disinfectants to control vegetative bacteria and nonlipid-containing viruses; however, they are not active against bacterial spores at typical concentrations (1:750). They have many and varied uses including food hygiene in hospitals, preoperative disinfection of unbroken skin, algal contamination control in swimming pools, and preservatives for eyedrop preparations and contact lens soaking solutions.

Phenolic compounds (0.5%–2%) are recommended for the killing of vegetative bacteria, including TB, fungi, and lipid-containing viruses. They are less effective against spores and nonlipid-containing viruses. They are often used for cleaning equipment and floors. Phenolics are derived from the tar by-product of destructive distillation of coal, solubilized with soaps. They have been implicated in depigmentation and can cause severe damage to unprotected skin on contact. Lysol(tm) is a cresol solubilized with a soap prepared from linseed oil and potassium hydroxide. It retains the corrosive nature of the phenol.

Ethylene oxide (EtO) is a highly toxic gas that inactivates all types of microorganisms, including endospores of bacteria and viruses. The action is influenced by concentration, temperature, duration of exposure, and water content of the microorganisms. EtO is widely used in hospital sterile supply departments and also by commercial suppliers of sterile hospital goods. Pure EtO is highly flammable, constituting a serious fire and explosion hazard. It has an extremely wide flammable range of approximately 3–100% in air. Also, it is mutagenic and potentially carcinogenic in humans. It is closely regulated in the US by OSHA under a chemical-specific standard.[69,80] While the sterilization process itself can be well-controlled with respect to fugitive airborne emissions of EtO, the off gassing of the sterile goods, especially plastics, may take several hours. Therefore, there is potential for worker exposure during load movements, in sterilizer rooms, and in areas for storage of sterile goods.

Chlorine dioxide is an antimicrobial agent recognized for its disinfectant properties since the early 1900s. Although it smells somewhat like chlorine bleach, it should not be confused with bleach or chlorine gas, as all three are distinct chemicals that react differently and so must be handled differently. In practice, sodium chlorite or stabilized ClO_2 are mixed with a reactant—usually an acid—to generate ClO_2 in a gaseous or liquid state. Liquid ClO_2 has been found to be sporocidal for anthrax at a concentration of 500 mg/l, given contact for 30 minutes; gaseous ClO_2 has been used at concentrations from 750–3000 ppm for up to 3 hours. Chlorine dioxide first gained widespread recognition among the industrial hygiene community when it was used in the federal decontamination response to the bioterrorism attacks that took place in October, 2001. In those instances, ClO_2 was used to decontaminate the Hart Senate Office Building, to treat mail packages, and to fumigate a Florida office building. Use of this agent is highly regulated owing to its health and safety hazards, and until Hurricane Katrina in 2005, only federal, state, or local governmental agencies had been permitted its use as described here. Since then, the application of gaseous ClO_2 to indoor mold and bacteria problems has been of increasing interest to industrial hygienists, but to date, its use in the U.S. is largely permitted only as a water purification additive.[81,82]

Biotechnology and Industrial Biohazards[10,83,84]

So far in this chapter, the real and potential hazards of biological agents—and strategies for their control—have been highlighted in both basic and clinical laboratory settings. Other texts have more fully described biosafety programs in academic, government, and other biological research laboratories.[85–88] This section will discuss biological hazards and the application of biosafety principles in commercial and industrial operations. Specifically, biotechnology R&D, large-scale biotechnology manufacturing, animal colonies, and enzymes in the detergent industry will be addressed. The definitions presented will serve adequately to describe most of the hazards and issues in these specialized endeavors, but some added explanations will be necessary given the tremendous rate of change in these pursuits. While the safe use of biohazardous materials in traditional settings has been well documented, as have failures in contamination control[89,90], the situation in commercial and industrial biohazards operations is quite different. With techniques such as gene replacement therapy from genetically modified organisms (GMOs) poised to find their way out of the laboratory and into production, and commercial accomplishments in biotechnology increasingly prevalent, possible hazards of such advances remain uncharted.[91] Although such hazards may prove to be minimal, given mankind's proven susceptibility to global epidemics prudent biohazards oversight in emerging biotechnologies is absolutely justified. For this reason the skill of the industrial hygienist to anticipate and recognize potential industrial biohazards is perhaps even more important than the ability to evaluate or control such new uses.

The word "biotechnology" describes processes that use organisms and their cellular, subcellular, or molecular components to provide goods, services, or environmental management. Biotechnology is still correctly considered a young industry, but the application of traditional genetic modification techniques has been used for decades to enhance food characteristics (e.g., hybrid corn, selective breeding); to manufacture food (e.g., bread, cheese, wine, vegetables, yogurt); for bacterial sewage treatment; in medicine (e.g., vaccines, hormones); for pesticides (e.g., *Bacillus thuringensis*); and for other uses. What is new and unique about the modern biotechnology industry is the ability to identify and locate specific genes (and their functions) and to manipulate the genetic materials intentionally and precisely within living cells, i.e., genetic engineering. Out of such abilities new commercial applications often present themselves, along with technical, safety, or ethical concerns.

There is little direct comparison between the stereotypical U.S. manufacturing plant of the 20th century and the modern biotechnology facility with its usual bioreactors. In these reactors modified cells are cultured, constituting *de facto* factories, to produce the desired product. The desired product (enzyme, factor, etc.) is then separated from the cells and nutrient broth in which they were cultured (by techniques such as centrifugation, filtration, etc.), purified (by techniques such as column chromatography), formulated, and packaged. In agriculture, plants themselves are genetically altered to add disease or insect resistance or other traits where they are not naturally present. Examples are strawberries that can grow at colder temperatures, tomatoes resistant to rot on the grocers' shelves, and adding nitrogen-fixing ability to rice, corn, and cereal grain crops to reduce the amount of nitrogen fertilizers necessary to produce the food. In environmental remediation applications Pseudomonas bacteria can break down a range of products including hydrocarbons contaminating soil and groundwater. DNA from several strains has been added to a single cell to produce a bacterium effective for oil spills. Mixtures of microbes and enzymes have also been designed to digest detergents and paper mill waste, including sulfite liquor.[83] Single- and multi-species BSL-1 biofilms are under development for bioremediation, wastewater treatment, fermentation, biotransformation, and fine chemical production.[92]

At present, biotechnology is a multidisciplinary laboratory-based production science incorporating many of the biohazards issues already discussed. Molecular and cellular biologists, immunologists, geneticists, virologists, protein and peptide chemists, biochemists, and biochemical engineers are most directly exposed to the real and potential hazards of rDNA technology. Other biotechnology workers with significant potential exposure to rDNA biohazards include maintenance and calibration technicians, glass-wash and housekeeping department workers, and operating engineers. In their survey of health and safety practitioners in the biotechnology industry, Lee and Ryan[84] found that scientific and support staff exposed to genetically engineered materials comprise only about 30%–40% of the total work force in those companies. The other 60–70% of biotechnology workers are found in academic, medical, and government research institutions.

In addition to genetically engineered organisms, biotechnology lab workers have potential exposures to a variety of more conventional hazards. Toxic chemicals, radioisotopes, repetitive stress injuries, confined space entry, temperature extremes, noise and vibration are integral hazards of the trade. The products of biotechnology are not necessarily viable organisms, but may present toxic or allergenic hazards similar to their chemically synthesized counterparts. There are ample references and resources pertaining to chemical and physical hazards in the R&D laboratory, in other chapters of this text, and elsewhere.[6,77,93–96] Aside from exposure to genetically engineered organisms per se, or the traditional workplace concerns just listed, other biological hazards are common in rDNA labs. These include human bloodborne pathogens concerns such as blood, body fluids, and human derived cell lines and reagents; communicable diseases, such as influenza; laboratory animal dander, allergens, and physical threats; and zoonotic illnesses that may be transferred from lab animals to humans.

Some of the better known zoonoses are rabies; the nonhuman primate counterpart to HIV (simian immunodeficiency virus, or SIV); Monkey B virus (*Herpesvirus simiae*); anthrax (*Bacillus anthracis*); psittacosis (*Chlamydia psittaci*); brucellosis (*Brucellosis abortus, B. suis, B. melitensis, B. canis*); and Q Fever and Rocky Mountain Spotted Fever (*Coxiella burnetii* and *Rickettsia rickettsii*, respectively). Except for SIV and Monkey B virus, which are hazards for biotechnology research workers in nonhuman primate centers, the most common zoonotic illnesses would be expected in agriculture or food processing facilities and not necessarily in biotechnology laboratories or animal research facilities.

The first biotechnology guidelines (on rDNA) were published in 1976 by NIH with the objective of ensuring that experimental DNA recombination would have no ill effects on those engaged in the work, on the general public, or on the environment. The 1976 NIHG were the product of extensive debate within the Recombinant Advisory Committee (RAC) convened by NIH. The essence of the NIHG is the subdivision of potential experiments by class, a decision as to which experiments should be permitted at present, and assignment to these of certain procedures for containment of recombinant organisms. No deliberate releases were allowed. Roles and responsibilities of the principal investigator (PI), the institution, the NIH and its staff were described, as well as the classification of organisms and containment levels for specific types of experiments.[97]

As scientific knowledge increased, it was expected that the NIHG would need periodic review and revision. Thus, the RAC now meets quarterly to consider and approve proposals for changes to the NIHG. For example, the NIHG no longer carry a blanket prohibition against deliberate release of genetically engineered organisms. Increasing numbers of proposals submitted for RAC approval involve specific human gene therapy experiments and corrections and reclassifications of organisms based on better characterized hazard potential. One very significant amendment to the NIHG was the creation of a large-scale containment category known as Good Large-Scale Practice (GLSP). It relaxed the containment requirements for non-pathogenic, non-toxigenic recombinant strains derived from host organisms that have an extended history of safe large scale use, or which have built in environmental limitations (i.e., biological containment) that permit optimum growth in the large scale setting but limited survival without adverse consequences in the environment.[98] Much has been learned about the relative safety of rDNA in the last several decades, as well as the benefits of the technology for individuals and society. That said, there continue to be general concerns by public interest groups about new applications and products of the technology.

In the 1980s, the first modern products of recombinant biotechnology emerged in the United States and Europe. Genetically engineered insulin was approved for use in 1982, as was a genetically engineered vaccine against the pig disease, scours.[99] Controversy began soon after with the creation of recombinant bovine somatotropin, which increases a cow's milk production and increases the weight of beef cattle. Concerns were raised about the public health and safety associated with the consumption of these products. Although the NIHG addressed protection for biotechnology workers and for the environment, they did not address product safety or public health issues arising from the recombinantly derived products. To assure the public that concerns about product safety were being addressed, in 1985 the U.S. Office of Science and Technology Policy published a comprehensive federal regulatory policy for ensuring the safety of biotechnology research and products.[100] Each covered agency—the Food and Drug Administration (FDA), OSHA, EPA, and the USDA—defined their policies applicable to rDNA activities within their jurisdictions. Where there were areas of overlapping authority, a lead agency was identified and the emerging regulatory framework coordinated by a new Biotechnology Science Coordinating Committee.

The potential risks of biotechnology and its products remain a matter of public concern in Europe as well as in the U.S. In April 1990, the European Community enacted two directives on the contained use and deliberate release into the environment of genetically modified organisms and microorganisms. Both directives require member states to ensure that all appropriate measures are taken to avoid adverse effects on human health or the environment that might arise from the contained use or deliberate release of genetically modified organisms and microorganisms. Under these rules the user bears responsibility for assessing all relevant risks in advance. In Germany the Genetic Technology Act was passed in 1990, partially in response to the EC directives, but also to respond to a need for legal authority to construct a trial recombinant insulin production facility.[101] More recently, the Australian government enacted its Gene Technology Act of 2000, to regulate biotechnology activities.[102]

To date, the earlier fears of genetically creating deleterious species or toxins have not materialized; however, the debate over the safety of genetic engineering and the products of biotechnology continues.[103,104] Products are one by one being integrated into modern society, especially in the forms of genetically modified (GM) foods and organisms. In 2006, over 250 million acres of transgenic crops were planted in over 20 countries by more than 10 million farmers.[105] Examples include herbicide- and insect-resistant soybeans, corn, cotton, canola, and alfalfa, sweet potatoes resistant to viruses, and rice varieties with vitamins to alleviate malnutrition. Recombinant vaccines are well received, and diagnostic kits based on rDNA technology are widely available. DNA fingerprinting is now commonplace forensic evidence, and can also be used to prove (technically, disprove) paternity. In an interesting paradox, it is increasingly true that rDNA may in fact promote public health rather than threaten it, given research into an experimental banana capable of producing human vaccines to Hepatitis B, and cows genetically modified to be resistant to mad cow disease.[105] The development of genetically modified organisms targeted to specific genes suited to reduce undesirable side-effects of live attenuated vaccines is also receiving great interest from a public health perspective.[106]

rDNA technology is also being applied in interesting and important areas such as human gene therapy (i.e., the use of genetic material to treat, cure, or prevent a disease or medical condition) to correct heritable diseases. Techniques have now advanced to include nonviral DNA/gene delivery systems, or vectors, which have the distinct advantage of being noninfectious.[107] The FDA's Center for Biologics Evaluation and Research (CBER) regulates all human gene therapies, which fall under the legal definition of a "biologic."[108] As such, approvals for any such products are subject to the investigational new drug (IND) process prior to use. It must be noted, however, that in contrast to the great promise of human gene therapies, the U.S. FDA has yet to approve for sale any such products (even though this may change by the time this chapter goes to press).[91]

With the exception of developmental processes or pilot scale activities, the vast majority of industrial rDNA applications use organisms of intrinsically low risk in systems employing large-scale physical containment technology. The physical plant in use is well-known to industry and has successfully been used to contain pathogenic organisms for years.[91] NIHG Appendix K specifically addresses containment in large-scale (>10 liters) operations such as manufacturing. Like the small-scale guidelines, the levels of physical containment are based primarily on the hazard potential of the organism. Thus, in addition to guidelines for GLSP, Biosafety Level 1 Large Scale (BSL-1-LS), BSL-2-LS and BSL-3-LS are referenced. Table 22.7 provides a summary of the large-scale containment guidelines, and Table 22.8 describes some of the most important industrial microorganisms found in such settings. Additional areas of industrial microbiology include quality assurance for the food, pharmaceutical, and chemical industries, oversight of air and plant contamination, baking, alcohol for beverages and in fuel production (gasohol), and products that range from organic acids to various sugars, amino acids, and detergents. Aspartame, for example, is derived from amino acids produced by microorganisms.[109]

The unit operations in a typical fermentation process are depicted in Figure 22.11, and serve to illustrate a common industrial microbiology application.[110] In the typical production environment, product protection, barriers to infection, and safeguards from exposure to process allergens are desirable. To accomplish these goals engineering containment of the rDNA manufacturing process is designed, especially at stages where aerosols might be generated. Inoculation and primary seed culture are two activities usually performed in dedicated rooms designed to accommodate both the requirement to avoid culture contamina-

Table 22.7 — Large Scale Guidelines Summary

Criteria	Containment Level[a] GLSP	BL1-LS	BL2-LS	BL3-LS
Formulate and implement institutional codes of practice for safety of personnel and adequate control of hygiene and safety measures.	X	X	X	X
Provide adequate written instructions and training of personnel to keep the workplace clean and tidy and to keep exposure to biological, chemical, or physical agents at a level that does not adversely affect health and safety of employees.	X	X	X	X
Provide changing and hand-washing facilities as well as protective clothing, appropriate to the risk, to be worn during work.	X	X	X	X
Prohibit eating, drinking, smoking, mouth pipetting, and applying cosmetics in the workplace.	X	X	X	X
Release of aerosols during sampling, addition of materials, transfer of cultivated cells, and removal of material, products, and effluents from the system is				
minimized by work practices and procedures	X			
minimized by engineering controls		X		
prevented by engineering controls			X	X
Internal accident reporting	X	X	X	X
Emergency plans required for handling large losses of cultures	X	X	X	X
Limited access to the workplace		X	X	X
Viable organisms should be handled in a system that physically separates the process from the external environment (closed system or other primary containment).		X	X	X
Culture fluids are not removed from the closed system until organisms are inactivated.		X	X	X
Minimize the release of untreated, viable exhaust gases.		X		
Prevent the release of untreated, viable exhaust gases.			X	X
Closed system is not to be opened until sterilized by a validated procedure.		X	X	X
Inactivate waste solutions and materials with respect to their biohazard potential.	X	X	X	X
Medical surveillance			X	X
Prevent leakage from rotating seals and other penetrations into the closed system.			X	X
Validate the integrity of the closed containment system.			X	X
Closed system shall be permanently identified for record-keeping purposes.			X	X
Universal Biosafety sign to be posted on each closed system.			X	X
Access to workplace is restricted.		X	X	X
Access to the controlled area is restricted.			X	
Closed system to be kept at as low pressure as possible to maintain integrity of containment features.				X

tion (HEPA-filtered supply air and positive pressure with respect to the anteroom or hall) and within a biological safety cabinet to protect the operator from exposure. The work is typically performed manually. Transfer of primary seed culture is done aseptically, usually by air pressure into the fermenter (bioreactor). There is potential for leakage and/or aerosolization at any transfer stage if the couplings or gaskets are faulty or not installed correctly, or if the transfer line ruptures. Depending on the specifics of the production system, fermentation may occur in batch or continuous processes. The only break in primary containment is at fermenter sample points where a degree of secondary containment, for example, a sample port in a cabinet, may be necessary. Primary containment during fermentation is important for product protection and demands detailed review of vessel design, validated monitoring of seals at all flange joints, continuous welded pipe, and absolute control of off-gases. At the completion of the fermentation stage, cell harvest represents a critical stage with respect to containment. Centrifugation can generate large aerosol masses and is a point where operator contact with microorganisms or cells is most likely. Membrane filtration is an alternative separation technique.

Downstream processing techniques do not differ significantly from standard purification steps except where a unique feature has been engineered into the cells. See Figure 22.12. In general, product must be released from the cell (by mechanical, chemical, enzymatic action, osmotic or temperature shock), separated and concentrated (by centrifugation or size specific filtration), purified (by any of several types of chromatography), and prepared into its final form (e.g., formulated, filled, lyophilized, depyrogenated, etc.). Cell breakage and separation of cell debris are the final activities where exposure to the recombinant organism is a risk, and these activities are typically conducted with some means of secondary containment.[111] Exposure to endotoxin (a component of the lipopolysaccharide layer of gram negative bacteria) is a recognized hazard during cell disruption activities. Leakage from centrifuges, sonicators, and so forth aerosolizes the cell debris, and inhalation exposures above about 300 ng/m³ can cause transient allergic type symptoms such

Table 22.8 — Some Biological Agents Important in Industrial Processes

Aspergillus niger is an asexual fungus commonly found degrading organic matter in nature. It is an opportunistic human pathogen, but has been used safely in the production of citric acid and several enzymes without causing toxic effects in workers.
Aspergillus oryzae is an asexual fungus found in nature and used in the production of soy sauce, miso, and sake without recorded incidents. A. oryzae does not colonize humans.
Bacillus licheniformis is a spore-forming bacterium, readily isolated from the environment, where it persists primarily as endospores. It has a history of safe use in the large-scale fermentation production of citric acid and detergent enzymes.
Bacillus subtilis is a spore-forming bacterium found naturally in terrestrial environments. It has a history of safe use in large-scale fermentation and is a source of single cell protein for human consumption in Asia.
Chinese hamster ovary cells are mammalian cells cultured in a variety of biopharmaceutical applications including the production of recombinant vaccines (e.g., hepatitis B); interferons (a, b, g); interleukins; coagulation factors; enzymes (e.g., glucose cerebrosidase for treatment of Gaucher's disease); and many genetically engineered mono- and polyclonal antibodies.
Clostridium acetobutylicum is isolated from soils, sediment, well water and from animal and human feces. It is distinguishable from closely related species that are known human pathogens. Used for the production of butanol and acetone from various feedstocks.
Escherichia coli K-12 is a bacterial strain readily distinguishable from close relatives that are human pathogens. It is a debilitated bacterium that does not normally colonize the human intestine.
Penicillium roqueforti is an asexual fungus that decomposes organic matter in nature. P. roqueforti's long history of use in the production of blue cheese has shown no adverse effects.
Saccharomyces cerevisiae is a yeast that survives well in the environment. It has a history of safe use in the commercial production of many products including beer.
Saccharomyces uvarum is a yeast that has a long history of safe use in the production (by fermentation) of alcoholic beverages and industrial ethanol.

Source: Reference 10

as fever, nausea, and headache.[112] The American Conference of Governmental Industrial Hygienists® (ACGIH®) has established a ceiling threshold limit value (TLV®) of 60 ng/m^3[113] for pure crystalline proteolytic enzymes (subtilisins), but not for biologically derived air contaminants such as endotoxin. NIOSH has a recommended exposure limit (REL), also 60 ng/m^3, but as a STEL for 60 minutes.[114] Evidence does not support a TLV for endotoxin, mycotoxins or antigens, although dose-response relationships for some assayable bioaerosols have been observed both in experimental and epidemiological studies. Accordingly, establishment of exposure limits for certain biologically derived airborne contaminants may be appropriate in the future.[115]

Once the product is in a soluble concentrated form, the emphasis turns to product protection from the surrounding environment, and work reverts into a positive pressure, clean-room type of operation. Although hazards related to the recombinant cells may no longer be at issue, it may still be necessary to control exposure to the product since it may be a highly biologically active molecule in concentrated form.[116]

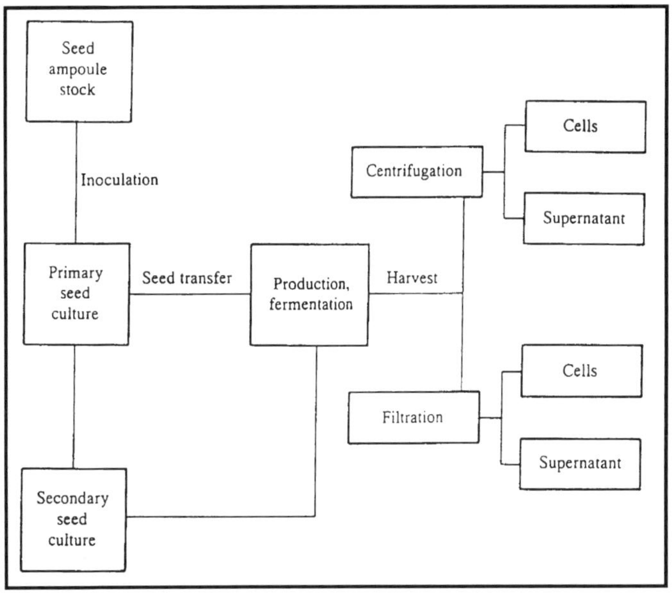

Figure 22.11 — Unit operations for fermentation and separation of recombinant organizations.

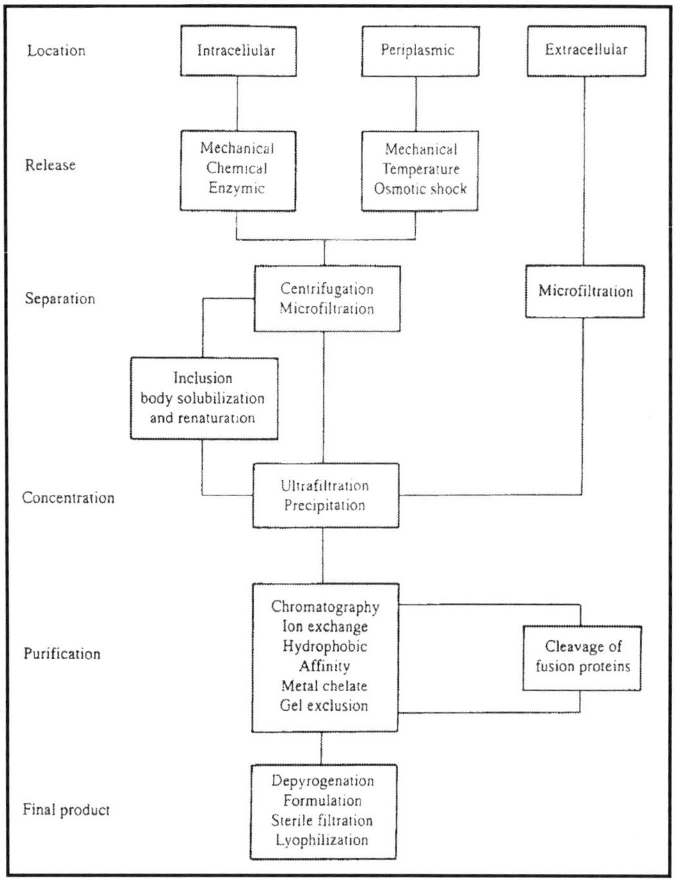

Figure 22.12 — Unit operations for downstream processing of recombinant products.

Enzymes in Industry[117]

Enzymes are complex proteins produced by virtually all living organisms to facilitate or accelerate chemical reactions necessary to maintain life. As used in detergents they catalyze the degradation of certain stains into basic components more easily removed by other ingredients in the detergent product. Used in the pharmaceutical industry, enzymes are created or purified to provide products where enzyme deficiencies may be present (e.g., human lactose intolerance). Enzymes have been used in cleaning applications since the early 1900s. They were widely introduced into detergent formulations in the early 1960s, after the industry solved production capacity and alkaline stability problems. By 1969, 80% of all laundry detergent products contained enzymes.

Although enzymes are biologically derived, the hazards and control strategies are quite similar to those for the bulk production and handling of chemical irritants and sensitizers. Routes of exposure are inhalation and direct contact with skin or eyes. If enough enzyme is inhaled, the body will begin to recognize the enzyme, produce allergic antibodies, and become sensitized to the material. Subsequent exposure may trigger allergic symptoms, including potentially serious occupational asthma. Upon dermal contact primary irritation is expected, and exposed areas should be protected by the use of gloves and other protective clothing where the potential for skin contact exists.[118] Primary irritation of the eye is also expected when detergents or enzymes come in direct contact, but the presence of enzymes in detergents does not necessarily increase the severity of the irritation. Enzymes have been demonstrated not to be skin sensitizers.

Control of exposure to enzymes in detergent manufacturing operations can be achieved by traditional industrial hygiene methods. These entail developing and using low-dust encapsulated formulations, implementing capital improvement of the manufacturing equipment (e.g., enclosed processes), local exhaust ventilation, and measuring and maintaining effectiveness through industrial hygiene monitoring and medical surveillance programs.

Treatment and Disposal of Infectious or Biohazardous Waste

Regardless of the workplace in which it is produced, waste is invariably generated from processes involving biological materials. To the extent such materials maintain one or more hazardous properties, their management will be prescribed by federal, state or local regulations. Under most such laws, biohazardous constituents of wastes assume secondary priority relative to any radioactive or chemical components. Unlike biohazardous materials, those waste components cannot be so easily decontaminated, neutralized, or otherwise legally treated on-site and made nonhazardous. It is therefore typically expected that the biohazardous properties of such mixed wastes will be eliminated first, prior to further processing of the material. Treatment and disposal of complex waste mixtures is beyond the scope of this chapter, and the reader is referred to the appropriate chapter of this text dealing with that issue. This section will address the basic principles for handling and disposal of single component biohazardous materials.

There are no federal regulations that definitively address biohazardous wastes, although EPA has considered regulations under the authority of the Resource Conservation and Recovery Act (RCRA) in past years. Under RCRA individual states can regulate hazardous waste, and several have included biohazardous materials within this authority. Congress passed the Medical Waste Tracking Act of 1988 to determine, on a trial basis, whether infectious waste should be controlled in a similar way to hazardous chemical wastes through a manifesting system. These regulations applied to several states, including New York, New Jersey, and Rhode Island. Ultimately, the trial period passed, the Act expired on June 21, 1999, and federal requirements have neither been continued nor expanded to other states.

Which waste streams are truly biohazardous or in need of heightened management oversight depends on a variety of qualitative factors, including the waste source, material age, state of contamination, the contaminating agent's pathogenicity, physical properties of waste contents (e.g., hypodermic needles or other sharp hazards) and the public's perception of risk. Because of the variable importance of these factors, biohazardous wastes may be defined categorically—on the basis of their potential hazard—and not on the basis of true biologic hazard. For example, surgically removed yet recognizable body parts (historically termed "pathological waste") will normally be regulated as infectious waste in most jurisdictions even if not infectious when removed, or even if preserved in formalin immediately upon autopsy. Since it is difficult or impossible to distinguish pathogenic contamination from nonpathogenic contamination by human senses, waste management systems typically consider all-or-none rules for identification and separation of the defined biohazard wastes. For logistical reasons as well as administrative concerns, health care facilities such as hospitals, nursing homes, walk-in clinics, and clinical laboratories are legally recognized generators of biohazardous waste contaminated with potentially infectious human blood and body fluids per OSHA.[55] Other wastes from industrial processes, R& D or clinical laboratories generating rDNA cultures, animal carcasses and bedding, and animal biohazardous agents may be regulated as infectious waste and require specified treatment(s) before disposal, depending on local laws.

In an attempt to address some of the (costly) uncertainties with potentially biohazardous wastes, EPA drafted a recommendation for the management of such materials. Consisting of 13 categories of infectious wastes[119], the draft manual for infectious waste management still serves as an adequate basis for the definition of biohazardous and infectious waste. The thirteen characteristics used by EPA are:

1. Isolation wastes: Generated by hospitalized patients who are isolated in separate rooms to protect others from their severe and communicable diseases.
2. Cultures and stocks of etiologic agents: All cultures and stocks are included because pathogenic organisms are present in high concentrations.
3. Blood and blood products: Included because of the possible presence of HIV, Hepatitis B, or other bloodborne pathogens.
4. Pathological wastes: Tissues, organs, body parts, blood, and body fluids from surgery and autopsy. EPA distinguished patients with infectious diseases from others, but considered it prudent to handle all pathological wastes as infectious because of the possibility of unknown infection in the patient or corpse.
5. Other wastes from surgery and autopsy: Soiled dressings, sponges, drapes, casts, lavage tubes, etc. The American Hospital Association recommends that all surgical dressings from patients be regarded as potentially infectious because of the possibility of unknown disease.
6. Contaminated laboratory waste: Materials that were in contact with pathogens in any type of laboratory work. This would include items such as culture dishes, pipettes, membrane filters, disposable gloves, lab coats and aprons, etc. The NIHG and CDC-BMBL guidelines for containment require that all wastes from BSL-3 or BSL-4 facilities be treated as infectious, necessitating that they be autoclaved

within the facility prior to removal and terminal disposal. There are compelling arguments against the need to handle all rDNA-contaminated solutions and equipment as infectious, yet common practice is to decontaminate rDNA wastes prior to disposal.

7. Sharps (e.g., hypodermic needles, syringes, Pasteur pipettes, broken glass, scalpel blades): Those items that present the hazard of physical injury via puncture or laceration, creating a portal of entry for an infectious agent contaminating the sharp object (assuming the object had been used in treatment of patients with an infectious disease).
8. Dialysis unit wastes: Infectious because they are in contact with the blood of dialysis patients, who as a group constitute a population with a documented high rate of hepatitis infection.
9. Carcasses and body parts of animals: This category includes animals exposed to pathogens in research, used in the production of biologicals, *in vivo* pharmaceutical test subjects, as well as those that died of known or suspected infectious disease. Biosafety experts recommend that all laboratory animals be considered potentially infectious because of the potential for acquiring zoonotic diseases.
10. Animal bedding and other waste from animal rooms: Similar to the previous category, these are included because pathogens may be secreted or excreted from animals contaminating these items.
11. Discarded biologicals: Materials produced by pharmaceutical companies for human or veterinary use. These may be discarded because of bad manufacturing lots, expired shelf life, or recall and removal from the market. It should be remembered that some drugs may contain heavy metals or other toxic ingredients, and so may also be considered hazardous waste.
12. Food and other products contaminated with etiologic agents: Includes canned foods being recalled because of the danger of intoxication resulting from the ingestion of botulinum, a toxic product of the *Clostridium botulinum* bacterium.
13. Equipment or machine parts contaminated with etiologic agents: These would include laboratory equipment and HEPA filters from biological safety cabinets, if not decontaminated *in situ*. Note that NSF-49 dictates that safety cabinet HEPA filters must be formaldehyde-decontaminated in place prior to removal.[60]

Once an item is defined by a biohazardous waste category, it is necessary to determine how waste streams containing such materials will be collected, treated and ultimately discarded. The nature of a biohazardous waste stream determines the most appropriate collection and storage conditions. "Double bags," "leakproof containers," and "red bag waste" are common terms used to describe some of the waste collection and storage requirements for biohazardous waste. For example, collection of sharps from hospital rooms and laboratories should be done in relatively small leakproof, puncture resistant, autoclavable containers. In the OSHA bloodborne pathogens standard, red bags or "BIOHAZARD" labels are required for waste contaminated with human blood or body fluids.[55] Storage temperatures and minimum holding times may need to be specified. Such is the case, for example, with isotope contaminated research animals whose carcasses must be stored frozen while the radioactive material within decays to acceptable levels. In the specific case of biotechnology effluents, validated kill methods are usually employed at the lab bench before terminal disposal.

Biohazardous waste handling and transportation is generally not a difficult undertaking to arrange on a routine basis, but special precautions must be exercised. Because of the nature of biohazard waste, prudent management is more costly than normal solid waste disposal. As such, minimization of all biohazardous waste streams is desirable from both a cost as well as risk-management perspective. Separation and segregation of the waste streams helps the minimization effort and also helps to ensure each specific waste stream is treated correctly. Procedures and equipment for transporting biohazard waste within a facility must anticipate the potential for spills as well as the risk of injury from direct contact with the material, such as cuts or puncture wounds from sharps. Rigid plastic containers protect workers from sharps, and double containment is recommended for spill prevention. In hospitals, covered carts are often preferred for aesthetic reasons as well as good infection control practice. Work practices and PPE also help to reduce the probability of injury to workers.

Terminal biohazard waste disposal methods are often a matter of local practice and jurisdiction as well as state control. Appropriate on-site treatments of biohazardous materials include autoclaving, the use of chemical disinfectants, and incineration (where permitted and cost-effective). Some of the most common on-site disinfectants are bleach (1:10 or 1:100 dilution of household bleach) to treat liquid biohazards, and glutaraldehyde or iodophors such as Wescodyne(tm) for ambient temperature disinfection of objects such as medical devices and reusable pipettes. Glutaraldehyde and formaldehyde are also recommended for more resilient agents such as spore forming anthrax. After on-site treatment biological waste remains may theoretically be disposed of as nonhazardous solid waste and placed in unregulated trash or discharged to drains. Local ordinances may bar such practices, however, requiring specific treatments, waste bag color, or labeling, before local landfills can receive such material. In some localities materials that are, or ever were, biohazardous wastes must be buried in secure cells of public landfills, or in more stringently operated industrial waste facilities. Owing to the variability of regional requirements, smaller or decentralized organizations in particular may find it more economical and operationally prudent to purchase turn-key services for biohazardous waste disposal. Such vendors package biohazardous materials to be shipped off-site for incineration, industrial sterilization, or other terminal disposal. The proper packaging is regulated by DOT for interstate transportation, and a manifest tracking system is routinely employed in such cases.

Management Issues

Typical Program Elements

If an organization is to effectively manage its biohazards certain components must be in place. Although there are certain to be noticeable differences among institutions, so too will there be a need for essentially similar functional groups or personnel. Various models for effective organizational structure exist[120–124] and the reader is directed to those for further details. For the sake of this chapter, three key fundamentals will be defined and considered. These basics of the biohazardous materials management program are effective organization, management support, and implementation and program maintenance.

In terms of organizational matters, biological hazards and risks are best managed and controlled locally by the technical specialists, line managers, and unit directors of the institution. Possible team members needed continuously or on occasion might include members from legal, risk management, facilities, custodial or environmental services, administration, academics/research, production, and senior management, in addition to specialists charged with categorical safety matters (e.g., fire safety, radiation safety, etc.). A competent example incorporating some of the functional duties of these positions is that of the NIHG.[125] Under these and similar guidelines, an institution should:

- Obtain management commitment for the establishment and oversight of a biosafety program. Executive management should adopt a written policy statement that describes this commitment as well as the specific principles important to the institution.
- Establish an Institutional Biosafety Committee (IBC, or simply "Biosafety Committee"). The IBC is required for federally supported biosafety programs encompassing rDNA activities, but its interests should not be limited to rDNA. The primary functions of the IBC should be to review and approve rDNA activities, define physical containment levels, assess facilities, procedures, practices, training, and expertise of personnel involved in rDNA research. The IBC can also adopt emergency plans covering spills and personnel contamination, and perform other functions as the institution requires, such as implementing a health surveillance program, serum banking, policies on personnel vaccinations, etc.

- Appoint a suitably credentialed Biological Safety Officer (BSO) even if not mandatory (as in the case of BSL-3, BSL-4, or large-scale production facilities). As much as for peer-acceptance as for demonstrated competency, this person should be educated in the sciences and experienced in the nature of the operations to be overseen. Under the NIHG, the BSO is a member of the IBC. His or her role is to inspect laboratories for compliance with the NIHG and report problems and violations to the IBC or laboratory manager/PI. The BSO is the technical expert advisor to the committee, PIs, and laboratory workers on matters of laboratory safety, risk assessment, emergency procedures, and laboratory security. Industrial hygienists are likely to be called on to be members of the IBC. With adequate education, training, and experience in microbiology and biosafety, an industrial hygienist may also serve as a BSO.
- Ensure that appropriate program requirements are implemented and that specific laboratory safety training is provided. Numerous training requirements exist in and out of the areas of biohazards per se, including the OSHA bloodborne pathogens requirements, hazardous waste disposal, hazard communication, and others.
- Determine the necessity for medical surveillance of personnel involved in work with bloodborne pathogens, rDNA, animal handling, etc.
- Report to the NIH (or authority having jurisdiction) any significant problems or violations of the NIHG, or any significant research-related accidents and illnesses.

Regardless of the organizational structure of a given biosafety program, for it to be truly effective, meaningful and visible management support is required. Such support is embodied in three generalized principles, and industrial hygienists may have a role in any or all of them. First, organizational direction starts at the top and so management commitment at the highest level is essential. Clear, unflinching, visible support enables the biohazards program initiatives by providing authority and resources (money, supplies, time, staff, facilities, and equipment), and assigning the roles and responsibilities for implementing the program. Second, respected specialized technical expertise is required to provide the scientific knowledge basis and peer-cooperation for the program. Senior level PIs, an organized biosafety committee chair, an informed and cooperative biosafety officer, an occupational health physician, industrial hygienists, and/or consultants may all be called on to perform risk assessments, provide training, plan for emergencies, and investigate accidents or incidents. Third, rational enforcement of rules and procedures is required to provide accountability and responsibility. NIHG assigns this function to the BSO, but many organizations prefer that line supervisors be responsible for their direct reports and staffs, enforcing rules through direct supervision and performance evaluations. In health care organizations the infection control practitioner may play the roles of both technical expert and enforcement officer.

Given an organizational structure that make sense for the institution or business, and committed management and support, the work of implementing and maintaining the biohazards function can most easily be accomplished. Steps necessary for this to occur are not unique to the health and safety function, and include:

- Defining the scope of the program based on hazards and risks;
- Developing policies and procedures;
- Training workers based on job functions, monitoring their work, and retraining as needed;
- Providing necessary and proper facilities and equipment;
- Performing the work safely; and
- Auditing the program on a periodic basis.

It is at the level of workers performing tasks that the effectiveness of the biosafety program is ultimately determined. This statement applies to safety and health employees, researchers, PIs, and line personnel alike. Each employee has the responsibility to comply with all health and safety rules that apply to his or her own actions and conduct.

Employees should participate in the development of health and safety programs, and have measurable goals and objectives that address compliance policies and procedures. They have the responsibility to report hazards to supervision, co-workers, and company health and safety representatives.

Emergency Planning and Risk Communication

Considerable information has been accumulated that identifies the major routes of exposure for laboratory acquired infections. The initial reviews of Sulkin and Pike[89,90] indicate that accidents with needles and syringes gave rise to many laboratory acquired infections. Despite new safety engineered needles and the like, the hazards of sharps are as prevalent today as they were years ago, perhaps more so. What has changed is the nature of some of the hazards common now, as well as the medical treatments available (or not, as the case may be). Accidental infections acquired in the 21st century are no longer primarily brucellosis, Q- fever, or Salmonella. Diseases of increasing risk include AIDS, hepatitis, E. coli 0157:H7, MRSA, and a re-emergence of tuberculosis, including multiple-drug resistant strains. Unfortunately, intentional exposures to biohazards are now also a very real possibility.[126–129]

With the specter of a global avian influenza A pandemic looming, many organizations have enlisted their industrial hygiene functions to participate in business continuation planning for such an eventuality. Influenza A (H5N1) virus — also called "H5N1 virus" — is an influenza A virus subtype that occurs in and mainly kills birds. H5N1 virus does not usually infect people, but confirmed cases of human infection have been reported since 1997. The risk from avian influenza is generally low to most people, but the public health concern is that the virus will mutate into a form that is highly infectious for humans.[130] Pathology of H5N1 is similar to that of the great influenza pandemic of 1918–19. In its present forms, overall mortality in reported H5N1 cases is high, at approximately 60%.[131] To date, there have been over 400 confirmed H5N1 cases worldwide, with more than 250 deaths.[132] The ongoing epizootic outbreak in Asia, Europe, the Near East, and Africa is not expected to diminish, and research suggests strains of H5N1 viruses are becoming more capable of causing disease in animals than were earlier H5N1 viruses.

Given the pandemic science portends, organizational continuity planning is essential. The CDC expects an H5N1 infection wave could last for 8–12 weeks, and occur in 2–3 waves several months apart. Clinics and hospitals would likely be overwhelmed, and because business could face a 40% absentee rate, plans are needed to deal with general staffing and the unavailability of key personnel. Employees may be deceased, sick, caring for a sick relative, caring for children unable to attend school, or simply afraid to come to work for fear of infection. Organizations need to be concerned about suppliers similarly affected. In-house response plans need to be rethought as well, and stockpiles of cleaning supplies should be held to ensure adequate hygiene in the event an employee or visitor falls ill. Depending on location, other materials might also need to be stockpiled including food, drinking water, cots, respirators, disinfectants, and gloves. Given the possibility the organization could come under quarantine, a process should be in place to feed and house employees. Finally, ongoing and emergency communication should be planned.[133]

Aside from catastrophic or community-based calamities, organizations must still plan for more routine yet infrequent incidents. All accidental exposures, whether overt or only suspected, which involve biological hazards should be immediately decontaminated and reported. Through routine employee in-service education or by those responsible for investigation and reporting of such incidents, employees should be trained to promptly seek medical evaluation for biohazardous agent exposures. It is conceivable that an initial accident report may need to be directed to several individuals, including the IBC chairperson. Such reporting permits the monitoring of frequency of accidents and near-misses, and helps in developing procedures or methods of prevention that make sense for the institution. It may also help by contributing to the body of knowledge concerning types of accidents that result in infection of laboratory workers. In determining the need for external reporting, the nature or identity of the agent, the amount involved, and the likelihood of exposure that might result in infection are important criteria. Depending on the pathogenicity and virulence of the agent, it may be prudent to make voluntary reports to state or federal officials even if such reports do not appear to be required.

Any organization using hazardous materials, including biohazards, should maintain an evergreen incident response plan to emergencies involving these items. Since all but a very few HAZMAT and rescue services are prepared to provide assistance in the event of a significant biological emergency, it is critically important for institutions that use biohazardous agents (including toxins) to have in place formal, practiced, internal response and assistance plans to handle potential biological emergencies. In essence, a facility biohazards incident response plan defines who is responsible and accountable for specified actions before, during, and after a biological event. When they exist, such plans not only serve as a formal guideline for internal response to biological emergencies, but also to provide rational assurances that the institution can addresses both its needs and those of the surrounding community. Basic information about the institution's mission, the type of work conducted, and an assessment of risks and methods for mitigating anticipated emergencies should be described in the plan, through language meaningful to the intended audience. In addition, the plan should provide a thorough discussion of the most probable events, worst case scenarios, and contingency based actions. Resources on-hand internally or externally available to mitigate all identified hazards should be listed in the plan, along with up-to-date contact information. Sections should provide flowcharts or otherwise unambiguously delineate communications and coordination between the institution and local, state, and/or federal authorities. Communications sections must define procedures to be followed to maintain on-site as well as community safety and environmental integrity.

With a response plan in place, employees listed in the document should be trained. Since biological spills or releases pose unique hazards, in-house emergency responders require special training in hazard evaluation and first aid, as well as decontamination and monitoring procedures. Optimally, the leader of the emergency response team would be trained in both biological and chemical safety. Under the NIHG, for example, the BSO is charged with developing emergency plans[125], and should function as the emergency response team leader unless incident command procedures dictate otherwise. Primary functions of the leader are to assess the scope of the accident, organize the remediation plans, and possibly to communicate with the public or press (although public communication may be reserved for more senior management or public affairs representatives). Core emergency response team members are on-site personnel trained in topics related to first aid, spill containment, decontamination procedures, selection and use of proper PPE, procedures for safe entry and egress from contaminated areas, and signs and symptoms of intoxication or infection.

Training of team members should be commensurate with the severity and probability of an incident for which they are trained and equipped to respond. Emergency response teams within organizations that use BSL-3 and BSL-4 pathogens should meet quarterly to participate in drills, discuss strategies for hypothetical accidents, review call listings, practice donning protective equipment, and review changes in agents on hand or to the facility. In some jurisdictions local emergency planning committees require biosafety to be included in the emergency planning required by the Emergency Planning and Community Right to Know Act.[134] Hospital emergency departments plan for community disasters as a part of their accreditation, and may wish to include elements of biohazards disasters in their efforts.[36] Radiological disaster scenarios are routinely practiced in areas near nuclear power plants, and depending on the local jurisdiction, hospital emergency departments may wish to prepare for biological emergencies as well.

Second only to the need to effectively mitigate the biohazardous incident, the organization should be prepared to communicate with the public about the risks, real or perceived, associated with an incident. In fact, a formalized risk communication dialog should be considered as part of the organization's overall public relations efforts. An open and sincere dialogue may help to foster trust and reduce any misconception about the biological risks within an institution or business. A strategy for risk communication should be developed based on the content and context of the message as well as the target audience. Sandman[135–138] and others[139] have described risk perceptions and how to effectively manage the process when dealing with sophisticated issues such as chemicals, biohazardous wastes, and other public hazards.

Individuals' perceptions of risk are determined by a number of factors, including past experience, values, and previously supplied information. Other intangible and nonquantifiable risk perceptions include voluntary versus involuntary participation, fair versus unfair treatment, immediate versus delayed health effects, reversible versus irreversible consequences, associated feelings of dread, availability of alternatives to taking the risk, and the reliability or trustworthiness of the source of information.[136] The general public is not likely to have a rational knowledge of biological hazards, and what they believe to be possible is likely to have been overly influenced by the popular press and entertainment industry (e.g., advanced cloning capabilities as portrayed in the movie *Jurassic Park*). The industrial hygienist should be aware that safety and health issues, while clearly important, may not be preeminent in community members' minds. Unanticipated outcomes only tangentially associated with the biohazards may be of more importance to them. A hypothetical scenario illustrating this circumstance would be the detrimental influence on property values in neighborhoods adjacent to a proposed medical waste incinerator. Where risk of illness or death is perceived as low, derivative concerns such as these may rise to the forefront in risk perception.

Careful consideration should be given to those who are assigned the duty of communicating risk. Risk can be communicated in a variety of ways including worst case scenario, reasonably foreseeable event, and most probable event. There is no one correct method or person for any given issue, and the optimal choice for both depends on the hazards and technicalities of the topic, the structure of the forum for discussion, and target audience. Communications following an unintentional release from the site will obviously be handled much differently than statements made at a public hearing in support of a biological materials permit, for example. Technical specialists such as biosafety professionals and industrial hygienists can be expected to effectively communicate risk assessments or recommendations to employees of an organization, and the PI should be prepared to discuss risk associated with his or her project when addressing the IBC. If communication is to take place in a public hearing, those holding the perception of a high degree of authority within the organization—the laboratory director, a public affairs officer, legal counsel, or a senior administrative officer—should be given measured consideration to make such presentations. Whatever the situation, it is wise to prospectively consult the public affairs or corporate communications department about the content and methods of communicating biological risk to the public.

Summary

Although industrial microbiology is hardly a new pursuit, because of significant molecular advances at the end of the last century some biotechnology processes are becoming increasingly important for industrial hygienists. The OSHA Bloodborne Pathogens Standard has focused attention on biological hazards for virtually all safety and health practitioners in that medical first aid, and its attendant hazards, is required in all places of employment under OSHA jurisdiction. Some industries and professions where biological agents may present recognized hazards are health care, police and emergency responder services, clinical laboratories, agriculture and veterinary science, in-vitro diagnostic laboratories, medical device manufacturers, biotechnology, biological R&D, detergent enzymes, and even construction or demolition of moldy infrastructure. While there are tremendous social and economic benefits derived from work with biological material, it is the ethical responsibility of the industrial hygienist to scientifically anticipate the biohazards to employees, and to work to safeguard employees and the community from them.

The primary goal of the biosafety program is not to prohibit work, but to enable safe work and the advancement of science and innovation. This is particularly important in light of emerging controls implemented in reaction to the general threat of terrorism. In this chapter the objectives were to provide industrial hygiene students and practitioners with an understanding of the uniqueness of biological hazards, and to present the basic principles, practices, and resources for biological safety. The essential and necessary elements defining engineering, administrative, and personal protective equipment were illustrated, and the constituents of an effective biological safety program described.

The field of biological safety is rapidly changing, being thrust forward by successes in genetic code interpretation and the refinement of techniques to create products from biological production systems. While expertise in biohazards control is not easily attained, this chapter has provided the foundation for additional reading and study for those desiring to enter into this complex and changing area.

Additional Internet Resources

American Biological Safety Association, Mundelein, IL. (www.absa.org)

American Industrial Hygiene Association®, Fairfax, VA. (www.aiha.org)

- Biosafety & Environmental Microbiology Committee
- Emergency Response Planning Committee
- Indoor Environmental Quality Committee
- Laboratory Health & Safety Committee

American Society of Microbiology, Washington, DC. (www.asm.org)

- Public and Scientific Affairs Board
- Laboratory Practices Committee
- Laboratory Safety Subcommittee

Association of Professionals in Infection Control and Epidemiology, Inc., Washington, DC. (www.apic.org)

Centers for Disease Control and Prevention, Atlanta, GA. (www.cdc.gov)

Joint Commission for the Accreditation of Healthcare Organizations, Oakbrook Terrace, IL. (www.jointcommission.org)

Occupational Safety and Health Administration, Washington, DC. (www.osha.gov)

National Sanitation Foundation (NSF International), Ann Arbor, MI. (www.nsf.org)

Society for Industrial Microbiology, Fairfax, VA. (www.simhq.org)

Acknowledgment

I would like to recognize the first edition authors of this chapter, Susan B. Lee and Barbara Johnson. Although I have significantly revised the organization, content, and flow of much of that earlier work, several of the figures and sections they created are so appropriate that I have included them essentially unchanged. Without their original efforts to build upon, the current chapter would have been a much more difficult undertaking and so I thank them for their efforts.

References

1. **Centers for Disease Control and Prevention (CDC):** Tracking a Mystery Disease: The Detailed Story of Hantavirus Pulmonary Syndrome, The "First" Outbreak. Available at http://www.cdc.gov/hantavirus/hps/history.html. [Accessed July 1, 2011.]
2. **Centers for Disease Control and Prevention (CDC):** All About Hantavirus, Navajo Medical Traditions and HPS. Available at http://www.cdc.gov/hantavirus/index.htm. [Accessed July 1, 2011.]
3. **South Coast Daily:** Two Arrested for Possession of Deadly Germs. Robert Macy. Updated February 19, 1998. Available at http://www.southcoasttoday.com/apps/pdcs.dll/article?AID=/19980220/news/302209958&cid=sitesearch. [Accessed July 1, 2011.]
4. Definition of Koch's postulates. Medicinenet.com. Updated October 19, 1998. Accessed July 1, 2011.
5. **Occupational Safety and Health Administration (OSHA):** OSHA Preambles, Section - IX. Summary and Explanation of the Standard Occupational Exposure to Bloodborne Pathogens. Code of Federal Regulations Title 29, Part 1910.1030. Federal Register 56: 64004. December 6, 1991.
6. **Centers for Disease Control and Prevention (CDC) and National Institutes of Health (NIOSH):** Biosafety in Microbiological and Biomedical Laboratories, 5th edition. Chosewood, L.C. and D.E. Wilson (eds.). Washington, DC: U.S. Government Printing Office, 2007.
7. **Heymann, D.L. (ed.):** *Control of Communicable Diseases Manual.* 19th edition. Washington, DC: American Public Health Association, 2008.
8. **American Biological Safety Association (ABSA):** Membership Directory. Mundelein, IL: ABSA, 2008.

9. **Tramont, E.C.:** Host Defense Mechanisms. In *Principles and Practices of Infectious Diseases*, 3rd edition. New York: Churchill Livingstone Inc., 1990. pp. 33-40.
10. **Lee, S.B. and B. Johnson:** Biohazards in the Work Environment. In *The Occupational Environment: Its Evaluation and Control.* Fairfax, VA: American Industrial Hygiene Association®, 1997. pp. 361–389.
11. **Bond, R.G., C.P. Straub, and R. Prober:** *CRC Handbook of Environmental Control.* West Palm Beach, FL: CRC Press, 1978. 103 pp.
12. **National Institutes of Health (NIH):** Guidelines for Research Involving Recombinant DNA Molecules (NIH Guidelines), Appendix B: Classification of Human Etiologic Agents on the Basis of Hazard. April, 2002.
13. Classification of Biological Agents. Article 18 and Annex. Council Directive of the European Communities (90/391/EEC), 1991.
14. **Centers for Disease Control and Prevention (CDC) and National Institutes of Health (NIH):** *Biosafety in Microbiological and Biomedical Laboratories*, 5th ed. Section VIII, Agent Summary Statements. Chosewood, L.C. and D.E. Wilson (eds.). Washington, DC: U.S. Government Printing Office, 2007.
15. **Centers for Disease Control and Prevention (CDC) and National Institutes of Health (NIH):** *Biosafety in Microbiological and Biomedical Laboratories*, 5th edition. Section II, Biological Risk Assessment. Chosewood, L.C. and D.E. Wilson (eds.). Washington, DC: U.S. Government Printing Office, 2007.
16. The Black Death: Bubonic Plague. TheMiddleAges.net. Available at http://www.themiddleages.net/plague.html. [Accessed July 1, 2011.]
17. John Snow. Available at http://www.ph.ucla.edu/epi/snow.html. Accessed July 1, 2011.
18. **Chin, J. (ed.):** *Control of Communicable Diseases Manual*, 17th edition. Washington, DC: American Public Health Association, 2000. p.103.
19. **Centers for Disease Control and Prevention (CDC) and the National Institute for Occupational Safety and Health (NIOSH):** NIOSH Topic Area: Severe Acute Respiratory Syndrome (SARS). Available at http://www.cdc.gov/ niosh/topics/SARS/. [Accessed on July 1, 2011.]
20. **Centers for Disease Control and Prevention (CDC):** Severe Acute Respiratory Syndrome Fact Sheet: Basic Information about SARS. Available at http://www.cdc.gov/ncidod/sars/factsheet.htm. [Accessed on July 1, 2011.]
21. **Centers for Disease Control and Prevention (CDC):** Cluster of Severe Acute Respiratory Syndrome Cases Among Protected Health-Care Workers—Toronto, Canada. *MMWR 52(19)*:433–436 (2003).
22. **Mackowiak, P.A.:** The normal microbial flora. *N. Engl. J. Med. 307*:83–86 (1982).
23. **Smith, H.W. and M.B. Huggins:** Further observations on the colicin V plasmid of Escherichia coli with pathogenicity and with survival in the alimentary tract. *J. Gen. Microbiol. 92*:335 (1976).
24. **Nicas, M.:** Modeling respirator penetration values with the beta distribution: an application to occupational tuberculosis transmission. *Am. Ind. Hyg. Assoc. J. 55*:515–524 (1994).
25. **Nardell, E.A., et al.:** Theoretical levels of protection achievable by building ventilation. *Am. Rev. Respir. Dis. 144*:302–306 (1991).
26. **Riley, C., et al.:** Infectiousness of air from a tuberculosis ward. *Am. Rev. Respir. Dis. 85*:511–525 (1962).
27. **Wells, W.F. (ed.):** Airborne Contagion and Air Hygiene. Cambridge, MA: Harvard University Press, 1955. pp. 15–17, 121–122.
28. **Centers for Disease Control and Prevention and National Institutes of Health:** *Biosafety in Microbiological and Biomedical Laboratories*, 5th edition. Section I, Introduction. Chosewood, L.C. and D.E. Wilson (eds.). Washington, DC: U.S. Government Printing Office, 2007.
29. Uniting and Strengthening America by Providing Appropriate Tools Required to Intercept and Obstruct Terrorism (USA PATRIOT) Act of 2001. Public Law 107-56, October 26, 2001.
30. Public Health Security and Bioterrorism Preparedness and Response Act of 2002. Public Law 107-188, June 12, 2002.
31. 42 CFR Parts 72 and 73. Federal Register 70 (52):13294-13325. March 18, 2005.
32. Guidelines for Research Involving Recombinant DNA Molecules (NIH Guidelines), Section I-D, Compliance with NIH Guidelines, p.10. April, 2002.
33. **Massachusetts Biotechnology Council:** Biotechnology Regulatory Guide for Communities. Cambridge, MA: Massachusetts Biotechnology Council, 1995. [Pamphlet].
34. OSHA Preambles, Section X. Authority and Signature. Code of Federal Regulations Title 29, Part 1910.1030. Federal Register 56: 64004 (Dec. 6, 1991).
35. **Centers for Disease Control and Prevention (CDC):** Update: Universal Precautions for Prevention of Transmission of Human Immunodeficiency Virus, Hepatitis B Virus and Other Bloodborne Pathogens in Healthcare Settings. MMWR 37:377–382, 387, 388 (1988).

36. **Joint Commission on Accreditation of Healthcare Organizations:** Environment of care standards 1.6, 2.5, 3.1. In *Comprehensive Accreditation Manual for Hospitals.* Chicago, IL: Joint Commission on Accreditation of Healthcare Organizations, 2008.
37. Effective Death Penalty and Public Safety Act of 1996. Public Law: 104-132, April 24, 1996.
38. Additional Requirements for Facilities Transferring or Receiving Select Infectious Agents. Code of Federal Regulations Title 42, Part 72. 1997.
39. **Centers for Disease Control and Prevention (CDC):** National Select Agent Registry. Available at http://www.selectagents.gov/index.html. [Accessed on July 1, 2011].
40. United States Code Annotated Title 42. Chapter 6A-Public Health Service. Part G – Quarantine and Inspections, paragraph 264. Regulations to Control Communicable Diseases.
41. **Ostroff, S.M.:** "Testimony before the U.S. House of Representative, Committee on Commerce, Subcommittee on Oversight and Investigations." Washington, D.C.: May 20, 1999.
42. Homeland Security Act of 2002. P.L. 107-296. November 5, 2002.
43. "Hazardous Materials Regulations" Code of Federal Regulations Title 49, Parts 171-180. 2005.
44. Publication 52 - Hazardous, Restricted and Perishable Mail. January, 2008. United States Postal Service. [Accessed]uly 1, 2011.]
45. **Hazardous Materials Regulations:** Editorial Corrections and Classifications; Final Rule. Federal Register 61:191 (1 October 1996). pp. 51333-51343.
46. Dangerous Goods Regulations. 50th edition. Montreal: International Air Transport Association, 2009.
47. "NAFTA Countries Seek Uniform Code." Chem. Reg. Rep. 20. August 9, 1996.
48. "Technical Instructions for the Safe Transport of Dangerous Goods by Air" (Doc. 9284-AN/905). Montreal: International Civil Aviation Organization, 2005-2006.
49. Hazardous Materials: Infectious substances; Harmonization with the United Nations Recommendations. 71 FR 32244, June 2, 2006.
50. Animal and Plant Products, Code of Federal Regulations Title 9, Parts 1-3, Subchapter A: Animal Welfare. 69 FR 42099, July 14, 2004.
51. Federal plant pest regulations, Code of Federal Regulations Title 7, Part 330. Available at http://www.access.gpo.gov/nara/cfr/. [Accessed July 1, 2011.]
52. Bureau of Industry and Security, Department of Commerce, Code of Federal Regulations Title 15, Parts 700-744, Defense Priorities and Allocation System. January 1, 2007.
53. Interstate Shipment of Etiological Agents, Code of Federal Regulations Title 42, Part 72.1. Revised October 1, 2006.
54. **Slavik, N.:** "Statement of the American Hospital Association before the Subcommittee on Regulation and Business Opportunities of the Small Business Committee of the U.S. House of Representatives on the Regulations of Infectious Waste." Washington, D.C. August 9, 1988.
55. Bloodborne pathogens, Code of Federal Regulations Title 29, Part 1910.1030. 73 FR 75586, December 12, 2008.
56. **Heinsohn, P.A., R.R. Jacobs, and B.A. Concoby (eds.):** Biosafety Reference Manual, 2nd edition. Fairfax, VA: American Industrial Hygiene Association, 1995.
57. **World Health Organization (WHO):** Laboratory Biosafety Manual, 3rd edition. Geneva, Switzerland: WHO, 2004.
58. **Department of Health and Human Services:** Primary Containment for Biohazards: Selection, Installation and Use of Biological Safety Cabinets. Chosewood, L.C. and D.E. Wilson, eds. Atlanta, GA: Centers for Disease Control and Prevention, 2007.
59. **Karabatsos, N. (ed):** *International Catalog of Arboviruses Including Certain Other Viruses of Vertebrates*, 3rd edition. San Antonio, TX: American Society for Tropical Medicine and Hygiene, 1985.
60. NSF Class II (Laminar Flow) Biosafety Cabinetry. 11th ed. NSF/ANSI Standard 49-2008. Ann Arbor, Mi: National Sanitation Foundation International. 2008.
61. **Vallat, B.:** Manual of Diagnostic Tests & Vaccines for Terrestrial Animals. 6th ed. Office International des Epizooties. Paris, France: OIE-World Organisation for Animal Health, 2008.
62. **Fox, J.C. and N.S. Lipman:** Infections transmitted by large and small laboratory animals. *Infect. Dis. Clin. N. Am. 5*:131–163 (1991).
63. **Miller, C.D., J.R. Songer, and J.F. Sullivan:** A 25-year review of laboratory-acquired human infections at the National Animal Disease Center. *Am. Ind. Hyg. Assoc. J. 48*:271–275 (1987).
64. **Jaxx, N., et al.:** Transmission of Ebola virus (Zaire strain) to uninfected control monkeys in a biocontainment laboratory. *Lancet 346*:1669–1671 (1995).
65. **Centers for Disease Control and Prevention (CDC):** Guidelines for the prevention of herpesvirus simiae (B virus) infection in monkey handlers. *MMWR 36*:680-682, 687-689 (1987).
66. **Richmond, J.Y.:** Hazard reduction in animal research facilities. *Lab. Anim. 20(2)*:23–29 (1991).

67. **Centers for Disease Control and Prevention and National Institutes of Health:** Biosafety in Microbiological and Biomedical Laboratories, 5th ed. Section V, Vertebrate Animal Biosafety Level Criteria for Vivarium Research Facilities. L.C. Chosewood and D.E. Wilson, eds. Washington, DC: U.S. Government Printing Office, 2007.
68. **National Institutes of Health (NIH):** Revised Guide for the Care and Use of Laboratory Animals (DHHS pub. no. NIH 86-23). Washington, DC: U.S. Government Printing Office, 1996.
69. **Hung, L.-L., Miller, J.D., and H.K. Dillon (eds.):** Field Guide for the Determination of Biological Contaminants in Environmental Samples, Second edition. Fairfax, VA: American Industrial Hygiene Association, 2005.
70. **Plog, B.A. and P.J. Quinlan (eds.):** Fundamentals of Industrial Hygiene, 5th edition. Chicago, IL: National Safety Council, 2001. pp. 422–424.
71. **Cole, E.C.:** "Environmental Decontamination." Presentation for Practicing Industrial Hygiene within the Biotechnology Industry at the American Industrial Hygiene Conference and Exposition professional development course. Salt Lake City, UT, May 19, 1991.
72. **Russell, A.D., W.B. Hugo, and G.A.J. Ayliffe (eds.):** Principles and Practice of Disinfection, Preservation, and Sterilization, 2nd edition. Oxford, U.K.: Blackwell Scientific Publications, 1992. pp. 9–43.
73. **Lawrence, C.A. and S.S. Block (eds.):** "Alcohols." In *Disinfection, Sterilization, and Preservation*. Philadelphia, PA: Lea and Febiger. 1968. pp. 237–252.
74. Occupational Exposure to Ethylene Oxide. *Federal Register 49*:122 (1984).
75. Occupational Exposure to Formaldehyde. *Federal Register 52*:233 (1987).
76. Hazard Communication, Code of Federal Regulations Title 29, Part 1200. 61 FR 5507, Feb. 13, 1996.
77. Occupational Exposure to Hazardous Chemicals in Laboratories, Code of Federal Regulation Title 29, Part 1450. 71 FR 16674, April 3, 2006.
78. **U.S. Environmental Protection Agency (EPA):** Should You Have the Air Ducts in Your Home Cleaned? Available at http://www.epa.gov/ iaq/pubs/airduct.html. [Accessed on July 1, 2011].
79. **U.S. Environmental Protection Agency (EPA):** Ozone Generators that are Sold as Air Cleaners. Available at http://www.epa.gov/iaq/pubs/ozonegen.html. [Accessed on July 1, 2011].
80. **Occupational Safety and Health Administration (OSHA):** Ethylene Oxide. Title 29 Code of Federal Regulations, Part 1910.1047. 2009.
81. **U.S. Environmental Protection Agency (EPA):** Anthrax spore decontamination using chlorine dioxide. Available at http://www.epa.gov/pesticides/factsheets/chemicals/chlorinedioxidefactsheet.htm. [Accessed on July 1, 2011].
82. **Webster, R.A.:** NY Decontamination service rids Pascal's Manale in New Orleans of toxic mold in one day. New Orleans CityBusiness. November 21, 2005. Available at http://findarticles.com/p/articles/mi_qn4200/is_20051121/ai_n15848581/. [Accessed on July 1, 2011].
83. **Sattelle, D.:** Biotechnology in Perspective. Washington, DC: IBA, Hobson Scientific, 1990. p. 4. [Pamphlet]
84. **Lee, S.B. and L.P. Ryan:** Occupational health and safety in the biotechnology industry-a survey of practicing professionals. *Am. Ind. Hyg. Assoc. J. 57*:381–386 (1996).
85. **Harris, R.L.:** *Patty's Industrial Hygiene*, 5th edition: Volume II: Recognition and Evaluation of Physical Agents, Biohazards, Engineering Control and Personal Protection. New York: John Wiley & Sons, 2000.
86. **Fleming, D.O., J.H. Richardson, J.J. Tulis, and D. Vesley (eds.):** *Laboratory Safety-Principles and Practices*, 2nd edition. Washington, D.C.: American Society of Microbiology Press, 1995.
87. **Rayburn, S.R. (ed.):** *The Foundations of Laboratory Safety: A Guide for the Biomedical Laboratory*. New York: Springer-Verlag, 1990.
88. **Fleming, D.O. and D.L. Hunt:** Biological Safety: Principles and Practices Washington, D.C.: ASM Press, 2006.
89. **Sulkin, S.E. and R.M. Pike:** Survey of laboratory acquired infections. J. Am. Med. Assoc. 147:1740–1745 (1951).
90. **Pike, R.M.:** Laboratory associated infections: summary and analysis of 3921 cases. *Health Lab. Sci. 13*:105–114 (1976).
91. **United States Department of Energy:** Human Gene Therapies: Novel Product Development Q&A with Celia M. Witten, Ph.D, M.D. Updated October 15, 2007. Available at http://www.fda.gov/ForConsumers/ConsumerUpdates/ucm103331.htm. [Accessed on July 1, 2011].
92. **Li, X.Z., B. Hauer, and B. Rosche:** Single-species microbial biofilm screening for industrial applications. *Appl. Microbiol. Biotech. 76*:1255–1262 (2007).
93. **Furr, A.K. (ed.):** *Handbook of Laboratory Safety*, 5th edition. Boca Raton, FL: CRC Press, Inc., 2000.

94. **Shapiro, J.:** *Radiation Protection, A Guide for Scientists and Physicians*, 4th edition. Cambridge, MA: Harvard University Press, 2002.
95. **National Research Council Committee on Prudent Practices for Handling, Storage, and Disposal of Chemicals in Laboratories:** Prudent Practices in the Laboratory: Handling and Disposal of Chemicals. Washington, D.C.: National Academy Press, 1995.
96. **National Fire Protection Association (NFPA):** Standard on Fire Protection for Laboratories Using Chemicals. Braintree, MA: NFPA, 2004.
97. Recombinant DNA Research. *Federal Register 41*:131 (1976). pp. 27903-27906.
98. Recombinant DNA Research Actions under the Guidelines. *Federal Register 56*:138 (1991). Appendix K-I.
99. **Sattelle, D.:** Biotechnology in Perspective. Washington, DC: IBA, Hobson Scientific, 1990. pp. 9, 28. [Pamphlet]
100. Coordinated Framework for Biotechnology Regulation. *Chem. Reg. Rep. 101*:0151-0158 (1993).
101. Genetic Technology Act. Austria. Bundesgesetzblatt für die Republik Österreich, No. 510, 12 July 1994, as amended. November 16, 1994.
102. Gene Technology Act of 2000. Act No. 169. Australia: Commonwealth Consolidated Acts, Canberra, Australia.
103. **Thomas, J.A. and L.A. Myers (eds.):** Biotechnology and Safety Assessment. New York: Raven Press, Ltd., 1993.
104. **Public Health Branch, Department of Human Services:** Statutory Review of the Gene Technology Act 2001. State Government of Victoria, Melbourne, Victoria. August 2006. pp. 1–2.
105. **United States Department of Energy:** Genetically Modified Foods and Organisms. Updated November 5, 2008. Available at http://www.ornl.gov/sci/techresources/Human_Genome/elsi/gmfood.shtml. [Accessed on July 1, 2011].
106. **Frey, J.:** Biological safety concepts of genetically modified live bacterial vaccines. *Vaccine 25*:5598–5605 (2007).
107. **Lambert, M.S.:** Molecular biosafety safety advance: transposon gene delivery systems. *Appl. Biosafety 12(3)*:194–46 (2007.
108. **United States Food and Drug Administration:** Human Gene Therapy and the Role of the Food and Drug Administration. September, 2000.
109. **Society for Industrial Microbiology, Education Committee:** Career Brochure. Society for Industrial Microbiology. 2007. Available at http://www.simhq.org/careers/ career-information/. [Accessed on July 1, 2011].
110. **Collins, C.H. and A.J. Beale (eds.):** Safety in Industrial Microbiology and Biotechnology. Oxford, U.K.: Butterworth-Heinemann Ltd., 1992. pp. 165–167.
111. **Collins, C.H. and A.J. Beale (eds.):** Safety in Industrial Microbiology and Biotechnology. Oxford, U.K.: Butterworth-Heinemann Ltd., 1992. p. 169.
112. **Balzer, K.:** "Strategies for Developing Biosafety Programs in Biotechnology Facilities." Paper presented to the 3rd National Symposium on Biosafety, Atlanta, GA, March 4, 1994.
113. **American Conference of Governmental Industrial Hygienists® (ACGIH®):** 2006 Two Thousand Six TLVs® and BEIs®. Threshold Limit Values® for Chemical Substances and Physical Agents & Biological Exposure Indices®. Cincinnati, OH: ACGIH®. p. 52.
114. **Centers for Disease Control and Disease Prevention and the National Institute for Occupational Safety and Health:** NIOSH Pocket Guide to Chemical Hazards. Subtilisins. September, 2005. Available at http://www.cdc.gov/niosh/npg/npgd0572.html. [Accessed February 1, 2009].
115. **American Conference of Governmental Industrial Hygienists® (ACGIH®):** 2002 TLVs® and BEIs®. Threshold Limit Values® for Chemical Substances and Physical Agents & Biological Exposure Indices®. Cincinnati, OH: ACGIH®. pp. 185–186.
116. **Collins, C.H. and A.J. Beale (eds.):** Safety in Industrial Microbiology and Biotechnology. Oxford, U.K.: Butterworth-Heinemann Ltd., 1992. pp. 167–169.
117. **Soap and Detergent Association:** Work Practices for Handling Enzymes in the Detergent Industry. New York: Soap and Detergent Association, 1995.
118. **Griffith, J.E., et al.:** Safety evaluation of enzyme detergents. Oral and coetaneous toxicity, irritancy and skin sensitization studies. *Food Cosmet. Toxicol. 7*:581–593 (1969).
119. **U.S. Environmental Protection Agency (EPA):** "Draft Manual for Infectious Waste Management." September 1982.
120. **Belasen, A.T.:** Leading the Learning Organization: Communication and Competencies for Managing Change. Albany, NY: State University of New York Press, 2000.
121. **Sharp, A.:** Workflow Modeling: Tools for Process Management and Application Development. Boston, MA: Artech House, 2001.
122. **Baker, J.J.:** Activity-based Costing and Activity-based Management for Health Care. Gaithersburg, MD: Aspen, 1998.
123. **Oakland, J.S.:** Total Organizational Excellence: Achieving World-class Performance. Oxford, U.K.: Butterworth-Heinemann, 1999.

124. **Cavaleri, S.A. and D.S. Fearon (eds.):** Managing in Organizations that Learn. Cambridge, Mass.: Blackwell, 1996.
125. Guidelines for Research Involving Recombinant DNA Molecule (NIH Guidelines), Section IV, Roles and Responsibilities. April, 2002.
126. **Centers for Disease Control and Prevention (CDC):** Update: investigation of anthrax associate with intentional exposure and interim public health guidelines, October 2002. *MMWR 50*:889–93 (2001).
127. **Kolavic, S.A., A. Kimura, S.L. Simons, L. Slutsker, S. Barth, and C.E. Haley:** Outbreak of Shigella dysenteriae type 2 among laboratory workers due to intentional food contamination. *JAMA 278*:396–98 (1997).
128. **Shane, S. and E. Lichtblau:** Scientist's Suicide Linked to Anthrax Inquiry. The New York Times. Available at http://www.nytimes.com/2008/08/02/washington/02anthrax.html. [Accessed on July 1, 2011].
129. **Sewell, D.L.:** Laboratory safety practices associated with potential agents of biocrime or bioterrorism. *J. Clin. Microb. 41(7)*:2801–09 (2003).
130. **Centers for Disease Control and Prevention (CDC):** Avian Influenza (Flu): Key Facts About Avian Influenza (Bird Flu) and Avian Influenza A (H5N1) Virus. Available at http://www.cdc.gov/flu/ avian/gen-info/facts.htm. [Accessed on July 1, 2011].
131. **Centers for Disease Control and Prevention (CDC):** Avian Influenza (Flu): Current H5N1 Situation. Available at http://www.cdc.gov/flu/avian/ outbreaks/current.htm. [Accessed on July 1, 2011].
132. World Health Organization (WHO: Cumulative Number of Confirmed Human Cases of Avian Influenza A/(H5N1) Reported to WHO. Updated January 27, 2009. Available at http://www.who.int/csr/disease/avian_influenza/country/cases_table_2009_01_27/en/index.html. [Accessed on January 30, 2009].
133. **Centers for Disease Control and Prevention (CDC):** Business Pandemic Influenza Planning Checklist. Available at http://www.flu.gov/professional/business/businesschecklist.html. [Accessed on July 1, 2011].
134. Title III Superfund Amendments and Reauthorization Act of 1986, Emergency Planning and Community Right to Know Act. Code of Federal Regulations Title 40, Parts 350, 355, 370, and 372.
135. **Sandman, P.M.:** *Responding to Community Outrage: Strategies for Effective Risk Communication.* Fairfax, VA: American Industrial Hygiene Association, 1993.
136. **Sandman, P.M.:** *Risk = Hazard + Outrage: A Formula for Effective Risk Communication.* Fairfax, VA: American Industrial Hygiene Association, 1993. [Video]
137. **Sandman, P.M.:** *Quantitative Risk Communication: Explaining the Data.* Fairfax, VA: American Industrial Hygiene Association, 1993. [Video]
138. **Sandman, P.M.:** *Implementing Risk Communication: Overcoming the Barriers.* Fairfax, VA: American Industrial Hygiene Association, 1993. [Video]
139. **Center for Environmental Communication (CEC):** Publications List. New Jersey Agricultural Experimental Station and the Edward J. Bloustein School of Planning and Public Policy. Brunswick, NJ: Cook College. May, 1993.

Outcome Competencies

After completing this chapter, the reader should be able to:

1. Describe the difference between nanomaterials and nanoparticles.
2. Describe differences and similarities between naturally occurring, incidental ultrafine and engineered nanoparticles.
3. Describe examples of various types of engineered nanoparticles and their applications.
4. Describe unique properties of engineered nanoparticles that may make them relatively more toxic than materials of larger size.
5. Describe the rationale for integrating the safe handling of nanomaterials into a comprehensive program.
6. Anticipate when and where nanomaterials may be present in the workplace.
7. Recognize specific situations where potential exposures to nanomaterials need to be managed.
8. Evaluate specific exposure situations to support application of the traditional Hierarchy of Control.
9. Control exposures through approaches that apply engineering and other controls appropriate for the hazard of the material and the potential for exposure.
10. Confirm risk management steps and controls through workplace measurements and epidemiological studies.
11. Describe the regulatory environment for nanomaterials.
12. Describe and apply training content and techniques for nanotechnology workers.

Key Terms

engineered nanoparticle • incidental ultrafine particle • nanofiber • nanoparticle • nanoplate • nanomaterial • nano-object • nanotechnology • nanotube • naturally occurring ultrafine particle • ultrafine particle

Prerequisite Knowledge

Prior to beginning this chapter, the user should review the following chapters:

Chapter Number	Chapter Topic
7	Principles of Evaluating Worker Exposure
8	Occupational and Environmental Health Risk Assessment/Risk Management
9	Comprehensive Exposure Assessment
39	Personal Protective Clothing
40	Respiratory Protection

Key Topics

I. Overview
II. Nanotechnology, Nanomaterials, and Nanoparticles
  A. Terminology
  B. Categories of Engineered Nanoparticles
  C. Unique Behavior at the Nanoscale
III. Environmental, Health, and Safety Impacts
  A. Absence of Occupational Exposure Limits
IV. Application of Risk Management Approaches to Protect Workers Handling Nanoparticles
  A. Anticipate Likely Hazards and Exposures Among Representative Worker Groups
  B. Recognize When Exposures are Occurring
  C. Evaluate Exposures
  D. Control Exposures
  E. Confirm that Risks are Adequately Managed
V. Hazard Communication for Nanoparticles
  A. Globally Harmonized System for Classification and Labeling of Chemicals (GHS)
VI. Regulatory and Voluntary Approaches Specific to Nanoparticles
  A. Government Regulatory Actions
  B. Voluntary Approaches
VII. Developing Effective Training Programs for Nanotechnology Workers
VIII. Conclusion
IX. Additional Resources

Engineered Nanomaterials

23

By Kristen Kulinowski, PhD and Bruce Lippy, PhD, CIH, CSP

Overview

The term nanotechnology describes a wide range of technologies, materials and applications that are affecting or will affect every sector of commerce including medicine, energy, construction, environmental remediation, automotive, and aerospace. Nanotechnology involves the manipulation of matter at the atomic level (e.g., Figure 23.1). Examples that exist today include photocatalytic particles that break down organic pollutants in contaminated groundwater, novel medical devices that demonstrate greater specificity for cancer cells, and fibers that improve mechanical strength while reducing mass in automobile parts. The aspects of nanotechnology that merit the attention of the occupational and environmental safety and health community are its impact across sectors, its novelty, and its potential for growth.

If the reader has read and understood other chapters in this text on *The Occupational Environment: Its Evaluation, Control, and Management*, they should have the foundation to successfully anticipate, recognize, evaluate, control, and confirm the appropriate management of occupational health and safety risks in a broad spectrum of situations.[1] Certain unique properties of engineered nanomaterials such as increased surface area, enhanced surface reactivity, or similarity to biological structures may make engineered nanomaterials relatively more toxic than materials of larger size. Development of an understanding of those properties is a work in progress and nanotechnology is an area of ongoing research, development, and applications. As such, changes are underway that must be continually assessed.

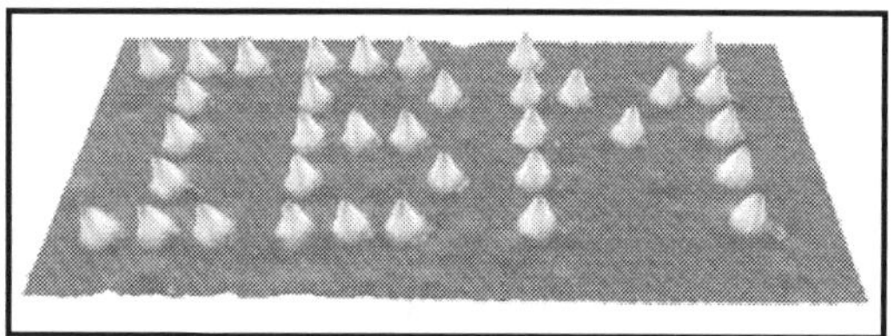

Figure 23.1 — Manipulation at the atomic level by IBM researcher Donald Mark Eigler. In 1989 he spelled IBM with individual xenon atoms using the Scanning Tunneling Electron Microscope. (Source: Wikimedia).

Concerns about health and safety are being addressed in research laboratories around the world but the application of this risk-relevant research to worker safety is still in the early stages. Peters and Grassian refer to the protection of workers who encounter nanomaterials as the "frontier of industrial hygiene."[2]

Nanotechnology, Nanomaterials and Nanoparticles

Not a single technology itself, nanotechnology offers a platform for improving existing materials, devices, and drugs by exploiting the novel properties that emerge when matter is taken down (or up) to the nanoscale. These new modes of action can significantly enhance the properties of the products in which they are used, leading to materials that are stronger, multifunctional, or more energy efficient. But novelty is a double-edged sword; the same unique properties that benefit a particular application could result in new risks to people or the environment.

Terminology

While precise definitions are still somewhat variable, most standard definitions recognize that nanotechnology involves science and engineering of matter at the nanoscale where properties may change with size or new properties may emerge. As defined by the National Nanotecholgy Inititative, the term *nanotechnology* refers to an emerging area of technology development involving the understanding and control of matter at the nanoscale, at dimension between approximately 1 and 100 nanometers (nm), where unique phenomena enable novel applications.[3]

Nanostructured materials, also called nanomaterials, have external or internal features that fall within the nanosize scale but may be larger than 100 nm as a whole. Examples of nanomaterials that are larger than 100 nm include microscale particles that have nanoscopic internal pores, or 300-nm diameter aggregates of 20-nm diameter primary particles. The terms nanomaterial and nanoparticle are often used interchangeably but have different meanings. Nanoparticles have one or more external dimensions between 1–100 nm such as a 4-nm quantum dot or a nanotube that is 2 nm in diameter. Thus, nanoparticles are a subset of nanomaterials.

The reader is advised to be aware of some differences in how terminology for nanotechnology is being developed and used in organizations such as the International Organization for Standardization Technical Committee 229 (Nanotechnologies). For example, according to ISO/TS 27687:2008, a nano-object is defined as material with one, two, or three external dimensions in the size range from approximately 1–100 nm. The precise definition of particle diameter depends on particle shape as well as how the diameter is measured. Subcategories of nano-object are (1) nanoplate, a nano-object with one external dimension at the nanoscale; (2) nanofiber, a nano-object with two external dimensions at the nanoscale with a nanotube defined as a hollow nanofiber and a nanorod as a solid nanofiber; and (3) *nanoparticle*, a nano-object with all three external dimensions at the nanoscale. Thus, nano-objects are commonly incorporated in a larger matrix or substrate referred to as a nanomaterial, and nano-objects may be suspended in a gas (as a nanoaerosol), suspended in a liquid (as a colloid or nanohydrosol), or embedded in a matrix (as a nanocomposite). For the most part, discussions in this chapter will use the term nanoparticles to refer to particles of any engineered nanomaterial.

The term ultrafine particle has traditionally been used by the aerosol research and occupational and environmental health communities to describe airborne particles smaller than 100 nm in diameter. As shown in Table 23.1, the terms naturally occurring ultrafine particle, incidental ultrafine particle, and engineered nanoparticle are sometimes used to differentiate among particles that are naturally occurring from sources such as volcanic eruptions (e.g., Figure 23.2), particles that are incidentally created during processes such as welding, and nanoparticles that are "engineered."

Particle morphologies may vary widely at the nanoscale. For instance, carbon fullerenes (Figure 23.3) represent nanoparticles with identical dimensions in all directions (i.e., spherical), whereas single-walled

Table 23.1 — Nanoparticle types by their mode of production

Nanoparticle Type	*Examples*
Naturally occurring (ultrafine)	Volcanic ash, sea spray, forest fire combustion products
Incidental (Ultrafine)	Welding fumes, diesel exhaust, combustion products from propane vehicles and direct-gas heaters
Engineered (Manufactured)	Nanotubes, nanoscale titanium dioxide

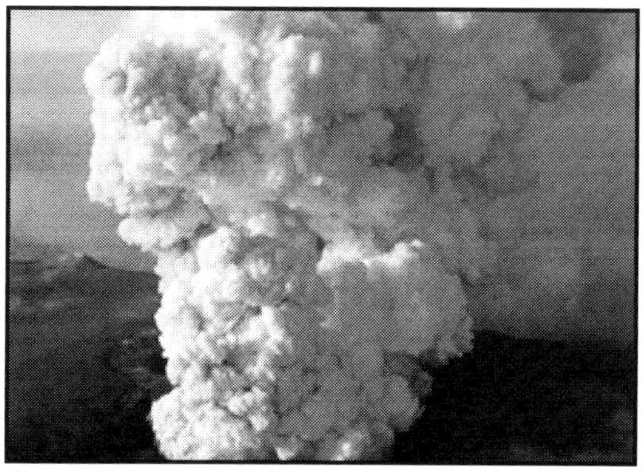

Figure 23.2 — Example of a dust plume including ultrafine particles from the Icelandic volcano, April 17, 2010. (Source: Wikimedia Commons)

carbon nanotubes (SWCNTs) (e.g., Figure 23.4) and multi-walled carbon nanotubes (MWCNTs) (e.g., Figure 24.5) represent nanofibers, which are typically found in convoluted bundles. Many regular but non-spherical particle morphologies can also be engineered at the nanoscale, including flower- and belt-like structures. Some nanostructures (e.g., the diamond nanodots shown in Figure 24.6) are attached to a substrate, rather than unbound. Other examples of nanoscale structures can be found online at sites such as www.nanoscience.gatech.edu/zlwang/research.html and www.nanoparticlelibrary.net.

Categories of Engineered Nanoparticles

Engineered nanoparticles can be made in many different forms from many different chemical substances. The types of nanoparticles in use today can be broadly classified into five categories: metals, metal oxides (ceramics), carbon-based, semiconducting (quantum dots), and organics. (See Table 23.2). Within these broad classifications there may be several subcategories each of which has its own set of properties. A nanoscale metal may be prized for its unique optical, electrical or catalytic properties or, in the case of silver, its antimicrobial activity. Metal oxides may have interesting magnetic, mechanical or catalytic behavior.

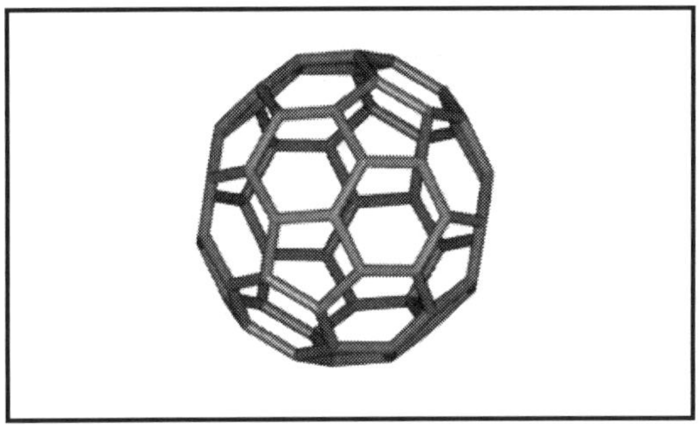

Figure 23.3 — Buckminster Fullerine (Bucky Ball) composed of 60 carbon atoms. (Source: Rice University).\

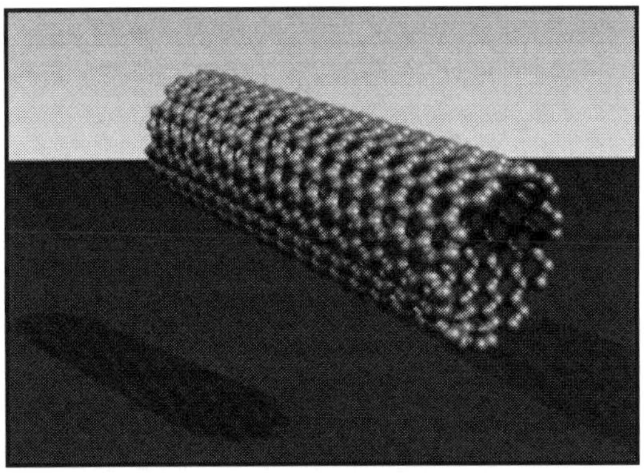

Figure 23.4 — Computer simulation of a nanotube. (Source: Wikimedia Commons)

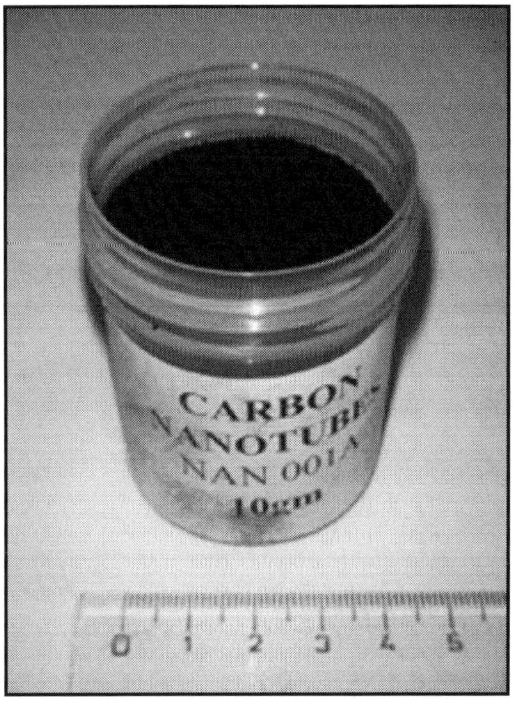

Figure 23.5 — Multiwalled carbon nanotubes as a black clumpy powder. 10 gram container, scale in centimeters. (Source: Shaddack, Wikimedia Commons)

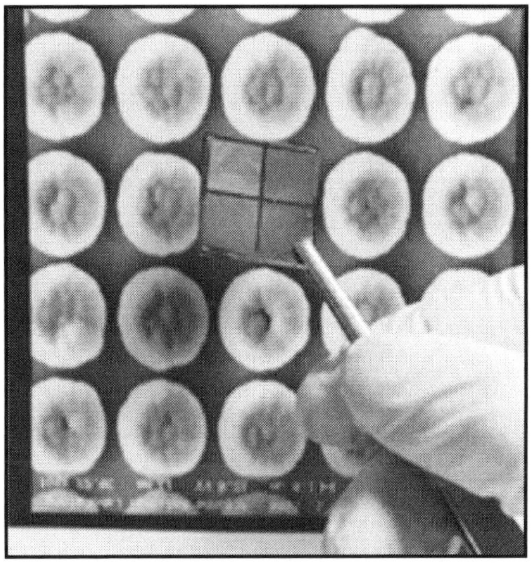

Figure 23.6 — Example of a silicon plate holding 40,000 diamond film dots for microelectronics, in comparison to a microscopic image of the individual dots. (Source: Lawrence Berkeley Laboratory)

Table 23.2 — Broad Categories of Nanoparticles

Broad category	Examples
Metals	Silver, Gold, Copper
Metal oxides (ceramics)	Titanium dioxide, Zinc oxide, Cerium oxide
Carbon-based	Fullerenes, Nanotubes
Semiconducting (quantum dots)	CdSe, CdS, ZnS
Organic	Polymer beads, Dendrimers

Carbon-based nanoparticles may impart mechanical strength and can be made to conduct electricity. Quantum dots have useful optical properties. Organic nanoparticles are especially useful in medical applications. While depictions of nanotechnology in science fiction abound, making it seem like something from the future, there are thousands of products already on the market today and many more in the pipeline. An inventory of nanotechnology-based consumer products on the market can be bound at www.nanotechproject.org/inventories/consumer/.

Unique Behavior at the Nanoscale

Smaller than microscale particles, yet larger than atoms and all but the largest molecules, nanoparticles occupy a transitional regime between classical and quantum physics where physical and chemical properties may depend on the nanoparticle's size, structure, composition, surface structure, or surface composition. Classical physics governs the behavior of objects in our everyday experience and thus is more intuitively. For example, an individual knows to duck (or raise a glove) when a baseball flies toward their head. The ball's trajectory, which is governed by the forces of gravity and friction, is easily predicted and can even be precisely calculated using the principles of classical physics. If that baseball were an object about 10 trillion times smaller, its behavior would be governed by quantum physics and classical ability to predict its location and path would be lost. Knowledge of when to duck would also be lost. Nanoparticles behave more like quantum objects than like baseballs, especially at the lower end of the size scale. This means that prior knowledge and experience with a substance may not always predict how that substance will behave when it is made at the nanoscale. As the nanoparticle's size increases, it acts more and more like a baseball, which is why there is an upper boundary on most definitions of the size scale.

One critical feature of nanoparticles is the tremendous surface area that is created for the same amount of mass. A thought experiment can illustrate how significant this can be for determining the nanomaterial's behavior. Consider a large cube of pure, solid gold that measures 1 meter on each side (Figure 23.7). This makes a surface area of 6 m^2. Now imagine that the cube is cut into smaller cubes that each measure ¼ m on a side; resulting in $4 \times 4 \times 4 = 64$ cubes with a total surface area of 24 m^2. Taking this thought experiment to the extreme, if the same cube of gold is divided into particles measuring 1 nm on each side, then there are $10^9 \times 10^9 \times 10^9 = 10^{27}$ cubes, with a total surface area of 6 billion m^2. That surface area is more than enough to cover the entire state of Delaware.

Color, magnetism, electrical conductivity and chemical reactivity are some of the properties that can change at and throughout the nanoscale. Gold affords a great example of the striking differences of materials between the macroscale and nanoscale, and within the nanoscale. Macroscale gold is prized for its chemical inertness as well as its luster. The shiny orange-yellow color of gold in coins and jewelry is a feature of the macroscale world. But nanoscale gold can appear quite different. Between 100 and about 30 nanometers, gold is purple and at 30 nm in size, a gold particle is bright red. Smaller particles become brownish in color.[4] Gold at the nanoscale can also be highly reactive, even being used as a catalyst in some chemical reactions.

Surface reactivity is also of concern for health effects: the same reactive surfaces that are prized for creating unique properties in new products appear to be implicated in much of the unwanted health effects. As the British Standards Institute correctly noted, "Altered chemical and/or physical properties might be expected to be accompanied by altered biological properties, some of which could imply increased toxicity."[5]

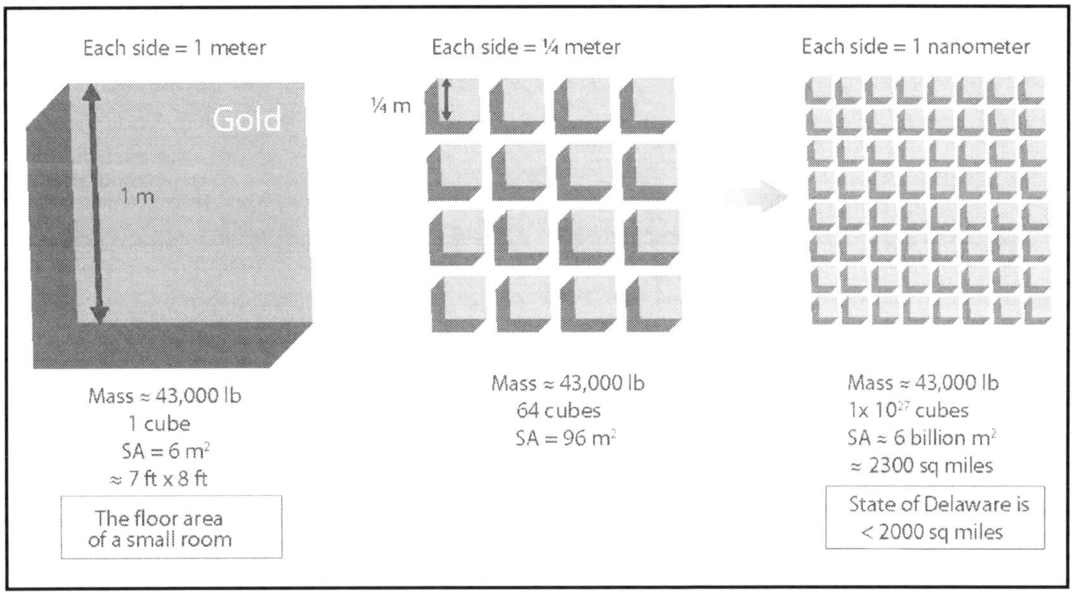

Figure 23.7 — Dividing a solid into nanometer-sized particles exposes a high fraction of the interior atoms to the surroundings, providing increased opportunity for chemical and biological interactions, and making surface area a critical metric for exposure assessment.

Environmental, Health, and Safety Impacts

Because of their small size and active surface chemistry nanoparticles may behave in different ways in the body than their non-nanoscale analogs. The majority of nano-EHS papers address some aspect of hazard, mostly acute toxicity tests done in cell culture.[6] Certain nanoparticles have been shown in animal studies to translocate along the olfactory nerve into the brain, cross the placenta and penetrate damaged or diseased skin. Once inside the body certain nanoparticles have induced inflammatory responses, cardiovascular effects, pulmonary fibrosis and genotoxicity. Certain carbon nanotubes, one of the most widely researched class of nanoparticles from both a technological and toxicological perspective, have even been shown to induce asbestos-like effects in rodents which raises concerns among occupational safety professionals.[7,8] Figure 23.8 shows evidence that multi-walled carbon nanotubes can migrate from the alveolar region of the lung in rodents and penetrate the pluera of the lung, which is the same site in which malignant mesothelioma can develop due to asbestos exposure.[9] It must be emphasized, however, that effects demonstrated by one type of nanoparticle in one laboratory study cannot be generalized to other nanoparticles.

In one carbon nanotube study, for example, only the long, straight, multiwalled forms acted in a manner similar to asbestos fibers when injected into the rodents' bodies. Other nanotube forms that were shorter and more flexible did not induce the harmful response, nor have other types of non-carbon-based nanotubes been shown to mimic toxic asbestos fibers.[10] Examples such as these serve to illustrate not that "nanoparticles are toxic" but that certain nanoparticles may pose a hazard under certain conditions.

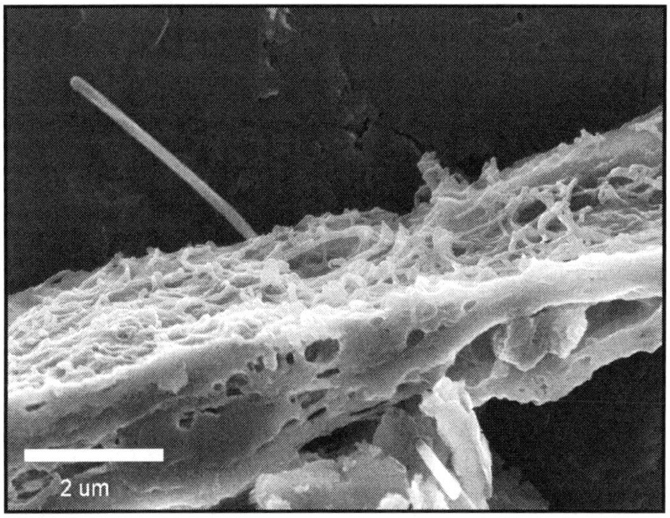

Figure 23.8 — A field emission scanning electron micrograph of a multi-walled carbon nanotube (MWCNT) penetrating the pleura of the lung. (Source: courtesy of Robert Mercer and Diane Schwegler-Berry, NIOSH)

The research community is working to develop a better understanding of how nanoparticles' physical and chemical characteristics can be correlated to their biological interactions. Without predictive models for linking measurable properties such as size, shape and surface area to biological interactions such as the production of reactive oxygen species, protein misfolding, cell death (apoptosis) and mutagenicity, the number of individual nanoparticle variants that would have to be tested is practically infinite. Experts recently concluded that predictive models are an important long-term goal requiring ten years of work or more.(11)

Nanotechnology environmental, health and safety (nano-EHS) research is still in an early phase with published findings scattered across dozens of different journals. The relevance of the nano-EHS hazard studies to real-life working conditions is unclear. Risk assessment relies upon an understanding of both hazard and exposure; when one is absent, the assessment is incomplete. Publications of relevance to this topic are collected, catalogued and indexed within the ICON Virtual Journal of Nano-EHS (http://icon.rice.edu/virtualjournal.cfm), an open web-based resource that contains citations to more than 4,000 papers. The Nano-EHS Database Analysis Tool permits users to sort this comprehensive resource by particle type, exposure target population, exposure pathway and other criteria.

Despite the large number of papers of the subject, it is difficult to draw robust conclusions about the risks engineered nanoparticles might pose to workers or the environment. The reasons for this are myriad, and include a lack of validated protocols for performing toxicology tests on nanoparticles, questions about the appropriate metric for measuring dose, lack of models for how nanoparticles are transformed in the body or the natural environment and the role of surface area and surface chemistry in controlling bio-interactions.(11) Despite these challenges, the large body of work does indicate that measures should be taken to protect nanotechnology workers.

Absence of Occupational Exposure Limits

As of 2011, there were no OSHA Permissible Exposure Limits for any nanoparticles. NIOSH, however, has proposed important draft Recommended Exposure Limits (RELs) for airborne carbon nanotubes (CNT)(12) and for ultrafine titanium dioxide (TiO_2).(13)

For CNT, NIOSH has proposed an 8-hour time weighted average of 7 micrograms per cubic centimeter of air (μg/m³) as respirable mass. NIOSH based this level on the risk of developing adverse respiratory health effects if exposed for a working lifetime at the upper limit of quantitation (LOQ) of NIOSH Method 5040 for elemental carbon, currently the recommended analytical method for measuring airborne CNT. The LOQ for detection of elemental carbon by NIOSH Method 5040 is 7 μg/m³.

For comparison purposes, the OSHA respirable nuisance dust standard of 5 mg/m³ is more than 700 times higher than the draft REL of 7 μg/m³ for carbon nanotubes.

In recommending use at this time of the mass-based analytical method, NIOSH has noted that other, more appropriate, methods such as electron micrographic methods for counting individual nanotubes or bundles of nanotubes, may become available. Part of the challenge is that there may be more than 10,000 combinations of carbon nanotubes possible.(13) It is also not clear how properties such as surface reactivity or the presence of residual catalyst materials such as cobalt from production of the CNT may affect the toxicity of CNT.

For titanium dioxide, NIOSH has recommended exposure limits of 2.4 mg/m³ for fine TiO_2 and 0.3 mg/m³ for ultrafine (including engineered nanoscale) TiO_2, as time-weighted average (TWA) concentrations for up to 10 hours per day during a 40-hour work week. NIOSH has determined that *ultrafine* TiO_2 is a potential occupational carcinogen but concluded that there were insufficient data at the time to classify *fine* TiO_2 as a potential occupational carcinogen.

Given the tentative nature of governmental action thus far, some private companies have begun to set exposure limits for their products. In November 2009, Bayer Material Science (BMS) announced an occupational exposure limit of 0.05 mg/m³ for Baytubes, a multi-wall carbon nanotube product. The company has incorporated this OEL in their Material Safety Data Sheets, which is an enlightened policy compared to the standard practice of referencing occupational exposure limit for graphite. The presence of a cobalt catalyst in the Baytubes provides a means of using detection of that metal as an indicator of the adequacy of control. Exposure assessment and verification of control based on measurement of cobalt as a surrogate for the nanotubes of interest is one of the few existing examples of the "routine monitoring" component of the graded approach to exposure assessment described below.

Given the lack of benchmarks for sampling, very few private organizations have reported monitoring their workplace for nanoparticles, although those that handle larger volumes of nanomaterials are more likely to do so.[14]

Application of Risk Management Approaches to Protect Workers Handling Nanoparticles

Nanoparticles may be new but hazardous substances are not. A risk management program for nanoparticles does not need to be constructed from scratch. What is important, however, is to carefully examine any assumptions and validate any existing tools when applying them to situations where nanoparticles are present. Many of the existing frameworks for dealing with toxic substances, especially the "anticipate, recognize, evaluate, control, and confirm" framework, may be applied to nanoparticles with little revision. Some special considerations are needed to account for details of the physical, chemical, and biological behavior of individual nanomaterials and classes of nanomaterials. As always, critical aspects of the risk management process are to anticipate and recognize the specific tasks that could bring or are bringing a worker into contact with a nanoparticle, to evaluate how best to control that exposure based on the expected toxicity of the material and the conditions of dispersion, to implement the controls, and finally to confirm that the controls are working and that health of the workers is being maintained. What follows here is a review of the currently existing approaches for anticipating, recognizing, evaluating, controlling, and confirming safe handling of nanoparticles in the workplace.

Anticipate Likely Hazards and Exposures among Representative Worker Groups

Because nanotechnology is a set of technology platforms that are applied across multiple sectors, it is difficult to quantify the nanotechnology "industry." There exists no North American Industry Classification System (NAICS) code for nanotechnology and a company may choose whether or not to disclose that it is engaged in commercial nanotechnology research, manufacture or use at its discretion. The federal government, working with the private sector, has attempted to identify the tasks that are most likely to generate worker exposures to nanoparticles. The following have been specifically noted:

- Generating nanoparticles in the gas phase in non-enclosed facilities;
- Handling nanostructured powders (e.g., Figure 23.9);
- Working with nanoparticles in liquid media without adequate protection, particularly gloves;
- Working with nanoparticles in liquid during pouring or mixing operations or where a high degree of agitation is involved;
- Conducting maintenance on equipment and processes used to produce or fabricate nanoparticles; and
- Cleaning up spills or waste materials.[15]

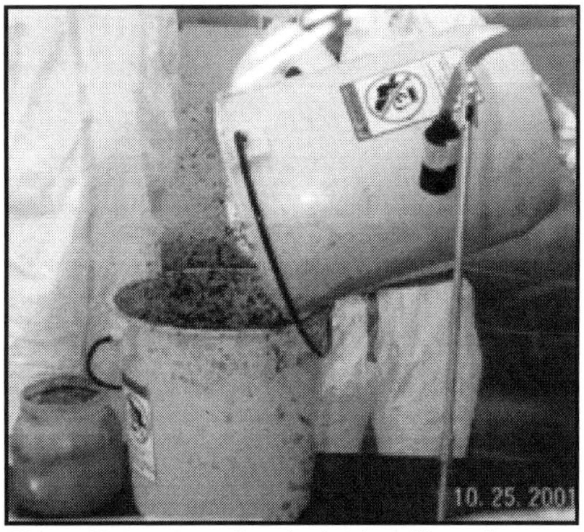

Figure 23.9 — Sampling during handling of carbon nanotubes. (Source: NIOSH)

Table 23.3 — Potential Exposures among Worker Populations. (Source: NIEHS Worker Education and Training Program)

Worker Population	*Types of Nanomaterials*	*Tasks*
Researchers, laboratory workers, and students	Wide range of nanomaterials	Receipt, handling, analytical assessments, experimentation, clean up, and disposal
Chemical plant industrial workers	Wide range of nanomaterials	Producing batches of nanoparticles in chemical plants
Manufacturing industry workers	Nanomaterials in electronics, aerospace, and auto parts	Machining parts and assembling cars
Stationary engineers	Nanosilver biocides	Adding biocides to cooling tower water and HVAC drip pans
Workers involved in construction, demolition and remediation	nano-scale zero-valent iron; photocatalytic concrete (which uses nano-scale TiO_2 as an additive)	Using nano-scale iron to treat soil contaminated with chlorinated solvents; demolishing structures containing photocatalytic concrete
Truck drivers	Suspensions of nanoparticles such as multiwalled carbon nanotubes and packaged dry nanoparticles	Driving trucks carrying packaged nanoparticles that may be involved in a spill on the highway
Industrial emergency responders	Wide range used in production of personal care products, paints and new ones daily	Spill cleanup and response
Municipal "first-on-scene" responders	Wide range of materials that may be spilled during transport	Spill cleanup and response
Firefighters	Wide range of nanomaterials	Responding to fires, explosions or leaks at firms producing, storing, or using nanomaterials
Cleanup workers	Nanoparticles in hazardous waste	Performing cleanup of waste sites
Waste treatment, storage, and disposal facility workers	Nanomaterials from a wide range of industrial and municipal sources	Receipt, treatment, transfer, repackaging, and disposal of waste
Nurses and physicians	Nanoparticles used in medicines	Preparing and injecting intravenous liquids
Environmental remediation site workers	Nanoremediation agents like nano iron oxide	Performing in situ injection of agents

Table 23.3 provides additional examples of worker populations, types of nanomaterials, and typical tasks that may lead to potential exposures.

If the size and scope of the industries involved in nanoparticle production or use are difficult to quantify, it is even harder to collect demographic information on the worker population. Such information would be invaluable in the development of a nanotechnology worker registry that would enable medical surveillance to identify potential problems early. The prospect of identifying the nanotech workforce is less daunting when considering a small-to-medium nanotechnology enterprise, as its core business most likely involves the manufacture or use of engineered nanoparticles. But for many large companies, nanoparticle production or use may constitute a small fraction of the total business and the employees who handle nanoparticles may not be distinguished from workers in other parts of the company. For this class of companies the nanotechnology workforce may not differ substantially in key demographic categories from workers in the chemicals industry.

NIOSH, in particular, is interested in gaining a greater understanding of the potentially affected workforce though it asserts, "there is insufficient scientific and medical evidence to recommend the specific medical screening of workers potentially exposed to engineered nanoparticles."[16] The European Agency for Safety and Health at Work unambiguously noted that, "At present, there is insufficient information on the number of workers exposed to nanomaterials in the work place or the effects on human health of such exposure."[17] This provides an impetus for readers of this chapter to assist in increasing awareness of when, where, and how exposures are occurring.

Recent studies indicated that the current number of workers who are directly involved with nanoparticles is probably relatively low. Research published in 2010 indicated that only 0.6% of manufacturing companies in Switzerland used nanomaterials, which led to an estimation of only 1,309 workers across the entire country, an average of 2.5 workers per company handling nanomaterials. An earlier study in England estimated 2,000 workers handling nanomaterials in that country, although the researcher's definition of a "nano" company was quite proscribed.[18] One market analysis estimates that the global workforce in nanotechnology industries will reach 2 million by the year 2018.[19] A better accounting of the potentially exposed workforce is needed to guide risk management.

In anticipating exposures from an industrial perspective, attention should be given to the potential dispersion of nanomaterial-containing droplets when fluids containing nanomaterials (e.g., as an additive to improve fluid performance of mineral oil-based coolants, as a catalyst, or as a process intermediate) are aerosolized. Oil and other liquid mists are common in many industrial environments due to the abundance of pressurized hydraulic and process lines. Even when nanomaterials are handled as liquid suspensions in contained and enclosed systems, a potential for respiratory exposure exists because process equipment can fail (e.g., breaches in transfer lines, leaks at interfaces between flanges and gaskets, and spills from damaged containers).

It is also prudent to anticipate limitations in the value of historical evaluations of workplace air quality for processes that are modified to include nanomaterials. For example, in many industrial environments, oil mist samples are periodically collected and the results are compared to the occupational exposure limit for highly refined mineral oil. If the results are below 10% of the limit, the process is considered contained and may not be re-sampled for several years. This could create the situation where an emerging exposure to nanomaterials is not assessed. Thus, process knowledge and informed anticipation are important tools to support effective recognition of situations where exposures may be occurring.

Given the increasing applications of nanoparticles in cleaning products, fabric treatments, or as additives in coolants, it is also prudent to anticipate that nanoparticles may enter the workplace in a manner that is not directly associated with "production line" creation or handling of nanoparticles. Failure to anticipate (and thereby establish procedures to track) such "secondary" introduction of nanoparticles into the workplace can complicate later steps to recognize, evaluate, and control exposures.

Recognize When Exposures are Occurring

Process knowledge and awareness of actual work being performed are critical to recognizing when exposures to nanoparticles may be occurring. This can be problematic in settings such as universities when laboratories and research activities can be dispersed over many buildings and locations, and where central purchasing and safety office coordination may be limited.

An approach adapted from the pharmaceutical industry can be used to facilitate recognition of situations where exposures may be occurring for a *specific compound*, in a *specific process*, in a *specific facility*.[20] As illustrated in Table 23.4, the approach draws together specific information relating to the material or compound characteristics that could lead to exposure, the process characteristics that may result in emissions, and the facility design nuances that might influence dispersion of emissions with the work areas.

Evaluate Exposures

The nanotechnology industrial hygiene community has been working to evaluate and

Table 23.4 — Pharmaceutical Industry Approach for Recognizing Exposures that might arise from Specific Characteristics of a Material, Process, and Facility.[20]

	Compound Characteristics	
Characteristic	*Low Risk Condition*	*High Risk Condition*
Physical form	Wet	Dry
Particle size	Large	Small
Particle density	Dense	Light
Particle shape	Spherical	Feathery
Electrostatic in nature	No	Yes
Routes of exposure	Limited	Unlimited
Bioavailability	Low	High
Acute/chronic toxicity	Fast/Reversible	Slow/Reversible
Mutagenicity / carcinogenicity, etc.	None	All
	Process Characteristics	
Characteristic	*Low Risk Condition*	*High Risk Condition*
Operation	Closed	Open
Process	Low energy / velocity	High energy / velocity
Pressure and temperature	Low	High
Transfers	None	Multiple
Training	Well	Poorly
Operator skill required	None required	High skill required
Task type	Routine	Non-routine
Duration	Short	Long
Frequency	One operation	Multiple operations
	Facility Characteristics	
Characteristic	*Low Risk Condition*	*High Risk Condition*
Room pressure differential	Low relative to corridors	High relative to corridors
Airlock	Two stage plus pressure differential	Single stage with no buffer
Engineering controls	Isolation	Local exhaust ventilation
Filtration	HEPA	No HEPA
Airflow	Away from worker access	Towards worker access

apply exposure assessment methods for use in a wide variety of situations, ranging from clean-room conditions in microelectronics, laboratory conditions in university or industrial research settings, industrial production conditions, to outdoor environmental conditions. A desirable graded approach to sampling would involve *initial screening and detection* of potential nanoparticle emissions, followed by *comprehensive characterization and assessment* of nanomaterials in locations of concern, and leading ultimately to the selection of sampling methods that are feasible and economical for *routine monitoring and control* (Figure 23.10).[21]

Level 1	Level 2	Level 3
Initial Screening and Detection	**Comprehensive Characterization and Assessment**	**Routine Monitoring and Control**
• Process knowledge • Gross mass or activity counting • Optical particle counting • Condensation particle counting • Microscopy	• Composition - Elemental and chemical • Particle size - Physical - Aerodynamic - Thermodynamic - Electrical mobility • Exposure Concentrations - Peaks, averages, variability • Biophysical properties - Shape, surface area, solubility • Other factors relevant to the assessment	• A necessary and sufficient subset of Level 1 and 2 methods for the material and situation of interest

Figure 23.10 — Illustration of a graded approach to exposure assessment and control.[1]

As Linda Abbott and Andrew Maynard have noted, "It is likely that no single metric will completely characterize exposure."[22] The standard model of industrial hygiene that has underpinned the profession as well as the OSHA regulatory approach since 1970 has been the measurement of exposures in the personal breathing zone of workers for comparison against established occupational exposure limits. Such limits have traditionally been established based on animal tests and, too often, upon human epidemiology, but given the decades of use of standard industrial solvents like toluene, the accumulated data were often impressive and persuasive for setting a limit that would arguably allow a working career of exposure without permanent, deleterious health effects. These numbers have generally been set to be an 8-hour time-weighted average. For dust exposures, the unit of measurement has historically been milligrams (or micrograms) per cubic meter of air.

Given the extraordinarily small size and weight of nanoparticles, however, these mass-based measurements may prove less meaningful for managing inhalation exposure risks for nanomaterials. As Peters and Grassian have noted,

> "The incredible structural and compositional variability of engineered nanoparticles virtually precludes the traditional measure-and-compare-to-the-OEL approach that has been the foundation of much of the field. Instead, the EHS professional must apply a more thoughtful and nuanced approach, an artfulness that is integral to the definition of industrial hygiene."[2]

Making risk comparisons solely based on weight ignores the importance of surface area and, consequently, may greatly underestimate the health hazards posed by nanoparticles. Referencing 40 year old "nuisance dust" standards, as most current Material Safety Data Sheets for carbon nanotubes do, is essentially saying that normal use of these carbon nanotube should generate less dust than a quarry or sawmill. Almost no other risk conclusion should be drawn from the use of old, mass-based standards. Even if the engineered nanoparticles are delivered suspended in solution, recent studies indicates that workers can be exposed to water droplets containing the particles during standard laboratory practices like sonicating the liquid to break up agglomeration, which is a common occurrence.[23]

Approaches Used by NIOSH to Count Particles and Measure Surface Area

Moving beyond traditional mass-based sampling, NIOSH has examined the following innovative approaches in its 2009 guidance document, "Approaches to Safe Nanotechnology."[24]

The first is counting particles. Fortunately, the industrial hygiene field has had access to affordable real-time instruments that count particles for a considerable time. The best known use of these instruments is for quantitative fit testing of respirators with instruments like the TSI Portacount. NIOSH researchers have used handheld condensation particle counters (CPCs) to count nanoparticles; these instruments use isopropyl alcohol to coat particles so they are large enough to be counted with a laser beam. CPCs report the total number of particles counted per cubic centimeter of air in the range of 10 nm to 1000 nm, but cannot identify the chemical makeup of the particles. Because the CPCs "grow" the size of the particles by condensing alcohol onto them to a size that can be observed by light scattering, the detected droplets are fairly homogeneous in size and do not provide information about the detailed particle size distribution.

In a variation on this technique, optical particle counters (OPCs) use laser light scattering to detect both the diameter and the total number of particles per liter of air. As with CPCs, it is not possible to identify the chemical makeup of the particles. OPCs are not able to report particles as small as those identified by CPCs, but they are able to report several discrete ranges of particle sizes. Consequently, CPCs and OPCs are often used together to provide a more complete picture of airborne particle concentrations. These instruments are generally used as screening tools to determine if processes might be releasing nanoparticles by comparing concentrations and size ranges before an operation starts with the numbers during operation.

Given the lack of chemical specificity associated with these CPCs and OPCs, it is critical for industrial hygienists to investigated other possible sources for elevated particles counts, such as propane-powered fork-lift vehicles, direct combustion gas heaters, oil mists, and ultrafine particles from electrical machinery and pumps. See, for example, the work by Heitbrink et al. for mapping of very fine particles concentrations in an engine machining and assembly facility.[25]

NIOSH conducted field studies at 12 sites including research and development laboratories, pilot plants, and manufacturing facilities using a new approach involving a battery of measurements that it has called the Nanoparticle Emission Assessment Technique (NEAT). NEAT is an example of the initial screening and detection step in a graded approach to exposure assessment. The field studies results have demonstrated the success of the sampling strategy, although the methods and equipment may not be readily available to the average industrial hygienist.[26] The results from the NIOSH field survey are the most comprehensive look at potential worker exposure published thus far. The authors concluded that the potential for release of engineered nanoparticles does exist during various processes."[27]

For the more detailed comprehensive characterization studies, a more complex and expensive instrument is the Particle Surface-Area Analyzer. These Instruments do not measure total active surface area, but indicate the surface area of particles that may be deposited in the lung in units of square micrometers per cubic centimeter, corresponding to either the tracheobronchial or alveolar regions of the lung. These devices are being evaluated by NIOSH and others for usefulness in conducting initial assessments.

Scanning Mobility Particle Sizers report particle diameter sizes and numbers, which can significantly enhance the capacity to identify releases of engineered nanoparticles, rather than naturally-occurring ultrafines. Instruments available can measure particles from 2.5 to 1000 nm in size and display data in many more size ranges than optical particle counters (up to 167 size channels in one instrument). The SMPS is widely used as a research tool for characterizing airborne nanoparticles, but hasn't been widely used to measure worker exposures because it is much more expensive and physically larger than other instruments. It also contains an internal radioactive source, which further complicates its use.

A cutting edge of real-time particle size and concentration measurement may be represented by the Fast Integrated Mobility Spectrometer (FIMS), which has been developed for rapid aerosol size distribution measurements including those aerosols with low particle number concentrations. Results from this instrument compared well with those measured by a scanning mobility particle sizer (SMPS) and total particle concentration measured by the FIMS agreed well with simultaneous measurements by a CPC. This device is also able to capture the size distribution of rapidly changing aerosol populations."[28]

Electron Microscopy (EM) is, arguably, the most definitive and widely used tool for analyzing nanoparticles in airborne, waterborne and surface wipe samples. At the time of this writing, there are no validated protocols for EM analysis, but the ASTM International has been developing a counting method that has much in common with the EPA's airborne asbestos protocol from the AHERA Method found in Appendix A to Subpart E of Part 763. This method collects samples on 0.45 micrometer porosity mixed cellulose ester filters held open-face in 25 mm. conductive cassettes. The laboratory uses a direct preparation so that the small portion of the filter observed under the electron microscope reveals particles as they were originally deposited on the filter, with a minimum of disturbance from the preparation.

The strength of EM is that it provides several tools for analyzing particles. The tremendous magnification capabilities of transmission electron microscopy (TEM) allow direct observation and measurement of nanoparticles. The ability to observe the raw nanoparticles under TEM prior to incorporation into products allows definitive identification of the engineered particles among the other airborne particles regularly found on filters collected in ambient air. Industrial hygienists should always consider submitting samples of the raw engineered nanoparticles to assist the lab in distinguishing the ENPs from the other particles in the air.

TEM also has a tool called energy dispersive spectroscopy (EDS) or energy dispersive x-ray analysis (EDXA). The electron beam that is directed down the column to enable the electron microscopist to visualize particles has the additional analytical benefit of causing the release of x-rays from any materials that are struck. The energy levels of these x-rays, measured in electron volts (eV), are characteristic for the elements in the materials. The beam can be focused very tightly onto an individual particle or fiber and determine its elemental composition. When these data are combined with visual observations, the microscopist is able to identify engineered nanoparticles with sufficient confidence.

Figure 23.11 illustrates how electron micrographic techniques can be used to establish a "source signature" based on the

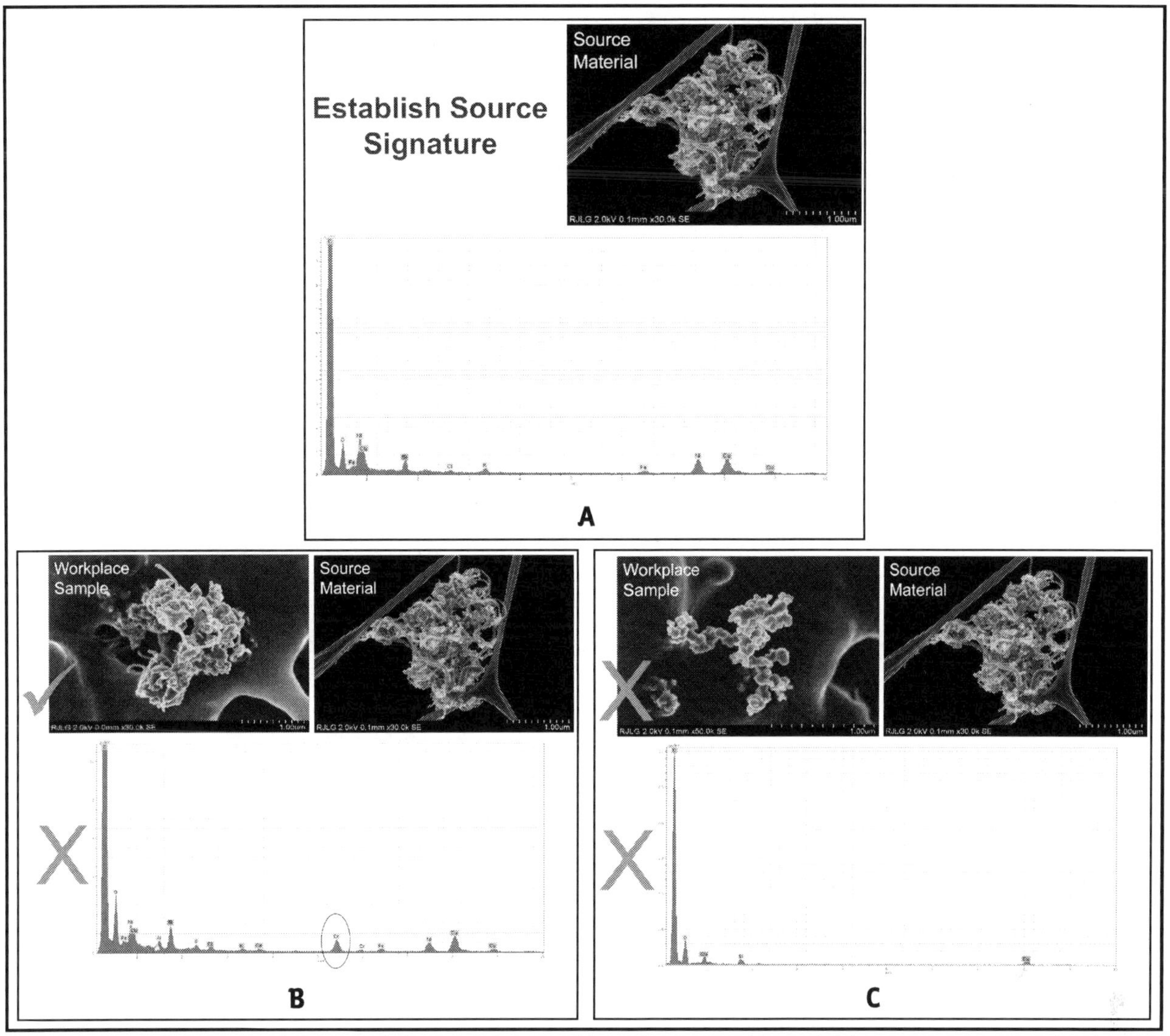

Figure 23.11 — Illustration of the use of electron micrographic techniques to (A) establish a source signature for the morphology and composition of a bulk sample of a carbon nanotube and catalyst material, (B) distinguish a workplace particle of other origin based on a difference in composition, and (C) distinguish a workplace particle of other origin based on differences in both morphology and composition. (Source: RJ Lee Group)

morphology and composition of a nanomaterial and then to use that signature to to distinguish between nanoparticles from the source material and those generated elsewhere.

Control Exposures

Hierarchy of Controls

The hierarchy of controls has served the industrial hygiene profession well for decades and works well in considering nanoparticles. The diagram from NIOSH researchers in Figure 23.12 describes the elements of the hierarchy and the application of the hierarchy in an overall company health and safety program.

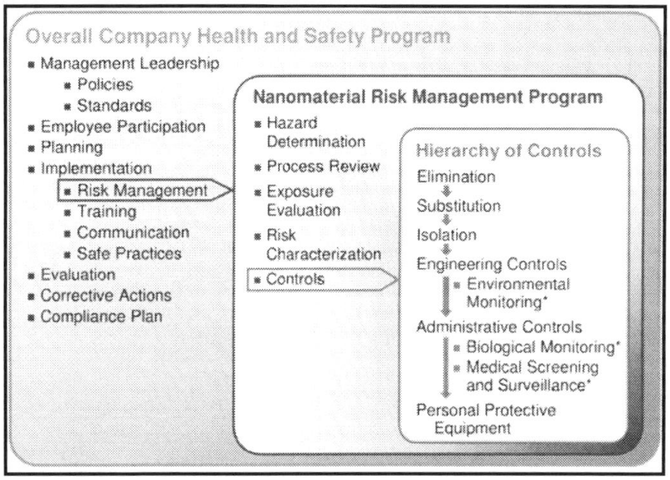

Figure 23.12 — Management system for nanotechnology.[15]

Detailed guidance on applying the hierarchy can be found in the *Canadian document, Best Practices Guide to Synthetic Nanoparticle Risk Management* (IRSST Report 599). The guide recommends that high-risk operations be isolated in separate rooms, ventilated and equipped with independent ventilation systems to avoid the possibility of workstation contamination and worker exposure. A closed circuit process was recommended as the main production method capable of effectively controlling emissions. Carbon black, silica fumes, nanoscaled TiO_2, metals and metal oxides are normally synthesized in closed circuit, according to the Canadian guidance.[29]

Control Banding Approaches

The lack of occupational exposure limits for nanoparticles, combined with the difficulties described above for measuring nanoparticles, complicates selection of "appropriate" controls. Control banding has been suggested as a viable option, particularly given its success controlling worker exposures in the absence of complete toxicological and exposure information in the pharmaceutical industry over the last 20 years.[30–32]

Control banding is a qualitative technique that uses categories or bands of health hazards that are combined with exposure potentials to determine desired levels of control.

A conceptual model was created by Andrew Maynard in 2007 using "impact" and "exposure" indices to combine elements like shape, size and surface area on the nanoparticles with their exposure availability (dustiness and amount in use.) This led to four control strategies:

1. General ventilation,
2. Fume hoods or local exhaust ventilation,
3. Containment, and
4. Seek specialist advice.[33]

A team of experts from Lawrence Livermore National Laboratory elaborated on that design to create a "CB Nanotool" that incorporated a Risk Level (RL) that was a combination of a severity score and a probability score in a standard 4 x 4 risk matrix. The model used the same four control categories as the Maynard model. The model was validated against the recommendations of independent industrial hygiene experts. A high level of consistency was found and the CB Nanotool tended towards over-control rather than under-control, which is preferable.[34] The tool, which is an Excel spreadsheet, has now been used internationally with good results. It represents an excellent teaching tool, as well. Hazmat instructors should consider having students, working in groups preferably, rate a nanomaterial with which they are familiar using either the electronic CB Nanotool or a paper copy.

The model requires assigning numerical weights to specific severity and probability factors. For instance, surface chemistry must be considered as a severity factor and assigned a score based on whether the surface activity is high (10 points), medium (5) or low (0). Similarly, points are assigned to particle shape, with fibrous forms getting the highest score.

The following severity factors are also scored for the nanoparticles:

- Particle diameter,
- Solubility,
- Carcinogenicity,
- Reproductive toxicity,
- Mutagenicity,
- Dermal toxicity, and
- Asthmagen.
- The probability factors that are weighted and must be reviewed include:
- Estimated amount used during the operation,
- Dustiness of the operation,
- Number of employees with similar exposure,
- Frequency of the operation, and
- Duration of the operation.

Total scores are calculated for severity and probability and a 4 x 4 matrix is used to determine the Risk Level (RL), which defines the appropriate control strategy (Figure 23.13). As the Risk Level increases, the control methods similarly increase in protectiveness from general ventilation (RL1), to fume hood or local exhaust ventilation (RL2), to containment (RL3), to seeking the advice of a specialist (RL4).[35]

Snapshot of Existing Control Practices

An international survey by the International Council on Nanotechnology (ICON) of manufacturing firms and research labs found that the principal means of controlling exposure are:

Severity	Probability: Extremely Unlikely (0-25)	Less Likely (26-50)	Likely (51-75)	Probable (76-100)
Very High (76-100)	RL 3	RL 3	RL 4	RL 4
High (51-75)	RL 2	RL 2	RL 3	RL 4
Medium (26-50)	RL 1	RL 1	RL 2	RL 3
Low (0-25)	RL 1	RL 1	RL 1	RL 2

Figure 23.13 — Example of a control banding approach.[35]

- 43% laboratory hoods,
- 32% glove boxes,
- 23% vacuum systems,
- 23% white rooms,
- 20% closed circuits,
- 15% laminar flow ventilation tables,
- 12% biosafety cabinets and
- 12% glove bag.

Most companies or laboratories use more than one means of emission control so the percent sums to greater than 100. The primary finding of the survey was that "actual reported EHS practices... do not significantly depart from conventional safety practices for handling chemicals."[16]

Ventilation

NIOSH, based on field sampling, considers the engineering controls that most employers have readily available useful in minimizing nanoparticle emissions.[36] However, the standard industrial ventilation approaches of general ventilation, fume hoods, and local exhaust ventilation must be carefully considered because of the buoyancy of nanoparticles (e.g., Figure 23.14).

For traditional laboratory fume hoods, totally enclosed on three sides, the universally recommended face velocity at the sash of 100 feet per minute air flow into the hood can cause nanoparticles being handled for operations such as weighing to be dispersed into the hood exhaust. Nevertheless, it is not advisable to work on an open bench outside a hood with dispersible nanoparticles in operations such as transferring or weighing simply because work conditions within traditional hoods have not been optimized for such work. It is advisable to use specially designed enclosures such as ventilated weighing balance enclosures to safely handle nanoparticles in a manner that will prevent them from being lost to the ventilation or release from the hood.

Selection of a well-designed hood, combined with good work practices (such as avoiding rapid arm movement into and out of the hood) is important. Studies have shown that handling dry nanoparticles inside laboratory fume hoods can cause a significant release from the hood.[37] Hood design affects the magnitude of release. With traditionally designed fume hoods, the airflow moves horizontally toward the hood, but becomes turbulent in the worker's wake, which can cause nanoparticles to be carried out with the circulating airflow.

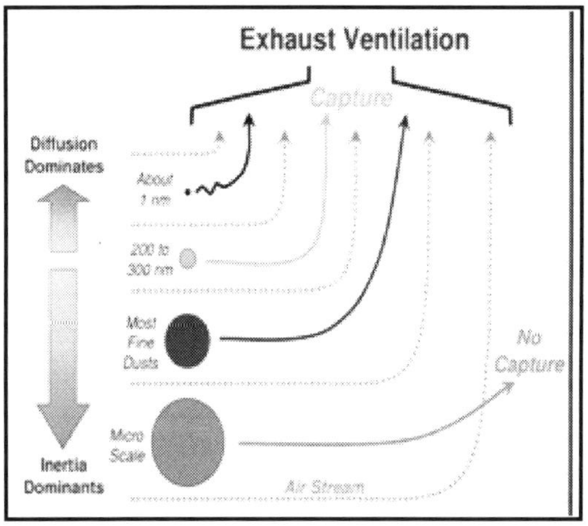

Figure 23.14 — Exhaust ventilation and particle size. (Source: Schulte et al. 2007)[15]

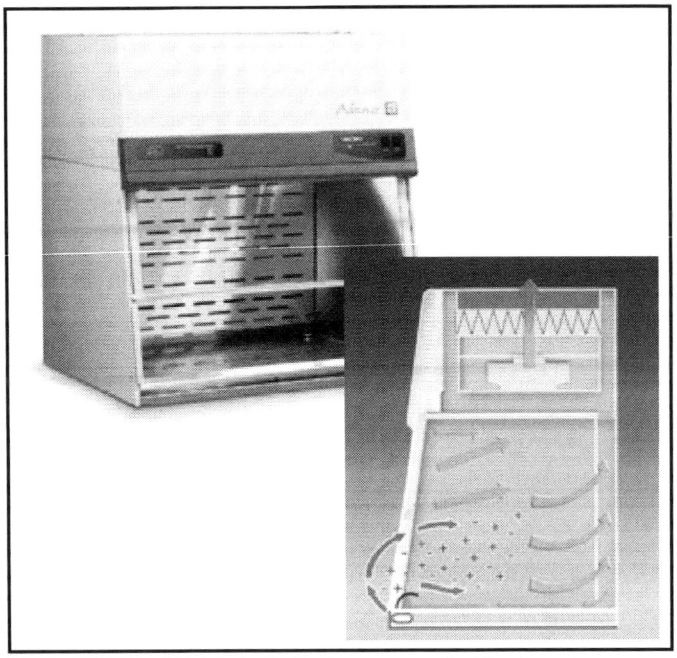

Figure 23.15 — Example enclosure front and side views: Xpert Nano Enclosure pulls room air into the enclosure through the front, directs air flow to the baffle and finally passes air through a 99.999% ULPA exhaust filter before returning the filtered air to the laboratory or cleanroom. (Source: Labconco)

Airborne particle concentrations were measured for three hood designs (constant-flow, constant-velocity, and air-curtain hoods) using manual handling of nanoalumina particles. The hood operator's airborne nanoparticle breathing zone exposure showed high variability for the constant-flow hood while the constant-velocity hood showed some variability, but was usually very low. The performance of the air-curtain hood, a new design with significantly different airflow pattern from traditional hoods, was consistent under all operating conditions and release was barely detected. Fog tests showed more intense turbulent airflow in traditional hoods, but not in the air-curtain hood.

Manufacturers are now making hoods recommended for use with nanoparticles (see, for example, Figure 23.15), but a worldwide survey of laboratories conducting nano-related research found that only 10 percent of researchers reported using nano-enabled hoods, and one in four did not use any type of general laboratory protection.[38]

HEPA Filtration

Given the extremely small size of nanoparticles there has been understandable (but technically unfounded) concern that they might be able to slip through even the highest efficiency filters. This unfounded concern is based on a common misconception that filters act as sieves. In reality, filters capture particles by a combination of physical processes, which include gravitational sedimentation, direct interception, inertial impaction, electrical attraction, and Brownian diffusion. Filtration efficiency is lowest in the particle size range where these combined effects (especially inertia and diffusion) are minimal. The most penetrating particle size (MPPS) is typically in the range of approximately 50 to 500 nm (0.05 to 0.5 μm). Particles above the MPPS are collected predominantly by impaction and interception and particles below the MPPS are collected predominantly by Brownian diffusion.

High Efficiency Particulate Air (HEPA) filters are tested and shown to be at least 99.97% efficient against monodispersed aerosols of 0.3 μm in aerodynamic diameter. This diameter was chosen because it typical of the most difficult size to capture, i.e. larger particles will be captured more easily through impaction and smaller ones through diffusion and electrostatic charges.

NIOSH has concluded that "a well-designed exhaust system with a high-efficiency particulate air (HEPA) filter should effectively remove nanoparticles."[39] Given that HEPA filters will collect nanoparticles at an efficiency of at least 99.97%, the challenge for industrial hygiene control of an operation with a given amount and dispersibility of material is to use an approach such as control banding to provide a level of control that is adequate to keep nanoparticle releases below acceptable limits. An informative set of studies has been conducted at Lawrence Berkeley National Laboratory to measure nanoparticle concentrations in work operations, use the measured concentrations as input to workplace and environmental release models to determine what concentrations would result within the workplace and offsite from release of nanoparticles from exhaust ventilation, and, thereby, to determine what level of filtration is required.[40]

Personal Protective Equipment (PPE)

Despite occupying the bottom rung on the hierarchy of controls, PPE against nanoparticles seems prudent even as other risk management strategies are put in place. Studies on the filtration performance of N-95 filtering-facepiece respirators have found that the mean penetration levels for 40 nm particles range from 1.4% to 5.2%, indicating that N-95 and higher performing respirator filters would be effective at capturing airborne nanoparticles at the expected efficiency of 95% or better.(41–42) A NIOSH-approved filtering-facepiece respirator or elastomeric half-face respirator equipped with a 95 or 100 series filter should provide protection at the assigned protection factor when properly fit-tested on the worker.(44) Thus, because respirator filters have been shown to "work" for nanoparticles, the standard NIOSH respirator selection logic(45) can be used to pick a type of respirator that will provide a level of protection that is adequate to reduce the expected airborne concentration of the nanoparticles to a concentration below appropriate occupational exposure limits (e.g., below the NIOSH recommendationed exposure limits of 7 µg/m³ for CNT or 30 µg/m³ for ultrafine TiO_2). The EPA, however, has been setting specific minimum respiratory protection requirements for specific nanoparticles under the Toxic Substances Control Act's Significant New Use of Chemical Substances Rule, 40 CFR Part 721. For instance, the EPA considers siloxane-modified alumina nanoparticles to be subject to reporting under the New Use Rule and requires manufacturers to provide, at a minimum, NIOSH-approved air-purifying, tight-fitting respirators equipped with N100 (if oil aerosols are absent), R100, or P100 filters (either half- or full-face).(46) The apparent premise is that the assigned protection factor for such respirators will provide protection that is adequate for the expected nanoparticle concentrations and characteristics. Under the same rule, EPA has determined that single-walled and multi-walled carbon nanotubes need to be reported as significant new uses and exposed workers needed to be provided NIOSH-approved air-purifying, tightfitting full-face respirators equipped with N100 filters.(47,48)

As for mitigation of any airborne hazard, selection of the appropriate respirator type should be based on knowledge of the hazard, the airborne exposure concentration, and whether an exposure limit exists for the engineered nanoparticle. In addition, the efficiency of the respirator is meaningless if the device isn't conscientiously worn. An international survey of nano-related laboratories found that nearly half of the researchers reported not using any type of respiratory protection.(38)

Nano-specific information on the performance of protective clothing is also emerging. One positive sign is that some clothing standards incorporate testing with nanoscale particles and therefore provide some indication of the effectiveness of protective clothing with regard to nanoparticles.(38) One governmental body recommended that outerwear be modified to reduce the production of static electricity, which increases the attraction of nanoparticles. They also recommended the use of disposable protective clothing because cleaning of garments to remove nanoparticles has not been sufficiently evaluated.(38)

The ICON 2006 survey of international firms and laboratories found that:

- 41 percent of the organizations said they used laboratory coats (7 percent of which were disposable);
- 26 percent used more protective coveralls (7% of them disposable),
- 11% used shoes reserved for the laboratory,
- 9% have their own laundry service, and
- The most common gloves were nitrile, latex and rubber.

Controlling Safety Hazards like Fire Potential

While most attention has rightly been given to the potential health effects of nanoparticles, there is clearly a need to focus on the safety issues, as well. OSHA has begun the process of holding hearings on a combustible dust standard because more than 130 workers have been killed and more than 780 injured in combustible dust explosions since 1980.(49)

It is common knowledge that explosive dust clouds can be created from most organic materials, many metals and even some non-metallic inorganic materials. The main element affecting the ease of ignition and explosive violence of airborne dust is the particle size and surface area, which are inversely related, i.e. for the same mass, as the particle size decreases, the surface area increases. The violence of the explosion and the ease of ignition generally increase as the particle size decreases. Consequently, many nanoparticle types have the potential to cause explosions, yet data on fire and explosion hazards of nanoparticles is almost nonexistent.[50]

Confirm that Risks are Adequately Managed

An important case study of the adequacy of control was the assessment of very fine particle number and mass concentrations in an engine machining and assembly facility.[25] A CPC and an OPC were used to measure particle number concentrations over a broad range. The OPC measurements were used to estimate the respirable mass concentration.

This study provided a baseline assessment of potential emission sources of engineered nanoparticles during a variety of operations, which showed that reactor cleanout was an uncontrolled source of emissions, apparently due to technicians brushing and scraping unwanted buildup from the inside of the reactor. This prompted an effort to minimize potential worker exposure, mainly through the use of PPE as well as consideration of other measures such as local exhaust ventilation systems (LEVs).

Sampling showed that "properly maintained LEV can be highly effective in controlling nanoparticle emissions. This finding, coupled with the current use of PPE, appears to be an acceptable method of reducing the potential for worker exposure."[51]

Overall confirmation of the adequacy of risk management for any situation can include a number of actions such as occupational epidemiologic studies that go beyond the basis evaluation of results from exposure assessment and verifications of control. Confirmation, documentation, and continuous improvement of the entire risk management process can ensure that all steps, beginning with anticipation, are scientifically grounded and appropriately applied. NIOSH has recommended prudent precautionary interim measures for reducing work-related exposures and assessing potential risk. Table 23.4 presents recommendations that NIOSH has proposed for employers and for workers handling carbon nanotubes (CNT) and carbon nanofibers (CNF).[12] NIOSH has also noted that In the hierarchy of prevention, it is important to consider where it may be of value to provide medical screening of workers who may be exposed to a potential health hazard, but who may be asymptomatic—that is, who have no identifiable symptom of an occupational disease. As research into the hazards of engineered nanoparticles continues, vigilant reassessment of available data is critical to determine whether specific medical screening is warranted for workers. In the interim, NIOSH has provided the following recommendations for workplaces where workers may be exposed to engineered nanoparticles in the course of their work:

- Take prudent measures to control exposures to engineered nanoparticles.
- Conduct hazard surveillance as the basis for implementing controls.
- Continue use of established medical surveillance approaches.

Until results from research studies can fully elucidate the physicochemical properties of CNT and CNF that define their inhalation toxicity, steps should be taken to minimize CNT and CNF exposures of all workers and to implement an occupational health surveillance program that includes elements of hazard and medical surveillance.

In its draft *Current Intelligence Bulletin on Occupational Exposure to Carbon Nanotubes and Nanofibers,* NIOSH has recommendation that employers and workers follow the steps listed in Table 23.4 to minimize potential health risks associated with exposure to CNT and CNF.

Hazard Communication for Nanoparticles

In the United States, the Occupational Safety and Health Administration's Hazard Communication Standard (29 CFR 1910.1200) requires that employers inform their workers of the chemical hazards to which they are exposed and how they should protect themselves. In Canada, the Workplace Hazardous Materials Information System (WHMIS) has the same requirement. The 2006 European REACH (Registration, Evaluation, Authorization and Restriction of Chemicals) initiative on chemical hazard communication is more comprehensive and ambitious than the OSHA requirements and requires chemical manufacturers to follow how their products are used by purchasers.

Globally Harmonized System for Classification and Labeling of Chemicals (GHS)

The most significant development in hazard communication in decades has been the international effort to create a harmonized system. In 2003, the United Nations adopted the Globally Harmonized System of Classification and Labeling of Chemicals (GHS), which includes criteria for classifying health, physical and environmental hazards; GHS also specifies what information should be included on labels of hazardous chemicals

Table 23.5 — Draft Recommendations for Employers and Workers to Minimize Potential Health Risks Associated with Occupational Exposure to Carbon Nanotubes (CNT) and Carbon Nanofibers (CNF). From NIOSH 2010.

Recommendations for employers	*Recommendations for workers*
• Use available information to continually assess current hazard potential related to CNT and CNF exposures in the workplace and make appropriate changes (e.g., sampling and analysis, exposure control) to protect workers health. • Identify and characterize processes and job tasks where workers come in contact with bulk ("free-form") CNT and CNT-containing materials (e.g., composites). • When possible, substitute a non-hazardous or less hazardous material for CNT and CNF when feasible. When substitution is not possible, use engineering controls as the primary method for minimizing worker exposure to CNT and CNF. • Establish criteria and procedures for selecting, installing, and evaluating the performance of engineering controls to ensure proper operating conditions. • Make sure workers are trained on how to check and use exposure controls (e.g., exhaust ventilation systems). • Routinely evaluate airborne exposures to ensure that control measures are working properly and that worker exposures are being maintained below the NIOSH REL of 7.0 μg/m³ using NIOSH Method 5040 or an equivalent method. • Follow exposure and hazard assessment procedures for determining the need for and selection of proper personal protective equipment, such as clothing, gloves, and respirators. • Educate workers on the sources and job tasks that may expose them to CNT and CNF and train them on how to use appropriate controls, work practices, and personal protective equipment to minimize exposure. • Provide facilities for hand-washing and encourage workers to make use of these facilities before eating, smoking, or leaving the worksite. • Provide facilities for showering and changing clothes, with separate facilities for storage of non-work clothing, to prevent the inadvertent cross contamination of non-work areas (including take-home contamination). • Use light-colored gloves, lab coats, and work bench surfaces to facilitate observation of contamination by dark CNT and CNF. • Develop and implement procedures to deal with clean-up of CNT and CNF spills and de-contamination of surfaces. • When respirators are provided for worker protection, the OSHA respiratory protection standard [29 CFR 1910.134] requires that a respiratory protection program be established that includes the following elements: – a medical evaluation of the worker's ability to perform the work while wearing a respirator, – regular training of personnel, – periodic workplace exposure monitoring, – respirator fit testing, and – respirator maintenance, inspection, cleaning, and storage.	• Ask your supervisor for training on how to protect yourself from the potential hazards associated with your job, including exposure to CNT and CNF. • Know and use the exposure control devices and work practices that keep CNT and CNF out of the air and off your skin. • Understand when and how to wear a respirator and other personal protective equipment (such as gloves, clothing, eye wear) that your employer might provide. • Avoid handling CNT and CNF in a 'free particle' state (e.g., powder form). • Store CNT and CNF, whether suspended in liquids or in a powder form, in closed (tightly sealed) containers whenever possible. • Clean work areas at the end of each work shift (at a minimum) using either a HEPA-filtered vacuum cleaner or wet wiping methods. • Do not store or consume food or beverages in workplaces where bulk CNT or CNF or where CNT- or CNF-containing materials are handled. • Dry sweeping or air hoses should not be used to clean work areas. • Prevent the inadvertent contamination of non-work areas (including takehome contamination) by showering and changing into clean clothes at the end of each work day.

and on safety data sheets. OSHA published a proposed rulemaking on September 30, 2009 to align OSHA's Hazard Communication standard (HCS) with the GHS.

The GHS provides consistency in format. Under the GHS, labels would include signal words, pictograms and precautionary statements. Safety data sheets would have a standardized format of 16 sections that is based on the ANSI Z400.1 consensus standard. It is valuable to ask if it the ANSI standard really is appropriate for nanomaterials. The last section of the GHS (and ANSI) format is called "other information" and is the only section that is not tightly prescribed and could, therefore, contain specific cautionary language about the nano-sized component in the product. One Hazcom expert offered an example of a warning he created: "Established exposure values do not address the small size of particles found in this product and may not provide adequate protection against occupational exposures."[52]

Material Safety Data Sheets (MSDSs) are required for nanoparticles that meet the definitions of hazardous chemicals under OSHA's Hazard Communication standard. According to a survey of firms in Massachusetts, MSDSs from suppliers are the preferred source of risk information for nanotechnology firms.[53]

Unfortunately, industry hasn't done a good job of communicating the hazards of standard industrial chemicals despite having two and a half decades since the promulgation of OSHA's Hazard Communication standard in 1983 to get it right. An OSHA-funded 1997 study of the peer-reviewed hazard communication literature indicated broad shortcomings with MSDSs, labels and warnings.[54] Three separate studies found that literate workers only comprehended roughly 60 percent of the health and safety information on sample MSDSs.[55–57]

A recent review of more current literature regarding the accuracy, comprehensibility and use of MSDSs unfortunately did not show improvements over the 1997 review. Accuracy and completeness were found to be relatively poor: the majority of studies showed that the MSDSs did not contain information on all the chemicals present and workers showed low comprehensibility because of overly complex language.[58]

NIOSH appears to maintain the most complete collection of MSDSs for engineered nanoparticles and recently analyzed 60 of them from 33 different manufacturers for technical sufficiency.[59] The researchers only rated 5 percent as "good" while 55 percent were rated as "in need of serious improvement." Over half contained Occupational Exposure Limits (OELs) for the bulk material without providing guidance that the OEL may not be protective for the nanoscale material. Eighty percent "failed to recognize the material as being nano in size or list a particle size distribution showing the nano size range" and a higher percentage "lacked toxicologic data specific to the nanoparticles." Eight percent failed to "suggest any type of engineering controls or mechanical ventilation."

These findings corroborated a similar analysis of a subset of the same MSDSs presented at an international conference sponsored by the EPA.[60] The earlier analysis also noted that of those MSDSs that recommended local exhaust ventilation, 25 percent recommended a face velocity greater than 100 feet per minute even though, as noted earlier, NIOSH has specifically warned against operating fume hoods at that rate because the turbulence can release nanoparticles. Additionally, not one of the MSDSs reported that nanoparticles pose a much greater flammability risk despite warnings from authoritative sources that "an increasing range of materials that are capable of producing explosive dust clouds are being produced as nanopowders."[61]

Regulatory and Voluntary Approaches Specific to Nanoparticles

Given the many unknowns regarding nanoparticles, a wide range of risk assessment approaches has been suggested for nanotechnology, going from recommendations for a total moratorium on any development and use of nanoparticles if and until they are proven to be safe to humans and the environment, to recommendations for relying on existing occupational safety and health laws and regulations.[62]

Development of safe and sustainable nanotechnology will require avoidance of the sad and repeated history of occupational diseases killing hundreds or thousands of workers before the federal government has acted to eliminate or curtail exposures. Asbestos is the most notorious example, but the list includes acrylonitrile, benzene, acetyl and lead. The latter is painfully illustrative. Austria, France and Belgium phased out lead in household paint in 1909. In this country, the trade association for lead paint agreed to take it out of paint used on children's toys in 1936, but it wasn't phased out completely until 1977. These additional 68 years of exposure have been credited with causing a population-wide IQ drop.[63] Even with the bans and existing regulations, products containing lead-based paint still surreptitiously enter the country.

The federal government has acknowledged this sordid history and publicly vowed to avoid a similar path with nanotechnology. The results thus far have been encouraging. Under the National Nanotechnology Initiative, all of the key agencies — EPA, OSHA, DOE, DoD, CPSC, FDA — and the White House have been working together in the Nanotechnology Environmental and Health Implications (NEHI) working group to identify the key research that should be conducted to protect workers and the environment.

Government Regulatory Actions

As a set of technologies, materials and devices, "nanotechnology" has been or will be determined to fall within several different regulatory frameworks. Each agency with regulatory authority over some form of nanotechnology has taken concrete steps to understand how best to apply its statutes to this new class of technologies. The actions taken by the key regulatory agencies are summarized in Table 23.4. For nanoparticles, the two federal statutes that have the most relevance today are the Toxic Substances Control Act (TSCA) and the Federal Insecticide, Fungicide and Rodenticide Act (FIFRA), both enforced by the Environmental Protection Agency (EPA).

Nanoparticles as Toxic Substances

Nanoparticles meet the definition of chemical substances under the Toxic Substances Control Act (TSCA).[64] At issue is whether they are considered new forms of existing chemicals, which would lower the burden on the manufacturer bringing that substance to market, or whether they are "new chemicals", which imposes greater reporting requirements. EPA's initial position that a nanoscale form of a chemical substance is not new solely by virtue of its size has garnered significant criticism. There are indications that EPA may be rethinking this, which could lead to big changes in how the agency regulates nanoparticles. If EPA were to deem nanoparticle forms new chemicals, the nanoparticles could be subject to reporting and testing that are not required for most nanoparticles being sold today.

Meanwhile, EPA is exercising its authority to regulate some nanoparticles using the significant new use rules (SNUR) under Section 5(a)(2) of TSCA. SNURs have already been issued on certain carbon nanotubes and siloxane nanoparticles, largely based on

Table 23.4 — Actions on Nanotechnology by Key Federal Regulatory Agencies

Agency	Primary Statutes	Actions
EPA	Toxic Substances Control Act (TSCA) Federal Insecticide, Fungicide and Rodenticide Act (FIFRA) CERCLA (Superfund) Clean Air Act Resource Conservation and Recovery Act	Implemented voluntary reporting program (TSCA) Published white paper (TSCA) Issued rules specific to nanoparticles (TSCA) Issued fines for noncompliance (FIFRA) Funded intramural and extramural research
FDA	Federal Food, Drug and Cosmetic Act	Created topics page at website Commenced internal research program Formed Task Force Issued white paper Published monograph on nanoscale sunscreen ingredients
OSHA	Occupational Safety and Health Act	Created topics page at website
CPSC	Consumer Product Safety Act Federal Hazardous Substances Act	Published white paper Commenced internal research program

the nanoscale form and influenced by publicly available toxicity data. The (siloxane) SNURs require manufacturers to notify EPA 90 days prior to sale and describe specific worker protection measures that must be taken when handling the materials.[65]

Nanoparticles as Pesticides

The Federal Insecticide, Fungicide, and Rodenticide Act (FIFRA) provides EPA the authority to control the distribution, sale and use of pesticides and pest control devices. Under FIFRA, EPA may determine the risks and benefits of pesticidal products incorporating nanotechnology ("nanopesticides") and may impose restrictions to limit potential risks. Some nanoscale materials such as titanium dioxide and nanoscale silver exhibit potent antimicrobial effects, which has been exploited in a growing number of consumer products. EPA has taken note of several products making antimicrobial claims on the label and leveled fines against the manufacturers for failing to register the products as pesticides or pest control devices as required by FIFRA. Examples of these include a $208,000 fine imposed on ATEN Technology, Inc. for the failure of its subsidiary IOGEAR to register several antimicrobial computer mouse and mouse/keyboard combination products and for making "unverified claims that coatings on keyboard and mouse accessories would eliminate pathogens and kill bacteria,"[66] and a fine of nearly $1 million against VF Corporation for failure to register 70 styles of footwear sold under the North Face brand that contain an AgION silver treated foot bed and claim to "inhibit the growth of disease-causing bacteria," "prevent bacterial and fungal growth" and continuously release antimicrobial agents.[67] In each case a nanoscale ingredient is believed to be the active antimicrobial agent.

How a washing machine became a pesticide: In everyday language a pesticide is something that kills cockroaches, ants, mosquitoes and other nuisance pests. In addition to insects the word 'pest' in EPA jargon includes another class of 'bugs': microbes. Therefore, any product that claims to kill bacteria, viruses, fungi or other unwanted microbes, is classified as a pesticide or pest control device by the EPA. A product that uses physical or mechanical means to control a pest is a pest control device (e.g., untreated flypaper and UV light disinfection systems) and does not require registration under FIFRA but if it uses a substance to control pests then it is a pesticide and must be registered if it makes a pesticidal claim.

In 2005, EPA advised a washing machine manufacturer (presumably Samsung) that its product (presumably the Silver NanoTM Silver Wash, Figure 23.16) would be classified as a pest control device. The Samsung Silver Wash product claims to kill odor-causing bacteria on fabrics by using electrolysis of a silver electrode to release silver ions into the wash water. Moreover, the product's marketing claims that the silver ions permeate the fabrics, providing anti-bacterial protection for up to one month.[1] Shortly after its decision became public, EPA received letters from waste water treatment facility operators urging it to reconsider its decision and classify the Samsung washing machine as a pesticide because it uses a compound (silver ions) to kill bacteria. The basis for the concern was the inevitable release of silver ion-containing water into sanitary sewer systems which could hamper efforts by plant operators to keep their effluents in compliance with federal limits on silver. Classification of the machine as a pesticide would permit EPA to request data on the potential impact of the machine on silver levels in the waste treatment system and open the door for mandatory restrictions on the sale of the product to avoid further bioaccumulation of silver in the environment. In 2007, EPA revised its ruling "because these items incorporate a substance or substances that accomplish their pesticidal function."[1] And that is how a washing machine became a pesticide.

Nanoparticles as Workplace Toxicants

Worker exposures have not been directly addressed in regulations, nor does OSHA have any plans to regulate nanoparticles. NIOSH has taken the lead by examining the measurement and control of exposures, and has exercised their powers under the OSHAct to create a recommended exposure limit for ultrafine titanium dioxide, and to prepare a current intelligence bulletin with a recommended exposure limit for carbon nanotubes.

When examining the regulatory tools available to OSHA, their 29 CFR 1910.120 Hazardous Waste Operation and Emergency Response (HAZWOPER) standard must be seen as extremely durable in its applicability over the 30 years of its history being applied to cleanup of drums of waste in the 70s and the response to terrorist attacks involving anthrax in 2001.

The HAZWOPER standard, which went into effect in 1990, protects the safety and health of employees involved in clean-up operations at hazardous waste sites; operations at hazardous waste treatment, storage and disposal facilities; and emergency responses to releases or potential releases of hazardous substances. Although created to protect workers dealing with uncontrolled industrial chemicals at that time, it takes little imagination to see the HAZWOPER connection to nanoparticles. Workers may encounter nanoparticles in the course of handling hazardous waste from a research lab or industrial operation or when cleaning up a large-scale spill in a factory or by the roadside. In addition to these more predictable scenarios for encountering nanoparticles, hazardous waste workers may find themselves purposefully introducing them as part of an EPA Superfund cleanup: nanoremediation is projected to be a major part of the overall cleanup strategy on governmental sites over the next 30 years, estimated to be between $87 and $98 billion in scope. The U.S. GAO has recently reviewed the EPA's regulatory options under CERCLA (Superfund) for regulating nanoparticles and noted that the EPA has the statutory authority to designate additional substances as hazardous under CERCLA if their release may present substantial danger to the public health or welfare or the environment.[17] The EPA's searchable database called Nanotechnology Project Profiles that can be found on its CLU-IN website.[68]

If HAZWOPER coverage involves some ambiguity, OSHA's Hazard Communication standard, 29 CFR 1910.1200, applies completely and importantly. It is hard to envision any population that has a more compelling issue of hazard communication than workers creating nanoparticles or adding them to the broad array of products currently on the market.

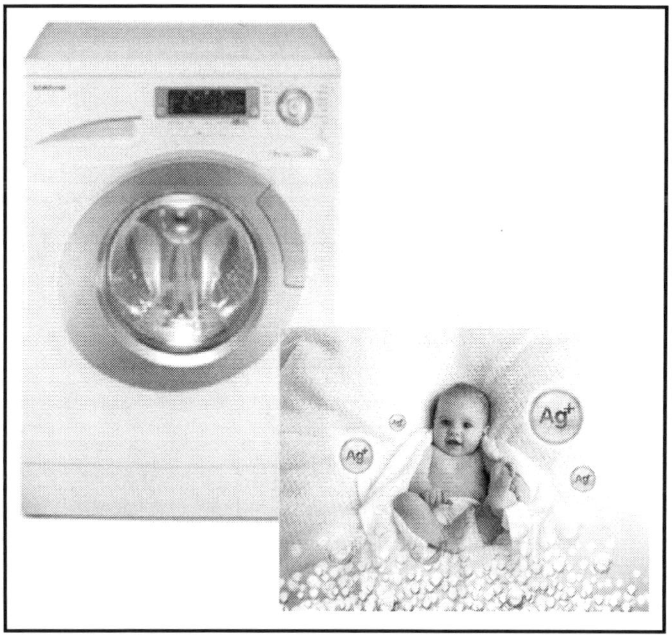

Figure 23.16 — (L) Samsung's patented Silver NanoTM Silver Wash machine as marketed by Samsung Electronics Australia Pty Ltd. (R) Samsung claims the product "protects sensitive skin and help prevent dermatitis." (Source: http://www.samsung.com/au/silvernano/site.html)

Going back to the earliest, contentious debates over the OSH Act, labor and management leaders at least agreed that occupational diseases presented the most serious case for government action.[69] With nanoparticles there are clear safety issues, particularly the risk of fire and explosions from reducing materials to extraordinarily small particle sizes that take exponentially less energy to ignite.[70] But the potential health risks posed by nanoparticles are an even more stark argument for government involvement.

Properly informing workers about the risks of nanoparticles requires a frank appraisal of the history and current state of industrial chemical regulation. OSHA has regulatory standards, called Permissible Exposure Limits (PELs), for approximately 600 chemical substances; the majority of these PELs are based on consensus standards set at least 40 years ago by volunteer members of the American Conference of Governmental Industrial Hygienists (ACGIH), many of whom were from the industries that produced the chemicals. During the past 40 years, the ACGIH® has lowered many of their recommended exposures limits based on continuing research, but OSHA continues to use the levels from 1969, despite an updating of the PELs in 1989 that the courts threw out in 1992.

The age of the OSHA PELs is a minor issue compared to the dearth of information on the overwhelming majority of chemicals in production. There is no definitive count of the number of chemicals in regular use today, but the EPA maintains a list of 83,000 chemicals under the Toxic Substances Control Act.[71] The Chemical Abstract Service had registered 52,122,026 organic and inorganic substances developed by industry as of February 12, 2010.[72] Scanning Tunneling Electron Microscopy allows the manipulation of individual atoms to create unique nanoparticles.

Given the 118 elements available for combination, a mind-numbing range of between 10200 to 10900 distinct nanoscale creations has been estimated as plausible; these are truly awe-inspiring numbers for regulators.[73] While federal regulators grapple with these large issues, local and state regulators are dealing with the direct impact of nanomaterials in their jurisdictions.

Regulations at the Local Level

In California, the city of Berkeley amended its hazardous-material reporting requirement in December 2006 to include a notification requirement regarding manufactured nanoparticles.[74] In 2009, the California Department of Toxic Substances Control (DTSC) exercised its authority under the Health and Safety Code, Chapter 699, to request information regarding analytical test methods, fate and transport in the environment, and other relevant information from manufacturers of carbon nanotubes.[75] DTSC has indicated its interest in expanding the data call-ins to other types of nanoparticles. Interest in other states could result in more actions in the future.

Voluntary Approaches

There is still a perception among many that guidance and existing regulation are not enough to address the knowledge gaps. In response, established international and intergovernmental bodies are engaging in their own processes, often with extensive participation from governments. Additionally, grassroots groups and consortia are developing interim strategies for managing risk while governments and other established bodies do their work. Several of these organizations have created guidance documents and consensus standards that can beused as resources. The importance of voluntary guidance was underscored by the international survey of research laboratories referenced previously that found nearly half of the labs had no internal rules on handling nanomaterials and another quarter of the respondents weren't aware of any internal regulations.[38]

Organization for Economic Co-operation and Development (OECD)

The Organization for Economic Co-operation and Development (OECD) is an intergovernmental organization in which representatives of 30 industrialized countries in North America, Europe and the Asia and Pacific region, as well as the European Commission, meet to co-ordinate and harmonize policies and work together to respond to international problems through more than 200 specialized committees and working groups.

The Working Party on Manufactured Nanomaterials was established in 2006 to help member countries address the safety challenges of nanomaterials by bringing together more than 100 experts from governments and other stakeholders. The Working Party is tackling the following important issues:

- Developing of a database on human health and environmental safety (EHS) research;
- Establishing EHS research strategies for manufactured nanomaterials;
- Testing the safety of a representative set of nanomaterials; and
- Cooperating on exposure measurement and exposure mitigation.[76]

International Organization for Standardization (ISO)

The International Organization for Standardization (ISO) is a non-governmental organization that develops and publishes voluntary consensus standards via a network of national standards institutes of 161 countries. ISO Technical Committee 229 Nanotechnologies (ISO/TC 229) was formed to develop consensus standards in nanotechnology and currently has four working groups. Working Group 3 is dedicated to developing standards in the health, safety and environmental aspects of nanotechnologies. ISO/TC 229 has published a Technical Report, ISO/TR 12885:2008, Health and safety practices in occupational settings relevant to nanotechnologies, which focuses on the manufacture and use of engineered nanomaterials. This report was produced in conjunction with the American National Standards Institute and "provides advice for companies, researchers, workers and other people to prevent adverse health and safety consequences during the production, handling, use and disposal of manufactured nanomaterials."[77] NIOSH personnel were heavily involved in creating this Technical Report.

ASTM International

ASTM International (ASTM) is another international non-governmental organization that develops and publishes voluntary consensus standards. Its Committee E56 on Nanotechnology produced an occupational health standard in 2007 titled, *Standard Guide for Handling Unbound Engineered Nanoscale Particles in Occupational Settings.*[78]

The guide outlines six elements for establishing a program to minimize exposures:

1. Establishing management commitment to the control principle;
2. identifying and communicating potential hazards;
3. assessing potential UNP exposures within the worksite;
4. identifying and implementing engineering and administrative controls for all relevant operations and activities;
5. establishing documentation and
6. periodically reviewing its adequacy.

ASTM International has premised its exposure control recommendations on the principle "that, as a cautionary measure, occupational exposures to unbound nanoscale particles should be minimized to levels that are as low as is reasonably practicable." The ALARA principle, As Low As Reasonably Achievable, is the foundation for radiation control and very familiar to the industrial hygiene community.

NanoRisk Framework

One of the most widely recognized voluntary approaches came from the unusual partnership of the DuPont company and the Environmental Defense Fund.[79] In June 2007, they jointly launched the Nano Risk Framework as a comprehensive, practical and flexible system to address the potential risks of nanoscale materials (see Figure 23.18). The Framework has been widely cited as best practice for industry and valuable input for government policy. In a manner similar to "anticipate, recognize, evaluate, control, and confirm", the framework includes a detailed output worksheet that companies can use to document each of the following six steps.

1. Describe Material and Its Applications;
2. Profile Lifecycles;
3. Evaluate Risk;
4. Assess Risk Management;
5. Decide, Document, and Act; and
6. Review and Adapt.

Developing Effective Training Programs for Nanotechnology Workers

There are many good sources available for creating effective training materials for workers. Arguably the guidance with the most substantial results to corroborate its value is the "Minimum Criteria" guidance of the National Institute of Environmental

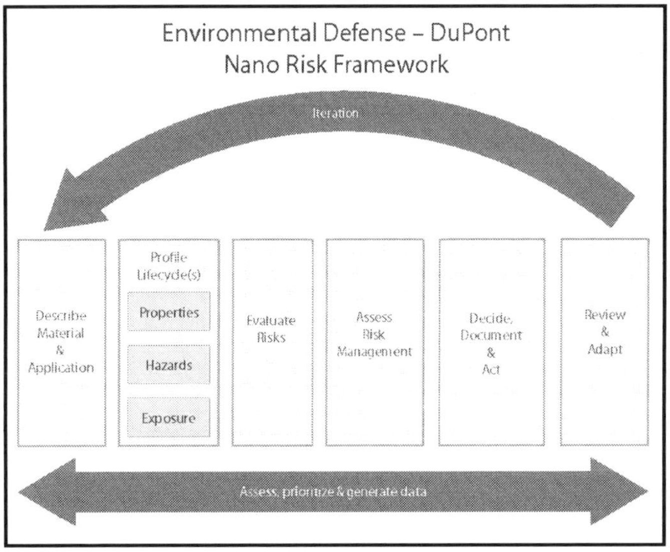

Figure 23.17 — Example of a Risk Management Framework for Nanotechnology. (Source: Environmental Defense – DuPont)

Health Sciences' Worker Education and Training Program (WETP). This guidance, which was updated in 2006, has provided the underlying principles for the creation, delivery and evaluation of training for over two million workers since the beginning of the program in 1987.The initial quality control for the program was developed through a participatory national technical workshop in 1990 and issued by the Program in 1991. This original "Minimum Criteria" was updated in 1994 as the "Interpretive Guidance" to the "Minimum Criteria." The guidance has served as the quality control basis for the WETP training grants program to the present time. It was also adopted by OSHA as a non-mandatory appendix to the HAZWOPER standard.

The following Minimum Criteria recommendations should be applied to any training program created to deal with nanoparticles:

- Provide peer-to-peer training with hands-on activities whenever possible.
- Fill at least one-third of the training program hours with hands-on training.
- Avoid making computer-based training methods the sole form of training, although they can greatly augment the effectiveness and reduce the cost of hazardous waste worker training.
- Make sure proven adult-learning techniques are the core of all worker training.
- Precede all worker safety and health training with a needs analysis to ensure the appropriate knowledge, skills and attitudes are being transmitted.
- Follow all training with a proper evaluation to document that the knowledge, skills or attitudes were acceptably transmitted and that the worker possesses the necessary abilities to perform the tasks.[80]

Despite the exploding literature on nanomaterials, only one article on training workers potentially exposed to nanoparticles was identified. The researchers distributed questionnaires to assess the training needs of safety and health personnel in nanotechnology industries in Taiwan.[81] Based on those results, they identified the three-tiered training hierarchy of I-Hazard Recognition, II-Hazard Evaluation, and III-Hazard Control that is presented in Table 23.6. An example approach for comprehensive initial and refresher training program for nanotechnology workers developed by Kulinowski and Lippy is presented in Table 23.7.[82]

Conclusion

In taking steps to anticipate, recognize, evaluate, control, and confirm appropriate management of nanotechnology-related hazards, it is useful to bear in mind the following observations from Bill Kojola, Industrial Hygienist for the AFL-CIO Health and Safety Department:

> "When the science is just developing — as it is for nanotechnology and its human health effects - it is a difficult call to know when to take action to protect or at least monitor workers. I think we learned from the impacts of asbestos exposure that if there is a technical uncertainty then precaution is well advised. We need to ensure that we make efforts to protect worker health and make sure all employers do so."

Additional Resources

There are many informational resources on nanotechnology and its potential impacts on human health and the environment. Many can be downloaded from the internet at no cost. There are also opportunities to participate in the various user groups, expert community activities, and voluntary standards organizations which are helping to develop and share new information. Given the growth of the field of nanotechnology in general and the explosion of information on nano-EHS issues, it is not practical to create an exhaustive list of web-based resources. Instead, the following sites either are themselves essential for all nanotechnology workers and worker trainers or aggregate relevant information from a broad set of sources.

A key message of this chapter is that you will need to assemble and assess a family of trusted sources to ensure that the methods described here are not obsolete, and to check for any applicable material-specific guidance. Example sources are:

- National Institute for Occupational Safety and Health (NIOSH): *Approaches to Safe Nanotechnology: Managing the*

Health and Safety Concerns Associated with Engineered Nanomaterials (Publication No. 2009-125). Cincinnati, Ohio: U.S. Department of Health and Human Services, 2009.
- NIOSH nanotechnology topic webpage, www.cdc.gov/niosh/topics/nanotech.
- U.S. Department of Energy Nanoscale Science Research Centers: *Approach to Nanomaterial ES&H*. Washington, DC: U.S. Department of Energy, 2008.
- ASTM International: *Standard Guide for Handling Unbound Engineered Nanoscale Particles in Occupational Settings* (ASTM E 2535-07). West Conshohocken, PA; ASTM International, 2007.
- National Academy of Sciences Committee on Prudent Practices in the Laboratory: An Update: *Prudent Practices in the Laboratory: Handling and Management of Chemical Hazards, Updated Version*. Washington, DC: The National Academies Press, 2011.

Table 23.6 — Example Approach for Training Nanotechnology Workers at the Introductory, Advanced, and Professional Levels[81]

	I. Hazard Recognition	
Introductory Level	*Advanced Level*	*Professional Level*
• Introduction to nanoparticle health-hazards	• Nanoparticle health-hazards of different exposure routes • Nanoparticle toxicities and their evaluation techniques	• Health-hazards for nanoparticle inhalation exposures • Health-hazards for nanoparticle dermal exposures • Nanoparticle toxicities and metabolisms • Nanoparticle toxicities evaluation techniques
	II. Hazard Evaluation	
Introductory Level	*Advanced Level*	*Professional Level*
• Introduction to nanoparticle exposure assessments	• Inhalation exposure assessment for nanoparticles • Dermal exposure assessment • Biological monitoring for nanoparticles • Sampling strategy for assessing nanoparticle exposure	• Techniques for assessing nanoparticle inhalation exposures • Instrumentation for assessing inhalation exposures • Principles and techniques used in biological monitoring for nanoparticles • Sampling strategy for assessing nanoparticle exposure • Data analysis techniques for assessing nanoparticle exposures
	III. Hazard Control	
Introductory Level	*Advanced Level*	*Professional Level*
• Introduction to the management and control of nanoparticle health hazards	• Control of nanoparticle health hazards • Management of nanoparticle health hazards	• Enclosure and isolation techniques for control of nanoparticles • Ventilation techniques for controlling nanoparticle exposures • Selection of PPE for protection from nanoparticles • Hazard communication techniques • Self-auditing techniques for nano-workplaces • Creation of standard operating procedures for nanoparticle operations • Medical surveillance concepts for nanoparticle exposures • Emergency response planning for nanoparticle operations

Table 23.7 — Example Approach for Comprehensive Initial and Refresher Training Program for Nanotechnology Workers[82]

Module 1: Introduction to Nanotechnology and Nanoparticles

Initial Training	*Refresher Training*	*Adult Learning Techniques*
• Define nanoparticles and nanomaterials. • Differentiate among nanoparticles, ultrafines, and engineered nanoparticles. • Explain the main classes of nanoparticles. • Describe carbon nanotubes and list some of their valuable properties. • Explain quantum dots and describe their properties. • Explain Dendrites and give examples of their properties. • Analyze the arguments raised about the risks versus the benefits of nanomaterials. • Describe the main difficulties with characterizing the exposed populations. • Analyze the importance of considering the life cycle of nanomaterials.	• An overview of the definition of nanoparticles, class of nanomaterials with an explanation of engineered versus naturally occurring and a discussion of the benefits, risks and life cycle of nanomaterials.	• Demonstration of commercially available models of nanoparticles. • Group discussions on whether the benefits exceed the risks and who bears the risks. • Class exercise of handling actual products (some nano and some not) and trying to determine if they contain nanoparticles. • Class discussion of operations in student workplaces where nanoparticles or nanomaterials are handled.

Module 2: Environmental, Health, and Safety Impacts of Nanoparticles

Initial Training	*Refresher Training*	*Adult Learning Techniques*
• Describe the difference between the amount of research on developing nanotechnologies and the amount on the health, safety and environmental impacts of nanotechnologies. • Describe the routes of entry for nanoparticles into the body. • Describe several of the health effects caused when nanoparticles enter the body.	• A facilitated discussion of routes of entry, known health effects, the value of control banding and areas where research is still needed.	• Group exercises analyzing historical occupational health problems in the workplace and their applicability to nanoparticles. • Demonstration using the Livermore Control Banding Nanotool

Module 3: Application of Traditional Risk Management Approaches to Protect Workers Handling Nanoparticles.

Initial Training	*Refresher Training*	*Adult Learning Techniques*
• List tasks that are most likely to generate worker exposures to nanoparticles. • Explain why the standard model of industrial hygiene sampling is of questionable value for airborne nanoparticles. • Explain the importance of the surface area of nanoparticles for biological activity. • Describe the specific needs for working with nanoparticles under local exhaust contamination. • Explain the current status of governmental and private efforts to develop occupational exposures limit and analyze the difficulties surrounding those efforts. • Review the hierarchy of controls and apply it to the management of risk associated with nanomaterials. • Define High Efficiency Particle Air (HEPA) filtration and describe the current understanding of the effectiveness of HEPA for capturing nanoparticles.	• Discussion of limitations of standard industrial hygiene approach to airborne measurement, status of development of occupational exposure limits, current understanding of ventilation effectiveness handling nanoparticles and respiratory protection recommendations by NIOSH. • Review of hazard communication issues.	• Facilitated discussion of the hierarchy of controls and its applicability to nanoparticles. • Group exercise reviewing actual MSDSs for nanomaterials. • Hands-on exercises with N-95 filtering facepiece respirators. • Hands-on exercises with industrial hygiene sampling equipment.

(continued on next page.)

Table 23.7 — Example Approach for Comprehensive Initial and Refresher Training Program for Nanotechnology Workers (continued)[82]

Module 3: Application of Traditional Risk Management Approaches to Protect Workers Handling Nanoparticles.		
Initial Training	*Refresher Training*	*Adult Learning Techniques*
• Discuss the current information available on the protection afforded by NIOSH-certified respirators against nanoparticles, including the use of N-95 filtering facepiece respirators. • Formulate a message for students on the effectiveness of protective garments against nanoparticles based on the current findings. • Describe safety hazards associated with nanomaterial production. • Characterize the international developments in hazard communication and their impact on informing workers about the risks of nanomaterials. • List several shortcomings of MSDSs for nanomaterials.		
Module 4: Regulatory and Voluntary Approaches Specific to Nanoparticles		
Initial Training	*Refresher Training*	*Adult Learning Techniques*
• Take an informed stance on whether the federal government is being sufficiently proactive managing the risks of nanotechnologies. • List several regulatory initiatives underway by federal agencies. • Discuss the difficulties faced by the EPA in regulating nanomaterials that enter the ecosystem. • Provide an overview of the scope of chemicals in use compared to the number regulated by OSHA and the potential number of chemicals that could be created at the nanoscale. • Describe several of the international voluntary guidance efforts underway. • Explain the steps of the NanoRisk Framework for identifying risks of nanoscale materials. • Explain the principles of control banding and why this approach is receiving serious consideration for assessing the risks of nanomaterials.	• Review of regulatory efforts across the federal government and internationally to protect workers from exposure to nanomaterials.	• Class internet exercise putting number of chemicals in perspective by checking current CAS numbers and potential number of nanoparticles versus EPA and OSHA regulated chemicals. • Group exercise applying Dupont/EDF NanoRisk Framework. • Group exercise applying control banding to a specific chemical familiar to the class. • Class discussion on the steps OSHA should be taking. • Class discussion on the value of the Precautionary Priniciple.

- **Peters, T.M., and V.H. Grassian:** Chapter 10, Engineered Nanomaterials. In V.E. Rose and B. Cohrssen, editors. *Patty's Industrial Hygiene*, 6th ed. New York: John Wiley & Sons, 2011.
- National Nanotechnology Initiative webpage, www.nano.gov.
- United Kingdom's Health and Safety Executive Website, http://www.hse.gov.uk/nanotechnology/.
- nanotechnology community resources at www.GoodNanoGuide.org.
- resources of the AIHA Nanotechnology Working Group at http://www.aiha.org/insideaiha/volunteergroups/Pages/NTWG.aspx.

Governmental

Environmental Protection Agency (EPA)

- National Center For Environmental Research (http://www.epa.gov/ncer/nano/index.html)
- Office of Pollution Prevention and Toxics (http://www.epa.gov/oppt/nano/)

- Office of Pesticide Programs (http://www.epa.gov/pesticides/about/intheworks/nanotechnology.htm)

Lawrence Livermore National Laboratory

- Control banding tool (http://control-banding.net/Services.html)

National Institute for Environmental Health Sciences (NIEHS)

- Clearinghouse for Worker Safety and Health Training page on nanotechnology (http://tools.niehs.nih.gov/wetp/)
- National Toxicology Program Nanotechnology Safety Initiative (http://ntp.niehs.nih.gov/)

National Institute for Occupational Safety and Health (NIOSH)

- Guidance, field studies, research, Nanoparticle Information Library (http://www.cdc.gov/niosh/topics/nanotech/)
- *Approaches to Safe nanotechnology: Managing the Health and Safety Concerns Associated with Engineered Nanomaterials.* Publication No. 2009-125. Cincinnati, OH: U.S. Dept. of Health and Human Services, 2009.

National Nanotechnology Initiative (NNI)

- US Government's nanotechnology portal (http://nano.gov)

Oak Ridge Institute for Science and Education (ORISE)

- Industrial Hygiene/ Occupational Safety Special Interest Group (http://orise.orau.gov/ihos/Nanotechnology/nanotech_safetyTraining.html)

Occupational Safety and Health Administration (OSHA)

- Standards for occupational practice (http://www.osha.gov/dsg/nanotechnology/nanotechnology.html)

U.S. Department of Energy

- U.S. Department of Energy Nanoscale Science Research Centers: *Approach to Nanomaterial ES&H.* Washington, D.C.: U.S. Department of Energy, 2008.

United Kingdom

- United Kingdom's Health and Safety Executive Website, http://www.hse.gov.uk/nanotechnology/.

Nongovernmental

GoodNanoGuide

- Information and protocols for safe handling (http://goodnanoguide.org)

International Council on Nanotechnology

- Aggregator of nano-EHS news, research, policy reports, industry survey, and backgrounders
    - Homepage (http://icon.rice.edu)
    - Database of research paper citations (http://icon.rice.edu/virtualjournal.cfm)
    - Survey of handling practices in the nanotech workforce (http://tinyurl.com/iconsurvey)

Wilson Center Project on Emerging Nanotechnologies

- Policy analysis and Consumer Product Inventory (http://www.nanotechproject.org/)

Nanoinformatics 2020 Roadmap

- Community-based nanoinformatics collaboration and pilot projects (http://eprints.internano.org/607/)

AIHA® Nanotechnology Working Group

- Technical information exchange and development and educational activities (http://www.aiha.org/insideaiha/volunteergroups/Pages/NTWG.aspx)

National Academy of Sciences Committee on Prudent Practices in the Laboratory: An Update

- *Prudent Practices in the laboratory: Handling and Management of Chemical Hazards,* Updated Version. Washington, D.C.: The National Academy Press, 2011.

Standards

ASTM International

- Technical Committee E56 on Nanotechnology (http://www.astm.org/COMMIT/COMMITTEE/E56.htm)
- Standard Guide for Handling Unbound Engineered Nanoscale Particles in Occupational Settings (ASTM E 2535-07). West Conshohocken, PA: ASTM International, 2007.

International Organization for Standardization (ISO)

- Technical Committee 229 Nanotechnologies (http://www.iso.org/iso/iso_technical_committee?commid=381983)

Educational Repositories and Books

- http://www.NanoEd.org (basic to intermediate)
- http://NanoHub.org (intermediate to advanced)
- Peters, T.M. and V.H. Grassian: Engineered Nanomaterials (Chapter 10). In *Patty's Industrial Hygiene*, 6th edition. Rose, V.E. and Cohrssen, B. (eds.). New York: John Wiley & Sons, 2011.

Acknowledgment

The authors gratefully acknowledge support they received from the National Clearinghouse for Worker Safety and Health Training under funding from the National Institute of Environmental Health Sciences' Worker Education and Training Program to write a report on Training Workers on Risks of Nanotechnology. That report drew heavily on authoritative research, recommendations, and guidance developed by the organizations such as the National Institute for Occupa-tional Safety and Health, and provided a primary basis for this chapter. The authors also gratefully acknowledge the invaluable input from experts in the NIOSH Nanotechnology Research Program, especially Charles L. Geraci, Jr., Laura Hodson, and Mark D. Hoover, and from experts in the AIHA® Nanotechnology Working Group, especially Gary Casuccio, Don Ewert, Ephraim Massawe, Randy Ogle, Tom Peters, Michael Rosenow, Keith Rickabaugh, Kevin Sheffield, and Betsy Shelton. The Clearinghouse is operated by MDB, Inc. The views, opinions, and content in this chapter are those of the authors and do not necessarily represent the views, opinions, or policies of their respective organizations. Mention of company names or products does not constitute endorsement by the authors or their respective organizations.

References

1. **Hoover, M.D., T. Armstrong, T. Blodgett, A.K. Fleeger, P.W. Logan, B. McArthur, and P.J. Middendorf:** Confirming our industrial hygiene decision-making framework. *The Synergist 22(1)*: 10 (2011).
2. **Peters, T.M., and V.H. Grassian:** Engineered Nanomaterials (Chapter 10). In *Patty's Industrial Hygiene*, 6th edition. Rose, V.E. and B. Cohrssen (eds.) New York: John Wiley & Sons, 2011.
3. **National Nanotechnology Initiative:** Nanotechnology 101. Available at http://www.nano.gov/nanotech-101. 2011. [Accessed on July 26, 2011].
4. **Fairbrothers, A.:** Managing the Risks of Manomaterials. *International Perspectives on Environmental Nanotechnology Applications and Implications Conference Proceedings*, Volume 2 – U.S. EPA Region 5. Chicago, IL, 2008.
5. **British Standards Institution:** Nanotechnologies Part 2: Guide to the safe handling and disposal of manufactured nanoparticles. PD 6699-2:2007.
6. **Ostrowski, A. D., et al.:** Nanotoxicology: characterizing the scientific literature, 2000–2007. *J. Nanoparticle Res. 11(2)*:251–57 (2009).
7. **Takagi, A., et al.:** Induction of mesothelioma in p53+/- mouse by intraperitoneal application of multi-wall carbon nanotube. *J. Tox. Sci. 33(1)*:105–16 (2008).
8. **Pacurari, M, et al.:** Raw single-walled carbon nanotube-induced cytotoxic effects in human bronchial epithelial cells: comparison to asbestos. *Tox. Env. Chem. 93(5)*: 1045–72 (2011).
9. **Mercer, R.R., et al:** Distribution and persistence of pleural penetrations by multi-walled carbon nanotubes. *Particle Fibre Tox. 7(28)*:1–11 (2010).
10. **Poland, C.A., et al.:** Carbon nanotubes introduced into the abdominal cavity of mice show asbestos-like pathogenicity in a pilot study. *Nature Nanotech. 3(7)*:423–28 (2008).
11. **International Council on Nanotechnology:** Towards predicting nano-biointeractions: An international assessment of nanotechnology environment, health and safety research needs. Available at http://bit.ly/dhphR2. 2008. [Accessed on May 10, 2010].
12. **National Institute for Occupational Safety and Health (NIOSH):** Draft NIOSH Current Intelligence Bulletin Occupational Exposure to Carbon Nanotubes and Nanofibers. Available at http://www.cdc.gov/niosh/docket/review/docket161a/pdfs/carbonNanotubeCIB_PublicReviewOfDraft.pdf. 2010, Nov. [Accessed July 22, 2011].

13. **National Institute for Occupational Safety and Health (NIOSH):** *Occupational Exposure to Titanium Dioxide.* Current Intelligence Bulletin 63. DHHS (NIOSH) Publication No. 2011–160. Cincinnati, OH: NIOSH, April 2011.
14. **International Council on Nanotechnology:** A Review of Current Practices in the Nanotechnology Industry — Phase Two Report: Survey of Current Practices in the Nanotechnology Workplace. Santa Barbara, CA: University of California - Santa Barbara. November 2006.
15. **Schulte, P., C. Geraci, R. Zumwalde, M. Hoover, and E. Kuempel:** Occupational risk management of engineered nanoparticles. *J. Occup. Env. Hyg.* 5:4, 240 (2008).
16. **Centers for Disease Control and Prevention (CDC), National Institute for Occupational Safety and Health (NIOSH):** Interim guidance for medical screening and hazardous surveillance for workers potentially exposed to engineered nanoparticles. (DHHS NIOSH Publication No. 02-2650). February 2009. Available at http://www.cdc.gov/niosh/docs/2009-116/pdfs/2009-116.pdf. [Accessed on July 22, 2011].
17. **U.S. Government Accountability Office:** *Report to the Chairman, Committee on Environment and Public Works, U.S. Senate. Nanotechnology: Nanomaterials are widely used in commerce, but EPA faces challenges in regulating risk.* GAO-10-549. May, 2010. p. 26.
18. **Schmid, K., B. Danuser, and M. Riediker:** Nanoparticle usage and protection measures in the manufacturing industry — A representative survey. *J. Occup. Env. Hyg.* *7*:224–32 (2010).
19. **Plunkett, J.W.:** Nanotechnology & MEMS Industry Almanac 2009 [Electronic version]. Houston, TX: Plunkett Research Ltd., 2009.
20. **Ewert, D.:** Personal Communication, OSO BioPharmaceuticals Manufacturing, Albuquerque, NM, July 2011.
21. **Hoover, M.D.:** Methods for Comprehensive Characterization of Radioactive Aerosols: A Graded Approach. In *Radioactive Air Sampling Methods.* Maiello, M.L. and M.D. Hoover (eds.). Boca Raton, FL: CRC Press, 2011.
22. **Abbott, L. and A. Maynard:** Exposure assessment approaches for engineered nanomaterials. *Risk Anal. 30*:1634–44 (2010).
23. **Johnson, D.R., M.M. Methner, A.J. Kennedy, and J.A. Steevens:** Potential for Occupational Exposure to Engineered Carbon-Based Nanomaterials in Environmental Laboratory Studies. *Env. Health Persp. 118(1)*:49-54 (2010).
24. **National Institute for Occupational Safety and Health (NIOSH): Approaches to Safe Nanotechnology:** An Information Exchange with NIOSH. 2009. http://www.cdc.gov/niosh/docs/2009-125/. [Accessed on July 22, 2011].
25. **Heitbrink, W.A., D.E. Evans, T.M. Peters, and T.J. Slavin:** Characterization and mapping of very fine particles in an engine machining and assembly facility. *J. Occup. Env. Hyg. 4(5)*:341–51 (2007).
26. **Methner, M., L. Hodson, A. Dames, and C. Geraci:** Nanoparticle Emission Assessment Technique (NEAT) for the Identification and Measurement of Potential Inhalation Exposure to Engineered Nanoparticles—Part B: Results from 12 Field Studies. *J. Occup. Env. Hyg. 7(3)*:163–76 (2010).
27. **Methner, M.M., M.E. Birch, D.E. Evans, B.-K. Ku, K. Crouch, and M.D. Hoover:** Case Study. *J. Occup. Env. Hyg. 4(12)*:D125–D130 (2007).
28. **Olfert, J.S., P. Kulkarni, and J. Wang:** Dynamic characteristics of a Fast-Response Aerosol Size
29. Spectrometer. *Aerosol Sci. Tech. 43(2)*:97–111 (2009).
30. **Ostiguy, L., B. Roberge, L. Ménard, and C. Endo:** *Best Practices Guide to Synthetic Nanoparticle Risk Management.* Institut de recherche Robert-Sauvé en santé et en sécurité du travail (IRSST). Available at http://www.irsst.qc.ca/files/documents/PubIRSST/R-599.pdf. 2009. [Accessed on July 22, 2011].
31. **Naumann, B.D., E.V. Sargent, B.S .Starkman, W.J. Fraser, G.T. Becker and D.L. Kirk:** Performance-based exposure control limits for pharmaceutical active ingredients. *Am. Ind. Hyg Assoc. J. 57*:33–42 (1996).
32. **American Industrial Hygiene Association (AIHA®):** *Guidance for Conducting Control Banding Analyses.* Fairfax, VA: AIHA®, 2007.
33. **National Institute for Occupational Safety and Health (NIOSH):** *Qualitative Risk Characterization and Management of Occupational Hazards: Control Banding (CB).* (DHHS NIOSH Publication No. 2009-152). Cincinnati, OH: NIOSH, 2009. Available at http://www.cdc.gov/niosh/docs/2009-152/. [Accessed on July 28, 2011].
34. **Maynard, A.:** Nanotechnology: the next big thing, or much ado about nothing? *Ann. Occup. Hyg. 51(1)*:1–12 (2007).
35. **Zalk, D.M., S.Y. Paik, and P. Swuste:** (2009, June). Evaluating the control banding nanotool: A qualitative risk assessment method for controlling nanoparticle exposures. *J. Nanoparticle Res. 11(7)*:1685–704 (2009).
36. **Zalk, D. and S. Paik:** Control banding and nanotechnology. *The Synergist 21(3)*:28 (2010).
37. **Methner, M., L. Hodson, A. Dames, and C. Geraci:** Nanoparticle Emission Assessment Technique (NEAT) for the Identification and Measurement of Potential Inhalation Exposure to Engineered Nanoparticles—Part B: Results from 12 Field Studies. *J. Occup. Env. Hyg. 7(3)*:163–76 (2010).

38. **Tsai, S.J., R.F. Huang, and M.J. Ellenbecker:** Airborne Nanoparticle Exposures while using constant-flow, constant-velocity, and air-curtain-isolated fume hoods. *Ann. Occup. Hyg. 54(1)*:78–87 (2010).
39. **Balas, F., M. Arruebo, J. Urrutia, and J. Santamaria:** Reported nanosafety practices in research laboratories worldwide. *Nature Nanotech. 5*:93–96 (2010).
40. **National Nanotechnology Initiative:** Precautionary measures for employers and workers handling engineered nanoparticles: NIOSH recommendations. [online]. 2007. http://www.nano.gov/html/society/occupational_safety/20070306_NIOSH_Precautionary_Measures.html. [Accessed February 10, 2010].
41. **Casuccio, G.R., et al.:** Worker and Environmental Assessment of Potential Unbound Engineered Nanoparticle Releases, Phase III Final Report, Validation of Preliminary Control Band Assignments, Lawrence Berkeley National Laboratory, September 2010.
42. **Dolez, P.I., N. Bodila, J. Lara, and G. Truchon:** Personal protective equipment against nanoparticles. *Internatl. J. Nanotech. 7(1)*:99–111 (2010).
43. **Balazy, A., M. Toivola, T. Reponen, A. Podgorski, A. Zimmer, and S.A. Grinshpun:** Manikin-based performance evaluation of N95 filtering-facepiece respirators challenged with nanoparticles. *Ann. Occup. Hyg. 50*:259–69 (2006).
44. **Rengasamy, S., R. Verbofsky, W.P. King, and R.E. Shaffer:** Nanoparticle penetration through NIOSH-approved N95 filtering-facepiece respirators. *J. Internatl. Soc. Resp. Prot. 24*:49–59 (2007).
45. **Rengasamy, S., W.P. King, B. Eimer, and R.E. Shaffer:** Filtration performance of NIOSH-approved N95 and P100 filtering facepiece respirators against 4-30 nanometer size nanoparticles. *J. Occup. Env. Hyg. 5(9)*:556–64 (2008).
46. **National Institute for Occupational Safety and Health (NIOSH):** Respirator Selection Logic 2004, National Institute for Occupational Safety and Health, Department of Health and Human Services, Publication No. 2005-100. Cincinnati, OH, NIOSH, October 2004. Available at: http://www.cdc.gov/niosh/docs/2005-100/ . [Accessed July 28, 2011].
47. **U.S. Environmental Protection Agency (EPA):** Siloxane-modified alumina nanoparticles (generic). 40 CFR 721.10120(a)(2)(i). Washington, D.C.: EPA, November 5, 2008.
48. **U.S. Environmental Protection Agency (EPA):** Multi-walled carbon nanotubes (generic). 40 CFR 721.10155(a)(2)(i). Washington, D.C.: EPA, September 17, 2010.
49. **U.S. Environmental Protection Agency (EPA):** Single-walled carbon nanotubes (generic). 40 CFR 721.10156(a)(2)(i). Washington, D.C.: EPA, September 17, 2010.
50. **Occupational Safety and Health Administration (OSHA):** (2010, Jan. 27). OSHA schedules informal stakeholder meetings on combustible dust. [online]. http://www.osha.gov/pls/oshaweb/owadisp.show_document?p_table=NEWS_RELEASES&p_id=17112. [Accessed February 8, 2010].
51. **British Standards Institute (BSI):** *Nanotechnologies — Part 2: Guide to Safe Handling and Disposal of Manufactured Nano-particles.* PD 6699-2:2007. London: BSI, 2007. p. 5.
52. **Methner, M.M.:** Engineering case reports. *J. Occup. Env. Hyg. 5(6)*:D63–D69 (2008).
53. **Levine, D.:** Personal communication. New York: Product Safety Solutions, September 15, 2006.
54. **Lindberg, J.E. and M.M. Quinn:** *A Survey of Environmental, Health and Safety Risk Management Information Needs and Practices among Nanotechnology Firms in the Massachusetts Region"* PEN Research Brief Number 1. Lowell, MA: The Project on Emerging Nanotechnologies, 2007.
55. **Sattler, B., Lippy, B. and T. Jordan:** Hazard Communication: A Review of the Science Underpinning the Art of Communication for Health and Safety. Washington, D.C.: OSHA, 1995. http://www.osha.gov/SLTC/hazardcommunications/otherresources.html.
56. **Kolp, P., B. Sattler, M. Blayney, and T. Sherwood:** Comprehensibility of Material Safety Data Sheets. *Am. J. Ind. Med. 23*:139 (1993).
57. **Phillips, C., B. Wallace, C. Hamilton, R. Pursley, G. Petty, and C. Bayne:** Efficacy of MSDSs and worker acceptability. J. Safety Res. (30):113–22 (1999).
58. **Printing Industries of America:** *Comments on the OSHA Hazard Communications Standard.* Docket H-022G. Sewickley, PA: Printing Industries of America, 1990.
59. **Nicol, A. M., Hurrell, A.C., Wahyuni, D., McDowall, W., and W. Chu.** (July, 2008) "Accuracy, Comprehensibility, and Use of Material Safety Data Sheets: A Review" Am. J. Industrial Medicine (51) 11 861-876.
60. **Crawford, C. and L. Hodson:** Guidance for preparing good MSDSs for engineered nanoparticles. Poster session presented at the American Industrial Hygiene Conference & Expo, Toronto, Ontario, Canada, 2009.
61. **Lippy, B.E.:** MSDSs fail to communicate the hazards of nanotechnologies to workers. Paper presented at the International Environmental Nanotechnology Conference, Chicago, IL. October 2008.

62. **Pritchard, D.K.:** Literature Review — Explosion Hazards Associated with Nanopowders. HSL/2004/12. Health and Safety Lab. Harpur Hill, Buxton, UK: Health and Safety Executive, 2004.
63. **Murashov, V. and J. Howard:** Essential features for proactive risk management. Commentary: Nature Nanotech. 4:469 (2009).
64. **Markowitz, G. and D. Rosner:** *Deceit and Denial: The Deadly Politics of Industrial Pollution.* Berkley and Los Angeles, CA: University of California Press, 2002.
65. **U.S. Environmental Protection Agency (EPA):** Concept paper for the Nanoscale Materials Stewardship Program under TSCA. 2008. http://www.regulations.gov/fdmspublic/component/main?main=DocumentDetail&d=EPA-HQ-OPPT-2004-0122-0058. [Accessed on May 11, 2010].
66. **U.S. Environmental Protection Agency (EPA):** Significant New Use Rules on Certain Chemical Substances. Federal Register 73(215): 65743-65766. Washington, D.C.: EPA, 2008.
67. **U.S. Environmental Protection Agency (EPA):** U.S. EPA fines Southern California technology company $208,000 for "nano coating" pesticide claims on computer peripherals. http://yosemite.epa.gov/opa/admpress.nsf/2dd7f669225439b78525735900400c31/16a190492f2f25d585257403005c2851!OpenDocument. [Accessed on August 4, 2011].
68. **U.S. Environmental Protection Agency (EPA):** The North Face' Clothing Parent Company Facing Nearly $1M in Federal Fines Following Unsubstantiated Product Claims. 2009. http://yosemite.epa.gov/opa/admpress.nsf/2dd7f669225439b78525735900400c31/bcbd9b468b9aaf67852576390055de2f!OpenDocument. [Accessed on December 23, 2009].
69. **U.S. Environmental Protection Agency (EPA):** CLU-IN Technology Innovation Program. http://www.clu-in.org/products/nano/search.cfm. [Accessed on August 4, 2011].
70. **Mendeloff, J.:** *Regulating Safety: An Economic and Political Analysis of Occupational Safety and Health Policy.* Cambridge, MA: The MIT Press, 1980.
71. **Pritchard, D.K.:** Literature review: explosion hazards associated with nanopowders. HSL/2004/12. Buxton, U.K.: Health and Safety Laboratory, March 2004.
72. **U.S. Environmental Protection Agency (EPA):** New Chemical Program under TSCA. 2010. [online] http://www.epa.gov/opptintr/newchems/pubs/invntory.htm. [Accessed on February 7, 2010].
73. **Chemical Abstract Service:** Registry Number and Substance Count. 2010. [online] http://www.cas.org/cgi-bin/cas/regreport.pl. [Accessed on February 7,2010].
74. **Frey, T.:** Nanotech and the Precautionary Principle. October, 2008. http://www.futuristspeaker.com/2008/10/nanotech-and-the-precautionary-principal/. [Accessed on August 4, 2011].
75. **City of Berkeley, California:** Manufactured Nanoscale Materials Health & Safety Disclosure. Toxics Management Division, Planning and Development Department. 2009.
76. **California Department of Toxic Substances Control:** Nanotechnology call-in. 2010. [online]. http://www.dtsc.ca.gov/TechnologyDevelopment/Nanotechnology/index.cfm. [Accessed February 10, 2010].
77. **Organisation for Economic Co-operation and Development (OECD):** Series on safety of manufactured nanomaterials, number 10. ENV/JM/MONO(2009)15. Paris, France: OECD, June 2009.
78. **International Organization for Standardization (ISO):** Health and safety practices in occupational settings relevant to nanotechnologies, ISO/TR 12885:2008. http://www.iso.org/iso/iso_catalogue/catalogue_tc/catalogue_detail.htm?csnumber=52093. [Accessed on July 29, 2011.]
79. **ASTM International:** *Standard Guide for Handling Unbound Engineered Nanoscale Particles in Occupational Settings.* ASTM E 2535-07. West Conshohocken, PA; ASTM International, 2007.
80. **Environmental Defense Fund and Dupont:** Nano Risk Framework. 2006. http://nanoriskframework.com/page.cfm?tagID=1095. [Accessed on July 27, 2011].
81. **National Institute of Environmental Health Sciences:** *Worker Education and Training Program. Minimum Health and Safety Training Criteria.* Research Triangle Park, NC: NIEHS, January 2006.
82. **Hsieh, F.M., P.J. Tsai, W.Y. Chen, C.P. Chang:** *Developing on-the-job Training Program for the occupational safety and health personnel in nanotechnology industries.* Proceedings of the 2009 IEEE IEEM, 2009.
83. **Kulinowski, K. and B. Lippy:** *Training Workers on Risks of Nanotechnology.* February 2011. Available at http://tools.niehs.nih.gov/wetp/index.cfm?id=537. [Accessed July 29, 2011.]

Index

A

B

C

D

E

F

G

H

I

J

K

L

M

N

O

P

Q

R

S

T

U

V

W

X

Y

Z